Drug Addiction

From Basic Research to Therapy

Rao S. Rapaka • Wolfgang Sadée
Editors

Drug Addiction

From Basic Research to Therapy

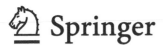 Springer

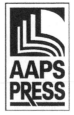

Editors
Dr. Rao S. Rapaka
National Institute on Drug Abuse
Bethesda, MD
USA

Dr. Wolfgang Sadée
College of Medicine and Public Health
Ohio State University
Columbus, OH
USA

ISBN 978-1-4419-2632-6   e-ISBN 978-0-387-76678-2
DOI: 10.1007/978-0-387-76678-2

Printed on acid-free paper

9 8 7 6 5 4 3 2 1

springer.com

Preface

This book affords a comprehensive overview of current research on drug addiction and related disciplines, with topical reviews written by eminent scientists in the field. It was inspired by a joint AAPS–NIDA symposium "Frontiers in Science: Drug Addiction – From Basic Research to Therapies", held in September 2004, at the NIH campus. Subsequently, we have invited leading scientists to contribute chapters on a broad range of topics, covering basic research (e.g. mechanisms of action of drugs of abuse, development of receptor-specific ligands, animal models), discovery and development of therapies, and other clinical applications. As neuronal circuits involved in drug addiction also impinge upon many other vital functions of the brain and peripheral tissues, we have broadened the scope to include pathophysiologies related to drug abuse/addiction. For example, the complex actions of opioids on pain, addiction liability, and other adverse effects have triggered an intensive search for non-addictive opioid pain medications and for non-opioid analgesics directed against novel targets. Other directions include treatment of stimulant addiction and toxicity, new therapies for gastrointestinal dysfunction, inflammation, cognitive and neurodegenerative disorders, and immunological diseases.

This book is divided into several portions, each addressing issues of importance in drug addiction or in scientific areas that have naturally evolved as research targets for addiction researchers:

1. General topics
2. Transporters and stimulants and hallucinogens
3. Drug design: nicotine, opioids, and related ligands
4. Opioids: general
5. Cannabinoids

The first section starts out with a detailed analysis of a principal addiction pathway involving DARPP32, a key regulator of dopamine signaling, presented by Greengard and colleagues. This is followed by drug discovery from natural sources (Kinghorn), antibodies, endogenous peptides, and small RNAs as drug candidates, and computational analysis of G protein coupled receptors (Reggio). The scope of basic topics further includes pharmacogenetics (Rutter), and addresses the role of chemokines, nicotinic receptors, and PDZ domains as protein–protein interaction modules.

The second section addresses issues related to neurotransmitter transporters and their role in mediating the effects of stimulants and hallucinogens. This focuses on monoamine synaptic reuptake transporters and cocaine, among other stimulants. A series of chapters further discuss the interaction of stimulants and hallucinogens with various receptors and their mechanisms of action.

The third section "Drug design: nicotine, opioids, and related ligands" critically assesses the molecular biology, physiology, and pharmacology of receptors and other targets for drugs of abuse. Focusing on drug design, several chapters address the basic tools for drug discovery such as crystallography and chemistry, with applications to opioid and nicotinic receptors. This leads to Sect. 4 with opioid ligands and their interaction with target receptors as the focus. Relevant issues include molecular modes of target interactions, opioid receptor regulation and tolerance, the relevance of receptor oligomerization, CNS drug delivery, homology modeling, and the serendipitous discovery of cell-permeable, mitochondrial-targeted peptide antioxidants – an example of a distinct application arising from addiction research.

The last section deals with cannabinoids, an area of tremendous recent growth because of the role cannabinoids play in multiple physiological systems, including those involved in pain modulation.

These diverse disciplines and technologies all converge on a more detailed understanding of addiction and the promise for developing improved treatment strategies for a spectrum of neurological disorders. This volume uniquely brings together seemingly disparate, but nevertheless complementary critical reviews that together paint a rather comprehensive picture of current efforts in drug addiction and its treatment. It also shows how one discipline reaches into many other areas, with the interplay among them yielding the promise for significant advances in understanding and treating drug addiction and related disorders.

Columbus, OH   Rao S. Rapaka
                                                                 Wolfgang Sadee

Contents

V Cannabinoid

Contributors

Ravikumar Aalinkeel
Department of Medicine, Division of Allergy, Immunology and Rheumatology,
State University of New York at Buffalo, Buffalo General Hospital, 100 High
Street, Buffalo, NY 14203

Martin W. Adler
Center for Substance Abuse Research, Temple University School of Medicine,
Philadelphia, PA 19140
and
Department of Pharmacology, Temple University School of Medicine,
Philadelphia, PA 19140

Richard S. Agnes
Department of Chemistry, University of Arizona, Tucson, AZ

Isabel Alves
Department of Chemistry, University of Arizona, Tucson, AZ
and
Departments of Biochemistry and Molecular Biophysics, University of Arizona,
Tucson, AZ

Subramaniam Ananthan
Department of Organic Chemistry, Southern Research Institute, Birmingham, AL

Jon R. Appel
Torrey Pines Institute for Molecular Studies, San Diego, CA

Marcy J. Balunas
Division of Medicinal Chemistry and Pharmacognosy, College of Pharmacy,
The Ohio State University, Columbus, OH 43210
and
Program for Collaborative Research in the Pharmaceutical Sciences, Department
of Medicinal Chemistry and Pharmacognosy, College of Pharmacy,
University of Illinois at Chicago, Chicago, IL 60612

Eric L. Barker
Department of Medicinal Chemistry and Molecular Pharmacology,
Purdue University School of Pharmacy, West Lafayette, IN 47907

Michael H. Baumann
Clinical Psychopharmacology Section, Intramural Research Program, National
Institute on Drug Abuse, National Institutes of Health, Department of Health
and Human Services, Baltimore, MD

B. Bindukumar
Department of Medicine, Division of Allergy, Immunology and Rheumatology,
State University of New York at Buffalo, Buffalo General Hospital, 100 High
Street, Buffalo, NY 14203

Bruce E. Blough
Chemistry and Life Sciences Group, Research Triangle Institute International,
Research Triangle Park, NC

Laura M. Bohn
Departments of Pharmacology & Psychiatry, The Ohio State University College
of Medicine and Public Health, Columbus, OH 43210

Marcus Brackeen
Research Triangle Institute, Research Triangle Park, NC 27709-2194

Sumner Burstein
Department of Biochemistry and Molecular Pharmacology, University of
Massachusetts Medical School, 364 Plantation Street, Worcester, MA 01605

Minying Cai
Department of Chemistry, University of Arizona, Tucson, AZ

F. Ivy Carroll
Center for Organic and Medicinal Chemistry, Research Triangle Institute,
Research Triangle Park, NC 27709

Hee Byung Chai
Division of Medicinal Chemistry and Pharmacognosy, College of Pharmacy,
The Ohio State University, Columbus, OH 43210

Xiaohong Chen
Center for Substance Abuse Research, Temple University School of Medicine,
Philadelphia, PA 19140

Steven R. Childers
Department of Physiology and Pharmacology, Center for the Neurobiological
Investigation of Drug Abuse, Wake Forest University School of Medicine,
Winston-Salem, NC 27157

Young-Won Chin
Division of Medicinal Chemistry and Pharmacognosy, College of Pharmacy,
The Ohio State University, Columbus, OH 43210

Andrew Coop
Department of Pharmaceutical Sciences, University of Maryland School
of Pharmacy, 20 Penn Street, Baltimore, MD 21201

Scott Cowell
Department of Chemistry, University of Arizona, Tucson, AZ

Peg Davis
Department of Pharmacology, University of Arizona, Tucson, AZ

Thomas P. Davis
Department of Medical Pharmacology, College of Medicine,
The University of Arizona, LSN 542, 1501 N. Campbell Avenue,
Tucson, AZ 85724

Fabien M. Décaillot
Department of Pharmacology and Biological Chemistry, Mount Sinai School
of Medicine, New York, NY 10029

Jeffrey R. Deschamps
Laboratory for the Structure of Matter, Naval Research Laboratory, Washington,
DC 20375

Dale G. Deutsch
Department of Biochemistry and Cell Biology, State University of New York
at Stony Brook, Stony Brook, NY

Lakshmi A. Devi
Department of Pharmacology and Biological Chemistry, Mount Sinai School
of Medicine, New York, NY 10029

Tobin J. Dickerson
The Skaggs Institute for Chemical Biology and Departments of Chemistry
and Immunology, The Scripps Research Institute, 10550 North Torrey
Pines Road, La Jolla, CA 92037

Geraldina Dominguez
Yerkes National Primate Research Center, Emory University, Atlanta, GA 30329

Colette T. Dooley
Torrey Pines Institute for Molecular Studies, San Diego, CA

David M. Ferguson
Department of Medicinal Chemistry, College of Pharmacy, University of
Minnesota, Minneapolis, MN 55455

Annette E. Fleckenstein
Department of Pharmacology and Toxicology, University of Utah, Salt Lake City,
Utah 84112

Barbara S. Fox
Addiction Therapies, Inc, Wayland, MA 01778

Lloyd D. Fricker
Department of Molecular Pharmacology, Albert Einstein College of Medicine,
1300 Morris Park Avenue, Bronx, NY 10461

Lorise C. Gahring
Geriatric Research Education and Clinical Center, Salt Lake City VAMC,
Salt Lake City, Utah 84132
and
The Department of Internal Medicine, University of Utah School of Medicine,
Salt Lake City, Utah 84132

Ellen B. Geller
Center for Substance Abuse Research, Temple University School of Medicine,
Philadelphia, PA 19140

Paul Greengard
Laboratory of Molecular and Cellular Neuroscience, The Rockefeller University,
New York, NY 10021

Achla Gupta
Department of Pharmacology and Biological Chemistry, Mount Sinai School
of Medicine, New York, NY 10029

Glen R. Hanson
Department of Pharmacology and Toxicology, University of Utah, Salt Lake City,
Utah 84112

Wayne W. Harding
Division of Medicinal & Natural Products Chemistry, College of Pharmacy,
The University of Iowa, Iowa City, IA 52242

Ralph L. Henry
Department of Biological Sciences, University of Arkansas, Fayetteville,
AR 72701

Anita Hermann
Department of Biochemistry and Cell Biology, State University of New York
at Stony Brook, Stony Brook, NY

Andrea G. Hohmann
Neuroscience and Behavior Program, Department of Psychology,
University of Georgia, Athens, GA 30602-3013

Richard A. Houghten
Torrey Pines Institute for Molecular Studies, San Diego, CA

James L. Howard
Howard Associates, LLC, Research Triangle Park, NC 27709

Leonard L. Howell
Yerkes Regional Primate Research Center, Emory University, Atlanta GA 30329

Victor J. Hruby
Department of Chemistry, University of Arizona, Tucson, AZ
and
Departments of Biochemistry and Molecular Biophysics, University of Arizona,
Tucson, AZ

George W. Hubert
Yerkes National Primate Research Center, Emory University, Atlanta, GA 30329

Kim D. Janda
The Skaggs Institute for Chemical Biology and Departments of Chemistry
and Immunology, The Scripps Research Institute, 10550 North Torrey Pines Road,
La Jolla, CA 92037

Jason N. Jaworski
Yerkes National Primate Research Center, Emory University, Atlanta, GA 30329

Lankupalle D. Jayanthi
Department of Neurosciences, Division of Neuroscience Research, Medical
University of South Carolina, Charleston, SC 29425

Faming Jiang
Biosciences Division, SRI International, Menlo Park, CA 94025

Martin Kaczocha
Department of Biochemistry and Cell Biology, State University of New York
at Stony Brook, Stony Brook, NY

Brian E. Kane
Department of Medicinal Chemistry, College of Pharmacy, University of
Minnesota, Minneapolis, MN 55455

Steven E. Kern
Department of Pharmaceutics and Pharmaceutical Chemistry, College
of Pharmacy, University of Utah, Salt Lake City, UT
and
Department of Anesthesiology, School of Medicine, University of Utah,
Salt Lake City, UT

Daniel E. Keyler
Minneapolis Medical Research Foundation, Department of Medicine,
University of Minnesota Medical School, Minneapolis, MN

A. Douglas Kinghorn
Division of Medicinal Chemistry and Pharmacognosy, College of Pharmacy,
The Ohio State University, Columbus, OH 43210

Michael J. Kuhar
Yerkes Regional Primate Research Center, Emory University, Atlanta GA 30329

Josephine Lai
Department of Pharmacology, University of Arizona, Tucson, AZ

Yeon Sun Lee
Department of Chemistry, University of Arizona, Tucson, AZ

Mark G. LeSage
Minneapolis Medical Research Foundation, Department of Medicine,
University of Minnesota Medical School, Minneapolis, MN

Anita H. Lewin
Chemistry and Life Sciences, Research Triangle Institute, Research Triangle
Park, NC

Anu Mahadevan
Organix, Inc, Woburn, MA 01801

Supriya D. Mahajan
Department of Medicine, Division of Allergy, Immunology and Rheumatology,
State University of New York at Buffalo, Buffalo General Hospital, 100 High
Street, Buffalo, NY 14203

S. Wayne Mascarella
Research Triangle Institute, Research Triangle Park, NC 27709-2194

Matthew D. Metcalf
Department of Pharmaceutical Sciences, University of Maryland School
of Pharmacy, 20 Penn Street, Baltimore, MD 21201

Dale F. Mierke
Department of Molecular Pharmacology, Division of Biology and Medicine,
Brown University, 171 Meeting Street, Providence, RI 02912
and
Department of Chemistry, Brown University, Providence, RI 02912

Henry I. Mosberg
Department of Medicinal Chemistry, College of Pharmacy, University of
Michigan, Ann Arbor, MI 48109

Madhavan P.N. Nair
Department of Medicine, Division of Allergy, Immunology and Rheumatology,
State University of New York at Buffalo, Buffalo General Hospital,
100 High Street, Buffalo, NY 14203

Angus C. Nairn
Laboratory of Molecular and Cellular Neuroscience, The Rockefeller University,
New York, NY 10021
and
Department of Psychiatry, Yale University School of Medicine, New Haven,
CT 06508

Cris Olsen
Biosciences Division, SRI International, Menlo Park, CA 94025

S. Michael Owens
Department of Pharmacology and Toxicology, College of Medicine,
University of Arkansas for Medical Sciences, Little Rock, AR 72205

Kevin M. Page
Research Triangle Institute, Research Triangle Park, NC 27709-2194

Paul R. Pentel
Minneapolis Medical Research Foundation, Department of Medicine,
University of Minnesota Medical School, Minneapolis, MN

Roger G. Pertwee
School of Medical Sciences, Institute of Medical Sciences,
University of Aberdeen, Foresterhill, Aberdeen AB25 2ZD, Scotland, UK

Eric Peterson
Department of Pharmacology and Toxicology, College of Medicine,
University of Arkansas for Medical Sciences, Little Rock, AR 72205

Kelly B. Philpot
Yerkes National Primate Research Center, Emory University, Atlanta, GA 30329

Andrea Piserchio
Department of Molecular Pharmacology, Division of Biology
and Medicine, Brown University, 171 Meeting Street, Providence, RI 02912

Irina D. Pogozheva
Department of Medicinal Chemistry, College of Pharmacy, University of
Michigan, Ann Arbor, MI 48109

Willma Polgar
Biosciences Division, SRI International, Menlo Park, CA 94025

Frank Porreca
Department of Pharmacology, University of Arizona, Tucson, AZ

Thomas E. Prisinzano
Division of Medicinal & Natural Products Chemistry, College of Pharmacy,
The University of Iowa, Iowa City, IA 52242

Magdalena J. Przydzial
Department of Medicinal Chemistry, College of Pharmacy, University of
Michigan, Ann Arbor, MI 48109

Kirsten M. Raehal
Departments of Pharmacology & Psychiatry, The Ohio State University College
of Medicine and Public Health, Columbus, OH 43210

Sammanda Ramamoorthy
Department of Neurosciences, Division of Neuroscience Research,
Medical University of South Carolina, Charleston, SC 29425

Suneetha Ramanujapuram
Division of Pharmaceutical Sciences, Mylan School of Pharmacy,
Duquesne University, Pittsburgh, PA 15282

Rao S. Rapaka
National Institute on Drug Abuse
Ohio State University

Raj K. Razdan
Organix, Inc, Woburn, MA 01801

Patricia H. Reggio
Center for Drug Design, Department of Chemistry and Biochemistry,
University of North Carolina Greensboro, Greensboro, NC

Soundar Regunathan
Department of Psychiatry and Human Behavior, Division of Neurobiology and
Behavior Research, University of Mississippi Medical Center, Jackson, MS

Jessica L. Reynolds
Department of Medicine, Division of Allergy, Immunology and Rheumatology,
State University of New York at Buffalo, Buffalo General Hospital,
100 High Street, Buffalo, NY 14203

Evan L. Riddle
Department of Pharmacology and Toxicology, University of Utah,
Salt Lake City, Utah 84112

William Roeske
Department of Pharmacology, University of Arizona, Tucson, AZ

Scott W. Rogers
Geriatric Research Education and Clinical Center, Salt Lake City VAMC,
Salt Lake City, Utah 84132
and
The Department of Neurobiology and Anatomy, University of Utah School
of Medicine, Salt Lake City, Utah 84132

Thomas J. Rogers
Center for Substance Abuse Research, Temple University School
of Medicine, Philadelphia, PA 19140
and
Fels Institute for Cancer Research and Molecular Biology,
Temple University School of Medicine, Philadelphia, PA 19140
and
Department of Pharmacology, Temple University School of Medicine,
Philadelphia, PA 19140

Richard B. Rothman
Clinical Psychopharmacology Section, Intramural Research Program, National
Institute on Drug Abuse, National Institutes of Health, Department of Health
and Human Services, Baltimore, MD

Joni L. Rutter
National Institute on Drug Abuse, National Institutes of Health, Department
of Health and Human Services, 6001 Executive Boulevard, Bethesda, MD 20892

Wolfgang Sadée
College of Medicine and Public Health, Ohio State University

Zdzislaw Salamon
Departments of Biochemistry and Molecular Biophysics, University of Arizona,
Tucson, AZ

Peter W. Schiller
Laboratory of Chemical Biology and Peptide Research, Clinical Research Institute
of Montreal, 110 Pine Avenue West, Montreal, Quebec, Canada H2W 1R7

Stanley A. Schwartz
Department of Medicine, Division of Allergy, Immunology and Rheumatology,
State University of New York at Buffalo, Buffalo General Hospital, 100 High
Street, Buffalo, NY 14203

Herbert H. Seltzman
Research Triangle Institute, Research Triangle Park, NC 27709-2194

Mark Spaller
Department of Chemistry, Wayne State University, Detroit, MI 48202

Richard L. Suplita, II
Neuroscience and Behavior Program, Department of Psychology,
University of Georgia, Athens, GA 30602-3013

Christopher K. Surratt
Division of Pharmaceutical Sciences, Mylan School of Pharmacy,
Duquesne University, Pittsburgh, PA 15282

Per Svenningsson
Laboratory of Molecular and Cellular Neuroscience, The Rockefeller University,
New York, NY 10021

Bengt Svensson
Department of Medicinal Chemistry, College of Pharmacy, University of
Minnesota, Minneapolis, MN 55455

Don Sykes
Department of Medicine, Division of Allergy, Immunology and Rheumatology,
State University of New York at Buffalo, Buffalo General Hospital, 100 High
Street, Buffalo, NY 14203

Hazel H. Szeto
Department of Pharmacology, Joan and Sanford I. Weill Medical College
of Cornell University, New York, NY

Brian F. Thomas
Research Triangle Institute, Research Triangle Park, NC 27709-2194

Kevin Tidgewell
Division of Medicinal & Natural Products Chemistry, College of Pharmacy,
The University of Iowa, Iowa City, IA 52242

Lawrence Toll
Biosciences Division, SRI International, Menlo Park, CA 94025

Gordon Tollin
Department of Chemistry, University of Arizona, Tucson, AZ
and
Departments of Biochemistry and Molecular Biophysics,
University of Arizona, Tucson, AZ

Okechukwu T. Ukairo
Division of Pharmaceutical Sciences, Mylan School of Pharmacy,
Duquesne University, Pittsburgh, PA 15282

Todd Vanderah
Department of Pharmacology, University of Arizona, Tucson, AZ

Eva Varga
Department of Pharmacology, University of Arizona, Tucson, AZ

Crystal C. Walline
Department of Medicinal Chemistry and Molecular Pharmacology,
Purdue University School of Pharmacy, West Lafayette, IN 47907

Harel Weinstein
Department of Physiology and Biophysics, and Institute for Computational
Biomedicine, Weill Medical College of Cornell University, New York, NY 10021

Kellie J. White
Department of Medicinal Chemistry and Molecular Pharmacology,
Purdue University School of Pharmacy, West Lafayette, IN 47907

Ken A. Witt
Pharmaceutical Sciences, School of Pharmacy, Southern Illinois University,
Edwardsville, 200 University Park Drive, Edwardsville, IL 62026, USA

Erica Wittwer
Department of Pharmaceutics and Pharmaceutical Chemistry,
College of Pharmacy, University of Utah, Salt Lake City, UT

Henry I. Yamamura
Department of Pharmacology, University of Arizona, Tucson, AZ

Nurulain Zaveri
Biosciences Division, SRI International, Menlo Park, CA 94025

Yanan Zhang
Research Triangle Institute, Research Triangle Park, NC 27709-2194

Part I
General Topics

Chapter 1
DARPP-32 Mediates the Actions of Multiple Drugs of Abuse

Per Svenningsson,[1] Angus C. Nairn,[1,2] and Paul Greengard[1]

Abstract Drugs of abuse share the ability to enhance dopaminergic neurotransmission in the dorsal and ventral striatum. The action of dopamine is modulated by additional neurotransmitters, including glutamate, serotonin and adenosine. All these neurotransmitters regulate the phosphorylation state of Dopaminal serine/threonine protein phosphatase, PP-1. Phosphorylatine- and cAMP-regulated phosphoprotein, Mr 32 kDa (DARPP-32). Phosphorylation at Thr^{34} by protein kinase A converts DARPP-32 into a potent inhibitor of the multifunction at Thr^{75} by Cdk5 converts DARPP-32 into an inhibitor of protein kinase A. The state of phosphorylation of DARPP-32 at Thr^{34} also depends on the phosphorylation state of Ser^{97} and Ser^{130}, which are phosphorylated by CK2 and CK1, respectively. By virtue of regulation of these 4 phosphorylation sites, and through its ability to modulate the activity of PP-1 and protein kinase A, DARPP-32 plays a key role in integrating a variety of biochemical, electrophysiological, and behavioral responses controlled by dopamine and other neurotransmitters. Importantly, there is now a large body of evidence that supports a key role for DARPP-32-dependent signaling in mediating the actions of multiple drugs of abuse including cocaine, amphetamine, nicotine, caffeine, LSD, PCP, ethanol and morphine.

Keywords protein phosphorylation, psychostimulants, dopamine, striatum

[1] Laboratory of Molecular and Cellular Neuroscience, The Rockefeller University, New York, NY 10021

[2] Department of Psychiatry, Yale University School of Medicine, New Haven, CT 06508

Corresponding Author: Paul Greengard, Laboratory of Molecular and Cellular Neuroscience, The Rockefeller University, New York, NY 10021. Tel: 212-327-840x; Fax: 212-327-7888; E-mail: greengard@rockefeller.edu

R.S. Rapaka and W. Sadée (eds.), *Drug Addiction.*
© American Association of Pharmaceutical Scientists 2008

DARPP-32, a Multifunctional Regulator of Protein Kinases and Protein Phosphatases

Dopamine- and cAMP-regulated phosphoprotein, Mr 32 kDa (DARPP-32), was initially discovered as a major target for dopamine-activated adenylyl cyclase and protein kinase A (PKA) in striatum.[1] Phosphorylation by PKA at Thr^{34} converts DARPP-32 into a potent high-affinity inhibitor of the multi-functional serine/threonine protein phosphatase, PP-1. The IC_{50} for inhibition of PP-1 is ~10^{-9} M.[2] Since DARPP-32 is expressed in very high concentration (~50 μM) in all medium spiny neurons,[3] including those in both the striatonigral and striatopallidal projection pathways (see below), and the concentration of all PP-1 isoforms is likely less than 20 μM,[4] a substantial proportion of PP-1 activity will be inhibited in response to even moderate increases in DARPP-32 phosphorylation.

Detailed structure-function studies have established that the first 40 amino acids at the NH_2-terminus of DARPP-32 are sufficient (when Thr^{34} is phosphorylated) for DARPP-32 to bind to and inhibit PP-1. Moreover, several different types of biochemical approaches have revealed that the remaining COOH-terminal portion of DARPP-32 serves an important role in the modulation of DARPP-32 function. In intact neurons, DARPP-32 is highly phosphorylated at Ser^{97} and Ser^{130} under basal conditions. Ser^{97} is phosphorylated by CK2 and Ser^{130} is phosphorylated by CK1. In vitro, phosphorylation of Ser^{97} of DARPP-32 increases the efficiency of phosphorylation of Thr^{34} by PKA.[5] In vitro, phosphorylation of Ser^{130} decreases the rate of dephosphorylation of Thr^{34} by PP-2B,[6] and in striatal slices, DARPP-32 phosphorylated at Ser^{130} is phosphorylated to a higher level at Thr^{34}.[7] The overall consequence of phosphorylation of DARPP-32 by CK1 or CK2 in intact cells is to increase the state of phosphorylation of Thr^{34}. The physiological role of these two phosphorylation events is to potentiate D1 dopaminergic signaling through the DARPP-32/PP-1 pathway.

A variety of recent studies have found that DARPP-32 is a physiological target for the proline-directed kinase, cdk5/p35, a cyclin-dependent kinase family member that is highly expressed in post-mitotic neurons where it is activated by the non-cyclin cofactor p35.[8] In vitro, phosphorylation of DARPP-32 at Thr^{75} does not alter the kinetics of phosphorylation by either CK1 or CK2. However, phosphorylation of Thr^{75} has a major inhibitory effect on the phosphorylation of Thr^{34} by PKA, and has a general inhibitory effect on phosphorylation of other PKA substrates. The resultant decrease in phosphorylation of Thr^{34} of DARPP-32 would act to inhibit D_1 dopamine signaling through the DARPP-32/PP-1 cascade.

DARPP-32 is Enriched in Dopaminoceptive Neurons

A prominent aspect of the distribution of DARPP-32 in the brain is its high enrichment in dopaminoceptive neurons in the striatum.[9] This distribution is very similar in all species studied, suggesting that it may be relevant to extrapolate functional data obtained in rodents to man. The highest levels of DARPP-32 are found in the striatum (caudate-putamen and nucleus accumbens), olfactory tubercle, bed nucleus of stria terminalis, and portions of the amygdaloid complex. These brain regions send projections to various target areas, including globus pallidus, ventral pallidum, the entopeduncular nucleus, and substantia nigra pars reticulata. Although concentrated in the striatum, it is important to note that moderate levels of DARPP-32 are found throughout the neocortex, with particular enrichment in layers II, III, and VI, in the dentate gyrus of the hippocampus and in the choroid plexus. There are also low levels of DARPP-32 in several other brain regions including hypothalamus and cerebellum. Within the striatum, DARPP-32 is found in medium-sized spiny neurons. Medium spiny neurons constitute the major cell type (95%) in the striatum, are inhibitory, and utilize GABA as their major neurotransmitter.[10] At the ultrastructural level, DARPP-32 has been found in most cytosolic subcellular compartments of medium spiny neurons, including dendrites, axons and axon terminals. Some nuclei also appear to contain DARPP-32 immunoreactivity.

Medium spiny neurons can be divided into two equally large subpopulations based on their peptide content and their projection areas.[11-13] One subpopulation contains substance P and dynorphin and projects directly to substantia nigra pars reticulata and the entopeduncular nucleus (the direct striatonigral pathway). The other subpopulation contains enkephalin and projects indirectly to these structures via relays in the globus pallidus and subthalamic nucleus (the indirect striatopallidal pathway). DARPP-32 is expressed at high levels in both striatonigral and striatopallidal neurons. Large-sized cholinergic interneurons and medium-sized GABAergic interneurons are devoid of DARPP-32 immunoreactivity.[14,15]

Regulation of the Phosphorylation of DARPP-32 by Dopamine, Glutamate, Serotonin and Adenosine

Within medium spiny neurons, a major role for dopamine is to modulate the actions of glutamate. Cross-talk between dopamine and glutamate plays important roles in the regulation of emotion, mood, reward, and cognition. Pertubations of these neurotransmitter systems are thought to contribute to the etiology of several common neuropsychiatric disorders, including schizophrenia, bipolar disorder and ADHD, and to play an important role in the actions of drugs of abuse. In addition to dopamine and glutamate, serotonin is also highly involved in the regulation of mood and reward and in the actions of several drugs of abuse. Indeed, the psychostimulants cocaine and amphetamine act on both dopamine and serotonin reuptake transporters and cause significant increases in the extracellular levels of these two monoamines in various regions of the brain, particularly in the striatum and nucleus accumbens.[16,17] We shall briefly review some of the studies of regulation of DARPP-32 by dopamine, glutamate and serotonin. As adenosine A_{2A} receptors are critical for the actions of caffeine and are important in the regulation of DARPP-32 phosphorylation in striatopallidal neurons, we will also briefly review the regulation of DARPP-32 by adenosine. For a more detailed discussion of these and other neurotransmitters, neuromodulators and neuropeptides see.[18]

Dopamine: Five different G protein-coupled dopamine receptors have been identified. D_1 receptor subtypes (D_1, D_5) stimulate adenylyl cyclase, whereas D_2 receptor subtypes (D_{2S}, D_{2L}, D_3, D_4) inhibit adenylyl cyclase.[19] In addition, both D_1-type and D_2-type receptors have been shown to regulate intracellular Ca^{2+} levels. D_1-type receptors can interact with calcyon and influence Ca^{2+}-dependent signaling via G_q-coupled release of Ca^{2+} from intracellular stores[20] D_2-type receptors are coupled directly to phospholipase C and the production of inositol triphosphate. As a result, activation of D_2-type receptors leads to activation of the Ca^{2+}/calmodulin-dependent protein phosphatase, calcineurin (also known as PP-2B).[21] D_2 receptors are found on dopaminergic nerve terminals, where they are thought to play an autoinhibitory role, and postsynaptically on medium spiny neurons. D_1 and D_3 receptors are predominantly expressed postsynaptically on medium spiny neurons. Anatomical studies have shown that striatonigral neurons contain high levels of D_1 receptors, whereas striatopallidal neurons predominantly express D_2 receptors.[22] However, biochemical and physiological evidence supports the idea that there is also a population of medium spiny neurons that express both D_1 and D_2 types of receptor.[23,24]

As a consequence of the actions of the different types of receptors, dopamine regulates the state of phosphorylation of DARPP-32 in a bidirectional manner. In striatal slices or whole animals, activation of D_1 receptors, via stimulation of PKA, results in phosphorylation of DARPP-32 at Thr^{34}.[21,25] This effect is counteracted by the activation of D_2 receptors via inhibition of adenylyl cyclase and via stimulation of Ca^{2+}-dependent activation of calcineurin.[21,26] Activation of D_1 receptors also decreases the phosphorylation state of DARPP-32 at Thr^{75} by a process that appears to involve the PKA-dependent activation of PP-2A.[27] Thus, enhanced dopaminergic transmission via D_1 receptors leads to a decreased phosphorylation of Thr^{75}-DARPP-32, which reduces inhibition of PKA and thereby facilitates signaling via the PKA/Thr^{34}-DARPP-32/PP-1 cascade.

Glutamate: The regulation of DARPP-32 phosphorylation by glutamate is complex and involves the actions of both ionotropic (NMDA and AMPA) and metabotropic (mGlu) glutamate receptors. Glutamate, released at glutamatergic nerve terminals, activates NMDA- and AMPA-type receptors, leading to a decrease in DARPP-32 Thr^{34} phosphorylation through the Ca^{2+}-dependent activation of calcineurin.[28,29] Activation of NMDA and AMPA receptors also results in a decrease in Thr^{75} phosphorylation.[29] Surprisingly, the regulation of Thr^{75} phosphorylation is not mediated through Ca^{2+}-dependent activation of calcineurin, but rather via Ca^{2+}-dependent activation of PP-2A, and involves a mechanism that is not yet fully understood. The primary action of glutamate through NMDA and AMPA receptors is to reduce phosphorylation of Thr^{34} and as a result to activate PP-1. However, under conditions where Thr^{34} phosphorylation is low, the dephosphorylation of Thr^{75} and the resulting disinhibition of PKA caused by glutamate may act to potentiate dopamine/D_1 receptor/PKA/phospho-Thr^{34} DARPP-32 signaling.

Metabotropic glutamate receptors are subdivided into three groups: group I (mGlu1 and mGlu5 receptors), group II (mGlu2 and mGlu3 receptors), and group

III (mGlu4, mGlu6, mGlu7, and mGlu8 receptors).[30] Group I mGlu receptors are expressed in both direct and indirect pathway neostriatal neurons,[31] and group II and III mGlu receptors are expressed on the terminals of corticostriatal afferents.[32] Activation of mGlu5 receptors in striatal slices stimulates DARPP-32 Thr^{34} phosphorylation, an effect that is dependent on activation of adenosine A_{2A} receptors by endogenous adenosine.[33] This study has further suggested that there is a synergistic interaction of mGlu5 receptors and adenosine A_{2A} receptors at the level of production of cAMP, and that this effect of mGlu5 receptors requires MAP kinase signaling.

Group I mGlu receptors also regulate the phosphorylation of DARPP-32 at Thr^{75} and Ser^{130}. Treatment of striatal slices with a group I mGlu receptor agonist stimulates the activity of CK1, leading to an increase in the phosphorylation of DARPP-32 at Thr^{75} and Ser^{130}.[34,35] Detailed analysis of the mechanism of CK1 activation revealed that group I mGlu receptors, coupled to G_q, activate phospholipase C and stimulate the generation of inositol triphosphate, leading to an increase in intracellular Ca^{2+}. The increased intracellular Ca^{2+} activates calcineurin, causing dephosphorylation of inhibitory autophosphorylation sites in CK1. Activation of CK1 causes phosphorylation of Ser^{130} and results in activation of Cdk5 and phosphorylation of Thr^{75} by an unknown mechanism.

The relative temporal contributions of ionotropic and metabotropic glutamate receptors in mediating effects of glutamate on phosphorylation of DARPP-32 at Thr^{34} and Thr^{75} have been recently studied.[36] Treatment with glutamate caused a complex change in DARPP-32 Thr^{34} phosphorylation. An initial rapid increase in Thr^{34} phosphorylation was NMDA/AMPA/mGlu5 receptor-dependent and was mediated through activation of a neuronal nitric oxide synthase/nitric oxide/cGMP/cGMP-dependent kinase signaling cascade. A subsequent decrease in phosphorylation was attributable to activation of an NMDA/AMPA receptor/Ca^{2+}/calcineurin signaling cascade. This decrease was followed by rephosphorylation via a pathway involving a mGlu5 receptor/phospholipase C and MAP kinase signaling cascade. Treatment with glutamate initially decreased Thr^{75} phosphorylation through activation of NMDA/AMPA receptor/Ca^{2+}/PP-2A signaling. Thereafter, glutamate slowly increased Thr^{75} phosphorylation through activation of mGlu1 receptor/phospholipase C signaling.

Serotonin: Various serotonin receptors, including 5-HT_{1B}, 5-HT_{1F}, 5-HT_{2A}, 5-HT_{2C}, 5-HT_{3}, 5-HT_{4}, and 5-HT_{6}, are expressed in medium spiny neurons in the striatum.[37] These receptors act primarily via the following second messenger systems: $5\text{-HT}_{1B/E}$ receptors decrease cAMP formation, $5\text{-HT}_{2A/C}$ receptors increase inositol triphosphate and diacylglycerol production, 5-HT_{3} receptors increase Na^+ and Ca^{2+} influx, and 5-HT_{4} and 5-HT_{6} receptors increase cAMP formation. Studies in striatal slices and whole animals have shown that serotonin stimulates phosphorylation of DARPP-32 at Thr^{34} and decreases phosphorylation at Thr^{75} primarily via activation of 5-HT_{4} and 5-HT_{6} receptors.[38] Serotonin stimulates phosphorylation of Ser^{130}–DARPP-32 primarily via 5-HT_{2} receptors. As a consequence of their actions on DARPP-32 phosphorylation, these three serotonin pathways act synergistically to inhibit PP-1.

Adenosine: Adenosine is found intra- and extracellularly in all organs of the body. Most adenosine is formed via breakdown of ATP intracellularly and transported to the extracellular space via equilibrative transporters. Extracellular adenosine acts via G-protein-coupled receptors of which two, A_1 and A_{2A} receptors, are abundantly expressed in the brain. Adenosine A_1 receptors inhibit, and A_{2A} receptors stimulate, adenylyl cyclase. A_1 receptors have a widespread distribution in the brain, with the highest levels in hippocampus and cerebellum, whereas A_{2A} receptors are almost exclusively found in striatum where they are restricted to striatopallidal neurons.[39] In striatal slices, the A_{2A} receptor agonist CGS21680 was found to increase the level of DARPP-32 phosphorylated at Thr[34] in a concentration-dependent manner.[40] When treatment with CGS 21680 was combined with treatment with SKF81297, a selective D_1 agonist, an additive response was observed both on cAMP levels and Thr[34]-DARPP-32 phosphorylation. In whole animals, in vivo, antagonists at A_{2A} and D_1 receptors had an additive effect in reducing DARPP-32 phosphorylation.[25] A_{2A} receptors are co-localized with D_2 receptors. Since A_{2A} receptors increase and D_2 receptors decrease cAMP levels, adenosine-dopamine interactions are in most instances antagonistic. Indeed, the A_{2A} antagonist, SCH 58261, significantly counteracted the increase in Thr[34]-DARPP-32 phosphorylation that was observed following treatment with selective D_2 receptor antagonists.[25] Likewise, the ability of D_2 antagonists to increase Thr[34]-DARPP-32 phosphorylation was dramatically reduced in A_{2A} receptor KO mice. These data provided further support for the notion that adenosine acting on A_{2A} receptors provides a basal tonic activity of the cAMP/PKA/Thr[34]-DARPP-32 pathway, which is necessary to mediate many of the effects of dopamine acting via D_2 receptors. It has also been shown that A_{2A} agonism, via cAMP-dependent mechanisms, decreases the phosphorylation at Thr[75]-DARPP-32.[41]

Role of DARPP-32 Phosphorylation in the Actions of Drugs of Abuse

It is well established that the dopaminergic system plays an important role in reward-related behaviors, and drugs with reinforcing properties share the ability to increase dopaminergic transmission.[42,43] By virtue of its regulation by dopamine, as well as by other neurotransmitters linked to the actions of drugs of abuse, DARPP-32 is positioned to play an important role in either mediating or modulating the short, and perhaps long, term actions of drugs of abuse. The generation of DARPP-32 knockout (KO) mice,[44] and the more recent generation of mice in which individual phosphorylation sites have been mutated,[45] have provided powerful animal models for use in studies of the role of DARPP-32 in the actions of drugs of abuse. A wide variety of approaches using these mouse models have demonstrated that DARPP-32 mediates many biochemical, electrophysiological, gene transcriptional, and behavioral effects of dopamine. A general feature of the results obtained is that DARPP-32 is required for the actions of physiological concentrations of dopamine, while the consequences of the lack of DARPP-32 are less pronounced at higher, supraphysiological, concentrations of dopamine. We will briefly summarize these recent studies of DARPP-32 mutant mice as well as summarize studies of the regulation of DARPP-32 phosphorylation by a variety of drugs of abuse.[18,46,47]

Cocaine and amphetamine: Cocaine inhibits reuptake of dopamine, whereas amphetamine promotes release of dopamine from nerve terminals through a weak-base-mediated reverse transport mechanism.[42,43] Acute treatment of mice with cocaine or amphetamine increases the phosphorylation of Thr[34]-DARPP-32 and Ser[130]-DARPP-32, but decreases the phosphorylation at Thr[75].[43,45] A recent immunohistochemical study[48] has demonstrated that the psychostimulant-induced phosphorylation of Thr[34]-DARPP-32 occurs primarily in striatonigral neurons. Chronic treatment with cocaine upregulates the expression of both Cdk5 and p35 in striatum, and this leads to increased phosphorylation of Thr[75] of DARPP-32 and consequently to decreased phosphorylation of Thr[34].[49] A well-known behavioral effect of repeated cocaine administration is the development of sensitization. Notably, intraaccumbal application of Cdk5 inhibitors was found to potentiate cocaine-induced behavioral sensitization,[49] indicating that Cdk5 is likely to be involved in counteracting this sensitization phenomenon.

From studies of DARPP-32 KO and phospho-site knockin mice, DARPP-32 is likely to be involved in changes in gene transcription that are important for maintaining altered synaptic function and for initiating adaptive morphological changes of the type believed to underlie the effects of various drugs of abuse. Treatment of animals with cocaine increases the phosphorylation state of CREB, ELK, and multiple immediate early genes.[42,43] CREB, c-Fos, Fras, and many other immediate early genes regulate gene transcription and may coordinate alterations in gene expression, leading to long-term changes in neuronal function. Dopamine, via activation of D_1 receptors and PKA, stimulates phosphorylation of CREB at Ser[133] in striatum,[50] and the dephosphorylation of CREB at Ser[133] is under the control of PP-1.[51] Other transcription factors, such as ELK, are regulated by the MAP kinase signaling cascade.[42] Notably, dopamine receptor-mediated activation of MAP kinase, CREB, c-Fos, and ΔFosB is strongly attenuated in DARPP-32 KO mice.[13,52,53]

A detailed study of the regulation of the MAP kinase signaling cascade by DARPP-32 showed a prominent role of Thr[34]-DARPP-32/PP-1 signaling.[48] Inhibition of PP-1 appears to be important at several levels for activating the ERK cascade. On the one hand, it prevents extracellular regulated kinase (ERK) dephosphorylation by striatal enriched phosphatase (STEP), by maintaining this tyrosine phosphatase in a phosphorylated, inactive, state. On the other hand, PP-1 is also critical upstream of ERK, because MEK phosphorylation in response to psychostimulants was dramatically reduced in DARPP-32 KO mice.

Several alterations in the behavioral responses to acute and chronic treatment with cocaine are exhibited in DARPP-32 KO mice. An attenuated locomotor responsiveness to a single injection of cocaine is found in DARPP-32 KO mice compared with wild-type mice.[44] In contrast, following chronic treatment with cocaine, DARPP-32 KO mice show increased locomotor sensitization as compared with wild-type mice.[54] The different involvement of DARPP-32 in acute and chronic responses to cocaine may be related to the differences in the relative levels of Thr[75]-DARPP-32 and Thr[34]-DARPP-32, which have been found following acute vs chronic treatment with cocaine, and the antagonistic relationship between these two sites.[27,49] The acquisition of place-preference is also significantly attenuated in DARPP-32 KO mice.[55,56]

The effects of D-amphetamine on two other behavioral parameters—sensorimotor gating and repetitive movements—were also greatly diminished in DARPP-32 KO, Thr[34]Ala-DARPP-32 and Ser[130]Ala-DARPP-32 mice.[45]

Opioids: Opiates regulate striatal function via an indirect action on mesencephalic dopamine neurons and a direct action on opioid receptors located within striatum.[43] There is a relatively abundant expression of all three opioid receptor sub-types (μ, δ, and κ) in striatum.[57,58] κ opioid receptors are expressed primarily on dopaminergic nerve terminals, whereas μ- and δ-receptors are expressed in medium spiny neurons. μ-receptors appear to be enriched in striatonigral neurons where they are colocalized with D_1 receptors. δ-receptors are highly expressed in cholinergic interneurons, but there is also some expression in striatopallidal neurons. Both μ- and δ-receptors are negatively coupled to adenylyl cyclase. In striatal slices, activation of opioid receptors was found to modulate the effects of dopamine and adenosine on DARPP-32 phosphorylation at Thr[34].[59] Thus, consistent with the cellular localization of its receptor, the μ-opioid receptor agonist, DAMGO, inhibits the increase in DARPP-32 phosphorylation induced by SKF 81,297, a D_1 receptor agonist, but not by CGS 21,680, an A_{2A} receptor agonist. Conversely, the δ-opioid receptor agonist, DPDPE, inhibits DARPP-32 phosphorylation induced by activation of A_{2A} receptors, but not by activation of D_1 receptors.

Nicotine: Nicotine has been shown to modulate dopaminergic neurotransmission mainly by enhancing dopamine release in nigrostriatal and mesolimbic dopaminergic systems.[60,61] Five types of α subunits ($\alpha2$-$\alpha6$) and three types of β subunits ($\beta2$-$\beta4$) constitute α and β type heteromeric nicotinic acetylcholine receptors (nAChRs), whereas $\alpha7$ subunits constitute homomeric nAChRs.[62] Four major populations of nAChRs are expressed at dopaminergic terminals in the striatum, with the major subtype containing $\alpha4\beta2$ subunits.[63] The other predominant subtype, $\alpha7$, is expressed at glutamatergic terminals in the striatum.[64]

Acute application of nicotine in mouse neostriatal slices produces a dose-dependent response, with a low concentration (1 μM) causing a sustained decrease in DARPP-32 Thr[34] phosphorylation, and a high concentration (100 μM) causing a transient increase in Thr[34] phosphorylation.[65] Using a variety of pharmacological reagents, nicotine at a low concentration (1 μM) has been found to stimulate $\alpha4\beta2$-containing nAChRs at dopaminergic terminals. Activation of $\alpha4\beta2$ nAChRs results in the release of dopamine, and the released dopamine selectively activates dopamine D_2 receptor signaling, leading to a reduction in phosphorylation at Thr[34]. Conversely, nicotine at a high concentration (100 μM) was found to stimulate both $\alpha4\beta2$ nAChRs at dopaminergic terminals and $\alpha7$ nAChRs at glutamatergic terminals. Activation of $\alpha7$ nAChRs results in the release of glutamate. Co-activation of $\alpha4\beta2$ nAChRs by nicotine, and of NMDA/AMPA receptors by glutamate, synergistically induces robust dopamine release, leading to the activation of dopamine D_1 receptors and phosphorylation of Thr^{34}. Thus, depending on the amount of dopamine released locally in response to low and high concentrations of nicotine, either dopamine D_2 receptor signaling in striatopallidal neurons or dopamine D_1 receptor signaling in striatonigral neurons is predominantly activated.

Lysergic acid diethylamide (LSD) and Phencyclidine (PCP): LSD and other related hallucinogens act via multiple serotonin receptors, including 5-HT_2, 5-HT_5 and 5-HT_6 receptors.[66,67] Behavioral studies using discrimination paradigms have suggested a major role for 5-HT_2 receptors in mediating the discriminative stimulus effects of hallucinogens.[68] Stimulation of 5-HT2 receptors increases Ser^{130}-DARPP-32 in slices and LSD also significantly increases phosphorylation of Ser^{130}-DARPP-32 in mice.[45] LSD had similar effects on Ser^{130}-DARPP-32 in slices prepared from striatum and in striata from whole animals. LSD also increased phosphorylation at Thr^{34}-DARPP-32. In slices, but not in striata from whole animals, LSD decreased Thr^{75}-DARPP-32.

PCP acts as a non-competitive antagonist at NMDA receptors and causes a complex behavioral response. In general, NMDA receptor antagonists can produce psychotic symptoms in humans that are indistinguishable from acute episodes of schizophrenia. As a result, glutamatergic dysfunction has been proposed as an underlying cause of the pathophysiology of schizophrenia.[69] Hence, NMDA receptor antagonists, such as PCP, have been used extensively to pharmacologically model psychosis in animals. However, PCP also potently regulates the reward system. Rats can be trained to self-administer PCP.[70] Interestingly, this effect appears to be largely dopamine-independent. Furthermore, PCP-induced locomotor stimulation and potentiation of cocaine reinforcement, can occur without a concomitant increase in dopamine release.[71,72] PCP as well as MK801, another NMDA antagonist, increases Thr^{34}-DARPP-32 phosphorylation.[21,45] PCP also increases Ser^{130}-DARPP-32, but has no effect on Thr^{75}-DARPP-32.[45]

The pattern of DARPP-32 phosphorylation induced by D-amphetamine, LSD, and PCP would be predicted to result in synergistic inhibition of PP-1. In accordance with these biochemical observations, the effects of LSD and PCP, as well as of D-amphetamine, on sensorimotor gating and repetitive movements were reduced in DARPP-32 KO mice and in mice with point mutations at Thr^{34} or Ser^{130} of DARPP-32.[45]

Caffeine: Caffeine, the most commonly used psychostimulant, acts as an antagonist at A_1 as well as A_{2A} adenosine receptors.[73] A role for A_1 adenosine receptors in the stimulatory actions of caffeine was initially suggested. However, it is now recognized that blockade of A_{2A} receptors is critical for the actions of caffeine.[73,74] Recent studies have provided strong evidence for an involvement of DARPP-32 in the stimulatory actions of caffeine. Systemic administration of caffeine, or of SCH58261, a selective A_{2A} receptor antagonist, causes an increase of Thr^{75}-DARPP-32 in wild-type mice.[41] The stimulatory effects of caffeine and SCH 58,261 on locomotor activity, seen in wild-type mice, were greatly reduced in DARPP-32 KO mice. The blockade of a basally active A_{2A}/PKA/PP-2A/Thr^{75}-DARPP-32 pathway may, therefore, play a critical role for the stimulatory actions of caffeine.

Ethanol: DARPP-32 appears to be involved in both acute and long-term responses to ethanol. Conditioned place preference studies of wild-type and DARPP-32 KO mice indicate a requirement for DARPP-32 in mediating ethanol reward.[75] DARPP-32 KO mice also exhibit a significant decrement in ethanol self-administration. However, DARPP-32 KO mice show a greater sensitivity to the motor stimulant effect produced by a single injection of ethanol. Another recent study has shown that DARPP-32 appears to play a role in ethanol reinforcement by acting to regulate the ability of ethanol to inhibit NMDA receptor function.[76] In the presence of ethanol, NMDA synaptic currents are generally reduced. In brain regions containing DARPP-32, dopamine, via D_1 receptors, stimulates the PKA-mediated phosphorylation of the NR1 subunit of the NMDA receptor at Ser^{897}. In DARPP-32 KO mice this regulation of NMDA receptors is absent, and activation of D_1 receptors does not prevent the ability of ethanol to inhibit NMDA receptors. Interestingly, moderate levels of ethanol increase phosphorylation of Thr^{34} in striatal slices, although the mechanism involved has not been determined.

Summary

A large body of work over the last two decades has found that DARPP-32, when phosphorylated at Thr^{34}, acts as an amplifier of PKA-mediated signaling through its ability to potently inhibit PP-1. This amplifying property of DARPP-32 is critical for dopaminergic signaling, but it is also utilized by multiple other neurotransmitters, including glutamate, serotonin and adenosine, in the striatum and other brain regions. In addition to its role as a PP-1 inhibitor, DARPP-32 when phosphorylated at Thr^{75} inhibits PKA. Upon dopaminergic neurotransmission, the phosphorylation state at Thr^{75} is reduced allowing disinhibition of PKA and further increasing phosphorylation at Thr^{34}. This complex positive feedback loop potentiates dopaminergic signaling.

An important component of our studies of DARPP-32 function, particularly those related to the actions of drugs of abuse, has been the use of DARPP-32 KO mice. More recently these studies have been complemented by generation of mice in which each of the 4 phosphorylation sites have been individually mutated. In future studies, these "phosphomutant" mice will be used to further dissect the precise roles played by Thr^{34}, Thr^{75}, Ser^{97} (the mouse equivalent of Ser^{102}) and Ser^{130} in the stimulatory and rewarding effects of drugs of abuse.

Other recent studies have indicated that the actions of dopamine and adenosine differ between sub-populations of striatal neurons. For example, a recent immuno-histochemical study,[48] demonstrated that amphetamine and cocaine increase levels of Thr^{34}-DARPP-32 phosphorylation mainly in striatonigral neurons. It will be important in the future to analyze DARPP-32 phosphorylation in either striatonigral or striatopallidal neurons in response to the actions of different drugs of abuse. We hope that these and other novel types of approach will enable us to identify protein kinases, protein phosphatases and phosphoprotein substrates that mediate the actions of drugs of abuse and that could be novel targets for development of treatments for drug dependence.

Acknowledgments This work was supported by National Institutes of Health Grant DA10044 (A.C.N, P.G) and DA018343 (A.C.N).

References

1. Walaas SI, Aswad DW, Greengard P. A dopamine- and cyclic AMP-regulated phosphoprotein enriched in dopamine-innervated brain regions. *Nature*. 1983;301:69-71.
2. Hemmings HC Jr, Greengard P, Tung HY, Cohen P. DARPP-32, a dopamine-regulated neuronal phosphoprotein, is a potent inhibitor of protein phosphatase-1. *Nature*. Aug 9-15, 1984;310(5977):503-505.
3. Ouimet CC, Langley-Gullion KC, Greengard P. Quantitative immunocytochemistry of DARPP-32-expressing neurons in the rat caudatoputamen. *Brain Res*. 1998;808:8-12.
4. da Cruz e Silva EF Fox CA, Ouimet CC, Gustafson E, Watson SJ, Greengard P. Differential expression of protein phosphatase 1 isoforms in mammalian brain. *J Neurosci*. 1995;15:3375-3389.
5. Girault JA Jr, Hemmings HC Jr, Williams KR, Nairn AC, Greengard P. Phosphorylation of DARPP-32, a dopamine- and cAMP-regulated phosphoprotein, by casein kinase II. *J Biol Chem*. 1989;264:21748-21759.
6. Desdouits F, Cohen D, Nairn AC, Greengard P, Girault JA. Phosphorylation of DARPP-32, a dopamine- and cAMP-regulated phosphoprotein, by casein kinase I in vitro and in vivo. *J Biol Chem*. 1995;270:8772-8778.
7. Desdouits F, Siciliano JC, Greengard P, Girault JA. Dopamine- and cAMP-regulated phosphoprotein DARPP-32: phosphorylation of Ser-137 by casein kinase I inhibits dephosphorylation of Thr-34 by calcineurin. *Proc Natl Acad Sci USA*. 1995;92:2682-2685.
8. Bibb JA, Snyder GL, Nishi A, et al. Phosphorylation of DARPP-32 by Cdk5 modulates dopamine signalling in neurons. *Nature*. 1999;402:669-671.
9. Ouimet CC Jr, Miller PE Jr, Hemmings HC Jr, Walaas SI, Greengard P. DARPP-32, a dopamine- and adenosine 3':5'-monophosphate-regulated phosphoprotein enriched in dopamine-innervated brain regions. III. Immunocytochemical localization. *J Neurosci*. 1984;4:111-124.
10. Yoshida M, Precht W. Monosynaptic inhibition of neurons of the substantia nigra by caudato-nigral fibers. *Brain Res*. 1971;32:225-228.
11. Beckstead RM, Cruz CJ. Striatal axons to the globus pallidus, entopeduncular nucleus and substantia nigra come mainly from separate cell populations in cat. *Neuroscience*. 1986;19:147-158.
12. Gerfen CR 3rd, Young WS 3rd. Distribution of striatonigral and striatopallidal peptidergic neurons in both patch and matrix compartments: an in situ hybridization histochemistry and fluorescent retrograde tracing study. *Brain Res*. 1988;460:161-167.
13. Kawaguchi Y, Wilson CJ, Emson PC. Projection subtypes of rat neostriatal matrix cells revealed by intracellular injection of biocytin. *J Neurosci*. 1990;10:3421-3438.
14. Anderson KD, Reiner A. Immunohistochemical localization of DARPP-32 in striatal projection neurons and striatal interneurons: implications for the localization of D1-like dopamine receptors on different types of striatal neurons. *Brain Res*. 1991;568:235-243.
15. Ouimet CC, Greengard P. Distribution of DARPP-32 in the basal ganglia: an electron microscopic study. *J Neurocytol*. 1990;19:39-52.
16. Carboni E, Imperato A, Perezzani L, Di Chiara G. Amphetamine, cocaine, phencyclidine and nomifensine increase extracellular dopamine concentrations preferentially in the nucleus accumbens of freely moving rats. *Neuroscience*. 1989;28:653-661.

17. Parsons LH, Koob GF, Weiss F. Serotonin dysfunction in the nucleus accumbens of rats during withdrawal after unlimited access to intravenous cocaine. *J Pharmacol Exp Ther.* 1995;274:1182-1191.
18. Svenningsson P, Nishi A, Fisone G, Girault JA, Nairn AC, Greengard P. DARPP-32: an integrator of neurotransmission. *Annu Rev Pharmacol Toxicol.* 2004;44:269-296.
19. Stoof JC, Kebabian JW. Opposing roles for D-1 and D-2 dopamine receptors in efflux of cyclic AMP from rat neostriatum. *Nature.* 1981;294:366-368.
20. Bergson C, Levenson R, Goldman-Rakic PS, Lidow MS. Dopamine receptor-interacting proteins: the Ca(2+) connection in dopamine signaling. *Trends Pharmacol Sci.* 2003;24:486-492.
21. Nishi A, Snyder GL, Greengard P. Bidirectional regulation of DARPP-32 phosphorylation by dopamine. *J Neurosci.* 1997;17:8147-8155.
22. Gerfen CR, Engber TM, Mahan LC, et al. D1 and D2 dopamine receptor-regulated gene expression of striatonigral and striatopallidal neurons. *Science.* 1990;250:1429-1432.
23. Surmeier DJ, Song WJ, Yan Z. Coordinated expression of dopamine receptors in neostriatal medium spiny neurons. *J Neurosci.* 1996;16:6579-6591.
24. Aizman O, Brismar H, Uhlen P, et al. Anatomical and physiological evidence for D1 and D2 dopamine receptor colocalization in neostriatal neurons. *Nat Neurosci.* 2000;3:226-230.
25. Svenningsson P, Lindskog M, Ledent C, et al. Regulation of the phosphorylation of the dopamine- and cAMP-regulated phosphoprotein of 32 kDa in vivo by dopamine D1, dopamine D2, and adenosine A2A receptors. *Proc Natl Acad Sci USA.* 2000;97:1856-1860.
26. Lindskog M, Svenningsson P, Fredholm BB, Greengard P, Fisone G. Activation of dopamine D2 receptors decreases DARPP-32 phosphorylation in striatonigral and striatopallidal projection neurons via different mechanisms. *Neuroscience.* 1999;88:1005-1008.
27. Nishi A, Bibb JA, Snyder GL, Higashi H, Nairn AC, Greengard P. Amplification of dopaminergic signaling by a positive feedback loop. *Proc Natl Acad Sci USA.* 2000;97:12840-12845.
28. Halpain S, Girault JA, Greengard P. Activation of NMDA receptors induces dephosphorylation of DARPP-32 in rat striatal slices. *Nature.* 1990;343:369-372.
29. Nishi A, Bibb JA, Matsuyama S, et al. Regulation of DARPP-32 dephosphorylation at PKA- and Cdk5-sites by NMDA and AMPA receptors: distinct roles of calcineurin and protein phosphatase-2A. *J Neurochem.* 2002;81:832-841.
30. Schoepp DD, Jane DE, Monn JA. Pharmacological agents acting at subtypes of metabotropic glutamate receptors. *Neuropharmacology.* 1999;38:1431-1476.
31. Tallaksen-Greene SJ, Kaatz KW, Romano C, Albin RL. Localization of mGluR1a-like immunoreactivity and mGluR5-like immunoreactivity in identified populations of striatal neurons. *Brain Res.* 1998;780:210-217.
32. Testa CM, Friberg IK, Weiss SW, Standaert DG. Immunohistochemical localization of metabotropic glutamate receptors mGluR1a and mGluR2/3 in the rat basal ganglia. *J Comp Neurol.* 1998;390:5-19.
33. Nishi A, Liu F, Matsuyama S, et al. Metabotropic mGlu5 receptors regulate adenosine A2A receptor signaling. *Proc Natl Acad Sci USA.* 2003;100:1322-1327.
34. Liu F, Ma XH, Ule J, et al. Regulation of cyclin-dependent kinase 5 and casein kinase 1 by metabotropic glutamate receptors. *Proc Natl Acad Sci USA.* 2001;98:11062-11068.
35. Liu F, Virshup DM, Nairn AC, Greengard P. Mechanism of regulation of casein kinase I activity by group I metabotropic glutamate receptors. *J Biol Chem.* 2002;277:45393-45399.
36. Nishi A, Watanabe Y, Higashi H, Tanaka M, Nairn AC, Greengard P. Glutamate regulation of DARPP-32 phosphorylation in neostriatal neurons involves activation of multiple signaling cascades. *Proc Natl Acad Sci USA.* 2005;102:1199-1204.
37. Barnes NM, Sharp T. A review of central 5-HT receptors and their function. *Neuropharmacology.* 1999;38:1083-1152.
38. Svenningsson P, Tzavara ET, Liu F, Fienberg AA, Nomikos GG, Greengard P. DARPP-32 mediates serotonergic neurotransmission in the forebrain. *Proc Natl Acad Sci USA.* 2002;99:3188-3193.

39. Schiffmann SN, Jacobs O, Vanderhaeghen JJ. Striatal restricted adenosine A2 receptor (RDC8) is expressed by enkephalin but not by substance P neurons: an in situ hybridization histochemistry study. *J Neurochem.* 1991;57:1062-1067.
40. Svenningsson P, Lindskog M, Rognoni F, Fredholm BB, Greengard P, Fisone G. Activation of adenosine A2A and dopamine D1 receptors stimulates cyclic AMP-dependent phosphorylation of DARPP-32 in distinct populations of striatal projection neurons. *Neuroscience.* 1998;84:223-228.
41. Lindskog M, Svenningsson P, Pozzi L, et al. Involvement of DARPP-32 phosphorylation in the stimulant action of caffeine. *Nature.* 2002;418:774-778.
42. Hyman SE, Malenka RC. Addiction and the brain: the neurobiology of compulsion and its persistence. *Nat Rev Neurosci.* 2001;2:695-703.
43. Nestler EJ. Molecular basis of long-term plasticity underlying addiction. *Nat Rev Neurosci.* 2001;2:119-128.
44. Fienberg AA, Hiroi N, Mermelstein PG, et al. DARPP-32: regulator of the efficacy of dopaminergic neurotransmission. *Science.* 1998;281:838-842.
45. Svenningsson P, Tzavara ET, Carruthers R, et al. Diverse psychotomimetics act through a common signaling pathway. *Science.* 2003;302:1412-1415.
46. Fienberg AA, Greengard P. The DARPP-32 knockout mouse. *Brain Res Brain Res Rev.* 2000;31:313-319.
47. Nairn AC, Svenningsson P, Nishi A, Fisone G, Girault JA, Greengard P. The role of DARPP-32 in the actions of drugs of abuse. *Neuropharmacology.* 2004;47:14-23.
48. Valjent E, Pascoli V, Svenningsson P, et al. Regulation of a protein phosphatase cascade allows convergent dopamine and glutamate signals to activate ERK in the striatum. *Proc Natl Acad Sci USA.* 2005;102:491-496.
49. Bibb JA, Chen J, Taylor JR, et al. Effects of chronic exposure to cocaine are regulated by the neuronal protein Cdk5. *Nature.* 2001;410:376-380.
50. Liu FC, Graybiel AM. Spatiotemporal dynamics of CREB phosphorylation: transient versus sustained phosphorylation in the developing striatum. *Neuron.* 1996;17:1133-1144.
51. Hagiwara M, Alberts A, Brindle P, et al. Transcriptional attenuation following cAMP induction requires PP-1-mediated dephosphorylation of CREB. *Cell.* 1992;70:105-113.
52. Yan Z, Feng J, Fienberg AA, Greengard P. D(2) dopamine receptors induce mitogen-activated protein kinase and cAMP response element-binding protein phosphorylation in neurons. *Proc Natl Acad Sci USA.* 1999;96:11607-11612.
53. Svenningsson P, Fienberg AA, Allen PB, et al. Dopamine D(1) receptor-induced gene transcription is modulated by DARPP-32. *J Neurochem.* 2000;75:248-257.
54. Hiroi N, Fienberg AA, Haile CN, et al. Neuronal and behavioural abnormalities in striatal function in DARPP-32-mutant mice. *Eur J Neurosci.* 1999;11:1114-1118.
55. Zachariou V, Benoit-Marand M, Allen PB, et al. Reduction of cocaine place preference in mice lacking the protein phosphatase 1 inhibitors DARPP 32 or Inhibitor 1. *Biol Psychiatry.* 2002;51:612-620.
56. Heyser CJ, Fienberg AA, Greengard P, Gold LH. DARPP-32 knockout mice exhibit impaired reversal learning in a discriminated operant task. *Brain Res.* 2000;867:122-130.
57. Schoffelmeer AN, Hansen HA, Stoof JC, Mulder AH. Blockade of D-2 dopamine receptors strongly enhances the potency of enkephalins to inhibit dopamine-sensitive adenylate cyclase in rat neostriatum: involvement of delta- and mu-opioid receptors. *J Neurosci.* 1986;6:2235-2239.
58. Georges F, Stinus L, Bloch B, Le Moine C. Chronic morphine exposure and spontaneous withdrawal are associated with modifications of dopamine receptor and neuropeptide gene expression in the rat striatum. *Eur J Neurosci.* 1999;11:481-490.
59. Lindskog M, Svenningsson P, Fredholm B, Greengard P, Fisone G. Mu- and delta-opioid receptor agonists inhibit DARPP-32 phosphorylation in distinct populations of striatal projection neurons. *Eur J Neurosci.* 1999;11:2182-2186.
60. Role LW, Berg DK. Nicotinic receptors in the development and modulation of CNS synapses. *Neuron.* 1996;16:1077-1085.

61. Wonnacott S. Presynaptic nicotinic ACh receptors. *Trends Neurosci.* 1997;20:92-98.
62. Ramirez-Latorre J, Crabtree G, Turner J, Role L. Molecular composition and biophysical characteristics of nicotinic receptors. In: Arneric SP, Brioni JD, eds. *Neuronal nicotinic receptors: pharmacology and therapeutic opportunities.* New York: Wiley-Liss, Inc; 1999:43-64.
63. Zoli M, Moretti M, Zanardi A, McIntosh JM, Clementi F, Gotti C. Identification of the nicotinic receptor subtypes expressed on dopaminergic terminals in the rat striatum. *J Neurosci.* 2002;22:8785-8789.
64. Nomikos GG, Schilstrom B, Hildebrand BE, Panagis G, Grenhoff J, Svensson TH. Role of alpha7 nicotinic receptors in nicotine dependence and implications for psychiatric illness. *Behav Brain Res.* 2000;113:97-103.
65. Hamada M, Higashi H, Nairn AC, Greengard P, Nishi A. Differential regulation of dopamine D1 and D2 signaling by nicotine in neostriatal neurons. *J Neurochem.* 2004;90:1094-1103
66. Aghajanian GK, Marek GJ. Serotonin and hallucinogens. *Neuropsychopharmacology.* 1999;21:16S-23S.
67. Grailhe R, Waeber C, Dulawa SC, et al. Increased exploratory activity and altered response to LSD in mice lacking the 5-HT(5A) receptor. *Neuron.* 1999;22:581-591.
68. Glennon RA, Titeler M, McKenney JD. Evidence for 5-HT2 involvement in the mechanism of action of hallucinogenic agents. *Life Sci.* 1984;35:2505-2511.
69. Sawa A, Snyder SH. Schizophrenia: diverse approaches to a complex disease. *Science.* 2002;296:692-695.
70. Carlezon WA Jr, Wise RA. Rewarding actions of phencyclidine and related drugs in nucleus accumbens shell and frontal cortex. *J Neurosci.* 1996;16:3112-3122.
71. Druhan JP, Rajabi H, Stewart J. MK-801 increases locomotor activity without elevating extracellular dopamine levels in the nucleus accumbens. *Synapse.* 1996;24:135-146.
72. Pierce RC, Meil WM, Kalivas PW. The NMDA antagonist, dizocilpine, enhances cocaine reinforcement without influencing mesoaccumbens dopamine transmission. *Psychopharmacology (Berl).* 1997;133:188-195.
73. Svenningsson P, Le Moine C, Fisone G, Fredholm BB. Distribution, biochemistry and function of striatal adenosine A2A receptors. *Prog Neurobiol.* 1999;59:355-396.
74. Ledent C, Vaugeois JM, Schiffmann SN, et al. Aggressiveness, hypoalgesia and high blood pressure in mice lacking the adenosine A2a receptor. *Nature.* 1997;388:674-678.
75. Risinger FO, Freeman PA, Greengard P, Fienberg AA. Motivational effects of ethanol in DARPP-32 knock-out mice. *J Neurosci.* 2001;21:340-348.
76. Maldve RE, Zhang TA, Ferrani-Kile K, et al. DARPP-32 and regulation of the ethanol sensitivity of NMDA receptors in the nucleus accumbens. *Nat Neurosci.* 2002;5:641-648.

Chapter 2
Drug Discovery From Natural Sources

Young-Won Chin,[1] Marcy J. Balunas,[1,2] Hee Byung Chai,[1]
and A. Douglas Kinghorn[1]

Abstract Organic compounds from terrestrial and marine organisms have extensive past and present use in the treatment of many diseases and serve as compounds of interest both in their natural form and as templates for synthetic modification. Over 20 new drugs launched on the market between 2000 and 2005, originating from terrestrial plants, terrestrial microorganisms, marine organisms, and terrestrial vertebrates and invertebrates, are described. These approved substances, representative of very wide chemical diversity, together with several other natural products or their analogs undergoing clinical trials, continue to demonstrate the importance of compounds from natural sources in modern drug discovery efforts.

Keywords natural products, drug discovery, terrestrial plants, terrestrial microorganisms, marine organisms, terrestrial vertebrates, terrestrial invertebrates, chemical diversity

Introduction

For thousands of years, natural products have played an important role throughout the world in treating and preventing human diseases. Natural product medicines have come from various source materials including terrestrial plants, terrestrial microorganisms, marine organisms, and terrestrial vertebrates and invertebrates.[1] The importance of natural products in modern medicine has been discussed in recent reviews and reports.[1-6] The value of natural products in this regard can be

[1] Division of Medicinal Chemistry and Pharmacognosy, College of Pharmacy, The Ohio State University, Columbus, OH 43210

[2] Program for Collaborative Research in the Pharmaceutical Sciences, Department of Medicinal Chemistry and Pharmacognosy, College of Pharmacy, University of Illinois at Chicago, Chicago, IL 60612

Corresponding Author: A. Douglas Kinghorn, Division of Medicinal Chemistry and Pharmacognosy, College of Pharmacy, The Ohio State University, Columbus, OH 43210. Tel: (614) 247-8094; Fax: (614) 247-8642; E-mail: kinghorn.4@osu.edu

assessed using 3 criteria: (1) the rate of introduction of new chemical entities of wide structural diversity, including serving as templates for semisynthetic and total synthetic modification, (2) the number of diseases treated or prevented by these substances, and (3) their frequency of use in the treatment of disease.

An analysis of the origin of the drugs developed between 1981 and 2002 showed that natural products or natural product-derived drugs comprised 28% of all new chemical entities (NCEs) launched onto the market.[2] In addition, 24% of these NCEs were synthetic or natural mimic compounds, based on the study of pharmacophores related to natural products.[1] This combined percentage (52% of all NCEs) suggests that natural products are important sources for new drugs and are also good lead compounds suitable for further modification during drug development. The large proportion of natural products in drug discovery has stemmed from the diverse structures and the intricate carbon skeletons of natural products. Since secondary metabolites from natural sources have been elaborated within living systems, they are often perceived as showing more "drug-likeness and biological friendliness than totally synthetic molecules,"[3] making them good candidates for further drug development.[5,7]

Scrutiny of medical indications by source of compounds has demonstrated that natural products and related drugs are used to treat 87% of all categorized human diseases (48/55), including as antibacterial, anticancer, anticoagulant, antiparasitic, and immunosuppressant agents, among others.[2] There was no introduction of any natural products or related drugs for 7 drug categories (anesthetic, antianginal, antihistamine, anxiolytic, chelator and antidote, diuretic, and hypnotic) during 1981 to 2002.[2] In the case of antibacterial agents, natural products have made significant contributions as either direct treatments or templates for synthetic modification. Of the 90 drugs of that type that became commercially available in the United States or were approved worldwide from 1982 to 2002, ~79% can be traced to a natural product origin.[2]

Frequency of use of natural products in the treatment and/or prevention of disease can be measured by the number and/or economic value of prescriptions, from which the extent of preference and/or effectiveness of drugs can be estimated indirectly. According to a study by Grifo and colleagues,[8] 84 of a representative 150 prescription drugs in the United States fell into the category of natural products and related drugs. They were prescribed predominantly as anti-allergy/pulmonary/respiratory agents, analgesics, cardiovascular drugs, and for infectious diseases. Another study found that natural products or related substances accounted for 40%, 24%, and 26%, respectively, of the top 35 worldwide ethical drug sales from 2000, 2001, and 2002.[9] Of these natural product-based drugs, paclitaxel (ranked at 25 in 2000), a plant-derived anticancer drug, had sales of $1.6 billion in 2000.[10,11] The sales of 2 categories of plant-derived cancer chemotherapeutic agents were responsible for approximately one third of the total anticancer drug sales worldwide, or just under $3 billion dollars in 2002; namely, the taxanes, paclitaxel and docetaxel, and the camptothecin derivatives, irinotecan and topotecan.[10,11]

This short review covers new drugs derived from natural sources launched in the 6-year period from 2000 to 2005, and drug candidates from natural sources in clinical trials during the same time period arranged according to their origin (terrestrial plants, terrestrial microorganisms, marine organisms, and other natural sources). For drug candidates in clinical trials,[12] only examples of new chemical templates of potential cancer chemotherapeutic drugs will be mentioned.

Drug Discovery From Terrestrial Plants

Terrestrial plants, especially higher plants, have a long history of use in the treatment of human diseases. Several well-known species, including licorice (*Glycyrrhiza glabra*), myrrh (*Commiphora* species), and poppy capsule latex (*Papaver somniferum*), were referred to by the first known written record on clay tablets from Mesopotamia in 2600 BC, and these plants are still in use today for the treatment of various diseases as ingredients of official drugs or herbal preparations used in systems of traditional medicine.[1] Furthermore, morphine, codeine, noscapine (narcotine), and papaverine isolated from *P. somniferum* were developed as single chemical drugs and are still clinically used. Hemisuccinate carbenoxolone sodium, a semi-synthetic derivative of glycyrrhetic acid found in licorice, is prescribed for the treatment of gastric and duodenal ulcers in various countries.[13]

Historical experiences with plants as therapeutic tools have helped to introduce single chemical entities in modern medicine. Plants, especially those with ethnopharmacological uses, have been the primary sources of medicines for early drug discovery. In fact, a recent analysis by Fabricant and Farnsworth showed that the uses of 80% of 122 plant-derived drugs were related to their original ethnopharmacological purposes.[14] Current drug discovery from terrestrial plants has mainly relied on bioactivity-guided isolation methods, which, for example, have led to discoveries of the important anticancer agents, paclitaxel from *Taxus brevifolia* and camptothecin from *Camptotheca acuminata*.[15] Other NCEs discovered or modified from terrestrial plants between 2000–2005 are summarized below (Fig. 2.1).[12]

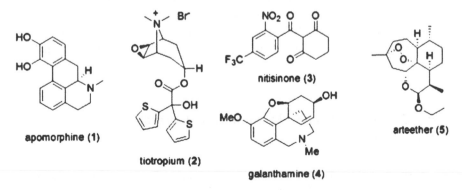

apomorphine (1)

tiotropium (2)

nitisinone (3)

galanthamine (4)

arteether (5)

Fig. 2.1 New drugs from terrestrial plants (2000 to 2005).

Approved Drugs

Apomorphine hydrochloride (**1**, Apokyn, Bertek, 2004), a short-acting dopamine D_1 and D_2 receptor agonist, is a potent dopamine receptor agonist used to treat Parkinson's disease, a chronic neurodegenerative disease caused by the loss of pigmented mesostriatal dopaminergic neurons linking the substantia nigra (pars compacta) to the neostriatum (caudate nucleus and putamen). Apomorphine is a derivative of morphine isolated from poppy (*Papaver somniferum*). Subcutaneous apomorphine is currently used for the management of sudden, unexpected and refractory levodopa-induced off states in fluctuating Parkinson's disease.[16]

Tiotropium bromide (**2**, Spiriva Handihaler, Boehringer Ingelheim, 2004) has been approved by the United States Food and Drug Administration (FDA) for the treatment of bronchospasm associated with chronic obstructive pulmonary disease (COPD). Tiotropium, a derivative of atropine from *Atropa belladonna* (Solanaceae) and related tropane alkaloids from other solanaceous plants, is a potent reversible nonselective inhibitor of muscarinic receptors. Tiotropium is structurally analogous to ipratropium, a commonly prescribed drug for COPD, but has shown longer-lasting effects.[17]

Nitisinone (**3**, Orfadin, Swedish Orphan, 2002) is a derivative of leptospermone, an important new class of herbicides from the bottlebrush plant (*Callistemon citrinus*), and exerts an inhibitory effect for *p*-hydroxyphenylpyruvate dioxygenase (HPPD) involved in plastoquinone synthesis.[18] This drug has been used successfully as a treatment of hereditary tyrosinaemia type 1 (HT-1), a severe inherited disease of humans caused by a deficiency of fumaryl acetoacetate hydrolase (FAH), leading to accumulation of fumaryl and maleyl acetoacetate, and progressive liver and kidney damage.[19]

Galantamine hydrobromide (**4**, Reminyl, Janssen, 2001) is an Amaryllidaceae alkaloid obtained from *Galanthus nivalis* that has been used traditionally in Bulgaria and Turkey for neurological conditions,[20,21] and was launched onto the market as a selective acetylcholinesterase inhibitor for Alzheimer's disease treatment, slowing the process of neurological degeneration by inhibiting acetylcholinesterase as well as binding to and modulating the nicotinic acetylcholine receptor.[5]

Arteether (**5**, Artecef, Artecef BV, 2000), an antimalarial agent, has been developed from artemisinin, a sesquiterpene lactone isolated from *Artemisia annua* (Asteraceae), a plant used in traditional Chinese medicine as a remedy for chills and fevers. Other derivatives of artemisinin are in various stages of clinical development as antimalarial drugs in Europe.[5,22]

Examples of Plant-derived Compounds Currently in Clinical Trials

From terrestrial plant-derived secondary metabolites, several new chemical entities (Fig. 2.2) are undergoing clinical trials including four that are derivatives of known anticancer drugs (camptothecin, paclitaxel, epipodophyllotoxin, and vinblastine).[12]

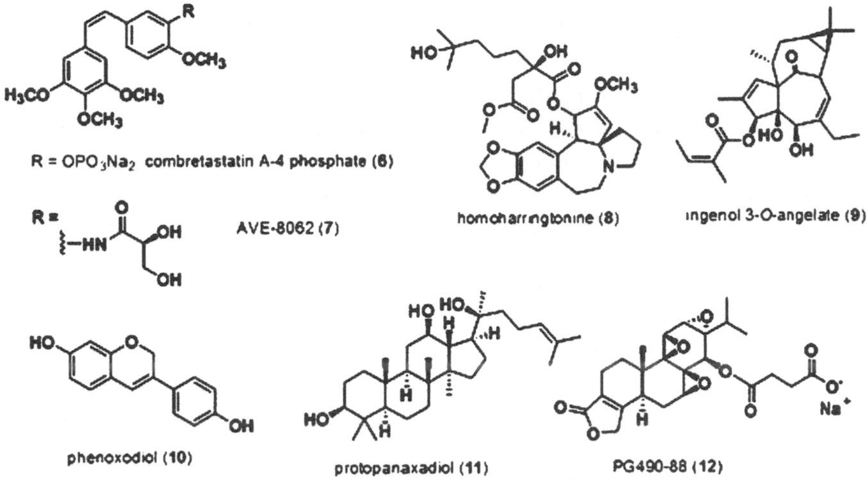

R = OPO$_3$Na$_2$ combretastatin A-4 phosphate (6)

AVE-8062 (7)

homoharringtonine (8)

ingenol 3-O-angelate (9)

phenoxodiol (10)

protopanaxadiol (11)

PG490-88 (12)

Fig. 2.2 Plant-derived drug candidates.

In addition, combretastatin A4, isolated from the South African medicinal tree, *Combretum caffrum* (Combretaceae), was derivatized to combretastatin A4 phosphate (**6**) and AVE-8062 (**7**).[23,24] These analogs bind to tubulin leading to morphological changes and then disrupt tumor vasculature, and are in phase II trials.[25,26] Homoharringtonine (**8**), a cephalotaxus alkaloid from the tree, *Cephalotaxus harringtonia* found in mainland China,[27] is an inhibitor of protein synthesis and is reported to have activity against hematologic malignances.[28] Ingenol 3-*O*-angelate (**9**), an analog of the polyhydroxy diterpenoid, ingenol, which was originally obtained from *Euphorbia peplus* (known as "petty spurge" in England or "radium weed" in Australia), is a potential topical chemotherapeutic agent for skin cancer and exhibits its action through activation of protein kinase C.[29,30] Phenoxodiol (**10**), a synthetic analog of daidzein, a well known isoflavone from soybean (*Glycine max*), is being developed as a therapy for cervical, ovarian, prostate, renal, and vaginal cancers, and induces apoptosis through inhibition of anti-apoptotic proteins including XIAP and FLIP.[31] Phenoxodiol is currently undergoing clinical studies in the United States and Australia.[32] Protopanaxadiol (**11**), a derivative of a triterpene aglycone of several saponins from ginseng (*Panax ginseng*), exhibits its apoptotic effects on cancer cells through various signaling pathways, and is also reported to be cytotoxic against multidrug resistant tumors.[33,34] Triptolide, a diterpene triepoxide, was isolated from *Tripterygium wilfordii*, and has been used for autoimmune and inflammatory diseases in the People's Republic of China.[35] PG490–88 (**12**, 14-succinyl triptolide sodium salt), a semisynthetic analog of triptolide, exerts antiproliferative and proapoptotic activities on primary human prostatic epithelial cells as well as tumor regression of colon and lung xenografts.[36]

Drug Discovery From Terrestrial Microorganisms

Until the development of penicillin in the early 1940s, most natural product-derived drugs were obtained from terrestrial plants. The success of penicillin in treating infection led to an expansion in the area of drug discovery from microorganisms. Terrestrial microorganisms are a plentiful source of structurally diverse bioactive substances, and have provided important contributions to the discovery of antibacterial agents including penicillins, cephalosporins, aminoglycosides, tetracyclines, and polyketides.[13] Current therapeutic applications of metabolites from microorganisms have expanded into immunosuppressive agents (eg, cyclosporins and rapamycin), cholesterol-lowering agents (eg, lovastatin and mevastatin), antihelmintic agents (eg, ivermectin), an antidiabetic agent (acarbose), and anticancer agents (eg, pentostatin, peplomycin, and epirubicin).[2,12,37] Recently approved drugs derived from terrestrial microorganisms are shown in Figs. 2.3, 2.4, and 2.5.

Approved Drugs

Micafungin sodium (**13**, Mycamine, Fujisawa, 2005) is an antifungal agent of the echinocandin type obtained from the culture broth of the fungus *Coleophoma empetri*, and inhibits β-(1,3)-D-glucan synthase of fungi.[38,39] Micafungin exhibited good antifungal activity against a broad range of *Candida* species, including azole-resistant strains, and *Aspergillus* species, during in vitro and animal studies.[38]

Tigecycline (**14**, Tygacil, Wyeth, 2005) is the 9-*tert*-butyl-glycylamido derivative of minocycline, which is a semi-synthetic product of chlortetracycline isolated from *Streptomyces aureofaciens*. Tigecycline exhibited antibacterial activity typical of other tetracyclines, but with more potent activity against tetracycline-resistant organisms. Tigecycline is only utilized in an injectable formulation for clinical use, unlike currently marketed tetracyclines that are available in oral dosage forms.[40]

Everolimus (**15**, Certican, Norvatis, 2004) is an orally active 40-*O*-(2-hydroxyethyl) derivative of rapamycin, originally produced from *Streptomyces hygroscopicus*. Everolimus exhibits its immunosuppressive effect by blocking growth factor (interleukin (IL)-2 and IL-15) mediated proliferation of hematopoietic (T cells and B cells), and non-hematopoietic (vascular smooth muscle cells) cells through inhibiting p70 S6 kinase, leading to arrest of the cell cycle at the G_1/S phase.[41]

Telithromycin (**16**, Ketek, Aventis, 2004) is a semi-synthetic derivative of the 14-membered macrolide, erythromycin A, isolated from *Saccharopolyspora erythraea*, and retains the macrolactone ring as well as a D-desosamine sugar moiety. It inhibits protein synthesis by interacting with the peptidyltransferase site of the bacterial 50S ribosomal subunit, and exhibits antibacterial effect on respiratory tract pathogens resistant to other macrolides.[42]

Miglustat (**17**, Zavesca, Actelion, 2003) has been approved for patients unable to receive enzyme replacement therapy as a therapeutic drug for type I Gaucher

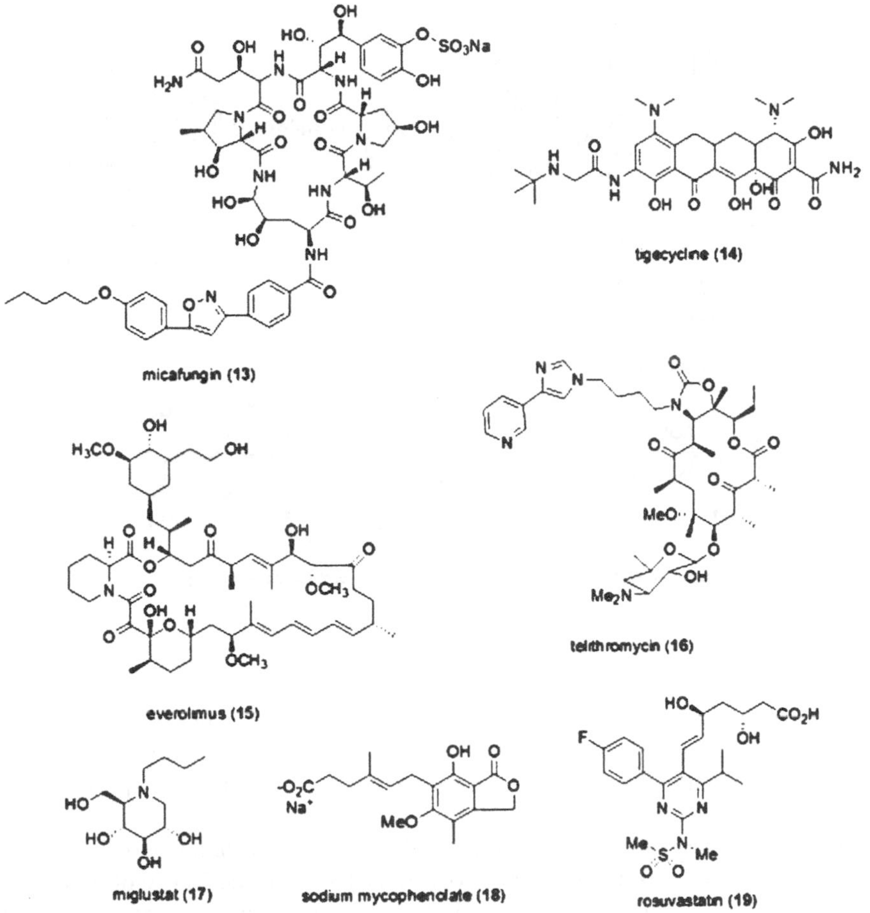

Fig. 2.3 New drugs from terrestrial microorganisms (2000 to 2005).

disease. Miglustat, an analog of nojirimycin isolated from the broth filtrate of *Streptomyces lavendulae*, reversibly inhibits glucosylceramide synthase, a ceramide-specific glucosyltransferase that catalyzes the formation of glucocerebroside, and thereby decreases tissue storage of glucosylceramide. Gaucher disease is a progressive lysosomal storage disorder associated with pathological accumulation of glucosylceramide in cells of the monocyte/macrophage lineage. Enzyme replacement therapy using human placenta-derived alglucerase (Ceredase) has been available for type I Gaucher disease since 1991.[43,44]

Mycophenolate sodium (**18**, Myfortic, Norvatis, 2003) is a selective, noncompetitive, reversible inhibitor of inosine monophosphate dehydrogenase (IMPDH), the rate-limiting enzyme in the de novo pathway of guanosine nucleotide synthesis. Thus, mycophenolic acid, originally purified from *Penicillium brevicompactum*,

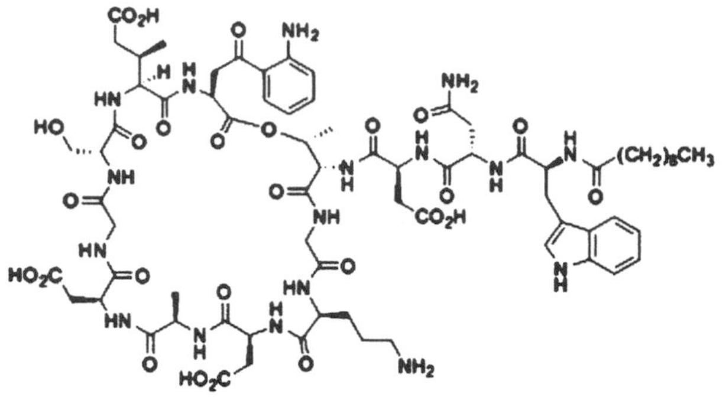

daptomycin (20)

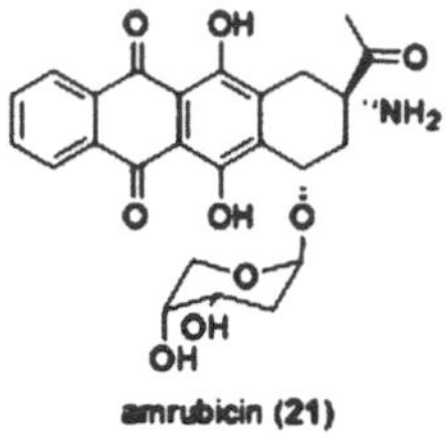

amrubicin (21)

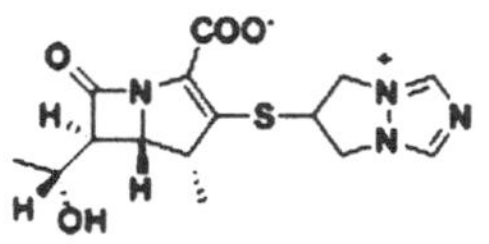

biapenem (22)

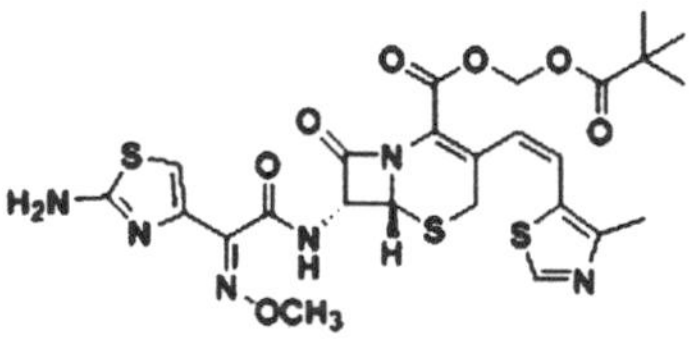

cefditoren pivoxil (23)

Fig. 2.4 New drugs from terrestrial microorganisms (2000 to 2005).

has a selective antiproliferative effect on lymphocytes that rely on the de novo synthesis of purine and is used for the prophylaxis of organ rejection in patients receiving allogeneic renal transplants treated with ciclosporin (cyclosporin A) and corticosteroids.[45,46]

Rosuvastatin calcium (**19**, Crestor, AstraZeneca, 2003), an inhibitor of 3-hydroxy-3-methylglutaryl coenzyme A (HMG-CoA) reductase and a derivative of mevastatin isolated from *Penicillium citrinum* and *P. brevicompactum*, is an effective lipid-lowering agent approved internationally (in most of Europe, the United States, and Canada) for the management of dyslipidemias.[47] Like other available HMG-CoA reductase inhibitors (atrovastatin, fluvastatin, lovastatin, pravastatin, and simvastatin), rosuvastatin competitively inhibits the rate-limiting step in the formation of endogenous cholesterol by HMG-CoA reductase. Consequently, hepatic intracellular stores of cholesterol are reduced, which results in reduced serum levels of low-density lipoprotein-cholesterol (LDL-C) and triglycerides, and increased serum levels of high-density lipoprotein-cholesterol (HDL-C), and thus improves the overall lipid profile of patients.[48]

Pitavastatin (Livalo, Sankyo/Kowa, 2003), an analog of mevastatin like rosuvastatin, has been approved for the treatment of dyslipidemia in Japan.[49]

Daptomycin (**20**, Cubicin, Cubist, 2003) is a cyclic lipopeptide antibacterial agent derived from *Streptomyces roseosporus*, which has been approved for the treatment of complicated skin and skin structure infections (cSSSIs). Daptomycin binds to bacterial cell membranes and then disrupts the membrane potential, leading to blocking of the synthesis of proteins, DNA, and RNA.[50]

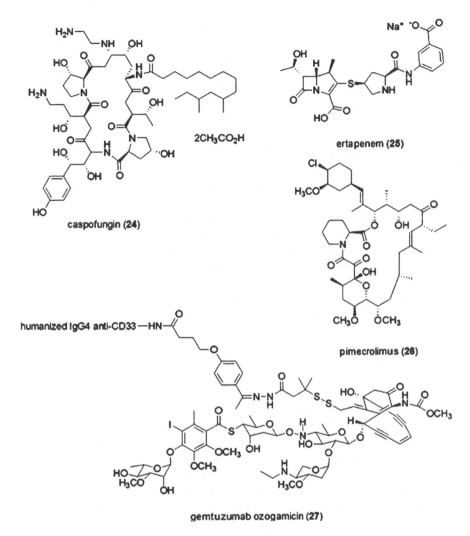

Fig. 2.5 New drugs from terrestrial microorganisms (2000 to 2005).

Amrubicin hydrochloride (21, Cased, Sumitomo Pharmaceuticals Co, 2002, Japan) is a completely synthetic 9-aminoanthracycline and converts to its active form in the body.[51] Amrubicin, a derivative of doxorubicin isolated from *Streptomyces peucetius* var *caesius*, demonstrated activity comparable to that of doxorubicin on transplantable animal tumors, including P388 leukemia, sarcoma 180, and Lewis lung carcinoma, and more potent antitumor activity against human tumor xenografts of breast, lung, and gastric cancer.[52]

Biapenem (22, Omegacin, Wyeth Lederle Japan, 2002, Japan) is a new analog of carbapenem based on thienamycin, isolated from *Streptomyces cattleya*, an antibacterial agent effective against both Gram-negative and Gram-positive bacteria including species producing β-lactamases. Biapenem is more stable to hydrolysis by human renal dehydropeptidase-I than imipenem, meropenem, and panipenem. The early carbapenems (eg, imipenem) are not stable to hydrolysis by human renal dihydropeptidase-I (DHP-I) and consequently are coadministered with a DHP-I inhibitor (eg, cilastatin). Biapenem can be administered as a single agent without a DHP-I inhibitor.[53]

Cefditoren pivoxil (**23**, Spectracef, TAP, 2001) is an oral prodrug of cefditoren, a derivative of cephalosporin isolated from *Cephalosporium* species, and is rapidly hydrolyzed by intestinal esterases to the microbiologically active form. Cefditoren has a broad spectrum of activity against both Gram-positive and Gram-negative bacteria, and is stable to hydrolysis in the presence of a variety of β-lactamases. This drug was approved in 2001 for acute bacterial exacerbation of chronic bronchitis (AECB), group A beta-hemolytic streptococcal pharyngotonsillitis, and uncomplicated skin/skin structure infections in adult and adolescent patients.[54]

Caspofungin acetate (**24**, Cancidas, Merck, 2001) is a semisynthetic lipopeptide derived from pneumocandin B_0, a fermentation product of *Glarea lozoyensis*. It inhibits the synthesis of the glucose homopolymer β-(1,3)-D-glucan, which is an essential component of the cell wall of many fungi but is absent in mammals. The noncompetitive inhibition of β-(1,3)-D-glucan synthase by caspofungin interferes with fungal cell wall synthesis, leading to osmotic instability and death of the fungal cell.[55-57]

Ertapenem (**25**, Invanz, Merck, 2001) is a new 1β-methylcarbapenem based on thienamycin, isolated from *Streptomyces cattleya*, with broad-spectrum antibacterial activity and improved stability to hydrolysis by renal dehydropeptidase enzymes located in the brush border of the kidneys.[58] Ertapenem exhibits excellent antibacterial activity against clinically relevant Enterobacteriaceae including *Escherichia coli*, *Klebsiella* species, *Citrobacter* species, *Enterobacter* species, *Morganella morganii*, *Proteus* species, and *Serratia marcescens*.[58]

Pimecrolimus (**26**, Elidel, Novartis, 2001) is a novel analog of ascomycin, isolated as a fermentation product of *Streptomyces hygroscopicus* var *ascomyceticus*. Its mechanism of action involves blocking T cell activation via the pimecrolimus-macrophilin complex that prevents the dephosphorylation of the cytoplasmic component of the nuclear factor of activated T cells (NF-AT). This drug was approved for the treatment of inflammatory skin diseases such as allergic contact dermatitis and atopic dermatitis.[59]

Gemtuzumab ozogamicin (**27**, Mylotarg, Wyeth-Ayerst, 2000) is a prodrug of calicheamicin bound to anti-CD33 monoclonal antibody. The calicheamicins (also known as the LL-E3328 antibiotics) were discovered from fermentation products produced by *Micromonospora echinospora* ssp. *calichensis*. Lysosomes in the cells cleave the covalent link between the monoclonal antibody and calicheamicin, allowing calicheamicin release. Calicheamicin is a hydrophobic member of the enediyne family of DNA-cleaving antibiotics and effective in treatment of patients with acute myeloid lymphoma.[60,61]

Examples of Terrestrial Microbial and Fungal-derived Compounds in Clinical Trials

As potential anticancer lead compounds from microorganisms, twenty-four substances with new chemical skeletons are undergoing clinical studies (Fig. 2.6 and 2.7).[12] Elsamitrucin (28, elsamicin A), which has a common chromophore with chartreusin from *Streptomyces chartreusis*, was isolated from the unidentified actinomycete strain J907–21. This compound binds to DNA but also inhibits activity of topo-isomerase II, leading to an antitumor effect.[62,63] Brostallicin (29), an α-bromoacryloyl derivative of distamycin A that was isolated from the culture mycelium of *Streptomyces distallicus*, is a DNA minor groove binding anticancer agent.[64,65]

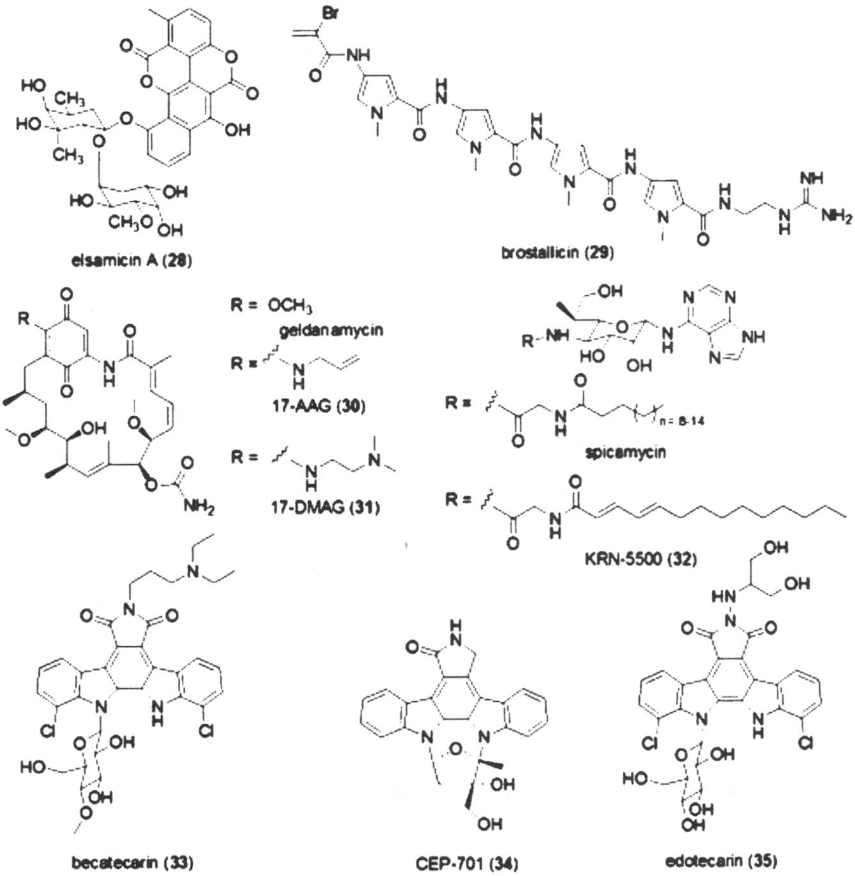

Fig. 2.6 Terrestrial microorganism-derived drug candidates.

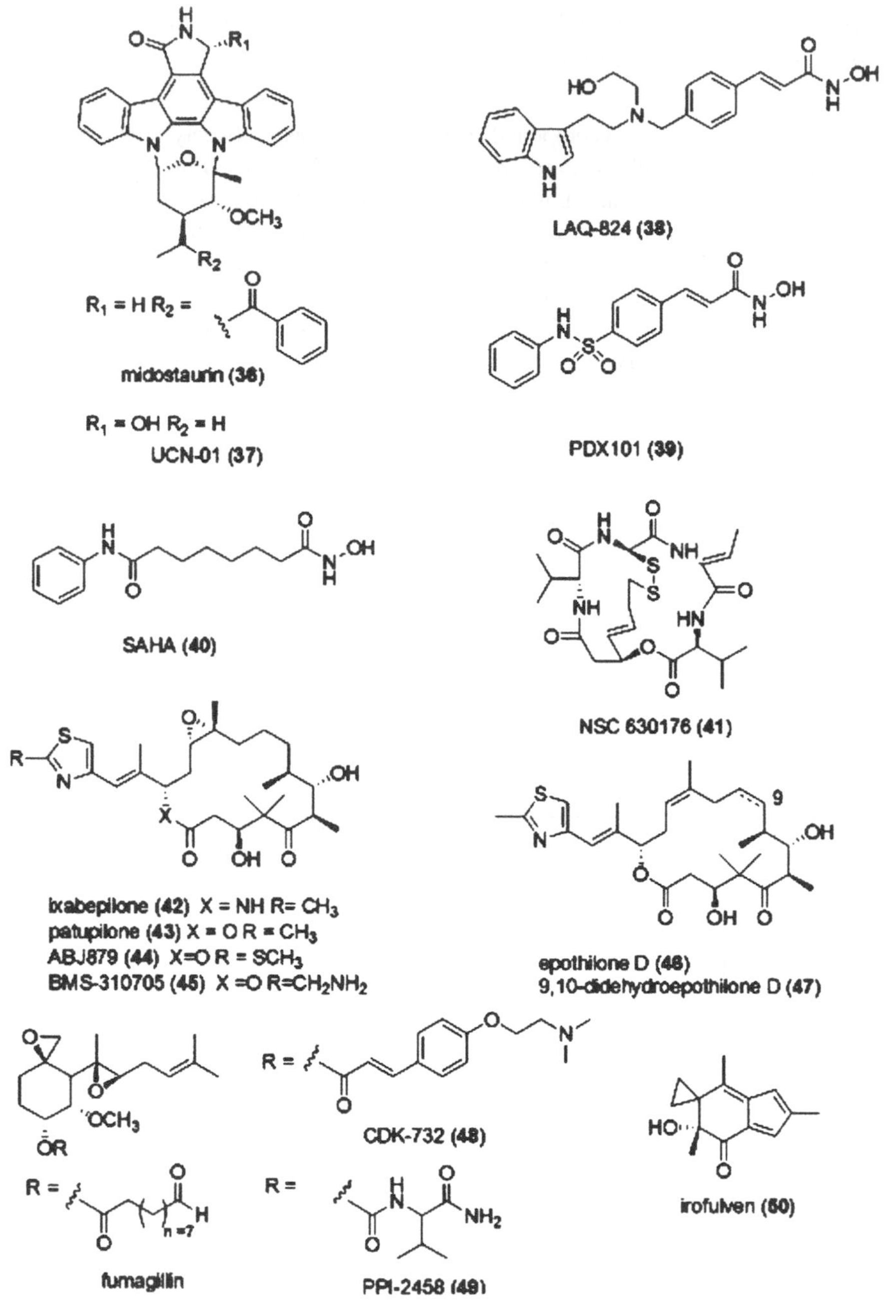

R₁ = H R₂ =

midostaurin (36)

R₁ = OH R₂ = H
UCN-01 (37)

LAQ-824 (38)

PDX101 (39)

SAHA (40)

NSC 630176 (41)

ixabepilone (42) X = NH R= CH₃
patupilone (43) X = O R = CH₃
ABJ879 (44) X=O R = SCH₃
BMS-310705 (45) X =O R=CH₂NH₂

epothilone D (46)
9,10-didehydroepothilone D (47)

R =

CDK-732 (48)

R =

R =

fumagillin

PPI-2458 (49)

irofulven (50)

Fig. 2.7 Terrestrial microorganism-derived drug candidates.

Its mechanism of action is associated with activation after binding to glutathione (GSH), catalyzed by glutathione-S-transferase (GST), and the relatively high GST/GSH levels of cancer cells have made them more susceptible to the antitumor effects of brostallicin than normal cells.[66] Geldanamycin, a polyketide natural product, was originally obtained from *Streptomyces hygroscopicus*,[67,68] and its analogs [17-AAG (**30**) and 17-DMAG (**31**)] are currently under clinical evaluation due to their inhibition of the protein chaperone heat shock protein (HSP) 90.[69,70] The spicamycins are a mixture of nucleoside-like antibiotics with an antitumor effect from *Streptomyces alanosinicus*, and an analog, KRN5500 (**32**), was reported to exhibit antitumor activity via inhibition of protein synthesis rather than the synthesis of DNA or RNA even though the mechanism of antiproliferative effect has not been established unequivocally.[71] Becatecarin (**33**), CEP-701 (**34**), edotecarin (**35**), midostaurin (**36**), and UCN01 (**37**), derivatives of staurosporine originally found in *Nocardiopsis* species, are being developed as anticancer drugs.[72-78] Their mechanism of action is known to involve inhibition of toposiomerase I or II, FLT3 (class III tyrosine kinase), and CDK1 (cyclin-dependent kinase I). Trichostatin, a metabolite of *Streptomyces hygroscopicus*,[79] and its analogs [LAQ-824 (**38**), PDX101 (**39**), and SAHA (**40**)] have demonstrated cytotoxicity against cancer cells and rely on inhibition of histone deacetylase (HDAC), causing growth arrest, differentiation, and apoptosis of tumor cells.[80-83] The depsipeptide (NSC 630176, **41**) from *Chromobacterium violaceum*, a bicyclic peptide containing a non-cysteine disulfide bond, is structurally distinct from other known HDAC inhibitors, and is currently in phase II clinical trials for the treatment of patients with peripheral or cutaneous T cell lymphoma. The antitumor effects of this compound are correlated with the expression of angiogenesis factors, such as vascular endothelial growth factor and basic fibroblast growth factor.[84,85] The epothilones, cytotoxic macrolides discovered from the myxobacterium *Sorangium cellulosum*, were identified as microtubule-stabilizing drugs, acting in a similar manner to the taxanes. Five analogs [ixabepilone (**42**), patupilone (**43**), ABJ879 (**44**), BMS-310705 (**45**), and ZK-EPO (structure apparently not available in the public domain)] of epothilone B, epothilone D (**46**), and 9,10-didehydroepothilone D (**47**) are now undergoing investigation as candidate anticancer drugs, and their preclinical studies have indicated a broad spectrum of antitumor activity including multidrug-resistant models.[12,86-89] Fumagillin, a natural antibiotic produced by *Aspergillus fumigatus fresenius*, along with its analogs, has been shown to exert its inhibitory activity against methionine aminopeptidase 2 (MetAP2).[90] CKD-732 (**48**) and PPI-2458 (**49**), derivatives of fumagillin, inhibited tumor growth and their mechanisms of action were correlated to the level of MetAP-2 inhibition. They have also shown in vivo anti-angiogenic efficacy, inhibiting the growth of cancers in animal models.[90,91] Illudin-S is a sesquiterpenoid from *Omphalotus illudens* (known as the Jack O' Lantern mushroom) with bioluminescent properties. Its analog, irofulven (**50**), has demonstrated efficacy against several tumors in preclinical and clinical trials through induction of DNA damage, activation of MAP kinase, and apoptosis.[92-94]

Drug Discovery From Marine Organisms

Unlike the long-standing historical medical uses of terrestrial plants, marine organisms have a shorter history of utilization in the treatment and/or prevention of human disease. Among the first bioactive compounds from marine sources, spongouridine and spongothymidine from the Caribbean sponge (*Cryptotheca crypta*), were isolated serendipitously in the early 1950s.[95] They were approved as an anticancer drug (cytosine arabinoside, Ara-C) and an antiviral drug (adenine arabinoside, Ara-A), respectively, 15 years later.[96] The secondary metabolites of marine organisms have been studied extensively over the past 30 years, since a small number of academic chemists began to isolate and elucidate novel compounds from marine sources in the 1970's. Drug discovery research from marine organisms has been accelerating and now involves interdisciplinary research including biochemistry, biology, ecology, organic chemistry, and pharmacology.[97,98] Recently, much attention has been given to marine organisms due to their considerable biodiversity that has been found in the widespread oceans that cover over 70% of the world.[99] Structurally unique secondary metabolites have been isolated and identified from marine organisms and, consequently, a compound based on new chemical template has been developed and launched in 2004, while numerous other candidates are in clinical trials (Figs. 2.8 and 2.9).[12,95,96]

Approved Drug

Ziconotide (51, Prialt, Elan, 2004), one of the ω-conotoxins, which were identified from cone snail (*Conus magus*) venom, and are 24–27 residue peptides members of the cyclic cysteine knot family. Ziconotide, known as ω-contotoxin MVIIA, selectively blocks the N-type voltage-gated calcium channel. As a novel non-opioid analgesic, ziconotide was developed for the treatment of severe chronic pain, and is currently used in pain management.[100]

Examples of Marine Organism-derived Compounds in Clinical Trials

Aplidine (**52**), an analog of the didemnins isolated from the Mediterranean tunicate, *Aplidium albicans*, has shown activity against certain tumor types (medullary thyroid carcinoma, renal carcinoma, melanoma, and tumors of neuroendocrine origin).[101] It has also been reported to inhibit the secretion of vascular endothelial growth factor (VEGF) related to angiogenesis and to arrest the cell cycle at the G_1 and G_2 phases.[101] Agelasphins, new glycosphingolipids, were isolated as antitumor agents from an Okinawan sponge, *Agelas mauritianus*.[102] Of their synthetic derivatives, KRN7000 (**53**) was selected as a candidate for clinical trials. The antitumor effect of KRN7000 has been attributed to natural killer cell activation by functioning as a

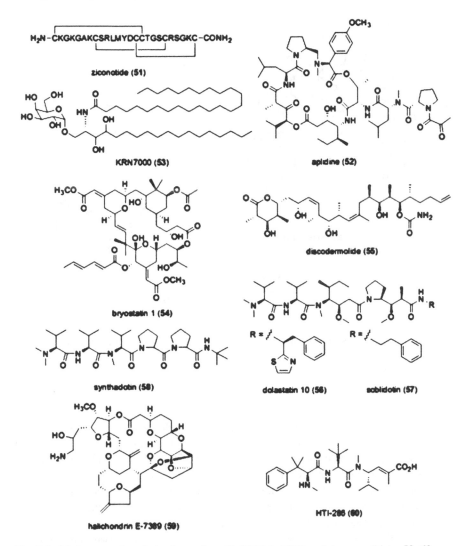

Fig. 2.8 Marine organism-derived new drug **51** (2000 to 2005) and drug candidates **52–60**.

ligand of VαT cell antigen receptor.[103] Bryostatin I (**54**) was isolated from the bryozoan, *Bulgula neritina,* and acts by binding to the same receptors as the phorbol esters, which were found to be tumor promoters, but bryostatin I has no tumor-promoting activity. The binding of bryostatin I to its receptors downregulates protein kinase C isoforms in various tumor cells, leading to inhibition of growth, alteration of differentiation, and/or cell death.[96,104] Discodermolide (**55**), isolated from the marine sponge, *Discodermia dissoluta,*[105] is a microtubule-stabilizing drug. This compound inhibits tumor cell growth in vitro, including against paclitaxel-and epothilone-resistant cells, and is also active in hollow fiber and xenograft mouse

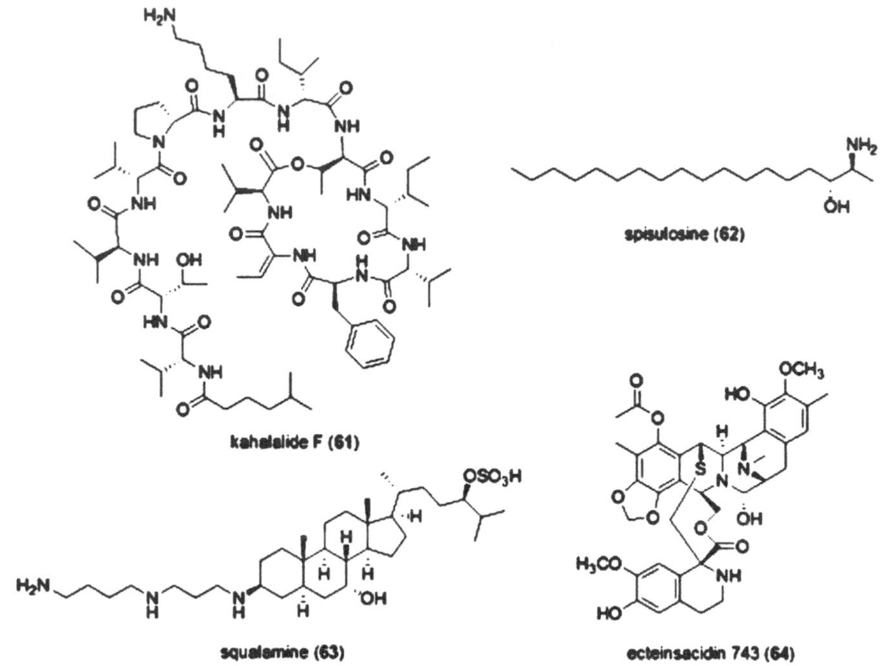

Fig. 2.9 Marine organism-derived drug candidates.

models.[97,98] Dolastatins 10 and 15, linear peptides isolated from the Indian Ocean sea hare *Dolabela auricularia*,[106,107] demonstrate antineoplastic activity through inhibition of microtubule assembly. Dolastatin 10 (**56**), soblidotin (**57**, a derivative of dolastatin 10), and synthadotin (**58**, an analog of dolastatin 15), are currently undergoing clinical trials.[108-111] Halichondrin E7389 (**59**), a derivative of the *Halichondria okadai* constituent, halichondrin B,[96] was found to inhibit tumor cell proliferation in association with the G_2/M arrest and microtubule polymerization.[112] HTI-286 (**60**), a synthetic analog of the tripeptide, hemiasterlin, originally isolated from the South African sponge *Hemiasterella minor*, depolymerizes microtubules and blocks cell growth. HTI-286 has also shown antitumor activity in human tumor xenograft murine models.[96,113] The cyclic depsipeptide, kahalalide F (**61**), isolated from the mollusk, *Elysia rufescens*, shows antitumor activity in patients with hepatoma, melanoma, and breast and pancreatic carcinomas. This compound did not affect bone marrow progenitors and was less sensitive to non-tumor cell lines.[114,115] Spisulosine (**62**), isolated from *Spisula polynyma*, has demonstrated antiproliferative activity against various human cancer cell lines (colon, gastric, pancreas, pharynx, and renal tumors), and inhibits tumor growth of human renal tumors, melanoma and prostate tumors in in vivo mouse studies.[116,117] Squalamine (**63**), an aminosterol purified from the dogfish shark, *Squalus acanthias*, is an inhibitor of growth factor-mediated endothelial cell proliferation and migration and angiogenesis.[118,119] Ecteinascidin 743 (**64**), a potent antitumor agent, was isolated from the marine tunicate *Ecteinascidia turbinata*.[120,121] Ecteinascidin 743 possesses potent cytotoxic activity against a variety of tumor cell lines in vitro and against several rodent tumors and human tumor xenografts in vivo.[121] It showed particularly high activity against advanced sarcomas that had relapsed or were resistant to conventional therapy.[122]

Drug Discovery From Terrestrial Vertebrates and Invertebrates

During the course of research on human physiology and pathology, many biochemical molecules have been discovered and their functions have been investigated. Since these biochemical compounds are related to biological action in the human body, an excess or deficiency of them has often caused pathological problems in humans. Neurohormones (adrenaline, levodopa, and histamine), peptide hormones (insulin and glucagons), sex hormones (estrogens, progesterone, and testosterone), other hormones (hydrocortisone and aldosterone), and prostaglandins (prostaglandin E_1 and E_2) are examples of compounds used for the treatment of diseases related to their physiological action.[37] Besides human biochemicals and their analogs, other drugs in this category have been discovered from various terrestrial vertebrates and invertebrates, including an inhibitor of angiotensin-converting enzyme (ACE) developed from teprotide, which was isolated from the venom of Brazilian viper (*Bothrops jararaca*) after the venom was found to cause a sudden and massive drop in blood pressure.[12] Two drugs from vertebrates and invertebrates have been approved from 2000 to the present (Fig. 2.10).

Approved Drugs

Exenatide (**65**, Byetta, Amylin and Eli Lilly, 2005) is a synthetic analog of exenadin-4, which was originally isolated as a 39 amino acid peptide from the saliva of the Gila monster (*Heloderma suspectum*), and the first insulin mimetic

ʟ-His-Gly-ʟ-Glu-Gly-ʟ-Thr-ʟ-Phe-ʟ-Thr-ʟ-Ser-ʟ-Asp-ʟ-Leu-ʟ-Ser-ʟ-Lys-.-Gln-ʟ-Met-ʟ-Glu-ʟ-Glu-.-Glu-ʟ-Ala-ʟ-Val-ʟ-Arg-ʟ-
Leu-.-Phe-ʟ-Ile-.-Glu-ʟ-Trp-ʟ-Leu-:-Lys-ʟ-Asn-Gly-Gly-.-Pro-ʟ-Ser-ʟ-Ser-Gly-.-Ala-ʟ-Pro-ʟ-Pro-ʟ-Pro-ʟ-Ser–NH₂

exenatide (**65**)

ᴅ-Phe-ʟ-Pro-ʟ-Arg-ʟ-Pro-Gly-Gly-Gly-Gly-ʟ-Asn-Gly-ʟ-Asp-ʟ-Phe-ʟ-Glu-ʟ-Glu-.-Ile-ʟ-Pro-ʟ-Glu-.-Glu-
.-Tyr-ʟ-Leu

bivalirudin (**66**)

Fig. 2.10 New drugs from terrestrial vertebrates and invertebrates (2000 to 2005).

found to improve glycemic control. Subcutaneous exenatide was launched in the United States for use in patients with type 2 diabetes who have failed in glycemic control by treatment with metformin and/or a sulfonylurea.[123,124]

Bivalirudin (66, Angiomax, MDCO, 2000) is a leech anti-platelet protein that is an inhibitor of collagen-induced platelet aggregation.[125] This compound is a new, genetically engineered form of hirudin, the substance in the saliva of the leech (*Haementeria officinalis*) and stops blood clotting. Bivalirudin is used to reduce the risk of blood clotting in adults with severe chest pain (unstable angina) who are undergoing a procedure to open blocked arteries in the heart.[126]

Conclusion

As shown above, 23 new drugs derived from natural sources have been launched on the market during 2000–2005, even though many pharmaceutical companies have discontinued their programs of drug discovery from natural sources. These new drugs have been approved for the treatment of cancer, neurological diseases, infectious diseases, cardiovascular and metabolic diseases, immunological, inflammatory and related diseases, and genetic disorders, which encompass many of the common human diseases. Besides new drugs launched on the market from 2000 to the present, there are a variety of new chemical entities from natural sources undergoing clinical trials. Further research on these compounds at industrial, governmental, and academic institutions is seen as vital for the enhancement of human health.

References

1. Newman DJ, Cragg GM, Snader KM. The influence of natural products upon drug discovery. *Nat Prod Rep.* 2000;17:215-234.
2. Newman DJ, Cragg GM, Snader KM. Natural products as sources of new drugs over the period 1981-2002. *J Nat Prod.* 2003;66:1022-1037.
3. Koehn FE, Carter GT. The evolving role of natural products in drug discovery. *Nat Rev Drug Discov.* 2005;4:206-220.
4. Paterson I, Anderson EA. The renaissance of natural products as drug candidates. *Science.* 2005;310:451-453.
5. Balunas MJ, Kinghorn AD. Drug discovery from medicinal plants. *Life Sci.* 2005;78:431-441.
6. Jones WP, Chin Y-W, Kinghorn AD. The role of pharmacognosy in modern medicine and pharmacy. *Curr Drug Targets.* 2006;7:247-264
7. Drahl C, Cravatt BF, Sorensen EJ. Protein-reactive natural products. *Angew Chem Int Ed Engl.* 2005;44:5788-5809.
8. Grifo F, Newman D, Fairfield A, Bhattacharya B, Grupenhoff J. The origins of prescription drugs. In: Grifo F, Rosenthal J, eds. *Biodiversity and Human Health*. Washington, DC: Island Press; 1997:131-163
9. Butler MS. The role of natural product chemistry in drug discovery. *J Nat Prod.* 2004;67:2141-2153.
10. Thayer A. Bristol-Myers to settle suits. *Chem Eng News.* 2003;81:6

11. Oberlies NH, Kroll DJ. Camptothecin and taxol: historic achievements in natural products research. *J Nat Prod.* 2004;67:129-135.
12. Butler MS. Natural products to drugs: natural products derived compounds in clinical trials. *Nat Prod Rep.* 2005;22:162-195.
13. Dewick PM. *Medicinal Natural Products: A Biosynthetic Approach.* 2nd ed. Chichester, UK: John Wiley & Sons; 2002
14. Fabricant DS, Farnsworth NR. The value of plants used in traditional medicine for drug discovery. *Environ Health Perspect.* 2001;109:69-75.
15. Kinghorn AD. The discovery of drugs from higher plants. In: Gullo VP, ed. *The Discovery of Natural Products with Therapeutic Potential.* Boston, MA: Butterworth-Heinemann; 1994:81-108
16. Deleu D, Hanssens Y, Northway MG. Subcutaneous apomorphine: an evidence-based review of its use in Parkinson's disease. *Drugs Aging.* 2004;21:687-709.
17. Koumis T, Samuel S. Tiotropium bromide: a new long-acting bronchodilator for the treatment of chronic obstructive pulmonary disease. *Clin Ther.* 2005;27:377-392.
18. Hall MG, Wilks MF, Provan WM, Eksborg S, Lumholtz B. Pharmacokinetics and pharmacodynamics of NTBC [2-(2-nitro-4-fluoromethyl-benzoyl)-1,3-cyclohexanedione] and mesotrione, inhibitors of 4-hydroxyphenyl pyruvate dioxygenase (HPPD) following a single dose to healthy male volunteers. *Br J Clin Pharmacol.* 2001;52:169-177.
19. Mitchell G, Bartlett DW, Fraser TEM, et al. Mesotrione: a new selective herbicide for use in maize. *Pest Manag Sci.* 2001;57:120-128.
20. Howes M-JR, Perry NSL, Houghton PJ. Plants with traditional uses and activities, relevant to the management of Alzheimer's disease and other cognitive disorders. *Phytother Res.* 2003;17:1-18.
21. Heinrich M, Teoh HL. Galanthamine from snowdrop—the development of a modern drug against Alzheimer's disease from local Caucasian knowledge. *J Ethnopharmacol.* 2004;92:147-162.
22. van Agtmael MA, Eggelte TA, van Boxtel CJ. Artemisinin drugs in the treatment of malaria: from medicinal herb to registered medication. *Trends Pharmacol Sci.* 1999;20:199-205.
23. Cirla A, Mann J. Combrestatins: from natural products to drug discovery. *Nat Prod Rep.* 2003;20:558-564.
24. Pinney KG, Jelinek C, Edvardsen K, Chaplin DJ, Pettit GR. The discovery and development of the combrestatins. In: Cragg GM, Kingston DGI, Newman DJ, eds. *Anticancer Agents from Natural Products.* Boca Raton, FL: CRC Press; 2005:23-46.
25. West CML, Price P. Combrestatin A4 phosphate. *Anticancer Drugs.* 2004;15:179-187.
26. Young SL, Chaplin DJ. Combrestatin A4 phosphate: background and current clinical status. *Expert Opin Investig Drugs.* 2004;13:1171-1182.
27. Powell RG, Weisleder D, Smith CR, Rohwedder WK. Structures of harringtonine, isoharringtonine, and homoharringtonine. *Tetrahedron Lett.* 1970;11:815-818.
28. Kantarjian HM, Talpaz M, Santini V, Murgo A, Cheson B, O'Brian SM. Homoharringtonine: history, current research, and future direction. *Cancer.* 2001;92:1591-1603.
29. Kedei N, Lundberg DJ, Toth A, Welburn P, Garfield SH, Blumberg PM. Characterization of the interaction of ingenol 3-angelate with protein kinase C. *Cancer Res.* 2004;64:3243-3255.
30. Ogbourne SM, Suhrbier A, Jones B, et al. Antitumor activity of ingenol 3-angelate: plasma membrane and mitochondrial disruption and necrotic cell death. *Cancer Res.* 2004;64:2833-2839.
31. Kamsteeg M, Rutherford T, Sapi E, et al. Phenoxodiol - an isoflavone analog - induces apoptosis in chemoresitant ovarian cancer cells. *Oncogene.* 2003;22:2611-2620.
32. Constantinou AI, Mehta R, Husband A. Phenoxodiol, a novel isoflavone derivative, inhibits dimethylbenz[a]anthracene (DMBA)-induced mammary carcinogenesis in female Sprague-Dawley rats. *Eur J Cancer.* 2003;39:1012-1018.
33. Shibata S, Tanaka O, Sado M, Tsushima S. The genuine sapogenin of ginseng. *Tetrahedron Lett.* 1963;4:795-800.
34. Jia W, Yan H, Bu X, Liu G, Zhao Y. Aglycone protopanaxadiol, a ginseng saponin, inhibits P-glycoprotein and sensitizes chemotherapy drugs on multidrug resistant cancer cells. *J Clin Oncol.* 2004;22:9663

35. Kiviharju TM, Lecane PS, Sellers RG, Peehl DM. Antiproliferative and proapoptotic of trip-tolide (PG490), a natural product entering clinical trials, on primary cultures of human prostatic epithelial cells. *Clin Cancer Res.* 2002;8:2666-2674.
36. Fidler JM, Li K, Chung C, et al. PG490-88, a derivative of triptolide, causes tumor regression and sensitizes tumors to chemotherapy. *Mol Cancer Ther.* 2003;2:855-862.
37. Sneader W. *Drug Discovery: A History.* Hoboken, NJ: John Wiley & Sons; 2005
38. Jarvis B, Figgitt DP, Scott LJ. Micafungin. *Drugs.* 2004;64:969-982.
39. Frattarelli DAC, Reed MD, Giacoia GP, Aranda JV. Antifungals in systemic neonatal candidiasis. *Drugs.* 2004;64:949-968.
40. Zhanel GG, Homenuik K, Nichol K, et al. The glycylcyclines: a comparative review with the tetracyclines. *Drugs.* 2004;64:63-88.
41. Chapman TM, Perry CM. Everolimus. *Drugs.* 2004;64:861-872.
42. Zhanel GG, Walters M, Noreddin A, et al. The ketolides: a critical review. *Drugs.* 2002; 62:1771-1804.
43. Pastores GM, Barnett NL, Kolodny EH. An open-label, noncomparative study of miglustat in type I Gaucher disease: efficacy and tolerability over 24 months of treatment. *Clin Ther.* 2005;27:1215-1227.
44. Weinreb NJ, Barranger JA, Charrow J, Grabowski GA, Mankin HJ, Mistry P. Guidance on the use of miglustat for treating patients with type 1 Gaucher disease. *Am J Hematol.* 2005;80:223-229.
45. Bardsley-Elliot A, Noble S, Foster RH. Mycophenolate mofetil: a review of its use in the management of solid organ transplantation. *BioDrugs.* 1999;12:363-410.
46. Curran MP, Keating GM. Mycophenolate sodium delayed release: prevention of renal transplant rejection. *Drugs.* 2005;65:799-805.
47. Carswell CI, Plosker GL, Jarvis B. *Drugs.* 2002;62:2075-2085.
48. Scott LJ, Curran MP, Figgitt DP. Rosuvastatin: a review of its use in the management of dyslipidemia. *Am J Cardiovasc Drugs.* 2004;4:117-138.
49. Mukhtar RYA, Reid J, Reckless JPD. Pitavastatin. *Int J Clin Pract.* 2005;59:239-252.
50. Fenton C, Keating GM, Curran MP. Daptomycin. *Drugs.* 2004;64:445-455.
51. Ogawa M. Novel anticancer drugs in Japan. *J Cancer Res Clin Oncol.* 1999;125:134-140.
52. Sugiura T, Ariyoshi Y, Negoro S, et al. Phase I/II study of amrubicin, a novel 9-aminoanthracycline, in patients with advanced non-small-cell lung cancer. *Invest New Drugs.* 2005;23:331-337.
53. Perry CM, Ibbotson T. Biapenem. *Drugs.* 2002;62:2221-2234.
54. Darkes MJM, Plosker GL. Cefditoren pivoxil. *Drugs.* 2002;62:319-336.
55. Keating G, Figgitt D. Caspofungin: a review of its use in oesophageal candidiasis, invasive candidiasis and invasive aspergillosis. *Drugs.* 2003;63:2235-2263.
56. Letscher-Bru V, Herbrecht R. Caspofungin: the first representative of a new antifungal class. *J Antimicrob Chemother.* 2003;51:513-521.
57. McCormack PL, Perry CM. Caspofungin A: review of its use in the treatment of fungal infections. *Drugs.* 2005;65:2049-2068.
58. Sader HS, Gales AC. Emerging strategies in infectious diseases: new carbapenem and trinem antibacterial agents. *Drugs.* 2001;61:553-564.
59. Gupta AK, Chow M. Pimecrolimus: a review. *J Eur Acad Dermatol Venereol.* 2003;17:493-503.
60. Lee MD, Dunne TS, Siegel MM, Chang CC, Morton GO, Borders DB. Calichemicins, a novel family of antitumor antibiotics. 1. Chemistry and partial structure of calichemicin γ_1. *J Am Chem Soc.* 1987;109:3464-3466.
61. Giles F, Estey E, O'Brien S. Gemtuzumab ozogamicin in the treatment of acute myeloid leukemia. *Cancer.* 2003;98:2095-2104.
62. Portugal J. Chartreusin, elsamicin A and related anti-cancer antibiotics. *Curr Med Chem Anticancer Agents.* 2003;3:411-420.
63. Lam KS, Veitch JA, Forenza S, Combs CM, Colson KL. Biosynthesis of elsamicin A, a novel antitumor antibiotic. *J Nat Prod.* 1989;52:1015-1021.
64. DiMarco A, Gaetani M, Orezzi P, Scotti T, Arcamone FF. Experimental studies on distamycin A - a new antibiotic with cytotoxic activity. *Cancer Chemother Rep.* 1962;18:15-19.

65. Broggini M, Marchini S, Fontana E, Moneta D, Fowst C, Geroni C. Brostacillin: a new concept in minor groove DNA binder development. *Anticancer Drugs*. 2004;15:1-6.
66. Geroni C, Marchini S, Cozzi P, et al. Brostalicin, a novel anticancer agent whose activity is enhanced upon binding to glutathione. *Cancer Res*. 2002;62:2332-2336.
67. DeBoer C, Meulman PA, Wnuk RJ, Peterson DH. Geldanamycin, a new antibiotic. *J Antibiot (Tokyo)*. 1970;23:442-447.
68. Sasaki K, Rinehart KL Jr, Slomp G, Grostic MF, Olson BC. Geldanamycin. I. Structure assignment. *J Am Chem Soc*. 1970;92:7591-7593.
69. Bisht KS, Bradbury M, Mattson D, et al. Geldanamycin and 17-allylamino-17-demethoxygeldanamycin potentiate the *in vitro* and *in vivo* radiation response of cervical tumor cells via the heat shock protein 90-mediated intracellular signaling and cytotoxicity. *Cancer Res*. 2003;63:8984-8995.
70. Kaur G, Belotti D, Burger AM, et al. Antiangiogenic properties of 17-(dimethylaminoethylamino)-17-demethoxygeldanamycin: an orally bioavailable heat shock protein 90 modulator. *Clin Cancer Res*. 2004;10:4813-4821.
71. Supko JG, Eder JP, Ryan DP, et al. Phase I clinical trial and pharmacokinetic study of the spicamycin analog KRN500 administered as a 1-hour intravenous infusion for five consecutive days to patients with refractory solid tumors. *Clin Cancer Res*. 2003;9:5178-5186.
72. Yoshinari T, Ohkubo M, Fukasawa K, et al. Mode of action of a new indolocarbazole anticancer agent, J-107088, targeting topoisomerase I. *Cancer Res*. 1999;59:4271-4275.
73. Zaugg K, Rocha S, Resch H, et al. Differential p53-dependent mechanism of radiosensitization *in vitro* and *in vivo* by the protein kinase C-specific inhibitor PKC412. *Cancer Res*. 2001;61:732-738.
74. Long BH, Rose WC, Vyas DM, Matson JA, Forenza S. Discovery of antitumor indolocarbazoles: rebeccamycin, NSC 655649, and fluoroindolocarbazoles. *Curr Med Chem Anticancer Agents*. 2002;2:255-266.
75. Chen J, De Angelo DJ, Kutok JL, et al. PKC412 inhibits the zinc finger 198-fibroblast growth factor receptor 1 fusion tyrosine kinase and is active in treatment of stem cell myeloproliferative disorder. *Proc Natl Acad Sci USA*. 2004;101:14479-14484.
76. Kondapaka SB, Zarnowski M, Yver DR, Sausville EA, Cushman SW. 7-Hydroxystaurosporine (UCN-01) inhibition of Akt Thr[308] but not Ser[473] phosphorylation: a basis for decreased insulin-stimulated glucose transport. *Clin Cancer Res*. 2004;10:7192-7198.
77. Smith BD, Levis M, Beran M, et al. Single-agent CEP-701, a novel FLT3 inhibitor, shows biological and clinical activity in patients with relapsed or refractory acute myeloid leukemia. *Blood*. 2004;103:3669-3676.
78. Marshall JL, Kindler H, Deeken J, et al. Phase I trial of orally administered CEP-701, a novel neurotrophin receptor-linked tyrosine kinase inhibitor. *Invest New Drugs*. 2005;23:31-37.
79. Tsuji N, Kobayashi M, Nagashima K, Wakisaka Y, Koizumi K. A new antifungal antibiotic, trichostatin. *J Antibiot (Tokyo)*. 1976;29:1-6.
80. Plumb JA, Finn PW, Williams RJ, et al. Pharmacodynamic response and inhibition of growth of human tumor xenografts by the novel histone deacetylase inhibitor PXD101. *Mol Cancer Ther*. 2003;2:721-728.
81. Arts J, Schepper S, Emelen K. Histone deacetylase inhibitors: from chromatin remodeling to experimental cancer therapeutics. *Curr Med Chem*. 2003;10:2343-2350.
82. Atadja P, Gao L, Kwon P, et al. Selective growth inhibition of tumor cells by a novel histone deacetylase inhibitor, NVP-LAQ824. *Cancer Res*. 2004;64:689-695.
83. Monneret C. Histone deacetylase inhibitors. *Eur J Med Chem*. 2005;40:1-13.
84. Sandor V, Bakke S, Robey RW, et al. Phase I trial of the histone deacetylase inhibitor, depsipetide (FR901228, NSC 630176), in patients with refractory neoplasms. *Clin Cancer Res*. 2002;8:718-728.
85. Shiraga T, Tozuka Z, Ishimura R, Kawamura A, Kagawama A. Identification of cytochrome P450 enzymes involved in the metabolism of FK228, a potent histone deacetylase inhibitor, in human liver microsomes. *Biol Pharm Bull*. 2005;28:124-129.

86. Kosmidis PA, Manegold C. Advanced NSCLC: new cytostatic agents. *Lung Cancer.* 2003;41:S123-S132.
87. Starks CM, Zhou Y, Liu F, Licari PJ. Isolation and characterization of new epothilone analogues from recombinant *Myxococcus xanthus* fermentation. *J Nat Prod.* 2003;66:1313-1317.
88. Goodin S, Kane MP, Rubin EH. Epothilones: mechanism of action and biologic activity. *J Clin Oncol.* 2004;22:2015-2025.
89. Rizvi N, Villalona-Calere M, Lynch T, et al. Phase II study of KOS-862 (epothilone D) as second-line therapy in non-small cell lung cancer. *Lung Cancer.* 2005;49:S266-S267.
90. Chun E, Han CK, Yoon JH, Sim TB, Kim Y-K, Lee K-Y. Novel inhibitors targeted to methionine aminopeptidase 2 (MetAP2) strongly inhibit the growth of cancers in xenografted nude model. *Int J Cancer.* 2005;114:124-130.
91. Bernier SG, Lazarus DD, Clark E, et al. A methionine aminopeptidase-2 inhibitor, PPI-2458, for the treatment of rheumatoid arthritis. *Proc Natl Acad Sci USA.* 2004;101:10768-10773.
92. McMorris TC, Anchel M. Fungal metabolites. The structures of the novel sesquiterpenoids illudin-S and -M. *J Am Chem Soc.* 1965;87:1594-1600.
93. McMorris TC, Kelner MJ, Wang W, Yu J, Estes LA, Taetle R. (Hydroxymethyl)acylfulvene: an illudin derivative with superior antitumor properties. *J Nat Prod.* 1996;59:896-899.
94. Wang J, Wiltshire T, Wang Y, et al. ATM-dependent CHK2 activation induced by anticancer agent, irlfulven. *J Biol Chem.* 2004;279:39584-39592.
95. Newman DJ, Cragg GM. Advanced preclinical and clinical trials of natural products and related compounds from marine sources. *Curr Med Chem.* 2004;11:1693-1713.
96. Newman DJ, Cragg GM. Marine natural products and related compounds in clinical and advanced preclinical trials. *J Nat Prod.* 2004;67:1216-1238.
97. Capon RJ. Marine bioprospecting-trawling for treasure and pleasure. *Eur J Org Chem.* 2001;2001:633-645.
98. Haefner B. Drugs from the deep: marine natural products as drug candidates. *Drug Discov Today.* 2003;8:536-544.
99. Jensen PR, Fenical W. Marine microorganisms and drug discovery: current status and future potential. In: Fusetani N, ed. *Drugs from the Sea.* New York: Karger; 2000:6-29.
100. Schroeder CI, Smythe ML, Lewis RJ. Development of small molecules that mimic the binding of ω-conotoxins at the N-type voltage-gated calcium channel. *Mol Divers.* 2004;8:127-134.
101. Taraboletti G, Poli M, Dossi R, et al. Antiangiogenic activity of aplidine, a new agent of marine origin. *Br J Cancer.* 2004;90:2418-2424.
102. Natori T, Morita M, Akimoto K, Koezuka Y. Agelasphins, novel antitumor and immunostimulatory cerebrosides from the marine sponge *Agelas mauritianus. Tetrahedron.* 1994;50:2771-2784.
103. Hayakawa Y, Rovero S, Forni G, Smyth MJ. α-Galactosylceramide (KRN7000) suppression of chemical- and oncogene-dependent carcinogenesis. *Proc Natl Acad Sci USA.* 2003;100:9464-9469.
104. Newman DJ. The bryostatins. In: Cragg GM, Kingston DGI, Newman DJ, eds. *Anticancer Agents from Natural Products.* Boca Raton, FL: CRC Press; 2005:137-150
105. Honore S, Kamath K, Braguer D, Wilson L, Briand C, Jordan MA. Suppression of microtubule dynamics by discodermolide by a novel mechanism is associated with mitotic arrest and inhibition of tumor cell proliferation. *Mol Cancer Ther.* 2003;2:1303-1311.
106. Pettit GR, Kamano Y, Herald CL, et al. The isolation and structure of a remarkable marine animal antineoplastic constituent: dolastatin 10. *J Am Chem Soc.* 1987;109:6883-6885.
107. Pettit GR, Kamano Y, Dufresne C, Cerny RL, Herald CL, Schmidt JM. Isolation and structure of the cytostatic linear depsipeptide dolastatin 15. *J Am Chem Soc.* 1989;54:6005-6006.
108. Kerbrat P, Dieras V, Pavlidis N, Ravaud A, Wanders J, Fumoleau P. Phase II study LU103793 (dolastatin analogue) in patients with metastatic breast cancer. *Eur J Cancer.* 2003;39:317-320.
109. Marks RS, Graham DL, Sloan JA, et al. A phase II study of the dolastatin 15 analogue LU 103793 in the treatment of advanced non-small-cell lung cancer. *Am J Clin Oncol.* 2003;26:336-337.

110. Kindler HL, Tothy PK, Wolff R, et al. Phase II trials of dolastatin-10 in advanced pancreaticobiliary cancers. *Invest New Drugs*. 2005;23:489-493.

111. Perez EA, Hillman DW, Fishkin PA, et al. Phase II trial of dolastatin-10 in patients with advanced breast cancer. *Invest New Drugs*. 2005;23:257-261.

112. Jordan MA, Kamath K, Manna T, et al. The primary antimiotic mechanism of action of the synthetic halichondrin E7389 is suppression of microtubule growth. *Mol Cancer Ther*. 2005;4:1086-1095.

113. Loganzo F, Hari M, Annable T, et al. Cells resistant to HT-286 do not overexpress P-glycoprotein but have reduced drug accumulation and a point mutation in α-tubulin. *Mol Cancer Ther*. 2004;3:1319-1327.

114. Suárez Y, González L, Cuadrado A, Berciano M, Lafarga M, Muñoz A. Kahalalide F, a new marine-derived compound, induces oncosis in human prostate and breast cancer cells. *Mol Cancer Ther*. 2003;2:863-872.

115. Janmaat ML, Rodriguez JA, Jimeno J, Kruyt FAE, Giaccone G. Kahalalide F induces necrosis-like cell death that involves depletion of ErB3 and inhibition of Akt signaling. *Mol Pharmacol*. 2005;68:502-510.

116. Jimeno JM, Garcia-Gravalos D, Avila J, Smith B, Grant W, Faircloth GT. ES-285, a marine natural product with activity against solid tumors. *Clin Cancer Res*. 1999;5:3792s.

117. Cuadros R, Garcini EM, Wandosell F, Faircloth G, Fernández-Sousa JM, Avila J. The marine compound spisulosine, an inhibitor of cell proliferation, promotes the disassembly of actin stress fibers. *Cancer Lett*. 2000;152:23-29.

118. Moore KS, Wehrli S, Roger H, et al. Squalamine: an aminosterol antibiotic from the shark. *Proc Natl Acad Sci USA*. 1993;90:1354-1358.

119. Hao D, Hammond LA, Eckhardt SG, et al. A phase I and pharmacokinetic study of squalamine, an aminosterol angiogenesis inhibitor. *Clin Cancer Res*. 2003;9:2465-2471.

120. Soares DG, Poletto NP, Bonatto D, Salvador M, Schwartsmann G, Henriques JAP. Low cytotoxicity of ecteinascidin 743 in yeast lacking the major endonucleolytic enzymes of base and nucleotide excision repair pathways. *Biochem Pharmacol*. 2005;70:59-69.

121. Rinehart KL. Antitumor compounds from tunicates. *Med Res Rev*. 2000;20:1-27.

122. Chen X, Chen J, De Paolis M, Zhu J. Synthetic studies toward ecteinascidin 743. *J Org Chem*. 2005;70:4397-4408.

123. Malhotra R, Singh L, Eng J, Raufman J-P. Exendin-4, a new peptide from *Heloderma suspectum* venom, potentiates cholecystokinin-induced amylase release from rat pancreatic acini. *Regul Pept*. 1992;41:149-156.

124. Keating GM. Exenatide. *Drugs*. 2005;65:1681-1692.

125. Gladwell TD. Bivalirudin: A direct thrombin inhibitor. *Clin Ther*. 2002;24:38-58.

126. Ledizet M, Harrison LM, Koskia RA, Cappello M. Discovery and pre-clinical development of antithrombotics from hematophagous invertebrates. *Curr Med Chem Cardiovasc Hematol Agents*. 2005;3:1-10.

Chapter 3
Computational Methods in Drug Design: Modeling G Protein-Coupled Receptor Monomers, Dimers, and Oligomers

Patricia H. Reggio[1]

Abstract G protein-coupled receptors (GPCRs) are membrane proteins that serve as very important links through which cellular signal transduction mechanisms are activated. Many vital physiological events such as sensory perception, immune defense, cell communication, chemotaxis, and neurotransmission are mediated by GPCRs. Not surprisingly, GPCRs are major targets for drug development today. Most modeling studies in the GPCR field have focused upon the creation of a model of a single GPCR (ie, a GPCR monomer) based upon the crystal structure of the Class A GPCR, rhodopsin. However, the emerging concept of GPCR dimerization has challenged our notions of the monomeric GPCR as functional unit. Recent work has shown not only that many GPCRs exist as homo- and heterodimers but also that GPCR oligomeric assembly may have important functional roles. This review focuses first on methodology for the creation of monomeric GPCR models. Special emphasis is given to the identification of localized regions where the structure of a GPCR may diverge from that of bovine rhodopsin. The review then focuses on GPCR dimers and oligomers and the bioinformatics methods available for identifying homo- and heterodimer interfaces.

Keywords GPCR modeling, GPCR dimer, GPCR oligomer

Introduction

G protein-coupled receptors (GPCRs) are membrane proteins that serve as very important links through which cellular signal transduction mechanisms are activated. Many vital physiological events such as sensory perception, immune defense, cell

[1] Center for Drug Design, Department of Chemistry and Biochemistry, University of North Carolina Greensboro, Greensboro, NC

Corresponding Author: Patricia H. Reggio, Center for Drug Design, Department of Chemistry and Biochemistry, University of North Carolina Greensboro, Greensboro, NC 27402.
Tel: (336) 334-5333; Fax: (336) 334-5402; E-mail: phreggio@uncg.edu

R.S. Rapaka and W. Sadée (eds.), *Drug Addiction.*
© American Association of Pharmaceutical Scientists 2008

communication, chemotaxis, and neurotransmission are mediated by GPCRs. Not surprisingly, GPCRs are major targets for drug development today. The total number of GPCRs with and without introns in the human genome has been estimated to be ~950, of which 500 are odorant or taste receptors and 450 are receptors for endogenous ligands.[1] Many of these GPCRs have been classified as orphan receptors because their endogenous ligands have not yet been identified. Based upon sequence homology, GPCRs have been classified into 6 families/classes (A-F).[2] Alternatively, the GPCRs have been broken down into a numerical system (1–5)[3] or the GRAFS (Glutamate, Rhodopsin, Adhesion, Frizzled/Taste2, and Secretion) system.[4] The rhodopsin family is the largest and forms 4 main groups with 13 subbranches. The rhodopsin-like family Class A (named 1 or rhodopsin in the GRAFS system) includes the cationic neurotransmitters and such receptors as the cannabinoid and EDG (Endothelial Differentiation Gene) receptors, which have lipid-derived endogenous ligands. It is this first family of receptors that has received the majority of attention thus far in the modeling literature. The other GPCR classes/families include the secretin-like Class B (or 2 or secretin) class/family; the metabotropic glutamate and pheromone Class C (3 or glutamate) family; the fungal pheromone Class D (or 4) family[5]; the cAMP receptor Class E family; and the frizzled/smoothened Class F (or 5 or frizzled) family.[2-4]

Ballesteros and Weinstein[6] have proposed a universal numbering scheme for Class A GPCRs. In this numbering system, the most highly conserved residue in each transmembrane (TM) helix is assigned a locant of .50. This number is preceded by the TM number and followed in parentheses by the sequence number. All other residues in a TM helix are numbered relative to this residue. In this numbering system, for example, the most highly conserved residue in TM2 of bovine rhodopsin is D2.50(83). The residue that immediately precedes it is A2.49(82). The Ballesteros-Weinstein numbering system will be used throughout this review.

GPCRs are expressed on cell membranes and are constructed to recognize specific ligands that can range in size from small organic molecules, such as dopamine, to much larger ligands, such as the peptide hormones. As revealed by the crystal structure of bovine rhodopsin at 2.8 Å,[7] 2.65 Å,[8] 2.6 Å,[9] and 2.2 Å resolution,[10] the general topology of a GPCR includes (1) an extracellular N terminus; (2) 7 TM alpha helices arranged to form a closed bundle; (3) loops connecting TM helices that extend intra- and extracellularly; and (4) an intracellular C terminus that begins with a short helical segment (Helix 8) oriented parallel to the membrane surface. Ligand binding in GPCRs is thought to occur within the binding site crevice formed by the TM helix bundle, to extracellular loops, or to a combination of extracellular loop and binding site crevice residues. Agonists are thought to bind and produce a conformational change that initiates coupling to the G protein that is located inside the cell. An agonist-bound receptor activates an appropriate G protein that promotes dissociation of GDP (guanosine diphosphate). Although the interactions between receptor and G protein are poorly understood, both mutagenesis and biochemical experiments with a variety of GPCRs suggest that, first, ligand-induced receptor activation causes a change in the relative orientations of TM3 and TM6. This modification then affects the conformation of the G protein-interacting intracellular loops of the receptor and thus uncovers previously masked G protein binding sites.[11] Second, as GDP is buried within the G protein, the receptor–G protein interaction must, in addition, promote changes in interdomain interactions.[12] Thus, to activate the G protein, the receptor has to deliver *2 pieces of information*: the first for the formation of the receptor/G protein complex and the second to induce the exchange of bound GDP (guanosine diphosphate) for GTP (guanosine triphosphate) on the heterotrimeric G protein, resulting in the dissociation of the G protein into active Gα-GTP and Gβγ subunits. Both the Gα-GTP and Gβγ subunits then interact with effectors to transduce the signal initiated by agonist binding.

Rhodopsin is the dim-light photoreceptor and is a prototypical member of the Class A GPCR family.[3] It consists of a 348-amino-acid protein, opsin, which binds the chromophore 11-cis-retinal via a protonated Schiff base linkage to Lys7.43(296), giving the ground state of the protein an absorption maximum at 498 nm.[13] Absorption of a photon by 11-cis-retinal triggers its isomerization to the all-trans form, converting light energy into molecular movement. Rhodopsin then thermally relaxes through a series of distinct photointermediates, each with characteristic UV/visible absorption maxima (λ_{max}). The early photointermediates include bathorhodopsin (batho, λ_{max} = 543 nm), a blue-shifted intermediate, and lumirhodopsin (lumi, λ_{max} = 497 nm).[14] An equilibrium is formed between the later photointermediates, metarhodopsin I (meta I, λ_{max} = 480 nm) and metarhodopsin II (meta II, λ_{max} = 380 nm). Meta II corresponds to the fully activated receptor, which binds to and activates the heterotrimeric G protein transducin.[13]

Rhodopsin has been crystallized in its ground state in 2 different space groups: a tetragonal $P4_1$[7,10] crystal form and a trigonal $P3_1$ packing arrangement.[8] The structures determined by x-ray crystallography from these 2 crystal forms are very similar within the TM domains but show differences in the G-protein binding region of the cytoplasmic surface, where the location of the third intracellular loop (IC-3 loop) between TM5 and TM6 is highly variable. Several additional water molecules are visible in the $P3_1$ structure, including a water molecule that crosslinks the kinks in TM6 and TM7 and a water molecule that is part of the complex counterion of the Schiff base. EM data show that the IC-3 loop adopts the same conformation as seen in the $P3_1$ structure (see Fig. 3.2d in Schertler[15]). Okada et al reported the rhodopsin structure with the highest resolution (2.2 Å) so far from tetragonal crystals.[10] However, in the tetragonal $P4_1$ crystal, there is a crystal contact between the IC-3 loops in neighboring molecules in the crystal. This contact distorts the loop structure seen in the 2.2 Å structure (PDB, Protein Data Bank, accession number 1U19). For this reason, the 2.65 Å structure (PDB accession number 1GZM)[8] may be the better structural template from which to start a homology model of a rhodopsin-like GPCR, particularly in the region of the IC-3 loop because there is no distortion of loop structures due to crystal packing in the 1GZM structure.

Modeling GPCR Monomers

Homology Modeling of the GPCR Inactive State

By far the most common way the inactive/ground state of a GPCR is modeled is by homology modeling based on the crystal structure of bovine rhodopsin.[7-10] The first step in homology modeling would be sequence alignment with the bovine rhodopsin sequence. There are numerous sequence alignment programs available (see http://helix.nih.gov/apps/bioinfo/msa.html and http://www.hku.hk/bruhk/sgaln.html for a sampling). One of the most commonly used alignment programs is ClustalW (http://www.ebi.ac.uk/clustalw/). ClustalW is a general-purpose multiple sequence alignment program for DNA or proteins. It produces biologically meaningful multiple sequence alignments of divergent sequences. It calculates the best match for the selected sequences and lines sequences up so that the identities, similarities, and differences can be seen. Evolutionary relationships can be seen via viewing cladograms or phylograms. However, a word of caution is in order. Such automatic sequence alignment programs work best when the GPCR sequence one wishes to align with bovine rhodopsin contains all of the highly conserved residues/ sequence motifs across Class A GPCRs. Using the Ballesteros and Weinstein numbering system,[6] these are N1.50 in TM1, D2.50 in TM2, (D/E)RY in TM3, W4.50 in TM4, P5.50 in TM5, CWXP in TM6, and NPXXY in TM7. Misalignment of a TM region can occur in a helix span for which the appropriate residue or motif is missing or where more than one residue of the same type is located in proximity to each other. As an example, the cannabinoid CB1 and CB2 receptors, which are Class A receptors, lack the highly conserved proline at 5.50. As detailed in an early paper,[16] the second most highly conserved residue in TM5 of most Class A GPCRs is a Tyr at position 5.58 in the C terminal portion of TM5. The CB1 and CB2 receptors have 2 Tyr in common in this region (CB1: YLMFWIGVTSVLLLFIVY**Y**AYM **Y**ILWKA; CB2: YLLSWLLFIAFLFSGII**Y**T**Y**GHVLWKA). Consequently, automatic alignment results for CB1/CB2 in the TM5 region can diverge from one another depending on the alignment program employed. To determine which of these would correspond to Tyr 5.58 in other GPCRs, we performed a manual "structural alignment."[6,16] In such an alignment, residues are aligned based upon their predicted interior or surface-exposed character. First, the cytoplasmic end of TM5 was predicted using the criterion that Arg/Lys patches at the intracellular end of a TM helix face the lipid domain and may anchor the helix in the membrane by interaction with the negatively charged phospholipid head groups.[17] The cytoplasmic end of TM5 predicted using the Arg/Lys criterion was used then to superimpose the predicted accessibility profile for TM5 of CB1 with the equivalent profile of the rest of the proteins used in the original alignment (see Bramblett et al[16]). By this method, Y294 in CB1 and Y210 in CB2 can be aligned with the highly conserved Tyr at 5.58 in other GPCRs. The Leu residue 8 residues back in the sequence, which normally is a Pro in Class A GPCRs, was assigned the locant 5.50 to preserve numbering system correspondence with other GPCRs.

Software such as MODELLER can be used for homology or comparative modeling of GPCR 3-dimensional structures.[18] The user provides an alignment of a sequence to be modeled with known related structures, and MODELLER automatically calculates a model containing all nonhydrogen atoms. MODELLER implements comparative protein structure modeling by satisfaction of spatial restraints[19] and can calculate loop segments for models of GPCRs.[20]

The bovine rhodopsin sequence also has sequence motifs that dictate local structure that may be absent in another GPCR. Ballesteros et al have proposed that the overall structures of rhodopsin and of aminergic receptors are very similar, although there are localized regions where the structure of these receptors may diverge. Furthermore, they have proposed that several of the highly unusual structural features of rhodopsin are also present in aminergic GPCRs, despite the absence of amino acids that might have been thought critical to the adoption of these features. Thus, different amino acids or alternate microdomains can support similar deviations from regular α-helical structure, thereby resulting in similar tertiary structure. Such structural mimicry may be a mechanism by which a common ancestor could diverge sufficiently to develop the selectivity necessary to interact with diverse signals, while still maintaining a similar overall fold. Through this process, the core function of signaling activation through a conformational change in the TM segments that alters the conformation of the cytoplasmic surface and subsequent interaction with G proteins is presumably shared by the entire Class A family of receptors, despite their selectivity for a diverse group of ligands.[21] In the Class A aminergic GPCRs (with the exception of most of the muscarinic receptor family) there is a Pro at 2.59 in TM2. In bovine rhodopsin, no Pro exists in TM2, but TM2 does have a GGXTT motif that begins at G2.57(89) and ends at T2.61(93). This GGXTT motif causes a local distortion in the TM2 helix backbone that may be mimicked by P2.59 in most of the aminergic GPCRs.

But in other Class A GPCRs, there is neither a GGXTT motif nor a P2.59. This was the case with the cannabinoid CB2 receptor. We were drawn to the study of TM2 by substituted cysteine accessibility method data obtained by our collaborator, Dr. Zhao-Hui Song, which indicated that C2.59 in CB2 can be labeled by methanethiosulfonate (MTS) reagents, indicating that this residue is accessible from within the binding site crevice.[22] Our original TM2 model had been modeled as a regular α-helix because CB2 TM2 lacked the GGXTT motif of rhodopsin. In this modeled helix, C2.59 faced lipid. So, we sought some other residue or motif in the CB2 sequence that could alter the conformation of CB2 TM2.

Both serines and threonines have been shown to be able to act as hinge residues to affect the conformation of an α helix via an intrahelical hydrogen bond between the Oγ atom of the Ser or Thr (in a g^- or $+60°$ $\chi 1$) and the i-3 or i-4 carbonyl oxygen of the helix backbone. This is of particular significance for membrane proteins.[23] Using the biased Monte Carlo/simulated annealing method Conformational Memories,[24] we tested the hypothesis that S2.54(84) in a $g^-(+60°)$ $\chi 1$ forms an intrahelical hydrogen bond that produces an alteration from normal α-helicity in CB2 TM2. We found that S2.54(84) can indeed influence the backbone conformation of TM2. This influence was extracellular to S2.54(84), allowing the highly conserved residue, D2.50, to remain oriented as in rhodopsin. While we did not see a statistically significant difference in TM2 helix bend angles, we did see a statistically significant difference in another measure of helix geometry, wobble angle. So our Conformational Memories calculations suggested that S2.54(84) introduces a distortion from normal α-helicity in TM2. As illustrated in Fig. 3.1, our Conformational Memories calculations predicted that the S2.54(84) effect on the TM2 conformation allowed a wobble in TM2 that places C2.59 in the TM2-TM3 interface, where it is accessible to MTS reagent. The corresponding residue in bovine rhodopsin, T2.59, faces lipid, as illustrated in Fig. 3.1. This result suggests that there is a localized region in TM2 (extracellular to S2.54) where the structure of CB2 and rhodopsin diverge.

Even when the GPCR to be modeled has the highly conserved GPCR motifs, there still may be sequence-dictated variability from the rhodopsin structure. The CWXP motif in TM6 is thought to act as a flexible hinge, permitting TM6 to straighten during GPCR activation.[25] So can one expect that the flexibility and the helix geometry of TM6 is the same for all helices that have the CWXP motif? A study of TM6 in the cannabinoid receptors is offered here to illustrate that one cannot assume a common geometry. Both the CB1 and the CB2 receptors have the CWXP motif in TM6. In CB1, the sequence is CWGP, and in CB2, it is CWFP. We undertook a Conformational Memories study of CB1 versus CB2 TM6 in isolation

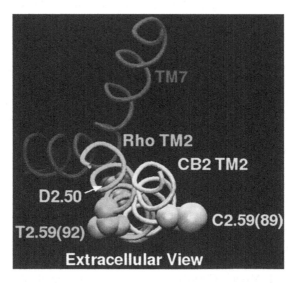

Fig. 3.1 A comparison of the relative positions of residue 2.59 in TM2 of Rho versus TM2 of CB2 (as predicted by Conformational Memories). TM2 of Rho and TM2 of CB2 have been superimposed at their intracellular ends to D2.50. It is clear here that the extracellular portions of TM2 of Rho versus CB2 differ significantly, resulting in a shift in the location of residue 2.59, for example. TM indicates transmembrane segment; CB, cannabinoid 2 receptor.[22]

to better understand the conformations possible for this important helix.[26] The Conformational Memories method employs multiple Monte Carlo/simulated annealing random walks and the Amber* force field. Conformational Memories has been shown to achieve complete sampling of the conformational space of flexible molecules, to converge in a very practical number of steps, and to be capable of overcoming energy barriers efficiently.[24] When Conformational Memories is used, the conformational properties of a helix can be fully characterized by the free energy of each conformation that the helix can adopt. This property includes not only the intrinsic energy of each conformational state but also the probability that the helix will adopt each conformation relative to all other ones accessible in an equilibrated thermodynamic ensemble. The calculation is performed in 2 phases. In the first phase, repeated runs of Monte Carlo/simulated annealing are performed to map the entire conformational space of the helix. In the second phase, new Monte Carlo/simulated annealing runs are performed in only the populated regions identified in the first phase of the calculation. The final output is 100 structures at 310 K. Conformers are grouped using X-Cluster (Schrödinger, Portland, OR) according to their increasing root mean square (rms) deviation from the first structure output at 310 K. Because X-Cluster rearranges the conformers so that the rms deviation between nearest neighbors is minimized, any large jump in rms deviation is indicative of a large conformational change and hence identifies a new conformational family or cluster.

The Conformational Memories results for TM6 in wildtype (WT) CB1 and CB2 indicated a dramatic difference in the range of conformations possible for each receptor subtype (Fig. 3.2A and 3.2B). Conformers were superimposed at their extracellular ends. For WT CB1 (Fig. 3.2A), 2 major clusters were identified (yellow and magenta in Fig. 3.2). For WT CB2 (Fig. 3.2B), a single cluster was identified (green in Fig. 3.2). The average proline kink and SD for all 100 conformers generated by Conformational Memories at 310 K are given at right in each Figure. For WT CB1, 2 clusters of conformers resulted. For all 100 conformers of WT CB1 generated by Conformational Memories, the average kink angle was 40.9° (SD ±16.9°; Fig. 3.2A). For CB2, a single cluster of less kinked structures resulted. The average kink angle for all 100 structures was 24.6° (SD ± 4.3°; Fig. 3.2B). The flexibility of WT CB2 TM6 was very consistent with the flexibility reported for TM6 in the β2-adrenergic receptor.[25] However, the results for WT CB1 suggested that CB1 TM6 has increased flexibility. We hypothesized that this difference in flexibility may be due to the size of the residue that immediately precedes P6.50 (ie, residue 6.49) in each receptor subtype. In the more flexible TM6 (CB1), residue 6.49 is small in size, a glycine. In the less flexible TM6 (CB2), residue 6.49 is much larger in size, a phenylalanine. To test this hypothesis, Conformational Memories was used to compare the range of conformations possible for the "switch mutants," CB1 G6.49F and CB2 F6.49G. The results appear in Fig. 3.2C and 3.2D. Here, conformers have been superimposed at their extracellular ends. For the CB1 G6.49F mutant, one population of moderately kinked helices with an average kink angle of 25.3° (SD ±5.7°; Fig. 3.2C) resulted. These results are similar to those for WT CB2 (Fig. 3.2B). For the CB2 F6.49G mutant, 2 clusters resulted. The average kink angle for all 100

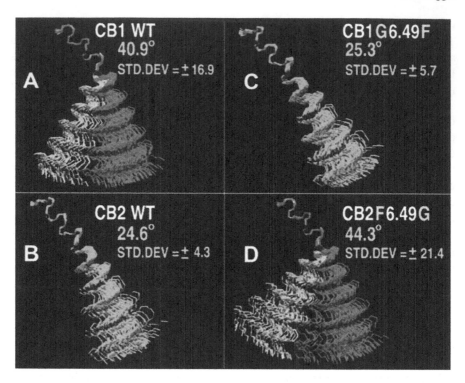

Fig. 3.2 CM results for (A) WT CB1, (B) WT CB2, (C) CB1 G6.49F, and (D) CB2 F6.49G TM6. Conformers have been superimposed at their extracellular ends. For (A) and (D), 2 major clusters were identified. For (B) and (C), a single cluster was identified by CM. The average proline kink and SD for all 100 conformers generated by CM at 310 K are given to the right in each Figure. It is clear here that WT CB1 TM6 has greater flexibility than WT CB2 TM6. The swap mutation results—(C) and (D)—suggest that this flexibility is due to the presence of a Gly at position 6.49 immediately preceding the Pro in TM6 of WT CB1. CM indicates Conformational Memories; WT, wildtype; CB, cannabinoid; TM, transmembrane segment.[26]

conformers was 44.3° (SD ±21.4°; Fig. 3.2D). These results are similar to those obtained for WT CB1 (Fig. 3.2A). Taken together, these results suggest that TM6 in CB1 has been engineered to have greater flexibility and ability to bend because of the small Gly residue in the flexible hinge motif, CWGP, in CB1. Clearly, many of the helices output by Conformational Memories for WT CB1 are too bent to be able to be accommodated in the TM bundle. We were able to use this output to choose an inactive state TM6 for CB1 (Pro kink angle = 53.1°) and an activated state (see below) TM6 (Pro kink angle = 21.8°). Another important outcome of the Conformational Memories studies was that while the wobble angle of CB2 TM6 is similar to that in rhodopsin (placing the extracellular end of TM6 close to TM5 in the context of the TM bundle), the wobble angle of TM6 in CB1 is quite different

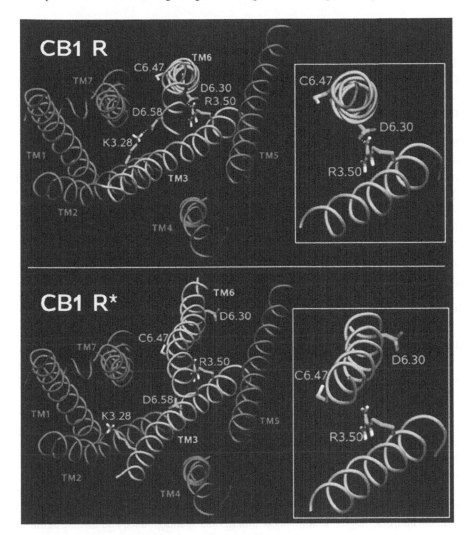

Fig. 3.3 (Top) An extracellular view of the CB1 TM bundle model of the inactive (R) state. In the R state, the wobble angle of TM6 causes the extracellular end to be close to TM3. As a result, a salt bridge is possible between D6.58 and K3.28. (Inset) A salt bridge between R3.50 and D6.30 brings the intracellular ends of TM3 and TM6 close in the inactive state. (Bottom) An extracellular view of the CB1 TM bundle model of the active (R*) state. In the R* state, TM6 has straightened and both TM3 and TM6 have rotated counterclockwise. (Inset) At the intracellular end, the salt bridge between R3.50 and D6.30 has broken. CB indicates cannabinoid; TM, transmembrane segment.

(pointing the extracellular end of TM6 toward TM3). As illustrated in our R model for CB1 in Fig. 3.3 below, the flexibility of TM6 and its different wobble angle enables a salt bridge to form between K3.28 and D6.58.

De Novo Modeling of the GPCR Inactive State

Before the publication of the bovine rhodopsin crystal structure in 2000,[7] many GPCR models were created de novo[6,16] using a Fourier transform analysis of sequence periodicity in a set of highly homologous sequences.[27,28] This approach permitted the identification of helical segments within the sequence and, through calculation of moment vectors, the correct orientation of each helix within the bundle.[29,30] Helix tilts were arranged based on the projection structure of rhodopsin available at that time.[31,32] Today there are methods available that create de novo models in much this same way. The Goddard group has developed a method, called Membstruk,[33] that has been used to create de novo models of the dopamine D2 and the β2-adrenergic receptors.[34,35] These de novo methods may be particularly useful for modeling non-Class A GPCRs that have divergences from the well-known sequence motifs present in rhodopsin and other Class A receptors.

Creating Models of GPCR Activated State Conformation(s)

Recent electron microscopy (EM) studies have allowed the investigation of the metarhodopsin I intermediate, revealing evidence about the early changes during the photolysis process.[36] Comparison of this map with x-ray structures of the ground state[7-10] reveals that metarhodopsin I formation does not involve large rigid-body movements of helices, but there is a rearrangement close to the bend of TM6, at the level of the retinal chromophore. There is no gradual buildup of the large conformational change known to accompany metarhodopsin II formation (see below). The protein remains in a conformation similar to that of the ground state until late in the photobleaching process.

To date, no crystal or EM structure of rhodopsin in its fully activated, Meta II state has been published. Yet knowledge of the structure of this state is critical for modeling studies. Pharmacological studies show that agonists, antagonists, and inverse agonists do not bind to a single receptor conformation.[37] Many models of GPCRs fail to distinguish this fact, opting to dock agonists, antagonists, and inverse agonists in the same receptor model, usually based on the rhodopsin (inactive state) crystal structure. In contrast, pharmacological, biophysical, and structural data, and data on constitutively active receptors, all demonstrate that GPCRs exist in distinguishable conformations and, hence, *a single model for any receptor can never be adequate*.

So, how can one obtain a model of the activated state of a GPCR of interest? It would seem that one way to approach obtaining a model of the activated state would be via molecular dynamics (MD) simulations that start with the agonist bound in the inactive state. The time scale for activation has been estimated to be milliseconds for light activation of rhodopsin[38] but seconds for activation of the β2-AR (adrenergic receptor) by its diffusible ligand.[39] It is not possible at the present time to perform MD simulations to study agonist-induced changes to the inactive (R) state to generate the activated (R*) state because GPCR activation takes much longer than the typical length of MD simulations (10–100 ns).

An alternate way to build an activated state model is to create a model that reflects the conformational changes suggested to occur during GPCR activation as deduced from biophysical studies. Such studies of rhodopsin activation and activation of the β2-adrenergic receptor have revealed important information about the conformational changes that occur upon activation of these GPCRs. These studies have suggested that activation is accompanied by rigid domain motions and rotations of TM helices 3 and 6 (counterclockwise from an extracellular perspective).[39-41] At their intracellular ends, TMs 3 and 6 in rhodopsin are constrained by an E3.49(134)/R3.50(135)/E6.30(247) salt bridge that limits the relative mobility of the cytoplasmic ends of TM3 and TM6 in the inactive state[7] and acts like an "ionic lock."[42,43] During activation, P6.50 of the highly conserved CWXP motif in TM6 of GPCRs may act as a flexible hinge, permitting TM6 to straighten upon activation, moving its intracellular end away from TM3 and upward toward the lipid bilayer.[44] In our work, we have chosen to create models of the activated state of the cannabinoid receptors based upon these documented changes that occur during the R to R* transition.[45] Fig. 3.3 illustrates our current CB1 R and CB1 R* bundles. The importance of the generation of such models has been discussed by Gouldson et al.[46]

To deduce the sequence-specific rotamer "toggle switch" within the binding pocket that leads to the R* state of individual GPCRs, initial R* models (see above) can be refined through a combination of computational and experimental studies. Klein-Seetharaman and coworkers[47] have reported that even in the dark (inactive) state of rhodopsin, only some strong constraints exist, whereas the majority of the molecule experiences conformational flexibility. Light activation of rhodopsin, therefore, does not require the breaking and forming of thousands of specific contacts within nanoseconds. Instead, activation requires only a few specific contacts restricting the inactive state, including indole side-chain contacts of tryptophan residues, to break on activation. These changes can then be transmitted through the entire membrane protein because of its dynamic plasticity. One of the tryptophan residues that Klein-Seetharaman and coworkers have reported to be restricted in rhodopsin is W6.48(265). In the dark (inactive) state of rhodopsin, the beta-ionone ring of 11-cis-retinal is close to W6.48(265) of the CWXP motif on TM6 and acts as a linchpin, constraining W6.48 in a χ_1 = g+ conformation.[7-9] In the light-activated state, the beta-ionone ring moves away from TM6 and toward TM4, where it resides close to A4.58(169).[48] This movement releases the constraint on W6.48(265), making it possible for W6.48(265) to undergo a conformational change. Lin and Sakmar[49] reported that perturbations in the environment of W6.48(265) of rhodopsin occur during the conformational change concomitant with receptor activation. This suggests that the conformation of W6.48(265) when rhodopsin is in its inactive/ground state (R; χ_1 = g+) changes during activation (ie, W6.48(265) χ_1 g+ → trans).[25] In the Class A aminergic receptors, a highly conserved cluster of aromatic amino acids is found on TM6 that faces the binding site crevice bracketing W6.48 (F6.44, W6.48, F6.51, and F6.52).[25] Shi and coworkers used mutation studies of the β2-adrenergic receptor combined with the biased Monte Carlo technique of Conformational Memories to propose that a C6.47 *trans*/W6.48 *g*+/F6.52 *g*+ → C6.47 *g*+/W6.48 *trans*/F6.52 *g*+ transition is the key switch within the binding site crevice that leads to the R* state of the β2-AR (adrenergic receptor).[25]

Restriction of W6.48 by a TM6 aromatic cluster is not possible in the cannabinoid receptors, as the CB1 receptor has leucines at 6.44, 6.51, and 6.52. Instead, the CB1 receptor contains a microdomain of aromatic residues that face into the ligand binding pocket in the TM3-4–5-6 region, including F3.25(189), F3.36(200), W4.64(255), Y5.39(275), W5.43(279), and W6.48(356). Singh and coworkers used the biased Monte Carlo technique of Conformational Memories combined with receptor modeling to suggest that the F3.36(200)/W6.48(356) interaction may act as a mimic of the 11-cis-retinal/W6.48 interaction in the rhodopsin dark state and may serve as the toggle switch for CB1 activation, with F3.36(200) χ1 *trans*/ W6.48(356) χ1 *g*+ representing the inactive (R) and F3.36(200) χ1 *g*+/W6.48(356) χ1 *trans* representing the active (R*) state of CB1.[50] Fig. 3.4 illustrates this, with F3.36 and W6.48 engaged in a direct aromatic stack in the R state and rotated away from each other in the R* state. A detailed functional analysis of mouse CB1 F3.36A and W6.48A mutants, undertaken to test this toggle switch hypothesis, showed statistically significant increases in ligand-independent stimulation of GTPγS binding for a F3.36A mutant versus WT mCB1, while basal levels for the W6.48A mutant were not statistically different from WT mCB1. These results suggested that F3.36 may function as a linchpin, restraining W6.48 from moving to an active state conformation in the CB1 receptor.[45]

It is important to note that there is accumulating experimental evidence for the existence of more than one "activated" state for a GPCR, with conformation influenced by the type of agonist bound.[51,52] So, the assumption of a single activated state for any GPCR is, admittedly, a simplifying assumption. However, in our hands, despite the fact that we may have created a single R* model for each cannabinoid receptor subtype in the absence of ligand, we see differences between agonist/R* complexes depending upon which agonist occupies the receptor (data not shown).

Modeling Loop Regions

In much of the literature, GPCR models have been built of the TM regions only, with the implicit assumption that agonist/antagonist interaction occurs with TM residues only and therefore models need not include the loop regions. This is a simplifying assumption that may need to be reconsidered in light of experimental results. For example, for the κ-opioid receptor, there is evidence that extracellular loop regions form part of the binding site for ligands.[53] Loop conformations can be generated using homology modeling, database searching, or *ab initio* computational methods. A comprehensive review of the loop modeling literature is beyond the scope of this article. However, some methods in use are discussed below.

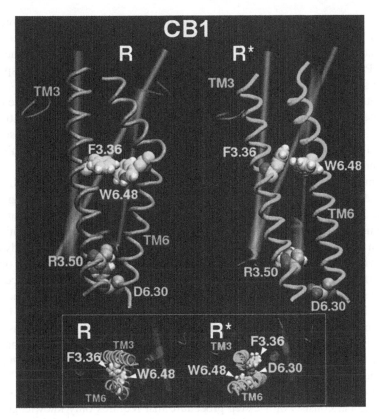

Fig. 3.4 The relationship between F3.36(201) and W6.48(357) in the inactive (R) and active (R*) states of CB1 as predicted by molecular modeling. The major view is from TM5 looking toward TM3/TM6. (Left) In the R state, W6.48(356) adopts a g+ χ1, whereas F3.36(200) adopts a trans χ1. In this arrangement, W6.48(356) and F3.36(200) are engaged in an aromatic stacking interaction that stabilizes the R state. By analogy with Rho, the CB1-inactive state is also characterized by a salt bridge between R3.50(214) and D6.30(338) at the intracellular side of CB1 that keeps the intracellular ends of TM3 and TM6 close. The TM6 kink extracellular to W6.48(357) permits a hypothesized salt bridge between K3.28(193) and D6.58(367) to form. This salt bridge is made possible by the profound flexibility in TM6 due to the presence of G6.49(357) in the CW*X*P motif of TM6. (Right) In the R* state, W6.48(356) and F3.36(200) have moved apart because of rotation of TM3 and TM6 during activation. W6.48(356) has adopted a trans χ1 and has moved toward the viewer, and F3.36(200) has adopted a g+ χ1 and has moved away from the viewer. The R3.50(214)/D6.30(338) salt bridge is broken, and the proline kink in TM6 has moderated. (Inset) An extracellular view of CB1. It is clear that in R, F3.36(200) and W6.48(356) are engaged in an aromatic stacking interaction, but in R*, F3.36(200) and W6.48(356) are no longer close enough to interact. CB indicates cannabinoid; TM, transmembrane segment.[45]

One approach to adding loop segments to GPCR TM bundle models is to search the Protein Data Bank (http://www.rcsb.org/pdb/) to identify loop conformations in the database with the highest sequence homology with each loop segment of the receptor to be modeled. Another approach is to use a protein structure predictor such as PredictProtein (http://www.predictprotein.org). PredictProtein is a service for sequence analysis and structure prediction. Users submit protein sequences, and PredictProtein retrieves similar sequences in the database and predicts aspects of protein structure.

Tosatto and coworkers have described an algorithm that uses a database of pre-calculated lookup tables, which represent a large set of possible conformations for loop segments of variable length. The target loop is recursively decomposed until the resulting conformations are small enough to be compiled analytically. The algorithm generates a ranked set of loop conformations.[54]

As mentioned earlier, the Sali lab has developed MODELLER, which can be used to add loops to GPCR models.[18,20] The Honig lab has developed a program for protein loop prediction, the *loopy* program (http://honiglab.cpmc.columbia.edu/programs/loop/intro.html). The program can also perform sequence mutation and addition of a missing protein segment.[55] If the segment to be predicted already exists, *loopy* will delete the original segment and predict a new one to assemble onto the stems. If the segment to be predicted does not exist, the residue sequence of the missing segment must be provided and *loopy* will predict a segment with those residues and assemble it onto the 2 end stems. The *loopy* program first builds multiple initial conformations using an *ab initio* method. Each of the conformations is then closed using a random tweak method. Fast energy minimization in torsional angle space is then performed and the side chain is assembled using the side-chain prediction program (scap). Colony energy is used to sort out the best predictions.[55]

Mehler and Weinstein[56,57] have developed an *ab initio* approach for loop segment modeling that consists of a 2-step procedure that requires only knowledge of the structure (experimental or model) of the domains to be connected. The method employs simulated annealing Monte Carlo simulations performed on the loop segment starting from a completely extended structure, combined with a biased scaled collective variables Monte Carlo technique designed to complete the closure of the segment. This method is based on the assumption that loop regions have an intrinsic propensity for a particular set of conformations based on their amino acid sequence, but this intrinsic folding has to be disrupted for the best fit of the loop segment within the tertiary structure of the native protein. Thus, the final folding of the loops in the context of the protein is a compromise between 2 opposite effects: the intrinsic tendency to adopt a specific folding pattern dictated by the amino acid sequence, and the partial unfolding that is imposed by the inclusion of the loop in the native conformation of the protein. The sampling methodology uses simulated annealing Monte Carlo simulations to find conformations that are representative of the segment structure in solution, as encoded in the primary sequence, and subsequently forces a slow unfolding of the segment to fit the final protein conformation using an adjustable force constant scheme and Monte Carlo simulations with a scaled collective variables technique. The scaled collective variables technique allows the Monte Carlo simulation to improve the efficiency of the search. Finally, since an accurate force field for the study of peptide and protein conformational preferences must account for the hydrophobic and electrostatic effects of the solvent, the method also uses a continuum electrostatic model developed by Hassan and coworkers. This method is based on screened Coulomb potentials and has been validated in several systems ranging in size from small molecules to large.[58]

GPCR Dimers and Oligomers

While it has been common to build models of GPCRs as monomers and some recent studies support monomeric GPCRs as functional units,[59] the emerging concept of GPCR dimerization has begun to challenge this notion. Recent work has shown not only that many GPCRs exist as homo- and heterodimers but also that GPCR oligomeric assembly may have important functional roles.[60,61] Terrillon and Bouvier have described the 5 stages of the GPCR life cycle that could be affected by dimerization: ontogeny, ligand-promoted regulation, pharmacological diversity, signal transduction, and internalization.[60] Studies have suggested that dimerization may be important in receptor maturation, as dimerization appears to occur early after biosynthesis. Dimerization may mask specific retention signals or hydrophobic patches that would cause receptor retention in the endoplasmic reticulum (ER).[62] The importance of dimerization to ontogeny has been clearly shown for the GPCR family C metabotropic γ-aminobutyric acid b receptor (GbR), which is composed of 2 subunits, GbR1 and GbR2.[63] When expressed alone, GbR1 is retained intracellularly as an immature protein because it has a carboxy-terminal ER retention motif,[64] whereas GbR2 reaches the cell surface but is not functional. Following their coexpression, heterodimerization masks the GbR1 ER retention signal (RXR(R) in the C terminus), allowing the proper targeting of a functional heterodimeric GbR to the plasma membrane.[64]

Experiments based on fluorescence resonance energy transfer (FRET) and bioluminescence energy transfer reveal that many GPCRs exist as oligomers, or at least as closely packed clusters, in the membranes of living cells.[60,65] Once a receptor has reached the cell surface, its oligomeric state could be dynamically regulated by a ligand. Whether receptor activation can promote or inhibit dimerization and/or favor exchanges between protomers is a key question with wide implications for the mechanisms of receptor activation and regulation. Unfortunately, there is no general consensus yet. Several studies suggest that ligand binding can regulate the dimer by either promoting or inhibiting its formation (see, eg, Roess and Smith[66] and Latif et al[67]); others conclude that homodimerization and heterodimerization are constitutive processes that are not modulated by ligand binding (see, eg, Terrillon et al[68]). In any case, the structural data available strongly suggest that at least some GPCRs can form dimers in the absence of ligand stimulation. For example, Palczewski and coworkers used atomic force spectroscopy to show that rhodopsin and opsin form constitutive dimers in dark-adapted native retinal membranes.[69,70]

Jordan and Devi's work on coexpressed δ- and κ-opioid receptors was the first evidence presented in the literature that GPCR heterodimerization could play a role in pharmacological diversity.[71] These investigators found that coexpression of both receptors led to the formation of a stable heterodimer with low affinity for δ- or κ-selective ligands when administered alone, but high affinity when these 2 agonists were administered together. Since these experiments, positive or negative ligand binding cooperativity that occurs after receptor coexpression has been interpreted as resulting from receptor heterodimerization for many other GPCRs.[72-76]

The first evidence that GPCR dimerization could have a crucial effect on signal transduction came from studies of the GPCR family C metabotropic GbR.[64] Heterodimerization has also been proposed to be crucial for the formation of functional taste receptors.[77,78] Heterodimer formation has been suggested to underlie signal potentiation in numerous receptors, including the chemokine CCR5/CCR2,[79] somatostatin SSTR5/dopamine D2,[75] and angiotensin AT1/bradykinin B2 receptors,[80] while signal attenuation has been described for other heterodimers such as adenosine A1/dopamine D1[81] and somatostatin SST2a/SST3 receptors.[82] Heterodimerization has also been proposed to promote changes in G protein selectivity. Kearn et al recently reported that a regulated association of cannabinoid CB1 and dopamine D2 receptors profoundly alters CB1 signaling, providing evidence that CB1/D2 receptor complexes exist, are dynamic, and are agonist regulated, with highest complex levels detected when both receptors are stimulated with subsaturating concentrations of agonist. The consequence of this interaction is a differential preference for signaling through a "nonpreferred" G protein. In this case, D2 receptor activation, simultaneously with CB1 receptor stimulation, results in the receptor complex coupling to Gs protein rather than to the expected Gi/o proteins.[83]

The emerging concept of GPCR dimerization has also challenged assumptions that one receptor interacts with one G protein. Several points of contact between G protein (G-α and G-βγ subunits) and receptor have been proposed.[84] However, the crystal structure of rhodopsin reveals that the receptor is too small to make all of these contacts simultaneously. It has been proposed that 2 receptors may be necessary to satisfy all proposed points of contact with G protein.[70,84] Baneres and Parello have shown that activated leukotriene B4 receptor (BLT1) and Gα12β1γ2 corresponds to a pentameric assembly of one G heterotrimeric protein and one dimeric receptor.[85]

Heterodimerization has also been suggested to affect agonist-promoted endocytosis. In many cases, stimulation of one of the protomers in a heterodimer promotes co-internalization of both receptors.[82,86-88]

The functional consequences of GPCR dimerization have been commonly studied in heterologous expression systems. It is possible in such systems to coexpress receptors that are actually never expressed together in vivo or to express receptors at such high levels that spurious interactions occur. However, the pharmacological relevance of heterodimerization has been demonstrated in cells that endogenously express the GPCRs under consideration. The potential physiological importance of heterodimerization is supported by studies in cells that endogenously coexpress the GPCRs under consideration. For example, blockade of either the AT1 receptor or the β2-adrenergic receptor with selective antagonists inhibits the signaling of both receptors simultaneously in freshly isolated mouse cardiomyocytes,[89] a phenomenon linked to the ability of the 2 receptors to heterodimerize.

Proposed Physical Models of Dimerization

Despite the fairly extensive literature on dimerization in GPCRs, there has been little discussion on the nature of the dimers. Two basic modes of dimerization have been proposed, contact dimers and domain-swapped dimers.

Contact Dimers

In *contact dimerization*, a dimer forms between 2 different TM bundles (monomers) with separate binding sites by packing at an interface that would face the lipid environment in the monomeric receptor (ie, by "touching" specific lipid faces). Experimental support for *contact dimers* can be found in the literature.[69,70,90-94] One example comes from Javitch and coworkers, who used cysteine cross-linking of the endogenous cysteine residue C4.58(168) to show that TM4 forms a symmetrical dimer interface in the dopamine D2 receptor.[95] More recently,[96] this same group mapped the homodimer interface in the dopamine D2 receptor over the entire length of TM4 by crosslinking of substituted cysteines. Residue susceptibilities to crosslinking were found to be differentially altered by the presence of agonists and inverse agonists. The TM4 dimer interface in the inverse agonist-bound conformation was consistent with the dimer of the inactive form of rhodopsin modeled with constraints from atomic force microscopy.[70] Crosslinking of a different set of engineered cysteines in TM4 was slowed by inverse agonists and accelerated in the presence of agonists; crosslinking of the latter set locks the receptor in an active state. These results suggest that a conformational change at the TM4 dimer interface is part of the receptor activation mechanism.[96]

Domain-Swapped Dimers

If, on the other hand, during dimerization, a hinge loop opens out, the domains could exchange to form a *domain-swapped dimer*. Gouldson and coworkers report that *domain-swapped dimers* are less common than *contact dimers* but have the major advantage that the interactions between the domains already present in the monomers can be reused to form the dimers; thus, domain swapping is an efficient way of forming dimerization interfaces. The length of the hinge loop is important in this process. For GPCRs, the hinge loop has been proposed to be IC-3, which connects TM5 and TM6 because it is frequently the longest loop in GPCRs.[97] The concept of domain-swapped dimers has also received experimental support.[98-105] One example is from the work of Maggio and coworkers, who found that muscarinic receptor heterodimerization was inhibited when the IC-3 loop was shortened. Maggio and coworkers concluded that their data suggested that an intermolecular interaction between muscarinic receptors, involving the exchange of amino-terminal (containing TM domains 1–5) and carboxyl-terminal (containing TM domains 6 and 7) receptor fragments (ie, the formation of a *domain-swapped dimer*), depended on the presence of a long IC-3 loop.[106]

Methodology for the Prediction of Dimer/Oligomer Interfaces

Bioinformatics techniques used to predict dimer and oligomer interfaces begin with multiple sequence alignments and share the assumption that proteins that are evolutionarily related might exhibit common structural and functional features corresponding to detectable patterns in their sequences. As a result, a suitable representation of the evolutionary relationships between proteins under study is an essential requirement for the prediction of dimer/oligomer interfaces.[107]

Correlated Mutation Analysis

The correlated mutation analysis (CMA) method is based upon sequence analyses and has been shown to provide information about interdomain contacts.[108] The correlation is the result of the tendency for amino acid positions in a sequence to mutate in a coordinated manner if the interface has to be preserved for structural or functional reasons. Sequence changes occurring over evolutionary time at the dimerization interface of monomer A would be compensated for by changes at the interacting face of monomer B to preserve the interaction interface.[107] Gouldson and coworkers recently used the CMA method to analyze candidate residues for the subtype-specific heterodimerization observed for the chemokine, opioid, and somatostatin receptors.[109]

Subtractive Correlated Mutation Method

Although CMA is a powerful bioinformatics tool that was demonstrated from specific tests to identify residues that are functionally essential, the original CMA method in itself does not usually achieve specific identification of the residue composition of the dimerization interfaces of GPCRs (eg, results of Gouldson et al,[109] which essentially show correlated mutations in all 7 TM helices). Filizola and coworkers have enhanced the CMA approach with filtering algorithms to enable identification of the likely hetero- and homo-oligomerization interfaces of family A GPCRs.[110,111] The new method, termed the subtractive correlated mutation (SCM) method,[110] consists of a modified version of an earlier algorithm[112] that provides a means to filter out the intramolecular pairs of correlated residues within each interacting monomer from the complete list of intra- and intermolecular pairs of correlated residues. Multiple sequence alignment of concatenated monomeric sequences of the 2 different GPCRs, obtained from the same organisms, is used to identify these correlated mutations. Concatenation is essential for the identification of the heterodimerization interface.[110] A similar approach was developed independently by Pazos et al.[108] Additional stringency criteria have been added for the application to GPCR homodimerization, to achieve reliable predictions of the dimerization/oligomerization interface of GPCRs.[107] To increase the chance of obtaining correctly predicted contacts, correlated pairs with a correlation index ≤ 0.7 are purged from the list. With the information contained in the crystal structure of rhodopsin,[7] residues are screened for lipid exposure. Only pairs of correlated residues where both positions have a surface exposure (to lipid) of more than $45 \, \text{Å}^2$ are considered as candidates for intermolecular contacts (the implicit assumption is that association of GPCRs occurs only via contact dimers/oligomers). Finally, only residues that are part of an interacting neighborhood (defined as at least 3 residues on the lipid face of the helix within i+7 of each other) are retained.[107]

We recently used the SCM method to identify the most likely homodimerization interface for the cannabinoid CB1 receptor. TM1 and TM4 contained the most predicted residues, but the residues identified for TM4 formed a continuous lipid-facing ridge (interaction neighborhood). Therefore, TM4 was chosen as the most likely homodimer interface for CB1. Fig. 3.5 illustrates a side view and an extracellular view of this proposed homodimer, with the gray residues contoured at their Van der Waals radii representing the residues identified by the SCM method. Only the TM regions of the CB1 dimer are illustrated here.[113]

Evolutionary Trace Method

The evolutionary trace (ET) method is another approach for determining functional sites in a protein given its 3-dimensional structure and a multiple sequence alignment. The ET method was first described by Lichtarge and coworkers as an approach to predict functionally important residues in proteins of known structure.[114-116] Based on the earlier hierarchical analysis of residue conservation in proteins developed by Livingstone and Barton,[117] the ET method has some similarities with the CMA method, as evolutionary trace residues may also be correlated, but the ET method has the advantage that conserved residues are also included in the analysis.[115,118] Built from the idea that proteins that have evolved from a common ancestor will show similar backbone structure,[119] the ET method assumes that within a multiple sequence alignment, the protein family retains its fold. The method also assumes that the protein family should conserve the location of functional sites and have a distinctly lower mutation rate at these sites, punctuated by mutation events that cause divergence.[115]

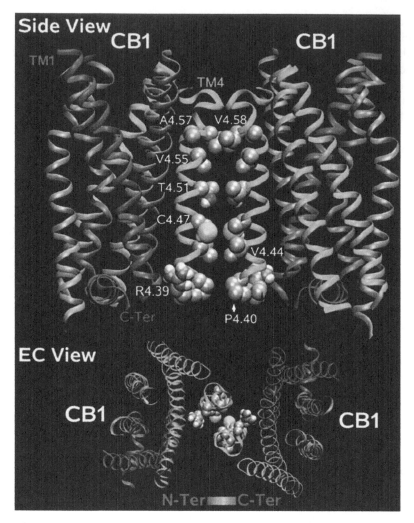

Fig. 3.5 A side view (top) and an EC view (bottom) of the CB1 homodimer predicted by the subtractive correlated mutation method. Residues predicted to be part of the homodimer interface at TM4 are shown in gray and are contoured at their Van der Waals radii. To determine the possible interface orientations for the homodimer, we looked for patches of continuous residues, or "interaction neighborhoods." Both TM1 and TM4 contained the most predicted residues. However, TM4 contained a continuous exterior ridge formed by the predicted residues. The TM bundles are illustrated here without loops to simplify the display. EC indicates extracellular; CB, cannabinoid; TM, transmembrane segment.[113]

Hidden-Site Class Model

Evolutionary relationships between proteins can be represented by a matrix indicating the rate at which every amino acid substitution occurs during evolution. Current models use a single substitution matrix for all locations in all sequences. This is a limitation of these models because the probability that an amino acid substitution at a particular location in the protein sequence would produce a functional effect is not the same at all locations.[107] The hidden-site class model has been proposed to overcome this limitation by using different substitution matrices to represent amino acid substitutions at different locations in a protein sequence.[120-122] It has been demonstrated that this method attains better phylogenic inferences by identifying locations in the sequences that are considered to be under similar selective pressure and by characterizing changes in selective pressure. Locations that are assigned to site classes with the slowest rate of substitution are expected to correspond to structurally or functionally important positions. This method has been applied recently to 199 Class A GPCR aminergic receptors. The method identified lipid-exposed evolutionarily conserved locations on TM4, TM5, and TM6 in different subfamilies.[123]

In their recent review, Filizola and Weinstein[107] point out that both the assumptions underlying the computational algorithms and the selection of sequences in the alignment determine the nature of the answers returned by the algorithm. *The statistical nature of the tools makes their success in predicting dimer/oligomer interfaces highly dependent on the number of sequences available for a family and subfamily.* As more sequences become available with the completion of the sequencing of more genomes, the power of these approaches can be expected to increase.[107]

GPCR Dimer Interface Predictions

Filizola and Weinstein have analyzed the occurrence of lipid-exposed residues in predictions from bioinformatics methods applied to search for dimerization/oligomerization interfaces of GPCRs (see Figure 3.3 in Filizola and Weinstein[107]).

These authors report that residues most frequently identified cluster in TM4, TM5, and TM6, indicating that the prediction of dimerization/oligomerization interfaces of GPCRs with various computational methods has thus far pointed to a specific role for the lipid-exposed regions of these 3 helices. Among the residues identified within each of these 3 helices, 4.58, 5.48, and 6.42 have the greatest number of occurrences. In TM6, residue 6.30 (at the boundary between TM6 and the IC-3 loop) had nearly the same frequency of occurrence as 6.42. The high occurrence of residue 6.30 in dimer/oligomer analyses can be explained by an involvement of this residue in a broader oligomerization scheme of GPCRs. This is suggested by the atomic force microscopy map of rhodopsin in native membranes,[70] which indicates that the cytoplasmic loop connecting TM5 and TM6 facilitates the formation of rows of rhodopsin dimers.

Conclusions

The x-ray crystal structure of the Class A GPCR, rhodopsin, in its inactive state has catalyzed the construction of computational models of many other GPCRs. Models of the activated states of GPCRs are now emerging in the literature based upon evidence from biophysical studies of the conformational changes that occur upon the activation of rhodopsin and other GPCRs. These models are proving useful as hypothesis generators for experimental studies aimed at deducing ligand binding sites and ligand-receptor activation mechanisms. Recent experimental work has shown not only that many GPCRs exist as homo- and heterodimers but also that GPCR oligomeric assembly may have important functional roles. In response to these findings, a whole new computational literature is emerging to address the creation of homodimer, heterodimer, and oligomeric models of GPCRs. The new dimeric and oligomeric models that emerge from computational studies should prove very valuable as hypothesis generators for studies of the functional significance of GPCR dimerization and oligomerization.

Acknowledgments The author wishes to thank Mr Dow Hurst for his technical assistance. This work was supported by National Institutes of Health/National Institute on Drug Abuse grants DA03934 and DA00489 (Patricia H. Reggio).

References

1. Takeda S, Kadowaki S, Haga T, Takaesu H, Mitaku S. Identification of G protein-coupled receptor genes from the human genome sequence. *FEBS Lett.* 2002;520:97-101.
2. Kolakowski LF, Jr. GCRDb: a G-protein-coupled receptor database. *Receptors Channels.* 1994;2:1-7.
3. Bockaert J, Pin JP. Molecular tinkering of G protein-coupled receptors: an evolutionary success. *EMBO J.* 1999;18:1723-1729.
4. Fredriksson R, Lagerstrom MC, Lundin LG, Schioth HB. The G-protein-coupled receptors in the human genome form five main families. Phylogenetic analysis, paralogon groups, and fingerprints. *Mol Pharmacol.* 2003;63:1256-1272.
5. Eilers M, Hornak V, Smith SO, Konopka JB. Comparison of class A and D G protein-coupled receptors: common features in structure and activation. *Biochemistry.* 2005;44:8959-8975.
6. Ballesteros JA, Weinstein H. Integrated methods for the construction of three dimensional models and computational probing of structure function relations in G protein-coupled receptors. In: Sealfon SC, Conn PM, eds. *Methods in Neurosciences.* vol. 25. San Diego, CA: Academic Press; 1995:366-428.
7. Palczewski K, Kumasaka T, Hori T, et al. Crystal structure of rhodopsin: a G protein-coupled receptor. *Science.* 2000;289:739-745.
8. Li J, Edwards PC, Burghammer M, Villa C, Schertler GF. Structure of bovine rhodopsin in a trigonal crystal form. *J Mol Biol.* 2004;343:1409-1438.
9. Okada T, Fujiyoshi Y, Silow M, Navarro J, Landau EM, Shichida Y. Functional role of internal water molecules in rhodopsin revealed by X-ray crystallography. *Proc Natl Acad Sci USA.* 2002;99:5982-5987.
10. Okada T, Sugihara M, Bondar AN, Elstner M, Entel P, Buss V. The retinal conformation and its environment in rhodopsin in light of a new 2.2 A crystal structure. *J Mol Biol.* 2004;342:571-583.
11. Wess J. G-protein-coupled receptors: molecular mechanisms involved in receptor activation and selectivity of G-protein recognition. *FASEB J.* 1997;11:346-354.
12. Iiri T, Farfel Z, Bourne HR. G-protein diseases furnish a model for the turn-on switch. *Nature.* 1998;394:35-38.
13. Menon ST, Han M, Sakmar TP. Rhodopsin: structural basis of molecular physiology. *Physiol Rev.* 2001;81:1659-1688.

14. Lewis JW, Kliger DS. Photointermediates of visual pigments. *J Bioenerg Biomembr.* 1992;24:201-210.
15. Schertler GF. Structure of rhodopsin and the metarhodopsin I photointermediate. *Curr Opin Struct Biol.* 2005;15:408-415.
16. Bramblett RD, Panu AM, Ballesteros JA, Reggio PH. Construction of a 3D model of the cannabinoid CB1 receptor: determination of helix ends and helix orientation. *Life Sci.* 1995;56:1971-1982.
17. Ballesteros JA, Weinstein H. Analysis and refinement of criteria for predicting the structure and relative orientations of transmembranal helical domains. *Biophys J.* 1992;62:107-109.
18. Marti-Renom MA, Stuart AC, Fiser A, Sanchez R, Melo F, Sali A. Comparative protein structure modeling of genes and genomes. *Annu Rev Biophys Biomol Struct.* 2000;29:291-325.
19. Sali A, Blundell TL. Comparative protein modelling by satisfaction of spatial restraints. *J Mol Biol.* 1993;234:779-815.
20. Fiser A, Do RK, Sali A. Modeling of loops in protein structures. *Protein Sci.* 2000;9:1753-1773.
21. Ballesteros JA, Shi L, Javitch JA. Structural mimicry in G protein-coupled receptors: implications of the high-resolution structure of rhodopsin for structure-function analysis of rhodopsin-like receptors. *Mol Pharmacol.* 2001;60:1-19.
22. Zhang R, Hurst DP, Barnett-Norris J, Reggio PH, Song ZH. Cysteine 2.59(89) in the second transmembrane domain of human CB2 receptor is accessible within the ligand binding crevice: evidence for possible CB2 deviation from a rhodopsin template. *Mol Pharmacol.* 2005;68:69-83.
23. Ballesteros JA, Deupi X, Olivella M, Haaksma EE, Pardo L. Serine and threonine residues bend alpha-helices in the chi(1) = g(−) conformation. *Biophys J.* 2000;79:2754-2760.
24. Guarnieri F, Weinstein H. Conformational memories and the exploration of biologically relevant peptide conformations: an illustration for the gonadotropin-releasing hormone. *J Am Chem Soc.* 1996;118:5580-5589.
25. Shi L, Liapakis G, Xu R, Guarnieri F, Ballesteros JA, Javitch JA. Beta 2 adrenergic receptor activation. Modulation of the proline kink in transmembrane 6 by a rotamer toggle switch. *J Biol Chem.* 2002;277:40989-40996.
26. Barnett-Norris J, Hurst DP, Buehner K, Ballesteros JA, Guarnieri F, Reggio PH. Agonist alkyl tail interaction with cannabinoid CB1 receptor V6.43/I6.46 groove induces a Helix 6 active conformation. *Int J Quantum Chem.* 2002;88:76-86.
27. Eisenberg D, Weiss RM, Terwilliger TC. The hydrophobic moment detects periodicity in protein hydrophobicity. *Proc Natl Acad Sci USA.* 1984;81:140-144.
28. Komiya H, Yeates TO, Rees DC, Allen JP, Feher G. Structure of the reaction center from Rhodobacter sphaeroides R-26 and 2.4.1: symmetry relations and sequence comparisons between different species. *Proc Natl Acad Sci USA.* 1988;85:9012-9016.
29. Donnelly D, Johnson MS, Blundell TL, Saunders J. An analysis of the periodicity of conserved residues in sequence alignments of G-protein coupled receptors: implications for the three-dimensional structure. *FEBS Lett.* 1989;251:109-116.
30. Donnelly D, Overington JP, Ruffle SV, Nugent JH, Blundell TL. Modeling alpha-helical transmembrane domains: the calculation and use of substitution tables for lipid-facing residues. *Protein Sci.* 1993;2:55-70.
31. Baldwin J. The probable arrangement of the helices in G protein-coupled receptors. *EMBO J.* 1993;12:1693-1703.
32. Schertler GF, Villa C, Henderson R. Projection structure of rhodopsin. *Nature.* 1993;362:770-772.
33. Trabanino RJ, 3rd, Hall SE, 3rd, Vaidehi N, 3rd, Floriano WB, 3rd, Kam VW, 3rd, Goddard WA, 3rd. First principles predictions of the structure and function of g-protein-coupled receptors: validation for bovine rhodopsin. *Biophys J.* 2004;86:1904-1921.
34. Kalani MY, Vaidehi N, Hall SE, et al. The predicted 3D structure of the human D2 dopamine receptor and the binding site and binding affinities for agonists and antagonists. *Proc Natl Acad Sci USA.* 2004;101:3815-3820.

35. Freddolino PL, Kalani MY, Vaidehi N, et al. Predicted 3D structure for the human beta 2 adrenergic receptor and its binding site for agonists and antagonists. *Proc Natl Acad Sci USA*. 2004;101:2736-2741.
36. Ruprecht JJ, Mielke T, Vogel R, Villa C, Schertler GF. Electron crystallography reveals the structure of metarhodopsin I. *EMBO J*. 2004;23:3609-3620.
37. Gether U, Kobilka BK. G protein-coupled receptors, II: mechanism of agonist activation. *J Biol Chem*. 1998;273:17979-17982.
38. Arnis S, Fahmy K, Hofmann KP, Sakmar TP. A conserved carboxylic acid group mediates light-dependent proton uptake and signaling by rhodopsin. *J Biol Chem*. 1994;269: 23879-23881.
39. Ghanouni P, Steenhuis JJ, Farrens DL, Kobilka BK. Agonist-induced conformational changes in the G-protein-coupling domain of the beta 2 adrenergic receptor. *Proc Natl Acad Sci USA*. 2001;98:5997-6002.
40. Farrens D, Altenbach C, Ynag K, Hubbell W, Khorana H. Requirement of rigid-body motion of transmembrane helices for light activation of rhodopsin. *Science*. 1996;274:768-770.
41. Gether U, Lin S, Ghanouni P, Ballesteros J, Weinstein H, Kobilka B. Agonists induce conformational changes in transmembrane domains III and VI of the beta2 adrenoceptor. *EMBO J*. 1997;16:6737-6747.
42. Ballesteros J, Jensen A, Liapakis G, et al. Activation of the b_2 adrenergic receptor involves disruption of an ionic link between the cytoplasmic ends of transmembrane segments 3 and 6. *J Biol Chem*. 2001;276:29171-29177.
43. Visiers I, Ebersole BJ, Dracheva S, Ballesteros J, Sealfon SC, Weinstein H. Structural motifs as functional microdomains in G-protein-coupled receptors: energetic considerations in the mechanism of activation of the serotonin 5-HT2a receptor by disruption of the ionic lock of the arginine cage. *Int J Quantum Chem*. 2002;88:65-75.
44. Jensen AD, Guarnieri F, Rasmussen SG, Asmar F, Ballesteros JA, Gether U. Agonist-induced conformational changes at the cytoplasmic side of transmembrane segment 6 in the beta 2 adrenergic receptor mapped by site-selective fluorescent labeling. *J Biol Chem*. 2001;276:9279-9290.
45. McAllister SD, Hurst DP, Barnett-Norris J, Lynch D, Reggio PH, Abood ME. Structural mimicry in class A G protein-coupled receptor rotamer toggle switches: the importance of the F3.36(201)/W6.48(357) interaction in cannabinoid CB1 receptor activation. *J Biol Chem*. 2004;279:48024-48037.
46. Gouldson PR, Kidley NJ, Bywater RP, et al. Toward the active conformations of rhodopsin and the beta2-adrenergic receptor. *Proteins*. 2004;56:67-84.
47. Klein-Seetharaman J, Yanamala NV, Javeed F, et al. Differential dynamics in the G protein-coupled receptor rhodopsin revealed by solution NMR. *Proc Natl Acad Sci USA*. 2004;101:3409-3413.
48. Borhan B, Souto ML, Imai H, Shichida Y, Nakanishi K. Movement of retinal along the visual transduction path. *Science*. 2000;288:2209-2212.
49. Lin S, Sakmar T. Specific tryptophan UV-absorbance changes are probes of the transition of rhodopsin to its active state. *Biochemistry*. 1996;35:11149-11159.
50. Singh R, Hurst DP, Barnett-Norris J, Lynch DL, Reggio PH, Guarnieri F. Activation of the cannabinoid CB1 receptor may involve a W6.48/F3.36 rotamer toggle switch. *J Pept Res*. 2002;60:357-370.
51. Ghanouni P, Gryczynski Z, Steenhuis JJ, et al. Functionally different agonists induce distinct conformations in the G protein coupling domain of the beta 2 adrenergic receptor. *J Biol Chem*. 2001;276:24433-24436.
52. Mukhopadhyay S, Howlett AC. Chemically distinct ligands promote differential CB1 cannabinoid receptor-Gi protein interactions. *Mol Pharmacol*. 2005;67:2016-2024.
53. Paterlini MG. The function of the extracellular regions in opioid receptor binding: insights from computational biology. *Curr Top Med Chem*. 2005;5:357-367.
54. Tosatto SC, Bindewald E, Hesser J, Manner R. A divide and conquer approach to fast loop modeling. *Protein Eng*. 2002;15:279-286.

55. Xiang Z, Soto CS, Honig B. Evaluating conformational free energies: the colony energy and its application to the problem of loop prediction. *Proc Natl Acad Sci USA*. 2002;99:7432-7437.
56. Mehler EL, Periole X, Hassan SA, Weinstein H. Key issues in the computational simulation of GPCR function: representation of loop domains. *J Comput Aided Mol Des*. 2002;16:841-853.
57. Hassan SA, Mehler EL, Weinstein H. Structure calculation of protein segments connecting domains with defined secondary structure: a simulated annealing Monte Carlo combined with biased scaled collective variables technique. In: Schlick T, Gan HH, eds. *Computational Methods for Macromolecules: Challenges and Applications. Vol 24*. New York, NY: Springer Verlag; 2002:197-231.
58. Hassan SA, Guarnieri F, Mehler EL. A general treatment of solvent effects based on screened coulomb potentials. *J Phys Chem B*. 2000;104:6478-6489.
59. Chabre M, le Maire M. Monomeric G-protein-coupled receptor as a functional unit. *Biochemistry*. 2005;44:9395-9403.
60. Terrillon S, Bouvier M. Roles of G-protein-coupled receptor dimerization. *EMBO Rep*. 2004;5:30-34.
61. Bulenger S, Marullo S, Bouvier M. Emerging role of homo- and heterodimerization in G-protein-coupled receptor biosynthesis and maturation. *Trends Pharmacol Sci*. 2005;26:131-137.
62. Reddy PS, Corley RB. Assembly, sorting, and exit of oligomeric proteins from the endoplasmic reticulum. *Bioessays*. 1998;20:546-554.
63. Marshall FH, Jones KA, Kaupmann K, Bettler B. GABAB receptors—the first 7TM heterodimers. *Trends Pharmacol Sci*. 1999;20:396-399.
64. Margeta-Mitrovic M, Jan YN, Jan LY. A trafficking checkpoint controls GABA(B) receptor heterodimerization. *Neuron*. 2000;27:97-106.
65. Milligan G. Oligomerisation of G-protein-coupled receptors. *J Cell Sci*. 2001;114: 1265-1271.
66. Roess DA, Smith SM. Self-association and raft localization of functional luteinizing hormone receptors. *Biol Reprod*. 2003;69:1765-1770.
67. Latif R, Graves P, Davies TF. Ligand-dependent inhibition of oligomerization at the human thyrotropin receptor. *J Biol Chem*. 2002;277:45059-45067.
68. Terrillon S, Durroux T, Mouillac B, et al. Oxytocin and vasopressin V1a and V2 receptors form constitutive homo- and heterodimers during biosynthesis. *Mol Endocrinol*. 2003;17:677-691.
69. Fotiadis D, Liang Y, Filipek S, Saperstein DA, Engel A, Palczewski K. Atomic-force microscopy: rhodopsin dimers in native disc membranes. *Nature*. 2003;421:127-128.
70. Liang Y, Fotiadis D, Filipek S, Saperstein DA, Palczewski K, Engel A. Organization of the G protein-coupled receptors rhodopsin and opsin in native membranes. *J Biol Chem*. 2003;278:21655-21662.
71. Jordan BA, Devi LA. G-protein-coupled receptor heterodimerization modulates receptor function. *Nature*. 1999;399:697-700.
72. Galvez T, Duthey B, Kniazeff J, et al. Allosteric interactions between GB1 and GB2 subunits are required for optimal GABA(B) receptor function. *EMBO J*. 2001;20:2152-2159.
73. Gomes I, Jordan BA, Gupta A, Trapaidze N, Nagy V, Devi LA. Heterodimerization of mu and delta opioid receptors: a role in opiate synergy. *J Neurosci*. 2000;20:RC110.
74. Maggio R, Barbier P, Colelli A, Salvadori F, Demontis G, Corsini GU. G protein-linked receptors: pharmacological evidence for the formation of heterodimers. *J Pharmacol Exp Ther*. 1999;291:251-257.
75. Rocheville M, Lange DC, Kumar U, Patel SC, Patel RC, Patel YC. Receptors for dopamine and somatostatin: formation of hetero-oligomers with enhanced functional activity. *Science*. 2000;288:154-157.
76. Franco R, Ferre S, Agnati L, et al. Evidence for adenosine/dopamine receptor interactions: indications for heteromerization. *Neuropsychopharmacology*. 2000;23:S50-S59.

77. Nelson G, Chandrashekar J, Hoon MA, et al. An amino-acid taste receptor. *Nature*. 2002;416:199-202.
78. Nelson G, Hoon MA, Chandrashekar J, Zhang Y, Ryba NJ, Zuker CS. Mammalian sweet taste receptors. *Cell*. 2001;106:381-390.
79. Mellado M, Rodriguez-Frade JM, Vila-Coro AJ, et al. Chemokine receptor homo- or heterodimerization activates distinct signaling pathways. *EMBO J*. 2001;20:2497-2507.
80. AbdAlla S, Lother H, Quitterer U. AT1-receptor heterodimers show enhanced G-protein activation and altered receptor sequestration. *Nature*. 2000;407:94-98.
81. Gines S, Hillion J, Torvinen M, et al. Dopamine D1 and adenosine A1 receptors form functionally interacting heteromeric complexes. *Proc Natl Acad Sci USA*. 2000;97:8606-8611.
82. Pfeiffer M, Koch T, Schroder H, et al. Homo- and heterodimerization of somatostatin receptor subtypes. Inactivation of sst(3) receptor function by heterodimerization with sst(2A). *J Biol Chem*. 2001;276:14027-14036.
83. Kearn CS, Blake-Palmer K, Daniel E, Mackie K, Glass M. Concurrent stimulation of cannabinoid CB1 and dopamine D2 receptors enhances heterodimer formation: a mechanism for receptor cross-talk? *Mol Pharmacol*. 2005;67:1697-1704.
84. Hamm HE. How activated receptors couple to G proteins. *Proc Natl Acad Sci USA*. 2001;98:4819-4821.
85. Baneres JL, Parello J. Structure-based analysis of GPCR function: evidence for a novel pentameric assembly between the dimeric leukotriene B4 receptor BLT1 and the G-protein. *J Mol Biol*. 2003;329:815-829.
86. Rocheville M, Lange DC, Kumar U, Sasi R, Patel RC, Patel YC. Subtypes of the somatostatin receptor assemble as functional homo- and heterodimers. *J Biol Chem*. 2000;275:7862-7869.
87. Xu J, He J, Castleberry AM, Balasubramanian S, Lau AG, Hall RA. Heterodimerization of alpha 2A- and beta 1-adrenergic receptors. *J Biol Chem*. 2003;278:10770-10777.
88. Stanasila L, Perez JB, Vogel H, Cotecchia S. Oligomerization of the alpha 1a- and alpha 1b-adrenergic receptor subtypes. Potential implications in receptor internalization. *J Biol Chem*. 2003;278:40239-40251.
89. Barki-Harrington L, Luttrell LM, Rockman HA. Dual inhibition of beta-adrenergic and angiotensin II receptors by a single antagonist: a functional role for receptor-receptor interaction in vivo. *Circulation*. 2003;108:1611-1618.
90. Schulz A, Grosse R, Schultz G, Gudermann T, Schoneberg T. Structural implication for receptor oligomerization from functional reconstitution studies of mutant V2 vasopressin receptors. *J Biol Chem*. 2000;275:2381-2389.
91. Lee SP, O'Dowd BF, Ng GY, et al. Inhibition of cell surface expression by mutant receptors demonstrates that D2 dopamine receptors exist as oligomers in the cell. *Mol Pharmacol*. 2000;58:120-128.
92. Hamdan FF, Ward SD, Siddiqui NA, Bloodworth LM, Wess J. Use of an in situ disulfide cross-linking strategy to map proximities between amino acid residues in transmembrane domains I and VII of the M3 muscarinic acetylcholine receptor. *Biochemistry*. 2002;41:7647-7658.
93. Hadac EM, Ji Z, Pinon DI, Henne RM, Lybrand TP, Miller LJ. A peptide agonist acts by occupation of a monomeric G protein-coupled receptor: dual sites of covalent attachment to domains near TM1 and TM7 of the same molecule make biologically significant domain-swapped dimerization unlikely. *J Med Chem*. 1999;42:2105-2111.
94. Overton MC, Blumer KJ. The extracellular N-terminal domain and transmembrane domains 1 and 2 mediate oligomerization of a yeast G protein-coupled receptor. *J Biol Chem*. 2002;277:41463-41472.
95. Guo W, Shi L, Javitch JA. The fourth transmembrane segment forms the interface of the dopamine D2 receptor homodimer. *J Biol Chem*. 2003;278:4385-4388.
96. Guo W, Shi L, Filizola M, Weinstein H, Javitch JA. Crosstalk in G protein-coupled receptors: changes at the transmembrane homodimer interface determine activation. *Proc Natl Acad Sci USA*. 2005;102:17495-17500.

97. Gouldson PR, Higgs C, Smith RE, Dean MK, Gkoutos GV, Reynolds CA. Dimerization and domain swapping in G-protein-coupled receptors: a computational study. *Neuropsychopharmacology*. 2000;23:S60-S77.

98. Maggio R, Vogel Z, Wess J. Coexpression studies with mutant muscarinic/adrenergic receptors provide evidence for intermolecular "cross-talk" between G-protein-linked receptors. *Proc Natl Acad Sci USA*. 1993;90:3103-3107.

99. Ridge KD, Lee SS, Abdulaev NG. Examining rhodopsin folding and assembly through expression of polypeptide fragments. *J Biol Chem*. 1996;271:7860-7867.

100. Kobilka BK, Kobilka TS, Daniel K, Regan JW, Caron MG, Lefkowitz RJ. Chimeric alpha 2-beta 2-adrenergic receptors: delineation of domains involved in effector coupling and ligand binding specificity. *Science*. 1988;240:1310-1316.

101. Schoneberg T, Liu J, Wess J. Plasma membrane localization and functional rescue of truncated forms of a G protein-coupled receptor. *J Biol Chem*. 1995;270:18000-18006.

102. Schoneberg T, Yun J, Wenkert D, Wess J. Functional rescue of mutant V2 vasopressin receptors causing nephrogenic diabetes insipidus by a co-expressed receptor polypeptide. *EMBO J*. 1996;15:1283-1291.

103. Gudermann T, Schoneberg T, Schultz G. Functional and structural complexity of signal transduction via G-protein-coupled receptors. *Annu Rev Neurosci*. 1997;20:399-427.

104. Nielsen SM, Elling CE, Schwartz TW. Split-receptors in the tachykinin neurokinin-1 system—mutational analysis of intracellular loop 3. *Eur J Biochem*. 1998;251:217-226.

105. Bakker RA, Dees G, Carrillo JJ, et al. Domain swapping in the human histamine H1 receptor. *J Pharmacol Exp Ther*. 2004;311:131-138.

106. Maggio R, Barbier P, Fornai F, Corsini GU. Functional role of the third cytoplasmic loop in muscarinic receptor dimerization. *J Biol Chem*. 1996;271:31055-31060.

107. Filizola M, Weinstein H. The study of G-protein coupled receptor oligomerization with computational modeling and bioinformatics. *FEBS J*. 2005;272:2926-2938.

108. Pazos F, Helmer-Citterich M, Ausiello G, Valencia A. Correlated mutations contain information about protein-protein interaction. *J Mol Biol*. 1997;271:511-523.

109. Gouldson PR, Dean MK, Snell CR, Bywater RP, Gkoutos G, Reynolds CA. Lipid-facing correlated mutations and dimerization in G-protein coupled receptors. *Protein Eng*. 2001;14:759-767.

110. Filizola M, Olmea O, Weinstein H. Prediction of heterodimerization interfaces of G-protein coupled receptors with a new subtractive correlated mutation method. *Protein Eng*. 2002;15:881-885.

111. Filizola M, Weinstein H. Structural models for dimerization of G-protein coupled receptors: the opioid receptor homodimers. *Biopolymers*. 2002;66:317-325.

112. Olmea O, Valencia A. Improving contact predictions by the combination of correlated mutations and other sources of sequence information. *Fold Des*. 1997;2:S25-S32.

113. Barnett-Norris J, Reggio PH. Identification of possible CB₁/dopamine D2 heterodimer interfaces using correlated mutation analysis. 2005 Symposium on the Cannabinoids; June 24-27; Clearwater Beach, FL. Burlington, VT: International Cannabinoid Research Society; 2005:101.

114. Lichtarge O, Bourne HR, Cohen FE. Evolutionarily conserved Galphabetagamma binding surfaces support a model of the G protein-receptor complex. *Proc Natl Acad Sci USA*. 1996;93:7507-7511.

115. Lichtarge O, Bourne HR, Cohen FE. An evolutionary trace method defines binding surfaces common to protein families. *J Mol Biol*. 1996;257:342-358.

116. Lichtarge O, Yamamoto KR, Cohen FE. Identification of functional surfaces of the zinc binding domains of intracellular receptors. *J Mol Biol*. 1997;274:325-337.

117. Livingstone CD, Barton GJ. Protein sequence alignments: a strategy for the hierarchical analysis of residue conservation. *Comput Appl Biosci*. 1993;9:745-756.

118. Madabushi S, Gross AK, Philippi A, Meng EC, Wensel TG, Lichtarge O. Evolutionary trace of G protein-coupled receptors reveals clusters of residues that determine global and class-specific functions. *J Biol Chem*. 2004;279:8126-8132.

119. Chothia C, Lesk AM. The relation between the divergence of sequence and structure in proteins. *EMBO J*. 1986;5:823-826.
120. Koshi JM, Mindell DP, Goldstein RA. Using physical-chemistry-based substitution models in phylogenetic analyses of HIV-1 subtypes. *Mol Biol Evol*. 1999;16:173-179.
121. Koshi JM, Goldstein RA. Models of natural mutations including site heterogeneity. *Proteins*. 1998;32:289-295.
122. Koshi JM, Goldstein RA. Context-dependent optimal substitution matrices. *Protein Eng*. 1995;8:641-645.
123. Soyer OS, Dimmic MW, Neubig RR, Goldstein RA. Dimerization in aminergic G-protein-coupled receptors: application of a hidden-site class model of evolution. *Biochemistry*. 2003;42:14522-14531.

Chapter 4
Symbiotic Relationship of Pharmacogenetics and Drugs of Abuse

Joni L. Rutter[1]

Abstract Pharmacogenetics/pharmacogenomics is the study of how genetic variation affects pharmacology, the use of drugs to treat disease. When drug responses are predicted in advance, it is easier to tailor medications to different diseases and individuals. Pharmacogenetics provides the tools required to identify genetic predictors of probable drug response, drug efficacy, and drug-induced adverse events—identifications that would ideally precede treatment decisions. Drug abuse and addiction genetic data have advanced the field of pharmacogenetics in general. Although major findings have emerged, pharmacotherapy remains hindered by issues such as adverse events, time lag to drug efficacy, and heterogeneity of the disorders being treated. The sequencing of the human genome and high-throughput technologies are enabling pharmacogenetics to have greater influence on treatment approaches. This review highlights key studies and identifies important genes in drug abuse pharmacogenetics that provide a basis for better diagnosis and treatment of drug abuse disorders.

Keywords Pharmacogenomics, addiction, treatment, psychiatric disease, SNP

Introduction

Pharmacogenetics/pharmacogenomics is the study of how genetic variation among individuals affects their capacity to metabolize drugs (pharmacokinetics) and the drugs' effects on the individuals (pharmacodynamics). Pharmacogenetics emerged several decades ago, but only recently have the tools been in place for the field to flourish, led in part by the availability of the human genome sequence and the improving genotyping technologies. Pharmacogenetics provides the foundation for scientists to identify biological predictors of drug response, drug efficacy, and drug-induced adverse

---

[1] National Institute on Drug Abuse, National Institutes of Health, Department of Health and Human Services, 6001 Executive Boulevard, Bethesda, MD 20892

Corresponding Author:
Joni L. Rutter; National Institute on Drug Abuse, NIH, DHHS, 6001 Executive Boulevard, Bethesda, MD 20892 Tel: (301) 443-1887; Fax: (301) 594-6043; Email: jrutter@mail.nih.gov

events to enable clinicians to use the information to make the best treatment decisions. The understanding of genetic variation may hold the most promise in clinically evaluating and predicting a drug's effects, and successfully treating a patient.

Substance abuse is a unique psychiatric disorder given that genetic vulnerability can lead to disease only if the substance (licit or illicit) is readily available and used. In addition to the public health burden, addiction disorders cost society over $500 billion per year.[1] The gene-environment interaction of substance abuse and addiction may provide scientific building blocks to advance the field of pharmacogenetics. Understanding the genetics of the pharmacokinetics and pharmacodynamics of drugs, whether or not they are abused, can provide relevant crossover concepts for tailoring drug treatments. Drug use triggers the onset of the addictive process and maintains the neuroplastic changes after chronic use.[2] Thus, the genetics of substance abuse and addiction, by nature, is pharmacogenetic. The current impetus is to predict actual individual differences in risk of drug abuse vulnerability, drug response, and response to treatments for drug abuse based upon knowledge about specific genes. Genetic differences could contribute to acute drug responses (aversive vs nonaversive) and may also predict drug use and/or drug response.

Environmental interventions are likely to be most effective in reducing the number of people who start to use drugs, including alcohol and tobacco; however, these interventions may not be as effective in helping those already addicted. To unravel and point to biological targets highlighting genetic variants important for understanding addiction, drug treatment, and drug response, genetic and neurobiological studies are needed; they will help clarify the complex nature of addiction, which has a 40% to 60% genetic variance.[3-5] Although genetic studies are critical to advancing the field, some misconceptions are that genetic information will be used solely to identify those at high risk of addiction by screening people for susceptibility alleles,[6] or that susceptibility alleles will be "replaced" through gene therapy.[7] These approaches are not likely to be effective or efficient. Instead, studies to understand gene variants that confer vulnerability and predict treatment response are needed to provide a comprehensive approach to treating addiction effectively and to inform prevention strategies that will have a significant public health impact.

This review highlights some of the research from the field of drug use, abuse, and addiction and the importance of pharmacogenetics/pharmacogenomics in working toward better treatments for these types of psychiatric disorders.

Pharmacogenetics of Metabolism, Drugs of Abuse, and Addiction Genetics

Pharmacogenetics of Drug Metabolism: Therapy Versus Toxicity

Drug treatment can result in effective therapy, can fail, and/or can create toxicities and other side effects. Administering the same dose of a given medication to individuals with different drug-metabolizing genotypes gives rise to differences in drug response phenotypes—namely, the drug's therapeutic and toxic effects.[8] Genetic variation in metabolism genes alters the activation of a drug, which can result in more potent metabolites, different metabolic patterns with varying half-lives, or inactive metabolites (eg, nicotine metabolized to inactive cotinine by CYP2A6). If certain drugs are not metabolized appropriately or are given at the wrong dose, they can cause liver damage, triggering certain enzymes normally found in the liver to be secreted into the bloodstream, signifying distress in liver function. Although plasma blood tests are used to assess high liver enzymes that indicate toxicity, this approach is crude since it does not indicate potential toxicities affecting other organs or take into account the reasons for the toxicity. Once liver toxicity is identified, the remedy often results in discontinued use of a needed medication, or a change in the medication to one that may be less effective.

Most drugs are metabolized in the liver by the cytochrome P450 (CYP450) system, with metabolizing enzymes CYP3A4 and CYP2D6 responsible for the largest contribution. The CYP450 enzymes are expressed in most cells and are particularly abundant in the liver.[8] Although the roles of these enzymes are known (eg, metabolism of compounds), there is little understanding of how genetic variation in metabolizing enzymes, transporters, and receptor targets can be used in the clinical environment. One of the central aspects of pharmacogenetics involves understanding the genetic variations within the CYP450 system and how the variations affect drug metabolism and ultimately contribute to treatment response.

Extrahepatic organs such as the brain, kidney, and lung also express CYP450 enzymes that metabolize drugs. For psychiatric diseases and drugs that act centrally, in the central nervous system, the brain is an important organ to consider. It is a heterogeneous organ, so drug metabolism in different cell types may create microenvironments with differing drug and metabolic levels, which would not necessarily be predicted by plasma drug monitoring. This concept is important for toxicity, since hepatic cells can regenerate but neurons cannot. Thus, single nucleotide polymorphisms (SNPs) or other types of genetic variations in metabolism genes as well as other genes involved in drug receptor/transporter pathways may account for variations in responses to centrally acting drugs and may affect receptor adaptation, toxicities, altered drug effects, and cross-tolerance.[9] The following Web page has a list of SNPs in the metabolism genes: http://www.genome.utah.edu/genesnps/cgi-bin/query.cgi?FunctionClass=2. Further pharmacogenetic studies are needed to establish connections between CYP450 expression in the liver and in specific brain regions to determine the consequences on drug effects and brain function.

Smoking

Nicotine is a psychoactive substance responsible for establishing and maintaining tobacco dependence. There are more than 1.1 billion smokers worldwide, each dictating nicotine intake through markedly different behavioral patterns.[10] Smoking is a highly regulated behavior; those addicted are precise in maintaining steady-state brain levels of nicotine.[11] A recent prospective study examining the health consequences of smoking concludes that smoking as little as 1 to 4 cigarettes per day engenders significantly higher risk for all causes of mortality, most notably, heart disease and lung cancer.[12] Relative risks associated with increased cigarette consumption are unclear.[13-15] However, evidence indicates that smoking fewer cigarettes does not provide much, if any, protection.

When heavy smokers (at least 20 cigarettes per day) reduced their nicotine intake to 5 cigarettes per day, so that they more closely resembled "chippers" (smokers who average 1–5 cigarettes a day but do not become dependent), the heavy smokers compensated by increasing their nicotine intake 3-fold by lengthening their puff duration, but the chippers did not.[16] Pinpointing the genetic variance accounting for the level of self-regulation among smokers is an important step toward understanding the risks of becoming addicted, the consequences of being addicted, and the treatment options for those already addicted. In addition to prevention efforts, smoking cessation therapies with tailored drug treatments are important in fighting the health consequences of smoking. This paradigm may also be applied to other drugs of abuse as well as to treatment medications for other disorders. The National Institute on Drug Abuse (NIDA) has initiated an emphasis on this important avenue of smoking cessation research.

Drug prevention efforts will continue to be a public health need, with emphasis on targeting adolescents through school programs. However, even though some of these programs have shown reductions in cigarette use rates of up to 20%, less than 10% of the school districts are using the programs.[17] Much of the success in decreasing the smoking prevalence since the 1950s has been realized through these types of preventive/educational programs (Fig. 4.1). The steady decrease in prevalence from 1970 to 1990 appears to have reached a plateau and looks to have fluctuated little since 1990 (Fig. 4.1 inset). This leveling off may indicate a significant

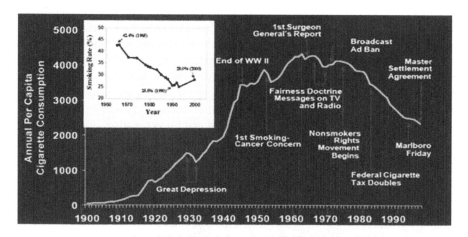

Fig. 4.1 Historical Events Affecting Smoking in the United States, 1900–2000. Adapted from the US Department of Agriculture and the US Department of Health and Human Services (DHHS), *1986 Surgeon General's Report* and *Morbidity and Mortality Weekly Report* (www.cdc.gov/tobacco/news/achievements99.htm) 1999.

preventive/educational role in decreasing the prevalence of smoking for a proportion of the population. The plateau may suggest that prevention may not be as effective in the actively smoking population, indicating that current smokers who cannot quit may represent a more genetically at-risk population. Understanding the genetics and pharmacogenetics of smoking may provide insight into the best treatments for those already addicted.

Smoking Pharmacogenetics

Data from twin studies provide consistent and strong evidence for the heritability of smoking addiction (estimates range from 0.4 to 0.6).[18-20] Although the precise genetic variants responsible are not clearly delineated, research has focused on genes in the dopamine, serotonin, glutamatergic, and norepinephrine receptor pathways, and the *CYP450* metabolism pathways, such as *DRD2-4, DAT1, TPH1, GABAB2, 5 HTT/SERT, MAO-A, CYP2A6, CYP2D6, CHRNA4,* and *ANKK1* (Table 4.1).[21-31]

Table 4.1 Selected Genes Associated With Addiction Genetics and Pharmacogenetics

Gene Symbol	Gene Name	Chromosomal Location	Drug Association	References
5HTT/SERT	5-hydroxy tryptamine transporter	17q11.1–q12	Nicotine, opioids	25,32
ANKK1	Ankyrin repeat and kinase domain containing 1	11q23.2	Nicotine	31
BCHE	Butyrylcholinesterase	3q26.1–q26.2	Cocaine	33
CGRP	Calcitonin/calcitonin-related polypeptide	11p15.2-p15.1	Opioids	34
CHRNA4	Nicotine acetylcholine receptor, alpha subunit	20q13.2–q13.3	Nicotine	35
CNR1	Cannabinoid receptor 1	6q14–q15	Nicotine, opioids	36,37
COMT	Catechol-o-methyltransferase	22q11–q21	Opioids, stimulants	38-40
CYP2A6	Cytochrome P450, family 2, subfamily A, polypeptide 6	19q13.2	Metabolism, nicotine	8,41,42
CYP2D6	Cytochrome P450, family 2, subfamily D, polypeptide 6	22q13.1	Metabolism, nicotine, opioids	8
CYP3A4	Cytochrome P450, family 3, subfamily A, polypeptide 4	7q21.1	Metabolism	8
DAT1	Dopamine transporter	5p15.3	Nicotine, opioids	24,27,43-47
DBH	Dopamine beta hydroxylase	9q34	Stimulants	32
DRD2	Dopamine receptor D2	11q23	Nicotine, opioids, stimulants	21,22,29,48-55
DRD3	Dopamine receptor D3	3q13.3	Nicotine, opioids, stimulants	55
DRD4	Dopamine receptor D4	11p15.5	Nicotine, opioids, stimulants	26,39,40,55,56

(continued)

Table 4.1   (continued)

Gene Symbol	Gene Name	Chromosomal Location	Drug Association	References
GABAB2	Gamma-aminobutyric acid (GABA) B receptor, subtype 2	9q22.1–q22.3	Nicotine	[23]
GABRG2	Gamma-aminobutyric acid (GABA) A receptor, gamma 2	5q31.1–q33.1	Methamphetamine	[57]
GSTP1	Glutathione-S-transferase P1	11q13	Stimulants	[58,59]
HOMER1	Homer homolog 1	5q14.2	Cocaine	[60]
HOMER2	Homer homolog 2	5q24.3	Cocaine	[60]
MAO-A	Monoamine oxidase-A	Xp11.3	Nicotine	[30]
MCR1	Melanocortin 1 receptor	16q24.3	Opioids	[61,62]
OPRD1	Opioid receptor, delta 1	1p36.1–p34.2	Opioids	[63]
OPRK1	Opioid receptor, kappa 1	8q11.2	Opioids	[32]
OPRM1	Opioid receptor, mu 1	6q24–q25	Nicotine, opioids	[64-73]
TPH1	Tryptophan hydroxylase 1	11p15.3–p14	Nicotine	[28]

Approximately 70% to 80% of nicotine is metabolized to an inactive metabolite by *CYP2A6*. There are several genetic polymorphisms within *CYP2A6* that have been associated with nicotine metabolism and consumption. Since each individual receives 2 copies of every gene—maternal and paternal—each individual may have different combinations of forms of the gene, depending on the genetic variation that was inherited. Several studies have shown that polymorphisms in *CYP2A6* account for high enzyme activity.[41,42] Individuals receiving 2 copies of this allele are able to metabolize nicotine rapidly, while individuals receiving only 1 copy of the allele or no copies are intermediate or slow metabolizers, respectively.[41]

Effective smoking cessation pharmacologic intervention strategies are currently in use, such as nicotine replacement therapies (NRTs) and some nonnicotine agents (eg, antidepressant medications like bupropion).[74] Nevertheless, up to 80% of cessation attempts using these medications result in relapse within the year.[75]

NRTs such as nicotine gum, patches, inhalers, and nasal sprays can significantly increase smoking cessation rates compared with behavioral counseling[76] and are the standard treatment for smoking dependence. NRTs seem to be most effective for treating the withdrawal symptoms accompanying cessation but are not as effective in reducing the craving for cigarettes, which often renders the quit attempt unsuccessful.[77,78] However, some NRTs work well, in part because of the genotypic profile of the individual taking them. Lerman et al examined the mu-opioid receptor variant *OPRM1* A118G (discussed in further detail below) in either the transdermal nicotine patch or nicotine nasal spray in 320 smokers.[64] Smokers who were given the transdermal nicotine and who had the G allele were more likely to be abstinent by the end of the treatment period (odds ratio [OR] = 2.4; 95% confidence interval [CI] = 1.14–5.06).[64] Although the sample size was small, this finding gives credence to future studies attempting to identify gene variants for predicting successful treatment.

Of other nonnicotine pharmacologic agents for smoking cessation, bupropion seems to be the most successful to date, offering further support for genetic profile–tailored agents, with some caveats. Swan et al indicate that women with at least one A1 allele of the *DRD2* gene reported early termination of the bupropion because of side effects (OR = 1.91, 95% CI = 1.01–3.60), but this result was not seen in men.[29] In 2 randomized clinical trials, Lerman et al examined *DRD2* variants in subjects given NRT or bupropion, respectively, for tobacco dependence. The bupropion trial showed that subjects homozygous for the ins C variant of the -141 C ins/del SNP responded better to bupropion compared with those carrying the del C allele (OR = 4.99; 95% CI = 1.42–17.62; *P* = 0.01).[48] The NRT trial, on the other hand, suggests that individuals carrying the ins C allele had fewer quit attempts than those with the del C (OR = 0.44; 95% CI = 0.25–0.79; *P* = .006). Thus, NRT may be most beneficial for those with the del C allele and bupropion best for those with the ins C allele.[48]

Newer drugs are showing early promise for more successful smoking cessation, including rimonabant and varenicline.[79] Rimonabant is a selective cannabinoid receptor 1 (CB1) blocker. CB1 is expressed in brain and adipose tissue and is known to regulate food intake. Upon chronic stimulation with nicotine, the endocannabinoid system (and CB1) become dysregulated and imbalanced.[36,37] By blocking CB1, rimonabant stabilizes the endocannabinoid system. In clinical trials, patients receiving up to 20 mg of rimonabant were twice as likely to quit smoking and stay abstinent for significantly longer (36.2%) than the placebo group (20.6%). Making the drug even more attractive is that on average, patients on rimonabant lost over a half-pound, while those on placebo gained 2.5 pounds.[80]

Varenicline is a partial nicotine agonist and selective nicotinic receptor modulator to the α4β2 nicotinic receptor. Genetic variants within the *CHRNA4* gene encoding the α4β2-containing nicotinic acetylcholine receptor seem to play a role in modulating the effects of nicotine and alcohol in mouse strains.[35] Varenicline appears to act on α4β2 receptors to remove feelings of reward from smoking and to prevent withdrawal symptoms.[79] Current NIDA-supported studies will further examine genetic variants known in metabolism and other targeted pathways of these medications. Although years away, a major goal is to determine a genetic profile that will result in high success rates for people given these medications.

Another treatment for smoking cessation is the nicotine vaccine. One vaccine, NicVAX, confers active immunity by inducing the formation of antibodies to nicotine.[81,82] The vaccine binds to nicotine prior to its crossing the blood-brain barrier and prevents it from entering the brain. In rats, NicVAX is effective in reducing nicotine's access to the brain more than it reduces nicotine's access to other tissues.[81] The vaccine had a good safety profile in a recent clinical trial. Healthy smokers receiving the vaccine did not smoke more cigarettes during the study period and did not experience cravings or withdrawal symptoms.[83] As the vaccine proves successful in some addicted smokers, pharmacogenetic studies may provide the evidence needed to prevent smoking addiction and expedite smoking cessation in vulnerable individuals.

NRTs and bupropion inhibit smoking for some smokers. However, many relapse, indicating that maintaining long-term abstinence is more difficult.[76,84] Although these 2 treatments are available, genetic information is not currently being used to pinpoint which treatment modality would be most effective. Emerging pharmacogenetic data, such as the *DRD2* -141C ins/del SNP and treatment response to NRT or bupropion, seem to support the notion that practitioners will eventually be able to individualize the choice of pharmacotherapies to be prescribed based on the genotypes of their patients who smoke. Perhaps this tailored treatment approach, along with the newer medications, will reduce the high rates of relapse.

Heroin and Other Opioid Substances

Heroin is an illicit opioid that is commonly abused. Genetic studies have revealed that heroin addiction disorder is highly heritable.[32,85-87] Several genes are associated with opioid addiction (*DRD2-4, CYP2D6, DAT1, 5HTT/SERT, GABRG2, OPRM1, OPRD1, OPRK1, CNR1*; see Table 4.1).[1,32] One recent study identified DRD2 as a strong susceptibility gene for heroin dependence in Chinese subjects (OR = 52.8; 95% CI = 7.2–382.5), but in a German sample this gene was associated with a low risk of heroin dependence.[49] These findings suggest that *DRD2* is a risk gene specific to heroin dependence in certain populations, as it has not been associated with disorders involving use of other substances, including alcohol and cocaine, in varying populations.[50-54,56] Also, the *DRD2* variant may be in linkage disequilibrium with another variant that is the actual functional variant. One possibility is the *ANKK1* gene, which is a serine/threonine kinase involved in signal transduction pathways.[31] Consequently, further clarification of the actual role in heroin addiction and potential roles in other drug and alcohol addictions is needed, including more dense SNP maps to reveal the underlying genetic architecture for *DRD2, ANKK1,* and other addiction candidate genes.

The *OPRM1* susceptibility gene is the primary site of action of the most commonly used opiates, including heroin, morphine, and most drugs used to treat opiate dependence, such as methadone, LAAM (levo-alpha-acetylmethadol), and buprenorphine. A polymorphism in *OPRM1* changes the more common allele at position 118 from an A to a G (A118G) and results in a functionally relevant coding change in the protein from an asparagine residue at amino acid position 40 to an aspartate residue. The literature is inconsistent regarding associations of the A118G polymorphism with addictions, possibly because of differences in minor allele frequencies among different populations,[32,65,66] the need for larger sample sizes to detect associations of small effect, or linkage disequilibrium associations with another allele. It has been suggested that the mu-opioid receptors encoded by the aspartate variant bind beta-endorphin and activate receptors more potently,[67] causing a gain of function, but this mechanism has not been replicated.[68-70] Zhang et al instead have shown by allele-specific expression in *OPRM1* mRNA that the G-allele is 1.5- to 2.5-fold less abundant than the A-allele, translating to ~10-fold lower protein levels.[70] These results suggest a loss of function rather than a gain of function. Either way, the functional data presented provide strong evidence supporting the importance of A118G for abuse and addiction susceptibility.[70]

Opioid Receptor Gene Variants in Opioid Pharmacogenetics

The A118G variant may be pharmacogenetically relevant as well. In a recent randomized, placebo-controlled clinical trial, Oslin et al[71] examined the A118G polymorphism among patients treated for alcohol dependence with either naltrexone or placebo. Naltrexone is an opioid receptor antagonist that was originally used to treat dependence on opioid drugs but has been beneficial for treating alcohol dependence. In survival analysis for time to relapse, naltrexone-treated subjects carrying a 118G allele showed significantly longer time to relapse (OR = 3.52; 95% CI = 1.03–11.96, P = .04).[71] These data, although preliminary, suggest that genotyping may be useful for identifying patients who may benefit from naltrexone more than they would from other treatment options. Since naltrexone's effects are mediated by the mu-opioid receptor, investigating the outcomes of subjects treated with other medications acting through this receptor will be valuable, as the A118G variant may be a key predictor of response to other μ-opioid receptor-mediated drugs.

Opioid Receptors and Pain

There is a large array of individual variability in sensitivity and perception of pain.[34,88] Morphine is the most commonly prescribed opioid, although only 10% to 30% of chronic pain patients do not respond or have intolerable side effects,[89] especially those with renal disease who have an accumulation of active metabolite that is normally cleared by the kidney. Opioid treatment has been a conundrum for many treatment providers trying to strike a balance between pain management on the one hand, and abuse and addiction liability on the other. Dose escalation based upon patient feedback has resulted in discrepancies in pain management that have often resulted in under- or overmedication. A small (10%) portion of morphine is metabolized to morphine-6-glucuronide (M6G), an opioid agonist that contributes to morphine's clinical effects.[90] In a study examining the effects of morphine and MG6 by measuring pupil diameters, heterozygous and homozygous individuals with the A118G variant had reduced M6G potency in constricting pupils, but this effect was not seen in variant carriers who were administered morphine.[72] This finding indicates that A118G carriers are at lower risk for renal side effects of morphine therapy,[72] especially in individuals with impaired renal function.

Heritability of pain perception has been reported to be in the range of 10% to 46%.[73,91] Other genes, such as OPRD1,[63]COMT,[38]CGRP,[34] and MCR1,[61,62] were shown to be associated with certain types of pain responses. COMT polymorphisms are associated with altering downstream responses of the mu-opioid neurotransmitter system, likely through changes in receptor concentration, binding affinity for beta-endorphin, or allele-specific expression, each of which can modulate pain perception.[92]

Work by Fillingim et al[73] supports the role of the dopamine system and the opioid receptor pathway in pain perception. Healthy subjects with at least 1 rare allele

(118G) exhibited lower sensitivity to pressure pain compared with subjects homozygous for the common allele (A118). Ross et al found no association with the A118G variant in cancer patients with chronic pain who were unable to tolerate morphine after dose escalation and switched to other opioid analgesics.[89] An association was found with beta-arrestin, a protein involved with desensitizing the mu-opioid receptor and internalized receptor trafficking.[89] These data suggest that other genes such as those involved with receptor signaling, receptor density, and receptor trafficking, in addition to those involved in the complex process of pain perception, require further study.

Pharmacogenetics has the potential to affect pain management by providing information on genetic variants that are associated with clinical effects and possibly by elucidating biological correlates of prescription opioid addiction risk. Research in this area is ongoing, and more studies are needed.

Amphetamines, Cocaine, and Other Stimulants

Abuse of amphetamine, especially methamphetamine, is a growing trend in the United States, with persistent abuse often causing a paranoid psychotic state.[93,94] Methamphetamine increases levels of dopamine in the brain and elicits euphoria, contributing to its addictive properties.[95] Heritability estimates for psychostimulants are around 66%.[86,96,97] Many of the genetic studies have concentrated on the contribution of variants within the dopamine system genes (*DAT1*, *DRD2*, and *DBH*; see Table 4.1) and *GABA* genes[57] to determine the association with abuse and treatment of cocaine and methamphetamine, but further studies focusing on other abused stimulants are needed. Glutamatergic transmission seems to be important for cocaine's effects of tolerance and withdrawal. The genes *HOMER1* and *HOMER2* have recently been identified as mediators of glutamate transmission and may be good targets for future genetic and pharmacogenetic study.[60]

Chen et al[55] examined the *DRD2*, *DRD3*, and *DRD4* gene variants in 851 methamphetamine subjects with and without psychosis (416 methamphetamine abusers and 435 controls). Results showed that the 7-repeat (exon III) *DRD4* polymorphism occurred more frequently in the methamphetamine abusers than in the controls (2% vs 0.6%; respectively, OR = 3.4; 95% CI = 1.2–9.4).[55] No other differences were noted. In a follow-up study, Li et al[39] examined the *DRD4* gene variants in combination with the Val158Met *COMT* gene variant. There was a modest interaction among the high-activity allele of *COMT* and *DRD4* genotypes (OR = 1.45; 95% CI = 1.1–1.8) among the methamphetamine abusers.[39] Another study showed significant main effects of these 2 genes but no interaction[40] suggesting that further studies are needed. If the interaction is upheld, it suggests that the lower-activity allele of *COMT* may be protective against methamphetamine abuse and that *DRD4* alleles may also contribute to the protective effects.[39]

The *DAT1* gene is associated with the effects of amphetamine and cocaine. Several studies support the notion that genetic variations in *DAT1* may contribute to the individual variability in response to these drugs. Gelernter et al demonstrated that the 9 allele of the *DAT1* gene was present in more subjects with cocaine-induced paranoia than without cocaine-induced paranoia ($P = .047$).[43] The 9-repeat allele results in reduced expression of *DAT1*,[44] but it is not yet clear how or whether the reduced expression explains the effect of cocaine-induced paranoia. The 9-repeat allele of *DAT1* contributes to reduced responsiveness to acute amphetamine administration,[45] suggesting that with amphetamine, the 9-repeat allele seems to protect individuals from dependence.[45] Indirectly supporting this finding is the finding that individuals with the 9-repeat allele showed a significantly reduced responsiveness to methylphenidate, an amphetamine-like compound used to treat attention deficit hyperactivity disorder.[46] If this finding is replicated, the 9-repeat allele may be an effective pharmacogenetic marker to predict who will not respond well to methylphenidate.

Mice with mutated *dat1* have shown reduced binding to cocaine and methylphenidate but not amphetamine or methamphetamine, indicating that the binding sites for cocaine and methylphenidate may overlap but are distinct from those for amphetamine and methamphetamine.[47] Clinical trials examining drugs that target *DAT1* have been somewhat disappointing, but some data suggest that genotyping for *DAT1* may help clinicians select appropriate treatments for psychostimulant addictions.

In a Japanese population study, the *GSTP1* I105V gene variant was associated with methamphetamine abusers with psychosis compared with controls (OR = 1.84; 95% CI = 1.13–2.97), but it was not associated with spontaneous relapse.[58] This variant results in a 30% decrease in enzyme activity,[59] which may contribute to reduced metabolism of methamphetamine and higher abuse risk.

Butyrylcholinesterase (BChE), an enzyme involved in cocaine hydrolysis, has genetic variants in the *BCHE* gene that affect the rate of cocaine detoxication.[33] The variant D70G in *BCHE* had a 10-fold lower binding affinity for cocaine, and individuals with this variant may not be able to metabolize cocaine as fast, resulting in severely toxic or fatal outcomes.[33] A pharmacogenetic approach would be to screen for this genetic variant in cocaine overdose victims so that treatment action for those with the G variant could be to provide them with exogenous BChE to attenuate the cocaine toxicity.

Conclusions

Pharmacogenetics may not yet be able to conclusively predict adverse events or ensure the most effective treatment, but it is contributing to the much-needed development of tailored care. In the future, an important part of the process of assigning an effective medication at an appropriate dose will be incorporating pharmacogenetic data that provide an understanding of how an individual's profile of genetic variation will best predict treatment response and outcome. For example, taking the medication less frequently, taking dosages adjusted for the rates of metabolism inferred from a genetic profile, or changing the medication to one better tailored to a patient's genetic makeup may prevent the onset of liver toxicities or other untoward side effects.

Addiction is a chronic brain disease[98] that is driven by 2 critical elements, genes and environment; neither can be ignored. Genetic studies have been invaluable in identifying addiction vulnerability loci and genetic variants that are important for understanding the neurobiology of the disease, pointing to potential drug targets, and identifying alleles that may be useful for tailored treatment interventions. Social and environmental elements such as family, peer, community, and social attitudes and beliefs are also important psychobehavioral domains that contribute to the complexity of addiction. Treatment and prevention interventions for substance abuse disorders and other complex diseases will have maximum benefit when multifaceted approaches, which incorporate genetic, pharmacologic, and environmental influences, are taken into account.[99] Management of drug abuse and addiction must be individualized according to the drugs involved and the specific problems of the individual patient. Effective treatment options for psychiatric diseases, which often include a high incidence of comorbidity or co-occurring disease, are still not well understood.[100,101] Many chronic disorders, such as addictions, diabetes, heart disease, and asthma, require behavioral intervention and/or long-term medication, but identifying the best treatment may involve trying several medications to determine which is most effective and has the fewest side effects. Some pharmacogenetics research suggests that pharmacogenetics may be a powerful tool for informing treatment options for those needing long-term pharmacotherapy.

This review highlighted many genetic targets for addiction vulnerability and treatment. However, the review is neither exhaustive nor complete. The genes reviewed in the article, listed in Table 4.1, are related to common pathways of addiction, such as dopamine, serotonin, glutamate, and metabolism. Many of the genes reviewed have overlapping roles for each class of drug discussed. Some of the genes may be associated with addiction in general, while some may be drug-specific.[102,103] When pharmacogenetic strategies to individualize the treatment of drug abuse and addiction are being designed, all of these genes, gene systems, and cell-type-specific expression of the genes must be considered.

The next step is to incorporate into the clinical setting those data that are reliably consistent. To this end, the US Food and Drug Administration is facilitating the use of pharmacogenetic data in drug development[104] and has issued several guidelines for industry as well as voluntary genomic data submissions from clinical trials (http://www.fda.gov/cder/genomics/regulatory.htm). Furthermore, analogous to the National Institutes of Health (NIH) Roadmap initiative, the neuroscience institutes within NIH have implemented the Blueprint Initiative (http://neuroscienceblueprint. nih.gov). One initiative is the NIH Blueprint Microarray Consortium, consisting of 4 microarray centers to serve the expression profiling and SNP genotyping needs of grantees within the neuroscience institutes. This resource will provide the most updated tools and allow investigations of many pharmacogenomic questions.

Other consortiums are in place and are making progress in incorporating pharmacogenetics into many areas of biological research. The Pharmacogenetics Research Network and Knowledge Base (http://www.pharmgkb.org), for example, is a relatively new initiative working toward correlating drug response phenotypes with genetic variation in various areas (eg, nicotine addiction and treatment, metabolism, transport, cancer and cancer treatment, asthma, cardiovascular disease). The idea is to create a valuable knowledge base populated with reliable information that links phenotypes to genotypes, and to promote interactive science to elevate the field of pharmacogenetics with knowledge, tools, and resources. For a more thorough mining of pharmacogenetic data in drug abuse, one can go to http://pharmdemo.stanford.edu/pharmdb/main.spy and search by drug name (eg, "heroin" or "cocaine").[105]

The NIDA Genetics Consortium (http://zork.wustl.edu/nida) is a group of investigators collecting samples (currently over 20 000) and comprehensive diagnostic information from individuals with smoking, cocaine, opioid, and polysubstance abuse and addictions. These resources are used to increase the understanding of addiction vulnerability and addiction treatment response, and most are available to the broad scientific community for further study.

Genetic data to date have pointed to pharmacodynamic genes involved in drug abuse and addiction, which have in turn elucidated genetic variants that may be helpful in identifying appropriate treatment medications for different individuals. These combined investments should begin to elucidate the importance of human genome variation on clinical treatment of addiction.

References

1. Uhl GR, Grow RW. The burden of complex genetics in brain disorders. *Arch Gen Psychiatry.* 2004;61:223-229.
2. Lichtermann D, Franke P, Maier W, Rao ML. Pharmacogenomics and addiction to opiates. *Eur J Pharmacol.* 2000;410:269-279.
3. Berrettini W, Bierut L, Crowley T, et al. Letter—Setting priorities for genomic research. *Science.* 2004;304:1445-1447.
4. Goldman D, Oroszi G, Ducci F. The genetics of addictions: uncovering the genes. *Nat Rev Genet.* 2005;6:521-532.
5. Lessov CN, Swan GE, Ring HZ, Khroyan TV, Lerman C. Genetics and drug use as a complex phenotype. *Subst Use Misuse.* 2004;39:1515-1569.
6. Hall WD. Will nicotine genetics and a nicotine vaccine prevent cigarette smoking and smoking-related diseases? *PLoS Med.* 2005;2:e266.
7. Merikangas KR, Risch N. Setting priorities for genomic research. *Science.* 2003;302:599-601.
8. Evans WE, Relling MV. Pharmacogenomics: translating functional genomics into rational therapeutics. *Science.* 1999;286:487-491.
9. Miksys S, Tyndale RF. Drug-metabolizing cytochrome P450s in the brain. *J Psychiatry Neurosci.* 2002;27:406-415.
10. Peto R. Smoking and death: the past 40 years and the next 40. *BMJ.* 1994;309:937-939.
11. Benowitz NL. Drug therapy: pharmacologic aspects of cigarette smoking and nicotine addiction. *N Engl J Med.* 1988;319:1318-1330.
12. Bjartveit K, Tverdal A. Health consequences of smoking 1–4 cigarettes per day. *Tob Control.* 2005;14:315-320.
13. Kawachi I, Colditz GA, Stampfer MJ, et al. Smoking cessation and time course of decreased risks of coronary heart disease in middle-aged women. *Arch Intern Med.* 1994;154:169-175.
14. Rosengren A, Wilhelmsen L, Wedel H. Coronary heart disease, cancer and mortality in middle-aged light smokers. *J Intern Med.* 1992;231:357-362.

15. Prescott E, Scharling H, Osler M, et al. Importance of light smoking and inhalation habits on risk of myocardial infarction and all cause mortality: a 22-year follow-up of 12,149 men and women in the Copenhagen City heart study. *J Epidemiol Community Health.* 2002;56:702-706.

16. Shiffman S, Fischer LB, Zettler-Segal M, Benowitz NL. Nicotine exposure among nondependent smokers. *Arch Gen Psychiatry.* 1990;47:333-336.

17. Ellickson PL, McCaffrey DF, Ghosh-Dastidar B, Longshore DL. New inroads in preventing adolescent drug use: results from a large-scale trial of project ALERT in middle schools. *Am J Public Health.* 2003;93:1830-1836.

18. Hall W, Madden P, Lynskey M. The genetics of tobacco use: methods, findings and policy implications. *Tob Control.* 2002;11:119-124.

19. Tyndale RF. Genetics of alcohol and tobacco use in humans. *Ann Med.* 2003;35:94-121.

20. Li MD, Cheng R, Ma JZ, Swan GE. A meta-analysis of estimated genetic and environmental effects on smoking behavior in male and female adult twins. *Addiction.* 2003;98:23-31.

21. Bierut LJ, Rice JP, Edenberg HJ, et al. Family-based study of the association of the dopamine D2 receptor gene (DRD2) with habitual smoking. *Am J Med Genet.* 2000;90:299-302.

22. Comings DE, Ferry L, Bradshaw-Robinson S, Burchette R, Chiu C, Muhleman D. The dopamine D2 receptor (DRD2) gene: a genetic risk factor in smoking. *Pharmacogenetics.* 1996;6:73-79.

23. Beuten J, Ma JZ, Payne TJ, et al. Single- and multilocus allelic variants within the $GABA_B$ receptor subunit 2 (GABAB2) gene are significantly associated with nicotine dependence. *Am J Hum Genet.* 2005;76:859-864.

24. Vandenbergh DJ, Kozlowski LT, Bennett CJ, et al. DAT's not all, but it may be more than we realize. *Nicotine Tob Res.* 2002;4:251-252.

25. Lerman C, Shields PG, Audrain J, et al. The role of the serotonin transporter gene in cigarette smoking. *Cancer Epidemiol Biomarkers Prev.* 1998;7:253-255.

26. Shields PG, Lerman C, Audrain J, et al. Dopamine D4 receptors and the risk of cigarette smoking in African-Americans and Caucasians. *Cancer Epidemiol Biomarkers Prev.* 1998;7:453-458.

27. Sabol SZ, Nelson ML, Fisher C, et al. A genetic association for cigarette smoking behavior. *Health Psychol.* 1999;18:7-13.

28. Sullivan PF, Jiang Y, Neale MC, Kendler KS, Straub RE. Association of the tryptophan hydroxylase gene with smoking initiation but not progression in nicotine dependence. *Am J Med Genet.* 2001;105:479-484.

29. Swan GE, Valdes AM, Ring HZ, et al. Dopamine receptor *DRD2* genotype and smoking cessation outcome following treatment with bupropion SR. *Pharmacogenomics J.* 2005;5:21-29.

30. McKinney EF, Walton RT, Yudkin P, et al. Association between polymorphisms in dopamine metabolic enzymes and tobacco consumption in smokers. *Pharmacogenetics.* 2000;10:483-491.

31. Neville MJ, Johnstone EC, Walton RT. Identification and characterization of *ANKK1*: a novel kinase gene closely linked to *DRD2* on chromosome band 11q23.1. *Hum Mutat.* 2004;23:540-545.

32. Kreek MJ, Bart G, Lilly C, Laforge KS, Nielsen DA. Pharmacogenetics and human molecular genetics of opiate and cocaine addictions and their treatments. *Pharmacol Rev.* 2005;57:1-26.

33. Xie W, Altamirano CV, Bartels CF, Speirs RJ, Cashman JR, Lockridge O. An improved cocaine hydrolase: the A328Y mutant of human butyrylcholinesterase is 4-fold more efficient. *Mol Pharmacol.* 1999;55:83-91.

34. Mogil JS, Miermeister F, Seifert F, et al. Variable sensitivity to noxious heat is mediated by differential expression of the *CGRP* gene. *Proc Natl Acad Sci USA.* 2005;102: 12938-12943.

35. Owens JC, Balogh SA, McClure-Begley TD, et al. Alpha 4 beta 2* nicotinic acetylcholine receptors modulate the effects of ethanol and nicotine on the acoustic startle response. *Alcohol Clin Exp Res.* 2003;27:1867-1875.

36. Cohen C, Kodas E, Griebel G. CB1 receptor antagonists for the treatment of nicotine addiction. *Pharmacol Biochem Behav.* 2005;81:387-395.
37. Castane A, Berrendero F, Maldonado R. The role of the cannabinoid system in nicotine addiction. *Pharmacol Biochem Behav.* 2005;81:381-386.
38. Zubieta JK, Heitzeg MM, Smith YR, et al. COMT val158met genotype affects mu-opioid neurotransmitter responses to a pain stressor. *Science.* 2003;299:1240-1243.
39. Li T, Chen CK, Hu X, et al. Association analysis of the DRD4 and COMT genes in methamphetamine abuse. *Am J Med Genet B Neuropsychiatr Genet.* 2004;129:120-124.
40. Vandenbergh DJ, Rodriguez LA, Hivert E, et al. Long forms of the dopamine receptor (DRD4) gene VNTR are more prevalent in substance abusers: no interaction with functional alleles of the catechol-o-methyltransferase (COMT) gene. *Am J Med Genet.* 2000;96:678-683.
41. Tyndale RF, Sellers EM. Variable CYP2A6-mediated nicotine metabolism alters smoking behavior and risk. *Drug Metab Dispos.* 2001;29:548-552.
42. Pianezza ML, Sellers EM, Tyndale RF. Nicotine metabolism defect reduces smoking. *Nature.* 1998;393:750.
43. Gelernter J, Kranzler HR, Satel SL, Rao PA. Genetic association between dopamine transporter protein alleles and cocaine-induced paranoia. *Neuropsychopharmacology.* 1994;11:195-200.
44. Fuke S, Suo S, Takahashi N, Koike H, Sasagawa N, Ishiura S. The VNTR polymorphism of the human dopamine transporter (DAT1) gene affects gene expression. *Pharmacogenomics J.* 2001;1:152-156.
45. Lott DC, Jr, Kim S-J, Jr, Cook EH, Jr, de Wit H. Dopamine transporter gene associated with diminished subjective response to amphetamine. *Neuropsychopharmacology.* 2005;30:602-609.
46. Stein MA, Waldman ID, Sarampote CS, et al. Dopamine transporter genotype and methylphenidate dose response in children with ADHD. *Neuropsychopharmacology.* 2005;30:1374-1382.
47. Chen R, Han DD, Gu HH. A triple mutation in the second transmembrane domain of mouse dopamine transporter markedly decreases sensitivity to cocaine and methylphenidate. *J Neurochem.* 2005;94:352-359.
48. Lerman C, Jepson C, Wileyto EP, et al. Role of Functional Genetic Variation in the Dopamine D2 Receptor (DRD2) in Response to Bupropion and Nicotine Replacement Therapy for Tobacco Dependence: Results of Two Randomized Clinical Trials. *Neuropsychopharmacology.* 2006;31:231-242.
49. Xu K, Lichtermann D, Lipsky RH, et al. Association of specific haplotypes of D2 dopamine receptor gene with vulnerability to heroin dependence in 2 distinct populations. *Arch Gen Psychiatry.* 2004;61:597-606.
50. Noble EP, Zhang X, Ritchie TL, Sparkes RS. Haplotypes at the DRD2 locus and severe alcoholism. *Am J Med Genet.* 2000;96:622-631.
51. Gelernter J, Kranzler H. D2 dopamine receptor gene (DRD2) allele and haplotype frequencies in alcohol dependent and control subjects: no association with phenotype or severity of phenotype. *Neuropsychopharmacology.* 1999;20:640-649.
52. Sander T, Ladehoff M, Samochowiec J, Finckh U, Rommelspacher H, Schmidt LG. Lack of an allelic association between polymorphisms of the dopamine D2 receptor gene and alcohol dependence in the German population. *Alcohol Clin Exp Res.* 1999;23:578-581.
53. Gelernter J, Kranzler H, Satel SL. No association between D2 dopamine receptor (DRD2) alleles or haplotypes and cocaine dependence or severity of cocaine dependence in European- and African-Americans. *Biol Psychiatry.* 1999;45:340-345.
54. Goldman D, Urbanek M, Guenther D, Robin R, Long JC. Linkage and association of a functional DRD2 variant [Ser311Cys] and DRD2 markers to alcoholism, substance abuse and schizophrenia in Southwestern American Indians. *Am J Med Genet.* 1997;74:386-394.
55. Chen CK, Hu X, Lin SK, et al. Association analysis of dopamine D2-like receptor genes and methamphetamine abuse. *Psychiatr Genet.* 2004;14:223-226.
56. Chang FM, Ko HC, Lu RB, Pakstis AJ, Kidd KK. The dopamine D4 receptor gene (DRD4) is not associated with alcoholism in three Taiwanese populations: six polymorphisms tested separately and as haplotypes. *Biol Psychiatry.* 1997;41:394-405.

57. Nishiyama T, Ikeda M, Iwata N, et al. Haplotype association between GABAA receptor gamma2 subunit gene (GABRG2) and methamphetamine use disorder. *Pharmacogenomics J.* 2005;5:89-95.
58. Hashimoto T, Hashimoto K, Matsuzawa D, et al. A functional glutathione *S*-transferase P1 gene polymorphism is associated with methamphetamine-induced psychosis in Japanese population. *Am J Med Genet B Neuropsychiatr Genet.* 2005;135:5-9.
59. Zimniak P, Nanduri B, Pikula S, et al. Naturally occurring human glutathione S-transferase GSTP1-1 isoforms with isoleucine and valine in position 104 differ in enzymic properties. *Eur J Biochem.* 1994;224:893-899.
60. Szumlinski KK, Abernathy KE, Oleson EB, et al. Homer isoforms differentially regulate cocaine-induced neuroplasticity. *Neuropsychopharmacology.* 2005;14.Epub ahead of print.
61. Mogil JS, Ritchie J, Smith SB, et al. Melanocortin-1 receptor gene variants affect pain and mu-opioid analgesia in mice and humans. *J Med Genet.* 2005;42:583-587.
62. Mogil JS, Wilson SG, Chesler EJ, et al. The melanocortin-1 receptor gene mediates female-specific mechanisms of analgesia in mice and humans. *Proc Natl Acad Sci USA.* 2003;100:4867-4872.
63. Kim H, Neubert JK, San MA, et al. Genetic influences on variability in human acute experimental pain sensitivity associated with gender, ethnicity and psychological temperament. *Pain.* 2004;109:488-496.
64. Lerman C, Wileyto EP, Patterson F, et al. The functional mu opioid receptor (OPRM1) Asn40Asp variant predicts short-term response to nicotine replacement therapy in a clinical trial. *Pharmacogenomics J.* 2004;4:184-192.
65. Gelernter J, Kranzler H, Cubells J. Genetics of two μ opioid receptor gene (OPRM1) exon 1 polymorphisms: population studies, and allele frequencies in alcohol- and drug-dependent subjects. *Mol Psychiatry.* 1999;4:476-483.
66. Bart G, Heilig M, LaForge KS, et al. Substantial attributable risk related to a functional mu-opioid receptor gene polymorphism in association with heroin addiction in central Sweden. *Mol Psychiatry.* 2004;9:547-549.
67. Bond C, LaForge KS, Tian M, et al. Single-nucleotide polymorphism in the human mu opioid receptor gene alters beta-endorphin binding and activity: possible implications for opiate addiction. *Proc Natl Acad Sci USA.* 1998;95:9608-9613.
68. Befort K, Filliol D, Decaillot FM, Gaveriaux-Ruff C, Hoehe MR, Kieffer BL. A single nucleotide polymorphic mutation in the human mu-opioid receptor severely impairs receptor signaling. *J Biol Chem.* 2001;276:3130-3137.
69. Beyer A, Kock T, Schroder H, Schulz S, Hollt V. Effect of the A118G polymorphism on binding affinity, potency and agonist-mediated endocytosis, desensitization, and resensitization of the human mu-opioid receptor. *J Neurochem.* 2004;89:553-560.
70. Zhang Y, Wang D, Johnson AD, Papp AC, Sadee W. Allelic expression imbalance of human mu opioid receptor (OPRM1) caused by variant A118G. *J Biol Chem.* 2005;280: 32618-32624.
71. Oslin DW, Berrettini W, Kranzler HR, et al. A functional polymorphism of the μ-opioid receptor gene is associated with naltrexone response in alcohol-dependent patients. *Neuropsychopharmacology.* 2003;28:1546-1552.
72. Lotsch J, Skarke C, Grosch S, Darimont J, Schmidt H, Geisslinger G. The polymorphism A118G of the human mu-opioid receptor gene decreases the pupil constrictory effect of morphine-6-glucuronide but not that of morphine. *Pharmacogenetics.* 2002;12:3-9.
73. Fillingim RB, Kaplan L, Staud R, et al. The A118G single nucleotide polymorphism of the mu-opioid receptor gene (OPRM1) is associated with pressure pain sensitivity in humans. *J Pain.* 2005;6:159-167.
74. Fiore MC. Treating tobacco use and dependence: an introduction to the US Public Health Service Clinical Practice Guideline. *Respir Care.* 2000;45:1196-1199.
75. National Institute on Drug Abuse. Research Report Series: Nicotine Addiction. NIH Publ No 01-4342. 2001. Bethesda, MD:NIDA. Available at: http://www.nida.nih.gov/researchreports/nicotine/nicotine.html. Accessed February 23, 2006.

76. Fiore MC, Smith SS, Jorenby DE, Baker TB. The effectiveness of the nicotine patch for smoking cessation: a meta-analysis. *JAMA*. 1994;271:1940-1947.
77. Paoletti P, Fornai E, Maggiorelli F, et al. Importance of baseline cotinine plasma values in smoking cessation: results from a double-blind study with nicotine patch. *Eur Respir J.* 1996;9:643-651.
78. Pickworth WB, Fant RV, Butschky MF, Henningfield JE. Effects of transdermal nicotine delivery on measures of acute nicotine withdrawal. *J Pharmacol Exp Ther*. 1996;279:450-456.
79. Foulds J, Burke M, Steinberg M, Williams JM, Ziedonis DM. Advances in pharmacotherapy for tobacco dependence. *Expert Opin Emerg Drugs*. 2004;9:39-53.
80. Anthenelli RM. Rimonabant helps for smoking cessation, weight loss. ACC 53rd Annual Scientific Session: Late-Breaking Clinical Trials; March 9, 2004; New Orleans, LA.
81. Heading CE. NicVAX Nabi Biopharmaceuticals. *IDrugs*. 2003;6:1178-1181.
82. Cerny T. Anti-nicotine vaccination: where are we now? *Recent Results Cancer Res.* 2005;166:167-175.
83. Hatsukami DK, Rennard S, Jorenby D, et al. Safety and immunogenicity of a nicotine conjugate vaccine in current smokers. *Clin Pharmacol Ther*. 2005;78:456-467.
84. Dale LC, Glover ED, Sachs DP, et al. Bupropion for smoking cessation: predictors of successful outcome. *Chest*. 2001;119:1357-1364.
85. Merikangas KR, Stolar M, Stevens DE, et al. Familial transmission of substance use disorders. *Arch Gen Psychiatry*. 1998;55:973-979.
86. Tsuang MT, Lyons MJ, Meyer JM, et al. Co-occurrence of abuse of different drugs in men: the role of drug-specific and shared vulnerabilities. *Arch Gen Psychiatry*. 1998;55:967-972.
87. Regier DA, Farmer ME, Rae DS, et al. Comorbidity of mental disorders with alcohol and other drug abuse: results from the Epidemiology Catchment Area (ECA) study. *JAMA*. 1990;264:2511-2518.
88. Ikeda K, Soichiro I, Han W, Hayashida M, Uhl GR, Sora I. How individual sensitivity to opiates can be predicted by gene analyses. *Trends Pharmacol Sci*. 2005;26:311-317.
89. Ross JR, Rutter D, Welsh K, et al. Clinical response to morphine in cancer patients and genetic variation in candidate genes. *Pharmacogenomics J*. 2005;5:324-336.
90. Tiseo PJ, Thaler HT, Lapin J, Inturrisi CE, Portenoy RK, Foley KM. Morphine-6-glucuronide concentrations and opioid-related side effects: a survey in cancer patients. *Pain.* 1995;61:47-54.
91. MacGregor AJ, Griffiths GO, Baker J, Spector TD. Determinants of pressure pain threshold in adult twins: evidence that shared environmental influences predominate. *Pain.* 1997;73:253-257.
92. Rainville P, Duncan GH, Price DD, Carrier B, Bushnell MC. Pain affect encoded in human anterior cingulate but not somatosensory cortex. *Science*. 1997;277:968-971.
93. Snyder SH. Amphetamine psychosis: a "model" schizophrenia mediated by catecholamines. *Am J Psychiatry*. 1973;130:61-67.
94. Sato M, Chen CC, Akiyama K, Otsuki S. Acute exacerbation of paranoid psychotic state after long-term abstinence in patients with previous methamphetamine psychosis. *Biol Psychiatry*. 1983;18:429-440.
95. Volkow ND. Message from the Director on Amphetamine Abuse. Available at: http://www.nida.nih.gov/about/welcome/messagemeth405.html. Accessed February 23, 2006.
96. Kendler KS, Karkowski LM, Neale MC, Prescott CA. Illicit psychoactive substance use, heavy use, abuse, and dependence in a US population-based sample of male twins. *Arch Gen Psychiatry*. 2000;57:261-269.
97. Tsuang MT, Lyons MJ, Eisen SA, et al. Genetic influences on DSM-III-R drug abuse and dependence: a study of 3,372 twin pairs. *Am J Med Genet*. 1996;67:473-477.
98. Leshner AI. Addiction is a brain disease, and it matters. *Science*. 1997;278:45-47.
99. Merikangas KR, Risch N. Will the genomics revolution revolutionize psychiatry? *Am J Psychiatry*. 2003;160:625-635.
100. Croghan TW, Tomlin M, Pescosolido BA, et al. American attitudes toward and willingness to use psychiatric medications. *J Nerv Ment Dis*. 2003;191:166-174.

101. Nunes EV, Levin FR. Treatment of depression in patients with alcohol or other drug dependence: a meta-analysis. *JAMA*. 2004;291:1887-1896.
102. Kendler KS, Jacobson KC, Prescott CA, Neale MC. Specificity of genetic and environmental risk factors for use and abuse/dependence of cannabis, cocaine, hallucinogens, sedatives, stimulants, and opiates in male twins. *Am J Psychiatry*. 2003;160:687-695.
103. Bierut LJ, Rice JP, Goate A, et al. A genomic scan for habitual smoking in families of alcoholics: common and specific genetic factors in substance dependence. *Am J Med Genet A*. 2004;124:19-27.
104. Frueh FW, Goodsaid F, Rudman A, Huang S-M, Lesko LJ. The need for education in pharmacogenomics: a regulatory perspective. *Pharmacogenomics J*. 2005;5:218-220.
105. Rubin DL, Thorn C, Klein TE, Altman RB. A statistical approach to scanning the biomedical literature for pharmacogenetics knowledge. *J Am Med Inform Assoc*. 2005;12:121-129.

Chapter 5
Monoclonal Antibody Form and Function: Manufacturing the Right Antibodies for Treating Drug Abuse

Eric Peterson,[1] S. Michael Owens,[1] and Ralph L. Henry[2]

Abstract Drug abuse continues to be a major national and worldwide problem, and effective treatment strategies are badly needed. Antibodies are promising therapies for the treatment of medical problems caused by drug abuse, with several candidates in preclinical and early clinical trials. Monoclonal antibodies can be designed that have customized affinity and specificity against drugs of abuse, and because antibodies can be designed in various forms, in vivo pharmacokinetic characteristics can be tailored to suit specific clinical applications (eg, long-acting for relapse prevention, or short-acting for overdose). Passive immunization with antibodies against drugs of abuse has several advantages over active immunization, but because large doses of monoclonal antibodies may be needed for each patient, efficient antibody production technology is essential. In this minireview we discuss some of the antibody forms that may be effective clinical treatments for drug abuse, as well as several current and emerging production systems that could bridge the gap from discovery to patient use.

Keywords antibody therapy, antibody production

Introduction

Antibody treatments are in preclinical and clinical development for addressing a wide range of medical problems caused by drug abuse. These treatments include vaccination to help prevent relapse to nicotine addiction,[1,2] and monoclonal antibodies (mAb) to (1) treat overdose from phencyclidine or methamphetamine,[3-5] or (2) prevent relapse to methamphetamine abuse.[6]

[1] Department of Pharmacology and Toxicology, College of Medicine, University of Arkansas for Medical Sciences, Little Rock, AR 72205

[2] Department of Biological Sciences, University of Arkansas, Fayetteville, AR 72701

Corresponding Author: Ralph L. Henry, Biological Sciences Department, 601 SCEN, Fulbright College of Arts and Sciences, University of Arkansas, Fayetteville, AR 72701. Tel: (479) 575-2529; Fax: (479) 575-4010; E-mail: rahenry@uark.edu

R.S. Rapaka and W. Sadée (eds.), *Drug Addiction.*
© American Association of Pharmaceutical Scientists 2008

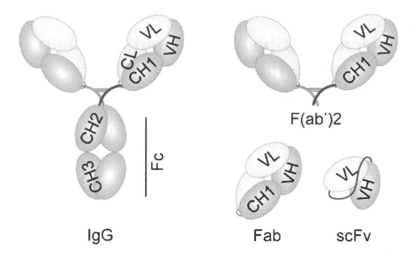

Fig. 5.1 Selected antibody forms relative to therapeutic applications. Each oval represents an immunoglobulin folding domain. Disulfide bonds are represented as thick gray lines, and the polypeptide linker of the scFv chain is represented by a black connecting ribbon. VL indicates variable domain light chain; VH, variable domain heavy chain; CL, constant domain light chain; CH, constant domain heavy chain; Fc, Fc fusion; IgG, immunoglobulin G; F(ab')2, dimeric antigen binding fragment; Fab, antigen binding fragment; scFv, single chain antigen binding fragment.

A considerable obstacle for mAb therapy (eg, immunoglobulin G [IgG], antigen binding fragment [Fab]; single chain antigen binding fragment [scFv]; Fig. 5.1) is that discovering potentially important mAb medications and then producing sufficient quantities for rigorous preclinical or clinical testing takes a while. This is a major hurdle that must be overcome if this new technology is to be taken to clinics in a timely manner. Because the early-stage manufacturing and formulation of mAb-based medications is both technologically challenging and expensive, this review will examine the production of these therapies at the levels needed for preclinical in vivo studies (eg, 0.5–10 g), with a special emphasis on alternative production systems, including plants.

Potential Advantages of mAb Therapy

Passive immunotherapy with mAb has important advantages over active immunization. First, significantly larger doses of mAb can be administered, and protection is immediate. Second, the duration of action of mAb is more predictable than antibody generated by active immunization and likely to be related to the biological half-life of the mAb. For example, currently approved mAb medications for treating other disease processes (eg, cancer) have half-lives of up to 28 days in humans.[7] Third, unlike with active immunizations, there is no immunological memory of the abused drug and the possibility of unexpected cross reactivity with endogenous ligands is less likely with mAb.

The frequency of mAb dosing should be based on the fundamental principles of clinical pharmacokinetics. For instance, dosing with mAb could occur once every mAb half-life, and loading dosing could be easily predicted for use in achieving rapid steady-state mAb concentrations. It is also important that administration of mAb could provide immediate protection to patients at critical times in the addictive disease process, when drug craving is high and relapse may be imminent. Rapid clinical effects would also be needed when using the mAb medications to treat drug overdose.

Another advantage of mAb medications is the ability to preselect for the affinity and specificity of the antibody, and thereby have the medication parameters be constant from one production lot to the next. The ideal specificity and affinity of each antibody can be selected for the intended purpose. For example, an antimethamphetamine antibody should be highly specific for the abused (+)-methamphetamine isomer, while having little affinity for (−)-methamphetamine, which is commonly used in over-the-counter inhalants, or endogenous molecules.

It is also possible to use the same mAb to produce other functional isoforms for treatment of other drug abuse–related medical applications. For instance, an IgG would be best suited for medical situations where a long duration of action is needed (eg, relapse prevention). Human IgG1, IgG2, and IgG4 have extended half-lives because of catabolic protection that is afforded by the so-called neonatal receptor (FcRn).[8,9] Human IgG3 has a much shorter half-life compared with the other human IgG isoforms because of a single amino acid difference in the FcRn binding domain[10]: at position 435 there is an arginine instead of a histidine.

Small antidrug binding fragments could also prove medically useful. The same IgG used for preventing relapse to drug abuse could be converted to a Fab or scFv. This would reduce the molecular weight of the protein from ~150 000 Da to ~50 000 Da for Fab and 27 000 Da for scFv. Since both Fab and scFv would be derived from the binding sites of the intact IgG, there would be no significant loss in affinity or specificity. The major change would be in the pharmacokinetic properties and routes of elimination. Instead of having a half-life of ~3 weeks for the IgG, the Fab and scFv half-life would be less than 1 day (eg, 0.5–21 hours),[7,11] because of rapid clearance of Fab and scFv by renal glomerular filtration.

Potential Disadvantages of mAb Therapy

Antibody-based therapies could potentially save lives and reduce the crippling effects of chronic drug abuse, but they will not be a magic bullet to cure addiction. In many ways the problems associated with treating drug abuse are analogous to the problems associated with treating a chronic infectious disease (eg, HIV). For instance, certain individuals and segments of the population are more susceptible to infectious diseases, and the best way to prevent epidemics is to stop the spread of the disease from individual to individual. By analogy, we need medical prevention to aid individuals and groups who are at an increased risk for addiction, and we need specific medications for treating key individuals who are important vectors for spreading drug abuse in the population.

Although mAb have significant promise as therapeutic agents, they are not without problems. The 3 major problems are the high cost, the risk of toxicity, and the potential for allergic-type reactions. The current cost for mAb medications for treating cancer and other health problems is thousands of dollars per month. Although this is a great deal of money, it is still significantly less than the cost of a day in a hospital emergency room or intensive care unit, or even time in prison, and the accompanying costs to society. Ideally, the cost of antibody production will continue to decrease with advances in technology.

Toxicity may also result from the expected pharmacological effects of the antibody treatment of drugs of abuse. For instance, if a patient is addicted to a drug like methamphetamine, rapid removal of the drug by the mAb could precipitate withdrawal, with subsequent clinical manifestations. Nonspecific toxicity may occur, including infusion reactions, cytokine release, and hypersensitivity to foreign immunoglobulins. Toxicity after treatment with mAb may be anticipated and prevented in some cases based on the pretesting of the mAb in immunohistochemical studies using human tissues. The US Food and Drug Administration requires this type of testing before human clinical trials begin.

Hypersensitivity reactions to the xenogeneic component of chimeric and humanized antibodies can occur upon the first dose of antibody and following repeated exposure. Development of an immune response to the mAb medication can adversely affect the antibody's pharmacokinetic, safety, and efficacy profile. All therapeutic antibodies approved to date have shown some degree of immunogenicity, even in immunosuppressed patients.[7] An antiglobulin response to an mAb medication may be anti-isotypic, anti-idiotypic, or anti-allotypic. An anti-isotypic response is directed against the constant regions of the heavy or light chains and may not directly impair antigen binding, although acceleration of mAb clearance through immune complexation may cause mAb serum concentrations to drop below effective levels. Anti-idiotypic antibodies develop against idiotypes of the mAb variable region and can block the antigen binding site in addition to accelerating mAb clearance. Anti-allotypic responses may occur in individuals who are homozygous for polymorphisms of the IgG constant regions. mAb immunogenicity may also be enhanced by aggregates in the dosing formulation or by posttranslational modifications, such as glycosylation, that may present antigenic determinants.

Antiglobulin responses to antibody products usually alter pharmacokinetic profiles. Immune complex formation accelerates clearance, reduces serum levels, and impairs targeting of the therapeutic antibodies.[7,12] Serious safety risks may be associated with immunogenicity. Adverse reactions may be local or systemic and may vary from mild injection site reactions to life-threatening anaphylaxis.[7,13] Accelerated clearance of therapeutic antibodies or neutralization of the antigen binding domain can result in loss of product efficacy, impaired antigen targeting, or interference with antibody-based diagnostic tests.[7,13,14]

Production Systems for mAb and Different mAb Forms

While different mAb forms (IgG, Fab, scFv) could provide distinct therapeutic advantages for the treatment of specific medical needs such as overdose or relapse, producing each of these different mAb forms in gram quantities suitable to conduct both in vitro and in vivo preclinical studies is extremely challenging, especially within a reasonable time frame (6 months or less). Each mAb and mAb form is a unique protein with distinct folding requirements as well as unique biochemical and biophysical characteristics that affect its ability to be expressed at high levels as a soluble, biologically active protein. To date, no single expression system appears ideal for the production of mAb or engineered mAb fragments. Even the rapid production of recombinant full-length mAb on an intermediate scale by traditional mammalian cell culture can be problematic because of the length of time (~1 year) required to identify and establish a high-producing stably transformed cell line.

To address time and protein production level requirements, alternative production systems or production strategies are being developed. These techniques show promise for the generation of mAb and mAb fragments at the intermediate levels needed to conduct preclinical studies. In addition, many of these approaches can then be scaled or adapted for eventual use in clinical applications. Alternative production systems include bacteria, yeast, insect cells, plants, and animals, including, most recently, eggs from chimeric chickens.

The use of plants or animals may hold little advantage over traditional mammalian cell culture for intermediate-level production. This is because of the amount of time required to establish a high-producing transgenic line (1 year or longer) and the diverse technical demands associated with adapting this technology. However, new transformation technologies are both reducing these time lines and simplifying the methods required to take advantage of plants and cultured mammalian cells for intermediate-level mAb production.

Production of scFv and Fab Antibody Fragments

Mammalian Cell Expression

While transgenic mammalian cells (eg, Chinese hamster ovary cells [CHO]) grown in culture are the industry standard for producing full-length mAb, work to date indicates that mammalian cells are less suited for high-level production of scFv, despite the less complex structure of these engineered fragments. Typical expression levels for an scFv in mammalian cells are on the order of 1 to 4 mg/L, which is tens to hundreds of times below the level of mAb achieved using mammalian cells.[15] Consequently, scFv production has been explored in prokaryotic and other eukaryotic expression systems.

Escherichia coli Expression

Results of these studies indicate that bacteria are well suited for accumulating properly folded scFv. Although bacteria lack a compartmentalized secretory pathway that in mammalian cells is required for proper folding, disulfide bond formation, and glycosylation, bacteria do possess the necessary protein machinery to promote disulfide bond formation. The disulfide bond proteins (or dsb proteins), which function in the periplasmic space surrounding the bacterial cytoplasm, promote efficient formation of disulfide bonds and the isomerization of incorrectly formed disulfide bonds.[16] Even scFv, which contains far fewer disulfide bonds than mAb and no interchain disulfide bonds, possesses an intrachain disulfide in each variable domain that must form for proper function.

Given the successful production of scFv in the bacterial periplasm, mAb production has also been attempted. Results of these studies indicate that multiple mAb assembly intermediates accumulate in the periplasm, with only a small percentage of recombinant protein representing fully assembled IgG.[17] Fab fragments, which are less complex than mAb but require the formation of a single interchain disulfide, accumulate to levels between what is observed for scFv and mAb. Whereas scFv accumulation as high as 100 to 130 mg/L of culture can be achieved (refolded from inclusion bodies), Fab levels are not typically greater than 10 to 30 mg/L.[18]

We have examined the ability of *Escherichia coli* to express both scFv and Fab fragments. For Fab production, both antimethamphetamine and antiphencyclidine mAb were cloned into dual expression plasmids suitable for simultaneous expression of the light chain (LC) and corresponding heavy chain (HC) Fab domain (Fd). When a Strep affinity tag was placed at the C-terminus of the LC and a 6-histidine tag was placed at the C-terminus of the HC Fd, it was possible to select for fully assembled Fab using sequential affinity chromatography steps. Purified antimethamphetamine and antiphencyclidine Fab exhibit the correct size (~50 kDa), lack detectable bacterial contaminants, and possess the same affinity as the parent mAb (Fig. 5.2). It should be noted that both the level of expression and the solubility of *E coli*–expressed scFv and Fab can vary greatly. Accumulation of soluble Fab required expression at 21 °C. We found that higher growth temperatures limited the accumulation of soluble Fab and favored the formation of insoluble inclusion bodies. In addition, a similar antimethamphetamine scFv expressed in *E coli* formed insoluble inclusion bodies regardless of culture conditions examined and required protein refolding to acquire antigen binding properties.

Yeast Expression

We have found that scFv insolubility can be overcome by expression in the methylotrophic yeast *Pichia pastoris*[15] (see Cereghino et al[19] for review), using the yeast's traditional eukaryotic secretory system to properly fold and export scFv into the culture media. This folding pathway employs the use of conserved chaperone and

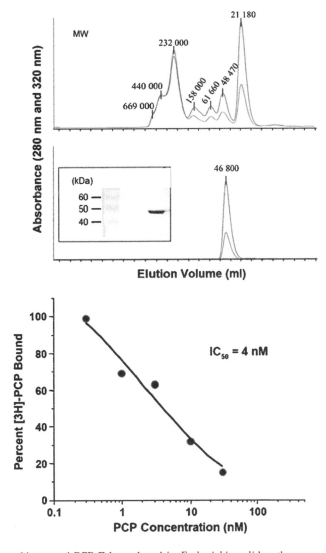

Fig. 5.2 Recombinant anti-PCP Fab produced in *Escherichia coli* has the same affinity as the parent mAb produced in mammalian cell culture. Left: Anti-PCP Fab purified from *E coli* assembles into a 46 800-Da heterodimer as judged by sizing chromatography and nonreducing PAGE (inset). Right: Binding of recombinant anti-PCP Fab to radiolabeled PCP was conducted in the presence of increasing unlabeled PCP. The concentration of PCP required to produce a 50% inhibition of [³H]-PCP binding (IC$_{50}$) mimics the binding characteristics of the parent mAb. PCP indicates phencyclidine; Fab, antigen binding fragment; mAb, monoclonal antibodies; PAGE, polyacrylamide gel electrophoresis; MW, molecular weight; IC, inhibitory concentration.

disulfide bond–forming proteins found in the *Pichia* endoplasmic reticulum that are absent in prokaryotes. Importantly, the affinity and specificity of scFv expressed in yeast appears identical to the parent mAb's.[20] Consistent with our observations, yeast-based expression provides high levels of correctly folded scFv (and Fab), which is recoverable in a single chromatographic step through the use of small affinity tags (eg, 6 histidine; Fig. 5.3). *P pastoris* is capable of extremely high cell densities in bioreactor cultures (≥400 g/L fresh cell weight), and protein levels on the order of 0.02 to 4 g/L of culture are reported.[21] An additional advantage of the *P pastoris* expression system is the ability to express therapeutic proteins in an organism that is free of animal viruses and endotoxin contamination.[22]

A potential drawback with the use of yeast-based expression systems compared with bacteria production is the added time required to develop cell lines with suitable expression levels (2–3 months). Unlike *E coli*–based systems, where expression is driven from complementary DNA (cDNA) harbored within replicating plasmids, yeast-based expression systems rely on genomic insertion of cDNA, which creates expression variability between cell lines. This is because expression levels are sensitive to the site of chromosomal insertion and the number of cDNA insertion events. Hence, yeast-based expression requires screening of different transformed cell lines in order to identify a cell line expressing suitable levels of a recombinant mAb fragment. For this reason, yeast-based expression is often explored only after attempting production in *E coli*. In some cases, antibody fragment–specific problems can be incurred using yeast-based expression systems—most notably, sensitivity to secreted proteases or the presence of a nonconserved glycosylation site in the HC variable region. This can lead to the addition of highly antigenic mannose-rich

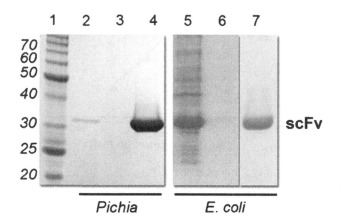

Fig. 5.3 scFv production in *Pichia pastoris* produced as a soluble protein that can be purified in 1 chromatography step. Coomassie-stained SDS-PAGE of 6-His tagged scFv produced in *Pichia* and *Escherichia coli* cells. Lane 1, MW marker. Lane 2, unclarified media from *Pichia* bioreactor run after 72 hours of production. Lane 3, flow through fraction from nickel-affinity chromatography column. Lane 4, elution of scFv from column. Lane 5, total cell lysate from the same scFv expressed in *E coli* after 18 hours. Lane 6, soluble fraction from *E coli* lysate. Lane 7, scFv after isolation from inclusion bodies, refolding, and nickel-affinity chromatography. scFv, single chain antigen binding fragment; SDS-PAGE, sodium dodecyl sulfate polyacrylamide gel electrophoresis; MW, molecular weight.

structures unique to yeast. However, proteolytic sensitivity can be circumvented using altered culture conditions,[23] and most scFv and Fab fragments lack glycosylation sites and are produced as aglycosylated proteins, as is done in *E coli*–based systems. In applications such as treatment of drug abuse with mAb-based medications, where glycosylation is not required to activate cell-based immunity, yeast could provide a suitable alternative to the production of full-length therapeutic mAb. This would require the replacement of Asn 297 in the HC with Ala or Gln to eliminate the conserved N-linked glycosylation site found in the Fc domain, which is not a prerequisite for proper antibody folding.

Plants as Antibody Factories

A large number of studies have established that plants can efficiently produce high levels of scFv or Fab,[24] partly because of the conserved nature of the secretory pathway in plants and animals. The pathway provides the proper folding and disulfide bond formation needed to assemble functional mAb fragments. Plant-based production systems possess several advantages over traditional mammalian-based production systems, including the lack of endotoxins and other potentially harmful agents (eg, prions, viruses). The scalability of plant production systems and the low cost associated with plant culture, compared with establishing and maintaining industrial-scale cell (bacterial, yeast, or mammalian) culture facilities, make plants an attractive production system for mAb-based therapies. Yet the time investment and technology needed to develop transgenic plant lines suitable for intermediate protein production levels have limited the adoption of this novel production system at the preclinical and clinical medications development level. This could well change with the advent of recently developed second-generation expression technology.

New expression technology in plants uses Agrobacterium to efficiently transfer many copies of recombinant DNA into leaf cells of intact plants. The transfer DNA, which contains the coding sequence and all of the elements for recombinant protein expression, supports transient expression of target protein in the leaf cells, eliminating the need for time-intensive tissue culture–based transformation methods. However, high levels of recombinant protein production come from coupling transient expression technology with the coexpression of viral replicons, which amplify the coding information for the recombinant target protein.[25-28] Used together, these technologies have led to levels of cytosolically expressed green fluorescent protein as high as 2.5 to 4 g/kg of leaf fresh weight in tobacco. This is even more impressive if you consider that a kilogram of leaves can be produced by only a few plants. Importantly, these recombinant protein levels were reached in only 8 days following transient transformation by Agrobacterium. The combined use of transient transfection and viral replicons has been termed magnifection. Neither scFv nor Fab has been reported to have been produced in plants by magnifection technology. However, this technology has been shown to support high-level plant-based production of recombinant secretory proteins. When routed to the secretory pathway in leaf cells of intact tobacco, human growth hormone accumulated in the leaf apoplast at levels that reached a stunning 1 g/kg fresh weight.[29] This provides a strong indication that magnifection or similar technology can be applied to the rapid high-level production of mAb forms required for preclinical or clinical applications since all of these mAb forms must pass through the secretory pathway in plants for proper folding and disulfide bond formation.

Production of Recombinant mAb

Could the same magnifection technology developed for high-level recombinant protein production in plants be applied to the rapid high-level production of full-length mAb in plants? While stably transformed plants have been shown in numerous studies to express and accumulate fully assembled and functional mAb, other factors may limit the immediate usefulness of plants for mAb production. Perhaps the greatest limitation to plant-based mAb production is the apparent high level of postassembly mAb degradation that takes place in plants. This problem appears to be substantially underrepresented in the literature and was once thought to be a protein assembly issue.

More recent data from a tobacco-based expression system indicate that half or more of the expressed mAb is degraded to its antigen binding fragments (mostly F(ab')2; Fig. 5.4).[30] Our own studies, which used tobacco to express a murine IgG1 (anti-phencyclidine mAb6B5), support these findings (Fig. 5.4). The vast majority of mAb6B5 recovered from soluble leaf extract by protein G affinity chromatography is found as 1 of 3 differently sized protein species observed by nonreducing gel electrophoresis (Fig. 5.4, left panel). Each of these proteins is recognized on Western blots with polyclonal antibodies directed against either murine IgG or murine kappa LC. These mAb fragments are observed even when protein extraction is conducted in the protective presence of protein denaturant, indicating that the fragments were formed in the plant prior to extraction and not by proteases released during the extraction process (results not shown). Importantly, the vast majority of plant-produced mAb6B5 is present as a F(ab')2-sized product (~70% of total mAb recovered) that contains an intact LC and an HC fragment lacking most of the Fc region in the HC (Fig. 5.4, right panel). Although it has been suggested that inefficient antibody assembly is a cause of the accumulation of mAb fragments in plants (eg, tobacco), more recent studies point to proteolytic cleavage of fully assembled mAb as the source of mAb fragments. Specifically, treatment of plant cells with an inhibitor of Golgi vesicle formation prevents IgG1 degradation.[30] Since antibodies reaching the Golgi network have already been assembled in the endoplasmic reticulum, proteolytic degradation of HC in plants must take place after antibody assembly, presumably at a step following residence in the Golgi. Given the robust ability of plants to produce engineered antibody fragments (eg, scFv), efforts to successfully eliminate proteolytic degradation of

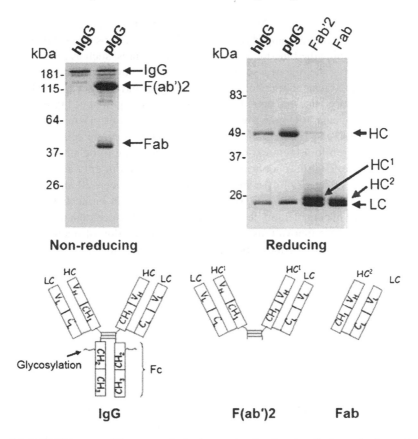

Fig. 5.4 IgG HC is susceptible to proteolytic cleavage in plant-based antibody production systems. Left: mAb6B5 murine IgG1 was recovered from tobacco leaves (pIgG) or cultured hybridoma cells (hIgG) by Protein G affinity chromatography and examined on nonreducing SDS-PAGE. Right: Bands corresponding to IgG, F(ab')2, and Fab were then excised from the gels and reexamined on SDS-PAGE reducing gels to identify individual polypeptides. Lower: Antibody models correspond to the most abundant mAb species identified in tobacco. IgG, immunoglobulin G; HC, heavy chain; SDS-PAGE, sodium dodecyl sulfate polyacrylamide gel electrophoresis; F(ab')2, dimeric antigen binding fragment; Fab, antigen binding fragment; mAb, monoclonal antibodies; LC, light chain; CH, constant domain heavy chain; CH_1, constant domain 1 of heavy chain; V_H, variable domain of heavy chain; V_L, variable domain of light chain; C_L, constant domain of light chain.

the HC Fc domain could help make plants a universal platform for the production of full-length mAb and engineered mAb fragments.

Unlike scFv and other mAb fragments, recombinant mAb can be produced at high levels by mammalian cells. The major drawback of current mammalian cell culture technologies is the time and cost associated with developing a stable mAb-producing cell line for each recombinant mAb. Hence, the technology is not well suited for situations where mAb-based medications that require large individual patient doses are being developed or where multiple renditions of a single mAb are desirable to examine the function of specific mAb features, such as the importance of glycosylation or the role of a specific residue in the binding pocket.

Advances in transient transfection technologies have begun to address the issue of production time and cost. Because of the development of highly efficient transfection reagents, it is now possible for many copies of plasmid DNA carrying the target LC and HC genes to be introduced into a single cell. The plasmid DNA can function in protein expression without needing to be stably integrated into the genome. High levels of protein can be produced in only a few days, and levels of mAb secreted into the media often range between 20 and 40 mg/L of mammalian cell culture.[31,32] Importantly, the process can be scaled to produce gram quantities in considerably less time than it takes to develop a transgenic cell line. However, these innovations in transient transformation of mammalian cells still do not address the financial bottleneck associated with the cost of mammalian cell cultures.

Conclusion

mAb and mAb engineered fragments present potentially effective therapies to treat drug abuse. The high affinity and exquisite specificity of these proteins to their drug targets and their customizable pharmacokinetic properties make them very attractive therapeutic candidates. However, like many protein-based pharmaceuticals, these medications are difficult to move from the bench to the clinic because of the large amounts needed for therapeutic doses. *E coli*, the prototypic protein production system for many proteins, is not able to produce intact IgG efficiently and often produces too few soluble antibody fragments. Thus, lower eukaryotes such as *P pastoris* are becoming more widely used for antibody fragment production, and the relative simplicity of their genetic manipulation make this system an attractive alternative to *E coli*. However, the potential for proteolytic degradation and unwanted glycosylation, as well as the need for special equipment (bioreactors), must be considered. Plants are emerging as a viable expression system for engineered mAb fragments and have enormous protein production capabilities. However, plant-based systems have until now been technically difficult to genetically modify and are plagued with IgG degradation problems. New advances in molecular technology and our understanding of these complex systems are beginning to overcome these issues and will eventually help stimulate cost-effective protein-based therapies for the treatment of drug abuse, so that these medications can become widely available.

Acknowledgments These studies were supported by National Institute on Drug Abuse grants PO1 DA14361, DA11560, and DA07610 and by National Institutes of Health grant P20 RR15569 from the COBRE Program of the National Center for Research Resources. We also thank Jon Hubbard and Huimin Liu for conducting studies with bacterial Fab and plant mAb production.

References

1. Pentel P, Malin D. A vaccine for nicotine dependence: targeting the drug rather than the brain. *Respiration (Herrlisheim)*. 2002;69:193-197.
2. Hieda Y, Keyler DE, Ennifar S, Fattom A, Pentel PR. Vaccination against nicotine during continued nicotine administration in rats: immunogenicity of the vaccine and effects on nicotine distribution to brain. *Int J Immunopharmacol*. 2000;22:809-819.
3. McClurkan MB, Valentine JL, Arnold L, Owens SM. Disposition of a monoclonal anti-phencyclidine Fab fragment of immunoglobulin G in rats. *J Pharmacol Exp Ther*. 1993;266:1439-1445.
4. Valentine JL, Mayersohn M, Wessinger WD, Arnold LW, Owens SM. Antiphencyclidine monoclonal Fab fragments reverse phencyclidine-induced behavioral effects and ataxia in rats. *J Pharmacol Exp Ther*. 1996;278:709-716.
5. Byrnes-Blake KA, Laurenzana EM, Carroll FI, et al. Pharmacodynamic mechanisms of monoclonal antibody-based antagonism of (+)-methamphetamine in rats. *Eur J Pharmacol*. 2003;461:119-128.
6. McMillan DE, Hardwick WC, Li M, Owens SM. Pharmacokinetic antagonism of (+)-methamphetamine discrimination by a low-affinity monoclonal anti-methamphetamine antibody. *Behav Pharmacol*. 2002;13:465-473.
7. Roskos LK, Davis CG, Schwab GM. The clinical pharmacology of therapeutic monoclonal antibodies. *Drug Dev Res*. 2004;61:108-120.
8. Brambell FW, Hemmings WA, Morris IG. A theoretical model of gamma-globulin catabolism. *Nature*. 1964;203:1352-1354.
9. Junghans RP. Finally! The Brambell receptor (FcRB). Mediator of transmission of immunity and protection from catabolism for IgG. *Immunol Res*. 1997;16:29-57.
10. Ghetie V, Ward ES. Transcytosis and catabolism of antibody. *Immunol Res*. 2002;25:97-113.
11. Trang J. Pharmacokinetics and metabolism of therapeutic and diagnostic antibodies. In: Ferraiolo B, Mohler M, Gloff C, eds. *Protein Pharmacokinetics and Metabolism*. New York, NY: Plenum Press; 1992:223-270.
12. Weiner LM. Monoclonal antibody therapy of cancer. *Semin Oncol*. 1999;26:43-51.
13. Stein KE. Immunogenicity: concepts/issues/concerns. *Dev Biol (Basel)*. 2002;109:15-23.
14. Kuus-Reichel K, Grauer LS, Karavodin LM, Knott C, Krusemeier M, Kay NE. Will immunogenicity limit the use, efficacy, and future development of therapeutic monoclonal antibodies? *Clin Diagn Lab Immunol*. 1994;1:365-372.
15. King DJ, Byron OD, Mountain A, et al. Expression, purification and characterization of B72.3 Fv fragments. *Biochem J*. 1993;290:723-729.
16. Kadokura H, Katzen F, Beckwith J. Protein disulfide bond formation in prokaryotes. *Annu Rev Biochem*. 2003;72:111-135. DOI: 10.1146/annurev.biochem.72.121801.161459.
17. Simmons LC, Reilly D, Klimowski L, et al. Expression of full-length immunoglobulins in *Escherichia coli*: rapid and efficient production of aglycosylated antibodies. *J Immunol Methods*. 2002;263:133-147.
18. Venturi M, Seifert C, Hunte C. High level production of functional antibody Fab fragments in an oxidizing bacterial cytoplasm. *J Mol Biol*. 2002;315:1-8.
19. Cereghino GP, Cereghino JL, Ilgen C, Cregg JM. Production of recombinant proteins in fermenter cultures of the yeast *Pichia pastoris*. *Curr Opin Biotechnol*. 2002;13:329-332.
20. Peterson EC, Farrance C, Henry R, Owens SM. Engineering of a single chain antibody for treatment of methamphetamine abuse. 2004 Experimental Biology meeting abstracts [on CD-ROM]. *FASEB J*. 2004;18.
21. Damasceno LM, Pla I, Chang HJ, et al. An optimized fermentation process for high-level production of a single-chain Fv antibody fragment in *Pichia pastoris*. *Protein Expr Purif*. 2004;37:18-26.
22. Joosten V, Lokman C, Van Den Hondel CA, Punt PJ. The production of antibody fragments and antibody fusion proteins by yeasts and filamentous fungi. *Microb Cell Fact*. 2003;2:1.

23. Murasugi A, Asami Y, Mera-Kikuchi Y. Production of recombinant human bile salt-stimulated lipase in *Pichia pastoris*. *Protein Expr Purif*. 2001;23:282-288.
24. Ma JK, Drake PM, Christou P. The production of recombinant pharmaceutical proteins in plants. *Nat Rev Genet*. 2003;4:794-805.
25. Gleba Y, Klimyuk V, Marillonnet S. Magnifection—a new platform for expressing recombinant vaccines in plants. *Vaccine*. 2005;23:2042-2048.
26. Gleba Y, Marillonnet S, Klimyuk V. Engineering viral expression vectors for plants: the 'full virus' and the 'deconstructed virus' strategies. *Curr Opin Plant Biol*. 2004;7:182-188.
27. Marillonnet S, Thoeringer C, Kandzia R, Klimyuk V, Gleba Y. Systemic Agrobacterium tumefaciens-mediated transfection of viral replicons for efficient transient expression in plants. *Nat Biotechnol*. 2005;23:718-723.
28. Santi L, Giritch A, Roy CJ, et al. Protection conferred by recombinant Yersinia pestis antigens produced by a rapid and highly scalable plant expression system. *Proc Natl Acad Sci USA*. 2006;103:861-866.
29. Gils M, Kandzia R, Marillonnet S, Klimyuk V, Gleba Y. High-yield production of authentic human growth hormone using a plant virus-based expression system. *Plant Biotechnol J*. 2005;3:613-620.
30. Sharp JM, Doran PM. Characterization of monoclonal antibody fragments produced by plant cells. *Biotechnol Bioeng*. 2001;73:338-346.
31. Derouazi M, Girard P, Van Tilborgh F, et al. Serum-free large-scale transient transfection of CHO cells. *Biotechnol Bioeng*. 2004;87:537-545.
32. Baldi L, Muller N, Picasso S, et al. Transient gene expression in suspension HEK-293 cells: application to large-scale protein production. *Biotechnol Prog*. 2005;21:148-153.

Chapter 6
Cocaine- and Amphetamine-Regulated Transcript Peptides Play a Role in Drug Abuse and Are Potential Therapeutic Targets

Michael J. Kuhar,[1] Jason N. Jaworski,[1] George W. Hubert,[1] Kelly B. Philpot,[1] and Geraldina Dominguez[1]

Abstract Cocaine- and amphetamine-regulated transcript (CART) peptides (55 to 102 and 62 to 102) are neurotransmitters with important roles in a number of physiologic processes. They have a role in drug abuse by virtue of the fact that they are modulators of mesolimbic function. Key findings supporting a role in drug abuse are as follows. First, high densities of CART-containing nerve terminals are localized in mesolimbic areas. Second, CART 55 to 102 blunts some of the behavioral effects of cocaine and dopamine (DA). This functional antagonism suggests that CART peptides be considered as targets for medications development. Third, CREB in the nucleus accumbens has been shown to have an opposing effect on cocaine self-administration. CREB may activate CART expression in that region, and, if so, CART may mediate at least some of the effects of CREB. Fourth, in addition to the effects of CART on DA, DA can influence CART in the accumbens. Thus a complex interacting circuitry likely exists. Fifth, in humans, CART is altered in the ventral tegmental area of cocaine overdose victims, and a mutation in the CART gene associates with alcoholism.

Overall, it is clear that there are functional interactions among CART, DA, and cocaine and that plausible cellular mechanisms exist to explain some of these actions. Future studies will clarify and extend these findings.

Keywords CART, cocaine, CREB, nucleus accumbens

Introduction

Cocaine- and amphetamine-regulated transcript (CART) peptides are peptide neurotransmitters and endocrine factors of physiologic importance. Several reviews have been written on various aspects of CART peptides.[1-4] This review focuses on the role of CART in drug abuse.

---

[1] Yerkes National Primate Research Center, Emory University, Atlanta, GA 30329

Corresponding Author: Michael J. Kuhar, Yerkes National Primate Research Center of Emory University, 954 Gatewood Rd NE, Atlanta, GA 30329; Tel: (404) 727-1737; Fax: (404) 727-3278; E-mail: michael.kuhar@emory.edu

R.S. Rapaka and W. Sadée (eds.), *Drug Addiction.*
© American Association of Pharmaceutical Scientists 2008

First, a note on nomenclature. Several fragments of pro-CART have been shown to be active;[5-7] two major fragments are rlCART 55 to 102 and rlCART 62 to 102, where "rl" refers to the long (l) form of the rat (r) transcript and its translated propeptide.[8] The identical peptides (except for one amino acid substitution at 55) in humans are written as hCART42–89 and hCART49–89, which reflects the finding that the human transcript is fully spliced to a smaller transcript yielding a shorter pro-CART of 89 amino acids compared with 102 for the rat long form (there is a rat short form of 89 amino acids as well). Most studies use rlCART 55 to 102 (or simply CART 55 to 102), which is commercially available, but other peptides have been examined, and we cannot rule out the idea that additional peptides may be shown to have activity as well.

The first demonstration of the existence of at least a fragment of CART peptide was in a publication by Spiess et al,[9] where the first 30 amino acids of CART 55 to 102 were sequenced and described as an "unknown" peptide with unknown function. In 1995, Douglass et al[10] reported that a transcript was increased in the striatum after acute cocaine or amphetamine administration (hence the name CART) and that the transcript coded for an apparent peptide neurotransmitter containing the 30 amino acid fragment of Spiess et al.[9] Additional key findings include the demonstration of CART peptide and its processing by Western blotting, immunoprecipitation, and sequencing;[6,11,12] its localization to neurons in the brain, gut, and other cells in the periphery;[13-23] its demonstrated electrophysiologic effects;[24-26] its ability to elicit expression of immediate early genes;[27] and its calcium-dependent release from hypothalamic explants.[28] A high-profile role for the CART peptide is its involvement in feeding; after noting the distribution of CART in the brain, our laboratory was the first to propose that CART regulates feeding,[13] and this was quickly confirmed using CART antibodies[29-31] and peptides.[31]

CART in Drug Abuse: A Modulator of Mesolimbic Neurons and Psychostimulants

Douglass et al[10] and others[32,33] reported that CART mRNA increased in the striatum after acute or binge administration of cocaine or amphetamine. This was an impetus to examine CART in the context of drug abuse. However, it has now become clear that this finding by Douglass et al[10] is not always easily reproduced, and some have published negative data.[34,35] Nevertheless, despite these conflicting reports, there is strong evidence implicating CART peptides in drug abuse, particularly in modulating mesolimbic function. In some cases, CART can affect dopamine (DA), and in other situations DA influences CART. Accordingly, we have developed a model with CART integrated into the mesolimbic circuitry (Fig. 6.1).

First, CART peptides are found in key brain regions associated with reward/reinforcement; these include the ventral tegmental area (VTA), ventral pallidum, amygdala, lateral hypothalamus, and nucleus accumbens.[14,15,33,36,37] In the accumbens, the peptides colocalize with gamma amino benzoic acid in medium spiny output

CART and the Mesolimbic Dopamine Circuit

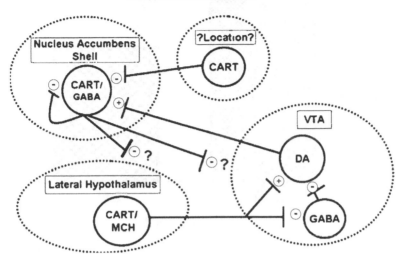

Fig. 6.1 Mesolimbic circuitry and the influence of CART peptide. High densities of CART-containing nerve terminals are found in the VTA, and many CART-containing cells and processes are found in the nucleus accumbens (see text). Many of the nerve terminals in the VTA derive from a CART input from the lateral hypothalamus, which may play a role in integrating food and drug reward. CART in the VTA can influence DA neurons directly or indirectly through gamma amino butyric acid neurons. In the accumbens, DA nerve terminals are found on CART neurons (GABAergic medium-spiny output neurons) suggesting that DA influences CART. CART synapses in the accumbens from recurrent collaterals or other sources additionally suggest that CART can influence accumbal output.

neurons and receive a DA input.[14,15,38] In the VTA, CART nerve terminals are found in all of the DAergic subnuclei, and some CART-containing nerve terminals synapse on DA-containing neurons and others on gamma amino butyric acid-containing neurons.[14,36] A major source of input to the VTA is from the lateral hypothalamus. Thus, CART is anatomically positioned to influence reward and reinforcement.

Second, CART is not only present in animals, as CART mRNA levels were changed in the VTA of cocaine overdose victims.[39,40] This is evidence that cocaine affects CART in animals and also in humans and supports a role for CART-cocaine interactions in humans.

Third, injection of CART into mesolimbic regions has behavioral effects related to psychostimulants. Kimmel et al[41] showed that injection of the CART peptide into the VTA caused a small increase in locomotor activity (which was blocked by haloperidol) and promoted conditioned place preference, suggesting that CART had psychostimulant-like effects. Our recent observation that intra-VTA CART causes an increase in the release of DA in the accumbens supports this (Fig. 6.2). But, the magnitude of the locomotor and DA release effects were small compared

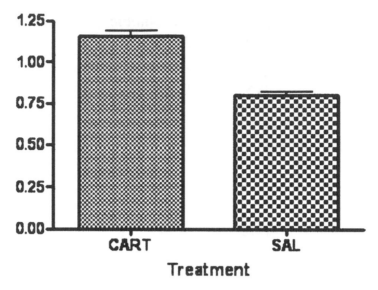

Fig. 6.2 Intra-VTA injection of CART peptide produces a small increase in DA efflux in the nucleus accumbens. Because CART injected into the VTA has weak behavioral psychostimulant-like effects (see text), its potential to increase DA efflux by in vivo microdialysis was examined. DA efflux, summed over time, was indeed increased significantly ($P < 0.01$). This effect could be attributable to direct stimulation of DA neurons, by disinhibition of gamma amino butyric acid neurons (both of which receive CART inputs), or both (see Fig. 6.1).

with those of cocaine, and we found recently that cotreatment of animals with both intra-VTA CART and systemic cocaine produced only partially additive effects. The additivity between CART and cocaine seemed to occur at lower concentrations of the drugs, but at higher doses, CART tended to oppose the locomotor activity induced by systemic cocaine (Jaworski et al, manuscript in preparation). This sounds like CART is a functional "partial agonist" in the VTA. Evidence supporting this has been found in the accumbens. When CART was injected into the nucleus accumbens, by itself there was no effect, but when combined with systemic cocaine or amphetamine, the injection of CART again blunted the locomotor increasing the effects of the drugs (Fig. 6.3).[42,43] Also, the CART peptide blunted the locomotor-increasing effects of DA injected into the accumbens, suggesting a downstream effect on the actions of DA (Fig. 6.4). Therefore, in either the VTA or the accumbens, CART may have some small psychostimulant-like effects, but then it tends to oppose the actions of psychostimulants at higher doses. Although speculative, it is possible that CART may, therefore, be homeostatic or restorative in that it tends to oppose the large changes caused by cocaine. A large number of controls for the active peptide and anatomic region were conducted in these experiments. CART, because it blunts at least some of the effects of psychostimulants, should be considered a target for medications development. The identification of the CART receptor would likely be essential for this.

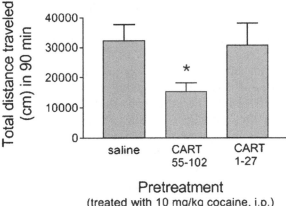

Fig. 6.3 Intraaccumbal injections of CART peptide reduce the locomotor-activating effects of systemic cocaine. CART 55 to 102 injected into the accumbens minutes before i.p. injection of cocaine reduces locomotor activity. However, saline does not, and an inactive CART fragment, CART 1 to 27, does not. Data from Jaworski et al. [42]

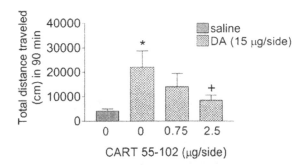

Fig. 6.4 CART blunts locomotor activity induced by intraaccumbal injection of DA. Direct injection of DA into the nucleus accumbens increases locomotor activity, but that is reduced when CART peptide is coinjected with the DA. Thus, CART can reduce the direct effects of DA, suggesting that it is blunting the actions of DA rather than its release. This effect of CART is dose-responsive. Data from Jaworski et al. [42]

Fourth, the intracerebroventricular injection of the CART peptide causes an increased turnover of DA in the nucleus accumbens.[44,45] This is an important functional counterpart of the observation that CART nerve terminals synapse on DA neurons in the VTA. Of course, the effect could be indirect, involving intervening neurons. Future experiments will be needed to resolve this.

Fifth, D3 DA receptors regulate the CART mRNA in accumbal cells.[2] D3 agonists deplete CART mRNA and the peptide in both the shell and the core (Hunter et al, manuscript in preparation). A reasonable hypothesis is that D3 receptors, which are well known to reduce cyclic adenosine monophosphate (cAMP) levels, could deplete CART by reducing active CREB in these cells. The effects of the D3 receptor are well known to interact with cocaine,[46-48] and our findings open the possibility that the D3 receptors may produce some of their effects through the CART peptides.

Sixth, other accumbal factors, such as cyclic AMP response element-binding protein (CREB), tend to have the same blunting effect on psychostimulants in that overexpression of CREB in the accumbens decreases the rewarding effects of cocaine.[49] It is relevant that CREB activates the promoter region of the CART gene[50-54] and may exert some of its effects through CART.

Seventh, whereas most genetic studies have focused on a connection between CART and human obesity, a recent study showed that a mutation in the CART gene was associated with alcoholism but not schizophrenia or bipolar disorder.[55] Again, CART is implicated in drug abuse not only in animals but also in humans.

Eighth, it has been shown that glucocorticoids are needed for cocaine to be self-administered.[56,57] We have found recently that corticosterone regulates CART levels in the nucleus accumbens. Perhaps CART somehow mediates the requirement for corticosterone.

In summary, DA, which is released/potentiated by drugs of abuse, can exert some control over CART peptide production and utilization, and CART peptides can, in turn, modulate mesolimbic DA function. The latter modulation can alter the effects of drugs of abuse. This hypothesized model (Fig. 6.1 and 6.5) is under current exploration in our laboratory from several viewpoints.

CART Is Involved in Other Physiologic Processes

All of the evidence for this is too extensive to be detailed here, but brief summaries can give the impressive picture of the importance of these peptides. This is an interesting example of how research in drug abuse can impact other areas.

In feeding, CART appears to play a major role in determining body weight in humans (reviewed in Ref.[4]). The human genetic data are very strong, and the animal studies are very supportive. A mutation in the human CART promoter causes increased girth.[58] Another mutation in the reading frame that appears to interfere with processing, sorting, and trafficking results in increased body weight.[59,60] Cells expressing the latter mutation produce altered levels of CART peptide; thus, the mutation has an actual effect on peptide levels.[52] Also, CART knockout mice exhibit a tendency to gain weight.[61] Because of the likely overlap of feeding reward mechanisms and drug reward mechanisms, studies of feeding mechanisms are likely to have some significance for drug abuse as well.

Stress is a risk factor for drug abuse, and CART peptides appear involved in stress. Hypothalamic CART mRNA and peptides are regulated by glucocorticoids,[62,63] and stress alters the levels of CART peptides in the arcuate nuclei (Balkan, manuscript in preparation). The blood levels of CART are also at least

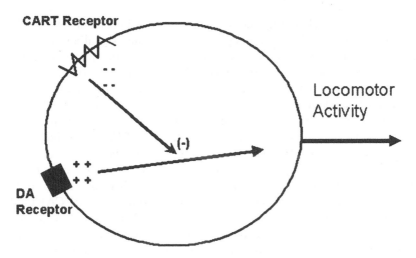

Fig. 6.5 Cell model of how CART peptide could blunt the effect of DA in the accumbens. DA receptor activation in the nucleus accumbens can increase locomotor activity. CART peptides by themselves have no effect but can reduce the effect of DA, perhaps through an intracellular mechanism. The exact intracellular change that occurs is not yet known.

partially affected by glucocorticoids.[23] Also, injection of CART 55 to 102 into the cerebral ventricles induces fos expression in cells in the paraventricular nucleus that contain CRF, suggesting that CART is involved in controlling the release of corticotropin-releasing factor (CRF).[64,65] Also, the CART promoter contains regulatory elements that could be involved in regulation by glucocorticoids as a result of interactions with transcription factors.[50] However, the precise and complete role of CART in stress is not yet fully known and is under current investigation. Of course, in this context, it is also important to note that glucocorticoids are critical factors for cocaine self-administration,[56,57] and the role of glucocorticoids in CART regulation is, therefore, important.

The CART peptide has antinociceptive effects,[66-68] although the precise nature of these effects is being clarified. In endocrine regulation, evidence for a role for CART is increasing. CART is found in the nuclei and regions historically associated with endocrine control, and CART peptides are found in the portal blood.[69] CART also caused changes in prolactin release and inhibited the release of thyroid-stimulating hormone from pituitary cells in culture.[70-72]

In development, CART has been found early in the brain and gut, as well as in the ovary and pancreas,[17,19-22,73] suggesting a role in development. CART has been shown to be neurotrophic in in vitro cell culture systems.[5] These are open areas of research where little has been published, but much is ongoing.

CART Is a Regulated mRNA and Peptide

Whether or not CART is regulated or simply produced constitutively is relevant. The peptides involved in physiologic regulation and signaling are routinely "regulated," that is, their synthesis is controlled by various physiologic factors. The CART levels are known to change fairly rapidly in a couple of hours in response to various stimuli. First, there was the initial observation that CART mRNA increased 1 hour after the acute injection of cocaine or amphetamine.[10] Although this has been repeated by some,[32,33] it has been challenged by others.[34,35] In our laboratory, we tend to get increases in CART mRNA levels, but only after high-binge doses of cocaine (data unpublished). Nevertheless, a regulation seems to occur at least under some conditions. Second, the D3 DA receptor agonists decrease the CART mRNA levels in the nucleus accumbens in a matter of hours, and this is blocked by D3 antagonists. In D3 knockout mice, the CART mRNA levels are up regulated in the accumbens.[74] Third, CART levels in the nucleus accumbens and in other regions undergo diurnal variations (Vicentic et al, in press); this and perhaps other rhythms may somehow cause or reflect the diurnal variation in cocaine intake.[75] Fourth, leptin has been shown to regulate CART mRNA in specific nuclei in the hypothalamus,[31,76] and the CART proximal promoter region contains a consensus signal transducer and activator of transcription site, which can be activated via leptin signaling.[50,54] Fifth, glucocorticoids, which can regulate drug intake,[56,57] also regulate CART levels in the peripheral blood[23,62,63] and in the brain.[62,63] Sixth, several studies in our laboratory and elsewhere show that changes in cAMP levels activate CREB, which, in turn, activates the CART gene,[50-54] and CREB plays a role in drug abuse.[49]

Whereas changes in levels may not always reflect transcriptional regulation, we assume that many of the above observations do indeed reflect it. Understanding the mechanisms regulating the CART promoter is key to understanding how CART is regulated and influenced. In several studies, we found that the CART proximal promoter contains a consensus cyclic adenosine monophosphate response element site that is functional in both GH3 (neuroendocrine-derived cell line) and CATH.a cells (neuronal-derived cell line) and is involved in CREB-mediated transcription.[50-54]

CATH.a cells are a neuronally derived cell line and express the type 1 CRF receptor (CRF-R1).[77] They are derived from locus coeruleus neurons, which are known to express CART.[13] CATH.a cells were transfected with −641 CART-LUC (a construct containing the proximal promoter region of the CART gene and the luciferase gene as a marker for promoter activity) and incubated in the presence of CRF alone or with combinations of H89 (an inhibitor of protein-kinase A) and CP154,526 (a selective antagonist to the CRF-R1). Luciferase expression was increased after CRF treatment, and the increase was reduced by H89. The response was CRF specific, because CP154,526 caused a significant reduction of luciferase activity after CRF treatment. Taken together, these data suggest that a naturally occurring peptide neurotransmitter (CRF) can influence CART expression in CATH.a cells and supports the hypothesis that CART transcriptional regulation occurs in neurons via the camp/protein kinase A pathway.[52] The utilization of a promoter-luciferase construct demonstrates true transcriptional regulation rather than simply showing a change in mRNA levels.

Acknowledgments This work is supported by National Institutes of Health grants RR00165, DA00418, DA10732, and DA15162.

References

1. Kuhar MJ, Adams S, Dominguez G, Jaworski J, Balkan B. CART peptides. *Neuropeptides*. 2002;36:1-8.
2. Hunter RG, Kuhar MJ. CART peptides as targets for CNS drug development. *Curr Drug Targets CNS Neurol Disord*. 2003;2:201-205.
3. Jaworski JN, Vicentic A, Hunter RG, Kimmel HL, Kuhar MJ. CART peptides are modulators of mesolimbic dopamine and psychostimulants. *Life Sci*. 2003;73:741-747.
4. Hunter RG, Philpot K, Vicentic A, Dominguez G, Hubert GW, Kuhar MJ. CART in feeding and obesity. *Trends Endocrinol Metab*. 2004;15:454-459.
5. Louis J, inventor. Methods of preventing neuron degeneration and promoting neuron regeneration.. Amgen, International Patent Application. Publication #WO96/34619. 1996
6. Thim L, Kristensen P, Larsen PJ, Wulff BS. CART, a new anorectic peptide. *Int J Biochem Cell Biol*. 1998;30:1281-1284.
7. Kimmel HL, Thim L, Kuhar MJ. Activity of various CART peptides in changing locomotor activity in the rat. *Neuropeptides*. 2002;36:9-12.
8. Kuhar MJ, Adams LD, Hunter RG, Vechia SD, Smith Y. CART peptides. *Regul Pept*. 2000;89:1-6.
9. Spiess J, Villarreal J, Vale W. Isolation and sequence analysis of a somatostatin-like polypeptide from ovine hypothalamus. *Biochemistry*. 1981;20:1982-1988.
10. Douglass J, McKinzie AA, Couceyro P. PCR differential display identifies a rat brain mRNA that is transcriptionally regulated by cocaine and amphetamine. *J Neurosci*. 1995;15:2471-2481.
11. Kuhar MJ, Yoho LL. CART peptide analysis by Western blotting. *Synapse*. 1999;33:163-171.
12. Dey A, Xhu X, Carroll R, Turck CW, Stein J, Steiner DF. Biological processing of the cocaine and amphetamine-regulated transcript precursors by prohormone convertases, PC2 and PC1/3. *J Biol Chem*. 2003;278:15007-15014.
13. Koylu EO, Couceyro PR, Lambert PD, Ling NC, DeSouza EB, Kuhar MJ. Immunohistochemical localization of novel CART peptides in rat hypothalamus, pituitary and adrenal gland. *J Neuroendocrinol*. 1997;9:823-833.
14. Koylu EO, Couceyro PR, Lambert PD, Kuhar MJ. Cocaine- and amphetamine-regulated transcript peptide immunohistochemical localization in the rat brain. *J Comp Neurol*. 1998;391:115-132.
15. Smith Y, Koylu EO, Couceyro P, Kuhar MJ. Ultrastructural localization of CART (cocaine- and amphetamine-regulated transcript) peptides in the nucleus accumbens of monkeys. *Synapse*. 1997;27:90-94.
16. Smith Y, Kieval J, Couceyro PR, Kuhar MJ. CART peptide-immunoreactive neurones in the nucleus accumbens in monkeys: ultrastructural analysis, colocalization studies, and synaptic interactions with dopaminergic afferents. *J Comp Neurol*. 1999;407:491-511.
17. Ekblad E, Kuhar M, Wierup N, Sundler F. Cocaine- and amphetamine-regulated transcript: distribution and function in rat gastrointestinal tract. *Neurogastroenterol Motil*. 2003;15:545-557.
18. Ellis LM, Mawe GM. Distribution and chemical coding of cocaine- and amphetamine-regulated transcript peptide (CART)-immunoreactive neurons in the guinea pig bowel. *Cell Tissue Res*. 2003;312:265-274.

19. Wierup N, Kuhar M, Nilsson BO, Mulder H, Ekblad E, Sundler F. Cocaine- and amphetamine-regulated transcript (CART) is expressed in several islet cell types during rat development. *J Histochem Cytochem.* 2004;52:169-177.

20. Wierup N, Yang S, McEvilly RJ, et al. Ghrelin is expressed in a novel endocrine cell type in developing rat islets and inhibits insulin secretion from INS-1 (832/13) cells. *J Histochem Cytochem.* 2004;52:301-310.

21. Kobayashi Y, Jimenez-Krassel F, Li Q, et al. Evidence that cocaine- and amphetamine-regulated transcript is a novel intraovarian regulator of follicular atresia. *Endocrinology.* 2004;145:5373-5383.

22. Dun SL, Castellino SJ, Yang J, Chang JK, Dun NJ. Cocaine- and amphetamine-regulated transcript peptide-immunoreactivity in dorsal motor nucleus of the vagus neurons of immature rats. *Brain Res Dev, Brain Res.* 2001;131:93-102.

23. Vicentic A, Dominguez G, Hunter RG, Philpot K, Wilson M, Kuhar MJ. CART peptide levels in blood exhibit a diurnal rhythm: regulation by glucocorticoids. *Endocrinology.* 2004;145:4119-4124.

24. Yermolaieva O, Chen J, Couceyro PR, Hoshi T. Cocaine- and amphetamine-regulated transcript peptide modulation of voltage-gated Ca2+ signaling in hippocampal neurons. *J Neurosci.* 2001;21:7474-7480.

25. Davidowa H, Li Y, Plagemann A. Altered responses to orexigenic (AGRP, MCH) and anorexigenic (alpha-MSH, CART) neuropeptides of paraventricular hypothalamic neurons in early postnatally overfed rats. *Eur J Neurosci.* 2003;18:613-621.

26. Chaki S, Kawashima N, Suzuki Y, Shimazaki T, Okuyama S. Cocaine- and amphetamine-regulated transcript peptide produces anxiety-like behavior in rodents. *Eur J Pharmacol.* 2003;464:49-54.

27. Vrang N, Tang-Christensen M, Larsen PJ, Kristensen P. Recombinant CART peptide induces c-Fos expression in central areas involved in control of feeding behaviour. *Brain Res.* 1999;818:499-509.

28. Murphy KG, Abbott CR, Mahmoudi M, et al. Quantification and synthesis of cocaine- and amphetamine-regulated transcript peptide (79-102)-like immunoreactivity and mRNA in rat tissues. *J Endocrinol.* 2000;166:659-668.

29. Lambert P, Couceyro P, Koylu E, Ling N, DeSouza E, Kuhar M. A role for novel CART peptide fragments in the central control of food intake. *Neuropeptides.* 1997;31:620-621.

30. Lambert PD, Couceyro PR, McGirr KM, Dall Vechia SE, Smith Y, Kuhar MJ. CART peptides in the central control of feeding and interactions with neuropeptide Y. *Synapse.* 1998;29:293-298.

31. Kristensen P, Judge ME, Thim L, et al. Hypothalamic CART is a new anorectic peptide regulated by leptin. *Nature.* 1998;393:72-76.

32. Brenz Verca MS, Widmer DA, Wagner GC, Dreyer J. Cocaine-induced expression of the tetraspanin CD81 and its relation to hypothalamic function. *Mol Cell Neurosci.* 2001;17:303-316.

33. Fagergren P, Hurd YL. Mesolimbic gender differences in peptide CART mRNA expression: effects of cocaine. *Neuroreport.* 1999;10:3449-3452.

34. Vrang N, Larsen PJ, Kristensen P. Cocaine-amphetamine regulated transcript (CART) expression is not regulated by amphetamine. *Neuroreport.* 2002;13:1215-1218.

35. Marie-Claire C, Laurendeau I, Canestrelli C, et al. Fos but not Cart (cocaine and amphetamine regulated transcript) is overexpressed by several drugs of abuse: a comparative study using real-time quantitative polymerase chain reaction in rat brain. *Neurosci Lett.* 2003;345:77-80.

36. Dallvechia-Adams S, Kuhar MJ, Smith Y. Cocaine- and amphetamine-regulated transcript peptide projections in the ventral midbrain: Colocalization with gamma-aminobutyric acid, melanin-concentrating hormone, dynorphin, and synaptic interactions with dopamine neurons. *J Comp Neurol.* 2002;448:360-372.

37. Beaudry G, Zekki H, Rouillard C, Levesque D. Clozapine and dopamine D3 receptor antisense reduce cocaine- and amphetamine-regulated transcript expression in the rat nucleus accumbens shell. *Synapse.* 2004;51:233-240.

38. Smith Y, Pare JF, Pare D. Cat intraamygdaloid inhibitory network: ultrastructural organization of parvalbumin-immunoreactive elements. *J Comp Neurol*. 1998;391:164-179.
39. Tang WX, Fasulo WH, Mash DC, Hemby SE. Molecular profiling of midbrain dopamine regions in cocaine overdose victims. *J Neurochem*. 2003;85:911-924.
40. Albertson DN, Pruetz B, Schmidt CJ, Kuhn DM, Kapatos G, Bannon MJ. Gene expression profile of the nucleus accumbens of human cocaine abusers: evidence for dysregulation of myelin. *J Neurochem*. 2004;88:1211-1219.
41. Kimmel HL, Gong W, Vechia SD, Hunter RG, Kuhar MJ. Intra-ventral tegmental area injection of rat cocaine and amphetamine- regulated transcript peptide 55-102 induces locomotor activity and promotes conditioned place preference. *J Pharmacol Exp Ther*. 2000;294:784-792.
42. Jaworski JN, Kozel MA, Philpot KB, Kuhar MJ. Intra-accumbal injection of CART (cocaine-amphetamine regulated transcript) peptide reduces cocaine-induced locomotor activity. *J Pharmacol Exp Ther*. 2003;307:1038-1044.
43. Kim JH, Creekmore E, Vezina P. Microinjection of CART peptide 55-102 into the nucleus accumbens blocks amphetamine-induced locomotion. *Neuropeptides*. 2003;37:369-373.
44. Shieh K. Effects of the cocaine- and amphetamine-regulated transcript peptide on the turnover of central dopaminergic neurons. *Neuropharmacology*. 2003;44:940-948.
45. Yang S-C, Pan J-T, Li H-Y. CART peptide increases the mesolimbic dopaminergic neuronal activity: A microdialysis study. *Eur J Pharmacol*. 2004;494:179-182.
46. Staley JK, Mash DC. Adaptive increase in D3 dopamine receptors in the brain reward circuits of human cocaine fatalities. *J Neurosci*. 1996;16:6100-6106.
47. Richtand NM, Logue AD, Welge JA, et al. The dopamine D3 receptor antagonist nafadotride inhibits development of locomotor sensitization to amphetamine. *Brain Res*. 2000;867:239-242.
48. Caine SB, Koob GF, Parsons LH, Everitt BJ, Schwartz JC, Sokoloff P. D3 receptor test in vitro predicts decreased cocaine self-adminstration in rats. *Neuroreport*. 1997;8:2373-2377.
49. Carlezon WA, Jr, Thome J, Olson VG, et al. Regulation of cocaine reward by CREB. *Science*. 1998;282:2272-2275.
50. Dominguez G, Lakatos A, Kuhar MJ. Characterization of the cocaine- and amphetamine-regulated transcript (CART) peptide gene promoter and its activation by a cyclic AMP-dependent signaling pathway in GH3 cells. *J Neurochem*. 2002;80:885-893.
51. Lakatos A, Dominguez G, Kuhar MJ. CART promoter CRE site binds phosphorylated CREB. *Brain Res Mol Brain Res*. 2002;104:81-85.
52. Dominguez G, Kuhar MJ. Transcriptional regulation of the CART promoter in CATH.a cells. *Brain Res Mol Brain Res*. 2004;126:22-29.
53. Barrett P, Morris MA, Moar KM, et al. The differential regulation of CART gene expression in a pituitary cell line and primary cell cultures of ovine pars tuberalis cells. *J Neuroendocrinol*. 2001;13:347-352.
54. Barrett P, Davidson J, Morgan P, et al. CART gene promoter transcription is regulated by a cyclic adenosine monophosphate response element: the differential regulation of CART gene expression in a pituitary cell line and primary cell cultures of ovine pars tuberalis cells. *Obes Res*. 2002;10:1291-1298.
55. Jung SK, Hong MS, Suh GJ, et al. Association between polymorphism in intron 1 of cocaine- and amphetamine-regulated transcript gene with alcoholism, but not with bipolar disorder and schizophrenia in Korean population. *Neurosci Lett*. 2004;365: 54-57.
56. Goeders NE. Stress and cocaine addiction. *J Pharmacol Exp Ther*. 2002;301:785-789.
57. Goeders NE. The HPA axis and cocaine reinforcement. *Psychoneuroendocrinology*. 2002;27:13-33.
58. Yamada K, Yuan X, Otabe S, Koyanagi A, Koyama W, Makita Z. Sequencing of the putative promoter region of the cocaine- and amphetamine-regulated-transcript gene and identification of polymorphic sites associated with obesity. *Int J Obes Relat Metab Disord*. 2002;26:132-136.
59. del Giudice EM, Santoro N, Cirillo G, D'Urso L, Di Toro R, Perrone L. Mutational screening of the CART gene in obese children: identifying a mutation (Leu34Phe) associated with

reduced resting energy expenditure and cosegregating with obesity phenotype in a large family. *Diabetes*. 2001;50:2157-2160.

60. Yanik T, Dominguez G, Kuhar MJ, Loh YP. Mutant Leu34Phe Pro-CART in obese humans is missorted, poorly processed and constituvely secreted in endocrine cells. *Annual Meeting the Endocrine Society, ENDO 2004*. 2004.

61. Asnicar MA, Smith DP, Yang DD, et al. Absence of cocaine- and amphetamine-regulated transcript results in obesity in mice fed a high caloric diet. *Endocrinology*. 2001;142:4394-4400.

62. Balkan B, Koylu EO, Kuhar MJ, Pogun S. The effect of adrenalectomy on cocaine and amphetamine-regulated transcript (CART) expression in the hypothalamic nuclei of the rat. *Brain Res*. 2001;917:15-20.

63. Balkan B, Koylu E, Pogun S, Kuhar MJ. Effects of adrenalectomy on CART expression in the rat arcuate nucleus. *Synapse*. 2003;50:14-19.

64. Vrang N, Larsen PJ, Kristensen P, Tang-Christensen M. Central administration of cocaine-amphetamine-regulated transcript activates hypothalamic neuroendocrine neurons in the rat. *Endocrinology*. 2000;141:794-801.

65. Sarkar S, Wittmann G, Fekete C, Lechan RM. Central administration of cocaine- and amphetamine-regulated transcript increases phosphorylation of cAMP response element binding protein in corticotropin-releasing hormone-producing neurons but not in prothyrotropin-releasing hormone-producing neurons in the hypothalamic paraventricular nucleus. *Brain Res*. 2004;999:181-192.

66. Damaj MI, Martin BR, Kuhar MJ. Antinociceptive effects of supraspinal rat cart (55–102) peptide in mice. *Brain Res*. 2003;983:233-236.

67. Damaj MI, Hunter RG, Martin BR, Kuhar MJ. Intrathecal CART (55–102) enhances the spinal analgesic actions of morphine in mice. *Brain Res*. 2004;1024:146-149.

68. Ohsawa M, Dun SL, Tseng LF, Chang J, Dun NJ. Decrease of hindpaw withdrawal latency by cocaine- and amphetamine- regulated transcript peptide to the mouse spinal cord. *Eur J Pharmacol*. 2000;399:165-169.

69. Larsen PJ, Seier V, Fink-Jensen A, Holst JJ, Warberg J, Vrang N. Cocaine- and amphetamine-regulated transcript is present in hypothalamic neuroendocrine neurones and is released to the hypothalamic-pituitary portal circuit. *J Neuroendocrinol*. 2003;15:219-226.

70. Baranowska B, Wolinska-Witort E, Chmielowska M, Martynska L, Baranowska-Bik A. Direct effects of cocaine-amphetamine-regulated transcript (CART) on pituitary hormone release in pituitary cell culture. *Neuroendocrinol Lett*. 2003;24:224-226.

71. Shieh KR. Effects of the cocaine- and amphetamine-regulated transcript peptide on the turnover of central dopaminergic neurons. *Neuropharmacology*. 2003;44:940-948.

72. Kuriyama G, Takekoshi S, Tojo K, Nakai Y, Kuhar MJ, Osamura RY. Cocaine- and amphetamine-regulated transcript Peptide in the rat anterior pituitary gland is localized in gonadotrophs and suppresses prolactin secretion. *Endocrinology*. 2004;145:2542-2550.

73. Brischoux F, Griffond B, Fellmann D, Risold PY. Early and transient ontogenetic expression of the cocaine- and amphetamine-regulated transcript peptide in the rat mesencephalon: correlation with tyrosine hydroxylase expression. *J Neurobiol*. 2002;52:221-229.

74. Hunter R, Kuhar M. Dopaminergic regulation of CART mRNA in the nucleus accumbens. *Soc Neurosci Abs*. 2003;889:21.

75. Abarca C, Albrecht U, Spanagel R. Cocaine sensitization and reward are under the influence of circadian genes and rhythm. *Proc Natl Acad Sci U S A*. 2002;99:9026-9030.

76. Elias CF, Lee C, Kelly J, et al. Leptin activates hypothalamic CART neurons projecting to the spinal cord. *Neuron*. 1998;21:1375-1385.

77. Thiel G, Cibelli G. Corticotropin-releasing factor and vasoactive intestinal polypeptide activate gene transcription through the cAMP signaling pathway in a catecholaminergic immortalized neuron. *Neurochem Int*. 1999;34:183-191.

Chapter 7
RNAi-Directed Inhibition of DC-SIGN by Dendritic Cells: Prospects for HIV-1 Therapy

Madhavan P.N. Nair,[1] Jessica L. Reynolds,[1] Supriya D. Mahajan,[1] Stanley A. Schwartz,[1] Ravikumar Aalinkeel,[1] B. Bindukumar,[1] and Don Sykes[1]

Abstract Drug-resistant human immunodeficiency virus (HIV) infections are increasing globally, especially in North America. Therefore, it is logical to develop new therapies directed against HIV binding molecules on susceptible host cells in addition to current treatment modalities against virus functions. Inhibition of the viral genome can be achieved by degrading or silencing posttranslational genes using small interfering (si) ribonucleic acids (RNAs) consisting of double-stranded forms of RNA. These siRNAs usually contain 21–23 base pairs (bp) and are highly specific for the nucleotide sequence of the target messenger RNA (mRNA). These siRNAs form a complex with helicase and nuclease enzymes known as "RNA-induced silencing complex" (RISC) that leads to target RNA degradation. Thus, siRNA has become a method of selective destruction of HIV now used by various investigators around the globe. However, given the sequence diversity of the HIV genomes of infected subjects, it is difficult to target a specific HIV sequence. Therefore, targeting nonvariable HIV binding receptors on susceptible cells or other molecules of host cells that are directly or indirectly involved in HIV infections may be an interesting alternative to targeting the virus itself. Thus, the simultaneous use of siRNAs specific for HIV and host cells may be a unique, new approach to the therapy of HIV infections. In this article, we present evidence that siRNA directed at the CD4 independent attachment receptor (DC-SIGN) significantly inhibits HIV infection of dendritic cells (DCs). This effect may be mediated by modulation of p38 mitogen activated protein kinase (MAPK).

Keywords siRNA, DC-SIGN, HIV-1, dendritic cells, co-stimulatory molecules, HIV-LTR/U5, MAPK

---

[1] Department of Medicine, Division of Allergy, Immunology and Rheumatology, State University of New York at Buffalo, Buffalo General Hospital, 100 High Street, Buffalo, NY 14203

Corresponding Author: Madhavan P.N. Nair, Professor, Department of Medicine, Division of Allergy, Immunology and Rheumatology, Buffalo General Hospital, 100 High Street, Buffalo, NY 14203. Tel: (716) 859-2985; Fax: (716) 859-2999; E-mail: mnair@buffalo.edu

R.S. Rapaka and W. Sadée (eds.), *Drug Addiction.*
© American Association of Pharmaceutical Scientists 2008

Introduction

RNA interference (i), using small interfering (si) RNAs,[1] provides a methodology for analyzing the role of cellular and viral regulatory factors in the human immuno-deficiency virus (HIV) life cycle. RNAi is an evolutionarily conserved mechanism that is operative in insects, nematodes, plants, and mammalian cells.[2-5] In this process, sequence-specific, posttranscriptional silencing is initiated by the introduction into cells of double-stranded, annealed, sense and antisense RNAs that are homologous to the sequence of the silenced gene.[6] The ultimate mediators of RNAi-induced degradation are 21-(mer) siRNAs generated by RNase III cleavage of double-stranded RNAs extending up to several hundred nucleotides that had been introduced into cells.[7,8] To use RNAi in mammalian systems, 21-mer sense and antisense RNA oligonucleotides homologous to a portion of the gene of interest are synthesized, annealed, and introduced into cells by transfection.[2,4,5] These siRNAs bind specifically to the cellular messenger (m) RNA of interest and activate an RNA degradation process that leads to an 80% to 90% decrease in the levels of the corresponding protein. Thus, RNAi can be used to silence the gene of interest but not other genes.[9] The exquisite selectivity of RNAi makes its clinical applications almost endless because virtually any gene whose expression may contribute to disease is a potential target. For RNA-based therapies, delivery, stability, and potency have been the most significant obstacles. Attempts to develop antisense drugs have been largely disappointing. Antisense is a single strand of RNA or deoxy-ribonucleic acid (DNA), complementary to a target mRNA sequence; pairing it up with the antisense strand prevents translation of the mRNA. Pairing of the antisense oligonucleotide with the mRNA prevents subsequent translation of the latter. Early studies suggested that antisense drugs effectively reduced viral loads in clinical trials. However, closer examination revealed that these results were largely due to an increase in production of interferons by the host in response to high doses of exog-enous RNA, rather than to specific silencing of any target genes. This realization led to disillusionment with antisense therapy. The emergence of the RNAi technology and the realization of its potential as a more effective way to silence gene expression have led to rapid progress in the evolution of this technology in recent years. The extraordinary selectivity of RNAi, combined with its potency (that is, only a few double-stranded RNAs are needed per cell), quickly made it the tool of choice for functional genomics and for targeted drug discovery and validation. By "knocking down" a gene with RNAi and determining the subsequent effect on cells, a researcher can, in the course of only a few days, develop significant insight into the function of the gene and determine if reducing its expression will be therapeutically useful. Whether or not RNAi has a better chance to succeed as a drug than the antisense therapy will ultimately be determined by clinical trials. RNAi technology is several orders of magnitude more potent at gene silencing than antisense technology because RNAi harnesses an endogenous, natural pathway.

Since RNAi was first recognized by Fire et al in 1998,[1] it has quickly become a powerful tool for HIV research. Several investigators have used siRNA specific for HIV genes to inhibit viral replication. These include siRNA specific for nef, gag, vif, tat, and rev genes.[10-14] However, given the significant sequence diversity of the HIV genome in infected subjects, it is difficult to target specific HIV sequences. Consequently, for potential therapeutic targets, investigators have turned to RNAi specific for critical genes of the host involved in the pathogenesis of HIV infections, such as the HIV receptor, CD4,[12,15,16] and the HIV co-receptors, CXCR4[15-18] and CCR5.[15,16,18,19] These studies have yielded some positive results in inhibiting HIV replication.

The novel dendritic cell (DC)–specific HIV-1 receptor, DC-SIGN, a C-type lectin, plays a key role in primary defense against HIV infection as well as in the dissemination of HIV-1 by DCs. DCs are essential for the early events of the immune response to HIV infection. Model systems of HIV sexual transmission show that DCs expressing DC-SIGN capture and internalize HIV at mucosal surfaces and are the first line of defense against HIV infection. Moreover, DCs efficiently transfer HIV to CD4+ T cells in lymph nodes, where subsequent viral replication occurs. DC-SIGN knockdown by siRNA in DCs selectively impairs infectious synapse formation between DCs and resting CD4+ T cells, but does not prevent the formation of DC–T cell conjugates. It was demonstrated that DC-SIGN is required downstream from viral capture for the formation of the infectious synapse between DCs and T cells.[20,21] DCs were unable to transfer HIV-1 infectivity to T cells in trans, demonstrating an essential role for the DC-SIGN receptor in transferring infectious viral particles from DCs to T cells.[20,21] Thus, the role of DC-SIGN in the transfer of HIV from DCs to T cells, a crucial step for HIV transmission and pathogenesis, is well established.

DCs also regulate the surface expression of the co-stimulatory molecules B7-1 and B7-2 (CD80 and CD86), which engage the CD28 molecule on the T cell. Optimal T-cell activation and viral replication occurs when the naive T cell receives 2 signals: the primary signal through the T-cell receptor recognizing foreign antigens; and the second signal through the B7-CD28 interaction.[22] Such a stimulus activates a cascade of genes, such as NFκB and mitogen activated protein kinase (MAPK), that lead to clonal expansion of antigen-specific T cells by binding to the viral promoter/enhancer (LTR), and driving high levels of transcription and consequently explosive virus production.[23] The current studies were undertaken to determine if DC-SIGN silencing modifies the expression of co-stimulatory molecules on the surface of DCs. In the present study, monocyte-derived, mature dendritic cells were transfected with siRNA specific for DC-SIGN. The kinetics of DC-SIGN gene suppression was investigated. Furthermore, the effects of DC-SIGN gene silencing on the expression of co-stimulatory molecules and HIV infectivity of DCs also were studied.

Materials and Methods

Purification of DCs

DCs were prepared as described by Dauer et al in 2002.[24] Briefly, human peripheral blood mononuclear cells (PBMCs) were isolated by density gradient centrifugation on Ficoll-Paque (Amersham Pharmacia Biotech, Piscataway, NJ). CD14$^+$ monocytes were separated from PBMCs using plastic adherence; the monocytes were cultured in RPMI 1640 with 1% human, AB serum, 500 U/mL recombinant human interleukin-4 (IL-4; R&D Systems, Minneapolis, MN), and 1000 U/mL recombinant human granulocyte-macrophage colony-stimulating factor (GMCSF; Amgen, Thousand Oaks, CA) for 24 hours. DCs were allowed to mature by culturing for an additional 2 days in the presence of interleukin-1β (IL-1β, R&D Systems), interleukin-6 (IL-6, R&D Systems), tumor necrosis factor (TNF, R&D Systems) and prostaglandin E$_2$ (PGE$_2$; Sigma-Aldrich, St Louis, MO). Maturation cytokines were added at final concentrations of IL-1β, 10 ng/mL; IL-6, 1000 U/mL; TNF, 10 ng/mL, and PGE$_2$, 1 μg/mL. Maturation of DCs was verified by CD83$^+$ and major histocompatibility complex (MHC-HLA-DR, DQ-DP) marker staining.

siRNA Sequences (DC-SIGN)

The following are the sequences of the various siRNAs used: DC-SIGN antisense, 5'- ATTTGTCGTCGTTCCAGCCAT-3'; DC-SIGN sense, 5'-ATGGCTGGAACG ACACAAA-3'; DC-SIGN antisense scrambled control, 5'-CACACCACATCTTT CCGTCAC-3': DC-SIGN sense scrambled control, 5'-GTGACGGAAAGATGT GGGTG-3. RNA oligonucleotides were custom synthesized by Dharmacon Research Inc (Lafayette, CO) with an overhang of 2 thymidine residues (dTdT) at the 3' end. The RNA oligonucleotides were dissolved in Tris-EDTA (10 mM Tris-HCl, pH 8.0; and 1 mM EDTA) as 200 μM solutions and were stored at −20°C. Double-stranded siRNA molecules were generated by mixing the corresponding pair of sense and antisense RNA oligonucleotides in annealing buffer (30 mM HEPES-KOH, pH 7.9; 100 mM potassium acetate; and 2 mM magnesium acetate) at 20 μM and then by incubating the reaction mixture at 95°C for 2 minutes, followed by gradually cooling to room temperature. The siRNAs were then aliquoted and stored at −20°C.

Transfection of siRNAs

Twenty-four hours before siRNA transfection, 1×10^5 DCs were seeded in 6-well plates in OPTI-minimal essential medium (OptiMEM; Invitrogen, Grand Island, NY) containing 10% Fetal Bovine Serum (FBS) with no antibiotics. Cells were seeded per 6-well plate to give 30% to 50% confluency at the time of the transfection. The siRNAs were transfected at a final concentration of 50 nM using Oligofectamine (Invitrogen) according to the manufacturer's recommendations. The control (untransfected) cells received either Oligofectamine alone or Oligofectamine plus scrambled sequence. The siRNAs added to control cells were incubated for 24, 48, and 72 hours, and the cells were harvested and RNA was extracted.

RNA Extraction

Cytoplasmic RNA was extracted by an acid guanidinium-thiocyanate-phenol-chloroform method as described.[25] Cultured DCs were centrifuged and resuspended in a 4 M solution of guanidinium thiocyanate. Cells were lysed by repeated pipetting and then phenol-chloroform extracted in the presence of sodium acetate. After centrifugation, RNA was precipitated from the aqueous layer by adding an equal volume of isopropanol and the mixture was kept at −20°C for 1 hour and then centrifuged to sediment the RNA. The RNA pellet was washed with 75% ethanol to remove any traces of guanidinium. The final pellet was dried and resuspended in diethyl pyrocarbonate (DEPC) water and the amount of RNA determined using a spectrophotometer at 260 nm. DNA contamination in the RNA preparation was removed by treating the RNA preparation with DNAse (1 IU/μg of RNA) for 2 hours at 37°C, followed by proteinase K digestion at 37°C for 15 minutes and subsequent extraction with phenol-chloroform and NH$_4$OAc/ETOH precipitation. DNA contamination of the RNA preparation was checked by including a control in which reverse transcriptase enzyme was not added in the polymerase chain reaction (PCR) amplification procedure. RNA devoid of any DNA contamination was used in subsequent experiments with semiquantitative PCR. The isolated RNA was stored at −70°C until used.

Real-Time Quantitative PCR

DC-SIGN, CD80, CD86, CD40, p38, and LTR- R/U5 gene expression were quantitated using real-time PCR using specific primers. Table 7.1 shows the primer sequences of the primers used in this study (All the primer sequences designed are

Table 7.1 List of Primer Sequences

Primer	PCR Product Size	Primer Sequence
β-Actin	[548 bp]	5' 5'-TGACGGGGTCACCCACACTGTGCCCATCTA-3'
		3' 5-AGTCATAGTCCGCCTAGAAGCATTTGCGGT-3'
DC-SIGN	[205 bp]	5' 5'-GAAGACTGCGCGGAATTTAG −3'
		3' 5'-TCGAAGGATGGAGAGAAGGA -3'
HIV-LTR-R/U5	[180 bp]	5' 5'-TCT CTC TGG TTA GAC CAG ATC TG-3'
		3' 5'-ACT GCT AGA GAT TTT CCA CAC TG-3'
p38 MAPK	[560 bp]	5' 5'-GGCAGGAGCTGAACAAGACAA-3'
		3' 5'-TTCAGCATGATCTCAGGAGCC -3'
CD80	[216 bp]	5'5'-GGGAAAGTGTACGCCCTGTA-3'
		3' 5'-GCTACTTCTGTGCCCACCAT-3'
CD86	[406 bp]	5'5'-ACAAAAAGCCCACAGGAATG-3'
		3' 5'-ATCCAAGGAATGTGGTCTGG-3'
CD40	[156 bp]	5'5'-CCACTGGGTATGGTGGTTTC-3'
		3' 5'-TCACCTTCTGCCTCCTGTCT-3'

proprietary). The relative abundance of each mRNA species was assessed using the SYBR green master mix from Stratagene (La Jolla, CA) to perform real-time quantitative PCR using the ABI Prism 5700 instrument that detects and plots the increase in fluorescence versus PCR cycle number, thus yielding a continuous measure of PCR amplification. To provide precise quantification of initial target in each PCR reaction, the amplification plot is examined at a point during the early log phase of product accumulation. This is accomplished by assigning a fluorescence threshold above background and determining the time point at which each sample's amplification plot reaches the threshold (defined as the threshold cycle number or C_T). Differences in threshold cycle number are used to quantify the relative amount of PCR target contained within each tube. Relative expression of mRNA species was calculated using the comparative C_T method as described.[26]

Infection of DCs with HIV-1 Isolates

DCs were infected with HIV-1$_{Ba-L}$ (NIH AIDS Research and Reference Reagent Program, Cat# 510) at a concentration of $10^{3.75}$ TCID$_{50}$/mL cells for 3 hours at 37°C. Cells were washed and cultured for an additional 24 hours, and supernatants were collected for p24 analysis and cells were collected for RNA analysis. The HIV-LTR-R/U5 region was amplified by real-time quantitative PCR using primers specific for a 180–base pair (bp) fragment of the region as described.[27] This method is designed to detect early stages of reverse transcription of HIV.

Results

Kinetics of DC-SIGN Silencing

DCs were transfected with DC-SIGN siRNA. Cells were harvested and RNA was extracted at 24, 48, and 72 hours following transfection. DC-SIGN gene expression was determined using real-time semiquantitative PCR. Results are expressed as the transcript accumulation index (TAI) with respect to the untransfected control. Data (Fig. 7.1) demonstrate a 76% (TAI = 0.24 ± 0.078; $P < .001$), 66% (TAI = 0.34 ± 0.66; $P < .001$), and 53% (TAI = 0.47 ± 0.17; $P < .001$) inhibition of DC-SIGN expression in DCs transfected for 24, 48, and 72 hours respectively, compared with control, scrambled siRNA transfected cells. Scrambled siRNA had no effect on DC-SIGN gene expression and was similar to the untreated control culture (data not shown). These results demonstrate that DC-SIGN siRNA was effective in silencing gene expression in a time-dependent manner.

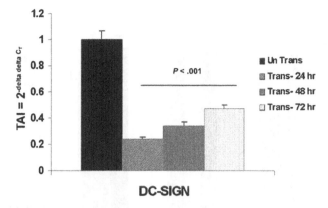

Fig. 7.1 Kinetics of DC-SIGN siRNA transfection of DCs on DC-SIGN gene expression. DCs $(1 \times 10^5$ cells/mL) were cultured in the absence or presence of DC-SIGN siRNA (50 nM) for 24, 48, and 72 hours. RNA was extracted and reverse transcribed, and DC-SIGN gene expression was analyzed by real-time quantitative PCR. Statistical significance was calculated by Student's 't' test (n = 2). (Un Trans indicates untransfected control; Trans indicates Transfected.)

Effect of DC-SIGN Silencing on Co-stimulatory Molecule Expression

We examined whether silencing DC-SIGN also modulates the expression of co-stimulatory molecules by DCs. DCs were transfected with DC-SIGN siRNA; RNA was extracted following transfection; and CD40, CD80, and CD86 gene expression was determined. Data presented in Figure 7.2 show that 24 hours following transfection with DC-SIGN–specific siRNA, a 43% inhibition of CD40 gene expression occurred (TAI = 0.57 ± 0.19, $P < .001$); while a 12% inhibition of CD40 gene expression was observed at 48 and 72 hours of incubation (TAI = 0.88 ± 0.01, 48 hours; 0.88 ± 0.21, 72 hours; $P < .05$). Inhibition of CD80 expression was 48% (TAI = 0.52 ± 0.04, $P < .001$) at 24 hours and 4% (TAI = 0.96 ± 0.03, $P = $ not significant [NS]) at 48 hours. Whereas, no inhibition of CD80 gene expression occurred at 72 hours, which was comparable to control values (TAI = 1.04 ± 0.07 vs TAI = 1.00 ± 0.04, $P = $ NS). A 26% (TAI = 0.74 ± 0.02, $P < .01$), 14% (TAI = 0.86 ± 0.04, $P < .05$), and 18% (TAI = 0.82 ± 0.04, $P < .05$) inhibition of CD86 gene expression occurred at 24, 48, and 72 hours, respectively (Fig. 7.2). Scrambled siRNA had no effect on CD40, CD80, and CD86 gene expression (data not shown). These results show that silencing of DC-SIGN gene expression with siRNA also decreased the gene expression of the co-stimulatory molecules, CD40, CD80, and CD86.

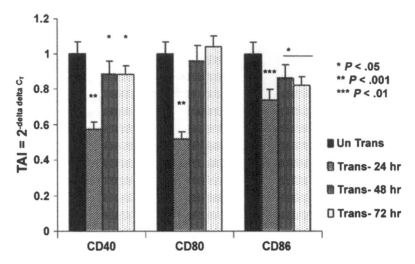

Fig. 7.2 Kinetics of DC-SIGN siRNA transfection of DCs on the gene expression of the co-stimulatory molecules, CD40, CD80, and CD86. DCs (1×10^5 cells/mL) were cultured with or without DC-SIGN siRNA (50 nM) for 24, 48, and 72 hours. RNA was extracted and reverse transcribed, and CD40, CD80, and CD86 gene expression was analyzed by real-time quantitative PCR. Statistical significance was calculated by Student's 't' test (n = 2). (Un Trans indicates untransfected control; Trans indicates Transfected.)

Effect of DC-SIGN Silencing on Signaling Molecule Expression

We investigated whether silencing DC-SIGN modulates the expression of the intracellular signaling protein, p38 MAPK in DCs. Data presented in Fig. 7.3 show the effect of DC-SIGN–specific siRNA on the gene expression of p38 MAPK by DCs at 24, 48, and 72 hours as determined by real-time semiquantitative PCR. Data demonstrate a 31% (TAI = 0.69 ± 0.06, $P < .05$) inhibition of p38 MAPK gene expression at 24 hours and a 28% (TAI = 0.72 ± 0.12, $P < .05$) inhibition at 48 hours. At 72 hours, the p38 MAPK gene expression was comparable to the untransfected, control culture (TAI = 1.05 ± 0.07 vs TAI =1.00 ± 0.13, P = NS). Scrambled siRNA had no effect on p38 MAPK gene expression (data not shown). These results demonstrate that silencing of DC-SIGN gene expression with specific siRNA also decreased the gene expression of the signaling molecule p38 MAPK.

Effect of DC-SIGN siRNA on p24 Levels and HIV-LTR-R/U5 Gene Expression

We examined whether siRNA-directed inhibition of DC-SIGN decreased the levels of p24 antigen production and HIV-LTR gene expression by HIV infected cells. DCs were transfected with DC-SIGN siRNA for 24 hours, then infected with HIV-1$_{BA-L}$.

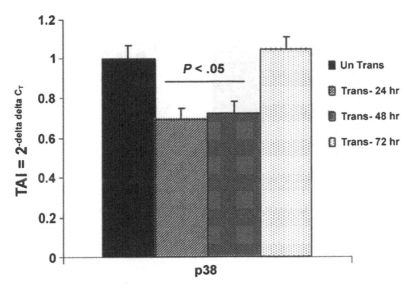

Fig. 7.3 Kinetics of DC-SIGN siRNA transfection of DCs on the gene expression of p38 MAPK. DCs (1×10^5 cells/mL) were cultured with or without DC-SIGN siRNA for 24, 48, and 72 hours. RNA was extracted and reverse transcribed, and p38 MAPK gene expression was analyzed by real-time quantitative PCR. Statistical significance was calculated by Student's 't' test (n = 2). (Un Trans indicates untransfected control; Trans indicates Transfected.)

Twenty-four hours after infection, culture supernatants were assayed for p24 using ELISA and HIV-LTR-R/U5 region gene expression by real-time semiquantitative PCR. A 76% inhibition of p24 levels (Fig. 7.4A) following DC-SIGN gene silencing was observed in harvested culture supernatants (3.95 pg/mL, $P < .009$) compared with untransfected, control cultures (17.4 pg/mL) infected with HIV. Furthermore, our results demonstrate (Fig. 7.4B) that silencing DC-SIGN gene expression also significantly (86%) inhibited HIV-LTR-R/U5 gene expression (TAI = 0.14 ± 0.07, $P < .001$) compared with untransfected control cultures infected with HIV (TAI = 1.00 ± 0.12) (Fig. 7.2). Scrambled siRNA had no effect on p24 levels or HIV-LTR-R/U5 region gene expression (data not shown). These data demonstrate that DC-SIGN–specific siRNA can inhibit significantly the production of HIV by infected DCs as demonstrated by decreases in p24 antigen production as well as HIV-LTR-R/U5 gene expression.

Discussion

Because of the sequence diversity of the HIV genome, current approaches to control HIV infection are problematic and incomplete. Although siRNA is highly specific, a change in the target mRNA by even 1 bp, can dramatically reduce the efficiency

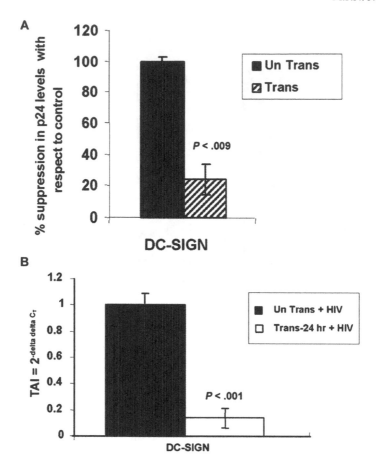

Fig. 7.4 Effects of DC-SIGN siRNA transfection on p24 levels and HIV-LTR-R/U5 region gene expression by DC. DCs (1×10^5 cells/mL) were transfected with or without DC-SIGN siRNA for 24 hours. DCs were then infected with HIV-1 $_{Ba-L}$ for 3 hours at 37°C, washed, and cultured for an additional 24 hours. (**A**) Culture supernatants were collected and assayed for p24. (**B**) RNA was extracted from cells and HIV-LTR-R/U5 gene expression was analyzed by real-time quantitative PCR. Statistical significance was calculated by Student's 't' test (n = 2). (Un Trans indicates untransfected control; Trans indicates Transfected.)

of degradation of the target mRNA. Because of the high error rate of HIV reverse transcriptase (1 in 1000 nucleotides per replication cycle), there is a high likelihood of generating siRNA escape mutants. Thus, an alternate approach is to target the stable molecules on the host cell that bind HIV-1 such as HIV-receptors, co-receptors, or CD4 independent binding structures. Furthermore, the simultaneous use of siRNA targeted at viral genes may increase the anti-HIV activities of siRNA. DC-SIGN has been shown to be the first molecule that facilitates HIV infection independent of CD4 or viral co-receptors[28-30] and thus may be an ideal target for

RNA interference. Arrighi et al[20,21] showed that DC-SIGN-negative DCs were unable to enhance transfer of HIV-1 infectivity to T cells in trans, demonstrating an essential role for DC-SIGN in the progression of HIV-1 infections. DCs increase the surface expression of the co-stimulatory molecules, CD80 and CD86, that engage the CD28 molecule on T cells.[29] Therefore, decreasing DC-SIGN gene expression also may alter the expression of these co-stimulatory molecules, further inhibiting DC–T cell interactions and the progression of HIV-1 infections. Our data demonstrate that silencing DC-SIGN decreases the gene expression of the co-stimulatory molecules CD40, CD80, and CD86 that, in turn, may inhibit the DC–T cell interactions needed for progression of HIV-1 infections.

CD80 (B7-1) and CD86 (B7-2) on DCs engage with the CD28 molecule on the T cell. This stimulus activates a cascade of genes such as MAPK, leading to clonal expansion of antigen-specific T cells and subsequently increased virus production.[23] Our studies show that siRNA induced–silencing of DC-SIGN and subsequent inhibition of co-stimulatory molecules and viral replication, as demonstrated by reduced p24 antigen production and LTR-RU- R/U5 gene expression, may be mediated by p38 MAPK inhibition.

Previous studies show that cytokines can induce differentiation or maturation of DCs.[31-34] Conflicting results were obtained on the replication of HIV-1 in DCs[35] because of differing stages of maturation. Immature DCs were found to be most susceptible to HIV infection and its progression. Frank et al[36] demonstrated that both mature and immature DCs pulsed with HIV-1 Ba-L were able to produce significant virus production as analyzed by p24 antigen expression. However, in co-cultures of DCs and T cells, virus replication was 3 times higher than in DCs alone. Ganesh et al[37] recently showed that DCs matured with poly(I-C) treatment could be transfected with HIV-1$_{ADA}$ vector. Our previous studies demonstrate that although immature DCs are a more susceptible target for HIV infection, mature DCs also show a basal level of infection with HIV and the efficiency of infection is associated with the stage of DC maturation.[38] Furthermore, we demonstrated that mature DCs transiently exposed to syngeneic T cells become highly susceptible to HIV infection (data not shown). Interestingly, RNAi against DC-SIGN decreases the gene expression of HIV-LTR-R/U5 and levels of p24 following infection with HIV BAL. These data demonstrate that for efficient HIV infection of DCs, DC-SIGN must be present, and the data further support the role of DC-SIGN in transferring infectious viral particles from DCs to T cells. Thus, designing drugs specifically silencing DC-SIGN gene expression likely will inhibit initial HIV infection of DCs and DC–T cell clustering, which, in turn, leads to subsequent infection of T cells. A long-term goal of our study is to develop novel therapeutic approaches to prevent initial binding of HIV-1 to primary target cells as a first step in inhibition of HIV-1.

Acknowledgments This work was supported in part by National Institute ib Drug Abuse (NIDA) grant numbers RO1-DA10632, RO-DA14218, RO1-DA12366 and the Margaret Duffy and Robert Cameron Troup Memorial Fund for Cancer Research of the Kaleida Health System, the Buffalo General Foundation, and the State University of New York at Buffalo.

References

1. Fire A, Xu S, Montgomery MK, Kostas SA, Driver SE, Mello CC. Potent and specific genetic interference by double-stranded RNA in Caenorhabditis elegans. *Nature.* 1998;391:806-811.
2. Caplen NJ, Parrish S, Imani F, Fire A, Morgan RA. Specific inhibition of gene expression by small double-stranded RNAs in invertebrate and vertebrate systems. *Proc Natl Acad Sci USA.* 2001;98:9742-9747.
3. Clemens JC, Worby CA, Simonson-Leff N, et al. Use of double-stranded RNA interference in Drosophila cell lines to dissect signal transduction pathways. *Proc Natl Acad Sci USA.* 2000;97:6499-6503.
4. Elbashir SM, Harborth J, Lendeckel W, Yalcin A, Weber K, Tuschl T. Duplexes of 21-nucleotide RNAs mediate RNA interference in cultured mammalian cells. *Nature.* 2001;411:494-498.
5. Elbashir SM, Lendeckel W, Tuschl T. RNA interference is mediated by 21- and 22-nucleotide RNAs. *Genes Dev.* 2001;15:188-200.
6. Bass BL. Double-stranded RNA as a template for gene silencing. *Cell.* 2000;101:235-238.
7. Hamilton AJ, Baulcombe DC. A species of small antisense RNA in posttranscriptional gene silencing in plants. *Science.* 1999;286:950-952.
8. Zamore PD, Tuschl T, Sharp PA, Bartel DP. RNAi: double-stranded RNA directs the ATP-dependent cleavage of mRNA at 21 to 23 nucleotide intervals. *Cell.* 2000;101:25-33.
9. Sodroski J, Patarca R, Rosen C, Wong-Staal F, Haseltine W. Location of the trans-activating region on the genome of human T-cell lymphotropic virus type III. *Science.* 1985;229:74-77.
10. Jacque JM, Triques K, Stevenson M. Modulation of HIV-1 replication by RNA interference. *Nature.* 2002;418:435-438.
11. Coburn GA, Cullen BR. Potent and specific inhibition of human immunodeficiency virus type 1 replication by RNA interference. *J Virol.* 2002;76:9225-9231.
12. Novina CD, Murray MF, Dykxhoorn DM, et al. siRNA-directed inhibition of HIV-1 infection. *Nat Med.* 2002;8:681-686.
13. Park WS, Miyano-Kurosaki N, Hayafune M, et al. Prevention of HIV-1 infection in human peripheral blood mononuclear cells by specific RNA interference. *Nucleic Acids Res.* 2002;30:4830-4835.
14. Hu WY, Bushman FD, Siva AC. RNA interference against retroviruses. *Virus Res.* 2004;102:59-64.
15. Anderson J, Banerjea A, Akkina R. Bispecific short hairpin siRNA constructs targeted to CD4, CXCR4, and CCR5 confer HIV-1 resistance. *Oligonucleotides.* 2003;13:303-312.
16. Anderson J, Banerjea A, Planelles V, Akkina R. Potent suppression of HIV type 1 infection by a short hairpin anti-CXCR4 siRNA. *AIDS Res Hum Retroviruses.* 2003;19:699-706.
17. Martinez MA, Gutierrez A, Armand-Ugon M, et al. Suppression of chemokine receptor expression by RNA interference allows for inhibition of HIV-1 replication. *AIDS.* 2002;16:2385-2390.
18. Qin XF, An DS, Chen IS, Baltimore D. Inhibiting HIV-1 infection in human T cells by lentiviral-mediated delivery of small interfering RNA against CCR5. *Proc Natl Acad Sci USA.* 2003;100:183-188.
19. Cordelier P, Morse B, Strayer DS. Targeting CCR5 with siRNAs: using recombinant SV40-derived vectors to protect macrophages and microglia from R5-tropic HIV. *Oligonucleotides.* 2003;13:281-294.
20. Arrighi JF, Pion M, Garcia E, et al. DC-SIGN-mediated infectious synapse formation enhances X4 HIV-1 transmission from dendritic cells to T cells. *J Exp Med.* 2004;200:1279-1288.
21. Arrighi JF, Pion M, Wiznerowicz M, et al. Lentivirus-mediated RNA interference of DC-SIGN expression inhibits human immunodeficiency virus transmission from dendritic cells to T cells. *J Virol.* 2004;78:10848-10855.

22. Smithgall MD, Wong JG, Linsley PS, Haffar OK. Costimulation of CD4+ T cells via CD28 modulates human immunodeficiency virus type 1 infection and replication in vitro. *AIDS Res Hum Retroviruses*. 1995;11:885-892.
23. Hiscott J, Kwon H, Genin P. Hostile takeovers: viral appropriation of the NF-kappaB pathway. *J Clin Invest*. 2001;107:143-151.
24. Dauer M, Obermaier B, Herten J, et al. Mature dendritic cells derived from human monocytes within 48 hours: a novel strategy for dendritic cell differentiation from blood precursors. *J Immunol*. 2003;170:4069-4076.
25. Chomczynski P, Sacchi N. Single-step method of RNA isolation by acid guanidinium thiocyanate-phenol-chloroform extraction. *Anal Biochem*. 1987;162:156-159.
26. Shively L, Chang L, LeBon JM, Liu Q, Riggs AD, Singer-Sam J. Real-time PCR assay for quantitative mismatch detection. *Biotechniques*. 2003;34:498-502, 504.
27. Secchiero P, Zella D, Curreli S, et al. Engagement of CD28 modulates CXC chemokine receptor 4 surface expression in both resting and CD3-stimulated CD4+ T cells. *J Immunol*. 2000;164:4018-4024.
28. Bashirova AA, Wu L, Cheng J, Kewal-Ramani VN, Hughes A, Carrington M. Novel member of the CD209 (DC-SIGN) gene family in primates. *J Virol*. 2003;77:217-227.
29. Steinman RM, Young JW. Signals arising from antigen-presenting cells. *Curr Opin Immunol*. 1991;3:361-372.
30. Steinman RM. DC-SIGN: a guide to some mysteries of dendritic cells. *Cell*. 2000;100:491-494.
31. Bender A, Sapp M, Schuler G, Steinman RM, Bhardwaj N. Improved methods for the generation of dendritic cells from nonproliferating progenitors in human blood. *J Immunol Methods*. 1996;196:121-135.
32. Cella M, Engering A, Pinet V, Pieters J, Lanzavecchia A. Inflammatory stimuli induce accumulation of MHC class II complexes on dendritic cells. *Nature*. 1997;388:782-787.
33. Romani N, Gruner S, Brang D, et al. Proliferating dendritic cell progenitors in human blood. *J Exp Med*. 1994;180:83-93.
34. Granelli-Piperno A, Delgado E, Finkel V, Paxton W, Steinman RM. Immature dendritic cells selectively replicate macrophagetropic (M-tropic) human immunodeficiency virus type 1, while mature cells efficiently transmit both M- and T-tropic virus to T cells. *J Virol*. 1998;72:2733-2737.
35. Cameron P, Pope M, Granelli-Piperno A, Steinman RM. Dendritic cells and the replication of HIV-1. *J Leukoc Biol*. 1996;59:158-171.
36. Frank I, Kacani L, Stoiber H, et al. Human immunodeficiency virus type 1 derived from cocultures of immature dendritic cells with autologous T cells carries T-cell-specific molecules on its surface and is highly infectious. *J Virol*. 1999;73:3449-3454.
37. Ganesh L, Leung K, Lore K, et al. Infection of specific dendritic cells by CCR5-tropic human immunodeficiency virus type 1 promotes cell-mediated transmission of virus resistant to broadly neutralizing antibodies. *J Virol*. 2004;78:11980-11987.
38. Nair MPN, Mahajan SD, Schwartz SA, et al. Cocaine modulates dendritic cell-specific C type intercellular adhesion molecule-3-grabbing nonintegrin expression by dendritic cells in HIV-1 patients. *J Immunol*. 2005;174:6617-6626.

Chapter 8
Viewing Chemokines as a Third Major System of Communication in the Brain

Martin W. Adler,[1,3] Ellen B. Geller,[1] Xiaohong Chen,[1] and Thomas J. Rogers[1,2,3]

Abstract There is irrefutable proof that opioids and other classes of centrally acting drugs have profound effects on the immune system. Evidence is mounting that products of the immune system, such as chemokines, can reciprocally alter the actions of these drugs and the endogenous ligands for their receptors. Chemokines are a family of small (8 to 12 kDa) proteins involved in cellular migration and intercellular communication. With a few exceptions, they act on more than one receptor. Although the chemokines and their G protein-coupled receptors are located in both glia and neurons throughout the brain, they are not uniformly distributed. They are found in such brain areas as the hypothalamus, nucleus accumbens, limbic system, hippocampus, thalamus, cortex, and cerebellum. Among the chemokines differentially localized in brain neurons and glia are CCL2/MCP-1, CXCL12/SDF-1α, CX3CL1/fractalkine, CXCL10/IP 10, CCL3/MIP-1α, and CCL5/RANTES. Functional roles for the chemokine system, composed of the chemokine ligands and their receptors, have been suggested in brain development and heterologous desensitization. The system can alter the actions of neuronally active pharmacological agents such as opioids and cannabinoids and interact with neurotransmitter systems. In this review, we propose that the endogenous chemokine system in the brain acts in concert with the neurotransmitter and neuropeptide systems to govern brain function. It can thus be thought of as the third major system in the brain.

Keywords opioids, cannabinoids, chemokines, brain, desensitization, neurotransmitters

[1] Center for Substance Abuse Research, Temple University School of Medicine, Philadelphia, PA 19140

[2] Fels Institute for Cancer Research and Molecular Biology, Temple University School of Medicine, Philadelphia, PA 19140

[3] Department of Pharmacology, Temple University School of Medicine, Philadelphia, PA 19140

Corresponding Author: Martin W. Adler, Center for Substance Abuse Research, Temple University School of Medicine, 3400 North Broad Street, Philadelphia, PA 19140. Tel: (215) 707-3242; Fax: (215) 707-1904; E-mail: baldeagl@temple.edu

R.S. Rapaka and W. Sadée (eds.), *Drug Addiction.*
© American Association of Pharmaceutical Scientists 2008

127

Neuroactive Compounds

Several groupings of compounds are used in an attempt to categorize chemicals that can affect neuronal activity. The common thread is that these agents not only affect the neuronal activity, but they play a functional role in regulating activity of the brain and nervous system in pathological and homeostatic states. A discussion of these agents may be found in many texts in neuropharmacology, neurophysiology, and neuroscience (for example, see Cooper et al[1] and Steward[2]). Moreover, it often depends on the particular situation as to which of the categories applies to a particular compound at a particular time. Among the most commonly used terms are neurotransmitter, neuromodulator, neuropeptide, and neurohormone. Even within these classes, overlap exists. For example, hypothalamic releasing factors are considered to be neurohormones, but they are a type of neuropeptide. Nevertheless, it is useful to consider some of the characteristics generally assigned to each of these categories in order to determine if chemokines fit into any of these categories.

1. Neurotransmitters are chemicals that are best understood in terms of how they function in interneuronal communication and in neuron-to-effector messaging. They are endogenous chemicals that are synthesized and released presynaptically following nerve stimulation and are found differentially distributed in the brain (as well as elsewhere). They are stored in a form ready to be released, and they can potentiate or block postsynaptic responses. There are mechanisms for inactivation or for removal from the synaptic cleft. Well-known examples are serotonin, dopamine, acetylcholine, and GABA.
2. Neuromodulators, unlike neurotransmitters, have no intrinsic activity but can modify synaptic activity, modulate transmission, and involve a second messenger system. Several neuropeptides have these characteristics. Although it is generally thought of as a neurotransmitter, serotonin has neuromodulator characteristics in certain areas such as the facial motor nucleus.
3. Neurohormones have intrinsic activity, are released from both neuronal and nonneuronal cells, and can travel and act at a site distant from their release site (eg, β-endorphin). In certain cases, neurotransmitters can also travel to other sites (eg, dopamine in the pituitary).
4. Neuropeptides generally target specific cells in the nervous system, including neurons and glia. Precursors are synthesized in the neuronal cell body (eg, proopiomelanocortin for β-endorphin and ACTH). Certain neuropeptides appear to act as neurotransmitters at certain sites (eg, Substance P at sensory afferents to the dorsal horn in the spinal cord). The mechanisms for inactivation in the synaptic cleft are not yet known for all members of the group. Examples of neuropeptides are enkephalins, dynorphin, cholecystokinin, substance P, endocannabinoids, and somatostatin.

Neuroscientists generally think of the systems of chemicals classified as neurotransmitters or neuropeptides as being responsible for neuronal transmission or modulation of neuronal events. The molar concentration of neuropeptides is 2 or 3 orders of magnitude lower than neurotransmitters and their receptors respond to the lower concentrations. Neurotransmitters and neuropeptides may be colocalized in individual synaptic terminals and may be coreleased. Like the neurotransmitter and neuropeptide systems, the chemokine system is widely but unevenly distributed in the brain and has both ligands and receptors located in neurons.[3,4]

Chemokines

A family of small (8–12 kDa) proteins found in the brain and the periphery, chemokines are involved in cellular migration and intercellular communication. Most chemokine ligands act on more than one receptor, although a few, such as CXCL12 and CX3CL1 have specificity for only one.[5,6] Chemokines and their G protein-coupled receptors are located in both microglia and neurons in such brain areas as the hypothalamus, nucleus accumbens, limbic system, hippocampus, thalamus, cortex, olfactory bulbs, and cerebellum.[3,7] Human neurons express multiple functional chemokine receptors and ligands.[8] Neural progenitor cells express chemokine receptors.[9] Among the chemokines having selective distribution in brain neurons and glia are CCL2/MCP-1, CXCL12/SDF-1α, CX3CL1/fractalkine, CXCL10/IP10, CCL3/MIP-1α, and CCL5/RANTES. (It should be noted that the official nomenclature is the first designation of each pair, with the final "L" denoting "ligand." The receptors are designated in a similar fashion, with the final letter "R"). As with neurotransmitter and neuropeptide systems, the differential distribution offers a clue as to possible functional roles.

Summary of Evidence for Chemokines in the Central Nervous System

Several reports have contributed to the hypothesis that chemokines play a major role in brain function. These include the following:

1. Receptors for several of the chemokines are expressed by brain neurons.[3,10]
2. Chemokines and their receptors are located selectively in areas throughout the brain.[4,7,10]
3. Chemokines show selective distribution in brain neurons and glia.[5,11]
4. Individual neurons appear to co-express multiple functional chemokine receptors and chemokines.[8,10]
5. CCR5 and CXCR4 in neurons are localized in the perikaryon in a vesicular or granular pattern and extend into the dendritic processes and axons.[12]
6. CXCR4 coexists with neurotransmitters in neurons in the caudate putamen and substantia nigra.[10] Coexistence with neurotransmitters may indicate an interaction of the 2 systems, especially if there is corelease.

Additional reports provide information supporting the idea of a functional role for chemokines in the brain:

1. Chemokines are involved in neuronal development.[6]
2. CXCL12 reduces the amplitude of evoked excitatory postsynaptic currents in Purkinje neurons in a dose-dependent manner.[13]
3. Functional chemokine receptors on astrocytes can release glutamate, which affects neuronal excitability.[14]
4. CXCR4 appears to be involved in the induction of neuronal apoptosis.[15]
5. CXCR4-mediated signal transduction may be involved in neuronal dysfunction during HIV-1-associated dementia.[16]
6. Chemokine receptor activation in neurons induces calcium transients and modulates ion channel activity,[14] indicating that there may be release of transmitters.
7. CXCL12 may be involved in neuronal communication,[17] and even cholinergic and dopaminergic neurotransmission.[10]

How Chemokines Interact With Opioids and Cannabinoids: Heterologous Desensitization

Most reports involved with chemokines in the brain focus on their role in inflammatory processes and in neurogenesis. The discovery that there is heterologous desensitization between opioids and the chemokines in vitro,[18,19] along with anatomical and immunohistochemical evidence about the chemokine system in the brain, led to a study designed to determine if such desensitization occurred in vivo. The concept of heterologous desensitization is illustrated in Fig. 8.1, using opioids, cannabinoids,

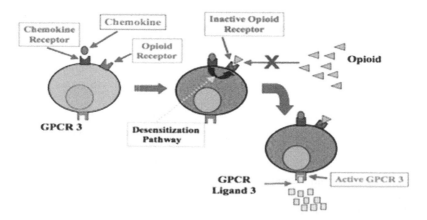

Fig. 8.1 Illustration of Heterologous Desensitization.

and chemokines as examples. In vitro evidence has demonstrated that the heterologous desensitization process is bidirectional, and chemokine receptor activation was shown to inactivate opioid receptor activity in vitro.[18,20,21] Of potential functional significance was the finding that cross-desensitization of CCR5 by opioids resulted in a decreased susceptibility to R5, but not X4 strains of HIV-1.[22]

To ascertain whether the in vitro findings had physiological relevance, in vivo experiments were conducted in male Sprague-Dawley rats. The aim was to determine if chemokine administration into the brain would block or diminish the antinociceptive effect of an opioid without producing an effect of its own. In these studies, the measure of analgesic response is the ability of a drug to increase the threshold to a noxious stimulus, in this case, exposure of the rat's tail to a cold water bath at $-3°C$. The end point is the rat's removal or flicking of its tail.[23] There is a cutoff time to prevent damage to the tail and the calculation is the percentage of the maximum possible analgesic response.

Animals were administered a range of doses of CXCL12, CCL5, or CX3CL1 directly into the periaqueductal gray (PAG), the area primarily involved in the antinociceptive effects of opioids, 30 minutes prior to morphine or D-Ala[2], NMe-Phe[4]-Glyol[5] (DAMGO), a selective agonist at the μ-opioid receptor. The chemokines blocked the expected analgesic response to the opioids.[18] The effects of the chemokines on opioid analgesia were dose-related and could be seen with doses as low as 1 ng. In another study, rats were given a PAG injection of a chemokine or saline before subcutaneous (sc) injection of 8 mg morphine (Fig. 8.2A). Pretreatment with CCL5/RANTES (100 ng) 30 minutes before morphine administration significantly reduced the antinociceptive effect of morphine. In a similar fashion, CXCL12/SDF-1 alpha (100 ng), 30 minutes before 8 mg/kg morphine, significantly reduced the antinociceptive effect (Fig. 8.2B). The lack of a total blockade is likely because the chemokines were injected directly into the PAG, whereas the morphine was sc. Since morphine also has analgesic actions that are outside the PAG, this is to be expected. Indeed, when both morphine and the chemokine are given into the PAG, no antinociception is seen (unpublished results, Chen et al, 2005).

The next question we explored was the time course of the desensitization. It was found that if the chemokine was given at the same time as the opioid, there was a marked attenuation of the expected opioid analgesia, but not a complete block (unpublished observations, Chen et al, 2005). If the chemokine was administered 60 minutes prior to the opioid, analgesia was only partially blocked, and if the interval was increased to 2 hours, the ability of CCL5 to desensitize the opioid receptor was abolished. Of interest was the finding that if the time interval was 2 hours or more and the chemokine was readministered, the blockade of the analgesic activity of DAMGO was restored.[18] Several possibilities exist as to why there was a restoration of the blockade. For example, the process might involve a reversible opioid receptor blockade, or the release of the ligand from the receptor and its subsequent metabolism. The blockade could then be reinstated with a second administration of the ligand, resulting in a recombination of receptor and ligand. It is also possible that new receptors are expressed on the cell surface, permitting additional ligand to bind. Formal proof regarding mechanisms has not been obtained, but we

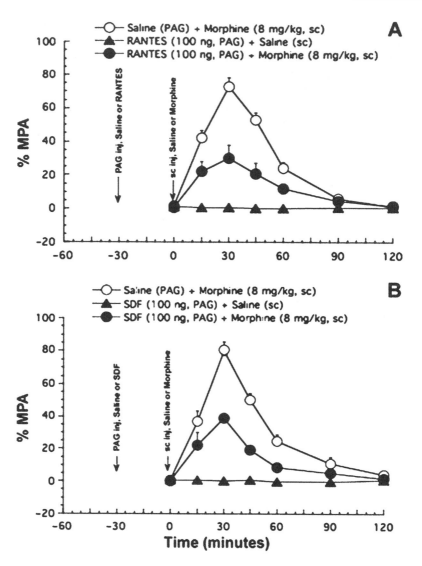

Fig. 8.2 Antagonistic effect of chemokines on antinociception induced by sc morphine: (A) 30-minute pretreatment with RANTES injected into PAG (n = 7–9); (B) 30-minute pretreatment with SDF-1 injected into PAG (n = 3–5). MPA indicates maximum possible analgesia; SDF, SDF-1∝ Each point represents the mean + SE.

have found that there is no detectable internalization of the chemokine or opioid receptor following cross-desensitization in either primary leukocytes or in several leukocyte and nonleukocyte cell lines.[18,24] It has also been shown that the receptor is phosphorylated and that heterodimers form.[24] It may be that the phosphorylation is reversible, as it is with many other types of receptors. Both RANTES and SDF-1 show a similar pharmacokinetic pattern.

The experiments cited above demonstrated that the μ-opioid receptor could be desensitized by chemokines. D-Pen^2, D-Pen^5-enkephalin (DPDPE), a selective δ agonist, and dynorphin A 1–17, the endogenous opioid that is a selective κ agonist, were used to determine if the δ-opioid and the κ-opioid receptors could also be cross-desensitized in vivo. As with the μ-opioid receptor, both the δ- and κ-opioid receptors were desensitized by CCL5 and CXCL12, indicating that there was a desensitization of all 3 types of opioid receptor by the CCR5 and CXCR4 chemokine receptors[18] (and unpublished results from our laboratories, 2005). These receptors are expressed on neurons in various areas of the brain, including the PAG.[10] In order to confirm that the chemokines act via their respective receptors, it is necessary to use a selective chemokine receptor antagonist. AMD 3100, an antagonist at the receptor for CXCL12, was tested. As expected, it prevented the desensitization of DAMGO, thus providing proof that the chemokine desensitization of the μ-opioid receptor was mediated via the chemokine receptor (unpublished observations, Chen et al, 2005).

Like CXCL12, CX3CL1 acts on a single receptor, has no antinociceptive action when administered into the PAG, and is expressed in the brain. In fact, it is the only chemokine reported to be expressed in higher concentrations in the central nervous system (CNS) than in the immune system and peripheral tissues.[6] CX3CL1, like CXCL12 and CCL5, was able to block the antinociceptive action of μ-, κ-, and δ-opioid receptor agonists (unpublished observations, Chen et al, 2005).

Receptors for CCL5, CXCL12, and CX3CL1, the chemokines that produced desensitization of the opioid receptors, have all been found in the PAG. However, CCR2 is a chemokine receptor not found in the PAG at a significant level.[4] As a consequence, injections of CCL2, the ligand for CCR2, into the PAG did not induce the cross-desensitization of the opioid receptors.

The in vitro results and the anatomical-type studies reported above suggest the importance of the chemokine system in the brain. Recent in vivo experiments indicate strongly that the chemokine system is important in brain function. Among those findings reported in abstracts and presented at meetings (manuscripts in preparation) are as follows:

1. CXCR4, CCR5, and CX3CR1 induce heterologous desensitization of μ-, κ-, and δ-opioid receptors in the PAG as demonstrated by effects on analgesia.
2. The desensitization is time- and dose-related, lasts for 60 to 90 minutes, and is reversible for μ-opioid receptors[18] and for δ- and κ-opioid receptors.
3. CXCR4 and CCR5 also desensitize cannabinoid receptors for analgesia, while CX3CR1 does not.

Hypothesis

The systems of neurotransmitters and neuropeptides in the brain are accepted as playing the major role in the functioning of the brain in maintaining homeostasis and reacting to perturbations of that homeostasis. *We propose that the endogenous chemokine system in the brain, consisting of ligands and receptors, is a third major system of the brain.* It is the third leg in the stool that supports brain function.

The chemokines have many of the characteristics discussed above under neuroactive compounds. They have important actions in the brain and they have both direct and indirect actions on neurons. In fact, Bajetto et al[15] suggested that chemokines might act as neuromodulators, and Tran and Miller[25] questioned whether chemokines might play some unexpected role in the physiology of the normal brain. Given the evidence that has accumulated in the past 5 to 7 years, it is reasonable to use the above hypothesis relating to the chemokine system in the brain to begin to make testable predictions.

The evidence cited above indicates that the chemokine system in the brain may well play a vital role in the functioning of the brain under both homeostatic and perturbed situations. Fig. 8.3 illustrates the concept being proposed in this review. It is known that glia can produce and release chemokines and that chemokines and

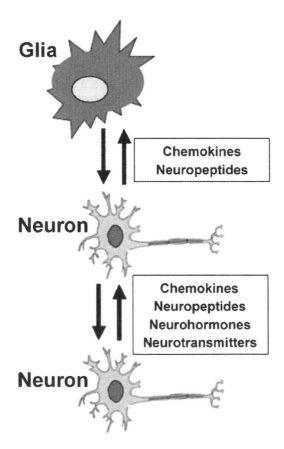

Fig. 8.3 Communication pathways in the nervous system.

their receptors are present in neurons. We are proposing that, in addition to their accepted role in glia-to-glia and glia-to-neuron communication, the chemokines function in neuron-to-glia communication. Even more important, perhaps, is our hypothesis that neuron-to-neuron communication, in many cases, involves the chemokine system of ligands and receptors. The neuropeptide and neurotransmitter systems function to transmit information between neurons, and we propose that chemokines also have this function. The fine control exercised by the brain under both normal and perturbed conditions is consonant with the idea of the chemokine system serving as an additional system of interacting molecules to explain how the neuronal system achieves such magnificent control of discrete physical, behavioral, and chemical action. It also allows one to anticipate new approaches to treat perturbations in homeostasis and enhance brain activity in nonpathological states.

Potential Therapeutic Significance

Several novel potential therapeutic applications can be envisioned by coupling the capacity for heterologous desensitization of the opioid and chemokine systems with knowledge about the neuronal function of the chemokine system. The in vivo finding that activation of the chemokine receptor CXCR4 or CCR5 in the PAG of the brain results in a rapid cross-desensitization of both the μ- and δ-opioid receptors,[18,20] depressing the analgesic function of the opioid receptors and enhancing perception of pain, has great implications. In situations where there is an elevation of chemokine levels in the brain (including most neuroinflammatory diseases such as multiple sclerosis and HIV encephalitis), a resulting loss of opioid receptor function could lead to greater sensitivity to painful stimuli.[18,26] Findings such as these, coupled with other evidence cited above about the chemokine system in the brain suggest the following therapeutic opportunities:

1. Alter treatment of pain associated with neuroinflammatory states by blocking heterologous desensitization of opioid receptors that may account for diminished efficacy of opioids in inflammatory pain.
2. Decrease certain unwanted side effects of opioids by chemokine desensitization of selected opioid pathways after determining neuronal localization of chemokine receptors.
3. Desensitize chemokine receptors that serve as coreceptors for entry of HIV in the CNS or periphery, resulting in reduced HIV susceptibility. The cross-desensitization of CCR5 and CXCR4 by other G protein-coupled receptors, including the opioid receptors, has been shown to result in the loss of HIV coreceptor function.[22]
4. Use the effects of chemokines to modify effects of drugs on behavior by altering the interactions of the neurotransmitter and neuropeptide systems involved in the behavioral effects of drugs abused or used therapeutically to treat mental disorders.

5. Bring new approaches to prevention and treatment of neurodegenerative diseases through blocking or enhancing the actions of chemokines.

Open Questions and Research Directions

As this review has put forth the postulate that chemokines function as transmitters in neuron-to-neuron, glia-to-neuron, and neuron-to-glia communication, it is vital that experiments be conducted to add to the body of information required to establish this role in the brain. Because the chemokine system has only recently been found to be involved in brain function, much remains to be discovered. As examples, the mechanism of release from neurons, the storage and the inactivation mechanisms, and their presence at excitatory or inhibitory synapses are not known. In addition, there are the questions as to whether the system is both pre- and postsynaptic, and whether the receptors endocytose. Little information exists as to specific functional systems in the brain linked to individual chemokines. However, despite the fact that neuropeptides have been known for over 30 years, not all the criteria have as yet been met[1] to allow neuropeptides to be called neurotransmitters. Nevertheless, there is general acceptance of their importance in interneuronal communication. The evidence that exists is consistent with the hypothesis that the chemokine system acts as a major system in the brain to facilitate or to be an actual chemical network of ligands and receptors that transmits information in a manner analogous to neurotransmitters and neuropeptides.

Conclusions

We propose that the endogenous chemokine system in the brain acts in concert with the neurotransmitter and neuropeptide systems to govern brain function. The chemokines are postulated to function as transmitters in neuron-to-neuron, glia-to-neuron, and neuron-to-glia communication. In addition, the system can alter the actions of neuronally active pharmacological agents such as opioids and cannabinoids and interact with neurotransmitter systems. Much remains to be discovered about the chemokine system in the brain. By understanding this system, therapeutic possibilities range from altering treatment of neuroinflammatory states to interfering with entry of HIV into cells to new treatment of degenerative diseases to modifying treatment of mental disorders to diminishing unwanted side effects of opioids.

Acknowledgments The authors wish to acknowledge the help of numerous members of the Temple University Center for Substance Abuse Research (CSAR) in conducting experiments and helping to develop the ideas that led to the hypothesis about the role of the chemokine system in brain function. Foremost among those is Dr Toby K. Eisenstein. In addition, the scientific help of the laboratories of Drs Lee-Yuan Liu-Chen, Ronald J. Tallarida, Alan Cowan, Ellen M. Unterwald, and Khalid Benamar and the technical help of Margy Deitz is gratefully acknowledged.

The research reported here from the laboratories of CSAR was supported by several grants, especially DA06650, DA07237, DA14230, and DA-P30-13429 from the National Institute on Drug Abuse (NIDA), National Institutes of Health (NIH), Bethesda, MD.

References

1. Cooper JR, Bloom FE, Roth RH. *The Biochemical Basis of Neuropharmacology.* New York, NY: Oxford University Press; 2003.
2. Steward O. *Functional Neuroscience.* New York, NY: Springer-Verlag; 2000.
3. van der Meer P, Ulrich AM, González-Scarano F, Lavi E. Immunohistochemical analysis of CCR2, CCR3, CCR5, and CXCR4 in the human brain: potential mechanisms for HIV dementia. *Exp Mol Pathol.* 2000;69:192-201.
4. Banisadr G, Quéraud-Lesaux F, Boutterin MC, et al. Distribution, cellular localization and functional role of CCR2 chemokine receptors in adult rat brain. *J Neurochem.* 2002;81:257-269.
5. Ambrosini E, Aloisi F. Chemokines and glial cells: a complex network in the central nervous system. *Neurochem Res.* 2004;29:1017-1038.
6. Bajetto A, Bonavia R, Barbero S, Florio T, Schettini G. Chemokines and their receptors in the central nervous system. *Front Neuroendocrinol.* 2001;22:147-184.
7. Horuk R, Martin AW, Wang Z, et al. Expression of chemokine receptors by subsets of neurons in the central nervous system. *J Immunol.* 1997;158:2882-2890.
8. Coughlan CM, McManus CM, Sharron M, et al. Expression of multiple functional chemokine receptors and monocyte chemoattractant protein-1 in human neurons. *Neuroscience.* 2000; 97:591-600.
9. Ji JF, He BP, Dheen ST, Tay SS. Expression of chemokine receptors CXCR4, CCR2, CCR5 and CX_3CR1 in neural progenitor cells isolated from the subventricular zone of the adult rat brain. *Neurosci Lett.* 2004;355:236-240.
10. Banisadr G, Fontanges P, Haour F, Kitabgi P, Rostène W, Parsadaniantz SM. Neuroanatomical distribution of CXCR4 in adult rat brain and its localization in cholinergic and dopaminergic neurons. *Eur J Neurosci.* 2002;16:1661-1671.
11. Mizuno T, Kawanokuchi J, Numata K, Suzumura A. Production and neuroprotective function of fractalkine in the central nervous system. *Brain Res.* 2003;979:65-70.
12. Westmoreland SV, Alvarez X, deBakker C, et al. Developmental expression patterns of CCR5 and CXCR4 in the rhesus macaque brain. *J Neuroimmunol.* 2002;122:146-158.
13 Ragozzino D, Renzi M, Giovannelli A, Eusebi F. Stimulation of chemokine CXC receptor 4 induces synaptic depression of evoked parallel fibers inputs onto Purkinje neurons in mouse cerebellum. *J Neuroimmunol.* 2002;127:30-36.
14 Cho C, Miller RJ. Chemokine receptors and neural function. *J Neurovirol.* 2002;8:573-584.
15. Bajetto A, Bonavia R, Barbero S, Schettini G. Characterization of chemokines and their receptors in the central nervous system: physiopathological implications. *J Neurochem.* 2002;82:1311-1329.
16. Zheng J, Thylin MR, Ghorpade A, et al. Intracellular CXCR4 signaling, neuronal apoptosis and neuropathogenic mechanisms of HIV-1-associated dementia. *J Neuroimmunol.* 1999;98:185-200.
17. Stumm RK, Rummell J, Junker V, et al. A dual role for the SDF-1/CXCR4 chemokine receptor system in adult brain: isoform-selective regulation of SDF-1 expression modulates CXCR4-dependent neuronal plasticity and cerebral leukocyte recruitment after focal ischemia. *J Neurosci.* 2002;22:5865-5878.
18. Szabo I, Chen XH, Xin L, et al. Heterologous desensitization of opioid receptors by chemokines inhibits chemotaxis and enhances the perception of pain. *Proc Natl Acad Sci USA.* 2002;99:10276-10281.

19. Zhang N, Rogers TJ, Caterina M, Oppenheim JJ. Proinflammatory chemokines, such as C-C chemokine ligand 3, desensitize μ-opioid receptors on dorsal root ganglia neurons. *J Immunol.* 2004;173:594-599.
20. Steele AD, Szabo I, Bednar F, Rodgers RJ. Interactions between opioid and chemokine receptors: heterologous desensitization. *Cytokine Growth Factor Rev.* 2002;13:209-222.
21. Rogers TJ, Steele AD, Howard OMZ, Oppenheim JJ. Bidirectional heterologous desensitization of opioid and chemokine receptors. *Ann N Y Acad Sci.* 2000;917:19-28.
22. Szabo I, Wetzel MA, Zhang N, et al. Selective inactivation of CCR5 and decreased infectivity of R5 HIV-1 strains mediated by opioid-induced heterologous desensitization. *J Leukoc Biol.* 2003;74:1074-1082.
23. Pizziketti RJ, Pressman NS, Geller EB, Cowan A, Adler MW. Rat cold water tail-flick: a novel analgesic test that distinguishes opioid agonists from mixed agonist-antagonists. *Eur J Pharmacol.* 1985;119:23-29.
24. Chen C, Li J, Bot G, Szabo I, Rogers TJ, Liu-Chen L-Y. Heterodimerization and cross-desensitization between the μ-opioid receptor and the chemokine CCR5 receptor. *Eur J Pharmacol.* 2004;483:175-186.
25. Tran PB, Miller RJ. Chemokine receptors in the brain: a developing story. *J Comp Neurol.* 2003;457:1-6.
26. Rogers TJ, Peterson PK. Opioid G protein-coupled receptors: signals at the crossroads of inflammation. *Trends Immunol.* 2003;24:116-121.

Chapter 9
Targeting the PDZ Domains of Molecular Scaffolds of Transmembrane Ion Channels

Andrea Piserchio[1], Mark Spaller[2], and Dale F. Mierke[1,3]

Abstract The family of multidomain proteins known as the synaptic associated proteins (SAPs) act as molecular scaffolds, playing an important role in the signaling and maintenance of several receptors and channels. The SAPs consist of 5 individual protein domains: 3 PDZ (PSD95, Disc Large, Zo1) domains, an SH3 domain, and an inactive guanyl kinase (GK) domain. The 3 PDZ domains bind the C-termini of specific receptors and channels, leading to the transient association with cytoskeletal and signaling proteins. Molecules targeting specific domains of the SAPs may provide a novel route for the regulation of channel and receptor function. Here we describe a structural-based approach for the development of such inhibitors for the PDZ domains of SAP90. The high sequence homology of the 3 domains has necessitated targeting regions outside the canonical binding pocket. The structural features of the PDZ domains with the C-termini of different receptors (GluR6), channels (Kv1.4), and cytoskeletal proteins (CRIPT) provide insight into targeting these regions.

Keywords PDZ domains, synaptic associated proteins, PSD95, SAP90, glutamate receptors, molecular scaffold, NMR, ligand binding

Introduction

PDZs (PSD95, Disc Large, Zo1) are small globular domains composed of ~90 amino acids exhibiting high sequential homology and functioning as protein-protein interaction modules. Typically PDZs adopt a β-sandwich fold including 2 α-helices

[1] Department of Molecular Pharmacology, Division of Biology and Medicine, Brown University, 171 Meeting Street, Providence, RI 02912

[2] Department of Chemistry, Wayne State University, Detroit, MI 48202

[3] Department of Chemistry, Brown University, Providence, RI 02912

Corresponding Author: Dale F. Mierke, Department of Molecular Pharmacology, Brown University, 171 Meeting Street, Providence, RI 02912. Tel: (401) 863-2139; Fax: (401) 863-1595; E-mail: dale_mierke@brown.edu

R.S. Rapaka and W. Sadée (eds.), *Drug Addiction.*
© American Association of Pharmaceutical Scientists 2008

and 2 β-sheets composed of 5/6 β-strands and recognize the C-termini of their protein targets, see Fig. 9.1. The binding contact occurs in a hydrophobic cleft delimited by the second α-helix, the second β strand, and the first loop. The ligand is normally inserted as an additional β-strand, in an anti-parallel fashion with respect to the second β-strand (β2), with the C-terminus inserted into a characteristic pocket formed by the β1/β2 loop. The most relevant side chains for PDZ selectivity are located at the 0 and −2 positions (employing a numbering scheme with the C-terminus 0, and proceeding −1, −2, toward the N terminus), which has been used for defining different classes of PDZ domains. However, all 6 C-terminal residues can play a role in modulating the binding affinity.[1] In some cases a contribution from residues located up to position −10 has been reported.[1]

The multidomain protein SAP90 (synapse-associated protein 90) contains 3 N-terminal PDZ domains followed by an SH3 and an inactive GK domain. SAP90, also known as PSD95 (post synaptic density protein-95) is concentrated in the post synaptic density of glutamatergic neurons and is one member of a super family of PDZ-containing proteins, including SAP97/hdlg, SAP102, and Chapsyn110/PSD93,[2-5] that play an important role in coupling the membrane ion channels with their signaling partners. The first 2 PDZ domains (PDZ1 and PDZ2) are responsible for the recognition of ion channels. For example, the PDZ1 domain selectively

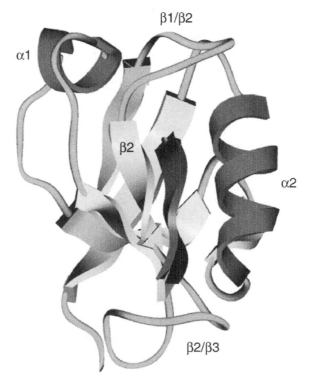

Fig. 9.1 Secondary structure elements of the PDZ1 of SAP90, illustrating the basic fold and the nomenclature of the secondary structural elements.

couples with the GluR6 subunit of kainate receptors,[6] while both PDZ1 and PDZ2 are capable of binding to receptors[7] and potassium channels.[8] The third PDZ domain (PDZ3) interacts preferentially with cytoskeleton proteins like CRIPT[9] or cell surface proteins, like neuroligins.[10] Furthermore, the PDZ2 domain is capable of binding the neuronal nitric oxide synthase (nNOS) protein,[11] catalyzing the synthesis of nitric oxide (NO). In this later case the SAP90 PDZ2 recognizes its partner through an internal motif located on a β-finger region of the nNOS protein.[12] The SAP90 PDZ domains, together with the GK domain, can bind several proteins (SynGAP,[13] SPAL,[14] and MAGUIN-1[15]) involved in the mitogen-activated protein kinase (MAPK) signaling cascade.[16]

Despite the different binding affinities, the 3 PDZ domains of SAP90 share a high sequence homology; binding C-termini with a hydrophobic residue at position 0 and serine/threonine in position −2 (defined as class I PDZ domains). Some differences outside these classification sites have been noted. The PDZ1 and PDZ2 domains prefer negatively charged residues in position −1 and −3,[1] while CRIPT,[9] binding to PDZ3, has serine and glutamine at −1 and −3, respectively. Here, we describe our efforts to develop structural insight into the specificity illustrated by the PDZ domains of SAP90. Using high-resolution nuclear magnetic resonance (NMR), we characterize the structure of different receptors (GluR6), channels (Kv1.4), and cytoskeletal proteins (CRIPT), while associated with PDZ1 of SAP90. Based on these structural features, coupled with results previously reported for the PDZ domains of SAP90,[17-19] several sites for development of PDZ domain-specific molecules are identified. A cyclic peptide, incorporating a side-chain to side-chain lactam-bridged system, targeting one site is described.

Methods

The 3 peptides were chosen based on their differing specificities for the PDZ domains of SAP90: GluR6 binds solely to PDZ1,[20] Kv1.4 displays affinity for both PDZ1 and PDZ2,[21] and CRIPT binds selectively to PDZ3.[9] The C-terminus of the GluR6 subunit of the kainite receptor was examined as a 15-residue peptide (His^{-14}-Thr^{-13}-Phe^{-12}-Gln^{11}-Asp^{-10}-Arg^{-9}-Arg^{-8}-Leu^{-7}-Pro^{-6}-Gly^{-5}-Lys^{-4}-Glu^{-3}-Thr^{-2}-Met^{-1}-Ala^0-OH). The Kv1.4 was examined as Tyr^{-5}-Lys^{-4}-Glu^{-3}-Thr^{-2}-Asp^{-1}-Val^0-OH, and was previously shown to bind tightly to PDZ1 of SAP90 (Table 9.1).[19] CRIPT, a cytoskeleton molecule that has been reported to target preferentially the PDZ3

Table 9.1 Peptide Sequences and Binding Affinities at PDZ1[19] and Relative PSD 95 PDZ Specificity

Peptide	Selectivity	Sequence	K_D (μM)
Kv1.4 (potassium channel)	PDZ1 and PDZ2	YKETDV-OH	1.5
CRIPT (microtubole associated protein)	PDZ3 (lower affinity to PDZ1 and PDZ2)	TKNYKQTSV-OH	15.0
GluR6 (kainite receptor)	PDZ1	HTFNDRRLPGKETMA-OH	160.0

domain, was examined as a 9-residue peptide[9] (Thr^{-8}-Ly^{-7}-Gln^{-6}-Tyr^{-5}-Lys^{-4}-Gln^{-3}-Thr^{-2}-Ser^{-1}-Val^{0}-OH).

The structures of the PDZ1 peptide complexes were determined by high-resolution NMR. The samples containing 1.0 mM ^{15}N,^{13}C-PDZ1 and 4.0 mM peptide were prepared in 10 mM phosphate buffer, 150 mM NaCl at a pH of 6.8. The ^{1}H and ^{15}N assignments were determined previously[19]; the ^{13}C assignments were determined employing standard methods.[22] Several 2- and 3-dimensional ^{15}N and ^{13}C filtered experiments were used to isolate the peptide resonances and to measure intramolecular and intermolecular nuclear Overhauser enhancements (NOEs) involving the peptide amide protons.

The structure refinement was achieved using dihedral angle constraints derived from TALOS[23] and a torsion angle simulated annealing using CNS.[24] For the resolved diastereotopic groups floating chirality was applied. Extensive molecular dynamics (MD) simulations were performed using the GROMACs package,[25,26] using a cubic box of $6.5 \times 6.5 \times 6.5$ nm^3 containing ~8500 molecules of water. The NOE-derived interproton distance restraints were applied with a constant of $10 \text{kJ mol}^{-1} \text{Ala}^{-2}$, and Arg^{-6} averaging was implemented on chemical equivalent and overlapped protons. The distance restraints were removed after 600 ps and the system was therefore freely evolving during the remaining 1.0 ns.

Results

The resulting structures of the complexes formed between the PDZ1 of SAP90 and the C-termini of GluR6, Kv1.4, and CRIPT are shown in Fig. 9.2. The structure of the PDZ1-Kv1.4 is delineated by an extremely large number of NOEs, both intramolecular and intermolecular. Interestingly, no intermolecular NOEs could be observed for the Lysecond^{-4} side chain, while the Tyr^{-5} aromatic ring is close to A80 methyl group. Noticeably, the β-protons of the N85 residue are close in space to the Tyr^{-5} Hα proton. In all of the refined structures, the isopropyl group of Val^{0} projects into a deep hydrophobic cavity between the β2 strand and the α2 helix formed by L75, F77, I79, and L137. The side chain of Thr^{-2} is located on the same side of the strand respect to Val^{0}. While the hydroxide hydrogen bonds with H130, the methyl group forms van der Waals contacts with the methyls of I79 and V134. On the opposite face of the strand, the side chain of Glu^{-3} is extended over the β-sheet surface and salt bridges with K98 on the β3 strand. The Lysecond^{-4} side chain appears relatively flexible, however in many NMR-derived structures the positively charged amino group is a short distance from the D84 carboxylic acid located on the top of the β2/β3 loop. The aromatic ring of Tyr^{-5} is accommodated in a pocket formed by the end of the β2 strand and the β2/β3 loop.

The structure of the PDZ1-CRIPT complex is similarly defined by a large number of NOEs, despite a lower binding affinity and therefore faster exchange rate of the ligand. Defining the mode of ligand binding there are intermolecular NOEs involving the methyl groups of both Val^{0} and Thr^{-2} with the β2 strand (F77, I79)

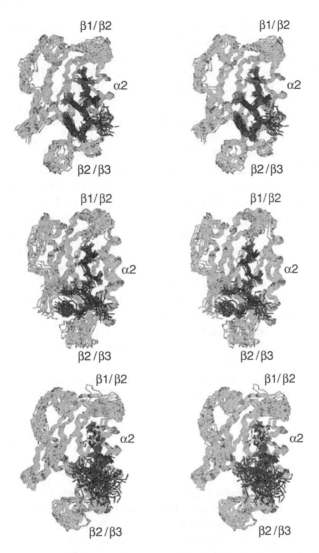

Fig. 9.2 Stereo views showing the NMR structures of the PDZ1 domain bound to Kv1.4 peptide (top), CRIPT (middle), and GluR6 (bottom). The conformers are superimposed for best fit of N, Cα, and carbonyl atoms. All the ligand's heavy atoms are shown for the fragment encompassing residues 0 and −5; carbons are depicted in dark green, oxygen in red, nitrogen in blue, sulfur in yellow. In the protein portion, only the superimposed atoms are shown as light green. (*See* also Color Insert).

and the α2 helix (V134, L137, K138). The side chains of Ser^{-1} and Gln^{-3} have NOEs with residues located on the β2 strand and on the β-sheet surface opposite to the α2 helix. The Lys in position −4 does not give detectable NOEs, while Tyr^{-5} gives several NOEs with the methyl of A80. No other intermolecular NOEs are detected for the remaining residues of the CRIPT peptide. The backbone of the

CRIPT peptide encompassing residues Val^0 and Thr^{-2} is well defined and shows the classical β-sheet insertion structural motif. Starting from Gln^{-3} the backbone is less ordered and moves away from the β2 strand by flanking the β2/β3 loop. The NOEs detected between the Tyr^{-5} side chain and the methyl of Ala^{80} places the aromatic ring at the conjunction of the β2 strand with the β2/β3 loop. Although the side chains of both Lysecond^{-4} and Lysecond^{-7} appear totally unordered, the backbone conformation would allow the positioning of the positively charged amino groups close to the negative charges located on the β2/β3 loop.

The structure of the GluR6-PDZ1 complex is defined by a much smaller number of NOEs, consistent with the weaker binding affinity. Indeed, no intermolecular NOEs are observed for Ala^0. Met^{-1} is well defined with backbone NOEs with S78 and I79 and side chain interactions with L75 or I100 located on the β3 strand. The Thr^{-2} methyl group gives NOEs with V134 on the α2 helix and with I79 on the β2 strand. Finally the Glu^{-3} side chain interacts with A80 and T97 on the β2 and β3 strand, respectively. A univocal family of structures for the GluR6/PDZ1 can be obtained if hydrogen bond restraints are introduced into the structure refinement calculation (Fig. 9.2, bottom). The variation in the chemical shifts of the amide protons in the carboxylic binding loop suggest the formation of hydrogen bonds with the C-terminus of GluR6. Similarly, the shifts of I79 can be explained with a hydrogen bond with the carbonyl of Thr^{-2}. The resulting structures are similar to PDZ1-Kv1.4 complex, where the C-terminal 3 residues are extending the β-sheet, with interactions to the β2 strand. The next 3 residues, Gly^{-5}-Lys^{-4}-Glu^{-3}, extend toward the β2/β3 loop. The remaining residues, further toward the N terminus, are unordered.

Discussion

The different binding affinities previously measured for the 3 ligands can be directly correlated to the quantity of the NMR restraints, and therefore to the resolution of the 3-dimensional models of the complexes. The best binder, the Kv1.4-derived peptide, leads to the better-defined structure, while a lower resolution is observed for the CRIPT and finally for the GluR6 ligands (see Fig. 9.2). Nevertheless, some common features can be extrapolated by comparing the 3 models. All of them in fact exhibit a similar extended conformation in the fragment encompassing positions 0 and −3. The peptides enhance the β-sheet surface in correspondence of the β2 strand in an antiparallel fashion (Fig. 9.3). The carboxylic C-terminal end enters the β1/β2 loop by hydrogen bonding the amides of residues L75, G76, and F77.

At the −4 position the peptide backbones deviates away from the β2 strand and interacts with the β2/β3 loop. The importance of this loop has been clearly demonstrated: the deletion of the loop in both PDZ1 and PDZ2 diminish the binding affinity to the Kv1.4 potassium channel.[21] The 3 ligands examined have different preferences for the 3 PDZ domains of SAP90 and a closer look of the sequences of

Fig. 9.3 Superposition of the last 6 C-terminal residues of Kv1.4 (dark green), CRIPT (blue), and GluR6 (magenta). The binding pocket of the PSD95/SAP90 PDZ1 domain is shown in light green. (*See* also Color Insert).

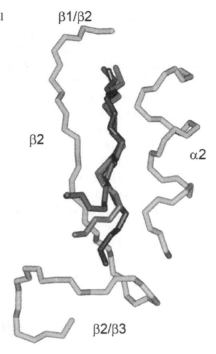

β1/β2

β2

α2

β2/β3

Fig. 9.4 Comparison of the β2/β3 loop of the PDZ1, PDZ2, and PDZ3 domains of SAP90.

```
PDZ1    GGTDNPHIGDDPSI

PDZ2    GGVGNQHIPGDNSI

PDZ3    GGED        GEGI

        **. *  **  .*  **
```

the β2/β3 loop illustrates several important features (Fig. 9.4) that may account for the range of binding affinities.

We previously reported that the PDZ2 domain closely resembles the PDZ1 domain in the canonical ligand-binding domain[19] and even the shape of the β2/β3 loops is similar. As the N85 residue is conserved in both domains, and its side chain undergoes chemical shift changes upon titration of the PDZ2 domain with the CAPON peptide,[18] it is probable that this residue mediates the ligand β-strand extension also in the PDZ2 domain. In the structure of PDZ2 from hPTP1 interacting with the C-terminus of the guanine nucleotide exchange factor RA-GEF-2,[27] an asparagine residue in the β2/β3 loop interacts a Asp^{-5} of the ligand. In contrast, the PDZ3 domain of SAP90 lacks 5 residues in the β2/β3 loop. Comparing our findings here with the x-ray structure of the CRIPT/PDZ3 complex demonstrates complete agreement for the C-terminal 4 residues (positions 0 to −3). Unfortunately, in the crystal the peptide does not diffract N-terminal of position −4, indicating that residues preceding this position are unordered in the crystal. In our NMR-derived structure of CRIPT bound to PDZ1, Tyr^{-5}-Lysecond^{-4} interact with the β2/β3 loop, particularly the abundant negatively charged residues within the loop. Given that these negative charges are not maintained in the PDZ2 of SAP90, in future design efforts we have targeted this region as a mode for enhancing the specificity for PDZ1.

In both structures of Kv1.4 and CRIPT bound to PDZ of SAP90, the side chain of the −3 residue projects out toward the β3 strand, placing a Glu^{-3} (Kv1.4) or Gln^{-3} (CRIPT) outside the canonical binding pocket. Comparison of the sequences of the 3 PDZ domains of SAP90 indicates an important difference in this region. Both PDZ1 and PDZ2 have a lysine (K98 and K193 for PDZ1 and PDZ2, respectively), while PDZ3 contains a phenylalanine, F340, at this position. One mode to target this difference is afforded by cyclization of the side chains at positions −1 and −3.[28] Previously we examined the cyclic peptide version of CRIPT, Tyr-Lys-c[-Lys-Thr-Glu(βAla)-]-Val-OH, while bound to the PDZ1 domain of SAP90 by NMR (Fig. 9.5).[29] The results from these studies clearly indicate that the lactam bond formed by the cyclization extends outside the canonical binding pocket to interact with the residues of the β3 strand.

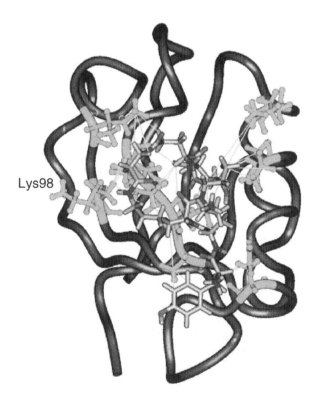

Lys98

Fig. 9.5 Structure of the cyclic peptide, Tyr-Lys-c[-Lys-Thr-Glu(βAla)-]-Val-OH, while bound to PDZ1 of SAP90. All of the residues in which intermolecular NOEs have been measured are shown in gray. The interaction of the cyclic, lactam ring system with K98 is illustrated.

Currently, we are modifying the linker to target the differences in the PDZ1/PDZ2 and PDZ3 domains of SAP90 in an effort to develop an analog with enhanced specificity for the different domains.

Conclusions

In conclusion we have solved the structure of PDZ1 of SAP90 bound to 3 peptides related to the C-terminus of Kv1.4, CRIPT, and GluR6. Our results allow for the detailed characterization of the structural determinants modulating affinity for the PDZ1 domain. Comparison of these data with the other known structures of the PDZ2 and PDZ3 of SAP90 provides several leads for the development of analogs with enhanced PDZ domain specificity.

References

1. Lim IAHD, Hell JW. Selectivity and promiscuity of the first and second PDZ domains of PSD-95 and synapse-associated protein 102. *J Biol Chem.* 2002; 277:21697-21711.
2. Garner CC, Kindler S. Synaptic proteins and the assembly of synaptic junctions. *Trends Cell Biol.* 1996; 6:429-433.
3. Garner CC, Nash J, Huganir RL. PDZ domains in synapse assembly and signalling. *Trends Cell Biol.* 2000; 10:274-280.
4. Craven SE, Bredt DS. PDZ proteins organize synaptic signaling pathways. *Cell.* 1998; 93:495-498.
5. Hirao K, Hata Y, Ide N, et al. A novel multiple PDZ domain-containing molecule interacting with N-methyl-D-aspartate receptors and neuronal cell adhesion proteins. *J Biol Chem.* 1998; 273:21105-21110.
6. Garcia EP, Mehta S, Blair LA, et al. SAP90 binds and clusters kainate receptors causing incomplete desensitization. *Neuron.* 1998; 21:727-739.
7. Kornau HC, Schenker LT, Kennedy MB, Seeburg PH. Domain interaction between NMDA receptor subunits and the postsynaptic density protein PSD-95. *Science.* 1995; 269:1737-1740.
8. Kim E, Niethammer M, Rothschild A, Jan YN, Sheng M. Clustering of Shaker-type K+ channels by interaction with a family of membrane-associated guanylate kinases. *Nature.* 1995; 378:85-88.
9. Niethammer M, Valtschanoff JG, Kapoor TM, et al. CRIPT, a novel postsynaptic protein that binds to the third PDZ domain of PSD-95/SAP90. *Neuron.* 1998; 20:693-707.
10. Irie M, Hata Y, Takeuchi M, et al. Binding of neuroligins to PSD-95. *Science.* 1997; 277:1511-1515.
11. Brenman JE, Chao DS, Gee SH, et al. Interaction of nitric oxide synthase with the postsynaptic density protein PSD-95 and alpha1-syntrophin mediated by PDZ domains. *Cell.* 1996; 84:757-767.
12. Hillier BJ, Christopherson KS, Prehoda KE, Bredt DS, Lim WA. Unexpected modes of PDZ domain scaffolding revealed by structure of nNOS-syntrophin complex. *Science.* 1999; 284:812-815.
13. Kim E, DeMarco SJ, Marfatia SM, Chishti AH, Sheng M, Strehler EE. Plasma membrane Ca2+ ATPase isoform 4b binds to membrane-associated guanylate kinase (MAGUK) proteins via their PDZ (PSD-95/Dlg/ZO-1) domains. *J Biol Chem.* 1998; 273:1591-1595.

14. Deguchi M, Hata Y, Takeuchi M, et al. BEGAIN (brain-enriched guanylate kinase-associated protein), a novel neuronal PSD-95/SAP90-binding protein. *J Biol Chem*. 1998; 273:26269-26272.

15. Yao I, Hata Y, Hirao K, et al. Synamon, a novel neuronal protein interacting with synapse-associated protein 90/postsynaptic density-95-associated protein. *J Biol Chem*. 1999; 274:27463-27466.

16. Martin KC, Michael D, Rose JC, et al. MAP kinase translocates into the nucleus of the presynaptic cell and is required for long-term facilitation in Aplysia. *Neuron*. 1997; 18:899-912.

17. Doyle DA, Lee A, Lewis J, Kim E, Sheng M, MacKinnon R. Crystal structures of a complexed and peptide-free membrane protein-binding domain: molecular basis of peptide recognition by PDZ. *Cell*. 1996; 85:1067-1076.

18. Tochio H, Hung F, Li M, Bredt DS, Zhang M. Solution structure and backbone dynamics of the second PDZ domain of postsynaptic density-95. *J Mol Biol*. 2000; 295:225-237.

19. Piserchio A, Pellegrini M, Mehta S, et al. The PDZ1 domain of SAP90. Characterization of structure and binding. *J Biol Chem*. 2002; 277:6967-6973.

20. Mehta S, Wu H, Garner CC, Marshall J. Molecular mechanisms regulating the differential association of kainate receptor subunits with sap90/psd-95 and sap97. *J Biol Chem*. 2001; 276:16092-16099.

21. Imamura F, Maeda S, Doi T, Fujiyoshi Y. Ligand binding of the second PDZ domain regulates clustering of PSD-95 with the Kv1.4 potassium channel. *J Biol Chem*. 2002; 277:3640-3646. Show: 3645 3610 3620 3650 3100 3200 3500 Sort Author Journal Pub Date Text File.

22. Grzesiek S, Bax A. Amino acid type determination in the sequential assignment procedure of uniformly 13C/15N-enriched proteins. *J Biomol NMR*. 1993; 3:185-204.

23. Cornilescu G, Delaglio F, Bax A. Protein backbone angle restraints from searching a database for chemical shift and sequence homology. *J Biomol NMR*. 1999; 13:289-302.

24. Brunger AT, Adams PD, Clore GM, et al. Crystallography & NMR system: A new software suite for macromolecular structure determination. *Acta Crystallogr D Biol Crystallogr*. 1998; 54:905-921.

25. Lindahl E, Hess B, van der Spoel D. GROMACS 3.0: A package for molecular simulation and trajectory analysis. *J Mol Mod*. 2001; 7:306-317.

26. Berendsen HJC, van der Spoel D, van Buuren R. GROMACS: A message passing parallel molecular dynamics implementation. *Comp Phys Comm*. 1995;91:43-56.

27. Kozlov G, Banville D, Gehring K, Ekiel I. Solution structure of the PDZ2 domain from cytosolic human phosphatase hPTP1E complexed with a peptide reveals contribution of the beta2-beta3 loop to PDZ domain-ligand interactions. *J Mol Biol*. 2002; 320:813-820.

28. Udugamasooriya G, Saro D, Spaller MR. Bridged peptide macrocycles as ligands for PDZ domain proteins. *Org Lett*. 2005; 7:1203-1206.

29. Piserchio A, Salinas GD, Li T, Marshall J, Spaller MR, Mierke DF. Targeting specific PDZ domains of PSD-95; structural basis for enhanced affinity and enzymatic stability of a cyclic peptide. *Chem Biol*. 2004; 11:469-473.

Chapter 10
Neuronal Nicotinic Acetylcholine Receptor Expression and Function on Nonneuronal Cells

Lorise C. Gahring[1,2] and Scott W. Rogers[1,3]

Abstract Of the thousands of proven carcinogens and toxic agents contained within a cigarette, nicotine, while being the addictive agent, is often viewed as the least harmful of these compounds. Nicotine is a lipophilic molecule whose effects on neuronal nicotinic acetylcholine receptors (nAChR) have been primarily focused on its physiologic impact within the confines of the brain and peripheral nervous system. However, recently, many studies have found neuronal nAChRs to be expressed on many different nonneuronal cell types throughout the body, where increasing evidence suggests they have important roles in determining the consequences of nicotine use on multiple organs systems and diseases as diverse as ulcerative colitis, chronic pulmonary obstructive disease, and diabetes, as well as the neurologic disorders of Parkinson's and Alzheimer's disease. This review highlights current evidence for the expression of peripheral nAChRs in cells other than neurons and how they participate in fundamental processes, such as inflammation. Understanding these processes may offer novel therapeutic strategies to approach inflammatory diseases, as well as precautions in the design of interventional drugs.

Keywords nicotine, inflammation, nicotinic receptors, nonneuronal

[1] Geriatric Research Education and Clinical Center, Salt Lake City VAMC, Salt Lake City, Utah 84132

[2] The Department of Internal Medicine, University of Utah School of Medicine, Salt Lake City, Utah 84132

[3] The Department of Neurobiology and Anatomy, University of Utah School of Medicine, Salt Lake City, Utah 84132

Corresponding Author: Lorise C. Gahring, Division of Geriatrics, SOM 2C110, Department of Internal Medicine, University of Utah School of Medicine, 50 North Medical Drive, Salt Lake City, UT 84132. Tel: (801) 585-6338; Fax: (801) 585-7327; E-mail: Lorise.Gahring@hsc.utah.edu

R.S. Rapaka and W. Sadée (eds.), *Drug Addiction.*
© American Association of Pharmaceutical Scientists 2008

149

Introduction

Neuronal nicotinic acetylcholine receptors (nAChR) are ligand-gated ion channels whose genetics and functional properties have been studied largely for their role in modulating neurotransmission. This receptor system has also been recognized as a participant in the progression of severe pathologies of the brain. For example, the high affinity nicotine receptors are among the first (if not the first) neurotransmitter system whose expression is diminished in Alzheimer's disease.[1] Subsequent studies[2-4] have suggested that chronic nicotine administration might in fact play a beneficial role in slowing the progression of this disease. While this finding is controversial, there is now ample evidence supporting a therapeutic benefit from nicotine in Parkinson's[5] disease, and as a neuroprotectant to toxic insults such as excitotoxins[6-10] or Beta-amyloid derived peptides.[10-12] Understanding the mechanistic basis for these and other similarly interesting findings,[13] including a cognitive benefit from nicotine,[2] would be of obvious importance. The name "neuronal" was based principally on the tissue source of the DNA libraries from which these receptors were first cloned, the brain,[14] but growing evidence indicates that cells other than neurons throughout the body express these receptors[15,16] including lymphocytes, macrophages, dendritic cells, adipocytes, keratinocytes, endothelial cells, and epithelial cells of the intestine and lung. This extended expression of nAChRs is of importance because, in addition to their regulation by endogenous agonists such as acetylcholine, choline, and the exogenous compound nicotine, their impact upon peripheral processes can be quite diverse as exemplified by their ability to in some cases enhance (Crohn's disease) disease or in other cases diminish (ulcerative colitis) progression.[17-20] These apparent contradictions in the effects of nicotine are not uncommon and understanding this complex biology will in turn optimize therapeutic benefit to ensure that neuroprotective therapy for one disease does not promote immune dysfunction and the survival of unwanted cells in other tissues.

Acetylcholine Receptors

Acetylcholine receptors (see Lindstrom[21] and Hogg et al[22]) consist of 2 major subtypes, the muscarinic-activated metabotropic receptors (second messenger coupled) and the fast-ionotropic cationic nicotine-activated channel receptors, both of which are activated by the endogenous neurotransmitter, acetylcholine. Receptors of the nicotinic subclass can be distinguished further as "muscle" or "neuronal." While the muscle and neuronal nicotinic receptors exhibit similar sensitivity to gating by acetylcholine, the muscle receptor is much less sensitive to nicotine. Hence, at physiological concentrations, the majority of nicotine's effects are through neuronal nicotinic acetylcholine receptors (nAChR), and, in fact, when nicotine levels are sufficiently high to act upon the muscle receptor (as might occur when smokers concurrently use the transdermal nicotine patch[23]), difficulties in breathing and muscle spasms that can result in death may occur.

The mammalian nAChR family (for review see Lindstrom[21] and Hogg et al[22] and references therein) is composed of multiple members (subunits) including 7 subunits that harbor the principal components of the ligand binding site ($\alpha2$, $\alpha3$, $\alpha4$, $\alpha6$, $\alpha7$, $\alpha9$, and $\alpha10$) and 4 structural subunits ($\alpha5$, $\beta2$, $\beta3$, and $\beta4$) that impart unique functional and pharmacological properties to the receptors. In general, nAChRs fall into 3 major subgroups, the high-affinity nicotine binding receptors harboring nAChR$\alpha4$, α-bungarotoxin binding proteins composed of nAChR$\alpha7$, and the receptors of the autonomic nervous system composed of nAChR$\alpha3$/$\beta4$ subunits. A particularly interesting aspect of nAChRs is that despite their being fast-excitatory ion channels, they may be localized in many parts of the cell including aggregates in the cell body (somal), presynaptic terminals (where they contribute to modulation of neurotransmitter release), and in or adjacent to the postsynaptic density. Because of these diverse locations, their participation in neurotransmission can be somewhat indirect as when they affect the amount of neurotransmitter released. This modulatory role directly contributes to the establishment and maintenance of tone between the excitatory and inhibitory systems.[24-31] Further, the relatively high calcium permeability of these receptors (especially nAChR$\alpha7$) appears to contribute to regulating second messenger signaling pathways such as the PI3-kinase/AKT pathway,[12,32] activation of transcriptional systems such as CREB,[33] and certain proteolytic processes.[34,35] Consequently, the placement of relatively small numbers of nAChRs at key regulatory sites can lead to multiple outcomes in terms of normal cell performance and susceptibility to exogenous challenges or participation in processes ranging from neurodegeneration to inflammation. Therefore, dysregulation or modification of the function of this system may be expected to be manifested more in modifying biological or metabolic "set-points" rather than having the often dramatic on-off effects seen with other neurotransmitter receptor systems.

Despite the importance of subunit composition to nAChR expression, function, and pharmacology, the rules governing subunit assembly of nAChRs in the brain into the mature pentameric receptor are not yet known, but it is well established that nAChRs of different subunit composition exhibit very different pharmacological and functional properties. For example, nAChRs composed of $\alpha7$ subunits (which bind α-bungarotoxin) exhibit almost a 10:1, Ca^{+2}:Na^+ permeability ratio, which exceeds that of the glutamate N-methyl-D-aspartate (NMDA) receptor and the ~4:1 ratio of most other nAChRs.[21,22] This finding suggests that the activation of nAChR$\alpha7$-type receptors, which also accumulate extrasynaptically, including in rafts,[36] impact upon free intracellular calcium and calcium-dependent mechanisms in a manner quite distinct from other ligand-activated ion channels as well as other nAChRs. In contrast, the majority of other nAChRs are composed of various combinations of α and β subunits. Prominent among these are receptors composed of at least nAChR$\alpha4$ and $\beta2$ subunits that form the high-affinity [^{3}H]nicotine binding receptor. A curiosity of nicotine's effect on this receptor is that when ligand is in excess and present chronically, as in a smoker, the number of binding sites actually increases in a process termed "up-regulation." While the mechanism underlying this process is controversial[21,22,37]; what is clear is that not all nAChR subtypes undergo upregulation,[38] and it is imminently associated with many of the characteristics of nAChR function such as those leading to addiction.[39]

Nicotine—Agonist or Antagonist?

Although nicotine is most often considered to be an agonist or activator of nAChRs, it has several effects on receptor function that complicate this assignment and require attention in any experimental design that employs this compound. Unlike the normal ligand such as acetylcholine or choline, which are either rapidly degraded or removed from the receptor vicinity, nicotine is not readily degraded or removed. Further, because it is lipophilic, it accumulates in certain tissues well beyond the concentration suggested by measuring the serum.[40] For example, concentrations of nicotine in the brain, owing to the drug's high hydrophobicity, can reach as high as 10 μM even though its serum concentration rarely exceeds high nanomolar and is more often in the low nanogram per milliliter range. Just as nicotine partitions and concentrates in the brain due to this lipophilic nature, other tissues also have elevated levels of nicotine compared with blood. It has been reported, using an animal model of nicotine infusion,[41] that the tissue-to-blood ratios of nicotine in different parts of the body are the following: brain 3.0, heart 3.7, muscle 2.0, adipose tissue 0.5, kidney 21.6, liver 3.7, lung 2.0, and gastrointestinal tissue 3.5. Therefore, several tissues can reach nicotine levels that approximate those achieved in the brain. As such, the duration and persistence of nicotine administration over time becomes an important pharmacological variable in the use and interpretation of this drug's actions.

These issues of concentration and duration of nicotine exposure lead to the important role that receptor desensitization, or closing of the receptor in the sustained presence of agonists, plays in understanding nicotine biology and also introduces the concept that nicotine can actually be a powerful antagonist of receptor function. Under normal conditions, desensitization is obviously a fortunate feature of this system since leaving a pore in the membrane open for prolonged periods of time would lead to death. Also, under normal conditions, desensitization is likely to be relatively brief and the receptor can reset to again be opened when a burst of agonist occurs. In contrast to this physiological state, the accumulation of nicotine and unceasing receptor binding results in sustained desensitization and in some cases can actually lead to complete receptor inactivation.[22] When lower concentrations of nicotine are present, receptor function may actually be a combination of both since different receptor subtypes also have very different sensitivities to both activation and desensitization. This phenomenon is readily demonstrated when comparing nAChRα7 receptors to nAChRα3/β4 receptors: nAChRα7 receptors are opened by relatively low nicotine concentrations but then rapidly desensitize, which is only very slowly reversible (possibly requiring complete receptor turnover); nAChRα3/β4 receptors, which populate autonomic ganglia, are relatively insensitive to low concentrations of nicotine and while slow to desensitize, they rapidly reverse this state when nicotine amounts decrease. Therefore, a great number of the effects of nicotine on a system may reflect receptor desensitization rather than activation. Further, when assessing the role of nicotine in the system it becomes critical to distinguish if the exposure is acute or chronic, what concentration of nicotine is actually achieved in the system, and whether or not nAChR subtype expression would suggest activation, desensitization, or both.

Peripheral Sites of nAChR Expression and the Anti-inflammatory Effects of Nicotine

The importance of discriminating between the effects of nicotine versus the effects of tobacco becomes apparent when examining the literature contributing to the developing concept of the "cholinergic anti-inflammatory pathway," where nAChRs could prove to be valuable targets of therapeutic agents directed toward mediators of inflammation. Pavlov and colleagues[42] and Wang et al[43] first reported that acetylcholine or nicotine pretreatment of human peripheral blood mononuclear cells acted through a posttranscriptional mechanism to reduce the amount of tumor necrosis factor alpha (TNFα) present in the media 2 hours following stimulation with the bacterial component lipopolysaccharide (LPS). The anti-inflammatory properties of nicotine were specific in that other inflammatory cytokine production such as IL-1β, IL-18, and IL-6 were inhibited but not the anti-inflammatory cytokine IL-10. Under normal conditions (ie, in the absence of nicotine), it would appear that the vagus nerve release of acetylcholine at sites of peripheral tissue innervation provides the source of agonist for the nAChR. This idea is supported by the observation that vagotomy followed by LPS stimulation resulted in greater levels of TNFα in serum compared with control animals receiving LPS alone or sham vagotomy. The nAChR responsible for this effect was pharmacologically determined to be the nAChRα7 homomeric receptor,[43] which was later supported by studies in mice, where the nAChRα7 subunit was genetically eliminated. This group has also suggested[44] that nAChRα7 stimulation results in the decreased production of high mobility group box 1 (HMGB1) protein, which is a late mediator of lethal sepsis.

Of note, Pavlov[42] and Wang[43] were not the first to identify an interaction between nicotine (acting through nAChRα7) and TNFα. Numerous tissue culture studies have identified interactions between these pathways that impart neuroprotection to neurons challenged with excitotoxins such as NMDA.[7,45] An interesting aspect of these studies is that while either nicotine or acutely administered TNFα were neuroprotective, when applied together, neuroprotection was abolished.[7] This apparent antagonism between nAChRα7 and TNFα pathways has been explored further and apparently does not require the NFκB system or caspase activation.[10] Rather, the possibility exists that interactions are through modifications of the sphingomyelinase system as revealed through restoration of the neuroprotective effect by supplementation with ceramides.[46] Whatever the case, these studies collectively suggest an interaction between the signaling pathways initiated by the pro-inflammatory cytokine TNFα and nicotine with the nAChRα7 subtype.

Intestinal Epithelium

One of the earliest noted effects of nicotine on a peripheral tissue was in inflammation of the intestine. Early reports discussed patients with ulcerative colitis who upon cessation of smoking experienced more severe disease progression, which was ameliorated by returning to smoking.[17,20] In contrast, patients with Crohn's disease experienced severe disease when smoking, requiring the immediate and complete cessation of any tobacco product use.[18,19] Nicotine appears to be the key mediator of these responses as has been demonstrated by the use of transdermal patches, where their use inhibits inflammation associated with ulcerative colitis.[47,48] While nicotine has anti-inflammatory properties in this disease, the therapeutic value of nicotine does not exceed that of more conventional treatments such as aminosalicylates.[48] The mechanism through which nicotine acts in either of these diseases has not been resolved, and while both diseases are considered autoimmune in origin and thought to be related to the overproduction of inflammatory cytokines, their different etiologies and highly specific impact of nAChR expression or function is of great interest.

A fascinating issue to be addressed is which nAChRs, or possibly their respective expression levels, might participate in these disease states and the differential response to nicotine. A recent report by Orr-Urtreger et al[49] has taken on this difficult issue and found that mice deficient in the structural nAChR subunit α5 are more susceptible to experimentally induced inflammatory bowel disease than their wild-type controls. However, the story is complicated since transdermal nicotine attenuated the disease process to a certain extent in both wild-type and knockout mice, albeit more so in the knockout. This result suggests that the absence of nAChRα5 alters (increases) the susceptibility to disease initiation and the presence of nAChRα5 in the wild-type animal appears to enhance therapeutic sensitivity to nicotine. Of course, this again brings up many questions including whether nAChR composition or function may differ between Crohn's and ulcerative colitis patients. An additional note is that while a great deal of attention has been given to nAChRα7 in peripheral disease and inflammation, this exciting result suggests that it is premature to assume that this receptor is alone in its participation in modulating the peripheral inflammatory status. In fact, nAChR subunit mRNA for α3, α5, β2, and β4[50] has been detected in multiple cell types of the intestine suggesting that, as in the brain, nicotine may impact upon different inflammatory processes with considerable specificity depending upon the nAChR subtypes present. Such speculation is supported by another interesting report regarding the possible role of nAChR in disease processes of the gut where Richardson et al[51] found the absence of nAChRα3, normally expressed by ganglion cells, muscle, and epithelium of the small bowel, to be associated with a rare intestinal disease of childhood. Further, Xu et al[52] report that mice lacking nAChRα3 or both nAChRβ2 and nAChRβ4 have similar autonomic dysfunction of the bowel. Whether direct interaction with nAChRs expressed by epithelium or receptor expression by ganglia contributes to these disease processes remains to be determined.

Lung

Expression of nAChR subunits by epithelial and endothelial cells in the lung has also been observed.[15,53-57] This includes primary cultures of human bronchial cultured epithelial cells (BEC) that have been tested for nAChR expression. These cells express nAChRα7 mRNA and α-bungarotoxin binding that is indicative of mature receptor expression.[58] Other nAChR subunits present include nAChRα3, α5, β2, and β4 as well as the other potentially homomeric receptors composed of α9 and α10 that have been found using reverse transcriptase-polymerase chain reaction (RT-PCR) on human airway cells.[59] BEC also express acetylcholine, choline acetyltransferase, and the choline high affinity transporter, suggesting that acetylcholine may function as an autocrine or paracrine hormone for bronchial epithelial cells. Another source of agonist could be choline,[60] a compound that is transiently made available either in serum or locally following ingestion of fatty foods or during membrane remodeling. Choline is a full agonist of nAChRα7 and at high concentrations can exhibit activity toward other nAChRs.[60]

What are the implications of nAChR expression in the lungs with regard to both smokers and nonsmokers? While smoking is a major causative factor for lung cancer, relatively few smokers generate chronic obstructive pulmonary disease (COPD), which has an incidence rate of ~20%, even among very heavy and long-term smokers.[61] In fact, while the lungs of healthy smokers contain elevated numbers of activated macrophages, pulmonary Langerhans' cells, and primed neutrophils,[62] these cells actually exhibit reduced surface expression of major histocompatibility complex (MHC) class II molecules and costimulatory T lymphocyte molecules relative to controls.[63] Therefore, while cells are present that are primed for activation, the immune and inflammatory response may be dampened, as has been observed in many smokers.[62] Expanding upon this possibility, Floto and Smith[64] suggested that the inflammatory response to the stimulatory components of tobacco may be counteracted by the anti-inflammatory effects of nicotine, which offers a rational explanation for why few smokers generate pulmonary Langerhans' cell histiocytosis. It has also been pointed out that there is a significantly lower incidence of sarcoidosis in smokers[65] and decreased incidence of immunoglobulin G (IgG) precipitins that develop during allergic alveolitis as occurs both in humans and guinea pigs.[66,67] Whether this is due to the anti-inflammatory effects of nicotine is a direction of future research, especially with regard to the genetics regulating expression of nAChRs or the individual's genetic background. An encouraging feature of dissecting these complex traits and interactions is the use of mouse model systems. Mice have proven to be an extremely valuable model for translational studies related to basic issues of immunological function and show considerable promise in bringing similar experimental enlightenment to both genetic and environmental aspects of sensitivity to peripheral and central effects of nicotine including COPD. Differential susceptibility of mouse strains to nicotine have been extensively studied by the Collins group.[68] Further, the expression of nAChRs in the central nervous system can differ substantially in both cell types expressing these receptors and their organization in the brain,[69] in a mouse strain-dependent manner. These studies, as well as familial studies of addiction, point to the very evident genetic regulation of responsiveness to nicotine. Similarly, there is a mouse strain-dependent response to the development of emphysema in cigarette smoke-exposed mice.[70] Of the mouse strains tested, NZW/Lac/J, C57BL/6, A/J, SJL, and AKR (which all differ in MHC haplotypes), the AKR mice demonstrated an enhanced susceptibility to the development of emphysema, while the C57BL/6, A/J, and SJL mice were mildly susceptible. The NZW/Lac/J mouse strain was resistant to emphysema and demonstrated a milder inflammation with reduced macrophage numbers and a remarkable lack of CD4+ or CD8+ T lymphocytes. Characterization of nAChR expression and function as they pertain to the genetics of these varied mouse strains would certainly enhance our understanding of these results.

Adipose Tissue

Smoking is a predisposing factor for insulin-resistance, which is associated with type 2 diabetes. Smokers are insulin-resistant and hyper-insulinaemic, and men who smoke are 4 times more likely to develop diabetes.[71] This is particularly interesting since type 2 diabetes is usually associated with obesity (excess adipose tissue) in adults; however, smokers are well established to be leaner, suggesting that simple explanations such as decreased eating is not the prime cause of this effect. In female smokers (but not necessarily in males), it is the fear of weight gain that often poses the greatest obstacle to smoking cessation.[72] Also of note is that exposure of mice to cigarette smoke for 6 months[70] resulted in weight loss in certain mouse strains (C57BL/6, AKR) but not others (A/J, SJL, NZW).

The role of the nAChRs in adipose tissue is only beginning to be explored as suggested by the limited and somewhat confusing literature. Miyazaki et al[73] have reported that smoking correlates significantly with decreased adiponectin levels in human plasma, which is usually associated with obesity and type 2 diabetes. Does a decrease in plasma adiponectin levels play a role in the generation of insulin-resistance in smokers even in the absence of obesity? Unfortunately, the function of adiponectin is not well understood. In a study to determine the role of nicotine on adipocytes, Liu et al[74] cultured rat adipocytes and found that mRNA for most of the neuronal and muscle nAChR were present in these cells, which were also found to bind [^{3}H]-nicotine. Further, pretreatment of these rat adipocytes with nicotine resulted in a reduced release of the pro-inflammatory cytokine TNFα as well as free fatty acids. Adiponectin levels in these adipocyte cultures, contrary to what might be expected from the in vivo studies, were elevated upon treatment with nicotine. Therefore, much remains to be explored in order to clarify the role of nAChR in the generation of smoke-induced insulin-resistance and metabolic syndrome with the occurrence of reduced adiposity.

Immune System

The relationship of nAChRs to immune function has 2 principal aspects. One resides in the realm of autoimmune attacks directed toward the expression of nAChRs, while the other addresses issues of nAChR expression by cells of the immune system and aspects of this relationship that are reflected in well-established observations such as the negative effect smoking has on the ability to fight infection. Autoimmune recognition of muscle nAChR at the neuromuscular junction resulting in myathenia gravis (MG)[75-77] continue to elucidate immune-mediated processes of this disease. While MG is the prototypical example of autoimmunity to the α1 subunit of the muscle nicotinic AChR, recent evidence suggests that other nAChR subunits[78] may also be targets in other autoimmune pathologies. One such subunit is α3, which when introduced into rabbits induced an autoimmune response with resulting autonomic neuropathy (AAN).[78] Further, this animal model replicates findings in some patients with idiopathic autonomic failure.[78] Such autoimmune recognition may also extend to nAChRα7, which contains amino acid sequences that are conditionally subject to proteolytic cleavage by granzyme B released from activated cytotoxic T cells.[79] Epitopes generated by cleavage of proteins with granzyme B tend to be autoantigenic.[80] Therefore, α7 cleavage by activated T cells is likely to be an excellent candidate as a target of presently unidentified autoimmune processes. While MG and AAN are peripheral pathologies, autoimmune processes against neuronal receptors may not be limited to peripheral diseases. For example, we have described[81] the presence and function of autoantibodies to a glutamate receptor (GluR3) in patients with Rasmussens encephalitis (RE), which is a rare pediatric seizure disorder characterized by intractable epilepsy. Many of these patients demonstrate anti-GluR3 antibodies that activate glutamate receptors on neurons. Further, GluR3 has a granzyme B site at the autoimmune epitope.[81] Lennon et al[82] have suggested that immune responses generated against nAChR may also result in seizure and dementia.

In the second arena of nAChR-immune cell interaction, chronic smoking affects both humoral and cell-mediated immune responses in rodents, monkeys, and humans.[62,83] Both thymic epithelium and thymocytes[84] express nAChR as do mature lymphocytes.[85,86] It has also been established that macrophages and dendritic cells also possess nAChR subunits. Exposure to cigarette smoke tends to suppress the response to infection.[87] For example, Kalra et al[88] demonstrated that smoking impairs antigen-mediated signaling in T cells and depletes IP3-sensitive Ca^{2+} stores, and van Dijk et al[89] have shown that transdermal nicotine (2 weeks on patch, normal volunteers) significantly reduced IL-2 production as well as a reduction in TNFα and IL-10 by blood cells stimulated with mitogen. A notable outcome of this effect may be that the anti-inflammatory properties of nicotine actually enhance the survival of influenza virus in mice and induce significantly higher titers of virus following infection.[63] Pneumonia caused by *Streptococcus pneumonia*, is also more frequent in smokers.[90]

Macrophages are critical effector cells for early recognition and destruction of organisms invading through most surfaces including the gut, skin, and lung. Matsunaga el al[91] have shown that nicotine treatment of a mouse alveolar macrophage cell line (expressing α4 and β2, but not α7) results in enhanced intracellular replication of *Legionella pneumophilia*. Further, the production of the inflammatory cytokines IL-6, TNFα, and IL-12 were down-regulated in these cells. While nicotine may inhibit macrophage function to promote pneumonia, it has also been reported that the generation of hypersensitivity pneumonia (HP) is lower in smokers than nonsmokers. HP is caused by inhalation of antigens such as *Saccharopolyspora rectivirgula,* which induces farmer's lung (once contracted, however, smoking worsens disease). Blanchet et al[92] observed that nicotine-induced inhibition of macrophage function may actually protect against inflammatory lung processes such as HP by decreasing the number of alveolar macrophages in the lungs of experimental animals and decreasing inflammatory cytokine production. Further, Shivji et al[93] reported recently that chronic nicotine exposure results in a reduction of lung S-adenosylmethionine (AdoMet), which is required for growth of *Pneumocystitis carinii*. As such, smoking and nicotine protect against *Pneumocystitis*. A clinical correlate of protection in humans against *Pneumocystitis*, which is closely associated with AIDS infection, has been reported by Saah et al.[94]

While macrophages initiate many inflammatory and innate immune functions, dendritic cells (DCs) are the principal antigen-presenting cells. Aicher et al[95] demonstrated that low doses of nicotine induced the expression of molecules with costimulatory activity toward antigen presentation and increased the secretion of IL-12 (pro-inflammatory) by TH1 T lymphocytes by 7-fold. This effect was mediated by PI3-kinase, AKT, and p38 MAPK. The overall effect observed was an increase in dendritic-cell stimulation of T-cell proliferation and cytokine secretion. They also report that DCs are increased in atherosclerotic plaques and that this effect of nicotine may contribute to progression of atherosclerotic lesions.

Skin

The relationship between smoking and skin has been a topic of investigation for a long period. This is in part because studies have suggested that smoking is a risk factor in development of premature facial wrinkling.[96,97] While not all studies necessarily agree with smoking contributing to increased wrinkling, they do conclude that smokers on average look older and suggest that smoking increases aging of the skin. Mechanistically, nicotine can impact upon epithelial keratinocytes (KC) that express nAChR receptor subunits as well as the enzymes for acetylcholine synthesis, which may act as cell signalling molecules ("cytotransmitters") as has been suggested for the lung.[53] Grando and colleagues[98] established that KCs express nAChRs and that these receptors respond functionally to nicotine. Kurzen et al[99] localized nAChR subunit expression in the skin and conclude that there is a very distinctive pattern of subunit expression in normal human epidermis. Perhaps more important than issues pertaining to premature wrinkling is the relationship between smoking (and nicotine use) and delayed wound healing. For example, nicotine inhibits keratinocyte migration[100,101] slowing wound healing. nAChRα7 expression by KC is implicated in underlying this observation, where it appears to play an important role in cell cycle progression, apoptosis, and differentiation.[102] This is particularly supported by studies of α7 knockout mice,[103] where the expression of pro-apoptotic proteins Bad and Bax are reduced, and an antagonist of muscarinic and nAChRα4/β4[104] cholinergic receptors (atropine) decreases the expression of desmoligein (Dsg), which is an important regulator of cell adhesion. How these results translate into biologic effects of nicotine on skin remains to be determined; however, the possibility exists that, through inhibition of apoptosis, tumorgenesis is also enhanced. Therefore, the reports of nicotine effects on the skin appear rather deleterious, although separating nicotine effects from those of cigarette smoke for skin effects has not been extensively examined in vivo. Future analysis of epidemiological data from subjects using nicotine delivery through the skin-patch will be of particular value in assessing these effects.

Oral Epithelium

The major preventable risk factor for periodontal disease is smoking, and there is a direct correlation between cigarette number and risk. Exposure to second-hand smoke has also been suggested to enhance periodontal risk by up to 20-fold,[105] and both smoking and nicotine have been reported to increase inflammation by reducing oxygen in gum tissue and initiating over-production of the inflammatory cytokines, which in excess are harmful to cells and tissue. Furthermore, when nicotine combines with oral bacteria, such as *Porphyromonas gingivalis*, the effect produces even greater levels of cytokines and eventually leads to periodontal connective-tissue breakdown.[106] Studies suggest that smokers are 11 times more likely than nonsmokers to harbor the bacteria that cause periodontal disease and 4 times more likely to have advanced periodontal disease. In one study, more than 40% of smokers lost their teeth by the end of their lives. Oral epithelial cells express nicotinic receptors. Arredondo et al[107] reported that both nicotine and environmental tobacco smoke (ETS) increased expression of regulators of the cell cycle and apoptosis. This up-regulation was inhibited by transfection into human keratinocytes from gingival of small interfering RNA for human nAChRα3. Further, the α3 knockout mouse did not generate these changes in gene expression with exposure to ETS or nicotine. These investigators[107] also report the presence of α5, α2, and the muscarinic receptors M2 and M3.

Endothelium

Smoking is a major risk factor for cardiovascular disease, and nicotine plays a role in some of the pathogenic processes involved. For example, Heeschen et al[108] have demonstrated that nicotine increases endothelial cell number, reduces apoptosis, increases capillary network formation, and accelerates the growth of atherosclerotic plaques. Growth of plaques is dependent on vascularization, which is increased in nicotine-treated mice. Macklin et al[54] find that human aortic endothelial cells that line blood vessels express functional nAChRs with α3 being a predominant subunit. These endothelial nAChR demonstrate similar ion-gating properties as those on ganglionic neurons. Further, these investigators have shown that acetylcholine is also produced by endothelial cells, suggesting that an autocrine mechanism of activation can occur. An intriguing discussion by these authors suggests that the effect of nicotine on desensitization (see above) of these receptors may make endothelial cells nonresponsive to the endogenously produced acetylcholine and that this nonresponsiveness should be considered in the pathogenesis of atherosclerosis. Intracellular mechanisms that are activated by nicotine in endothelial cells have been demonstrated by Di Luozzo et al[109] and include MAPKs p38 and p44/p42. The receptors present on rat endothelial cells, as revealed[110] by RT-PCR include nAChRs α2, α3, α4, α5, α7, β2, and β4 but not β3. Saeed et al[111] have demonstrated that nicotine inhibits the expression of endothelial adhesion molecules, suggesting that the effect of nicotine on these cells is anti-inflammatory. Therefore, both pro- and anti-inflammatory mechanisms may be involved in nicotine-mediated effects on endothelium and again points to the need for determination of the nAChR receptor subunits involved.

Conclusion

A frequently reported influence of nAChR expression and function by tissues of the periphery is on inflammation. Because the inflammatory response is an integral and specialized process in all tissues, this suggests that an equally broad and specific range of nAChR-related outcomes can be expected that may be both beneficial and harmful to the host. For example, controlling the inflammatory response in ulcerative colitis would ameliorate tissue damage. In contrast, suppressing the inflammatory response during an innate (or adaptive) immune response through chronic nAChR activation/desensitization would dampen this reaction and impact in a negative way on the rate of clearing of a microbial infection or the efficacy of long-term protection against recurrent challenges by foreign substances. In addition to the direct influence of chronically activated/desensitized nicotinic receptors, it is also important to consider that the many inflammatory processes as well as responses to nicotine are highly predisposed to genetic background as witnessed by the broad diversity of the influence of nicotine on mice of differing strain background. The effective usefulness of nAChR-based strategies will ultimately depend upon a clear understanding of the collective biological consequences of peripheral nAChR expression on inflammation, and it should also be considered that they will have the possibility of meeting with undesirable side-effects. For example, the anti-inflammatory properties of nicotine that promote neuronal survival in the aging brain could also encourage survival of proliferating cells in the periphery that should otherwise die, produce immune suppression, or even influence metabolism and insulin resistance. However, coupled to this complexity is the exciting prospect that a detailed understanding of how nAChRs impart these diverse effects will be rewarded with many novel therapeutic strategies.

Acknowledgments This mini-review undoubtedly and regrettably does not include many excellent papers in the literature regarding the peripheral expression of nAChR. The authors' research into nAChRs is funded by grants from the National Institutes of Health (NIH), Bethesda, MD (P01-HL72903, DA018930, and DA015148). Continued support by the Val A. Browning Foundation of Salt Lake City, Utah is greatly appreciated.

References

1. Kellar KJ, Whitehouse PJ, Martino-Barrows AM, Marcus K, Price DL. Muscarinic and nicotinic cholinergic binding sites in Alzheimer's disease cerebral cortex. *Brain Res*. 1987;436: 62-68.
2. Rezvani AH, Levin ED. Cognitive effects of nicotine. *Biol Psychiatry*. 2001;49:258-267.
3. Sabbagh MN, Lukas RJ, Sparks DL, Reid RT. The nicotinic acetylcholine receptor, smoking, and Alzheimer's disease. *J Alzheimers Dis*. 2002;4:317-325.
4. O'Neill MJ, Murray TK, Lakics V, Visanji NP, Duty S. The role of neuronal nicotinic acetylcholine receptors in acute and chronic neurodegeneration. *Curr Drug Targets CNS Neurol Disord*. 2002;1:399-411.
5. Quik M. Smoking, nicotine and Parkinson's disease. *Trends Neurosci*. 2004;27:561-568.
6. Shimohama S, Akaike A, Kimura J. Nicotine-induced protection against glutamate cytotoxicity. Nicotinic cholinergic receptor-mediated inhibition of nitric oxide formation. *Ann N Y Acad Sci*. 1996;777:356-361.
7. Carlson NG, Bacchi A, Rogers SW, Gahring LC. Nicotine blocks TNF-alpha-mediated neuroprotection to NMDA by an alpha-bungarotoxin-sensitive pathway. *J Neurobiol*. 1998;35:29-36.
8. Carlson NG, Wieggel WA, Chen J, Bacchi A, Rogers SW, Gahring LC. Inflammatory cytokines IL-1alpha, IL-1beta, IL-6, and TNF-alpha impart neuroprotection to an excitotoxin through distinct pathways. *J Immunol*. 1999;163:3963-3968.
9. Dajas-Bailador FA, Lima PA, Wonnacott S. The alpha7 nicotinic acetylcholine receptor subtype mediates nicotine protection against NMDA excitotoxicity in primary hippocampal cultures through a Ca(2+) dependent mechanism. *Neuropharmacology*. 2000;39:2799-2807.
10. Gahring LC, Meyer EL, Rogers SW. Nicotine-induced neuroprotection against N-methyl-D-aspartic acid or beta-amyloid peptide occur through independent mechanisms distinguished by pro-inflammatory cytokines. *J Neurochem*. 2003;87:1125-1136.
11. Kihara T, Shimohama S, Urushitani M, et al. Stimulation of alpha4beta2 nicotinic acetylcholine receptors inhibits beta-amyloid toxicity. *Brain Res*. 1998;792:331-334.
12. Kihara T, Shimohama S, Sawada H, et al. Alpha7 nicotinic receptor transduces signals to phosphatidylinositol 3-kinase to block A beta-amyloid-induced neurotoxicity. *J Biol Chem*. 2001;276:13541-13546.
13. Pauly JR, Charriez CM, Guseva MV, Scheff SW. Nicotinic receptor modulation for neuroprotection and enhancement of functional recovery following brain injury or disease. *Ann N Y Acad Sci*. 2004;1035:316-334.
14. Boulter J, O'Shea-Greenfield A, Duvoisin RM, et al. Alpha3, alpha5, and beta 4: 3 members of the rat neuronal nicotinic acetylcholine receptor-related gene family form a gene cluster. *J Biol Chem*. 1990;265:4472-4482.

15. Conti-Fine BM, Navaneetham D, Lei S, Maus AD. Neuronal nicotinic receptors in non-neuronal cells: new mediators of tobacco toxicity? *Eur J Pharmacol.* 2000;393:279-294.
16. Sharma G, Vijayaraghavan S. Nicotinic receptor signaling in nonexcitable cells. *J Neurobiol.* 2002;53:524-534.
17. Birtwistle J, Hall K. Does nicotine have beneficial effects in the treatment of certain diseases? *Br J Nurs.* 1996;5:1195-1202.
18. Rubin DT, Hanauer SB. Smoking and inflammatory bowel disease. *Eur J Gastroenterol Hepatol.* 2000;12:855-862.
19. Hilsden RJ, Hodgins DC, Timmer A, Sutherland LR. Helping patients with Crohn's disease quit smoking. *Am J Gastroenterol.* 2000;95:352-358.
20. Wolf JM, Lashner BA. Inflammatory bowel disease: sorting out the treatment options. *Cleve Clin J Med.* 2002;69:621-626, 629-631.
21. Lindstrom J. Neuronal nicotinic acetylcholine receptors. *Ion Channels.* 1996;4:377-450.
22. Hogg RC, Raggenbass M, Bertrand D. Nicotinic acetylcholine receptors: from structure to brain function. *Rev Physiol Biochem Pharmacol.* 2003;147:1-46.
23. Woolf A, Burkhart K, Caraccio T, Litovitz T. Self-poisoning among adults using multiple transdermal nicotine patches. *J Toxicol Clin Toxicol.* 1996;34:691-698.
24. Alkondon M, Albuquerque EX. The nicotinic acetylcholine receptor subtypes and their function in the hippocampus and cerebral cortex. *Prog Brain Res.* 2004;145:109-120.
25. Alkondon M, Albuquerque EX. Nicotinic acetylcholine receptor alpha7 and alpha4 beta2 subtypes differentially control GABAergic input to CA1 neurons in rat hippocampus. *J Neurophysiol.* 2001;86:3043-3055.
26. Alkondon M, Pereira EF, Albuquerque EX. Mapping the location of functional nicotinic and gamma-aminobutyric acidA receptors on hippocampal neurons. *J Pharmacol Exp Ther.* 1996;279:1491-1506.
27. Hasselmo ME, Hay J, Ilyn M, Gorchetchnikov A. Neuromodulation, theta rhythm and rat spatial navigation. *Neural Netw.* 2002;15:689-707.
28. Ji D, Dani JA. Inhibition and disinhibition of pyramidal neurons by activation of nicotinic receptors on hippocampal interneurons. *J Neurophysiol.* 2000;83:2682-2690.
29. Ji D, Lape R, Dani JA. Timing and location of nicotinic activity enhances or depresses hippocampal synaptic plasticity. *Neuron.* 2001; 31:131-141.
30. McGehee DS. Nicotinic receptors and hippocampal synaptic plasticity: it's all in the timing. *Trends Neurosci.* 2002;25:171-172.
31. Shao Z, Yakel JL. Single channel properties of neuronal nicotinic ACh receptors in stratum radiatum interneurons of rat hippocampal slices. *J Physiol.* 2000;527:507-513.
32. West KA, Brognard J, Clark AS, et al. Rapid Akt activation by nicotine and a tobacco carcinogen modulates the phenotype of normal human airway epithelial cells. *J Clin Invest.* 2003;111:81-90.
33. Brunzell DH, Russell DS, Picciotto MR. In vivo nicotine treatment regulates mesocorticolimbic CREB and ERK signaling in C57Bl/6J mice. *J Neurochem.* 2003;84:1431-1441.
34. Minana MD, Montoliu C, Llansola M, Grisolia S, Felipo V. Nicotine prevents glutamate-induced proteolysis of the microtubule-associated protein MAP-2 and glutamate neurotoxicity in primary cultures of cerebellar neurons. *Neuropharmacology.* 1998;37:847-857.
35. Meyer EL, Gahring LC, Rogers SW. Nicotine preconditioning antagonizes activity-dependent caspase proteolysis of a glutamate receptor. *J Biol Chem.* 2002;277:10869-10875.
36. Oshikawa J, Toya Y, Fujita T, et al. Nicotinic acetylcholine receptor alpha7 regulates cAMP signal within lipid rafts. *Am J Physiol Cell Physiol.* 2003;285:C567-C574.
37. Vallejo YF, Buisson B, Bertrand D, Green WN. Chronic nicotine exposure upregulates nicotinic receptors by a novel mechanism. *J Neurosci.* 2005;25:5563-5572.
38. Xiao Y, Kellar KJ. The comparative pharmacology and up-regulation of rat neuronal nicotinic receptor subtype binding sites stably expressed in transfected mammalian cells. *J Pharmacol Exp Ther.* 2004;310:98-107.
39. Tapper AR, McKinney SL, Nashmi R, et al. Nicotine activation of alpha4* receptors: sufficient for reward, tolerance, and sensitization. *Science.* 2004;306:1029-1032.

40. Department of Health and Human Services. Nicotine: pharmacokinetics, metabolism, and pharmacodynamics. *The Health Consequences of Smoking: Nicotine Addiction. A Report of the Surgeon General.* 1988; Available at: http://www.cdc.gov/tobacco/sgr/sgr_1988/. Accessed January 6, 2006.
41. Benowitz NL. Clinical pharmacology of nicotine. *Annu Rev Med.* 1986;37:21-32.
42. Pavlov VA, Wang H, Czura CJ, Friedman SG, Tracey KJ. The cholinergic anti-inflammatory pathway: a missing link in neuroimmunomodulation. *Mol Med.* 2003;9:125-134.
43. Wang H, Yu M, Ochani M, et al. Nicotinic acetylcholine receptor alpha7 subunit is an essential regulator of inflammation. *Nature.* 2003;421:384-388.
44. Wang H, Liao H, Ochani M, et al. Cholinergic agonists inhibit HMGB1 release and improve survival in experimental sepsis. *Nat Med.* 2004;10:1216-1221.
45. Wright SC, Zhong J, Zheng H, Larrick JW. Nicotine inhibition of apoptosis suggests a role in tumor promotion. *FASEB J.* 1993;7:1045-1051.
46. Gahring LC, Carlson NG, Wieggel WA, Howard J, Rogers SW. Alcohol blocks TNFalpha but not other cytokine-mediated neuroprotection to NMDA. *Alcohol Clin Exp Res.* 1999;23:1571-1579.
47. Coulie B, Camilleri M, Bharucha AE, Sandborn WJ, Burton D. Colonic motility in chronic ulcerative proctosigmoiditis and the effects of nicotine on colonic motility in patients and healthy subjects. *Aliment Pharmacol Ther.* 2001;15:653-663.
48. McGrath J, McDonald JW, Macdonald JK. Transdermal nicotine for induction of remission in ulcerative colitis. *Cochrane Database Syst Rev.* 2004;(4):CD004722.
49. Orr-Urtreger A, Kedmi M, Rosner S, Karmeli F, Rachmilewitz D. Increased severity of experimental colitis in alpha5 nicotinic acetylcholine receptor subunit-deficient mice. *Neuroreport.* 2005;16:1123-1127.
50. Glushakov AV, Voytenko LP, Skok MV, Skok V. Distribution of neuronal nicotinic acetylcholine receptors containing different alpha-subunits in the submucosal plexus of the guinea-pig. *Auton Neurosci.* 2004;110:19-26.
51. Richardson CE, Morgan JM, Jasani B, et al. Megacystis-microcolon-intestinal hypoperistalsis syndrome and the absence of the alpha3 nicotinic acetylcholine receptor subunit. *Gastroenterology.* 2001;121:350-357.
52. Xu W, Gelber S, Orr-Urtreger A, et al. Megacystis, mydriasis, and ion channel defect in mice lacking the alpha3 neuronal nicotinic acetylcholine receptor. *Proc Natl Acad Sci USA.* 1999;96:5746-5751.
53. Zia S, Ndoye A, Nguyen VT, Grando SA. Nicotine enhances expression of the alpha3, alpha4, alpha5, and alpha7 nicotinic receptors modulating calcium metabolism and regulating adhesion and motility of respiratory epithelial cells. *Res Commun Mol Pathol Pharmacol.* 1997;97:243-262.
54. Macklin KD, Maus AD, Pereira EF, Albuquerque EX, Conti-Fine BM. Human vascular endothelial cells express functional nicotinic acetylcholine receptors. *J Pharmacol Exp Ther.* 1998;287:435-439.
55. Maus AD, Pereira EF, Karachunski PI, et al. Human and rodent bronchial epithelial cells express functional nicotinic acetylcholine receptors. *Mol Pharmacol.* 1998;54:779-788.
56. Plummer HK, 3rd, Dhar M, Schuller HM. Expression of the alpha7 nicotinic acetylcholine receptor in human lung cells. *Respir Res.* 2005;6:29.
57. Reynolds PR, Hoidal JR. Temporal-spatial expression and transcriptional regulation of alpha7 nicotinic acetylcholine receptor (nAChR) by TTF-1 and EGR-1 during murine lung development. *J Biol Chem.* 2005;280:32548-32554.
58. Wang Y, Pereira EF, Maus AD, et al. Human bronchial epithelial and endothelial cells express alpha7 nicotinic acetylcholine receptors. *Mol Pharmacol.* 2001;60:1201-1209.
59. Carlisle DL, Hopkins TM, Gaither-Davis A, et al. Nicotine signals through muscle-type and neuronal nicotinic acetylcholine receptors in both human bronchial epithelial cells and airway fibroblasts. *Respir Res.* 2004;5:27.
60. Albuquerque EX, Alkondon M, Pereira EF, et al. Properties of neuronal nicotinic acetylcholine receptors: pharmacological characterization and modulation of synaptic function. *J Pharmacol Exp Ther.* 1997;280:1117-1136.

61. Mannino DM. Chronic obstructive pulmonary disease: definition and epidemiology. *Respir Care.* 2003;48:1185-1191.
62. Sopori M. Effects of cigarette smoke on the immune system. *Nat Rev Immunol.* 2002;2:372-377.
63. Sopori ML, Kozak W, Savage SM, Geng Y, Kluger MJ. Nicotine-induced modulation of T cell function: implications for inflammation and infection. *Adv Exp Med Biol.* 1998;437:279-289.
64. Floto RA, Smith KG. The vagus nerve, macrophages, and nicotine. *Lancet.* 2003;361: 1069-1070.
65. Hance AJ, Basset F, Saumon G, et al. Smoking and interstitial lung disease: the effect of cigarette smoking on the incidence of pulmonary histiocytosis X and sarcoidosis. *Ann N Y Acad Sci.* 1986;465:643-656.
66. Baur X, Richter G, Pethran A, Czuppon AB, Schwaiblmair M. Increased prevalence of IgG-induced sensitization and hypersensitivity pneumonitis (humidifier lung) in nonsmokers exposed to aerosols of a contaminated air conditioner. *Respiration.* 1992;59:211-214.
67. Cormier Y, Gagnon L, Berube-Genest F, Fournier M. Sequential bronchoalveolar lavage in experimental extrinsic allergic alveolitis: the influence of cigarette smoking. *Am Rev Respir Dis.* 1988;137:1104-1109.
68. Marks MJ, Stitzel JA, Collins AC. Genetic influences on nicotine responses. *Pharmacol Biochem Behav.* 1989;33:667-678.
69. Gahring LC, Persiyanov K, Dunn D, Weiss R, Meyer EL, Rogers SW. Mouse strain-specific nicotinic acetylcholine receptor expression by inhibitory interneurons and astrocytes in the dorsal hippocampus. *J Comp Neurol.* 2004;468:334-346.
70. Guerassimov A, Hoshino Y, Takubo Y, et al. The development of emphysema in cigarette smoke-exposed mice is strain dependent. *Am J Respir Crit Care Med.* 2004;170:974-980.
71. Nakanishi N, Nakamura K, Matsuo Y, Suzuki K, Tatara K. Cigarette smoking and risk for impaired fasting glucose and type 2 diabetes in middle-aged Japanese men. *Ann Intern Med.* 2000;133:183-191.
72. Filozof C, Fernandez Pinilla MC, Fernandez-Cruz A. Smoking cessation and weight gain. *Obes Rev.* 2004;5:95-103.
73. Miyazaki T, Shimada K, Mokuno H, Daida H. Adipocyte-derived plasma protein, adiponectin, is associated with smoking status in patients with coronary artery disease. *Heart.* 2003;89:663.
74. Liu RH, Mizuta M, Matsukura S. The expression and functional role of nicotinic acetylcholine receptors in rat adipocytes. *J Pharmacol Exp Ther.* 2004;310:52-58.
75. Lindstrom JM. Acetylcholine receptors and myasthenia. *Muscle Nerve.* 2000;23:453-477.
76. Vincent A, Drachman DB. Myasthenia gravis. *Adv Neurol.* 2002;88:159-188.
77. Navaneetham D, Jr, Penn A, Jr, Howard J, Jr, Conti-Fine BM. Expression of the alpha7 subunit of the nicotinic acetylcholine receptor in normal and myasthenic human thymuses. *Cell Mol Biol (Noisy-le-grand).* 1997;43:433-442.
78. Vernino S, Low PA, Lennon VA. Experimental autoimmune autonomic neuropathy. *J Neurophysiol.* 2003;90:2053-2059.
79. Gahring L, Carlson NG, Meyer EL, Rogers SW. Granzyme B proteolysis of a neuronal glutamate receptor generates an autoantigen and is modulated by glycosylation. *J Immunol.* 2001;166:1433-1438.
80. Casciola-Rosen L, Andrade F, Ulanet D, Wong WB, Rosen A. Cleavage by granzyme B is strongly predictive of autoantigen status: implications for initiation of autoimmunity. *J Exp Med.* 1999;190:815-826.
81. Gahring LC, Rogers SW. Autoimmunity to glutamate receptors in the central nervous system. *Crit Rev Immunol.* 2002;22:295-316.
82. Lennon VA, Ermilov LG, Szurszewski JH, Vernino S. Immunization with neuronal nicotinic acetylcholine receptor induces neurological autoimmune disease. *J Clin Invest.* 2003;111:907-913.
83. Mills CM. Cigarette smoking, cutaneous immunity, and inflammatory response. *Clin Dermatol.* 1998;16:589-594.

84. Mihovilovic M, Denning S, Mai Y, et al. Thymocytes and cultured thymic epithelial cells express transcripts encoding alpha-3, alpha-5, and beta-4 subunits of neuronal nicotinic acetylcholine receptors. Preferential transcription of the alpha-3 and beta-4 genes by immature CD4+8+ thymocytes and evidence for response to nicotine in thymocytes. *Ann N Y Acad Sci.* 1998;841:388-392.

85. Kawashima K, Fujii T. The lymphocytic cholinergic system and its biological function. *Life Sci.* 2003;72:2101-2109.

86. Peng H, Ferris RL, Matthews T, Hiel H, Lopez-Albaitero A, Lustig LR. Characterization of the human nicotinic acetylcholine receptor subunit alpha (alpha) 9 (CHRNA9) and alpha (alpha) 10 (CHRNA10) in lymphocytes. *Life Sci.* 2004;76:263-280.

87. Sopori ML, Kozak W. Immunomodulatory effects of cigarette smoke. *J Neuroimmunol.* 1998;83:148-156.

88. Kalra R, Singh SP, Savage SM, Finch GL, Sopori ML. Effects of cigarette smoke on immune response: chronic exposure to cigarette smoke impairs antigen-mediated signaling in T cells and depletes IP3-sensitive Ca(2+) stores. *J Pharmacol Exp Ther.* 2000;293:166-171.

89. van Dijk AP, Meijssen MA, Brouwer AJ, et al. Transdermal nicotine inhibits interleukin 2 synthesis by mononuclear cells derived from healthy volunteers. *Eur J Clin Invest.* 1998;28:664-671.

90. Nuorti JP, Butler JC, Farley MM, et al. Cigarette smoking and invasive pneumococcal disease. Active Bacterial Core Surveillance Team. *N Engl J Med.* 2000;342:681-689.

91. Matsunaga K, Klein TW, Friedman H, Yamamoto Y. Involvement of nicotinic acetylcholine receptors in suppression of antimicrobial activity and cytokine responses of alveolar macrophages to Legionella pneumophila infection by nicotine. *J Immunol.* 2001;167:6518-6524.

92. Blanchet MR, Israel-Assayag E, Cormier Y. Inhibitory effect of nicotine on experimental hypersensitivity pneumonitis in vivo and in vitro. *Am J Respir Crit Care Med.* 2004;169:903-909.

93. Shivji M, Jr, Burger S, Jr, Moncada CA, Jr, Clarkson AB, Jr, Merali S. Effect of nicotine on lung S-adenosylmethionine and development of *Pneumocystis* pneumonia. *J Biol Chem.* 2005;280:15219-15228.

94. Saah AJ, Hoover DR, Peng Y, et al. Predictors for failure of *Pneumocystis carinii* pneumonia prophylaxis. Multicenter AIDS Cohort Study. *JAMA.* 1995;273:1197-1202.

95. Aicher A, Heeschen C, Mohaupt M, Cooke JP, Zeiher AM, Dimmeler S. Nicotine strongly activates dendritic cell-mediated adaptive immunity: potential role for progression of atherosclerotic lesions. *Circulation.* 2003;107:604-611.

96. Kadunce DP, Burr R, Gress R, Kanner R, Lyon JL, Zone JJ. Cigarette smoking: risk factor for premature facial wrinkling. *Ann Intern Med.* 1991;114:840-844.

97. Misery L. Nicotine effects on skin: are they positive or negative? *Exp Dermatol.* 2004;13:665-670.

98. Grando SA. Biological functions of keratinocyte cholinergic receptors. *J Investig Dermatol Symp Proc.* 1997;2:41-48.

99. Kurzen H, Berger H, Jager C, et al. Phenotypical and molecular profiling of the extraneuronal cholinergic system of the skin. *J Invest Dermatol.* 2004;123:937-949.

100. Zia S, Ndoye A, Lee TX, Webber RJ, Grando SA. Receptor-mediated inhibition of keratinocyte migration by nicotine involves modulations of calcium influx and intracellular concentration. *J Pharmacol Exp Ther.* 2000;293:973-981.

101. Chernyavsky AI, Arredondo J, Marubio LM, Grando SA. Differential regulation of keratinocyte chemokinesis and chemotaxis through distinct nicotinic receptor subtypes. *J Cell Sci.* 2004;117:5665-5679.

102. Arredondo J, Nguyen VT, Chernyavsky AI, et al. Central role of alpha7 nicotinic receptor in differentiation of the stratified squamous epithelium. *J Cell Biol.* 2002;159:325-336.

103. Arredondo J, Nguyen VT, Chernyavsky AI, et al. Functional role of alpha7 nicotinic receptor in physiological control of cutaneous homeostasis. *Life Sci.* 2003;72:2063-2067.

104. Zwart R, Van Kleef RG, Vijverberg HP. Physostigmine and atropine potentiate and inhibit neuronal alpha4 beta4 nicotinic receptors. *Ann N Y Acad Sci.* 1999;868:636-639.

105. Bergstrom J. Tobacco smoking and chronic destructive periodontal disease. *Odontology.* 2004;92:1-8.
106. Wendell KJ, Stein SH. Regulation of cytokine production in human gingival fibroblasts following treatment with nicotine and lipopolysaccharide. *J Periodontol.* 2001;72:1038-1044.
107. Arredondo J, Chernyavsky AI, Marubio LM, et al. Receptor-mediated tobacco toxicity: regulation of gene expression through alpha3beta2 nicotinic receptor in oral epithelial cells. *Am J Pathol.* 2005;166:597-613.
108. Heeschen C, Jang JJ, Weis M, et al. Nicotine stimulates angiogenesis and promotes tumor growth and atherosclerosis. *Nat Med.* 2001;7:833-839.
109. Di Luozzo G, Pradhan S, Dhadwal AK, Chen A, Ueno H, Sumpio BE. Nicotine induces mitogen-activated protein kinase-dependent vascular smooth muscle cell migration. *Atherosclerosis.* 2005;178:271-277.
110. Moccia F, Frost C, Berra-Romani R, Tanzi F, Adams DJ. Expression and function of neuronal nicotinic ACh receptors in rat microvascular endothelial cells. *Am J Physiol Heart Circ Physiol.* 2004;286:H486-H491.
111. Saeed RW, Varma S, Peng-Nemeroff T, et al. Cholinergic stimulation blocks endothelial cell activation and leukocyte recruitment during inflammation. *J Exp Med.* 2005;201:1113-1123.

Part II
Transporters & Stimulants
& Hallucinogens

Chapter 11
Role of Monoamine Transporters in Mediating Psychostimulant Effects

Evan L. Riddle,[1] Annette E. Fleckenstein,[1] and Glen R. Hanson[1]

Abstract Monoamine transporters such as the dopamine (DA) transporter (DAT) and the vesicular monoamine transporter-2 (VMAT-2) are critical regulators of DA disposition within the brain. Alterations in DA disposition can lead to conditions such as drug addiction, Parkinson's disease, and schizophrenia, a fact that underscores the importance of understanding DAergic signaling. Psychostimulants alter DAergic signaling by influencing both DAT and VMAT-2, and although the effects of these drugs result in increased levels of synaptic DA, the mechanisms by which this occurs and the effects that these drugs exert on DAT and VMAT-2 vary. Many psychostimulants can be classified as releasers (ie, amphetamine analogs) or uptake blockers (ie, cocaine-like drugs) based on the mechanism of their acute effects on neurotransmitter flux through the DAT. Releasers and uptake blockers differentially modulate the activity and subcellular distribution of monoamine transporters, a phenomenon likely related to the neurotoxic potential of these drugs to DAergic neurons. This article will review some of the recent findings whereby releasers and uptake blockers alter DAT and VMAT-2 activity and how these alterations may be involved in neurotoxicity, thus providing insight on the neurodegeneration observed in Parkinson's disease.

Keywords dopamine transporter, vesicular monoamine transporter-2, amphetamine, cocaine, methylphenidate, Parkinson's disease

Introduction

Dopamine (DA) is a monoamine neurotransmitter important for many physiological processes such as motor movement, reward, motivation, and cognition. Accordingly, DAergic dysfunction can lead to a variety of disease states including drug addiction,

[1] Department of Pharmacology and Toxicology, University of Utah, Salt Lake City, Utah 84112

Corresponding Author: Glen R. Hanson, University of Utah, Department of Pharmacology and Toxicology, 30 South 2000 East, Room 201, Salt Lake City, Utah 84112. Tel: (801) 581-3174; Fax: (801) 585-5111; E-mail: glen.hanson@pharm.utah.edu

R.S. Rapaka and W. Sadée (eds.), *Drug Addiction.*
© American Association of Pharmaceutical Scientists 2008

Parkinson's disease, and schizophrenia. Consequently, appreciation of regulatory mechanisms relevant to the functioning of DA systems is critical to the elucidation of the etiology of these disorders and the development of more effective therapeutics.

Under normal physiological conditions, the DA transporter (DAT) and vesicular monoamine transporter-2 (VMAT-2) are key components in the regulation of DA disposition in the synapse and cytosol. Following vesicular DA release into the synapse, the DAT transports DA from the perisynaptic area into the cytosol of the presynaptic nerve terminal of DA neurons. The VMAT-2 transports cytosolic and newly synthesized DA into synaptic vesicles. Sequestration of DA into these vesicles makes the transmitter available for synaptic release in response to appropriate stimulation. It also provides an environment to protect against the intracellular production of reactive oxygen species that can result from DA oxidation.

Psychostimulants are potent modulators of DAergic signaling; therefore, it is not surprising that alterations in DAT and VMAT-2 function are caused by psychostimulant treatment, and that unique effect profiles exist for different drug types in this pharmacological category. It has long been known that psychostimulants alter DAT function; however, more recently, novel responses of DAT to these drugs as well as unexpected effects on VMAT-2 function have been observed. For example, our group and other researchers have recently observed heretofore unreported effects of the psychostimulants on monoamine transporters that help distinguish between 2 principal types of psychostimulants and provide insight into the physiological regulation of these proteins and their potential roles in both etiology of pathology and therapeutic targets. This review will focus on some of the recent findings elucidating mechanisms whereby amphetamine- and cocaine-like drugs alter DAT and VMAT-2 function. In addition, the clinical relevance of such alterations will be discussed.

Psychostimulants and Mechanisms of Action

Psychostimulants promote increased extracellular DA concentrations; however, there are 2 primary mechanisms by which these agents affect the DAT. Psychostimulants can be separated into "uptake blockers" and "releasers" based on the mechanism of their acute effects on neurotransmitter flux through the DAT. Although uptake blockers can have releasing properties[1,2] and releasers may also have some uptake blocking ability,[3] the general separation of drugs into these 2 classes helps to functionally distinguish the pharmacological profiles of some of the most commonly used psychostimulants.

In addition to effects on the DAT, other researchers[4,5] and we[6-8] have reported data indicating that uptake blockers and releasers differentially regulate the VMAT-2. These changes are associated with a redistribution of VMAT-2, and presumably VMAT-2-containing vesicles, within striatal presynaptic nerve terminals. Through the use of DA receptor agonists and antagonists, it is clear that this psychostimulant-induced vesicular redistribution is mediated by DA receptors. However, DA receptor-mediated vesicular trafficking is not sufficient to explain all of the psychostimulant-induced vesicular trafficking, suggesting that DA receptor-independent pathways also contribute to these psychostimulant effects.

Uptake Blockers

Cocaine and methylphenidate (MPD) are among the best-characterized uptake blockers with respect to effects on DAT and VMAT-2. Cocaine and MPD bind common sites on the DAT[9] and in most cases, their mechanisms of action on DA systems appear to be similar. However, with respect to VMAT-2, differences have been observed and will be discussed below.

DAT

Cocaine and MPD are classified as DA uptake blockers because their primary mechanism of action is by directly binding and inhibiting the transport of DA through the DAT.[10] Blockade of DAT activity leads to increased extracellular DA levels and is not associated with selective long-term toxicity to the nigrostriatal DA pathway.[11] Of interest, blockade of DAT by cocaine leads to a rapid increase in DA uptake in synaptosomes prepared from treated rats,[12] a preparation from which the drug has been presumably been washed out. Perhaps this occurs via enhanced recruitment of DATs to the plasma membrane.[13] These acute increases in DA uptake and plasmalemmal surface expression, observed in rodents and cell lines, respectively, after cocaine administration likely represent efforts to maintain normal synaptic DA functions. In humans who have repeatedly increased synaptic DA levels through the use of cocaine, increased DAT function is also observed, as assessed in synaptosomes from cryoprotected human brain.[14] The combination of an initial DAT blockade and a subsequent increase in DA uptake could contribute to the development and expression of cocaine addiction. It is possible that an over-abundance of extracellular DA during DAT blockade triggers this compensatory increase in DAT activity, which would ultimately produce a deficit in extracellular DA, perhaps contributing to drug dependence.

VMAT-2

In addition to blocking DAT, cocaine and MPD administrations alter the subcellular localization of VMAT-2-containing synaptic vesicles (Fig. 11.1).[7,8] Even though distinct patterns are observed with differential centrifugation techniques, suggesting that trafficking is readily regulated and likely has important functional consequences,[7,8,15]

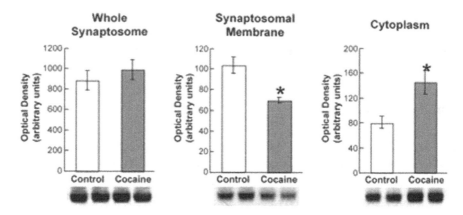

Fig. 11.1 Western blots demonstrating that cocaine redistributes VMAT-2 immunoreactivity from the synaptosomal membrane to the cytoplasm. Rats received a single injection of saline vehicle (1 mL/kg, intraperitoneally [ip]) or cocaine (30 mg/kg, ip) and were killed 1 hour later. Immunoreactivity was assessed as described by Riddle et al.[7] Columns represent the mean optical density, and error bars represent the SEM of determinations in 6 treated rats. *Values for cocaine-treated rats that are significantly different from saline-treated controls; $P \leq .05$.

it is unclear precisely which pool(s) of synaptic vesicles are altered as a consequence of exposure to these DAT inhibitors.

Although precise details are lacking, it appears that increased extracellular DA caused by the uptake blockers causes the redistribution of VMAT-2-containing vesicles from a plasmalemmal membrane fraction to a nonmembrane associated (presumably cytosolic) fraction because cocaine-induced vesicular trafficking can be blocked with DA D2 receptor antagonists.[16] In contrast, MPD-induced trafficking involves both D2 and D1 receptors since D1 and D2 antagonists are required to block the effects of MPD.[8] Consistent with a role for D2 receptors in these effects caused by DAT inhibitors is the finding that administration of D2 agonists causes vesicle trafficking in a manner similar to uptake blockers.[8,17-19] This finding suggests that in response to DAT blockade, the increased extracellular concentrations of DA in the synapse stimulates DA receptors causing vesicles to move into the cytosol. Implications of vesicular trafficking into the cytosol will be discussed subsequently.

Releasers

Amphetamine analogs such as amphetamine, methamphetamine (METH), and 3,4-methylenedioxymethamphetamine (MDMA) are classified as "releasers." Releasing drugs such as these likely promote DA release by disrupting vesicular pH gradients allowing vesicular DA to redistribute into the cytoplasm.[20,21] Subsequently, as cytoplasmic DA levels rise, DA exits the neuron via reverse transport and/or channel-like activity of the DAT,[22,23] leading to a dramatic increase in synaptic DA levels.

DAT

In rats, a single high-dose injection (10 mg/kg) of METH rapidly (within 1 hour) and reversibly decreases the amount of DA taken up into synaptosomes prepared from treated rodents.[24] Data from cell lines expressing the DAT demonstrate that exposure to amphetamine rapidly reduces plasma membrane-associated DAT, an effect likely representing a significant shift of this protein to the cytosolic fraction.[25] For in vivo relevance, it is difficult to extrapolate the time course of DA release through the DAT and a reduction of DAT on the cell surface; however, releasing drugs probably promote initial DA release followed by a removal of DAT from the cell surface.

The effects of releasing drugs become more complicated with higher doses (such as 4 × 10 mg/kg/injection of METH at 2-hour intervals) that cause persistent deficits in striatal DA systems. As with a single injection of METH, multiple high-dose administrations cause a rapid (within 1 hour after final METH injection) decrease in DAT activity; however, this decrease in DAT is substantially greater and may be linked to persistent DAergic deficits. Although the mechanisms of releaser-induced toxicity is not completely understood, DA, hyperthermia, and oxygen radicals contribute to this phenomenon.[26]

In addition to releaser-induced changes in DAT activity, our laboratory has recently demonstrated physical alterations in DAT caused by high doses of these drugs. More specifically, neurotoxic regimens of METH induce DAT complex formation.[27] At present, it is unclear whether these complexes are homomeric or heteromeric at their site of production, but these protein complexes only occur when neurotoxic regimens of METH are administered. These complexes appear to be linked to toxicity as their formation is dependent on DA, hyperthermia, and reactive species,[28] requisite factors for the METH-induced persistent DA deficits in the striatum. The functional consequences of METH-induced DAT complex formation remain to be determined.

VMAT-2

Like the uptake blockers, releaser psychostimulants appear to alter the subcellular localization of VMAT-2-containing synaptic vesicles. As with uptake blockers, it remains unclear which precise pool(s) of synaptic vesicles are altered and to what cellular location(s) they traffic; however, releaser drugs at high doses appear to redistribute vesicles from the cytoplasm to a subcellular region not retained in a synaptosomal preparation (Fig. 11.2).[7] Of interest, similar to uptake blockers, these VMAT-2-related effects are also prevented by pretreatment with D2 antagonists,[6]

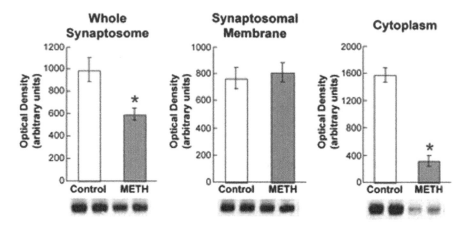

Fig. 11.2 Western blots demonstrating that METH redistributes VMAT-2 immunoreactivity from the cytoplasm to a location not retained in a synaptosomal preparation. Rats received multiple high-dose injections of METH (4 × 10 mg/kg, subcutaneously [sc], at 2-hour intervals) or saline vehicle (1 mL/kg, sc per injection) and were killed 1 hour after the final injection. Immunoreactivity was assessed as described by Riddle et al.[7] Columns represent the mean optical density, and error bars represent the SEM of determinations in 6 treated rats. *Values for METH-treated rats that are significantly different from saline-treated controls; $P \leq .05$.

which demonstrates that D2 activation is critical for releaser-induced vesicular trafficking. Thus D2 activation is required, but releasers employ heretofore unidentified mechanisms that result in vesicular trafficking in a manner different (and perhaps "opposite" with respect to the cytoplasmic pool) than that observed with D2 receptor agonists.

The effect of releaser psychostimulants to cause neurotoxicity may be related to the effect of these drugs on vesicular trafficking. The basis for this possibility is that neurotoxic effects of releasers likely require buildup of DA in the cytosol.[29] Under normal circumstances, VMAT-2 sequesters cytosolic DA, thus preventing the cytotoxic effects of oxidized DA. However, when exposed to releasers, the ability of VMAT-2 to sequester DA is compromised, allowing DA to be redistributed from inside the synaptic vesicle into the cytoplasm.[21] In addition, it is possible that after redistribution of DA into the cytosol, releasers cause vesicles to be moved far from the site of leakage, increasing the duration of cytosolic DA buildup. With this in mind, experiments were designed to determine if the effect of the uptake blocker, MPD, could protect against METH-induced toxicity.[15] Theoretically, if METH caused DA to leak into the cytoplasm and then removed VMAT-2-containing vesicles from the cytoplasm, MPD could protect against toxicity by trafficking vesicles into the cytoplasm to sequester the cytosolic DA. Indeed, posttreatment with methylphenidate of animals that received a neurotoxic dosing regimen of METH protected against METH-induced neurotoxicity. These data are consistent with previous findings that posttreatment with another uptake inhibitor, amfonelic acid, protects against the persistent DA deficits caused by METH.[30]

Discussion

During normal DAergic neurotransmission, the DAT regulates extracellular concentrations of DA, while VMAT-2 directly regulates cytosolic concentrations of DA and indirectly regulates extracellular DA by determining how much DA is released from each vesicle in response to action potential-linked release. It is likely that DA receptors allow the cell to monitor the levels of extracellular DA and provide a feedback mechanism to regulate DAT and VMAT-2 function, permitting the cell to respond to varying conditions. However, because of the reactive nature of DA, abnormal modifications in normal DAergic signaling and regulations may cause drastic consequences that can lead to damage of DA cells.

A common feature of most psychostimulants is that their administration increases synaptic DA concentrations. Psychostimulants achieve this primarily by their effects on DAT and/or VMAT-2 function; however, the mechanisms by which subclasses of psychostimulants (ie, uptake blockers and releasers) act are distinct and as a result produce important physiological and functional differences. For example, uptake blockers cause little or no persistent DA deficits, whereas releasers (at high doses) can cause persistent deficits in monoaminergic neurons. The mechanistic differences between uptake blockers and releasers provide clues on how neurotoxicity occurs and also suggest potential targets for therapeutic interventions. This is of great importance for degenerative diseases such as Parkinson's disease, since the cause of the age-related decline in nigrostriatal DAergic nerve terminals associated with this degenerative condition has not been fully elucidated. The selective toxicity of some releasers to specific DAergic neurons allows researchers the means to discover why and how DAergic neurodegeneration in vulnerable systems occurs and provides models to test ways to prevent it. Insights into DAergic neurotoxicity have been gained by advances in our understanding of the "opposite" nature of uptake blockers versus releasers. The releaser, METH, is neurotoxic to nigrostriatal DA neurons when administered at high doses, the same neurons that are lost in Parkinson's disease. Perhaps treatments that prevent METH toxicity have the potential to be useful in the treatment of Parkinson's disease; thus uptake blockers (and perhaps D2 agonists) are protective against METH-induced DA neurodegeneration and therefore should be considered as candidates for slowing the progression of Parkinson's disease.

Acknowledgments This work was supported by Grants DA00378, DA00869, DA13367, DA11389, DA04222 and Johnson and Johnson Focused Giving Gift (New Brunswick, NJ).

References

1. Butcher SP, Liptrot J, Aburthnott GW. Characterisation of methylphenidate and nomifensine induced dopamine release in rat striatum using in vivo microdialysis. *Neurosci Lett.* 1991;122:245-248.
2. Russell V, de Villiers A, Sagvolden T, Lamm M, Taljaard J. Differences between electrically-, Ritalin-, and D-amphetamine-stimulated release of [3H]dopamine from brain slices suggest

impaired storage of dopamine in an animal model of attention-deficit hyperactivity disorder. *Behav Brain Res.* 1998;94:163-171.

3. Horn AS, Coyle JT, Snyder SH. Catecholamine uptake by synaptosomes from rat brain: structure-activity relationships of drugs with differential effects on dopamine and norepinephrine neurons. *Mol Pharmacol.* 1971;7:66-80.

4. Hogan KA, Staal RG, Sonsalla PK. Analysis of VMAT2 binding after methamphetamine or MPTP treatment: disparity between homogenates and vesicle preparations. *J Neurochem.* 2000;74:2217-2220.

5. Eyerman DJ, Yamamoto BK. Lobeline attenuates methamphetamine-induced changes in vesicular monoamine transporter 2 immunoreactivity and monoamine depletions in the striatum. *J Pharmacol Exp Ther.* 2005;312:160-169.

6. Brown JM, Riddle EL, Sandoval V, et al. A single methamphetamine administration rapidly decreases vesicular dopamine uptake. *J Pharmacol Exp Ther.* 2002;302:497-501.

7. Riddle EL, Topham MK, Haycock JW, Hanson GR, Fleckenstein AE. Differential trafficking of the vesicular monoamine transporter-2 by methamphetamine and cocaine. *Eur J Pharmacol.* 2002;449:71-74.

8. Sandoval V, Riddle EL, Hanson GR, Fleckenstein AE. Methylphenidate redistributes vesicular monoamine transporter-2: role of dopamine receptors. *J Neurosci.* 2002;22:8705-8710.

9. Wayment HK, Deutsch H, Schweri MM, Schenk JO. Effects of methylphenidate analogues on phenethylamine substrates for the striatal dopamine transporter: potential as amphetamine antagonists. *J Neurochem.* 1999;72:1266-1274.

10. Ritz MC, Lamb RJ, Goldberg SR, Kuhar MJ. Cocaine receptors on dopamine transporters are related to self-administration of cocaine. *Science.* 1987;237:1219-1223.

11. Yeh SY, De Souza EB. Lack of neurochemical evidence for neurotoxic effects of repeated cocaine administration in rats on brain monoamine neurons. *Drug Alcohol Depend.* 1991;27:51-61.

12. Fleckenstein AE, Haughey HM, Metzger RR, et al. Differential effects of psychostimulants and related agents on dopaminergic and serotonergic transporter function. *Eur J Pharmacol.* 1999;382:45-49.

13. Daws LC, Callaghan PD, Moron JA, et al. Cocaine increases dopamine uptake and cell surface expression of dopamine transporters. *Biochem Biophys Res Commun.* 2002;290: 1545-1550.

14. Mash DC, Pablo J, Ouyang Q, Hearn WL, Izenwasser S. Dopamine transport function is elevated in cocaine users. *J Neurochem.* 2002;81:292-300.

15. Sandoval V, Riddle EL, Hanson GR, Fleckenstein AE. Methylphenidate alters vesicular monoamine transport and prevents methamphetamine-induced dopaminergic deficits. *J Pharmacol Exp Ther.* 2003;304:1181-1187.

16. Brown JM, Hanson GR, Fleckenstein AE. Cocaine-induced increases in vesicular dopamine uptake: role of dopamine receptors. *J Pharmacol Exp Ther.* 2001;298:1150-1153.

17. Truong JG, Rau KS, Hanson GR. Fleckenstein. Pramipexole increases vesicular dopamine uptake: implications for treatment of Parkinson's neurodegeneration. *Eur J Pharmacol.* 2003;474:223-226.

18. Truong JG, Hanson GR, Fleckenstein AE. Apomorphine increases vesicular monoamine transporter-2 function: implications for neurodegeneration. *Eur J Pharmacol.* 2004a ;492: 143-147.

19. Truong JG, Newman AH, Hanson GR, Fleckenstein AE. Dopamine D2 receptor activation increases vesicular dopamine uptake and redistributes vesicular monoamine transporter-2 protein. *Eur J Pharmacol.* 2004b ;504:27-32.

20. Sulzer D, Rayport S. Amphetamine and other psychostimulants reduce pH gradients in midbrain dopamine neurons and chromaffin granules: a mechanism of action. *Neuron.* 1990;5:797-808.

21. Sulzer D, Chen TK, Lau YY, Kristensen H, Rayport S, Ewing A. Amphetamine redistributes dopamine from synaptic vesicles to the cytosol and promotes reverse transport. *J Neurosci.* 1995;15:4102-4108.
22. Liang NY, Rutledge CO. Evidence for carrier-mediated efflux of dopamine from corpus striatum. *Biochem Pharmacol.* 1982;31:2479-2484.
23. Kahlig KM, Binda F, Khoshbouei H, et al. Amphetamine induces dopamine efflux through a dopamine transporter channel. *Proc Natl Acad Sci USA.* 2005;102:3495-3500.
24. Fleckenstein AE, Metzger RR, Gibb JW, Hanson GR. A rapid and reversible change in dopamine transporters induced by methamphetamine. *Eur J Pharmacol.* 1997;323:R9-10.
25. Saunders C, Ferrer JV, Shi L, et al. Amphetamine-induced loss of human dopamine transporter activity: an internalization-dependent and cocaine sensitive mechanism. *Proc Natl Acad Sci USA.* 2000;97:6850-6855.
26. Fleckenstein AE, Gibb JW, Hanson GR. Differential effects of stimulants on monoaminergic transporters: pharmacological consequences and implications for neurotoxicity. *Eur J Pharmacol.* 2000;406:1-13.
27. Baucum AJ, Rau KS, Riddle EL, Hanson GR, Fleckenstein AE. Methamphetamine increases dopamine transporter higher molecular weight complex formation via a dopamine- and hyperthermia-associated mechanism. *J Neurosci.* 2004;24:3436-3443.
28. Baucum AJ, Cook GA, Hanson JE, Hanson GR, Fleckenstein AE. Reactive oxygen species contribute to dopamine transporter oligomerization [abstract]. *Exp Biol.* 2005; Abstract 312.6.
29. Cubells JF, Rayport S, Rajendran G, Sulzer D. Methamphetamine neurotoxicity involves vacuolation of endocytic organelles and dopamine-dependent intracellular oxidative stress. *J Neurosci.* 1994;14:2260-2271.
30. Marek GJ, Vosmer G, Seiden LS. Dopamine uptake inhibitors block long-term neurotoxic effects of methamphetamine upon dopaminergic neurons. *Brain Res.* 1990;513:274-279.

Chapter 12
Development of the Dopamine Transporter Selective RTI-336 as a Pharmacotherapy for Cocaine Abuse

F. Ivy Carroll,[1] James L. Howard,[2] Leonard L. Howell,[3] Barbara S. Fox,[4] and Michael J. Kuhar[3]

Abstract The discovery and preclinical development of selective dopamine reuptake inhibitors as potential pharmacotherapies for treating cocaine addiction are presented. The studies are based on the hypothesis that a dopamine reuptake inhibitor is expected to partially substitute for cocaine, thus decreasing cocaine self-administration and minimizing the craving for cocaine. This type of indirect agonist therapy has been highly effective for treating smoking addiction (nicotine replacement therapy) and heroin addiction (methadone). To be an effective pharmacotherapy for cocaine addiction, the potential drug must be safe, long-acting, and have minimal abuse potential. We have developed several 3-phenyltropane analogs that are potent dopamine uptake inhibitors, and some are selective for the dopamine transporter relative to the serotonin and norepinephrine transporters. In animal studies, these compounds substitute for cocaine, reduce the intake of cocaine in rats and rhesus monkeys trained to self-administer cocaine, and have demonstrated a slow onset and long duration of action and lack of sensitization. The 3-phenyltropane analogs were also tested in a rhesus monkey self-administration model to define their abuse potential relative to cocaine. Based on these studies, 3β-(4-chlorophenyl)-2β-[3-(4'-methylphenyl)isoxazol-5-yl]tropane (RTI-336) has been selected for preclinical development.

Keywords RTI-336, dopamine transporter, cocaine abuse, pharmacotherapy, 3-aryltropanes

---

[1] Center for Organic and Medicinal Chemistry, Research Triangle Institute, Research Triangle Park, NC 27709

[2] Howard Associates, LLC, Research Triangle Park, NC 27709

[3] Yerkes Regional Primate Research Center, Emory University, Atlanta GA 30329

[4] Addiction Therapies Inc, Wayland, MA 01778

Corresponding Author: F. Ivy Carroll, Research Triangle Institute, PO Box 12194, Research Triangle Park, NC 27709. Tel: (919) 541-6679; Fax: (919) 541-8868; E-mail: fic@rti.org

Introduction

Drug abuse, addiction, and dependence represent a major and increasing threat to public health. Cocaine abuse has been an epidemic in the United States since the introduction of crack in the mid-1980s. The 2003 National Survey on Drug Use and Health (NSDUH) estimated that 34.9 million Americans, aged 12 and older, have used cocaine at least once in their lifetime, that 5.9 million used cocaine in the past year, and that 2.3 million Americans are current users—some frequently, others occasionally (NSDUH report).[1] In 2002, the estimated number of cocaine-related emergency episodes totaled over 199 000.[2] While these numbers on use and cost show the magnitude of the drug abuse problem, the human suffering is incalculable. Illness, crime, domestic violence, reduced productivity, and lost opportunity are direct consequences of drug abuse. There is an increasing understanding that drug abuse is a physiologic disorder and that the need for medications for the treatment of drug abuse is tremendous. Even though several pharmacological agents have been tried on the basis of various hypotheses, none of the pharmacotherapeutic approaches has proven effective.[3-6] To address this critical deficiency, National Institute on Drug Abuse (NIDA) has made the development of an anticocaine medication a high priority.

In vitro studies have demonstrated that cocaine blocks the presynaptic uptake of dopamine, serotonin, and norepinephrine. However, it is the dopamine transporter (DAT) that is believed to be the critical recognition site for cocaine, mediating the behavioral and reinforcing effects that contribute to its abuse liability.[7-11] Numerous cocaine-discrimination and self-administration studies in laboratory animals support this conclusion.

A dopamine reuptake inhibitor would be expected to partially substitute for cocaine, thus decreasing cocaine self-administration and minimizing the craving for cocaine. This type of substitution pharmacotherapy has been highly effective for treatment of nicotine addiction (nicotine gum and patch) and heroin addiction (methadone). The development of a comparable drug for cocaine addiction would allow control of the behavior of the abuser until a strategy for long-term abstinence could be developed. We have discovered novel 3-phenyltropane analogs that are dopamine-selective reuptake inhibitors. It is hoped that one of these compounds will be useful as a medication for treating cocaine addicts without deleterious side effects.[12]

Over the last several years, we synthesized several 3-phenyltropane analogs and evaluated them for binding at the dopamine, serotonin, and norepinephrine transporters (DAT, 5-HTT, and NET, respectively). Forty-seven compounds showed selectivity for the DAT relative to the 5-HTT and NET, based on their relative IC_{50} values.[12,13] The binding affinities of these compounds are compared with cocaine and 3-phenyltropane 2-carboxylic acid methyl ester (WIN 35,065-2) in Tables 12.1-12.4. The compounds possess either a 4-chloro or 4-methylphenyl group at the 3β-position of the tropane ring and have an ester, amide, isoxazole, oxadiazole, benzthiazole, benzimidazole, or thiazole group in the 2β-position. The 15 RTI compounds shown in Table 12.1 have various ester groups in the 2β position of the tropane ring. The affinity for the dopamine transporter varies from 0.96 nM for

RTI-190 to 9.6 nM for RTI-145. The affinities for the ten 2β amides listed in Table 12.2 vary from 0.75 nM for RTI-227 to 6.95 nM for RTI-156. Note the very high DAT selectivity for RTI-147, RTI-214, and RTI-218. The affinities for the 2β-isoxazoles listed in Table 12.3 vary from 0.50 nM for RTI-334 to 8.7 nM for RTI-371. Table 12.4 compares the inhibition of radioligand binding at the dopamine, norepinephrine, and serotonin transporters to those of cocaine and WIN 35,065-2 for 6 different other 2β heterocyclic analogs. Together, these compounds possess sufficient structural diversity to provide considerable variation in

Table 12.1 3β-Phenyltropane 2-Ester Analogs Selective for the DAT

Compound RTI-4229-	X	R	DA [3H]WIN 35,428	NE [3H] Nisoxetine	5-HT [3H] Paroxetine	NE/DA[a] Ratio	5-DA* HT/ Ratio
			IC$_{50}$, nM (K$_i$, nM)				
Cocaine	—	—	89.1	3298 (1987)	1045 (95)	37	12
WIN 35,065-2	H	CO$_2$CH$_3$	23	920 (554)	2000 (182)	40	87
190	Cl	CO$_2$C$_2$H$_5$	0.96	235 (142)	168 (15.3)	245	175
114	Cl	CO$_2$CH(CH$_3$)$_2$	1.40	778 (469)	1400 (122)	555	1000
193	CH$_3$	CO$_2$C$_2$H$_5$	1.68	644 (388)	1070 (92)	383	637
113	Cl	CO$_2$C$_6$H$_5$	1.98	2960 (1783)	2340 (212)	1490	1180
436	C$_6$H$_5$CH=CH	CO$_2$CH$_3$	3.09	1960 (1181)	335 (31)	634	108
120	CH$_3$	CO$_2$C$_6$H$_5$	3.26	5830 (3512)	24,500 (2227)	1788	7515
150	CH$_3$	CO$_2$C$_4$H$_7$	3.74	4740 (2855)	2020 (134)	1267	540
204	Cl	CO$_2$C$_6$H$_4$CH$_3$(2')	3.91	4780 (2880)	3770 (342)	1223	964
277	NO$_2$	CO$_2$C$_6$H$_5$	5.94	5700 (3434)	2910 (265)	960	490
430	C$_6$H$_5$(CH$_2$)$_2$C≡C-	CO$_2$CH$_3$	6.28	1470 (886)	2182 (198)	234	348
117	CH$_3$	CO$_2$CH(CH$_3$)$_2$	6.45	1930 (1153)	6090 (554)	299	944
278	NO$_2$	CO$_2$CH(CH$_3$)$_2$	8.14	4100 (2170)	2150 (196)	504	264
205	CH$_3$	CO$_2$C$_6$H$_4$CH$_3$(3')	8.19	2130 (1283)	5240 (427)	260	640
203	Cl	CO$_2$C$_6$H$_4$CH$_3$(3')	9.37	2740 (1651)	2150 (196)	292	230
145	Cl	CH$_2$OCO$_2$CH$_3$	9.6	1480 (892)	2930 (266)	154	305

*Ratios of IC$_{50}$ values.

Table 12.2 3β-Phenyltropane 2β-Amide Analogs Selective for the DAT

Compound RTI-4229-	X	R	IC$_{50}$ nM (K$_i$, nM)			NE/DA* Ratio	5-HT/DA* Ratio
			DA [^{3}H]WIN 35,428	NE [^{3}H] Nisoxetine	5-HT [^{3}H] Paroxetine		
Cocaine	—	—	89.1	3298 (1906)	1045 (95)	37	12
WIN 35,065-2	H	CO$_2$CH$_3$	23	920 (555.6)	2000 (182)	40	87
227	I	CONOCH$_2$CH$_2$CH$_2$	0.75	357 (275)	129 (11.7)	476	172
218	Cl	CONCH$_3$(OCH$_3$)	1.19	8563 (5158)	1910 (174)	7200	1605
129	Cl	CON(CH$_3$)$_2$	1.38	942 (568)	1079 (98.1)	683	781
147	Cl	CON(CH$_2$)$_4$	1.38	3950 (2375)	12,400 (1120)	2862	8985
208	Cl	CONOCH$_2$CH$_2$CH$_2$	1.47	1080 (650)	2470 (225)	735	1680
186	CH$_3$	CONCH$_3$(OCH$_3$)	2.55	442 (266)	3400 (309)	173	1333
214	Cl	CONCH$_2$CH$_2$OCH$_2$CH$_2$	2.90	8550 (5750)	88,800 (8070)	2948	30,620
217	Cl	CONHC$_6$H$_4$OH(2')	4.78	31,000 (7867)	16,800 (1530)	6485	3515
215	Cl	CON(C$_2$H$_5$)$_2$	5.48	5530	9430 (857)	1009	1720
156	Cl	CON(CH$_2$)$_5$	6.95	1750 (1054)	3470 (315)	252	499

*Ratios of IC$_{50}$ values.

Table 12.3 3β-Phenyltropane 2β-Isoxazole Analogs Selective for the DAT

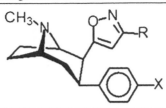

Compound RTI-4229-	X	R	DA [³H]WIN 35,428	NE [³H] Nisoxetine	5-HT [³H]Paroxetine	NE/DA* Ratio	5-HT/ DA* Ratio
			IC$_{50}$, nM (K$_i$, nM)				
Cocaine	—	—	89.1	3298 (1986)	1045 (45)	37	12
WIN 35,065-2	H		23	920 (554)	2000 (182)	40	87
334	Cl	–C₂H₅	0.50	120 (72)	3090 (281)	240	6180
165	Cl	–CH₃	0.59	181 (109)	572 (52)	307	970
171	CH₃	–CH₃	0.93	254 (153)	3820 (348)	273	4110
335	Cl	–CH(CH₃)₂	1.19	954 (575)	2320 (216)	801	1950
177	Cl	–C₆H₅	1.28	504 (304)	2420 (220)	394	1890
346	Cl	–C₆H₄OCH₃(4')	1.57	762 (454)	5880 (535)	485	3740
176	CH₃	–C₆H₅	1.58	398 (239)	5110 (465)	252	3230
354	CH₃	–C₂H₅	1.62	299 (180)	6400 (582)	185	3950
347	Cl	–C₆H₄F(4')	1.86	918 (553)	7256 (660)	494	3901
386	CH₃	–C₆H₄OCH₃(4')	3.93	756 (450)	4027 (380)	194	3600
336	Cl	–C₆H₄CH₃(4')	4.09	1714 (1033)	5741 (522)	419	1171
366	CH₃	–CH(CH₃)₂	4.5	2523 (1550)	42,900 (3900)	561	9533
345	Cl	–C₆H₄Cl(4')	6.42	5290 (3790)	>76 000 (6910)	824	>11,800
387	CH₃	–C₆H₅F(4')	6.45	917 (546)	>100 000 (9400)	141	>15,400
337	Cl	–C(CH₃)₃	7.31	6320 (3807)	36 800 (3346)	863	865
371	CH₃	–C₆H₄Cl(4')	8.74	>100,000 (60 200)	>100 000 (9090)	>11 400	>11 400

*Ratio of IC$_{50}$ values.

physicochemical properties. Furthermore, given their close structural similarity to other RTI compounds with known behavioral activity (RTI-32, −55, −113, −121, and −130),[14,15] it was expected that these compounds would both cross the blood-brain barrier and possess behavioral activity.

In designing a potential pharmacotherapy for cocaine abuse, other pharmacological activities must also be considered. Evidence from both animal and human studies suggests that the pharmacokinetic and pharmacodynamic properties of cocaine are important in reinforcement.[16-22] It is well known that cocaine gets into the brain quickly after peripheral administration and produces a "high" in 1 to 4 minutes.[16-18] This relatively rapid onset of action apparently contributes to cocaine's high efficacy

Table 12.4 3β-Phenyltropane 2β-Heterocyclic Analogs Selective for the DAT

Compound RTI-4229-	X	R	IC$_{50}$ nM (K$_i$, nM)			NE/DA* ratio	5-HT/DA* ratio
			DA [³H]WIN 35,428	NE [³H]Nisoxetine	5-HT [³H]Paroxetine		
cocaine			89	3298 (1986)	1045 (45)	37	12
WIN 35,065-2	H	CO$_2$CH$_3$	23	920 (554)	2000 (182)	40	87
470	Cl		0.094	1590 (994)	1080 (98)	16 900	11 500
202	Cl		1.37	403 (250)	1120 (202.1)	294	818
451	CH$_3$		1.53	476 (287)	7120 (647)	311	4700

439	CH$_3$		1.57	1320 (795)	>100 000 (>909)	841	>64 000
141	Cl	C$_6$H$_4$OCH$_3$(4')	1.81	835 (503)	357 (32.4)	461	186
219	Cl	C$_6$H$_5$	5.71	8560 (5157)	10 000 (909)	1500	1800

*Ratio of IC$_{50}$ values.

as a reinforcer. Therefore, to minimize the possibilities of abuse, an ideal indirect agonist clinical candidate for cocaine addiction would have a slow onset of action. Samaha and Robinson[23] have demonstrated that differences in the rate at which cocaine is administered determine its ability to produce psychomotor sensitization and presumably the associated adaptation in the brains of rats. Thus, a clinical candidate should also show low sensitization. In addition, a long duration of action would be desirable. Volkow et al[24] used positron emission tomography (PET) studies to show that the rate of clearance for the relatively more potent methylphenidate was significantly slower than for cocaine and suggested that this could account for the much lesser abuse of methylphenidate than cocaine despite their otherwise similar pharmacological properties. Furthermore, in selecting a candidate for further development, it is preferable for the compound to be orally available and no more stimulatory than cocaine at peak doses. As a direct test of the compound's potential efficacy in humans, the compound should substitute for cocaine in animal models and should block cocaine self-administration in both rats and rhesus monkeys.

In order to identify 3-phenyltropane analogs that possessed pharmacological properties suitable for further consideration, the compounds listed in Tables 12.1 to 12.4 were first evaluated for locomotor activity in mice[25] and cocaine discrimination in rats; several compounds were also tested in in vitro toxicity assays listed in Table 12.5. The 5 compounds listed in Tables 12.6 and 12.7 showed the most

Table 12.5 In Vitro Toxicity Assays*

Mutagenicity
NovaScreen
Cytochrome, P450
Sheep Isolated Cardiac Purkinje Fibers
HERG (ChanTest)

*HERG indicates human ether-a-go-go-related gene.

Table 12.6 Percentage Change From Vehicle in Locomotor Activity in Mice (intraperitoneal) for Compounds Selected for Further Evaluation*

Compound	Dose mg/kg	Hour 1	Hour 2	Hour 3	Hour 4	ED_{50} in Peak Hour mg/kg	First Hour: Ratio to Cocaine
Cocaine	5.6	+5	−26	−53	−1	18.8	
	17	+179[†]	−7	−53	−26		
	56	+452[†]	+201[†]	−47	−24		
RTI-177	1	+11	+27	+45	+76	3.4	1.1
	3	+331[†]	+456[†]	+377[†]	+378		
	10	+513[†]	+402[†]	+485[†]	+924[†]		
RTI-176	1	+48	+139	+89	+154	2.5	1.2
	3	+244[†]	+369	+283	+329		
	10	+526[†]	+663[†]	+363	+141		

(continued)

Table 12.6 (continued)

Compound	Dose mg/kg	Hour 1	Hour 2	Hour 3	Hour 4	ED_{50} in Peak Hour mg/kg	First Hour: Ratio to Cocaine
RTI-354	0.3	+34	+99	+173	−72	0.9	1.4
	1	+449†	+489†	+222	+48		
	3	+613†	+893†	+725†	+81		
RTI-336	1	+8	+44	−49	+170	3.9	0.7
	3	+23	+153	+265	+119		
	10	+308†	+1034†	+1024†	+493		
RTI-386	3	+73	+32	+27	+30	12.8	0.6
	10	+187†	+115†	+65	+34		
	30	+290†	+235†	+430†	+483†		

*Table adapted from Carroll et al.[25]
†Different from vehicle by Newman-Keuls following 1-way analysis of variance, $P < .05$.

Table 12.7 Drug Discrimination Effects of Compounds Selected for Further Evaluation in Rats (intraperitoneal)*

Compound	Percentage of Rats Choosing the Cocaine Lever											ED_{50} mg/kg
	0.1	0.17	0.3	0.56	1	1.7	3	5.6	10	17	30	
Cocaine					21	32	59	82	97			2.64
RTI-177						29	63	75				4.73
RTI-176							0	75	86			4.88
RTI-354			0	14	75	100						0.82
RTI-336					14		14	50	88			5.95
RTI-386							0			43	83	11.00

*Table adapted from Carroll et al.[25]

favorable overall balance of pharmacological properties and toxicity results. It is interesting to note that all 5 compounds are 3β-phenyltropane 2β-1,2-(isoxazole) analogs (see Table 12.3 for structures). Examination of the data in Table 12.6 shows that cocaine produced its greatest stimulation in hour 1, and that by hour 3 the effect was gone. In contrast, all 2β-1,2-(isoxazoles) had their largest effect in hours 2 to 4. The ED_{50} values for the 2β-1,2-(isoxazoles) ranged from 0.9 mg/kg for RTI-354 to 12.8 mg/kg for RTI-386. RTI-176 and RTI-354 produced greater stimulation than cocaine in their peak hours; RTI-177 had about the same stimulation as cocaine; and RTI-336 and RTI-386 were less stimulatory than cocaine.

All five 3β-(1,2-isoxazoles) selected for further evaluation showed full generalization to the cocaine cue (≥75% of rats choosing the cocaine lever), with the ED_{50} values ranging from 0.82 mg/kg for RTI-354 to 11.0 mg/kg for RTI-386; the ED_{50} for cocaine was 2.64 mg/kg.

3β-(4-Chlorophenyl)-2β̃ (3-phenylisoxazol-5-yl)tropane (RTI-177), which possessed
ED_{50} values of 4.7 and 5.7 mg/kg in the locomotor activity and drug-discrimination
test after oral administration (unpublished results, Carroll 2004) and also reduced
cocaine self-administration after oral administration in a rat model of self-administration, was studied for its effect on cocaine self-administration in rhesus monkeys.
Pretreatment intravenously (IV) with RTI-177 produced a dose-related reduction in
cocaine self-administration in rhesus monkeys trained to self-administer cocaine
(0.1 and 0.3 mg/kg) under a second-order schedule of IV drug delivery. The ED_{50}
was 0.11 mg/kg, which is an order of magnitude more potent than GBR 12909,
which has an ED_{50} of 1.29 mg/kg (Table 12.8).[26] PET neuroimaging studies revealed
that the ED_{10} doses of RTI-177 and GBR 12909 resulted in DAT occupancies
below the threshold (<10%) of detection, whereas ED_{50} doses resulted in DAT
occupancies of 73% and 67%, respectively.[26] RTI-177 and GBR 12909 were
substituted for cocaine in drug self-administration studies in order to characterize their
reinforcing effects. Both RTI-177 and GBR 12909 reliably maintained drug
self-administration at levels greater than those maintained by saline in all subjects (Fig. 12.1). Moreover, the shape of the dose-effect curves resembled an
inverted U-shape function typical of psychomotor stimulants. However, rates of
responding were lower than those maintained by the training dose of cocaine
(0.1 mg/kg/infusion) in 2 of 3 subjects substituted with GBR 12909 and in all 3
subjects substituted with RTI-177.

In acute toxicity studies in male rats, 3β-(4-chlorophenyl)-2β-[3-(4'-
methylphenyl)isoxazol-5-yl]tropane (RTI-336) possessed an LD_{50} of 180 mg/kg
after oral administration, compared with 49 mg/kg for RTI-177 (unpublished
results, Howell 2005; Table 12.9). These results suggested that RTI-336 was a better
candidate than RTI-177 for further preclinical development. Similar to RTI-177,
RTI-336 showed oral activity in the locomotor activity and drug-discrimination

Table 12.8 Relationship Between Reductions in Cocaine Self-administration and Dopamine
Transporter Occupancy

Subject	ED_{10}		ED_{50}	
	Dose mg/kg	Occupancy %	Dose mg/kg	Occupancy %
GBR 12909				
ROu-4	0.74	*	1.20	62
RLk-4	0.61	*	1.32	68
	0.52	*	1.45	71
Average ± SD	0.62 ± 0.11	*	1.29 ± 0.13	67 ± 4.6
RTI-177				
RMk-3	0.09	*	0.14	77
RMv-3	0.05	*	0.09	73
RLk-4	0.05	*	0.10	68
Average ± SD	0.06 ± 0.02	*	0.11 ± 0.03	73 ± 4.5

*Occupancy values that were below the limit of detection.

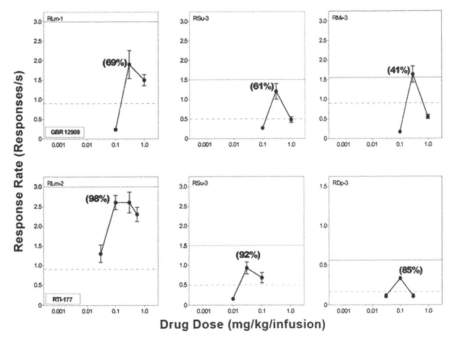

Fig. 12.1 Self-administration of GBR 12909 and RTI-177. Response rates (responses per second) for GBR 12909 and RTI-177 as a function of drug dose under a second-order schedule of IV drug self-administration in individual subjects. The unbroken lines indicate mean rates of responding maintained by the training dose of cocaine (0.1 mg/kg/infusion). Dashed lines indicate the upper limit for responding during saline extinction. Each data point was determined on a single occasion and is the mean (±SD) of the last 5 sessions in a condition. Numbers in parentheses indicate percentage of DAT occupancy at doses that maintained peak rates of responding. Modified from Lindsey et al.[26]

Table 12.9 Comparison of ED_{50}/LD_{50} Values and Minimum Lethal Dose for RTI-177 and RTI-336*

| RTI No. | Drug Discrimination and Lethality, Rat (PO) | | | Minimum Lethal, PO mg/kg |
	ED_{50} (mg/kg)	LD_{50} (mg/kg)	TI (LD_{50}/ED_{50})	
336	3.54	180	51	100
177	5.7	48.9	8.57	40–60

*PO indicates by mouth.

test with ED_{50}s of 14.4 and 3.54 mg/kg, respectively. Of importance, RTI-336 showed very low sensitization relative to cocaine. RTI-336 reduced cocaine self-administration in a rat model of self-administration (unpublished results, Howell 2004), and in preliminary rhesus monkey studies, RTI-336 produced dose-dependent reductions in cocaine self-administration in 4 subjects and was equally effective at both maintenance doses of cocaine (0.1 and 0.3 mg/kg/injection). Food-maintained behavior was suppressed at the same doses of RTI-336 that suppressed cocaine-maintained behavior. Positron emission tomography (PET) imaging was conducted in the same subjects to determine the level of DAT occupancy associated with behaviorally-relevant doses of RTI-336. Doses of RTI-336 that reduced cocaine-maintained behavior by 50% (ED_{50}) resulted in 90% DAT occupancy for the group of 4 subjects. Daily food intake, body weight, and behavior were normal.

Conclusion

In summary, RTI-336 showed locomotor activity less than that of cocaine with no sensitization. It was orally active in both the locomotor assay in mice and drug discrimination tests in rats and possessed an excellent therapeutic ratio. RTI-336 reduced cocaine self-administration in both rat and rhesus monkey models and showed slow onset and long duration of action in rodent and monkey models. These preliminary studies in rhesus monkeys showed that RTI-336 was effective in suppressing cocaine self-administration at doses that had no obvious adverse behavioral effects. Varying the maintenance dose of cocaine had no influence on the effectiveness of drug pretreatments. There was no evidence of selective reductions in cocaine self-administration compared with food-maintained behavior. High levels of DAT occupancy were required to produce robust reduction in cocaine use.

Acknowledgments This research was supported by the National Institute on Drug Abuse, National Institutes of Health, Bethesda, MD, grant No. DA05477.

References

1. Substance Abuse and Mental Health Services Administration. *2003 National Survey on Drug Use and Health.* Washington, DC: Department of Health and Human Services; 2003.
2. Substance Abuse and Mental Health Services Administration. *Drug Abuse Warning Network (DAWN) Publications (1994–2002).* Washington, DC: Department of Health and Human Services; 2004.
3. Carroll FI, Howell LL, Kuhar MJ. Pharmacotherapies for treatment of cocaine abuse: preclinical aspects. *J Med Chem.* 1999;42:2721-2736.
4. Howell LL, Wilcox KM. The dopamine transporter and cocaine medication development: drug self-administration in nonhuman primates. *J Pharmacol Exp Ther.* 2001;298:1-6.
5. Newman AH, Kulkarni S. Probes for the dopamine transporter: new leads toward a cocaine-abuse therapeutic: a focus on analogues of benztropine and rimcazole. *Med Res Rev.* 2002;22:429-464.
6. Carrera MR, Meijler MM, Janda KD. Cocaine pharmacology and current pharmacotherapies for its abuse. *Bioorg Med Chem.* 2004;12:5019-5030.
7. Ritz MC, Lamb RJ, Goldberg SR, Kuhar MJ. Cocaine receptors on dopamine transporters are related to self-administration of cocaine. *Science.* 1987;237:1219-1223.

8. Bergman J, Madras BK, Johnson SE, Spealman RD. Effects of cocaine and related drugs in nonhuman primates. III. Self-administration by squirrel monkeys. *J Pharmacol Exp Ther.* 1989;251:150-155.
9. Kuhar MJ, Ritz MC, Boja JW. The dopamine hypothesis of the reinforcing properties of cocaine. *Trends Neurosci.* 1991;14:299-302.
10. Wise RA, Jr, Newton P, Jr, Leeb K, Jr, Burnette B, Jr, Pocock D, Jr, Justice JB, Jr. Fluctuations in nucleus accumbens dopamine concentration during intravenous cocaine self-administration in rats. *Psychopharmacology (Berl).* 1995;120:10-20.
11. Wilcox KM, Rowlett JK, Paul IA, Ordway GA, Woolverton WL. On the relationship between the dopamine transporter and the reinforcing effects of local anesthetics in rhesus monkeys: practical and theoretical concerns. *Psychopharmacology (Berl).* 2000;153:139-147.
12. Carroll FI. 2002 Medicinal Chemistry Division Award address: monoamine transporters and opioid receptors. Targets for addiction therapy. *J Med Chem.* 2003;46:1775-1794.
13. Carroll FI, Runyon SP, Abraham P, et al. Monoamine transporter binding, locomotor activity, and drug discrimination properties of 3-(4-substituted-phenyl)tropane-2-carboxylic acid methyl ester isomers. *J Med Chem.* 2004;47:6401-6409.
14. Balster RL, Carroll FI, Graham JH, et al. Potent substituted-3b-phenyltropane analogs of cocaine have cocaine-like discriminative stimulus effects. *Drug Alcohol Depend.* 1991;29:145-151.
15. Fleckenstein AE, Kopajtic TA, Boja JW, Carroll FI, Kuhar MJ. Highly potent cocaine analogs cause long-lasting increases in locomotor activity. *Eur J Pharmacol.* 1996;311:109-114.
16. Fowler JS, Volkow ND, Logan J, et al. Measuring dopamine transporter occupancy by cocaine in vivo: radiotracer considerations. *Synapse.* 1998;28:111-116.
17. Volkow ND, Wang GJ, Fischman MW, et al. Effects of route of administration on cocaine induced dopamine transporter blockade in the human brain. *Life Sci.* 2000;67:1507-1515.
18. Zernig G, Giacomuzzi S, Riemer Y, Wakonigg G, Sturm K, Saria A. Intravenous drug injection habits: drug users' self-reports versus researchers' perception. *Pharmacology.* 2003;68:49-56.
19. Balster RL, Schuster CR. Fixed-interval schedule of cocaine reinforcement: effect of dose and infusion duration. *J Exp Anal Behav.* 1973;20:119-129.
20. Woolverton WL, Wang Z. Relationship between injection duration, transporter occupancy and reinforcing strength of cocaine. *Eur J Pharmacol.* 2004;486:251-257.
21. Lile JA, Morgan D, Birmingham AM, et al. The reinforcing efficacy of the dopamine reuptake inhibitor 2beta-propanoyl-3beta-(4-tolyl)-tropane (PTT) as measured by a progressive-ratio schedule and a choice procedure in rhesus monkeys. *J Pharmacol Exp Ther.* 2002;303:640-648.
22. Woolverton WL, Ranaldi R, Wang Z, et al. Reinforcing strength of a novel dopamine transporter ligand: pharmacodynamic and pharmacokinetic mechanisms. *J Pharmacol Exp Ther.* 2002;303:211-217.
23. Samaha AN, Robinson TE. Why does the rapid delivery of drugs to the brain promote addiction? *Trends Pharmacol Sci.* 2005;26:82-87.
24. Volkow ND, Fowler JS, Wang GJ, Swanson JM. Dopamine in drug abuse and addiction: results from imaging studies and treatment implications. *Mol Psychiatry.* 2004;9:557-569.
25. Carroll FI, Pawlush N, Kuhar MJ, Pollard GT, Howard JL. Synthesis, monoamine transporter binding properties, and behavioral pharmacology of a series of 3beta-(substituted phenyl)-2beta-(3'-substituted isoxazol-5-yl)tropanes. *J Med Chem.* 2004;47:296-302.
26. Lindsey KP, Wilcox KM, Votaw JR, et al. Effects of dopamine transporter inhibitors on cocaine self-administration in rhesus monkeys: relationship to transporter occupancy determined by positron emission tomography neuroimaging. *J Pharmacol Exp Ther.* 2004;309:959-969.

Chapter 13
Serotonin Transporters: Implications for Antidepressant Drug Development

Kellie J. White,[1] Crystal C. Walline,[1] and Eric L. Barker[1]

Abstract Due to the complexity of the disease, several hypotheses exist to explain the etiology of depression. The monoamine theory of depression suggests that disruptions in the serotonergic and noradrenergic systems result in depressive symptoms. Therefore, the serotonin transporter (SERT) has become a pharmacological target for treating these symptoms. This review will discuss what is known about the molecular interactions of antidepressants with SERT. The effects of antidepressants on SERT regulation and expression in addition to the receptors that may be involved in mediating these effects will be addressed. Specifically, how changes to SERT expression following chronic antidepressant treatment may contribute to the therapeutic benefits of antidepressants will be discussed. Furthermore, the effects of *SERT* gene polymorphisms on antidepressant efficacy will be examined. Finally, a brief overview of other hypotheses of depression will be addressed as well as factors that must be considered for future antidepressant development.

Keywords SSRIs, antidepressant, serotonin transporter, depression, reuptake

Monoamine Theory of Depression

Functional deficiencies in serotonin (5-hydroytryptamine, 5-HT) and norepinephrine (NE) have been implicated in the pathophysiology of depressive syndromes, and restoring the normal function of 5-HT- and NE-associated signaling pathway has been the target of antidepressants. Restoration of monoamine deficiencies to normal levels as a therapeutic strategy is based on the monoamine hypothesis of depression.[1]

[1] Department of Medicinal Chemistry and Molecular Pharmacology, Purdue University School of Pharmacy, West Lafayette, IN 47907

Corresponding Author: Eric L. Barker, Dept. of Medicinal Chemistry and Molecular Pharmacology, Purdue University School of Pharmacy, 575 Stadium Mall Drive, West Lafayette, IN 47907. Tel: (765) 494-9940; Fax: (765) 494-1414; E-mail: ericb@pharmacy.purdue.edu

R.S. Rapaka and W. Sadée (eds.), *Drug Addiction*.
© American Association of Pharmaceutical Scientists 2008

The oldest antidepressants, the monoamine oxidase inhibitors (MAOIs), increase synaptic levels of 5-HT and NE by inhibiting the enzymatic degradation of these neurotransmitters. The tricyclic antidepressants (TCAs), as well as newer selective 5-HT reuptake inhibitors (SSRIs) and 5-HT/NE reuptake inhibitors (SNRIs), all increase synaptic levels of 5-HT or NE by inhibiting reuptake via the 5-HT transporter (SERT) or NE transporter (NET), respectively. Emerging evidence indicates that the monoamine hypothesis of 5-HT and NE modulation fails to explain the whole mechanism of antidepressants. Other hypotheses, including the cytokine hypothesis of depression, the hypothalamic-pituitary-thyroid hypothesis of depression, as well as the role of brain-derived neurotrophic factor and cyclic AMP response element binding protein will be considered later in this review.

Antidepressant Development

The development of antidepressants began in the early 1950s with the fortuitous discovery that the antitubercular drug iproniazid, which functioned as an inhibitor of monoamine oxidase the enzyme responsible for breaking down 5-HT, had mood-elevating effects.[2] Subsequently, compounds with antihistamine activity such as imipramine and chlorpromazine were discovered to confer mood-elevating effects.[2] These discoveries led to the development of the first 2 classes of drugs used to treat depressed patients: the MAOIs and the TCAs. The first generation MAOIs (iproniazid, tranylcypromine, and phenelzine) were nonselective, irreversible inhibitors of MAO leading to increased levels of dopamine, 5-HT, and NE in patients. However, these drugs had dangerous and life-threatening side effects including hepatotoxicity and hypertensive crisis due to interactions with food high in tyramine. The risks of side effects and necessity for strict patient compliance led to the eventual disuse of these drugs. Nonetheless, MAOIs have seen a resurgence in recent years, particularly for the treatment of atypical and drug-resistant forms of depression.[3]

The first tricyclic antidepressant, imipramine, elicited antidepressant effects by inhibiting NE and 5-HT transport (Table 13.1). These compounds act as antagonists for SERT or NET and block neurotransmitter uptake, thus increasing synaptic concentrations of 5-HT or NE, respectively. However, imipramine was not without unfavorable side effects due to antihistaminic, antiadrenergic, and anticholinergic effects.[5,6] The development of second generation TCAs led to more selective inhibitors of NE uptake (desipramine, nortriptyline, maprotiline) and 5-HT uptake (clomipramine), but demonstrated no significant improvements in side effect profiles. More recently, the development of the SSRIs has consumed the mental health market (Table 13.1). The introduction of fluoxetine in 1988 provided clinicians with a safer treatment alternative to the MAOIs and the TCAs since the side effect profile was considerably improved. A meta-analysis of 36 double-blind clinical trials of TCAs and SSRIs found that patients taking a TCA were more likely to drop out of a study due to an adverse side effect (22.4%) than those prescribed an SSRI (15.9%).[7] However, despite the improvement in side effects and drug interactions, the SSRIs are generally no more clinically efficacious at treating depression than any previous therapy.[8] Increasing response rates to the SSRIs are paralleled with increases in the placebo effect.[5] For example, response rates as measured by a 50% or greater decrease in the total depression score on the Hamilton Rating Scale for Depression were 79% and 60% for sertraline and fluoxetine, respectively. However, the corresponding placebo effect was 48% for sertraline, compared with only 33% for fluoxetine indicating a similar (~30%) response rate to these SSRIs.[5] Additionally, approximately 30% to 45% of patients fail to attain an adequate response to their initial pharmacotherapy.[9]

The failure of the SSRIs to treat some depressed patients led to the development of less selective agents. These SNRIs are inhibitors of both 5-HT and NE uptake. The SNRIs may have increased clinical utility over the SSRIs at treating refractory depression and anxiety indicating the need to target both the serotonergic and noradrenergic uptake systems in some patients.[10] Additionally, the SNRIs may have efficacy in reducing the physical symptoms associated with depression, including muscle tension, fatigue, appetite changes, and body aches, in addition to an alternative use as a treatment for fibromyalgia.[11] Drugs in this class include venlafaxine and duloxetine and although they are less selective than the SSRIs with regard to targeting specific transporters, they have limited affinity for the muscarinic, adrenergic, and histaminergic receptors, resulting in a favorable side-effect profile.[12] Finally, the shift from focusing completely on the 5-HT system to the NE system was complete with the development of 2 selective NE reuptake inhibitors, reboxetine and atomoxetine. Reboxetine is indicated for major depressive disorder, whereas atomoxetine is prescribed for attention-deficit/hyperactivity disorder.

The discussion of drugs used to treat affective disorders would not be complete without mentioning the atypical antidepressants. These drugs do not fall into a specific class and affect a wide range of physiological targets. Clinically used agents include the $5HT_{2A}$ receptor antagonists such as trazadone and its second generation compound nefazodone, the NE/dopamine reuptake inhibitor bupropion, and the $5\text{-}HT_{1A}$ receptor agonist and D2 dopamine receptor antagonist buspirone.

Molecular Interactions of Antidepressants with SERT

Antidepressants are represented by many structurally distinct classes of compounds each of which may interact with SERT in a unique manner (Table 13.1). Although the 3-dimensional structure of SERT and other monoamine transporters such as the dopamine transporter and NET has not been solved, experimental assays correlating functional potency data to structural changes provide some clues into the binding sites of these different drug classes as well as possible distinct binding. Species-scanning mutagenesis has also been employed to identify residues that contribute to inhibitor binding. This method exploits the differences in inhibitor potencies between variants of SERT (ie, human versus rat). Similarly, cross-species chimeras can be generated to determine the influences of specific

Table 13.1 Structures of Commonly Prescribed Antidepressants and K_i Values for Inhibition at hSERT and hNET*

Structure	Antidepressants	hSERT K_i (nM), [³H]5-HT Uptake Inhibition	hNET K_i (nM), [³H]NE Uptake Inhibition
	Amitriptyline	36 ± 1	102 ± 9
	Nortriptyline	279 ± 20	21 ± 0.77
	Desipramine	163 ± 5	3.5 ± 0.6
	Imipramine	20 ± 2	142 ± 8
	Venlafaxine	102 ± 9	1644 ± 84
	Sertraline	3.3 ± 0.4	1716 ± 151

(continued)

Table 13.1 (continued)

Structure	Antidepressants	hSERT K_i (nM), [^{3}H]5-HT Uptake Inhibition	hNET K_i (nM), [^{3}H]NE Uptake Inhibition
	Fluoxetine	20 ± 2	2186 ± 142
	Citalopram	8.9 ± 0.7	30,285 ± 1600
	Paroxetine	0.83 ± 0.06	328 ± 25

*Data were Obtained in HEK cells Heterologously Expressing hSERT or hNET.[4]

transmembrane domain (TMD) regions on drug potencies. For example, Barker
and colleagues[13] generated cross-species chimeras between the human and
Drosophila SERT (hSERT and dSERT, respectively) homologs to determine the
regions of the SERT responsible for the divergent pharmacology of SERT inhibitors at the *Drosophila* species as compared with hSERT. The inhibitor potency
data from human/*Drosophila* SERT chimeras led to the observation that residues
distal to the second TMD conferred potency specificities for most inhibitors
including paroxetine and fluoxetine. Conversely, the region including TMDs I and
II contained key sites for species discrimination of citalopram and mazindol.
Further investigation revealed that mutation of tyrosine 95 in the hSERT to the
corresponding dSERT phenylalanine residue altered mazindol and citalopram
potency values nearly equivocal to those for dSERT.[12] Furthermore, computational
modeling of the SERT-citalopram interaction suggests a dipole-dipole interaction
of the nitril group of *S*-citalopram with Y95 providing further support for a specific
molecular interaction with this amino acid.[14]

Additionally, an aspartate in the first TMD of the dopamine transporter has been implicated as a key residue for dopamine transport and cocaine analog recognition.[15] To determine the role of this residue in SERT, several mutations were generated in rat SERT (rSERT). The carboxylic acid of the D98E mutant was identified as an essential point of interaction for the amine in 5-HT, indicating this residue was important for substrate recognition. Furthermore, this mutation caused a significant decrease in citalopram potency for inhibiting 5-HT transport.[16] Therefore, this aspartate may be important for antidepressant recognition as well. In addition to the D98 residue in TMD I, key residues in the third TMD of hSERT appear critical for the recognition of cocaine, amphetamine, and antidepressants (C. Walline, unpublished data).

Other key residues have been implicated in antidepressant recognition in NET within the TMD V-IX region.[17-19] Although discussion of other transporters within the monoamine family is outside the scope of this review, 2 of these amino acids (P418 and S375) are sites of sequence divergence between hSERT and dSERT. Therefore, these residues were ideal candidates for species-scanning mutagenesis in order to confirm their importance in antagonist recognition. Both P418 and S375 were independently mutated to the equivalent dSERT amino acid (serine and alanine, correspondingly).[20] Unfortunately, both mutants failed to show any statistically significant potency differences as compared with hSERT for a panel of TCA and SSRI antidepressants suggesting that these amino acids may not be critical sites for antidepressant recognition by SERT.[20]

Residues in SERT have also been discovered that confer high potency interaction with tricyclic antidepressants. Using species-scanning mutagenesis, F586 in hSERT was mutated to the corresponding valine in rSERT. The F586V hSERT mutant demonstrated a phenotype similar to the rSERT with regard to TCA potency.[21] The complementary rSERT mutation V586F showed hSERT-like potencies for the tricyclics imipramine, desipramine, and nortriptyline.[21] Taken together, these studies suggest that SERT TMD XII may contain distinct molecular determinants for binding of the TCAs. A more complete understanding of antidepressant recognition by SERT at the molecular level will be revealed by future efforts focused on elucidation of SERT structure.

Acute Regulation of SERT Expression by Antidepressants

Alterations to the serotonergic system are thought to partially explain the therapeutic benefits of antidepressants. Since the discovery that antidepressants work in part by potentiating the actions of 5-HT within the serotonergic system (for review see Schloss and Williams[22] and Vetulain and Nalepa[23]), the effects these drugs elicit on the SERT protein have been an area of active research. Specifically, antidepressants are thought to initially function by acting as SERT antagonists resulting in an immediate increase in the synaptic 5-HT concentration.[22] Changes to the expression level of SERT in response to drugs could contribute to neuroadaptive changes associated with chronic antidepressant administration (see below). Surprisingly, the effects of antidepressants on regulation of SERT expression remain largely unevaluated.

Regulation of SERT activity by kinases seems plausible as SERT contains putative phosphorylation sites for protein kinase C (PKC), cAMP-dependent protein kinase (PKA), and cGMP-dependent protein kinase (PKG). Early studies in human embryonic kidney (HEK) cells heterologously expressing hSERT (HEK-hSERT) identified SERT as a phosphoprotein sensitive to rapid internalization following activation of PKC concurrent with a decrease in SERT activity.[24,25] Further studies in the HEK-hSERT cells showed that antidepressants alone could not affect the ability of PKC to phosphorylate SERT. The ligand 5-HT, however, caused a reduction in PKC-induced phosphorylation.[26] Therefore, in the presence of substrate, SERT would not become phosphorylated, the signal necessary for internalization. Interestingly, acute treatment of HEK-hSERT cells with 5-HT in the presence of the SERT-selective anti-depressants, imipramine, paroxetine, and citalopram, but not the NET-selective nisoxetine, resulted in SERT phosphorylation by PKC.[26] The ability of antidepressants to counteract the action of 5-HT suggests a mechanism that would further increase the synaptic concentration of 5-HT by reducing the number of transporters at the cell surface available to eliminate 5-HT from the synapse.[26]

Although phosphorylation of SERT by acute PKC activation results in rapid changes in SERT activity and cellular distribution, regulation of SERT expression at the plasma membrane by PKA or PKG does not occur after acute kinase activation despite an increase in SERT phosphorylation.[25] One explanation for these results would be that although phosphorylation of SERT occurs through numerous kinase pathways, changes to SERT activity and expression due to PKA or PKG phosphory-lation occur over a longer period of time than PKC regulation. Another explanation is that HEK cells do not contain the proteins necessary to affect SERT expression following phosphorylation by PKA or PKG. Interestingly, chronic treatment with antidepressants increases the production of intracellular cAMP due to an increased coupling between the G protein Gs_{α} and adenylyl cyclase (for review see Donati and Rasenick[27]). Elevation of intracellular cAMP would result in increased translocation and activity of PKA suggesting a potential mechanism for PKA regulation of SERT after extended antidepressant administration. This effect could occur through changes to unidentified protein interactions facilitated by alterations in the phospho-rylation state of SERT. Studies in human placental choriocarcinoma (JAR) cells, a cell line that endogenously expresses SERT, suggest that increases in cAMP should lead to an increase in SERT activity due to an increase in both SERT mRNA and protein levels.[28] This study is in conflict, however, with numerous studies that have reported a decrease in SERT levels following chronic antidepressant administration (see below) despite the increase in cAMP production explained above. Further inves-tigation will be required to determine if this conflict is due to cell type-dependent variability in the role of PKA phosphorylation in SERT regulation under normal and antidepressant-treated conditions.

Not surprisingly, kinase pathways that increase the activity of SERT have also been reported. Studies have identified a mechanism for up-regulation of SERT expression through PKG-dependent pathways.[29] Previously, Miller and Hoffman[30] reported that the A_3 adenosine receptor regulated SERT in rat basophilic leukemia (RBL-2H3) cells through cGMP and nitric oxide, subsequently increasing the V_{max} value for 5-HT transport. This regulation of SERT could occur under physiological conditions as RBL-2H3 cells endogenously express both the A_3 adenosine receptor and SERT. Interestingly, the increase in 5-HT transport was not associated with an increased expression of SERT at the cell surface.[30] One caveat of these experiments is that the cell-surface binding was performed using a membrane permeable ligand, thus, limiting the conclusions that can be drawn. Zhu et al,[29] however, reported that an up-regulation of SERT surface expression occurred when activating A_3 adenosine receptors in RBL-2H3 cells as measured by specific binding of the cocaine analog [125I]RTI-55. Because SERT protein levels are low in RBL-2H3 cells, Chinese hamster ovary (CHO) cells were transiently transfected with A_3 adenosine receptor and SERT cDNAs to confirm these results. Similar increases in SERT protein surface expression levels following A_3 adenosine receptor activation occurred in the transfected CHO cells suggesting a common signaling pathway for SERT up-regulation within the 2 cell types.[29] Moreover, these studies extended those of Miller and Hoffman[30] by showing that activation of the PKG pathway required the upstream activity of phospholipase C, calcium, and guanylyl cyclase.[29] Additionally, investigation into other proteins involved in the PKG-signaling cascade led to the identification of p38 mitogen-activated protein kinase (MAPK) regulation of intrinsic SERT activity. Inhibition of p38 MAPK did not affect A_3 adenosine receptor-activated changes to SERT plasma membrane expression levels in RBL-2H3, thus suggesting that changes to SERT by the PKG activation of p38 MAPK occur independently of changes caused directly by PKG.[29] Interestingly, the studies of Samuvel et al[31] showed that application of the p38 MAPK-specific inhibitor PD169316 resulted in decreases in the activity, phosphorylation, and plasma membrane expression of SERT isolated in rat synaptosomes. Reduction of p38 MAPK by siRNA in HEK cells transiently expressing hSERT produced a reduction in SERT at the cell surface, and inhibition of p38 MAPK by PD169316 decreased delivery of SERT to the plasma membrane. Moreover, activation of either p38 MAPK or PKC also inhibited interaction of SERT with syntaxin 1.[31] Syntaxin 1 is a SNARE protein that has previously been found to interact with and regulate SERT's expression.[32-34] Therefore, p38 MAPK appears to influence SERT expression via regulation of plasma membrane insertion potentially by affecting SERT's interaction with syntaxin 1.[31] Additional investigations into the role of p38 MAPK regulation of SERT surface expression are necessary before the effects of antidepressants on these interactions can be investigated.

    In addition to interactions with numerous kinases that control SERT availability at the plasma membrane, SERT forms a complex with protein phosphatase 2A (PP2A) in HEK-hSERT cells.[35] Previously, inhibitors targeting PP2A and protein phosphatase 1 were found to down-regulate SERT activity.[25] Furthermore, p38 MAPK appears to regulate the interaction between SERT and PP2A.[31] Additional research must be performed to elucidate the complex network of kinase and phosphatase activity involved in controlling SERT expression. Moreover, the extent of SERT-regulating phosphorylation that occurs in vivo remains unresolved.

Further studies are necessary both in vivo and in vitro to establish the role of kinase phosphorylation on SERT expression under antidepressant-treated conditions both acutely and after chronic administration. Interestingly, an evaluation of kinase mRNA levels in rat brain following 21 days of fluoxetine or citalopram treatment showed a decrease in numerous kinases including PKC and PKA.[36] The effect this down-regulation confers on kinase protein levels and subsequent SERT regulation requires further analysis.

Effects of Chronic Antidepressant Exposure on SERT

Although antidepressants function to rapidly increase synaptic 5-HT concentrations, this initial effect does not instantly alleviate the symptoms of depression. In fact, a maximal clinical response to antidepressants will not become apparent until several weeks of continuous treatment (for review see Gelenberg and Chesen[37]). Thus, the acute blockade of SERTs to increase 5-HT signaling does not account for the typical delay in symptom improvement. Current thought proposes that the neuroadaptive changes necessary for the therapeutic benefits of some antidepressants results in part from down-regulation of postsynaptic β-adrenergic receptors.[38] Similar changes, however, are not characteristic for SSRIs and other antidepressants that act on SERT.[38] Therefore, neuroadaptive changes in SERT expression could be necessary for antidepressants to be effective. Reports of changes to SERT expression after treatment with antidepressants vary.

The effects of chronic antidepressant treatment on the expression level of SERT have been explored in few in vitro systems. Horschitz et al[39] treated HEK cells heterologously expressing rSERT with increasing concentrations of citalopram before determining the effects of treatment on [^{3}H]5-HT uptake and [^{3}H]-citalopram binding. Following a 3-day incubation with 500 nM citalopram, the maximal transport activity (V_{max} value) decreased to approximately 40% without a subsequent change in the K_m value for 5-HT. A similar reduction (~50%) in [^{3}H]-citalopram binding to rSERT at the plasma membrane occurred after this treatment; although a reduction in binding of approximately 25% was evident with as little as 20 nM citalopram. Moreover, a similar decrease in rSERT expression was not evident in cells chronically treated with the antidepressant, desipramine, a NET inhibitor.[39] Unfortunately, the precise mechanism for citalopram-induced down-regulation of SERT in HEK cells remains unclear as well as how these results will translate to neuronal cell lines.

Although the above results were obtained in a heterologous expression system, similar patterns of SERT down-regulation have been documented after chronic treatment of rats and humans with antidepressants. Specifically, Benmansour and colleagues[40,41] reported that chronic treatment (15 or 21 days) with paroxetine or sertraline in rats reduced the number of SERT binding sites by as much as 80% in the CA3 region of the hippocampus without long-term changes to SERT mRNA levels. Furthermore, chronoamperometry measurements of 5-HT levels revealed an increase in the time necessary to clear 5-HT in chronic sertraline-treated rats compared with the time required following an acute fluvoxamine block of SERT in saline-treated rats.[41] These data show that an overall decrease in the expression level of SERT induced by chronic antidepressant exposure results in 5-HT remaining in the synapse longer than observed with acute blockade of SERT alone. Additionally, Gould et al[42] reported a 75% to 80% decrease in the lateral nucleus of the amygdala, dentate gyrus, and dorsal raphe SERT binding sites after 6 weeks of paroxetine administration to rats. Similar treatment with the selective NET inhibitor, reboxetine, did not result in a change to SERT binding.[42] A study of 17 healthy humans administered 40 mg/day of citalopram found a reduction in diencephalon and brainstem SERT binding following 8 days of treatment.[43] Surprisingly, no further reduction in SERT binding occurred after an additional 8 days of treatment.[43] Changes in platelet 5-HT and SERT have been suggested as possible biomarkers for psychiatric illness (for review see Plein and Berk[44]). Interestingly, Alvarez et al[45] reported a decrease in platelet SERT binding sites in depressed versus healthy individuals that was further reduced following 12-week administration of clomipramine or fluoxetine. Furthermore, a greater drop in platelet SERT binding sites was evident in antidepressant treatment responders versus nonresponders.[45] These data support a possible link between SERT expression and responsiveness to antidepressant treatment. Interestingly, the responders showed an initial increase in platelet inositol triphosphate levels that returned to normal following chronic antidepressant treatment. In nonresponders, the inositol triphosphate levels remained elevated. An increase in inositol triphosphate indicates an increase in the phosphoinositide signaling pathway that would also lead to an increase in 1,2-diacylglycerol (DAG). Activation of PKC by DAG could then regulate SERT surface expression.[45] A more complex system for regulation of SERT expression is suggested by these data, however, since a decrease in DAG, in addition to inositol triphosphate, should result in a decrease in PKC activity. Therefore, an increase in SERT expression would be expected if PKC alone were responsible for SERT regulation.

Not all studies of chronic antidepressant treatments report a decrease in SERT expression levels. Hébert et al[46] described no significant changes to brain SERT binding sites in rats treated 21 days with numerous antidepressants with the exception of decreased SERT levels in the entorhinal cortex induced by both fluoxetine and venlafaxine. Interestingly, treatment with the tricyclic antidepressants trimipramine or desipramine appeared to increase SERT binding in several cortical brain regions compared with the transporter inhibitors fluoxetine and venlafaxine.[46] Moreover, an increase in hippocampal SERT binding sites occurred after a 10-week treatment with amitriptyline in 24-month-old rats. The treatment did not change the SERT levels in 10-month-old rats.[47] An increase in SERT following antidepressant treatment could contribute to age-related differences in therapeutic effectiveness of antidepressants.[47] Finally, a study of depressed versus healthy individuals showed an initial decrease in lymphocyte SERT binding sites in depressed individuals compared with controls that increased after chronic fluoxetine treatment concurrent with a clinical improvement in depressed symptoms.[48] Further studies are necessary to confirm the link between clinical response and changes in SERT expression in areas outside of the brain as regulatory mechanisms could differ substantially between neuronal and non-neuronal cells.

Although the above-mentioned studies only represent a small portion of the studies examining the effects of chronic antidepressant treatment on SERT binding sites (for further review see Schloss and Silliams[22] and Schloss and Henn[49]), the disparities described could be reflective of the systems used to measure SERT levels. For instance, differences in the specificity and cell permeability of the radiolabels used for these studies could account for variability of the results. Moreover, different antidepressants may elicit unique effects on SERT availability due to differences in recognition of the antidepressants by SERT. Additionally, the dose of antidepressant administered as well as the route of antidepressant administration could affect the local concentration of drug in the brain. Benmansour et al[40,41] and Gould et al[42] used osmotic minipumps to continuously dispense the drugs to the rats, whereas Hébert et al[46] administered the drugs to the rats through a single daily ip injection. In addition, the region of the brain under examination could account for differences in expression levels.[46] Finally, the population size, ethnicity, and age of subjects in human studies must be considered before generalizing the results.

Receptor Regulation of SERT

As described earlier, SERT is subject to regulation through kinase and phosphatase activity. These signaling proteins themselves are regulated by the activity of neurotransmitter receptors. Thus, the effect of chronic antidepressant treatment on various receptors and the subsequent effect the receptors confer on SERT is an area of active investigation. Unfortunately, specific receptor-mediated regulation of SERT remains poorly understood. One area of exploration involves the serotonin 5-HT$_{1A}$ receptor. The 5-HT$_{1A}$ receptor is believed to be important in the therapeutic effects observed upon chronic antidepressant treatment because this receptor is responsible for regulating firing of serotonergic neurons.[50] The increase in extracellular 5-HT caused by blockade of SERT by antidepressants results in a decrease in vesicular 5-HT release due to activation of the negative feedback mechanism facilitated by presynaptic 5-HT$_{1A}$ receptors. Desensitization of the presynaptic 5-HT$_{1A}$ receptor must then occur to return serotonergic neuronal firing to normal.[50,51] In the median and dorsal raphe, chronic treatment with fluoxetine leads to a decrease in presynaptic 5-HT$_{1A}$ receptor G-protein coupling without a decrease in receptor binding sites. These findings suggest that receptor desensitization occurs at the level of effector coupling.[52] Currently, no data support a direct role for 5-HT$_{1A}$ receptor regulation of SERT, although SERT expression is decreased in 5-HT$_{1A}$ receptor knockout mice,[53] an effect that could be a result of disrupting serotonergic signaling.

Recent exploration of the 5-HT$_{1B}$ receptor suggests a role for this receptor in regulating SERT activity in vivo.[54] Specifically, activating presynaptic 5-HT$_{1B}$ receptors results in increased clearance of 5-HT by SERT independent of 5-HT$_{1A}$ receptor activity.[55] In agreement with these findings, studies in 5-HT$_{1B}$ receptor knockout mice report a larger increase in extracellular ventral hippocampus 5-HT concentration following a single ip injection of fluoxetine compared with wild-type mice, although an alteration in SERT levels in the knockout mice could explain these results.[56] Interestingly, no significant change to extracellular 5-HT concentrations was evident in the frontal cortex suggesting differences in SERT regulation between the 2 brain areas.[56] Additionally, treatment of rats for 21 days with fluoxetine decreased 5-HT$_{1B}$ receptor mRNA levels in the dorsal raphe nucleus.[57] No concurrent measurement of changes to presynaptic 5-HT$_{1B}$ receptor protein levels was assessed in this study. If a decrease in 5-HT$_{1B}$ receptors were to occur, however, a decrease in SERT function would be considered likely since presynaptic 5-HT$_{1B}$ receptors regulate 5-HT uptake.[55]

The therapeutic benefits of antidepressants may rely in part on desensitization of 5-HT$_{1A}$ and 5-HT$_{1B}$ receptors.[50] Interestingly, co-administration of the 5-HT$_{1A}$ receptor antagonist pindolol with an SSRI increased the SSRI efficacy and decreased the lag between the start of drug treatment and a clinical response.[58] Studies by Shalom et al[59] showed that repeated application of a 5-HT$_{1B}$ receptor antagonist in the rat frontal cortex prevents fluoxetine-induced 5-HT$_{1B}$ receptor desensitization. Because of the importance of receptor desensitization in mediating the therapeutic benefits of chronic SSRI treatment, co-administration of an SSRI and a 5-HT$_{1B}$ receptor antagonist may not be more effective over an extended period of time than an SSRI alone.[59] Further investigation into the mechanism behind 5-HT$_{1B}$ receptor control of SERT activity could help with designing drug regimens for depressed individuals.

The role of the α_2-adrenergic receptor in the noradrenaline system, and the subsequent changes to the receptor's expression and function during depressed episodes are currently under intensive investigation. Specifically, changes to α_2-adrenergic receptors are known to occur when examining antidepressants that specifically inhibit NET with changes being dependent on the type of antidepressant.[49] Interestingly, Ansah and colleagues[60] recently reported that α_2-adrenergic receptor activation could inhibit SERT activity both in vitro and in vivo, and the presence of Ca^{2+} was essential for this inhibition. Application of an α_2-adrenergic receptor agonist at a concentration that resulted in maximal SERT inhibition in synaptosomal preparations did not decrease SERT activity in transfected cell lines suggesting activation of a pathway in vivo that was unavailable in transfected cells rather than a direct interaction of the receptor or drug with SERT. Furthermore, when analyzing the effects of the α_2-adrenergic receptor agonist UK14304 in vivo an increase in the amount of time necessary to clear 5-HT was evident. UK14304 did not change SERT phosphorylation or the V_{max} value, but did decrease the apparent K_m value for 5-HT.[60] Thus, regulation of SERT caused by the activation of α_2-adrenergic receptors does not appear to be changing the surface expression of SERT. Activation of α_2-adrenergic receptors, however, could influence the interaction of an ancillary protein with SERT that affects recognition of 5-HT. The influence that α_2-adrenergic receptors have on SERT expression and activity requires further investigation to determine what, if any, role these receptors play on changing SERT levels during antidepressant treatment.

SERT Polymorphisms and Antidepressant Response

Although the interplay between SERT, receptors, and signaling proteins must be considered for the current antidepressants, development of future drugs for the treatment of depression should not only consider these interactions, but also genetic polymorphisms of the *SERT* gene. Ramamoorthy and colleagues[61] isolated a single human *SERT* gene to chromosome *17q11.1-q12*. Later studies revealed a polymorphism in the promoter region of the human *SERT* gene that resulted in a deletion of a 44-basepair repeat.[62] Further investigation into the functional implications of the promoter deletion showed a 3-fold decrease in activity of the short (*s*) versus the long (*l*) promoter in JAR cells as measured by luciferase-promoter fusion constructs. Moreover, PKC- and cAMP-activated transcription was significantly greater at the *l SERT* gene promoter versus the *s* promoter.[62] Prevalence of the *s* versus the *l* alleles in 505 subjects revealed that 19% of the individuals were homozygous for the *s/s* genotype whereas 49% were *l/s* and the remaining subjects were *l/l*.[63] Basal transcriptional activity of the promoters were ascertained from lymphoblasts cultured from individuals with *l/l*, *l/s*, and *s/s* genotypes. Similar transcriptional activity to that shown in JAR cells was reported; a concurrent decrease in SERT protein expression was evident in lymphoblasts containing the *s/s* and *l/s* genotypes compared with the *l/l* genotype.[63]

Because these initial studies confirm that differences exist in the activities of the promoter as well as the distribution of the polymorphism in humans, the consequences of these allelic variations on antidepressant efficacy and response has become a subject of active inquiry. Rausch and colleagues[64] determined the SERT promoter polymorphism in 51 individuals diagnosed with major depression and examined the effects of fluoxetine on depression symptoms. Interestingly, patients with an *l* allele (either as *l/l* or *l/s*) exhibited an increase in the response to both fluoxetine and placebo as measured by a decrease in the Hamilton depression score compared with individuals with the *s/s* genotype.[64] In agreement with these findings, Chinese patients with the *l/l* genotype also showed a greater decrease in Hamilton scores after fluoxetine treatment compared with their *s/s* and *l/s* genotype counterparts.[65] Moreover, a more rapid onset of responsiveness for elderly people with the *l/l* genotype has been reported. Pollock et al[66] showed that after a week of treatment with paroxetine, *l/l* elderly patients had a decrease in the Hamilton depression score compared with both the *l/s* and *s/s* genotypes suggesting a faster rate of onset for the clinical effect. There was no change in onset of response in patients treated with nortriptyline suggesting a response unique to SERT-selective antidepressants.[66] Similar results indicating a faster rate of onset for response in *l/l* genotypes were obtained in a study of 176 elderly subjects treated with sertraline with no change in response to placebo-treated subjects.[67] Interestingly, neither study reported a further change in response subsequent to the initial response at the end of either a 12-week or 8-week study.[66,67] Thus, these data suggest a link between response to SSRIs and the age of the depressed subject.

Another polymorphism of the SERT gene results in a mutation in the eighth TMD of the SERT protein. This rare polymorphism was initially identified in 2 families with multiple neuropsychiatric illnesses.[68] The hSERT I425V mutation results in increased 5-HT transport in human cervical epitheloid carcinoma and COS-7 cells transfected with the I425V hSERT cDNA. The change in transport was accompanied with a decrease in the K_m value and an increase in the V_{max} value without a change in the surface expression suggesting a mutation-induced alteration to the transporter's activity.[69] Additionally, as previously shown with activation of SERT through the A_3 adenosine receptor,[30] a nitric oxide donor increased wild-type SERT activity. The increase in SERT activity following nitric oxide stimulation was equivalent to the activity of the I425V hSERT mutant in the absence of nitric oxide. hSERT I425V activity, however, was insensitive to nitric oxide. Therefore, hSERT I425V functions at a level equivalent to wild-type SERT after activating cGMP-signaling pathways.[69] Furthermore, the hSERT I425V polymorphism exists on the *l* allele.[68] Thus, individuals with this polymorphism would have increased expression of a catalytically enhanced transporter. Interestingly, individuals with the hSERT I425V polymorphism were resistant to antidepressant treatment.[68]

Although the present research strongly suggests genetic links to differences in response rates as well as overall response to antidepressants, specifically SSRIs, further investigation is necessary to determine how the changes in the *SERT* gene promoter alter the expression, regulation, and activity of the SERT protein. Rausch et al[64] reported a difference in the initial 5-HT K_m value by platelet SERT between subjects who responded to fluoxetine treatment versus nonresponders. This change in 5-HT interactions did not appear to be dependent on the allelic variant, although subjects with the *l* allele and an initial increase in the 5-HT K_m value did exhibit the most favorable response to treatment.[64] Furthermore, investigation into how the I425V polymorphism disrupts SERT regulation by PKG is necessary to further the understanding of how antidepressants affect SERT activity and expression. Such information could lead to the development of therapies for individuals who do not respond to common antidepressants.

Cytokines and Depression

In addition to antidepressants acting on the biogenic amine neurotransmitters, other signaling pathways may be involved with antidepressant action as well as the pathophysiology of affective disorders. One alternative to the monoamine hypothesis of depression is the macrophage hypothesis of depression developed by RS Smith in 1991.[70] Smith hypothesized that gross secretion of macrophage cytokines such as interleukin-1, tumor necrosis factor-α, and interferon-α (IFN-α) are responsible for some cases of major depression. Increases in these substances may elicit a hypersecretion of corticotrophin-releasing factor, resulting in hypercortisolemia, which may play a role in depressive diseases as a result of defects in negative feedback mechanisms controlling these substances.[71] In fact, a recent study has indicated that patients suffering from depressive syndromes with a history of suicidal attempts were associated with lowered adrenocorticotropin and cortisol levels, particularly after a recent suicide attempt.[72] Additionally, cancer patients receiving IFN-α or interleukin-2 therapy had significant decreases in serum tryptophan, the amino acid precursor to 5-HT.[73] Decreased serum tryptophan upon cytokine treatment may be due to induced tryptophan catabolism leading to increases in kynurenine and quinolinic acid. Patients who received IFN-α treatment for malignant melanoma showed significant increases in kynurenine as well as decreases in tryptophan and approximately half of these patients developed major depression during treatment.[74] However, patients who received paroxetine 2 weeks prior to IFN-α treatment did not develop major depression despite increases in kynurenine and quinolinic acid.[74] Although major depression frequently occurs in patients receiving cytokine therapy, these depressive symptoms can be attenuated with antidepressant treatment. Although a detailed discussion of cytokines and their purported link to depression via the hypothalamic-pituitary-adrenal axis is outside the scope of this review, it has been reviewed in detail elsewhere.[71,75]

Hypothalamic-pituitary-thyroid Axis

The hypothalamus is directly responsible for regulating the pituitary, which in turn secretes thyroid-stimulating hormone (TSH). Dysregulation of this tightly controlled system can result in thyroid dysfunction. Interestingly, hypothyroidism and depression share many of the same psychological and physical symptoms including anhedonia, fatigue, depressed mood, and cognitive disturbances, as well as sleep disturbances and weight change. Depression, in addition to hypothyroidism, may be a result of an imbalance of the regulatory functions of the hypothalamic-pituitary-thyroid (HPT) axis. Recently, Bschor and colleagues[76] reported a relationship between thyroid function and lithium pharmacotherapy. Although lithium therapy is one of the oldest treatments for mood disorders and remains a useful strategy for the treatment of refractory depression, the mode of lithium action has been poorly understood. Following lithium treatment, Bschor et al[76] reported significantly higher serum TSH levels, as well as significantly decreased triiodothyronine (T_3) and thyroxine (T_4) levels, resulting in a significant reduction of HPT system activity. Although the study did not provide evidence that thyroid status would predict responses to lithium therapy, it does provide support for a relationship between the HPT and depression.

Direct effects of psychotropic therapy on the HPT axis have been difficult to assess. Many studies are inconclusive and have considerable methodological differences making the results difficult to interpret. At the molecular level, in vitro studies have shown that incubation of thyroid cells with chlorpromazine causes a decrease of ^{131}I uptake, an important step in thyroid hormone synthesis.[77] Additionally, many antipsychotics and antidepressants with an alkylamino side chain (alimemazine, chlorpromazine, clomipramine, imipramine, and desipramine) can have a strong donor/acceptor interaction with iodine that could lead to iatrogenic hypothyroidism or thyroiditis.[77]

The possible interactions between antidepressants and thyroid metabolites are less clearly interpreted in clinical studies. Shelton and colleagues[78] reported that T_3 levels decreased transiently for both desipramine and fluoxetine treatment groups whereas desipramine treatment caused a significant increase in total T_4. Also, no significant treatment effects on free T_4, TSH, or TSH response to a thryrotropin-releasing hormone test were observed.[78] A similar study determined the antidepressant effects on thyroid function while controlling for the circadian activity of the thyrotrophs. Depressed patients had a significantly lower TSH response to protirelin, free T_4, and free T_3 than control patients.[79] The authors concluded that significant changes in thyroid function tests were associated with clinical recovery and not due to a direct effect of the antidepressant drug treatment.

Conversely, thyroid hormone levels could exert a positive influence on antidepressant treatment of depressive disorders. Sauvage et al[77] postulated that T_3 may enhance the effects of antidepressants through a potentiation of the β-adrenergic receptor system. Co-administration of T_3 during an antidepressant regimen may accelerate a response to antidepressant treatment to improve the overall treatment outcome.[77] Overall, depression and the HPT axis seem to be intimately linked, although this link remains to be clearly defined.

G-proteins, cAMP Response Element Binding Protein

Several hypotheses regarding the mechanism of action of antidepressants have been developed, including the monoamine, cytokine, and HPT hypotheses. However, all of these hypotheses fail to address the significant lag time (approximately 2 to 4 weeks) between initiating a treatment regimen and detecting a clinical response. Molecular interactions of antidepressants at targets such as transporters and receptors are well studied and these interactions are known to take place following the first dose of drug treatment. Additional mechanisms must account for the lengthy response time. One such mechanism proposed is an increase in G-protein coupled signaling.[27] An increase in the coupling of the heterotrimeric G-protein subunit Gs_α to adenylyl cyclase results in increased cAMP, cAMP-dependent activation of protein kinase A, and subsequent phosphorylation and activation of a multitude of downstream targets. The up- or down-regulation of these targets is dependent on transcriptional and translational events that require days or even weeks for full molecular and cellular effects to be achieved and may contribute to the lag time between initiation of pharmacotherapy and evidence of a clinical response. These targets may include the cAMP response element binding protein (CREB), a nuclear transcription factor that up-regulates gene expression. Chronic antidepressant treatment has been linked to the up-regulation of CREB in the hippocampus, cortex, and amygdala.[80,81] Wallace and coworkers[81] demonstrated that overexpression of CREB in the basolateral amygdala after training in the learned helpless model of depression caused a decrease in escape failures, an antidepressant response. In contrast, induction of CREB before training caused an increase in escape failures, a converse effect, as well as increased immobility in the forced swim test, indicating a prodepressive effect. Although the temporal expression of CREB was critical in determining antidepressant outcomes, it nonetheless implicates CREB as a key player in depression, learning, and memory, and signifies the need for controlled regulation.

Brain-derived Neurotrophic Factor

Brain-derived neurotrophic factor (BDNF) is a neurotrophin (ie, a peptide that regulates growth and survival of neurons) that functions as a neurotransmitter modulator and a regulator of plasticity mechanisms.[82] Human studies have shown that serum BDNF levels in antidepressant-naïve depressed patients are lower than those in antidepressant-treated patients or healthy controls. These findings indicate that decreased BDNF may be important in the pathophysiology of depression.[82] Shimizu et al[82] hypothesized that a decrease in BDNF may reduce the neuroprotective effect and cause stress-induced neuronal damage, leading to biological vulnerability and susceptibility to depressive diseases.[82] Several studies have reported robust increases in BDNF mRNA levels in several parts of the brain including the cortex and hippocampus after various (SSRI, TCA, MAOI) antidepressant treatments.[83] Coppell and coworkers[84] replicated this finding in rats with repeated administration of tranylcypromine, fluoxetine, paroxetine, or sertraline. Their data show BDNF mRNA levels were up-regulated in the hippocampus after long-term drug treatment. However, 4 hours after the last injection BDNF mRNA levels were down-regulated indicating that BDNF expression is differentially regulated in acute and chronic drug treatments. Interestingly, desipramine, maprotiline, and mianserin did not increase BDNF levels 24 hours post-injection.[84] Therefore, the regulation of BDNF may be drug specific as well as temporally regulated. Finally, CREB-deficient mice, unlike wild-type controls, do not exhibit increases in BDNF mRNA levels upon chronic desipramine administration.[85] Conti and colleagues[85] were unable to detect increased levels of BDNF mRNA after chronic fluoxetine administration in either control or CREB-deficient mice providing further evidence that this regulatory effect may be antidepressant specific. In summary, the data demonstrate that CREB may act upstream of BDNF and is necessary for antidepressant-induced alterations in BDNF mRNA expression.

Future Horizons of Antidepressant Development

Future treatments for depression will likely diverge further from the single target specificity of the SSRIs or the tricyclic antidepressants. Currently, novel 5-HT_{1D} and 5-HT_{1B} receptor antagonists that block presynaptic autoreceptors are under development. These agents would reverse the inhibitory role of the autoreceptors resulting in the subsequent release of 5-HT.[86] In addition, selective, reversible inhibitors of MAOs (RIMAs) such as befloxatone, teloxantrone, moclobemide, and brofaromine are being redeveloped.[11] If taken at low to moderate doses, RIMAs can be displaced from the enzyme and do not require the dietary restrictions of conventional MAOIs.[11] The emergency contraceptive mifepristone (RU-486) in addition to antagonizing progesterone receptors also antagonizes glucocorticoid receptors. Blocking the toxic effects of cortisol on glucocorticoid receptors may have therapeutic benefits in treating psychotic depression and bipolar disorder by enhancing neurocognitive function.[11,87] Furthermore, novel peptides that act as antagonists for the corticotropin-releasing factor are under development.[11] In fact, a recent study found that patients with mood disorders had a statistically significant increased number of corticotrophin-releasing hormone immunoreactive (CRH-IR) neurons in the paraventricular nucleus of the hypothalamus as well as a significantly higher number of CHR-IR neurons expressing the estrogen receptor alpha.[88] Finally, antagonists for the neurokinin receptors are being developed as inhibitors of substance P and other neurokinins. Antagonizing the effects of these peptides may have efficacy in treating mood disorders, psychosis, and anxiety.[11] Indeed, several neurokinin receptor antagonists have demonstrated the same antidepressant effect as amitriptyline and desipramine in a rodent forced-swim test model.[89]

Conclusion

Clinical depression is thought to result in part from disruptions in the serotonergic system. Numerous studies have identified SERT as a pharmacological target for treating these symptoms. Not surprisingly, an interaction of antidepressants with SERT alone is not sufficient for immediate therapeutic benefit. Although a preponderance of research has focused on determining the regulation of SERT expression, the exact mechanisms responsible remain undefined. Thus, until the normal processes of SERT regulation are delineated, the implications of discrepancies in SERT levels and function due to chronic antidepressant treatment cannot be ascertained. Furthermore, development of new antidepressants with greater therapeutic benefits will be hindered without knowing the contribution of the various receptors and signaling proteins to this regulation as well as the contribution of non-amine systems to the etiology of depression. Finally, recent evidence shows that allelic differences exist in the responsiveness to current antidepressants. Due to the prevalence of depression in society, further investigation into why the *l/l* genotype of SERT allows for faster onset of therapeutic response to antidepressants and how drugs can be designed to increase the responsiveness of the *s/s* SERT genotype must be addressed.

References

1. Heninger GR, Delgado PL, Charney DS. The revised monoamine theory of depression: a modulatory role for monoamines, based on new findings from monoamine depletion experiments in humans. *Pharmacopsychiatry.* 1996;29:2-11.
2. Nutt DJ. The neuropharmacology of serotonin and noradrenaline in depression. *Int Clin Psychopharmacol.* 2002;17:S1-12.
3. Rush A, Ryan N. Current and emerging therapeutics for depression. In: Davis K, Charney D, Coyle J, Nemeroff C, eds. *Neuropsychopharmacology: The Fifth Generation of Progress.* New York, NY: Raven Press; 2002:1081-1095.
4. Owens MJ, Morgan WN, Plott SJ, Nemeroff CB. Neurotransmitter receptor and transporter binding profile of antidepressants and their metabolites. *J Pharmacol Exp Ther.* 1997;283: 1305-1322.
5. Ban TA. Pharmacotherapy of depression: a historical analysis. *J Neural Transm.* 2001; 108:707-716.
6. Richelson E. The clinical relevance of antidepressant interaction with neurotransmitter transporters and receptors. *Psychopharmacol Bull.* 2002;36:133-150.
7. Steffens DC, Krishnan KR, Helms MJ. Are SSRIs better than TCAs? Comparison of SSRIs and TCAs: a meta-analysis. *Depress Anxiety.* 1997;6:10-18.
8. Song F, Freemantle N, Sheldon TA, et al. Selective serotonin reuptake inhibitors: meta-analysis of efficacy and acceptability. *BMJ.* 1993;306:683-687.
9. Fava M. New approaches to the treatment of refractory depression. *J Clin Psychiatry.* 2000;61: 26-32.
10. Gutierrez MA, Stimmel GL, Aiso JY. Venlafaxine: a 2003 update. *Clin Ther.* 2003;25:2138-2154.
11. Stahl SM, Grady MM. Differences in mechanism of action between current and future antidepressants. *J Clin Psychiatry.* 2003;64:13-17.
12. Shelton RC. The dual-action hypothesis: does pharmacology matter? *J Clin Psychiatry.* 2004;65:5-10.
13. Barker EL, Perlman MA, Adkins EM, et al. High affinity recognition of serotonin transporter antagonists defined by species-scanning mutagenesis. An aromatic residue in transmembrane domain I dictates species-selective recognition of citalopram and mazindol. *J Biol Chem.* 1998;273:19459-19468.
14. Ravna AW, Sylte I, Dahl SG. Molecular mechanism of citalopram and cocaine interactions with neurotransmitter transporters. *J Pharmacol Exp Ther.* 2003;307:34-41.
15. Kitayama S, Shimada S, Xu H, Markham L, Donovan DM, Uhl GR. Dopamine transporter site-directed mutations differentially alter substrate transport and cocaine binding. *Proc Natl Acad Sci USA.* 1992;89:7782-7785.
16. Barker EL, Moore KR, Rakhshan F, Blakely RD. Transmembrane domain I contributes to the permeation pathway for serotonin and ions in the serotonin transporter. *J Neurosci.* 1999;19: 4705-4717.
17. Paczkowski FA, Bryan-Lluka LJ. Tyrosine residue 271 of the norepinephrine transporter is an important determinant of its pharmacology. *Brain Res Mol Brain Res.* 2001;97:32-42.
18. Roubert C, Cox PJ, Bruss M, Hamon M, Bonisch H, Giros B. Determination of residues in the norepinephrine transporter that are critical for tricyclic antidepressant affinity. *J Biol Chem.* 2001;276:8254-8260.
19. Paczkowski FA, Bonisch H, Bryan-Lluka LJ. Pharmacological properties of the naturally occurring Ala(457)Pro variant of the human norepinephrine transporter. *Pharmacogenetics.* 2002;12:165-173.
20. Roman DL, Walline CC, Rodriguez GJ, Barker EL. Interactions of antidepressants with the serotonin transporter: a contemporary molecular analysis. *Eur J Pharmacol.* 2003;479:53-63.
21. Barker EL, Blakely RD. Identification of a single amino acid, phenylalanine 586, that is responsible for high affinity interactions of tricyclic antidepressants with the human serotonin transporter. *Mol Pharmacol.* 1996;50:957-965.

22. Schloss P, Williams DC. The serotonin transporter: a primary target for antidepressant drugs. *J Psychopharmacol.* 1998;12:115-121.

23. Vetulani J, Nalepa I. Antidepressants: past, present and future. *Eur J Pharmacol.* 2000;405:351-363.

24. Qian Y, Galli A, Ramamoorthy S, Risso S, DeFelice LJ, Blakely RD. Protein kinase C activation regulates human serotonin transporters in HEK-293 cells via altered cell surface expression. *J Neurosci.* 1997;17:45-57.

25. Ramamoorthy S, Giovanetti E, Qian Y, Blakely RD. Phosphorylation and regulation of antidepressant-sensitive serotonin transporters. *J Biol Chem.* 1998;273:2458-2466.

26. Ramamoorthy S, Blakely RD. Phosphorylation and sequestration of serotonin transporters differentially modulated by psychostimulants. *Science.* 1999;285:763-766.

27. Donati RJ, Rasenick MM. G protein signaling and the molecular basis of antidepressant action. *Life Sci.* 2003;73:1-17.

28. Ramamoorthy S, Cool DR, Mahesh VB, et al. Regulation of the human serotonin transporter. Cholera toxin-induced stimulation of serotonin uptake in human placental choriocarcinoma cells is accompanied by increased serotonin transporter mRNA levels and serotonin transporter-specific ligand binding. *J Biol Chem.* 1993;268:21626-21631.

29. Zhu CB, Hewlett WA, Feoktistov I, Biaggioni I, Blakely RD. Adenosine receptor, protein kinase G, and p38 mitogen-activated protein kinase-dependent up-regulation of serotonin transporters involves both transporter trafficking and activation. *Mol Pharmacol.* 2004;65: 1462-1474.

30. Miller KJ, Hoffman BJ. Adenosine A3 receptors regulate serotonin transport via nitric oxide and cGMP. *J Biol Chem.* 1994;269:27351-27356.

31. Samuvel DJ, Jayanthi LD, Bhat NR, Ramamoorthy S. A role for p38 mitogen-activated protein kinase in the regulation of the serotonin transporter: evidence for distinct cellular mechanisms involved in transporter surface expression. *J Neurosci.* 2005;25:29-41.

32. Haase J, Killian AM, Magnani F, Williams C. Regulation of the serotonin transporter by interacting proteins. *Biochem Soc Trans.* 2001;29:722-728.

33. Quick MW. Role of syntaxin 1A on serotonin transporter expression in developing thalamocortical neurons. *Int J Dev Neurosci.* 2002;20:219-224.

34. Quick MW. Regulating the conducting states of a mammalian serotonin transporter. *Neuron.* 2003;40:537-549.

35. Bauman AL, Apparsundaram S, Ramamoorthy S, Wadzinski BE, Vaughan RA, Blakely RD. Cocaine and antidepressant-sensitive biogenic amine transporters exist in regulated complexes with protein phosphatase 2A. *J Neurosci.* 2000;20:7571-7578.

36. Rausch JL, Gillespie CF, Fei Y, et al. Antidepressant effects on kinase gene expression patterns in rat brain. *Neurosci Lett.* 2002;334:91-94.

37. Gelenberg AJ, Chesen CL. How fast are antidepressants? *J Clin Psychiatry.* 2000;61:712-721.

38. Potter WZ, Hollister LE. Antidepressant agents. In: Katzung BG, ed. *Basic & Clinical Pharmacology.* New York, NY: Lange Medical Books/McGraw-Hill; 2004:482-496.

39. Horschitz S, Hummerich R, Schloss P. Down-regulation of the rat serotonin transporter upon exposure to a selective serotonin reuptake inhibitor. *Neuroreport.* 2001;12:2181-2184.

40. Benmansour S, Cecchi M, Morilak DA, et al. Effects of chronic antidepressant treatments on serotonin transporter function, density, and mRNA level. *J Neurosci.* 1999;19:10494-10501.

41. Benmansour S, Owens WA, Cecchi M, Morilak DA, Frazer A. Serotonin clearance in vivo is altered to a greater extent by antidepressant-induced downregulation of the serotonin transporter than by acute blockade of this transporter. *J Neurosci.* 2002;22:6766-6772.

42. Gould GG, Pardon MC, Morilak DA, Frazer A. Regulatory effects of reboxetine treatment alone, or following paroxetine treatment, on brain noradrenergic and serotonergic systems. *Neuropsychopharmacology.* 2003;28:1633-1641.

43. Kugaya A, Seneca NM, Snyder PJ, et al. Changes in human *in vivo* serotonin and dopamine transporter availabilities during chronic antidepressant administration. *Neuropsychopharmacology.* 2003;28:413-420.

44. Plein H, Berk M. The platelet as a peripheral marker in psychiatric illness. *Hum Psychopharmacol.* 2001;16:229-236.
45. Alvarez JC, Gluck N, Arnulf I, et al. Decreased platelet serotonin transporter sites and increased platelet inositol triphosphate levels in patients with unipolar depression: effects of clomipramine and fluoxetine. *Clin Pharmacol Ther.* 1999;66:617-624.
46. Hébert C, Habimana A, Élie R, Reader TA. Effects of chronic antidepressant treatments on 5-HT and NA transporters in rat brain: an autoradiographic study. *Neurochem Int.* 2001;38:63-74.
47. Yau JL, Kelly PA, Olsson T, Noble J, Seckl JR. Chronic amitriptyline administration increases serotonin transporter binding sites in the hippocampus of aged rats. *Neurosci Lett.* 1999;261:183-185.
48. Lima L, Urbina M. Serotonin transporter modulation in blood lymphocytes from patients with major depression. *Cell Mol Neurobiol.* 2002;22:797-804.
49. Schloss P, Henn FA. New insights into the mechanisms of antidepressant therapy. *Pharmacol Ther.* 2004;102:47-60.
50. Piñeyro G, Blier P. Autoregulation of serotonin neurons: role in antidepressant drug action. *Pharmacol Rev.* 1999;51:533-591.
51. Celada P, Puig M, Amargos-Bosch M, Adell A, Artigas F. The therapeutic role of 5-HT1A and 5-HT2A receptors in depression. *J Psychiatry Neurosci.* 2004;29:252-265.
52. Hensler JG. Differential regulation of 5-HT1A receptor-G protein interactions in brain following chronic antidepressant administration. *Neuropsychopharmacology.* 2002;26:565-573.
53. Ase AR, Reader TA, Hen R, Riad M, Descarries L. Regional changes in density of serotonin transporter in the brain of 5-HT1A and 5-HT1B knockout mice, and of serotonin innervation in the 5-HT1B knockout. *J Neurochem.* 2001;78:619-630.
54. Daws LC, Gerhardt GA, Frazer Λ. 5 HT1B antagonists modulate clearance of extracellular serotonin in rat hippocampus. *Neurosci Lett.* 1999;266:165-168.
55. Daws LC, Gould GG, Teicher SD, Gerhardt GA, Frazer A. 5-HT(1B) receptor-mediated regulation of serotonin clearance in rat hippocampus in vivo. *J Neurochem.* 2000;75:2113-2122.
56. Malagié I, David DJ, Jolliet P, Hen R, Bourin M, Gardier AM. Improved efficacy of fluoxetine in increasing hippocampal 5-hydroxytryptamine outflow in 5-HT1B receptor knock-out mice. *Eur J Pharmacol.* 2002;443:99-104.
57. Neumaier JF, Root DC, Hamblin MW. Chronic fluoxetine reduces serotonin transporter mRNA and 5-HT1B mRNA in a sequential manner in the rat dorsal raphe nucleus. *Neuropsychopharmacology.* 1996;15:515-522.
58. Artigas F, Perez V, Alvarez E. Pindolol induces a rapid improvement of depressed patients treated with serotonin reuptake inhibitors. *Arch Gen Psychiatry.* 1994;51:248-251.
59. Shalom G, Gur E, Van de Kar LD, Newman ME. Repeated administration of the 5-HT(1B) receptor antagonist SB-224289 blocks the desensitisation of 5-HT(1B) autoreceptors induced by fluoxetine in rat frontal cortex. *Naunyn Schmiedebergs Arch Pharmacol.* 2004;370:84-90.
60. Ansah TA, Ramamoorthy S, Montanez S, Daws LC, Blakely RD. Calcium-dependent inhibition of synaptosomal serotonin transport by the alpha 2-adrenoceptor agonist 5-bromo-N-[4,5-dihydro-1H-imidazol-2-yl]-6-quinoxalinamine (UK14304). *J Pharmacol Exp Ther.* 2003;305:956-965.
61. Ramamoorthy S, Bauman AL, Moore KR, et al. Antidepressant- and cocaine-sensitive human serotonin transporter: molecular cloning, expression, and chromosomal localization. *Proc Natl Acad Sci USA.* 1993;90:2542-2546.
62. Heils A, Teufel A, Petri S, et al. Allelic variation of human serotonin transporter gene expression. *J Neurochem.* 1996;66:2621-2624.
63. Lesch KP, Bengel D, Heils A, et al. Association of anxiety-related traits with a polymorphism in the serotonin transporter gene regulatory region. *Science.* 1996;274:1527-1531.
64. Rausch JL, Johnson ME, Fei YJ, et al. Initial conditions of serotonin transporter kinetics and genotype: influence on SSRI treatment trial outcome. *Biol Psychiatry.* 2002;51:723-732.
65. Yu YW, Tsai SJ, Chen TJ, Lin CH, Hong CJ. Association study of the serotonin transporter promoter polymorphism and symptomatology and antidepressant response in major depressive disorders. *Mol Psychiatry.* 2002;7:1115-1119.

66. Pollock BG, Ferrell RE, Mulsant BH, et al. Allelic variation in the serotonin transporter promoter affects onset of paroxetine treatment response in late-life depression. *Neuropsychopharmacology.* 2000;23:587-590.
67. Durham LK, Webb SM, Milos PM, Clary CM, Seymour AB. The serotonin transporter polymorphism, 5HTTLPR, is associated with a faster response time to sertraline in an elderly population with major depressive disorder. *Psychopharmacology (Berl).* 2004;174:525-529.
68. Ozaki N, Goldman D, Kaye WH, et al. Serotonin transporter missense mutation associated with a complex neuropsychiatric phenotype. *Mol Psychiatry.* 2003;8:933-936.
69. Kilic F, Murphy DL, Rudnick G. A human serotonin transporter mutation causes constitutive activation of transport activity. *Mol Pharmacol.* 2003;64:440-446.
70. Smith RS. The macrophage theory of depression. *Med Hypotheses.* 1991;35:298-306.
71. Connor TJ, Leonard BE. Depression, stress and immunological activation: the role of cytokines in depressive disorders. *Life Sci.* 1998;62:583-606.
72. Pfennig A, Kunzel HE, Kern N, et al. Hypothalamus-pituitary-adrenal system regulation and suicidal behavior in depression. *Biol Psychiatry.* 2005;57:336-342.
73. Capuron L, Ravaud A, Neveu PJ, Miller AH, Maes M, Dantzer R. Association between decreased serum tryptophan concentrations and depressive symptoms in cancer patients undergoing cytokine therapy. *Mol Psychiatry.* 2002;7:468-473.
74. Capuron L, Neurauter G, Musselman DL, et al. Interferon-alpha-induced changes in tryptophan metabolism: relationship to depression and paroxetine treatment. *Biol Psychiatry.* 2003;54:906-914.
75. Schiepers OJ, Wichers MC, Maes M. Cytokines and major depression. *Prog Neuropsychopharmacol Biol Psychiatry.* 2005;29:201-217.
76. Bschor T, Baethge C, Adli M, Lewitzka U, Eichmann U, Bauer M. Hypothalamic-pituitary-thyroid system activity during lithium augmentation therapy in patients with unipolar major depression. *J Psychiatry Neurosci.* 2003;28:210-216.
77. Sauvage MF, Marquet P, Rousseau A, Raby C, Buxeraud J, Lachatre G. Relationship between psychotropic drugs and thyroid function: a review. *Toxicol Appl Pharmacol.* 1998;149:127-135.
78. Shelton RC, Winn S, Ekhatore N, Loosen PT. The effects of antidepressants on the thyroid axis in depression. *Biol Psychiatry.* 1993;33:120-126.
79. Duval F, Mokrani MC, Crocq MA, et al. Effect of antidepressant medication on morning and evening thyroid function tests during a major depressive episode. *Arch Gen Psychiatry.* 1996;53:833-840.
80. Nibuya M, Nestler EJ, Duman RS. Chronic antidepressant administration increases the expression of cAMP response element binding protein (CREB) in rat hippocampus. *J Neurosci.* 1996;16:2365-2372.
81. Wallace TL, Stellitano KE, Neve RL, Duman RS. Effects of cyclic adenosine monophosphate response element binding protein overexpression in the basolateral amygdala on behavioral models of depression and anxiety. *Biol Psychiatry.* 2004;56:151-160.
82. Shimizu E, Hashimoto K, Okamura N, et al. Alterations of serum levels of brain-derived neurotrophic factor (BDNF) in depressed patients with or without antidepressants. *Biol Psychiatry.* 2003;54:70-75.
83. Duman RS. Role of neurotrophic factors in the etiology and treatment of mood disorders. *Neuromolecular Med.* 2004;5:11-25.
84. Coppell AL, Pei Q, Zetterstrom TS. Bi-phasic change in BDNF gene expression following antidepressant drug treatment. *Neuropharmacology.* 2003;44:903-910.
85. Conti AC, Cryan JF, Dalvi A, Lucki I, Blendy JA. cAMP response element-binding protein is essential for the upregulation of brain-derived neurotrophic factor transcription, but not the behavioral or endocrine responses to antidepressant drugs. *J Neurosci.* 2002;22:3262-3268.
86. Pullar IA, Boot JR, Broadmore RJ, et al. The role of the 5-HT1D receptor as a presynaptic autoreceptor in the guinea pig. *Eur J Pharmacol.* 2004;493:85-93.

87. Young AH, Gallagher P, Watson S, Del-Estal D, Owen BM, Nicol Ferrier I. Improvements in neurocognitive function and mood following adjunctive treatment with mifepristone (RU-486) in bipolar disorder. *Neuropsychopharmacology*. 2004;29:1538-1545.
88. Bao AM, Hestiantoro A, Van Someren EJ, Swaab DF, Zhou JN. Colocalization of corticotropin-releasing hormone and oestrogen receptor-{alpha} in the paraventricular nucleus of the hypothalamus in mood disorders. *Brain*. 2005.
89. Dableh LJ, Yashpal K, Rochford J, Henry JL. Antidepressant-like effects of neurokinin receptor antagonists in the forced swim test in the rat. *Eur J Pharmacol*. 2005;507:99-105.

Chapter 14
Recent Advances for the Treatment of Cocaine Abuse: Central Nervous System Immunopharmacotherapy

Tobin J. Dickerson[1] and Kim D. Janda[1]

Abstract Cocaine addiction continues to be a major health and societal problem in spite of governmental efforts devoted toward educating the public of the dangers of illicit drug use. A variety of pharmacotherapies and psychosocial programs have been proposed in an effort to provide a method for alleviation of the physical and psychological symptoms of cocaine abuse. Unfortunately, these methods have been met with limited success, illustrating a critical need for new effective approaches for the treatment of cocaine addiction. Recently an alternative cocaine abuse treatment strategy was proposed using intranasal administration of an engineered filamentous bacteriophage displaying cocaine-sequestering antibodies on its surface. These phage particles are an effective vector for CNS penetration and are capable of binding cocaine, thereby blocking its behavioral effects in a rodent model. The convergence of phage display and immunopharmacotherapy has allowed for an investigation of the efficacy of protein-based therapeutics acting within the CNS on the effects of cocaine in animal models and has uncovered a new tool in the battle against cocaine addiction.

Keywords cocaine, central nervous system, immunopharmacotherapy, virus, phage display

The Problem of Cocaine Addiction

The addiction syndrome is remarkably similar across different drug classes, primarily characterized by a chronic relapsing brain disorder with associated neurobiological changes that lead to a compulsion to take a drug without regard for drug intake.[1,2]

[1] The Skaggs Institute for Chemical Biology and Departments of Chemistry and Immunology, The Scripps Research Institute, 10550 North Torrey Pines Road, La Jolla, CA 92037

Corresponding Author: Kim D. Janda, Department of Chemistry and The Skaggs Institute for Chemical Biology, The Scripps Research Institute, 10550 North Torrey Pines Road, La Jolla, CA 92037. Tel: (858) 784-2516; Fax: (858) 784-2595; E-mail: kdjanda@scripps.edu

The dopamine hypothesis of reward, a common pathway of addiction, has recently been evolving, with the mesocorticolimbic dopaminergic system now viewed as central to both natural rewards and drug-seeking behavior, though perhaps having a more minor role in the maintenance of such behavior.[3-5] Cocaine, a powerful psychostimulant, triggers mechanisms in the brain as fundamental as those activated by food, water, and sexual activity. In essence, the effects of drug consumption are euphoric and stimulating, while the absence of the drug leads to dysphoria and depression. However, this does oversimplify the phenomenon as the transition from drug use to drug abuse is exceedingly complex since both positive and negative reinforcement phenomena are involved. Nonetheless, it is surprising that the most sought and abused drugs of abuse comprise a small set of naturally occurring molecules and closely related derivatives; among these compounds are such drugs as cocaine, nicotine, amphetamines, and opiates.

Cocaine (Fig. 14.1) is a tropane alkaloid extracted from the leaves of the native South American plant *Erythroxylon coca*. Although the most prevalent instances of the problems associated with cocaine have emerged in modern civilization, human cocaine use has likely occurred for thousands of years.[6] Cocaine is purified from coca leaves (containing between 0.6% and 1.8% alkaloidal cocaine) using a relatively simple method by which it is extracted from the leaves with an organic solvent (often kerosene), resulting in a coca paste containing approximately 80% cocaine. The alkaloids are passed through an acidic aqueous solution based on hydrochloric acid; the solution is neutralized and the cocaine is extracted by recrystallization. Cocaine hydrochloride (HCl) is the pharmaceutical form used as a local anesthetic, and abused by drug addicts. It is vulnerable to pyrolysis, resulting in a poor rewarding effect when smoked. However, upon transformation into cocaine freebase (popularly termed "crack" or "rock" cocaine) by dissolving it in an alkaline solution followed by precipitation, the hydrochloride salt transforms into a smokable, pyrolysis-resistant material. Most frequently, cocaine is used in the form of a powder. It can be introduced into the body by sniffing, swallowing, or injecting to produce its characteristic effects as cocaine is readily absorbed by all mucous membranes, such as the lining of the mouth, nasal passages, and gastrointestinal tract.

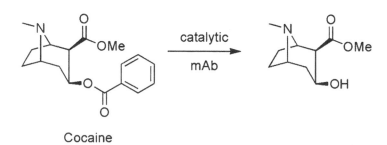

Cocaine

Fig. 14.1 Structure of cocaine and its nonpsychoactive metabolite methyl ecgonine. Antibodies capable of catalyzing this reaction have been a topic of significant interest for various research groups in an effort to design biocatalysts for the treatment of cocaine addiction.

The abuse of cocaine is maintained by the drug's effects on brain reward systems, and mediated at least in part by its dopaminergic action. The patterns and consequences of use are best understood by considering the pharmacokinetics (rapid absorption and delivery to the brain, relatively short half-life), the pharmacodynamics (intense central and peripheral neural stimulation), and the route of drug administration. Cocaine is used therapeutically as a topical and local anesthetic. Toxicity occurs primarily in cocaine abusers, but also occasionally after therapeutic dosing. Medical complications reflect primarily excessive central nervous system (CNS) stimulation and excessive vasoconstriction, the latter resulting in severe hypertension and/or organ ischemia with associated organ injury. Most deaths that result from medical complications of cocaine intoxication are sudden and occur before medical intervention is possible. Other complications of cocaine abuse with severe personal and social consequences include traumatic deaths and injuries, reproductive disturbances, and transmission of infectious diseases, especially AIDS. Recent surveys for cocaine abuse in the United States have indicated that more than 23 million people have tried cocaine, nearly 400 000 use it daily, and 5000 new users are added each day, despite the listing of this compound by the Drug Enforcement Agency as a Schedule II agent.[7] Although abuse appears to be stabilizing relative to the more rampant use of cocaine observed in the 1980s, as much as 0.3% of the population may be dependent on the drug.[8] A myriad of medical problems, including death, often accompany cocaine use and the association of the drug with the spread of AIDS is of great concern.[9,10] Furthermore, the detrimental effects are especially tragic for pregnant women where "crack" has been reported the most abused illicit drug.[11] From the behavioral pharmacology, it has been evident that cocaine is highly addictive and may be the most reinforcing of all commonly abused drugs.[12]

Cocaine Pharmacotherapy

Cocaine addiction represents a serious social and health problem, which has led the National Institute on Drug Abuse (NIDA) to urge the scientific research community for the development of an effective pharmacological treatment for this condition. However, pharmacotherapies of cocaine addiction that typically target the monoaminergic neurochemical substrates implicated in its reward properties, have as yet been unsuccessful, and often generate adverse side effects.

Extensive research efforts have been devoted to the development of an effective pharmacotherapy for the treatment of cocaine abuse. However, unlike the historically successful methadone treatment for heroin addiction, there is no proven pharmacotherapy for cocaine abuse.[13] In recent years, more than 2 dozen medications have been tested as potential therapeutic agents in the treatment of cocaine dependence.[14] A significant component of this effort is to rapidly screen currently marketed drugs to identify potential lead compounds for further testing. Of the compounds tested, 4 (cabergoline,[15] reserpine,[16] sertraline,[17] and tiagabine[18]) have been advanced to further phase II clinical trials, and 2 others (disulfiram[19] and selegiline[20]) have proceeded or are soon expected to proceed to phase III trials. Other compounds, including baclofen,[21] topiramate,[22] and modafinil[23] have also advanced into midstage clinical development. The approaches underlying these compounds can be divided into 3 key areas[15]: (1) Those compounds that can be used in a substitution-based treatment as a cross-tolerant stimulant; (2) medications that serve as antagonists by blocking the binding of cocaine to its cognate receptors; and (3) compounds that function by acting at other sites distinct from the cocaine site of action but functionally antagonize the effects of cocaine. Several biopsychosocial models have been proposed and evaluated to address addiction and relapse prevention.[24] Unquestionably, an improved pharmacotherapy would increase the effectiveness of such programs and alternative strategies for treating cocaine addiction are needed if progress is to be made.

The use of protein-based therapeutics has been employed as a strategy for the treatment of cocaine addiction. In this approach, proteins are designed to bind cocaine, thereby blocking its effects and/or degrading the drug, rendering it less psychoactive.[25] Over the past decade, our group and later additional laboratories have reported the successful blocking of the psychostimulant effects of cocaine by anticocaine antibodies with both active and passive immunization in rodent models. These results demonstrate that anticocaine antibodies bind to cocaine in circulation, retarding its ability to enter the brain.[26-30] Additionally, behavioral studies into cocaine-induced locomotor activity and self-administration have revealed that both strategies have some efficacy in rats. A related antibody-based approach to cocaine addiction treatment used catalytic antibodies specific for cocaine and the cleavage of its benzoyl ester (Fig. 14.1).[31-36] The efficiency of catalytic antibodies has been demonstrated in rodent models of cocaine overdose and reinforcement, but kinetic constants for all reported antibody catalysts are marginal and thus improved rates will be required before clinical development is warranted.[37] The development of cocaine vaccines using both active and passive immunization strategies and the advancement of these vaccines into clinical trials has been recently reviewed.[37,38] Finally, groups using butyrylcholinesterase (BChE),[39,40] the major cocaine-metabolizing enzyme present in the plasma of humans and other mammals, have reported that intravenous pretreatment with either wild-type or genetically engineered BChE can mitigate the behavioral and physiological effects of cocaine and accelerate its metabolism.[41-43] The main drawback common to all of these protein-based approaches is that none acts directly within the CNS; thus, their success depends solely on peripheral contact between the enzyme or antibody with ingested cocaine.

Bacteriophage and Its Therapeutic Application

Bacteriophage are viruses that infect bacteria, and are distinct from the animal and plant viruses in that they lack intrinsic tropism for eukaryotic cells.[43] There are an estimated $>10^{30}$ phages in the biosphere and since phage particles typically outnumber prokaryotic cells by approiximately 10-fold in environmental samples, phages probably constitute an absolute majority of organisms on our planet. In particular, filamentous bacteriophage can be produced at high titer in bacterial culture, making production simple and economical. Additionally, they are extremely stable under a variety of harsh conditions, including extremes in pH and treatment with nucleases or proteolytic enzymes.[44] But perhaps the most significant advantage is the genetic flexibility of filamentous phage. This property was exemplified in the seminal paper of Smith in which a method was reported that physically linked genotype and phenotype in a protein display system, now known as phage display.[45] In this work, foreign cDNA was fused to the gene encoding the surface protein pIII; thus, the foreign cDNA was transcribed and translated as a fusion protein with pIII and displayed on the phage surface. This enabled the researcher to actually select displayed proteins for specific properties and to recover the gene encoding this protein.

The filamentous phage M13 is approximately 895 nm long and 9 nm in diameter. Its single-stranded DNA genome contains 6407 bases that encode 10 different proteins. The DNA is enclosed in a protein coat composed of approximately 2800 copies of the gene VIII protein (pVIII). A viable phage also expresses 3 to 5 copies of pIII on its tip. Unlike most other bacteriophage, M13 does not produce a lytic infection in *Escherichia coli,* but rather induces a state in which infected host cells produce and secrete phage particles without undergoing lysis. Using this powerful technology, a wide variety of proteins, antibodies, and peptides can be displayed on the phage coat (Fig.14.2).

Over the past 2 decades, many important developments in the field of phage display have occurred. Very large libraries of proteins of assorted sizes, ranging from small peptides and antibody fragments to functional enzymes, can now be displayed on various coat proteins of the phage particle, allowing for the identification of natural or artificial ligands for a wide range of receptors, the selection of antibodies with high specificity and affinity against a given antigen, the targeted delivery of foreign DNA into cells, and the selection of enzymes with improved functionality, just to name a few possibilities of phage display technology.

The use of bacteriophage as a therapeutic agent has been known since the 1920s, when lytic phage were administered as antibacterial agents.[46] Their further

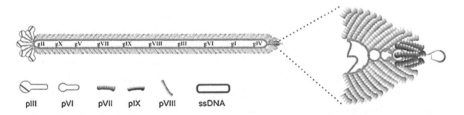

Fig. 14.2 Filamentous phage *fd* architecture. The phage coat contains 2800 copies of the major coat protein pVIII, whereas there are 5 molecules of each of the minor coat proteins pIII, pVII, and pIX.

application was hampered by several factors, of which the inability to remove endotoxins from preparations was predominant. More recently, animal studies have demonstrated that bacteriophage can rescue animals from a variety of fatal infections,[47] while studies conducted in Eastern Europe have shown that phage can be effective in treating drug-resistant infections in humans.[48,49] These encouraging findings have resulted in the emergence of several biotechnology companies embracing the use of phage technology as a therapeutic option, and the US Food and Drug Administration may soon issue regulatory guidelines for phage therapy.

The use of filamentous phage in vivo has been previously reported by Pasqualini and Ruoslahti.[50] In this work, bacteriophage displaying a random peptide library was intravenously injected into mice and subsequently rescued from the internal organs, showing that the integrity of the phage was not compromised.[51] The ability of bacteriophage to penetrate a wide range of vertebrate tissues without detrimentally affecting the host has also been recently reviewed.[52] Furthermore, the ability of filamentous phage to penetrate the CNS has also been reported.[53] Here, Frenkel and Solomon were able to deliver phage-displayed anti-β-amyloid antibodies via intranasal administration into the brains of mice. Frenkel and Solomon's report was significant as it provided the following findings: (1) filamentous phage can easily access the CNS; (2) phage can display foreign proteins on its surface and still penetrate the CNS; (3) bacteriophage can be injected intranasally multiple times into the same animals without visible toxic effects as evidenced by brain histology; and (4) the behavior and life span of all treated animals was monitored for 1 year and no harmful effects were found.

Previously, we have shown that sequestration of cocaine by anticocaine antibodies can suppress the psychomotor and reinforcing actions of the drug.[26-28] From these studies, a murine monoclonal antibody termed GNC92H2 emerged that has exquisite affinity and specificity to cocaine (K_d = 40 nM; while for its hydrolysis product benzoyl ecgonine K_d = 1.4 μM).[26] Within our laboratories, we have also demonstrated that antibody libraries can be displayed on the filamentous phage coat proteins pIII, pVII, and pIX for the selection of high-affinity antibodies to a wide variety of antigens.[54,55] Combining the results of Frenkel and Solomon with our previous studies in cocaine immunopharmacotherapy, we hypothesized that antibodies or enzymes specific for cocaine that are displayed on filamentous phage will have an unprecedented ability to access the CNS. Consequently, this enables for the first time, an investigation of how protein-based therapeutics acting in the CNS can influence the effects of cocaine in rat models.[56] In contrast to more traditional methods such as active or passive immunization, intranasal administration of bacteriophage-derived protein therapeutics provides a direct route for entry into the CNS. The advantage to this method stems from the fact that although antibodies may bind cocaine effectively, these biomacromolecules are unable to quantitatively remove cocaine from the bloodstream prior to CNS entry. Thus, the presence of a bacteriophage-bound cocaine-binding molecule within the CNS would allow for enhanced removal of the drug from the user's system.

Treating Cocaine Addiction with Viruses

To achieve a greater number of anticocaine antibodies on the phage surface, we chose the major coat protein pVIII as fusion partner for the scFv antibody molecule (Fig. 14.3), thus hoping to generate a "molecular sponge" to absorb cocaine. The affinity of GNC 92H2-pVIII for cocaine was determined by equilibrium dialysis to be between 50 nM and 5 μM, depending on the number of scFv 92H2 antibodies displayed on each phage particle. Thus, we surmised that the phage-displayed scFv 92H2 construct possessed comparable cocaine affinity to free scFv in solution.

To assess the efficacy of immunization with phage display antibodies within the CNS the psychostimulant effects of cocaine were measured in the rat. This psychostimulant effect is a dose-dependant increase in locomotor activity and stereotyped behavior as a result of cocaine's actions on dopaminergic neurons in the brain. Three different doses of cocaine were chosen for study: 10, 15, and 30 mg/kg. These doses of cocaine represent a broad range of both locomotor and behavioral responses. Thus, the lowest dose produces little locomotor and virtually no stereotyped behavior, whereas the medium dose produces a significant locomotor activation and modest stereotyped behavior and the highest dose produces less locomotor activity but more robust stereotyped behavior.

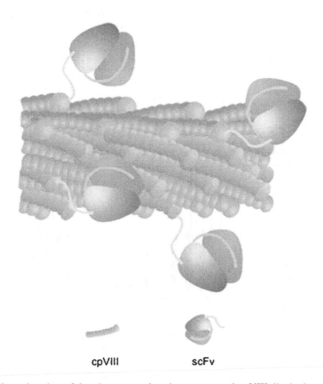

cpVIII   scFv

Fig. 14.3 Enlarged region of the phage coat showing coat protein pVIII displaying a single-chain antibody (scFv).

Animals were treated twice per day by intranasal administration for 3 consecutive days with phage displaying single chain antibodies on their pVIII surfaces. In these experiments, the antibodies used included GNC 92H2-pVIII and RCA$_{60}$28-pVIII, a control antibody that has excellent affinity (400 nM) and selectivity to RCA$_{60}$ (*Ricinus communis* agglutinin, "ricin").[54] In comparison to gene pIII, which can only exhibit up to 5 copies on the surface of a phage, the pVIII gene was chosen as it contains 2800 copies and was anticipated to provide an overall higher concentration of protein on the phage surface.[57] Protein surface concentration is a key element in success of this approach as the antibodies displayed were not catalytic; hence, sequestering was the only means of inhibiting cocaine from reaching its target. Monoclonal antibody GNC 92H2 has previously been shown to have excellent avidity and specificity to cocaine and has yielded outstanding results in previous passive immunization behavioral studies.[26-28]

Over 4 consecutive days, the immunized animals received daily intraperitoneal (IP) cocaine challenges of 1 of 3 doses of the drug, 4 days after the onset of the phage-infusion regime. Intranasal administration of phage GNC 92H2-pVIII versus RCA$_{60}$28-pVIII resulted in significant psychomotor differences between groups in response to cocaine (Fig. 14.4). At the 10 mg/kg dose, a 30% reduction in ambulatory

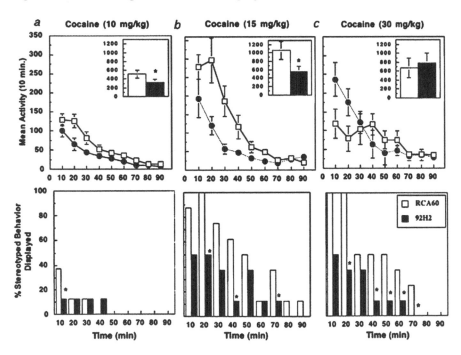

Fig. 14.4 Locomotor activity (crossovers; *Upper*) and stereotyped behavior (sniffing and rearing; *Lower*) after IP injection of cocaine after nasal immunization with GNC 92H2-pVIII (•) or RCA$_{60}$28-pVIII (□). The Fig. shows the response to postnasal immunization cocaine challenge at 10 (a), 15 (b), and 30 (c) mg/kg. *Upper* values represent means ± SEM of 16 animals (n = 8). * $P < .05$ ANOVA, significant difference between groups. *Lower* data represent the percentage of incidence of the observed behavior. *$P < .05$.

behavior (crossovers) compared with baseline values was observed in the GNC 92H2-pVIII group but not in controls and this difference was reflected in the stereotypy measurement during the first 10 minutes of the session. This modest difference in ambulation is not surprising given the tenuous hypermotility elicited at this dose. Furthermore, the paucity of the observed stereotypy is consistent with previous reports using a low dose of cocaine.[57] In contrast, a marked 47% decrease in locomotor activity was measured in GNC 92H2-pVIII-treated animals versus baseline values, while controls increased their overall responses by 11%. This quantitative trend was also observed in the percent stereotypy displayed, where the behavior was rated in controls up to 70 minutes into the session, as opposed to 50 minutes in the GNC 92H2-pVIII group. These results have a striking similarity to our previously reported results using both active immunization with 2 different cocaine conjugates[26-28] and passive immunization with the mAb GNC 92H2.[28] This similarity probably is contingent upon 2 main experimental factors. First, the same cocaine dose was used, therefore, the patterns of hyperactivity are congruent. Second, the cocaine-blocking mechanism, albeit central versus peripheral, still obeys an immune-mediated dynamic, which is subject to the same elements of affinity and titer surmountability. This so-called element of surmountability is most evident in the data depicted by Fig. 4C. At the 30-mg/kg cocaine dose, a reversal of behavioral profile was obtained, whereby control animals showed diminishing levels of locomotion compared with both their own baseline values and GNC 92H2-pVIII-treated rats during the first 30 minutes of the session (Fig. 4C). Interestingly, stereotyped behavior was sustained by controls significantly longer and at higher percentages than by the GNC 92H2-pVIII group (Fig. 4C) reflecting the typical emergence of increased levels of this measure at the higher doses of cocaine.[58] Therefore, the apparent absence of a blunting effect in locomotor activity in the GNC 92H2-pVIII-treated animals versus controls may instead be interpreted as an absence of group differences by virtue of a decrease in ambulation by control animals as their repetitive (stereotypic) behavior increased and endured.

Confirmation of the basis of the behavioral suppression was next studied by measuring the phage titer in the brain before, during, and after the time span of animal behavioral studies. The earliest time point at which phage were observed in the brain was at day 2, while the highest titer of phage observed in the brain was at day 4. Although high phage titers dropped precipitously from day 5 to day 7 (10^3), this level was maintained until day 15 and was not subsequently undetectable by day 17. Thus, upon subsequent challenges, (ie, day 4 and beyond), there were no significant differences in either motor measure between groups.

In understanding the role of any nasal vaccine, we felt it was important to investigate potential limitations. The CNS is considered an immune privileged site, however, the possibility of phage entering the periphery cannot be discounted. Filamentous phage in itself, and with displayed proteins on its surface, comprises a foreign entity to the immune system. Additionally, there is a growing body of research wherein nasal vaccination has become increasingly popular.[59,60] Gratifyingly, enzyme-linked immunosorbent assay (ELISA) analysis of rat serum from vaccinated animals showed no appreciable antibody titer to phage and thus provided further indication that potential toxic side effects are not being manifested in animals that were administered filamentous phage.[50,52,53]

Conclusions

The compilation of these studies has demonstrated a promising new strategy in the continuing effort to develop effective treatments for cocaine addiction. One of the key strengths of this approach in relation to previous immunopharmacotherapeutic strategies is the direct delivery of the therapeutic protein into the CNS, the primary site of drug action. Thus, convergence of phage display and immunopharmacotherapy has enabled, for the first time, an investigation of how a protein-based therapeutic acting within the CNS can influence the effects of cocaine in animal models. Future investigations in the context of cocaine abuse could include the combination of this phage-based approach with either passive or active immunization protocols to determine whether any synergistic benefits can be obtained from simultaneous peripheral and central immunization. Furthermore, prior to the advancement of this technology into a clinical scenario, a long-term study of intranasal phage administration is essential to assess the effect of chronic phage administration on brain structure and/or function.

As with all other pharmacotherapeutic approaches, a significant concern lies in the ability of a cocaine user to surmount the effects of a given medication by simply administering higher doses of the drug, with potentially lethal consequences. Furthermore, although cocaine-binding antibodies may prevent the effects of cocaine, this treatment does not abrogate the psychological need to take the drug. Clearly, in order to successfully recover from cocaine addiction, any pharmacotherapeutic approach should be performed under controlled conditions under the supervision of a medical professional in conjunction with suitable psychological treatment (eg, counseling). However, encouraging recent data have emerged suggesting that the issue of overcoming a vaccine may prove manageable in humans.[38]

However, this does not imply that intranasal administration of protein-based therapies for drug abuse treatment is limited to binding antibodies or peptide ligands only. Catalytic antibodies could be effective in cocaine abuse treatment as one equivalent of catalytic antibody can turnover many times; thus less protein would be required for a given pharmacological effect relative to binding antibodies. Furthermore, enzymes such as the bacterial cocaine esterase[61] (CocE) or butyryl-cholinesterase (BChE) show great promise in this area. CocE is the most efficient biocatalyst known for cocaine degradation. However, direct administration of this enzyme would result in both extensive proteolysis prior to action and a likely immune response directed against the enzyme. Based on our results, display on phage should attenuate this immune response and allow these proteins to become viable therapeutics. The combination of catalysis and the potentially large protein concentration attainable on the phage surface using gene pVIII could provide a powerful weapon in the treatment of cocaine addiction. Furthermore, we anticipate that other enzymes relevant to the metabolism and degradation of drugs of abuse could also be applied to this system.

References

1. Koob GF. Neurobiology of addiction. Toward the development of new therapies. *Ann N Y Acad Sci.* 2000;909:170-185.
2. Weiss F, Koob GF. Drug addiction: functional neurotoxicity of the brain reward systems. *Neurotoxic Res.* 2001;3:145-156.
3. Melichar JK, Daglish MRC, Nutt DJ. Addiction and withdrawal–current views. *Curr Opin Pharmacol.* 2001;1:84-90.
4. Spanagel R, Weiss F. The dopamine hypothesis of reward: past and current status. *Trends Neurosci.* 1999;22:521-527.
5. Di Chiara G. The role of dopamine in drug abuse viewed from the perspective of its role in motivation. *Drug Alcohol Depend.* 1995;38:95-137.
6. Johanson C-E, Fischman MW. The pharmacology of cocaine related to its abuse. *Pharmacol Rev.* 1989;41:3-52.
7. Blaine JD, Ling W. Psychopharmacologic treatment of cocaine dependence. *Psychopharmacol Bull.* 1992;28:11-14.
8. Substance Abuse and Mental Health Services Administration, Office of Applied Studies. *Preliminary estimates from the 1992 Household Survey on Drug Abuse, Advance Report No. 3.* Washington, DC: US Department of Health and Human Services, Public Health Service; June 1993.
9. Cregler LL, Herbert M. Medical complications of cocaine abuse. *N Engl J Med.* 1986;315:1495-1500.
10. Des Jarlais DC, Friedman SR. AIDS and i.v. drug use. *Science.* 1989;245:578-579.
11. Lee JH, Bennett G. Substance abuse in adulthood. In: Bennett G, Woolf D, eds. *Substance Abuse: Pharmacologic, Developmental and Clinical Perspectives.* Albany: Delman Publishing; 1991:157-170.
12. Walsh SL. Behavioral pharmacology of cocaine. In: Tarter RE, Ammerman RT, Ott PJ, eds. *Handbook of Substance Abuse: Neurobehavioral Pharmacology.* New York: Plenum; 1998:187-200.
13. Mendelson JH, Mello NK. Management of cocaine abuse and dependence. *N Engl J Med.* 1996;334:965-972.
14. Gorelick DA. Pharmacologic interventions for cocaine, crack, and other stimulant addiction. In: Graham AW, Schultz TK, eds. *Principles of Addiction Medicine.* Chevy Chase, MD: American Society of Addiction Medicine; 2003:89-111.
15. Gorelick DA, Gardner EL, Xi Z-X. Agents in the development for the management of cocaine abuse. *Drugs.* 2004;64:1547-1573.
16. Leiderman DB, Shoptaw S, Montgomery A, et al. Cocaine rapid efficacy screening trial (CREST). A paradigm for the controlled evaluation of candidate medications for cocaine dependence. *Addiction.* 2005;100:1-11.
17. Winhusen TM, Somoza EC, Harrer JM, et al. A placebo-controlled screening trial of tiagabine, sertraline and donepezil as cocaine dependence treatments. *Addiction.* 2005;100:68-77.
18. Gonzalez G, Sevarino K, Sofuoglu M, et al. Tiagabine increases cocaine-free urines in cocaine-dependent methadone-treated patients: results of a randomized pilot study. *Addiction.* 2003;98:1625-1632.
19. Carroll KM, Fenton LR, Ball SA, et al. Efficacy of disulfiram and cognitive behavior therapy in cocaine-dependent outpatients: a randomized placebo-controlled trial. *Arch Gen Psychiatry.* 2004;61:264-272.

20. Houtsmuller EJ, Notes LD, Newton T, et al. Transdermal selegiline and intravenous cocaine: safety and interactions. *Psychopharmacology (Berl).* 2004;172:31-40.
21. Shoptaw S, Yang X, Rotheram-Fuller EJ, et al. Randomized placebo-controlled trial of baclofen for cocaine dependence: preliminary effects for individuals with chronic patterns of cocaine use. *J Clin Psychiatry.* 2003;64:1440-1448.
22. Kampman KM, Pettinati H, Lynch KG, et al. A pilot trial of topiramate for the treatment of cocaine dependence. *Drug Alcohol Depend.* 2004;75:233-240.
23. Kampman KM, Volpicelli JR, Mulvaney F, et al. Effectiveness of propranolol for cocaine dependence treatment may depend on cocaine withdrawal symptom severity. *Drug Alcohol Depend.* 2001;63:69-78.
24. Hoffman JA, III, Caudill BD, III, Koman JJ, III, Luckey JW, Flynn PM, Hubbard RL. Comparative cocaine abuse treatment strategies: enhancing client retention and treatment exposure. *J Addict Dis.* 1994;13:115-128.
25. Cashman JR. Biocatalysts in detoxication of drugs of abuse. *NIDA Res Monogr.* 1997;173:225-258.
26. Carrera MRA, Ashley JA, Parsons LH, Wirsching P, Koob GF, Janda KD. Suppression of psychoactive effects of cocaine by active immunization. *Nature.* 1995;378:727-730.
27. Carrera MRA, Ashley JA, Zhou B, Wirsching P, Koob GF, Janda KD. Cocaine vaccines: antibody protection against relapse in a rat model. *Proc Natl Acad Sci USA.* 2000;97:6202-6206.
28. Carrera MRA, Ashley JA, Wirsching P, Koob GF, Janda KD. A second-generation vaccine protects against the psychoactive effects of cocaine. *Proc Natl Acad Sci USA.* 2001;98:1988-1992.
29. Fox BS, Kantak KM, Edwards MA, et al. Efficacy of a therapeutic cocaine vaccine in rodent models. *Nat Med.* 1996;2:11129-11132.
30. Kantak KM, Collins SL, Lipman EG, Bond J, Giovanoni K, Fox BS. Evaluation of anti-cocaine antibodies and a cocaine vaccine in a rat self-administration model. *Psychopharmacology (Berl).* 2000;148:251-262.
31. Landry DW, Zhao K, Yang GX-P, Glickman M, Georgiadis TM. Antibody-catalyzed degradation of cocaine. *Science.* 1993;259:1899-1901.
32. Cashman JR, Berkman CE, Underiner GE. Catalytic antibodies that hydrolyze (–)-cocaine obtained by a high-throughput procedure. *J Pharmacol Exp Ther.* 2000;293:952-961.
33. Yang G, Chun J, Arakawa-Uramoto H, et al. Anti-cocaine catalytic antibodies: a synthetic approach to improved antibody diversity. *J Am Chem Soc.* 1996;118:5880-5890.
34. Baird TJ, Deng S-X, Landry DW, Winger G, Woods JH. Natural and artificial enzymes against cocaine. I. Monoclonal antibody 15A10 and the reinforcing effects of cocaine in rats. *J Pharmacol Exp Ther.* 2000;295:1127-1134.
35. Matsushita M, Hoffman TZ, Ashley JA, Zhou B, Wirsching P, Janda KD. Cocaine catalytic antibodies: the primary importance of linker effects. *Bioorg Med Chem Lett.* 2001;11:87-90.
36. Isomura S, Hoffman TZ, Wirsching P, Janda KD. Synthesis, properties, and reactivity of cocaine benzoylthioester possessing the cocaine absolute configuration. *J Am Chem Soc.* 2002;124:3661-3668.
37. Meijler MM, Matsushita M, Wirsching P, Janda KD. Development of immunopharmacotherapy against drugs of abuse. *Curr Drug Discov Tech.* 2004;1:77-89.
38. Haney M, Kosten TR. Therapeutic vaccines for substance dependence. *Expert Rev Vaccines.* 2004;3:11-18.
39. Gorelick DA. Enhancing cocaine metabolism with butyrylcholinesterase as a treatment strategy. *Drug Alcohol Depend.* 1997;48:159-165.
40. Mattes CE, Belendiuk GW, Lynch TJ, Brady RO, Dretchen KL. Butyrylcholinesterase: an enzyme antidote for cocaine intoxication. *Addict Biol.* 1998;3:171-188.
41. Nachon F, Nicolet Y, Viquie N, Masson P, Fontecilla-Camps JD, Lockridge O. Engineering of a monomeric and low-glycosylated form of human butyrylcholinesterase: expression, purification, characterization and crystallization. *Eur J Biochem.* 2002;269:630-637.

42. Mattes CE, Lynch TJ, Singh A, et al. Therapeutic use of butyrylcholinesterase for cocaine intoxication. *Toxicol Appl Pharmacol*. 1997;145:372-380.
43. Sun H, Pang Y-P, Lockridge O, Brimijoin S. Re-engineering butyrylcholinesterase as a cocaine hydrolase. *Mol Pharmacol*. 2002;62:220-224.
44. Larocca D, Burg MA, Jensen-Pergakes K, Ravey PE, Gonzales AM, Baird A. Evolving phage vectors for cell targeted gene delivery. *Curr Pharm Biotechnol*. 2002;3:45-57.
45. Smith GP. Filamentous fusion phage; novel expression vectors that display cloned antigens on the virion surface. *Science*. 1985;228:1315-1317.
46. Carlton RM. Phage therapy: past history and future prospects. *Arch Immunol Ther Exp (Warsz)*. 1999;47:267-274.
47. Smith HW, Huggins RB. Successful treatment of experimental E coli infections in mice using phage: its general superiority over antibiotics. *J Gen Microbiol*. 1982;128:307-318.
48. Slopek S, Weber-Dabrowska B, Dabrowski M, Kucharewicz-Krukowski A. Results in bacteriophage treatment of suppurative bacterial infections in the years 1981-1986. *Arch Immunol Ther Exp (Warsz)*. 1986;35:569-583.
49. Stone R. Stalin's forgotten cure. *Science*. 2002;298:728-731.
50. Pasqualini R, Ruoslahti E. Organ targeting in vivo using phage display peptide libraries. *Nature*. 1996;380:364-366.
51. Essler M, Ruoslahti E. Molecular specialization of breast vasculature: a breast-homing phage-displayed peptide binds to aminopeptidase P in breast vasculatures. *Proc Natl Acad Sci USA*. 2002;99:2252-2257.
52. Dabrowska K, Switala-Jelen K, Opolski A, Weber-Dabrowska B, Gorski A. Bacteriophage penetration in vertebrates. *J Appl Microbiol*. 2005;98:7-13.
53. Frenkel D, Solomon B. Filamentous phage as vector-mediated antibody delivery to the brain. *Proc Natl Acad Sci USA*. 2002;99:5675-5679.
54. Gao C, Mao S, Lo C-HL, Wirsching P, Lerner RA, Janda KD. Making artificial antibodies: a format for phage display of combinatorial heterodimeric arrays. *Proc Natl Acad Sci USA*. 1999;96:6025-6030.
55. Gao C, Mao S, Kaufmann G, Wirsching P, Lerner RA, Janda KD. A method for the generation of combinatorial antibody libraries using pIX phage display. *Proc Natl Acad Sci USA*. 2002;99:12612-12616.
56. Carrera MRA, Kaufmann GF, Mee JM, Meijler MM, Koob GF, Janda KD. Treating cocaine addiction with viruses. *Proc Natl Acad Sci USA*. 2004;101:10416-10421.
57. Barbas CF, Burton DR, Scott JK, Silverman GJ. *Phage Display: A Laboratory Manual*. Tuebingen, Germany: Cold Spring Harbor Laboratory Press; 2001.
58. Lyon M, Robbins TW. The action of central nervous system stimulant drugs: a general theory concerning amphetamine effects. In: Essman W, Valzelli L, eds. *Current Developments in Psychopharmacology*. vol. 4. New York: Spectrum; 1975:79-163.
59. Illum L, Davis SS. Polymeric lamellar substrate particles for intranasal vaccination. *Adv Drug Deliv Rev*. 2001;51:97-111.
60. Jones N. The nose and paranasal sinuses physiology and anatomy. *Adv Drug Deliv Rev*. 2001;51:5-19.
61. Bresler MM, Rosser SJ, Basran A, Bruce NC. Gene cloning and nucleotide sequencing and properties of a cocaine esterase from *Rhodococcus* sp strain MB1. *Appl Environ Microbiol*. 2000;66:904-908.

Chapter 15
κ Opioids as Potential Treatments for Stimulant Dependence

Thomas E. Prisinzano,[1] Kevin Tidgewell,[1] and Wayne W. Harding[1]

Abstract Stimulant abuse is a major problem in the United States and the development of pharmacological treatments for stimulant abuse remains an important therapeutic goal. Classically, the "dopamine hypothesis" has been used to explain the development of addiction and dependence of stimulants. This hypothesis involves the direct increase of dopamine as the major factor in mediating the abuse effects. Therefore, most treatments have focused on directly influencing the dopamine system. Another approach, which has been explored for potential treatments of stimulant abuse, is the use of κ opioid agonists. The κ receptor is known to be involved, via indirect effects, in synaptic dopamine levels. This review covers several classes of κ opioid ligands that have been explored for this purpose.

Keywords kappa, opioid, self-administration, stimulant

Introduction

Drug dependence is a chronic, relapsing disorder in which compulsive drug-seeking and drug-taking behavior persists despite serious negative consequences.[1] The chronic use of abused drugs, such as central nervous system (CNS) stimulants, causes adaptive changes that lead to drug tolerance, physical dependence, drug craving, and relapse.[2] At present, there is no single theory to explain all aspects of drug dependence. Generally, addictive substances are able to act as positive reinforcers

[1] Division of Medicinal & Natural Products Chemistry, College of Pharmacy,
The University of Iowa, Iowa City, Iowa 52242

Corresponding Author: Thomas E. Prisinzano, Division of Medicinal & Natural Products Chemistry, College of Pharmacy, The University of Iowa, Iowa City, Iowa 52242. Tel: (319) 335-6920; Fax: (319) 335-8766; E-mail: thomas-prisinzano@uiowa.edu

R.S. Rapaka and W. Sadée (eds.), *Drug Addiction.*
© American Association of Pharmaceutical Scientists 2008

(producing pleasurable effects) or as negative reinforcers (relieving withdrawal symptoms).[1] However, environmental effects associated with drug use are also able to produce conditioned responses in the absence of drug.

Among the most widely abused substances in the world are the CNS stimulants cocaine (1) and methamphetamine (METH) (2) (Fig. 15.1). The abuse of these compounds has had great effects on public health.[3,4] The National Drug Threat Survey data for 2003 indicates that 37.0% of state and local law enforcement agencies nationwide identify cocaine (both powder and crack) as their greatest drug threat, higher than any other drug type.[5] In addition to the problems associated with cocaine abuse, a rise in the abuse of METH has been noted in West Coast cities.[6] In less than 10 years, METH has grown from a problem limited to the Southwestern and Midwestern United States to one of nationwide concern.[7-9] The number of METH laboratory seizures increased from 8577 in 2001 to 9188 in 2002, to 9815 in 2003.[5] More than 51.0 kg of METH was seized in Iowa alone.[10] This highlights the growing problem of METH dependence. The primary market areas for METH are Los Angeles, Phoenix, San Diego, San Francisco, and the central states (Arkansas, Illinois, Indiana, Missouri, and Iowa).[5] State and local law enforcement agencies in the central states identify METH as their greatest drug threat.[5] These facts further illustrate the problem of METH dependence, as well as the pressing need for the development of stimulant abuse therapeutics in the central states such as Iowa.

Currently, there are various compounds being pursued as possible stimulant abuse therapeutics based on the "dopamine hypothesis."[11-15] The dopamine hypo thesis considers the ability of stimulants to increase extracellular dopamine (DA) as being of primary importance in mediating the addictive effects of stimulants. The dopamine hypothesis explains some aspects of stimulant addiction, but other neurochemical mechanisms appear to be involved.[16-19] For example, cocaine has similar affinity for the dopamine transporter (DAT), serotonin transporter (SERT), and

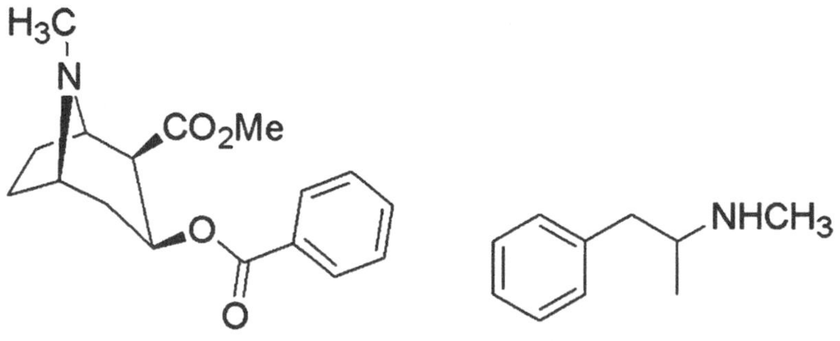

Fig. 15.1 Structures of cocaine (1) and methamphetamine (2).

norepinephrine transporter (NET).[20] Importantly, several studies indicate that the SERT and the NET also play a role in the pharmacological effects of cocaine.[21-24]

At present, there are no United States Food and Drug Administration (FDA)-approved therapeutic agents available for the treatment of stimulant abuse or for the prevention of its relapse. However, various agonist-like, replacement type of medications are currently being pursued.[11,25-28] This helps to support the hypothesis that agonist-substitution pharmacotherapy is a reasonable approach to developing pharmacotherapies for stimulant dependence.[28] However, additional approaches need to be explored.

A large body of evidence indicates that κ opioid receptors may be involved in the modulation of some abuse-related effects of CNS stimulants.[29,30] Administration of cocaine or methamphetamine upregulates κ receptors.[31,32] Like other opioid receptors, κ receptors have a role in the modulation of immune responses,[33] as well as some effects on human immunodeficiency virus (HIV) in vitro.[34-36] Interestingly, κ receptors have a role in the modulation of dopamine levels.[37-44] In particular, κ receptor activation modulates DA uptake in the nucleus accumbens[45] and κ agonists directly inhibit dopamine neurons in the midbrain.[43] Repeated treatment with κ agonists alters D2 receptor density[46] and function,[47] as well as attenuating the locomotor effects of cocaine in rats.[48] Furthermore, administration of κ agonists in rats alters levels of the dopamine transporter,[49,50] decreases cocaine-induced dopamine levels, blocks cocaine-induced place preference, and attenuates cocaine-induced locomotor activity.[51,52] Furthermore, κ agonists also attenuated the reinstatement of extinguished drug-taking behavior.[53] These findings indicate that the κ opioid receptors may be involved in the antagonism of some abuse-related effects of cocaine, offering a pharmacological approach to treat cocaine abuse. However, κ opioid receptor agonists, while being effective in reducing cocaine self-administration in monkeys, produce side effects including sedation and vomiting.[29] It has been speculated that the addition of μ agonist/antagonist activity to the κ agonist might lessen the incidence of side effects and encompass a useful treatment for cocaine abuse.[54]

Previous pharmacological approaches identified apparent subtypes of κ opioid receptors.[55-60] The opioid receptors κ_1 and κ_2 were identified due to their preferential binding to arylacetamides and benzomorphans, respectively.[61,62] In addition, these subtypes show differences in the affinity and selectivity of the κ antagonist nor-BNI.[55,63-65] However, only one κ opioid receptor clone has been identified at the present time.[66] Recent work has suggested that the apparent receptor subtypes may actually be different affinity states of the same receptor.[67] The relevance of the proposed subtypes and/or different affinity states in reducing cocaine abuse has not been fully elucidated.

The present review focuses on κ agonists explored as potential stimulant abuse therapeutics. Interestingly, a selective partial κ agonist has not been evaluated as a potential stimulant abuse therapeutic. This type of compound has the potential to antagonize the effects of CNS stimulants like a full κ agonist but likely without the psychotomimetic side effects. This hypothesis, however, awaits further testing.

κ Opioid Receptor Agonists

The endogenous ligand for the κ receptor is dynorphin A (Dyn A).[68,69] It binds with subnanomolar affinity at κ receptors but is quite active at all 3 opioid receptors. Dyn A has been shown to significantly decrease basal dopamine levels, as well as block increases in dopamine levels, block the formation of conditioned place preference, and attenuate locomotion induced by 15 mg/kg of cocaine in mice.[52] There are also several classes of nonpeptide κ agonists that have been investigated as potential stimulant abuse therapeutics.[70,71] These include the benzomorphans, arylaceta-mides, epoxymorphinans, and natural products such as the *Iboga* alkaloids and neoclerodane diterpenes.

Cyclazocine, Bremazocine, and 8-CAC

Cyclazocine (Fig. 15.2) is a benzomorphan originally synthesized in 1962 with mixed κ agonist and μ antagonist activity.[72] The treatment of rats with (±)-cyclazo-cine showed a dose dependent decrease in cocaine intake with no alteration of water intake.[73] In addition, (±)-cyclazocine significantly attenuated the increased dopamine levels induced by nicotine infusion and enhanced nicotine-induced increases in dopamine metabolites.[74] However, cyclazocine did not significantly alter cocaine self-administration in rhesus monkeys.[29] Interestingly, bremazocine, a structural analog and mixed κ agonist and μ antagonist, produced a significant and dose-dependent decrease in cocaine self-administration.[29] A recent study of cyclazocine in humans found that cocaine effects were consistently lower on the last administration following 4 days of pretreatment with cyclazocine compared with the first administration.[75] This study is suggestive of the utility of κ opioids to diminish acute effects of cocaine in humans.

As mentioned earlier, bremazocine has been shown to reduce cocaine-maintained behavior in rhesus monkeys.[29] An additional study found that pretreatment of

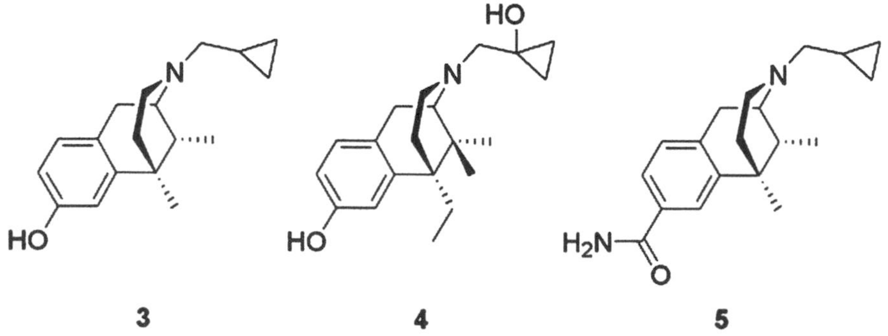

Fig. 15.2 Structures of cyclazocine (**3**), bremazocine (**4**), and 8-CAC (**5**).

bremazocine dose dependently decreased self-administration of cocaine, ethanol, and PCP.[76] This work also indicates that κ agonists attenuate self-administration of drug and nondrug reinforcers to smoked cocaine base, oral ethanol, PCP, and saccharin in rhesus monkeys. Furthermore, bremazocine reduces unrestricted free-choice ethanol self-administration in rats without affecting sucrose consumption.[77] This indicates the potential utility of bremazocine for ethanol dependence.

More recently, 8-CAC was synthesized to obtain a benzomorphan with a longer duration of action for potential use in treating cocaine abuse.[78] Additional testing showed that 8-CAC does not act as a μ opioid antagonist and that it is significantly longer acting than cyclazocine (15 hours vs 2 hours).[79] Acute administration of 8-CAC was found to reduce cocaine-maintained responding over a 10-fold range of cocaine unit doses.[80] However, doses of 8-CAC that decreased cocaine self-administration were similar to doses that decreased food-maintained responding. The results, however, suggest that mixed action κ/μ agonists might decrease cocaine self-administration with a lower incidence of undesirable effects. Other mixed κ/μ agonists also appear to offer advantages over selective κ agonists.[81]

U50,488, U69,593, and R-84760

Several highly κ selective arylacetamides,[82-84] U50,488, U69,593, and R-84760 (Fig. 15.3), have also been examined as potential stimulant abuse therapeutics. The first findings that κ agonists may be useful as functional cocaine antagonists were based on the actions of U50,488 in an in vivo microdialysis experiment in rats.[85] Maisonneuve et al showed that pretreatment with U50,488 attenuated the cocaine induced elevation of dopamine levels and that this phenomenon could be reversed by the κ opioid antagonist nor-BNI. Later work showed that U50,488 and fentanyl do not alter the discriminative stimulus effects of cocaine but U50,488 attenuates the cocaine induced responses.[86] Similarly, U50,488 produced dose-related decreases in self-administration of both morphine and cocaine.[87] A higher dose of U50,488 was needed to decrease the rate of water self-administration and the

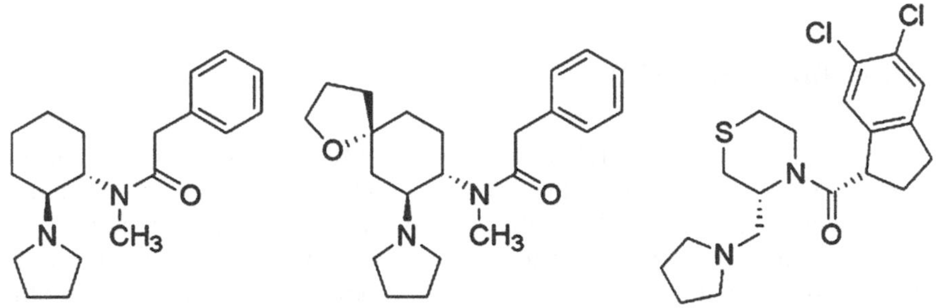

Fig. 15.3 Structures of U50,488 (6), U69,593 (7), and R-84760 (8).

effect was fully reversible by treatment with nor-BNI. Furthermore, U50,488 significantly blocks intravenous (IV) administration of cocaine and decreases morphine intake in rats.[88] These results also indicate that κ activation seems to increase the sensitivity for drug reward. Interestingly, U50,488 was found to attenuate the discriminative effects of low-dose (3.0 mg/kg) but not high-dose (10.0 mg/kg) cocaine.[89] These results suggest that cocaine-opioid interactions are dependent on the training dose of cocaine. In addition, chronic administration of U50,488 produces a dose-dependent, κ–receptor-mediated, and often sustained decrease in cocaine self-administration of 2 different doses of cocaine in rhesus monkeys.[90] However, doses that decrease self-administration also produce decreases in food-maintained responding, emesis, and sedation. Further work with U50,488 showed variable results in rhesus monkeys trained to discriminate cocaine (0.4 mg/kg) from saline.[91] Recent behavioral work indicates that U50,488 produces a κ opioid–receptor-mediated increase in the relative reinforcing effects of cocaine compared with food.[92] This study suggests that chronic κ agonist treatment may mimic some effects of stress that modulate the reinforcing effects of abused drugs.

Various studies have shown arylacetamide 7 to modulate the neurochemical and behavioral effects of cocaine. The administration of U69,593 attenuates cocaine's discriminative stimulus properties, its conditioned reinforcing effects, its self-administration, and the reinstatement of extinguished drug-taking behavior.[53,93] In addition, U69,593 attenuates the psychomotor stimulant effects of amphetamine and cocaine and modulates neurotoxic effects of METH.[94,95] Furthermore, U69,593 attenuates the discriminative stimulus effects of amphetamine in squirrel monkeys.[96] However, this study also suggests that there are large individual differences in the ability of κ opioids to alter the discriminative effects of amphetamine.

Recently, the effects of R-84760 on basal levels of dopamine, cocaine-induced conditioned place preference, and cocaine-induced locomotor activity in mice were evaluated.[51] Arylacetamide R-84760 was found to decrease levels of dopamine in a dose-dependent manner. In addition, 0.1 mg/kg, i.p. of R-84760 blocked cocaine-induced conditioned place preference and also significantly attenuated cocaine-induced locomotion. Interestingly, R-84760 did not produce conditioned place aversion seen with other arylacetamides, such as U50,488 or U69,593.

Nalfurafine (TRK-820)

Currently, the novel epoxymorphinan nalfurafine (TRK-820) is under investigation as an antipruritic.[97] Nalfurafine (Fig. 15.4) is a high-affinity κ agonist.[98,99] Further pharmacological testing has shown this compound to produce potent antinociception in nonhuman primates[100] and to be more potent than U50,488H in mice.[101] Interestingly, nalfurafine does not produce the psychotomimetic effects in healthy human volunteers seen with other κ agonists[102] and develops lower tolerance in comparison to other κ agonists.[103] Behavioral testing in rats found nalfurafine to significantly attenuate the discriminative and rewarding effects of cocaine and that

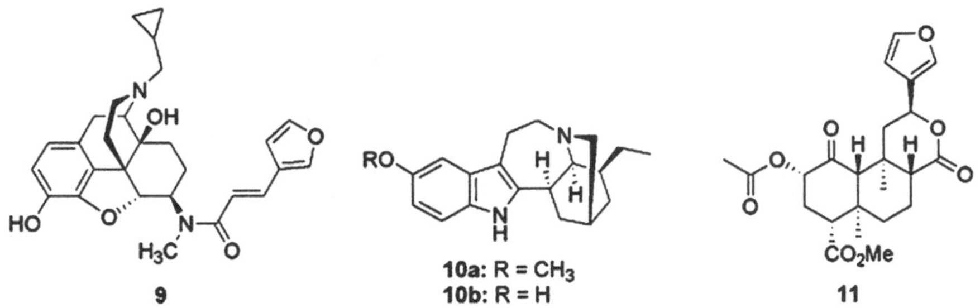

Fig. 15.4 Structures of nalfurafine (**9**), ibogaine (**10a**), 12-hydroxyibogamine (**10b**), and salvinorin A (**11**).

these effects were blocked by nor-BNI.[104] A low dose of nalfurafine (10–40 μg/kg) was found not to induce place preference or place aversion. However, a large dose (80 μg/kg) significantly induced place aversion. Further work has shown nalfurafine to attenuate the rewarding and locomotor effects of morphine in mice.[105] Additionally, nalfurafine decreased the mecamylamine-precipitated nicotine withdrawal aversive effect in rats chronically treated with nicotine.[105] Interestingly, nalfurafine did not completely substitute for U50,488 in rats trained to discriminate U50,488 from saline.[106] In cross substitution experiments, U50,488 was found to substitute for nalfurafine. These findings suggest that there are qualitative differences between the discriminative effects of U50,488 and nalfurafine.

Ibogaine

Ibogaine is a naturally occurring indole alkaloid isolated from the root, rootbark, stems, and leaves of the African shrub *Tabernanthe iboga*.[107] This plant has been used by indigenous peoples in low doses to combat fatigue and hunger and in higher doses as a sacrament in religious rituals.[108,109] Interest in ibogaine as a drug abuse therapeutic has been based on anecdotal reports of its efficacy in eliminating, in a single dose, the withdrawal symptoms and long-term drug craving for cocaine and heroin.[108] The psychopharmacology of ibogaine is complex due to its affinity for several receptors, transporters, and ion channels.[107] In addition, its primary metabolite, 12-hydroxyibogamine, is also biologically active.[110,111] Among these are the dopaminergic, serotonergic, adrenergic, muscarinic, NMDA, and opioidergic receptor systems.[112] The mechanism by which ibogaine exerts its anti-addictive effects is presently unknown although several receptor systems have been implicated in its activity.[113,114] However, it has been speculated that its κ agonist actions contribute to its effects on stimulant self-administration.[115,116]

In self-administration studies in rats, a single injection of ibogaine (40 mg/kg, i.p.) produced a significant decrease in cocaine intake.[117,118] Cocaine-induced locomotor activity is decreased by ibogaine in rodents.[119,120] Pretreatment of ibogaine has been shown to reduce the neuroadaptations produced by chronic cocaine administration in rats.[121] Under open label conditions of opioid detoxification in 33 human subjects, ibogaine eliminated signs of opioid withdrawal and drug seeking behavior in 25 cases.[122] This effect was sustained throughout the 72-hour period of posttreatment. The potential neurotoxic effects of ibogaine have raised concerns over its clinical use.[123] However, analogs of ibogaine are currently being explored as potentially safer medications.[124-128]

Salvinorin A

Recently, salvinorin A, the presumed active component of the hallucinogenic Mexican mint *Salvia divinorum*, was found to be a potent and selective κ agonist in vitro using a screen of 50 receptors, transporters, and ion channels.[129] Functional studies also demonstrated that salvinorin A is a potent and selective agonist at both cloned κ and native κ opioid receptors expressed in guinea pig brain. Surprisingly, salvinorin A was found to be more efficacious than U50,488 or U69,593 and similar in efficacy to Dyn A as a κ opioid receptor agonist.[130] A recent report compared the activity of salvinorin A to epoxymorphinan nalfurafine.[99] Binding affinities using [^{3}H]diprenorphine at κ receptors found nalfurafine (K_i = 75 pM) to have higher affinity than salvinorin A (K_i = 7.9 nM). Both compounds were found to be full agonists in the [^{35}S]GTP-γ-S binding assay with nalfurafine (EC$_{50}$ = 25 pM) >> salvinorin A (EC$_{50}$ = 2.2 nM). Interestingly, salvinorin A was found to be 40-fold less potent in promoting internalization of the hKOR compared with U50,488 and showed little anti-scratching activity and no antinociception in mice.[99]

There has been only one report of behavioral testing of salvinorin A in nonhuman primates.[131] All subjects (n = 3) dose-dependently emitted ≥90% U69,593-appropriate responding after subcutaneous injection of salvinorin A (0.001–0.032 mg/kg). Quadazocine (0.32 mg/kg), an opioid antagonist, blocked the effects of salvinorin A. However, the long-lasting κ selective antagonist GNTI (1 mg/kg; 24 hours pretreatment) antagonized the effects of salvinorin A in 2 of 3 monkeys. These findings are consistent with the in vitro characterization of salvinorin A as a κ agonist. Therefore, based on its similar mechanism of action to the previously described compounds, salvinorin A has the potential to reduce cocaine self-administration. However, the ability of salvinorin A to block cocaine self-administration has not been reported to date.

Conclusion

At present, there are no FDA-approved therapeutic agents available for the treatment of stimulant abuse or for the prevention of its relapse. Many types of medications are currently being pursued based on the "dopamine hypothesis." However, additional approaches need to be explored. κ Opioid receptor agonists offer an indirect approach to the modulation of some abuse-related effects of CNS stimulants. Both selective and nonselective κ opioids have been shown to attenuate stimulant self-administration in a variety of animal models. A selective partial κ agonist, however, has not been evaluated to date. While highly selective κ agonists attenuate stimulant self-administration in nonhuman primates, they are associated with behavioral side effects such as sedation and emesis. Mixed-action κ agonists decrease stimulant self-administration with a lower incidence of undesirable effects. The full extent to which κ agonists antagonize stimulant self-administration remains to be determined.

Acknowledgments   The authors wish to thank the College of Pharmacy and the Biological Sciences Funding Program of the University of Iowa for financial support of our research program.

References

1. Cami J, Ferre M. Drug addiction. *N Engl J Med*. 2003;349:975-986.
2. Nestler EJ. Molecular basis of long-term plasticity underlying addiction. *Nat Rev Neurosci*. 2001;2:119-128.
3. Mitscher LA, Baker W. Tuberculosis: a search for novel therapy starting with natural products. *Med Res Rev*. 1998;18:363-374.
4. McCoy CB, Inciardi JA. *Sex, Drugs, and the Continuing Spread of AIDS*. Los Angeles: Roxbury Publishing Co; 1995.
5. National Drug Intelligence Center. *National Drug Threat Assessment 2004*. Washington, DC: US Department of Justice; 2004.
6. Howell LL, Wilcox KM. The dopamine transporter and cocaine medication development: drug self-administration in nonhuman primates. *J Pharmacol Exp Ther*. 2001;298:1-6.
7. National DI. C. *National Drug Threat Assessment* Johnston, PA: US Department of Justice; 2001.
8. Anglin MD, Burke C, Perrochet B, Stamper E, Dawud-Noursi S. History of the methamphetamine problem. *J Psychoactive Drugs*. 2000;32:137-141.
9. Rawson RA, Anglin MD, Ling W. Will the methamphetamine problem go away? *J Addict Dis*. 2002;21:5-19.
10. Rood L. 2005.
11. Carroll FI, Howell LL, Kuhar MJ. Pharmacotherapies for treatment of cocaine abuse:preclinical aspects. *J Med Chem*. 1999;42:2721-2736.
12. Kuhar MJ, Ritz MC, Boja JW. The dopamine hypothesis of the reinforcing properties of cocaine. *Trends Neurosci*. 1991;14:299-302.
13. Koob GF, Bloom FE. Cellular and molecular mechanisms of drug dependence. *Science*. 1988;242:715-723.
14. Robinson TE, Berridge KC. The neural basis of drug craving: an incentive-sensitization theory of addiction. *Brain Res Brain Res Rev*. 1993;18:247-291.
15. Kuhar MJ, Pilotte NS. Neurochemical changes in cocaine withdrawal. *Trends Pharmacol Sci*. 1996;17:260-264.
16. Callahan PM, Cunningham KA. Modulation of the discriminative stimulus properties of cocaine: comparison of the effects of fluoxetine with 5-HT1A and 5-HT1B receptor agonists. *Neuropharmacology*. 1997;36:373-381.
17. Callahan PM, Cunningham KA. Modulation of the discriminative stimulus properties of cocaine by 5-HT1B and 5-HT2C receptors. *J Pharmacol Exp Ther*. 1995;274:1414-1424.

18. McMahon LR, Cunningham KA. Antagonism of 5-Hydroxytryptamine2A receptors attenuates the behavioral effects of cocaine in rats. *J Pharmacol Exp Ther*. 2001;297:357-363.

19. Kelley AE, Lang CG. Effects of GBR 12909, a selective dopamine uptake inhibitor, on motor activity and operant behavior in the rat. *Eur J Pharmacol*. 1989;167:385-395.

20. Carroll FI, Kotian P, Dehghani A, et al. Cocaine and 3β-(4'-Substituted phenyl)tropane-2β-carboxylic acid ester and amide analogues. New high-affinity and selective compounds for the dopamine transporter. *J Med Chem*. 1995;38:379-388.

21. Belej T, Manji D, Sioutis S, Barros HM, Nobrega JN. Changes in serotonin and norepinephrine uptake sites after chronic cocaine: pre- vs post-withdrawal effects. *Brain Res*. 1996;736:287-296.

22. Sora I, Hall FS, Andrews AM, et al. Molecular mechanisms of cocaine reward. Combined dopamine and serotonin transporter knockouts eliminate cocaine place preference. *Proc Natl Acad Sci USA*. 2001;98:5300-5305.

23. Baumann MH, Rothman RB. Alterations in serotonergic responsiveness during cocaine withdrawal in rats: similarities to major depression in humans. *Biol Psychiatry*. 1998;44:578-591.

24. Rothman RB, Baumann MH, Dersch CM, et al. Amphetamine-type central nervous system stimulants release norepinephrine more potently than they release dopamine and serotonin. *Synapse*. 2001;39:32-41.

25. Kulkarni SS, Newman AH, Houlihan WJ. Three-dimensional quantitative structure-activity relationships of mazindol analogues at the dopamine transporter. *J Med Chem*. 2002; 45:4119-4127.

26. Kreek MJ, LaForge KS, Butelman E. Pharmacotherapy of addictions. *Nat Rev Drug Discov*. 2002;1:710-726.

27. Prisinzano T, Rice KC, Baumann MH, Rothman RB. Development of neurochemical normalization ("agonist substitution") therapeutics for stimulant abuse: focus on the dopamine uptake inhibitor, GBR 12909. *Curr Med Chem CNS Agents*. 2004;4:47-59.

28. Grabowski J, Shearer J, Merrill J, Negus SS. Agonist-like, replacement pharmacotherapy for stimulant abuse and dependence. *Addict Behav*. 2004;29:1439-1464.

29. Mello NK, Negus SS. Interactions between kappa opioid agonists and cocaine. Preclinical studies. *Ann N Y Acad Sci*. 2000;909:104-132.

30. Shippenberg TS, Chefer VI, Zapata A, Heidbreder CA. Modulation of the behavioral and neurochemical effects of psychostimulants by kappa-opioid receptor systems. *Ann N Y Acad Sci*. 2001;937:50-73.

31. Collins SL, Kunko PM, Ladenheim B, et al. Chronic cocaine increases kappa-opioid receptor density: lack of effect by selective dopamine uptake inhibitors. *Synapse*. 2002;45:153-158.

32. Tzaferis JA, McGinty JF. Kappa opioid receptor stimulation decreases amphetamine-induced behavior and neuropeptide mRNA expression in the striatum. *Brain Res Mol Brain Res*. 2001;93:27-35.

33. McCarthy L, Wetzel M, Sliker JK, Eisenstein TK, Rogers TJ. Opioids, opioid receptors, and the immune response. *Drug Alcohol Depend*. 2001;62:111-123.

34. Chao CC, Gekker G, Hu S, et al. Kappa opioid receptors in human microglia downregulate human immunodeficiency virus 1 expression. *Proc Natl Acad Sci USA*. 1996;93:8051-8056.

35. Peterson PK, Gekker G, Lokensgard JR, et al. Kappa opioid receptor agonist suppression of HIV-1 expression in CD4+ lymphocytes. *Biochem Pharmacol*. 2001;61:1145-1151.

36. Gekker G, Hu S, Wentland MP, et al. κ-Opioid receptor ligands inhibit cocaine-induced HIV-1 expression in microglial cells. *J Pharmacol Exp Ther*. 2004;309:600-606.

37. Werling L, Frattali A, Portoghese P, Takemori A, Cox B. Kappa receptor regulation of dopamine release from striatum and cortex of rats and guinea pigs. *J Pharmacol Exp Ther*. 1988;246:282-286.

38. Di Chiara G, Imperato A. Opposite effects of mu and kappa opiate agonists on dopamine release in the nucleus accumbens and in the dorsal caudate of freely moving rats. *J Pharmacol Exp Ther*. 1988;244:1067-1080.

39. Di Chiara G, Imperato A. Drugs abused by humans preferentially increase synaptic dopamine concentrations in the mesolimbic system of freely moving rats. *Proc Natl Acad Sci USA*. 1988;85:5274-5278.

40. Spanagel R, Herz A, Shippenberg TS. The effects of opioid peptides on dopamine release in the nucleus accumbens: an in vivo microdialysis study. *J Neurochem.* 1990;55:1734-1740.
41. Spanagel R, Herz A, Shippenberg T. Opposing tonically active endogenous opioid systems modulate the mesolimbic dopaminergic pathway. *Proc Natl Acad Sci USA.* 1992;89: 2046-2050.
42. Jackisch R, Hotz H, Hertting G. No evidence for presynaptic opioid receptors on cholinergic, but presence of kappa-receptors on dopaminergic neurons in the rabbit caudate nucleus: involvement of endogenous opioids. *Naunyn Schmiedebergs Arch Pharmacol.* 1993;348:234-241.
43. Margolis EB, Hjelmstad GO, Bonci A, Fields HL. κ-Opioid agonists directly inhibit midbrain dopaminergic neurons. *J Neurosci.* 2003;23:9981-9986.
44. Suzuki T, Kishimoto Y, Ozaki S, Narita M. Mechanism of opioid dependence and interaction between opioid receptors. *Eur J Pain.* 2001;5:63-65.
45. Thompson AC, Jr, Zapata A, Jr, Justice JB, Jr, et al. κ-Opioid receptor activation modifies dopamine uptake in the nucleus accumbens and opposes the effects of cocaine. *J Neurosci.* 2000;20:9333-9340.
46. Izenwasser S, French D, Carroll FI, Kunko PM. Continuous infusion of selective dopamine uptake inhibitors or cocaine produces time-dependent changes in rat locomotor activity. *Behav Brain Res.* 1999;99:201-208.
47. Acri JB, Thompson AC, Shippenberg T. Modulation of pre- and postsynaptic dopamine D2 receptor function by the selective kappa-opioid receptor agonist U69593. *Synapse.* 2001;39:343-350.
48. Heidbreder CA, Schenk S, Partridge B, Shippenberg TS. Increased responsiveness of mesolimbic and mesostriatal dopamine neurons to cocaine following repeated administration of a selective kappa-opioid receptor agonist. *Synapse.* 1998;30:255-262.
49. Collins SL, Gerdes RM, D'Addario C, Izenwasser S. Kappa opioid agonists alter dopamine markers and cocaine-stimulated locomotor activity. *Behav Pharmacol.* 2001;12:237-245.
50. Collins SL, D'Addario C, Izenwasser S. Effects of κ-opioid receptor agonists on long-term cocaine use and dopamine neurotransmission. *Eur J Pharmacol.* 2001;426:25-34.
51. Zhang Y, Butelman ER, Schlussman SD, Ho A, Kreek MJ. Effect of the kappa opioid agonist R-84760 on cocaine-induced increases in striatal dopamine levels and cocaine-induced place preference in C57BL/6J mice. *Psychopharmacology (Berl).* 2004;173:146-152.
52. Zhang Y, Butelman ER, Schlussman SD, Ho A, Kreek MJ. Effect of the endogenous κ opioid agonist dynorphin A(1-17) on cocaine-evoked increases in striatal dopamine levels and cocaine-induced place preference in C57BL/6J mice. *Psychopharmacology (Berl).* 2004;172:422-429.
53. Schenk S, Partridge B, Shippenberg TS. Reinstatement of extinguished drug-taking behavior in rats: effect of the kappa-opioid receptor agonist, U69593. *Psychopharmacology (Berl).* 2000;151:85-90.
54. Neumeyer JL, Gu XH, van Vliet LA, et al. Mixed kappa agonists and mu agonists/antagonists as potential pharmacotherapeutics for cocaine abuse: synthesis and opioid receptor binding affinity of N-substituted derivatives of morphinan. *Bioorg Med Chem Lett.* 2001;11: 2735-2740.
55. Zukin RS, Eghbali M, Olive D, Unterwald EM, Tempel A. Characterization and visualization of rat and guinea pig brain kappa opioid receptors: evidence for kappa 1 and kappa 2 opioid receptors. *Proc Natl Acad Sci USA.* 1988;85:4061-4065.
56. Butelman ER, Ko MC, Sobczyk-Kojiro K, et al. kappa-Opioid receptor binding populations in rhesus monkey brain: relationship to an assay of thermal antinociception. *J Pharmacol Exp Ther.* 1998;285:595-601.
57. Caudle RM, Finegold AA, Mannes AJ, et al. Spinal kappa$_1$ and kappa$_2$ opioid binding sites in rats, guinea pigs, monkeys and humans. *Neuroreport.* 1998;9:2523-2525.
58. Wollemann M, Benyhe S, Simon J. The kappa-opioid receptor: evidence for the different subtypes. *Life Sci.* 1993;52:599-611.
59. Ni Q, Xu H, Partilla JS, et al. Selective labeling of κ$_2$ opioid receptors in rat brain by [^{125}I]IOXY: interaction of opioid peptides and other drugs with multiple κ$_{2a}$ binding sites. *Peptides.* 1993;14:1279-1293.

60. Rothman RB, Bykov V, Xue BG, et al. Interaction of opioid peptides and other drugs with multiple kappa receptors in rat and human brain. Evidence for species differences. *Peptides*. 1992;13:977-987.
61. Lahti RA, Mickelson MM, McCall JM, Von Voigtlander PF. [^{3}H]U-69593 a highly selective ligand for the opioid kappa receptor. *Eur J Pharmacol*. 1985;109:281-284.
62. Romer D, Buscher H, Hill RC, et al. Bremazocine: a potent, long-acting opiate kappa-agonist. *Life Sci*. 1980;27:971-978.
63. Portoghese PS, Lipkowski AW, Takemori AE. Binaltorphimine and nor-binaltorphimine, potent and selective kappa-opioid receptor antagonists. *Life Sci*. 1987;40:1287-1292.
64. Portoghese PS, Garzon-Aburbeh A, Nagase H, Lin CE, Takemori AE. Role of the spacer in conferring kappa opioid receptor selectivity to bivalent ligands related to norbinaltorphimine. *J Med Chem*. 1991;34:1292-1296.
65. Clark JA, Liu L, Price M, et al. Kappa opiate receptor multiplicity: evidence for two U50,488-sensitive kappa1 subtypes and a novel kappa3 subtype. *J Pharmacol Exp Ther*. 1989;251:461-468.
66. Raynor K, Kong H, Chen Y, et al. Pharmacological characterization of the cloned kappa-, delta-, and mu-opioid receptors. *Mol Pharmacol*. 1994;45:330-334.
67. Rusovici DE, Negus SS, Mello NK, Bidlack JM. Kappa-opioid receptors are differentially labeled by arylacetamides and benzomorphans. *Eur J Pharmacol*. 2004;485:119-125.
68. Goldstein A, Tachibana S, Lowney LI, Hunkapiller M, Hood L. Dynorphin-(1-13), an extraordinarily potent opioid peptide. *Proc Natl Acad Sci USA*. 1979;76:6666-6670.
69. Chavkin C, James IF, Goldstein A. Dynorphin is a specific endogenous ligand of the kappa opioid receptor. *Science*. 1982;215:413-415.
70. Casy AF, Parfitt RT. *Opioid Analgesics: Chemistry and Receptors*. New York: Plenum Press; 1986.
71. Eguchi M. Recent advances in selective opioid receptor agonists and antagonists. *Med Res Rev*. 2004;24:182-212.
72. Archer S, Glick SD, Bidlack JM. Cyclazocine revisited. *Neurochem Res*. 1996;21:1369-1373.
73. Glick SD, Visker KE, Maisonneuve IM. Effects of cyclazocine on cocaine self-administration in rats. *Eur J Pharmacol*. 1998;357:9-14.
74. Maisonneuve IM, Glick SD. (+/−)Cyclazocine blocks the dopamine response to nicotine. *Neuroreport*. 1999;10:693-696.
75. Preston KL, Umbricht A, Schroeder JR, et al. Cyclazocine: comparison to hydromorphone and interaction with cocaine. *Behav Pharmacol*. 2004;15:91-102.
76. Cosgrove KP, Carroll ME. Effects of bremazocine on self-administration of smoked cocaine base and orally delivered ethanol, phencyclidine, saccharin, and food in rhesus monkeys: a behavioral economic analysis. *J Pharmacol Exp Ther*. 2002;301:993-1002.
77. Nestby P, Schoffelmeer AN, Homberg JR, et al. Bremazocine reduces unrestricted free-choice ethanol self-administration in rats without affecting sucrose preference. *Psychopharmacology (Berl)*. 1999;142:309-317.
78. Wentland MP, Lou R, Ye Y, et al. 8-Carboxamidocyclazocine analogues: redefining the structure-activity relationships of 2,6-methano-3-benzazocines. *Bioorg Med Chem Lett*. 2001;11:623-626.
79. Bidlack JM, Cohen DJ, McLaughlin JP, et al. 8-Carboxamidocyclazocine: a long-acting, novel benzomorphan. *J Pharmacol Exp Ther*. 2002;302:374-380.
80. Stevenson GW, Wentland MP, Bidlack JM, Mello NK, Negus SS. Effects of the mixed-action kappa/mu opioid agonist 8-carboxamidocyclazocine on cocaine- and food-maintained responding in rhesus monkeys. *Eur J Pharmacol*. 2004;506:133-141.
81. Bowen CA, Negus SS, Zong R, et al. Effects of mixed-action kappa/mu opioids on cocaine self-administration and cocaine discrimination by rhesus monkeys. *Neuropsychopharmacology*. 2003;28:1125-1139.
82. Szmuszkovicz J, Von Voigtlander PF. Benzeneacetamide amines: structurally novel non-mμ opioids. *J Med Chem*. 1982;25:1125-1126.

83. Szmuszkovicz J. U-50,488 and the kappa receptor: a personalized account covering the period 1973 to 1990. *Prog Drug Res*. 1999;52:167-195.
84. Szmuszkovicz J. U-50,488 and the kappa receptor. Part II: 1991-1998. *Prog Drug Res*. 1999;53:1-51.
85. Maisonneuve IM, Archer S, Glick SD. U50,488, a kappa opioid receptor agonist, attenuates cocaine-induced increases in extracellular dopamine in the nucleus accumbens of rats. *Neurosci Lett*. 1994;181:57-60.
86. Broadbent J, Gaspard TM, Dworkin SI. Assessment of the discriminative stimulus effects of cocaine in the rat: lack of interaction with opioids. *Pharmacol Biochem Behav*. 1995; 51:379-385.
87. Glick SD, Maisonneuve IM, Raucci J, Archer S. Kappa opioid inhibition of morphine and cocaine self-administration in rats. *Brain Res*. 1995;681:147-152.
88. Kuzmin AV, Semenova S, Gerrits MA, Zvartau EE, Van Ree JM. Kappa-opioid receptor agonist U50,488H modulates cocaine and morphine self-administration in drug-naive rats and mice. *Eur J Pharmacol*. 1997;321:265-271.
89. Kantak KM, Riberdy A, Spealman RD. Cocaine-opioid interactions in groups of rats trained to discriminate different doses of cocaine. *Psychopharmacology (Berl)*. 1999;147:257-265.
90. Negus SS, Mello NK, Portoghese PS, Lin C-E. Effects of *kappa* opioids on cocaine self-administration by rhesus monkeys. *J Pharmacol Exp Ther*. 1997;282:44-55.
91. Negus SS, Mello NK. Effects of kappa opioid agonists on the discriminative stimulus effects of cocaine in rhesus monkeys. *Exp Clin Psychopharmacol*. 1999;7:307-317.
92. Negus SS. Effects of the kappa opioid agonist U50,488 and the kappa opioid antagonist nor-binaltorphimine on choice between cocaine and food in rhesus monkeys. *Psychopharmacology (Berl)*. 2004;176:204-213.
93. Schenk S, Partridge B, Shippenberg TS. U69593, a kappa-opioid agonist, decreases cocaine self-administration and decreases cocaine-produced drug-seeking. *Psychopharmacology (Berl)*. 1999;144:339-346.
94. Vanderschuren LJ, Schoffelmeer AN, Wardeh G, De Vries TJ. Dissociable effects of the kappa-opioid receptor agonists bremazocine, U69593, and U50488H on locomotor activity and long-term behavioral sensitization induced by amphetamine and cocaine. *Psychopharmacology (Berl)*. 2000;150:35-44.
95. El Daly E, Chefer V, Sandill S, Shippenberg TS. Modulation of the neurotoxic effects of methamphetamine by the selective κ opioid receptor agonist U69593. *J Neurochem*. 2000; 74:1553-1562.
96. Powell KR, Holtzman SG. Modulation of the discriminative stimulus effects of d-amphetamine by mu and kappa opioids in squirrel monkeys. *Pharmacol Biochem Behav*. 2000;65:43-51.
97. Sorbera L, Castaner J, Leeson P. Nalfurafine hydrochloride. Antipruritic, analgesic, kappa opioid agonist. *Drugs of the Future*. 2003;28:237-242.
98. Nagase H, Hayakawa J, Kawamura K, et al. Discovery of a structurally novel opioid κ-agonist derived from 4,5-epoxymorphinan. *Chem Pharm Bull (Tokyo)*. 1998;46:366-369.
99. Wang Y, Tang K, Inan S, et al. Comparison of pharmacological activities of three distinct κ-ligands (Salvinorin A, TRK-820 and 3FLB) on κ opioid receptors in vitro and their antipruritic and antinociceptive activities in vivo. *J Pharmacol Exp Ther*. 2004;312:220-230.
100. Endoh T, Tajima A, Izumimoto N, et al. TRK-820, a selective κ-opioid agonist, produces potent antinociception in cynomolgus monkeys. *Jpn J Pharmacol*. 2001;85:282-290.
101. Endoh T, Matsuura H, Tajima A, et al. Potent antinociceptive effects of TRK-820, a novel κ-opioid receptor agonist. *Life Sci*. 1999;65:1685-1694.
102. Endoh T, Tajima A, Suzuki T, et al. Characterization of the antinociceptive effects of TRK-820 in the rat. *Eur J Pharmacol*. 2000;387:133-140.
103. Suzuki T, Izumimoto N, Takezawa Y, et al. Effect of repeated administration of TRK-820, a κ-opioid receptor agonist, on tolerance to its antinociceptive and sedative actions. *Brain Res*. 2004;995:167-175.
104. Mori T, Nomura M, Nagase H, Narita M, Suzuki T. Effects of a newly synthesized κ-opioid receptor agonist, TRK-820, on the discriminative stimulus and rewarding effects of cocaine in rats. *Psychopharmacology (Berl)*. 2002;161:17-22.

105. Hasebe K, Kawai K, Suzuki T, et al. Possible pharmacotherapy of the opioid κ receptor agonist for drug dependence. *Ann N Y Acad Sci*. 2004;1025:404-413.
106. Mori T, Nomura M, Yoshizawa K, et al. Differential properties between TRK-820 and U-50,488H on the discriminative stimulus effects in rats. *Life Sci*. 2004;75:2473-2482.
107. Levi MS, Borne RF. A review of chemical agents in the pharmacotherapy of addiction. *Curr Med Chem*. 2002;9:1807-1818.
108. Mash DC, Kovera CA, Pablo J, et al. Ibogaine: complex pharmacokinetics, concerns for safety, and preliminary efficacy measures. *Ann N Y Acad Sci*. 2000;914:394-401.
109. Mash DC, Kovera CA, Buck BE, et al. Medication development of ibogaine as a pharmacotherapy for drug dependence. *Ann N Y Acad Sci*. 1998;844:274-292.
110. Baumann MH, Pablo JP, Ali SF, Rothman RB, Mash DC. Noribogaine (12-hydroxyibogamine): a biologically active metabolite of the antiaddictive drug ibogaine. *Ann N Y Acad Sci*. 2000;914:354-368.
111. Baumann MH, Rothman RB, Pablo JP, Mash DC. In vivo neurobiological effects of ibogaine and its O-desmethyl metabolite, 12-hydroxyibogamine (noribogaine), in rats. *J Pharmacol Exp Ther*. 2001;297:531-539.
112. Sweetnam PM, Lancaster J, Snowman A, et al. Receptor binding profile suggests multiple mechanisms of action are responsible for ibogaine's putative anti-addictive activity. *Psychopharmacology (Berl)*. 1995;118:369-376.
113. He D-Y, McGough NNH, Ravindranathan A, et al. Glial cell line-derived neurotrophic factor mediates the desirable actions of the anti-addiction drug ibogaine against alcohol consumption. *J Neurosci*. 2005;25:619-628.
114. Leal MB, Michelin K, Souza DO, Elisabetsky E. Ibogaine attenuation of morphine withdrawal in mice: role of glutamate N-methyl-aspartate receptors. *Prog Neuropsychopharmacol Biol Psychiatry*. 2003;27:781-785.
115. Glick SD, Maisonneuve IS. Mechanisms of antiaddictive actions of ibogaine. *Ann N Y Acad Sci*. 1998;844:214-226.
116. Glick SD, Maisonneuve IM, Pearl SM. Evidence for roles of kappa-opioid and NMDA receptors in the mechanism of action of ibogaine. *Brain Res*. 1997;749:340-343.
117. Cappendijk SL, Dzoljic MR. Inhibitory effects of ibogaine on cocaine self-administration in rats. *Eur J Pharmacol*. 1993;241:261-265.
118. Glick SD, Kuehne ME, Raucci J, et al. Effects of iboga alkaloids on morphine and cocaine self-administration in rats: relationship to tremorigenic effects and to effects on dopamine release in nucleus accumbens and striatum. *Brain Res*. 1994;657:14-22.
119. Sershen H, Hashim A, Harsing L, Lajtha A. Ibogaine antagonizes cocaine-induced locomotor stimulation in mice. *Life Sci*. 1992;50:1079-1086.
120. Maisonneuve IM, Jr, Rossman KL, Jr, Keller RW, Jr, Glick SD. Acute and prolonged effects of ibogaine on brain dopamine metabolism and morphine-induced locomotor activity in rats. *Brain Res*. 1992;575:69-73.
121. Szumlinski KK, Maisonneuve IM, Glick SD. Differential effects of ibogaine on behavioural and dopamine sensitization to cocaine. *Eur J Pharmacol*. 2000;398:259-262.
122. Alper KR, Lotsof HS, Frenken GM, Luciano DJ, Bastiaans J. Treatment of acute opioid withdrawal with ibogaine. *Am J Addict*. 1999;8:234-242.
123. O'Hearn E, Molliver ME. The olivocerebellar projection mediates ibogaine-induced degeneration of Purkinje cells: a model of indirect, trans-synaptic excitotoxicity. *J Neurosci*. 1997;17:8828-8841.
124. Bandarage UK, Kuehne ME, Glick SD. Chemical synthesis and biological evaluation of 18-methoxycoronaridine (18-MC) as a potential anti-addictive agent. *Curr Med Chem CNS Agents*. 2001;1:113-123.
125. Kuehne ME, He L, Jokiel PA, et al. Synthesis and biological evaluation of 18-methoxycoronaridine congeners. Potential antiaddiction agents. *J Med Chem*. 2003;46:2716-2730.
126. Glick SD, Maisonneuve IM, Szumlinski KK. 18-Methoxycoronaridine (18-MC) and ibogaine: comparison of antiaddictive efficacy, toxicity, and mechanisms of action. *Ann N Y Acad Sci*. 2000;914:369-386.

127. Glick SD, Maisonneuve IM, Dickinson HA. 18-MC reduces methamphetamine and nicotine self-administration in rats. *Neuroreport.* 2000;11:2013-2015.
128. Glick SD, Maisonneuve IM, Szumlinski KK. Mechanisms of action of ibogaine: relevance to putative therapeutic effects and development of a safer iboga alkaloid congener. *Alkaloids Chem Biol.* 2001;56:39-53.
129. Roth BL, Baner K, Westkaemper R, et al. Salvinorin A: a potent naturally occurring nonnitrogenous kappa opioid selective agonist. *Proc Natl Acad Sci USA.* 2002;99:11934-11939.
130. Chavkin C, Sud S, Jin W, et al. Salvinorin A, an active component of the hallucinogenic sage *Salvia divinorum* is a highly efficacious κ-opioid receptor agonist: structural and functional considerations. *J Pharmacol Exp Ther.* 2004;308:1197-1203.
131. Butelman ER, Harris TJ, Kreek MJ. The plant-derived hallucinogen, salvinorin A, produces kappa-opioid agonist-like discriminative effects in rhesus monkeys. *Psychopharmacology (Berl).* 2004;172:220-224.

Chapter 16
Regulation of Monoamine Transporters: Influence of Psychostimulants and Therapeutic Antidepressants

Lankupalle D. Jayanthi[1] and Sammanda Ramamoorthy[1]

Abstract Synaptic neurotransmission in the central nervous system (CNS) requires the precise control of the duration and the magnitude of neurotransmitter action at specific molecular targets. At the molecular level, neurotransmitter signaling is dynamically regulated by a diverse set of macromolecules including biosynthetic enzymes, secretory proteins, ion channels, pre- and postsynaptic receptors and transporters. Monoamines, 5-hydroxytryptamine or serotonin (5-HT), norepinephrine (NE), and dopamine (DA) play an important modulatory role in the CNS and are involved in numerous physiological functions and pathological conditions. Presynaptic plasma membrane transporters for 5-HT (SERT), NE (NET), and DA (DAT), respectively, control synaptic actions of these monoamines by rapidly clearing the released amine. Monoamine transporters are the sites of action for widely used antidepressants and are high affinity molecular targets for drugs of abuse including cocaine, amphetamine, and 3,4-methylenedioxymetamphetamine (MDMA) "Ecstasy." Monoamine transporters also serve as molecular gateways for neurotoxins. Emerging evidence indicates that regulation of transporter function and surface expression can be rapidly modulated by "intrinsic" transporter activity itself, and antidepressant and psychostimulant drugs that block monoamine transport have a profound effect on transporter regulation. Therefore, disregulations in the functioning of monoamine transporters may underlie many disorders of transmitter imbalance such as depression, attention deficit hyperactivity disorder, and schizophrenia. This review integrates recent progress in understanding the molecular mechanisms of monoamine transporter regulation, in particular, posttranscriptional regulation by phosphorylation and trafficking linked to cellular protein kinases, protein phosphatases, and transporter interacting proteins. The review also discusses the possible role of psychostimulants and antidepressants in influencing monoamine transport regulation.

Keywords phosphorylation, trafficking, interacting proteins, substrates, and ligands

[1] Department of Neurosciences, Division of Neuroscience Research,
Medical University of South Carolina, Charleston, SC 29425

Corresponding Author: Lankupalle D. Jayanthi, Department of Neurosciences, Medical University of South Carolina, Charleston, SC 29425. Tel: (843) 792-8542; Fax: (843) 792-4423; E-mail: jayanthi@musc.edu

R.S. Rapaka and W. Sadée (eds.), *Drug Addiction*.
© American Association of Pharmaceutical Scientists 2008

Neurobiology of Monoamine Transporters

The catecholamines dopamine (DA) and norepinephrine (NE) derived from tyrosine and the indolamine 5-hydroxytryptamine or serotonin (5-HT) derived from tryptophan, packaged into synaptic vesicles and released into synapse in response to depolarizing stimuli, activate pre- and postsynaptic receptors and elicit synaptic responses. Presynaptic plasma membrane transporters for 5-HT (SERT), NE (NET), and DA (DAT), respectively, control synaptic actions of these monoamines by rapidly clearing the released amine, thereby dictating the kinetics of postsynaptic responses and receptor desensitization. Drugs that modulate the activity of biogenic monoamine transporters produce profound behavioral effects, leading to their therapeutic use in depression, obsessive-compulsive disorder, and other mental diseases and also to their abuse as stimulants.

SERT

Altered serotonergic neurotransmission and serotonin (5-HT) have long been associated with psychiatric disorders including depression, suicide, impulsive violence, and alcoholism.[1,2] Presynaptic plasma membrane SERT controls serotonergic neurotransmission by rapid clearance of released 5-HT. Reduced binding of imipramine and paroxetine to brain and platelet SERTs in patients with depression and suicide victims indicates that altered SERT function might contribute to aberrant behaviors. Drugs that block SERT, including tricyclic antidepressants such as imipramine, and selective serotonin reuptake inhibitors (SSRIs) such as fluoxetine (Prozac), paroxetine (Paxil), sertraline (Zoloft), and citalopram (Celexa) are successfully used in the treatment of depression. SSRIs rapidly inhibit the uptake of 5-HT. However, the therapeutic efficacy of antidepressants develops slowly during several weeks of continuous treatment. These observations suggest that the elevation of synaptic 5-HT induces alterations in compensatory or intracellular regulatory pathways impacted by 5-HT signaling and hence neural plasticity. Therefore, changes in SERT kinetics and number will strongly influence the efficacy of antidepressants in the treatment of depression. Studies from DAT knockout (KO)[3] and SERT-DAT double knockout[4] mice demonstrate the involvement of the serotonergic system in the reward response and suggest that the interaction of cocaine with SERT might be necessary to initiate and maintain cocaine reward in DAT KO mice. Two polymorphic regions have been identified in the SERT promoter and implicated in anxiety, mood disorders, alcohol abuse, and in various neuropsychiatric disorders.[5,6] Recent studies indicate that an Ile to Val mutation at position 425 of hSERT found in obsessive compulsive disorder (OCD)-rich pedigrees leads to an increase in transport activity and insensitivity to stimulation by nitric oxide (NO) donors.[7,8] Thus, studies are just emerging to support the notion that impaired regulations might contribute to human disease conditions such as that seen in human variants of SERT coding region.

NET

Noradrenergic signaling is intimately linked with behavioral arousal[9] and is affected in stress-related paradigms linked to depression.[10] NE is an important chemical messenger in the nervous system and regulates affective states, learning and memory, endocrine, and autonomic functions. It has been implicated in depression, aggression, addiction, and cardiac and thermal regulation. NE acutely inhibits nociceptive transmission mediated by substance P (NK1), potentiates opioid analgesia, and underlies part of antinociceptive effects of tricyclic antidepressants.[11,12] NE transporter regulates noradrenergic signaling in central and peripheral nervous systems by mediating the clearance of NE and is an important target for antidepressants and psychostimulants.[13-16] Various biologic stimuli are known to regulate NE signaling, and alterations in NE signaling including NE clearance and NET density are observed in cardiovascular diseases and brain disorders.[17-20] Since reuptake into presynaptic nerve terminals is the predominant mechanism for terminating the action of released NE, changes in the activity of NET should have a significant impact on the concentration and duration of NE present in the synaptic cleft and consequently alter NE signaling. The psychostimulant supersensitivity[21] and potentiated opioid analgesia[22] in NET K/O animals indicate the importance of NET expression under physiological circumstances. A point mutation in the coding region of human NET is associated with peripheral orthostatic intolerance (OI), high plasma NE levels, and reduced systemic NE clearance.[23] This study demonstrates the impact of hNET coding variant on NE clearance contributing to a human disease condition.

DAT

DA signaling regulates many crucial functions, such as movement, emotion, and cognition.[24,25] DAT terminates dopaminergic neurotransmission by re-uptake of DA in presynaptic neurons and plays a key role in DA recycling. DAT can also provide reverse transport of DA under certain circumstances. Psychostimulants such as cocaine, and amphetamine and drugs used for ADHD such as methylphenidate exert their actions via DAT.[26,27] Recent molecular and pharmacological analyses using monoamine transport knockout mice have confirmed the physiological importance and requirement of presynaptic amine transporter expression for normal transmitter clearance, presynaptic transmitter homeostasis, postsynaptic response and response to drugs.[21,28,29] In particular, functional loss of DAT either through pharmacological inhibition[30,31] or gene knockout[32] results in profound physical, physiological, and behavioral changes. Altered DAT function or density has been implicated in various types of psychopathology, including depression, suicide, anxiety, aggression, and schizophrenia.[24,33-35] Associations between DAT gene polymorphisms and human disorders with possible links to DA system, including attention deficit hyperactivity disorder (ADHD) and consequences of cocaine and alcohol abuse have been reported.[2,36] Altered transport properties associated with some of the coding variants of DAT suggest that individuals with these DAT variants could display altered DA system.[37]

Monoamine Transporters and Addiction

Monoamine transporters are also of interest in the field of addiction because they constitute high affinity molecular targets mediating the cellular and behavioral effects of psychostimulants such as cocaine and amphetamine.[38,39] Given the importance of monoamine transmission in various aspects of addiction, and the profound influence that monoamine transport has on the extracellular levels of monoamines, as well as intracellular monoamine homeostasis, long-term changes in transporter level, kinetics, or regulation would be expected to greatly influence spontaneous and drug-induced behaviors. This possibility is clearly evidenced by the large effects on drug-induced behaviors, as well as on neurotransmitter synthesis, storage, and release by removing monoamine transporter genes in mutant mice.[27,32,40,41] Receptors that are known to influence amine transporter functions, such as 5-HT1B (SERT), D2, opioid, and mGluR5 (DAT) have been implicated in cocaine sensitization.[42,43] Such changes in receptor-linked signaling cascades could influence the transporter phosphorylation and transport activity. Since the second messenger-linked pathways can be linked to presynaptic receptors, these pathways may provide positive/negative feedback mechanisms in control of DA, 5-HT, and NE clearance in vivo.

Monoamine Transporters and Their Functional Regulation

Monoamine transporters belong to the Na^+, Cl^- -dependent, gamma-amino butyric acid (GABA)/norepinephrine transporter (GAT1/NET) gene family that also includes transporters for proline (PROT), taurine (TauT), glycine (GLYT), creatine (CreaT), betaine (BGT), and other "orphan" transporters. Monoamine transporters, in general, function by sequestering monoamines from specific nerve terminals. However, in several brain regions and under certain conditions, monoamine transporter functions can overlap.[44-46] Pharmacological and behavioral studies in genetic animal models with targeted disruption of monoamine transporters suggest functional overlap between these transporters. Consequently, pharmacological and physiological characterizations to distinguish their role in psychiatric illnesses and drug abuse require proper understanding of the mechanisms regulating monoamine transporter function.

Neural activity, hormones, growth factors, environmental factors, and pharmacological agents have been reported to regulate monoamine uptake, specific radioligand binding, and mRNA levels. These studies suggest the presence of endogenous regulatory mechanisms and such regulation could influence transporter expression and function at the level of gene transcription and translation (long-term or chronic regulation) or posttranslational protein modifications (short-term or acute regulation).

Regulation at the Gene Level

Structural analysis of transporters gene promoter region reveals several canonical transcription binding sites that may be important in controlling the responses of the transporter genes to regulatory factors. Notably, binding sites for transcription factors including TATA-like motif, an AP1 site, an element for CREB binding (CRE), AP-2, NF-IL6, NF-Kß, and SP1 sites have been identified for SERT. Relevant investigations performed on JAR cells have shown that activation of cAMP-dependent and independent pathways increase 5-HT uptake.[47-49]

The long-term modulation of SERT activity both in vivo and in vitro has been studied extensively and reviewed elsewhere.[50-52] Unlike SERT, very little is known about NET and DAT gene regulation. Earlier in vivo and in vitro studies demonstrate modulation of NE uptake by several factors such as insulin, atrial natriuretic peptide (ANP), angiotensine (ANG II), dexamethasone and nerve growth factor (NGF), and pharmacological substances such as desipramine and cocaine. Altered NET mRNA levels are shown for the NET modulation by insulin, dexamethasone, NGF, desipramine, and cocaine.[53-56] Recent reports showed an upregulation in the expression of DAT and NET genes following cocaine treatment. During pregnancy, cocaine exposure results in increased DAT mRNA levels in the fetal rhesus monkey brain.[57] Another study showed increased levels of NET binding sites in the placentas of rats treated with cocaine reflecting increased NET mRNA levels.[58] NET binding sites are also increased in stria terminalis of cocaine self-administered monkeys.[59] Although the actual cellular signaling pathways responsible for such regulation at the genetic level are yet to be identified, these studies suggest a significant functional role for the monoamine transporters not only in the monoaminergic neurotransmission, but also in the fetal development.

Regulation at the Protein Level

Reuptake of monoamine neurotransmitters into presynaptic terminals via the transporters is the principle mechanism for terminating the monoaminergic neurotransmission. Therefore, changes in the transporter activity or expression should have a significant impact on the duration and concentration of monoamines present in the synaptic cleft. These changes resulting in the regulation of transport function, in turn, would influence pre- and postsynaptic responses to released monoamines. The regulation of monoamine transporter function and expression reviewed here suggests that signaling proteins such as kinases, phosphatases, and transporter interacting proteins, as well as transporter ligands have a potential role in the regulation of transporters for appropriate transporter function and expression.

Amino acid sequence analysis of SERT, DAT, and NET proteins reveal numerous consensus sites for protein kinases as well as putative interactive motifs in cytoplasmic domains suggesting that second messengers are able to play a role in posttranslational regulation of monoamine transporters. Prior to the cloning of monoamine transporters, evidence suggests a pivotal role for second messenger-linked pathways in acute modulation of neurotransmitter uptake.[52] Potential pathways linked to second messenger-linked pathways might regulate transporter function acutely. Regulation of transport function can occur directly by phosphorylation of transporter protein. Phosphorylation of transporter protein might in turn change its intrinsic transport activity, turnover rate, plasma membrane insertion by modulating exocytic fusion, or sequestration from the plasma membrane by modulating endocytic machinery. Alternatively, transporters can be regulated through their association with other interacting proteins by phosphorylation dependent/or independent pathways. Substrate or antagonist binding may also modulate transport activity via its influence on transporter phosphorylation, trafficking, and interaction with transporter-interacting proteins.

Mechanisms of Acute Monoamine Transporter Regulation

Posttranslational modifications such as glycosylation and phosphorylation regulate monoamine transporter function and expression levels.[60-63] In addition, variations in monoamine transporter gene sequences known as polymorphisms may also alter transporter expression levels, activity, and/or regulation. Recent studies demonstrate that the activity and expression of monoamine transporters are regulated by phosphorylation and dephosphorylation of the transporter proteins. Thus, monoamine transporters are dynamically regulated by intracellular and extracellular regulation of phosphorylation state, which in turn should have a significant impact on the duration and concentration of monoamines present in the synaptic cleft.

Altered Transporter Surface Expression and Intrinsic Activity

Among various stimuli that acutely regulate monoamine transporters, the majority regulate transport function by altering transporter surface expression. In a variety of preparations, including synaptosomes and cell lines, application of protein kinase C (PKC) activator phorbol 12-myristate 13-acetate (β-PMA) selectively reduces the transport capacity (Vmax) for transport of DA, NE, and 5-HT.[61-65] The most consistent finding is that activators of PKC or the agents that maintain phosphorylation state such as phosphatase inhibitors rapidly reduce amine transport capacity. The major kinetic alterations typically observed in acute modulation paradigms are changes in Vmax, with little or no significant change in substrate affinity (Km). The reduction in Vmax values suggests silencing of plasma membrane resident amine transport protein or changing cell surface expression levels by regulating endocytosis or recycling or plasma membrane insertion of transporter proteins. First evidence for altered cell surface expression for monoamine transporter as the result of PKC activation has come from studies of human SERT stably expressed in human embryonic kidney (HEK-293) cells. Protein phosphatase inhibitor, okadaic acid, also regulates SERT activity, which suggests that cellular phosphatases monitor phosphorylation-dependent SERT regulation.[66] PKC activation by β-PMA also leads to a decrease in 5-HT transport capacity and SERT currents under voltage clamp.[67] Analogous kinase-mediated transporter redistribution has been detected for DAT and NET.[63-65,68,69] Of interest, dominant negative mutant of dynamin 1, which is shown to block clathrin-mediated endocytosis, is able to block PKC-dependent DAT internalization.[70] These observations suggest that PKC regulates DAT internalization by clathrin-mediated and dynamin-dependent cellular mechanisms. They also provide evidence that internalized DAT is targeted to endosomal/lysomal pathways for degradation. However, other studies show that internalized DAT is directed to recycling pool,[71] and plasma membrane DAT sequestration can occur due to a combination of accelerated internalization or reduced recycling.[72] However, the molecular mechanisms responsible for different PKC-dependent DAT internalization pathways (recycling endosomes vs degradative lysosomes) between these studies are unknown. Recently, clathrin-dependent mechanisms were demonstrated for both constitutive and PKC-mediated DAT internalization.[73] Nonclassical, distinct endocytic signals drive constitutive and PKC-regulated DAT internalization.[74] The DAT internalization signal is conserved across SLC6 neurotransmitter carriers and is functional in the homologous norepinephrine transporter. Together, the above studies suggest the involvement of unconventional mechanisms in DAT and NET internalization.

Recent studies from our laboratory provided the first evidence for lipid raft localization and raft-mediated internalization of NET and SERT.[63,75] SERT and NET are also expressed in nonneuronal tissues such as placenta and intestinal epithelial cells.[76-78] PKC activation stimulates lipid raft-mediated internalization of native NETs expressed in placental trophoblasts.[63] Of interest, PKC-, but not mitogen-activated protein kinase (p38 MAPK)-mediated SERT regulation in rat brain involves raft-mediated distribution.[75] The presence of NET and SERT in lipid rafts suggests that signaling machinery specific to lipid rafts may be linked to PKC-mediated transporter downregulation. Raft-associated sorting has been proposed to underlie several cellular processes including signal transduction, protein sorting, and membrane trafficking.[79] Receptors such as NK1R and TrkB, several channel proteins, many components of G protein coupled receptor (GPCR) signal transduction proteins such as, adenylyl cyclase, Akt1, PLC, activated PKC, PP2Ac, nonreceptor tyrosine kinases, and other signaling molecules such as syntaxin 1A (a SNARE protein), α-synuclein, and the PKC binding protein PICK1 (protein interacting with C kinase) have been shown to be associated with lipid rafts.[79,80] The localization of receptors such as NK1R that regulate monoamine transporter function and potential transporter-interacting proteins (syntaxin 1A, PP2Ac, PKC), as well as transporters in lipid raft microdomains, raises the possibility that lipid rafts may *act as morphological "conveners" of signal transduction* by placing various signal transduction molecules near the transporter molecule. For example, transporter-interacting proteins may *"guide"* targeting the transporter to lipid rafts and that phosphorylation of a *"motif/site"* within the transporter may act as a *"signal"* for fostering protein-protein interactions and redistribution. Thus, protein redistribution from plasma membrane microdomains may be one of the several mechanisms by which synaptic plasticity and neurotransmitter homeostasis are maintained.[81,82]

NET,[83] DAT,[84,85] and SERT[75,86] are also regulated by MAPKs. While studies on DAT[85] and SERT[75] implicate MAPK effects on transporter trafficking, other studies on NET and SERT indicate modulation of transporter catalytic activity. In our study,[75] p38 MAPK-mediated SERT redistribution involves enhanced plasma membrane insertion of the transporter. Numerous studies have indicated alterations in the 5-HT levels, SERT binding sites, and serotonergic neuronal firing in response to numerous stressors.[87] Thus, the regulation of SERT by p38 MAPK, a stress-induced kinase, may provide a novel presynaptic mechanism in maintaining appropriate synaptic 5-HT levels during stressful conditions. Several studies indicate that SERT is upregulated by cGMP/PKG-mediated pathway through altered surface expression.[8,86,88] Of interest, MAPK effects on SERT intrinsic activity are also sensitive to PKG activity.[86] Together, these studies suggest that transporters are subject to multiple, interacting modes of kinase- dependent modulation via trafficking-dependent and independent mechanisms.

Altered Transporter Phosphorylation

DAT, SERT, and NET proteins are phosphorylated in response to PKC activation.[61-63] DAT proteins become phosphorylated in transfected cells and synaptosomal preparations following treatment with PKC activators and PP2A inhibitors.[61,89] SERTs are also phosphorylated following PKC and PKA activation and PP2A inhibition. The PKC-dependent phosphorylation shows a close temporal correlation with reduction in transport capacity.[62,90] SERT substrates and antagonists influence PKC-dependent SERT phosphorylation and surface redistribution.[90] Our recent studies indicate that while PKC activation increases SERT basal phosphorylation, p38 MAPK inhibition decreases SERT basal phosphorylation indicating a role for p38 MAPK-induced phosphorylation in constitutive SERT expression.[75]

DAT is phosphorylated on N-terminal serine residues.[91] The PKC-mediated internalization of monoamine transporters occurs in parallel to an enhanced phosphorylation of the transporter. Although the transporters undergo phosphorylation in response to PKC activation or PP1/2A inhibition, it is not known whether phosphorylation of the transporter leads to its internalization. However, recent studies using phospho-site mutants of transporters provided positive as well as negative correlations between phosphorylation and transporter functional regulation.[92-95] Studies demonstrate that tyrosine kinase activity is also critical in maintaining NET,[83] DAT,[96] and GAT[97,98] cell surface levels. Phosphorylation of Y107 and Y317 on GAT1 is required for tyrosine kinase-mediated GABA transport regulation.[98] Of interest, the reciprocal relationship between PKC- and tyrosine kinase-mediated GAT1 phosphorylation suggests that a balance between these 2 states of phosphorylation may dictate relative abundance of GAT1 on the cell surface.[99]

While a part of N-terminal domain appears to interact with syntaxin 1A involved in PKC-mediated regulation,[100] determinants within the C-terminus of human NET (hNET) dictate NET trafficking, stability, and activity.[101] Of interest, nonclassical endocytic signals dictate constitutive and PKC-regulated internalization of DAT.[73,74] These signals are conserved in NET. However, it is not known whether there is a relationship between NET phosphorylation and PKC-induced transporter regulation. NET protein contains multiple consensus sites for several kinases including PKC that are distinct from those present in DAT or SERT, and therefore, NET may be regulated by mechanisms that are different for those of DAT and SERT. Recent work from our laboratory (Jayanthi et al, unpublished data, 2005) demonstrates that a PKC-site mutant of hNET is resistant to PKC-mediated downregulation and phosphorylation. This study provides the first evidence that phosphorylation of a PKC motif on a monoamine transporter is linked to transporter internalization. In addition, this PKC-site mutant of hNET exhibits altered transport properties such as increased affinity for NE and substrate-like ligand D-amphetamine, and decreased affinity for inhibitory ligands such as cocaine, desipramine, and nisoxetine. Phospho-site mutations could contribute to altered NE transport process due to physical conformational changes occurring as the result of mutation or altered phosphorylation state itself. Such changes can result in altered binding or recognition of the ligands. Recent studies on DAT harboring mutations in the second intracellular loop reported altered ligand binding properties attributed to structural changes in physical conformation of DAT protein.[102-105] Such investigations would prove useful in developing antidepressant drugs with higher efficacy and reduced potential side effects.

Altered Protein-Protein Interactions

As described earlier, agents that maintain phosphorylated state modulate amine transporter activity. For example, protein phosphatase 1/2A (PP1/PP2A) inhibitor, okadaic acid (OK), downregulates SERT, DAT, and NET activity. Phosphorylation state and regulation of amine transporter is a balance between the actions and localization of protein kinases and protein phosphatases. The pronounced effect of PP1/PP2A inhibition on amine uptake and amine transporter phosphorylation suggests the possible physical association of PP1/PP2A as a regulatory complex with amine transporter proteins. Indeed, physical complexes containing biogenic amine transporter and PP2Ac proteins were recently demonstrated.[66] SERT/PP2A complex is disrupted by PP1/PP2A inhibitors as well as PKC activators and can be stabilized by SERT substrate 5-HT, suggesting that modulation of SERT/phosphatase association is involved in regulated transporter phosphorylation and trafficking. Similar transporter and PP2Ac associations were found for DAT and NET proteins. Analogous to SERT studies, PP2Ac association with NET in vas deferens is also decreased by PKC activation and PP1/PP2A inhibition.

While direct phosphorylation and/or dephosphorylation of transporters by cellular protein kinases and phosphatases is involved in the dynamic regulation and expression of transporters, other integral membrane proteins also appear to play an important role in trafficking and catalytic function of transporters. First evidence for the physical association of GAT1 GABA transporter with atachment protein receptor (t)-SNARE protein syntaxin-1A as a complex comes from studies by Quick and his coworkers.[106,107] Of interest, this association is modulated by PKC-dependent manner and the interaction of GAT1 with syntaxin-1 is required for GAT1 regulation by PKC activation. Syntaxin-1A association not only regulates PKC-dependent trafficking of GAT1 but also appears to influence catalytic function of the transporter.[108] Recently, it has been shown that syntaxin-1A interacts with N-terminal cytoplasmic domain of GAT1 GABA transporter and decreases transport rates.[108] Like GAT1, SERT and NET are also physically associated with syntaxin-1A.[100,109] Using noradrenergic tissues such as vas deferens and transfected cell lines, Sung et al[100] reported that syntaxin-1A is found in NET immunoprecipitates. Activation of PKC or phosphatase inhibition decreases syntaxin-1A level with NET. Altering intracellular Ca^{2+} also regulates syntaxin-1A/NET interaction. Together these findings suggest an important role for syntaxin-1A in neurotransmission by regulating both transmitter release and reuptake.

Signals following presynaptic receptor stimulation may influence transporter function and expression by regulating the stability of transporter heteromeric complexes. Studies by Torres et al show the interaction of PDZ domain containing protein PICK1 with C-terminal cytoplasmic domains of DAT and NET.[110] Co-expression of DAT and PICK1 in HEK-293 cells enhances DAT activity and PICK1 co-immunoprecipitates with DAT. Confocal microscopy analysis reveals colocalization of both DAT and PICK1 in heterologous system and in dissociated dopaminergic neurons. Since PICK1 is a PKC binding protein, it is possible that PICK1 acts like an adaptor to bring PKC near DAT proteins, which in turn could regulate PKC-evoked DAT phosphorylation, trafficking, and function. Lee and coworkers recently identified the interaction of C-terminal cytoplasmic domain of DAT with α-synuclein.[111] α-Synuclein is enriched in dopaminergic nerve terminals and has been implicated in Parkinson's and other neurodegenerative disorders.[112] α-Synuclein binds directly to C-terminal region of DAT and facilitates the plasma membrane clustering and increase in DAT activity.[113] This study suggests that α-synuclein/DAT complex regulates normal dopaminergic neurotransmission, and altered interactions may result in abnormal DAT function causing dopaminergic neurodegeneration seen in Parkinson's disease. DAT also interacts with LIM domain-containing adapter protein, Hic-5.[114] Hic-5 is known to interact with signaling molecules such as nonreceptor protein tyrosine kinases FAK and FYN. This raises the possibility that Hic-5 may be involved in tyrosine kinase-mediated DAT regulation. Together, these studies indicate that protein-protein interactions play an important role in influencing transporter phosphorylation, trafficking, and intrinsic activity.

Influence of Substrates and Antagonists on Monoamine Transport Regulation

Another important observation is that the amine transporter substrates and antagonists influence transporter trafficking and plasma membrane residency. Since transporters are subjected to phosphorylation by multiple kinase-dependent modulations, it is possible that substrates may also influence transporter surface expression by regulating kinase-mediated transporter phosphorylation. For example, Ramamoorthy and Blakely provided the evidence that SERT substrates such as serotonin, amphetamines, fenfluramine, and antagonists such as antidepressants and cocaine control PKC-dependent SERT phosphorylation and surface redistribution.[90] SERT transporting substrates, 5-HT, amphetamine, and fenfluramine, protect SERT from PKC-linked phosphorylation and sequestration. The effect of 5-HT is SERT-dependent but not 5-HT receptor-dependent, and the nontransported ligands such as cocaine and antidepressants block the effect of 5-HT. Amphetamines substitute for substrates in suppressing PKC-mediated SERT phosphorylation. Such action could override homeostatic transporter sequestration processes and provide for psychostimulant sensitization by increasing the number of psychostimulant targets available to a subsequent stimulus. On the other hand, nonpermeant SERT ligands including SSRIs and cocaine that prevent 5-HT permeation block the effect of 5-HT, thus SSRIs may have therapeutic utility in disease states, not only by preventing 5-HT uptake but also by shifting the cellular distribution of SERT. Amphetamines trigger DAT internalization,[115] and while acute cocaine exposure increases DAT surface levels,[116,117] amphetamine-induced DAT internalization is blocked by cocaine.[115] This inverse relationship between antagonist binding and substrate translocation suggests that various transporter conformational states may promote or preclude their engagement with cellular endocytic machinery dictating transporter surface levels.

Transporter substrates are known to regulate transporter function and expression.[75,118-120] Substrate-induced upregulation of GAT1 requires tyrosine phosphorylation and acute substrate exposure slows down the transporter internalization rate, resulting in increased surface levels from continued delivery to the plasma membrane.[98,118] D-amphetamine, which is also a substrate for SERT, increases SERT basal phosphorylation that is sensitive to p38 MAPK inhibition suggesting that p38 MAPK may govern substrate-mediated effects on SERT basal phosphorylation.[75] Substrate translocation or ligand occupancy may influence the equilibrium of protein conformation required for transporter phosphorylation or transporter association with other regulators. Thus, a feedback loop may exist providing a mechanism by which changes in extracellular neurotransmitter concentrations could rapidly modulate neurotransmitter transport capacity. This way, the control of transporter cell surface expression by its substrates or ligands would provide a novel homeostatic mechanism in the neuron to fine-tune transport capacity to match demands imposed by fluctuating levels of the neurotransmitter. Signaling pathways linked to presynaptic auto- and hetero-receptors could provide a positive/negative feedback control and provide a mechanism by which changes in synaptic neurotransmitters could rapidly modulate transport capacity of the transporter.

Conclusions

In summary, evidence suggests that amine transporters may be modulated by various biologic stimuli as well as pharmacological agents. The intracellular second-messenger systems mimic cellular protein kinases and phosphatases and subsequently regulate amine transporter gene and protein expression. The past few years of active research on transporter function, structure, expression, and regulation strongly support the idea that amine transporters are principle players in regulating normal and abnormal amine signaling in the central nervous system (CNS) and periphery and hence complex behavioral and physiological functions. An even more exciting discovery is that the regulation of transporter phosphorylation by kinases or phosphatases indeed plays a major role in dictating transporter function. Recent studies that demonstrate altered response to second-messenger and/or kinase-mediated regulations in human variants of monoamine transporters[8,121,122] signify the search for underlying mechanisms of transporter phosphorylation regulating amine transport in normal physiology and pathophysiology. Another important lead in the monoamine transporter research is that intrinsic transport capacity of a transporter molecule governs its own plasma membrane expression and function. There appear to be multiple mechanisms by which transporter substrates and antagonists can influence transporter function and expression. The variations in the transporter response to different signals and the various mechanisms they adopt to regulate transporter function suggest a need for future research to focus on physiologically relevant events. The capacity of transporter to fine-tune its function in response to extracellular neurotransmitter would maintain a constant level of neurotransmitter at the synaptic cleft. Altered pattern or a disturbance in the pre- and post-synaptic regulatory mechanisms could lead to abnormal neurotransmission and hence abnormal behavior or brain disorders. Drugs of abuse such as cocaine and amphetamines bind and inhibit biogenic amine transporters and might interfere with activity-dependent regulatory mechanisms and cause or initiate drug addiction or sensitization. Along with information delineating cis/trans acting elements and signals for acute and chronic amine transporter regulation, over the next few years, we will expect rapid progress in understanding the role of cellular regulation of amine transporters in amine signaling and behavior. These developments add further impetus to the drive for psychotherapeutic innovation and a better understanding of mechanisms of monoamine transporter regulation in drug addiction.

Acknowledgments The support from the National Institutes of Health, Bethesda, MD, (grant no. DA016753) and (grant nos. MH062612 and P50DA015369) is greatly appreciated.

References

1. Heinz A, Mann K, Weinberger DR, Goldman D. Serotonergic dysfunction, negative mood states, and response to alcohol. *Alcohol Clin Exp Res.* 2001;25:487-495.
2. Hahn MK, Blakely RD. Monoamine transporter gene structure and polymorphisms in relation to psychiatric and other complex disorders. *Pharmacogenomics J.* 2002;2:217-235.
3. Rocha BA, Fumagalli F, Gainetdinov RR, et al. Cocaine self-administration in dopamine-transporter knockout mice. *Nat Neurosci.* 1998;1:132-137.
4. Sora I, Hall FS, Andrews AM, et al. Molecular mechanisms of cocaine reward: combined dopamine and serotonin transporter knockouts eliminate cocaine place preference. *Proc Natl Acad Sci USA.* 2001;98:5300-5305.
5. Flattem NL, Blakely RD. Modified structure of the human serotonin transporter promoter. *Mol Psychiatry.* 2000;5:110-115.
6. McCauley JL, Olson LM, Dowd M, et al. Linkage and association analysis at the serotonin transporter (SLC6A4) locus in a rigid-compulsive subset of autism. *Am J Med Genet B Neuropsychiatr Genet.* 2004;127:104-112.
7. Ozaki N, Goldman D, Kaye WH, et al. Serotonin transporter missense mutation associated with a complex neuropsychiatric phenotype. *Mol Psychiatry.* 2003;8:895-936.
8. Kilic F, Murphy DL, Rudnick G. A human serotonin transporter mutation causes constitutive activation of transport activity. *Mol Pharmacol.* 2003;64:440-446.
9. Astier B, Van Bockstaele EJ, Aston-Jones G, Pieribone VA. Anatomical evidence for multiple pathways leading from the rostral ventrolateral medulla (nucleus paragigantocellularis) to the locus coeruleus in rat. *Neurosci Lett.* 1990;118:141-146.
10. Pavcovich LA, Cancela LM, Volosin M, Molina VA, Ramirez OA. Chronic stress-induced changes in locus coeruleus neuronal activity. *Brain Res Bull.* 1990;24:293-296.
11. Holden JE, Naleway E. Microinjection of carbachol in the lateral hypothalamus produces opposing actions on nociception mediated by alpha(1)- and alpha(2)-adrenoceptors. *Brain Res.* 2001;911:27-36.
12. Jasmin L, Tien D, Weinshenker D. The NK1 receptor mediates both the hyperalgesia and the resistance to morphine in mice lacking noradrenaline. *Proc Natl Acad Sci USA.* 2002;99:1029-1034.
13. Axelrod J, Kopin IJ. The uptake, storage, release, and metabolism of noradrenaline in sympathetice nerves. *Prog Brain Res.* 1969;31:21-32.
14. Iversen LL. Uptake processes for biogenic amines. In: Iversen I, ed. *Handbook of Psychopharmacology.* 3rd ed. New York, NY: Prenum Press; 1978:381-442.
15. Pacholczyk T, Blakely RD, Amara SG. Expression cloning of a cocaine- and antidepressant-sensitive human noradrenaline transporter. *Nature.* 1991;350:350-354.
16. Amara SG, Arriza JL. Neurotransmitter transporters: three distinct gene families. *Curr Opin Neurobiol.* 1993;3:337-344.

17. Klimek V, Stockmeier C, Overholser J, et al. Reduced levels of norepinephrine transporters in the locus coeruleus in major depression. *J Neurosci.* 1997;17:8451-8458.
18. Ganguly PK, Dhalla KS, Innes IR, Beamish RE, Dhall NS. Altered norepinephrine turnover and metabolism in diabetic cardiomyopathy. *Circ Res.* 1986;59:684-693.
19. Merlet P, Dubois-Rande J-L, Adnot S, et al. Myocardial b-adrenergic desensitization and neuronal norepinephrine uptake function in idiopathic dilated cardiomyopathy. *J Cardiovasc Pharmacol.* 1992;19:10-16.
20. Robertson D, Flattem N, Tellioglu T, et al. Familial orthostatic tachycardia due to norepinephrine transporter deficiency. *Ann N Y Acad Sci.* 2001;940:527-543.
21. Xu F, Gainetdinov RR, Wetsel WC, et al. Mice lacking the norepinephrine transporter are supersensitive to psychostimulants. *Nat Neurosci.* 2000;3:465-471.
22. Thompson AC, Zapata A, Justice JB, Vaughan RA, Sharpe LG, Shippenberg TS. Kappa-opioid receptor activation modifies dopamine uptake in the nucleus accumbens and opposes the effects of cocaine. *J Neurosci.* 2000;20:9333-9340.
23. Hahn MK, Robertson D, Blakely RD. A mutation in the human norepinephrine transporter gene (SLC6A2) associated with orthostatic intolerance disrupts surface expression of mutant and wild-type transporters. *J Neurosci.* 2003;23:4470-4478.
24. Carlsson A, Waters N, Holm-Waters S, Tedroff J, Nilsson M, Carlsson ML. Interactions between monoamines, glutamate, and GABA in schizophrenia: new evidence. *Annu Rev Pharmacol Toxicol.* 2001;41:237-260.
25. Greengard P. The neurobiology of slow synaptic transmission. *Science.* 2001;294:1024-1030.
26. Sulzer D, Chen TK, Lau YY, Kristensen H, Rayport S, Ewing A. Amphetamine redistributes dopamine from synaptic vesicles to the cytosol and promotes reverse transport. *J Neurosci.* 1995;15:4102-4108.
27. Sora I, Wichems C, Takahashi N, et al. Cocaine reward models: conditioned place preference can be established in dopamine- and in serotonin-transporter knockout mice. *Proc Natl Acad Sci USA.* 1998;95:7699-7704.
28. Rioux A, Fabre V, Lesch KP, et al. Adaptive changes of serotonin 5-HT2A receptors in mice lacking the serotonin transporter. *Neurosci Lett.* 1999;262:113-116.
29. Carboni E, Spielewoy C, Vacca C, Nosten-Bertrand M, Giros B, Di Chiara G. Cocaine and amphetamine increase extracellular dopamine in the nucleus accumbens of mice lacking the dopamine transporter gene. *J Neurosci.* 2001;21:1-4.
30. Kula NS, Baldessarini RJ. Lack of increase in dopamine transporter binding or functions in rat brain tissue after treatment with blockers of neuronal uptake of dopamine. *Neuropharmacology.* 1991;30:89-92.
31. Giros B, El Mestikawy S, Godinot N, et al. Cloning, pharmacological characterization, and chromosome assignment of the human dopamine transporter. *Mol Pharmacol.* 1992;42:383-390.
32. Giros B, Jaber M, Jones SR, Wightman RM, Caron MG. Hyperlocomotion and indifference to cocaine and amphetamine in mice lacking the dopamine transporter. *Nature.* 1996;379:606-612.
33. Eichelman BS. Neurochemical and psychopharmacologic aspects of aggressive behavior. *Annu Rev Med.* 1990;41:149-158.
34. Comings DE. Clinical and molecular genetics of ADHD and Tourette syndrome: two related polygenic disorders. *Ann NY Acad Sci.* 2001;931:50-83.
35. Meyer JH, Goulding VS, Wilson AA, Hussey D, Christensen BK, Houle S. Bupropion occupancy of the dopamine transporter is low during clinical treatment. *Psychopharmacology (Berl).* 2002;163:102-105.
36. Miller GM, II, De La Garza RD, II, Novak MA, Madras BK. Single nucleotide polymorphisms distinguish multiple dopamine transporter alleles in primates: implications for association with attention deficit hyperactivity disorder and other neuropsychiatric disorders. *Mol Psychiatry.* 2001;6:50-58.
37. Lin Z, Uhl GR. Dopamine transporter mutants with cocaine resistance and normal dopamine uptake provide targets for cocaine antagonism. *Mol Pharmacol.* 2002;61:885-891.

38. Reith MEA, Meisler BE, Sershen H, Lajtha A. Structural requirements for cocaine congeners to interact with dopamine and serotonin uptake sites in mouse brain and to induce stereotyped behavior. *Biochem Pharmacol.* 1986;35:1123-1129.
39. Seiden LS, Sabol KE, Ricaurte GA. Amphetamine: effects on catecholamine systems and behavior. *Annu Rev Pharmacol Toxicol.* 1993;33:639-677.
40. Bengel D, Murphy DL, Andrews AM, et al. Altered brain serotonin homeostasis and locomotor insensitivity to 3,4-methylenedioxymetamphetamine ("ecstasy") in serotonin transporter-deficient mice. *Mol Pharmacol.* 1998;53:649-655.
41. Rocha BA, Scearce-Levie K, Lucas JJ, et al. Increased vulnerability to cocaine in mice lacking the serotonin-1B receptor. *Nature.* 1998;393:175-178.
42. Nestler EJ, Aghajanian GK. Molecular and cellular basis of addiction. *Science.* 1997;278:58-63.
43. Pierce RC, Kalivas PW. Repeated cocaine modifies the mechanism by which amphetamine releases dopamine. *J Neurosci.* 1997;17:3254-3261.
44. Cases O, Lebrand C, Giros B, et al. Plasma membrane transporters of serotonin, dopamine, and norepinephrine mediate serotonin accumulation in atypical locations in the developing brain of monoamine oxidase A knock-outs. *J Neurosci.* 1998;18:6914-6927.
45. Pan Y, Gembom E, Peng W, Lesch KP, Mossner R, Simantov R. Plasticity in serotonin uptake in primary neuronal cultures of serotonin transporter knockout mice. *Brain Res Dev Brain Res.* 2001;126:125-129.
46. Moron JA, Brockington A, Wise RA, Rocha BA, Hope BT. Dopamine uptake through the norepinephrine transporter in brain regions with low levels of the dopamine transporter: evidence from knock-out mouse lines. *J Neurosci.* 2002;22:389-395.
47. Ramamoorthy S, Cool DR, Mahesh VB, et al. Regulation of the human serotonin transporter: cholera toxin-induced stimulation of serotonin uptake in human placental choriocarcinoma cells is accompanied by increased serotonin transporter mRNA levels and serotonin transporter-specific ligand binding. *J Biol Chem.* 1993;268:21626-21631.
48. Ramamoorthy JD, Ramamoorthy S, Papapetropoulos A, Catravas JD, Leibach FH, Ganapathy V. Cyclic AMP-independent up-regulation of the human serotonin transporter by staurosporine in choriocarcinoma cells. *J Biol Chem.* 1995;270:17189-17195.
49. Ramamoorthy S, Ramamoorthy JD, Prasad P, et al. Regulation of the human serotonin transporter by interleukin-1b. *Biochem Biophys Res Commun.* 1995;216:560-567.
50. Blakely RD, Ramamoorthy S, Qian Y, Schroeter S, Bradley C. Regulation of antidepressant-sensitive serotonin transporters. In: Reith MEA, ed. *Neurotransmitter Transporters: Structure, Function, and Regulation.* Totowa, NJ: Humana Press; 1997:29-72.
51. Bradley CC. *Structure, Regulation, and Expression of the Human Serotonin Transporter Gene [Doctoral dissertation].* [thesis]. Atlanta, GA: Anatomy and Cell Biology, Emory University; 1998.
52. Ramamoorthy S. *Regulation of monoamine transporters: Regulated phosphorylation, dephosphorylation, and trafficking.* Totowa, NJ: Humana Press Inc; 2002.
53. Wakade AR, Wakade TD, Poosch M, Bannon MJ. Noradrenaline transport and transporter mRNA of rat chromaffin cells are controlled by dexamethasone and nerve growth factor. *J Physiol.* 1996;494:67-75.
54. Figlewicz DP, Szot P, Israel PA, Payne C, Dorsa DM. Insulin reduces norepinephrine transporter mRNA in vivo in rat locus coeruleus. *Brain Res.* 1993;602:161-164.
55. Meyer JS, Shearman LP, Collins LM. Monoamine transporters and the neurobehavioral teratology of cocaine. *Pharmacol Biochem Behav.* 1996;55:585-593.
56. Ikeda T, Kitayama S, Morita K, Dohi T. Nerve growth factor down-regulates the expression of norepinephrine transporter in rat pheochromocytoma (PC12) cells. *Brain Res Mol Brain Res.* 2001;86:90-100.
57. Fang Y, Ronnekleiv OK. Cocaine upregulates the dopamine transporter in fetal rhesus monkey brain. *J Neurosci.* 1999;19:8966-8978.
58. Shearman LP, Meyer JS. Cocaine up-regulates norepinephrine transporter binding in the rat placenta. *Eur J Pharmacol.* 1999;386:1-6.

59. Macey DJ, Smith HR, Nader MA, Porrino LJ. Chronic cocaine self-administration upregulates the norepinephrine transporter and alters functional activity in the bed nucleus of the stria terminalis of the rhesus monkey. *J Neurosci.* 2003;23:12-16.
60. Li LB, Chen N, Ramamoorthy S, et al. The role of N-glycosylation in function and surface trafficking of the human dopamine transporter. *J Biol Chem.* 2004;279:21012-21020.
61. Vaughan RA, Huff RA, Uhl GR, Kuhar MJ. Protein kinase C-mediated phosphorylation and functional regulation of dopamine transporters in striatal synaptosomes. *J Biol Chem.* 1997;272:15541-15546.
62. Ramamoorthy S, Giovanetti E, Qian Y, Blakely RD. Phosphorylation and regulation of antidepressant-sensitive serotonin transporters. *J Biol Chem.* 1998;273:2458-2466.
63. Jayanthi LD, Samuvel DJ, Ramamoorthy S. Regulated internalization and phosphorylation of the native norepinephrine transporter in response to phorbol esters: evidence for localization in lipid rafts and lipid raft mediated internalization. *J Biol Chem.* 2004;279:19315-19326.
64. Apparsundaram S, Galli A, DeFelice LJ, Hartzell HC, Blakely RD. Acute regulation of norepinephrine transport. I. PKC-linked muscarinic receptors influence transport capacity and transporter density in SK-N-SH cells. *J Pharmacol Exp Ther.* 1998;287:733-743.
65. Apparsundaram S, Schroeter S, Blakely RD. Acute regulation of norepinephrine transport. II. PKC-modulated surface expression of human norepinephrine transporter proteins. *J Pharmacol Exp Ther.* 1998;287:744-751.
66. Bauman AL, Apparsundaram S, Ramamoorthy S, Wadzinski BE, Vaughan RA, Blakely RD. Cocaine and antidepressant-sensitive biogenic amine transporters exist in regulated complexes with protein phosphatase 2A. *J Neurosci.* 2000;20:7571-7578.
67. Qian Y, Galli A, Ramamoorthy S, Risso S, DeFelice LJ, Blakely RD. Protein kinase C activation regulates human serotonin transporters in HEK-293 cells via altered cell surface expression. *J Neurosci.* 1997;17:45-57.
68. Kitayama S, Dohi T, Uhl G. Phorbol esters alter functions of the expressed dopamine transporter. *Eur J Pharmacol.* 1994;268:115-119.
69. Zhang L, Coffey LL, Reith MEA. Regulation of the functional activity of the human dopamine transporter by protein kinase C. *Biochem Pharmacol.* 1997;53:677-688.
70. Daniels G, Amara SG. Regulation trafficking of the human dopamine transporter clathrin-mediated internalization and lysosomal degradation in response to phorbol esters. *J Biol Chem.* 1999;274:35794-35801.
71. Melikian HE, Buckley KM. Membrane trafficking regulates the activity of the human dopamine transporter. *J Neurosci.* 1999;19:7699-7710.
72. Loder MK, Melikian HE. The dopamine transporter constitutively internalizes and recycles in a protein kinase C-regulated manner in stably transfected PC12 cell lines. *J Biol Chem.* 2003;278:22168-22174.
73. Sorkina T, Hoover BR, Zahniser NR, Sorkin A. Constitutive and protein kinase C-induced internalization of the dopamine transporter is mediated by a clathrin-dependent mechanism. *Traffic.* 2005;6:157-170.
74. Holton KL, Loder MK, Melikian HE. Nonclassical, distinct endocytic signals dictate constitutive and PKC-regulated neurotransmitter transporter internalization. *Nat Neurosci.* 2005;8:881-888.
75. Samuvel DJ, Jayanthi LD, Bhat NR, Ramamoorthy S. A role for p38 mitogen-activated protein kinase in the regulation of the serotonin transporter: evidence for distinct cellular mechanisms involved in transporter surface expression. *J Neurosci.* 2005;25:29-41.
76. Ramamoorthy S, Prasa PD, Kulanthaivel P, Leibach FH, Blakely RD, Ganapathy V. Expression of a cocaine-sensitive norepinephrine transporter in the human placental syncitiotrophoblast. *Biochemistry.* 1993;32:1346-1353.
77. Ramamoorthy JD, Ramamoorthy S, Leibach FH, Ganapathy V. Human placental monoamine transporters as targets for amphetamines. *Am J Obstet Gynecol.* 1995;173:1782-1787.
78. Jayanthi LD, Prasad PD, Ramamoorthy S, Mahesh VB, Leibach FH, Ganapathy V. Sodium- and chloride-dependent, cocaine-sensitive, high-affinity binding of nisoxetine to the human placental norepinephrine transporter. *Biochemistry.* 1993;32:12178-12185.

79. Chamberlain LH, Gould GW. The vesicle- and target-SNARE proteins that mediate Glut4 vesicle fusion are localized in detergent-insoluble lipid rafts present on distinct intracellular membranes. *J Biol Chem*. 2002;277:49750-49754.
80. Simons K, Toomre D. Lipid rafts and signal transduction. *Nat Rev Mol Cell Biol*. 2000;1:31-39.
81. Simons K, Ikonen E. Functional rafts in cell membranes. *Nature*. 1997;387:569-572.
82. Parton RG, Richards AA. Lipid rafts and caveolae as portals for endocytosis: new insights and common mechanisms. *Traffic*. 2003;4:724-738.
83. Apparsundaram S, Sung U, Price RD, Blakely RD. Trafficking-dependent and -independent pathways of neurotransmitter transporter regulation differentially involving p38 mitogen-activated protein kinase revealed in studies of insulin modulation of norepinephrine transport in SK-N-SH cells. *J Pharmacol Exp Ther*. 2001;299:666-677.
84. Carvelli L, Moron JA, Kahlig KM, et al. PI 3-kinase regulation of dopamine uptake. *J Neurochem*. 2002;81:859-869.
85. Moron JA, Zakharova I, Ferrer JV, et al. Mitogen-activated protein kinase regulates dopamine transporter surface expression and dopamine transport capacity. *J Neurosci*. 2003;23:8480-8488.
86. Zhu CB, Hewlett WA, Feoktistov I, Biaggioni I, Blakely RD. Adenosine receptor, protein kinase G, and p38 mitogen-activated protein kinase-dependent up-regulation of serotonin transporters involves both transporter trafficking and activation. *Mol Pharmacol*. 2004;65:1462-1474.
87. Chaouloff F, Berton O, Mormede P. Serotonin and stress. *Neuropsychopharmacology*. 1999;21:28S-32S.
88. Miller KJ, Hoffman BJ. Adenosine A$_3$ receptors regulate serotonin transport via nitric oxide and cGMP. *J Biol Chem*. 1994;269:27351-27356.
89. Huff RA, Vaughan RA, Kuhar MJ, Uhl GR. Phorbol esters increase dopamine transporter phosphorylation and decrease transport V$_{max}$. *J Neurochem*. 1997;68:225-232.
90. Ramamoorthy S, Blakely RD. Phosphorylation and sequestration of serotonin transporters differentially modulated by psychostimulants. *Science*. 1999;285:763-766.
91. Foster JD, Pananusorn B, Vaughan RA. Dopamine transporters are phosphorylated on N-terminal serines in rat striatum. *J Biol Chem*. 2002;277:25178-25186.
92. Bonisch H, Hammermann R, Bruss M. Role of protein kinase C and second messengers in regulation of the norepinephrine transporter. *Adv Pharmacol*. 1998;42:183-186.
93. Whitworth TL, Quick MW. Upregulation of gamma-aminobutyric acid transporter expression: role of alkylated gamma-aminobutyric acid derivatives. *Biochem Soc Trans*. 2001;29:736-741.
94. Granas C, Ferrer J, Loland CJ, Javitch JA, Gether U. N-terminal truncation of the dopamine transporter abolishes phorbol ester- and substance P receptor-stimulated phosphorylation without impairing transporter internalization. *J Biol Chem*. 2003;278:4990-5000.
95. Lin Z, Zhang PW, Zhu X, et al. Phosphatidylinositol 3-kinase, protein kinase C, and MEK1/2 kinase regulation of dopamine transporters (DAT) require N-terminal DAT phosphoacceptor sites. *J Biol Chem*. 2003;278:20162-20170.
96. Doolen S, Zahniser NR. Protein tyrosine kinase inhibitors alter human dopamine transporter activity in Xenopus oocytes. *J Pharmacol Exp Ther*. 2001;296:931-938.
97. Law RM, Stafford A, Quick MW. Functional regulation of gamma-aminobutyric acid transporters by direct tyrosine phosphorylation. *J Biol Chem*. 2000;275:23986-23991.
98. Whitworth TL, Quick MW. Substrate-induced regulation of gamma-aminobutyric acid transporter trafficking requires tyrosine phosphorylation. *J Biol Chem*. 2001; 276:42932-42937.
99. Quick MW, Hu J, Wang D, Zhang HY. Regulation of a gamma-aminobutyric acid transporter by reciprocal tyrosine and serine phosphorylation. *J Biol Chem*. 2004;279:15961-15967.
100. Sung U, Apparsundaram S, Galli A, et al. A regulated interaction of syntaxin 1A with the antidepressant-sensitive norepinephrine transporter establishes catecholamine clearance capacity. *J Neurosci*. 2003;23:1697-1709.
101. Bauman PA, Blakely RD. Determinants within the C-terminus of the human norepinephrine transporter dictate transporter trafficking, stability, and activity. *Arch Biochem Biophys*. 2002;404:80-91.
102. Uhl GR, Lin Z. The top 20 dopamine transporter mutants: structure-function relationships and cocaine actions. *Eur J Pharmacol*. 2003;479:71-82.

103. Goldberg NR, Beuming T, Soyer OS, Goldstein RA, Weinstein H, Javitch JA. Probing conformational changes in neurotransmitter transporters: a structural context. *Eur J Pharmacol.* 2003;479:3-12.
104. Loland CJ, Granas C, Javitch JA, Gether U. Identification of intracellular residues in the dopamine transporter critical for regulation of transporter conformation and cocaine binding. *J Biol Chem.* 2004;279:3228-3238.
105. Fornes A, Nunez E, Aragon C, Lopez-Corcuera B. The second intracellular loop of the glycine transporter 2 contains crucial residues for glycine transport and phorbol ester-induced regulation. *J Biol Chem.* 2004;279:22934-22943.
106. Deken SL, Beckman ML, Boos L, Quick MW. Transport rates of GABA transporters: regulation by the N-terminal domain and syntaxin 1A. *Nat Neurosci.* 2000;3:998-1003.
107. Horton N, Quick MW. Syntaxin 1A up-regulates GABA transporter expression by subcellular redistribution. *Mol Membr Biol.* 2001;18:39-44.
108. Wang D, Deken SL, Whitworth TL, Quick MW. Syntaxin 1A inhibits GABA flux, efflux, and exchange mediated by the rat brain GABA transporter GAT1. *Mol Pharmacol.* 2003;64:905-913.
109. Haase J, Killian AM, Magnani F, Williams C. Regulation of the serotonin transporter by interacting proteins. *Biochem Soc Trans.* 2001;29:722-728.
110. Torres GE, Yao WD, Mohn AR, et al. Functional interaction between monoamine plasma membrane transporters and the synaptic PDZ domain-containing protein PICK1. *Neuron.* 2001;30:121-134.
111. Lee FJ, Liu F, Pristupa ZB, Niznik HB. Direct binding and functional coupling of alpha-synuclein to the dopamine transporters accelerate dopamine-induced apoptosis. *FASEB J.* 2001;15:916-926.
112. Polymeropoulos MH, Lavedan C, Leroy E, et al. Mutation in the a-synuclein gene identified in families with Parkinson's disease. *Science.* 1997;276:2045-2047.
113. Wersinger C, Vernier P, Sidhu A. Trypsin disrupts the trafficking of the human dopamine transporter by alpha-synuclein and its A30P mutant. *Biochemistry.* 2004;43:1242-1253.
114. Carneiro AM, Ingram SL, Beaulieu JM, et al. The multiple LIM domain-containing adaptor protein Hic-5 synaptically colocalizes with the dopamine transporter. *J Neurosci.* 2002;22:7045-7054.
115. Saunders C, Ferrer JV, Shi L, et al. Amphetamine-induced loss of human dopamine transporter activity: an internalization-dependent and cocaine-sensitive mechanism. *Proc Natl Acad Sci USA.* 2000;97:6850-6855.
116. Daws LC, Callaghan PD, Moron JA, et al. Cocaine increases dopamine uptake and cell surface expression of dopamine transporters. *Biochem Biophys Res Commun.* 2002;290:1545-1550.
117. Little KY, Elmer LW, Zhong H, Scheys JO, Zhang L. Cocaine induction of dopamine transporter trafficking to the plasma membrane. *Mol Pharmacol.* 2002;61:436-445.
118. Bernstein EM, Quick MW. Regulation of gamma-aminobutyric acid (GABA) transporters by extracellular GABA. *J Biol Chem.* 1999;274:889-895.
119. Munir M, Correale DM, Robinson MB. Substrate-induced up-regulation of Na(+)-dependent glutamate transport activity. *Neurochem Int.* 2000;37:147-162.
120. Quick MW. Substrates regulate gamma-aminobutyric acid transporters in a syntaxin 1A-dependent manner. *Proc Natl Acad Sci USA.* 2002;99:5686-5691.
121. Hahn MK, Mazei-Robison M, Blakely RD. Single nucleotide polymorphisms in the human norepinephrine transporter gene impact expression, trafficking, antidepressant interaction and protein kinase C regulation. *Mol Pharmacol.* 2005;68:457-466.
122. Prasad HC, Zhu C, McCauley JL, et al. Human serotonin transporter variants display selective insensitivity to protein kinase G and p38 mitogen activated kinase. *Proc Natl Acad Sci USA.* 2005;102:11545-11550.

Chapter 17
Hallucinogen Actions on 5-HT Receptors Reveal Distinct Mechanisms of Activation and Signaling by G Protein-Coupled Receptors

Harel Weinstein[1]

Abstract We review the effect of some key advances in the characterization of molecular mechanisms of signaling by G protein-coupled receptors (GPCRs) on our current understanding of mechanisms of drugs of abuse. These advances are illustrated by results from our ongoing work on the actions of hallucinogens on serotonin (5-HT) receptors. We show how a combined computational and experimental approach can reveal specific modes of receptor activation underlying the difference in properties of hallucinogens compared with nonhallucinogenic congeners. These modes of activation—that can produce distinct ligand-dependent receptor states—are identified in terms of structural motifs (SM) in molecular models of the receptors, which were shown to constitute conserved functional microdomains (FM). The role of several SM/FMs in the activation mechanism of the GPCRs is presented in detail to illustrate how this mechanism can lead to ligand-dependent modes of signaling by the receptors. Novel bioinformatics tools are described that were designed to support the quantitative mathematical modeling of ligand-specific signaling pathways activated by the 5-HT receptors targeted by hallucinogens. The approaches for mathematical modeling of signaling pathways activated by 5-HT receptors are described briefly in the context of ongoing work on detailed biochemical models of 5-HT2A, and combined 5-HT2A/ 5-HT1A, receptor-mediated activation of the MAPK 1,2 pathway. The continuing need for increasingly more realistic representation of signaling in dynamic compartments within the cell, endowed with spatio-temporal characteristics obtained from experiment, is emphasized. Such developments are essential for attaining a quantitative understanding of how the multiple functions of a cell are coordinated and regulated, and to evaluate the specifics of the perturbations caused by the drugs of abuse that target GPCRs.

Keywords molecular modeling, molecular dynamics simulations, membrane proteins, signaling, mathematical modeling, bioinformatics tools

[1] Department of Physiology and Biophysics, and Institute for Computational Biomedicine, Weill Medical College of Cornell University, New York, NY 10021

Corresponding Author: Harel Weinstein, Department of Physiology and Biophysics, Box 75, Weill Medical College of Cornell University, 1300 York Avenue, New York, NY 10021 Tel: (212) 746-6358; Fax: (212) 746-8690; E-mail: haw2002@med.cornell.edu

Introduction

The rapid advances in the characterization of molecular mechanisms of signaling by G protein-coupled receptors (GPCRs) have enhanced the understanding of mechanisms of drugs of abuse. In particular, the recognition that the translation of intra-receptor mechanisms of activation into intracellular signaling through protein-protein interactions can take diverse forms that are ligand–dependent, is beginning to explain the special properties exhibited by drugs of abuse targeting this type of receptors. This relation is illustrated here by recent results from our ongoing work on the actions of hallucinogens on serotonin receptors, which are members of the rhodopsin-like GPCR family. The findings are reviewed briefly in the context of broader advances in understanding GPCR signaling to clarify the effect on the emerging understanding of cellular mechanisms of the hallucinogenic drugs of abuse that target these receptors.

A very recent review of the structures, pharmacology, and neurophysiology of hallucinogens provides a thorough and thoughtful analysis of the current information and understanding regarding the mechanisms underlying hallucinogen action.[1] The review illustrates as well how many of the fundamental questions regarding these mechanisms remain unanswered, despite the abundance of information available in the literature from work at all the levels accessible to physiological, pharmacological, and behavioral approaches. The understanding of the involvement of the 5-HT2 receptors targeted by the hallucinogens in these mechanisms, and the molecular and structural requirements for the function of these GPCRs in cellular signaling, are equally incomplete.

To change this situation, we have undertaken a coordinated collaborative effort that brings together experimental and computational approaches. The research effort is supported by the National Institute on Drug Abuse (Bethesda, MD) and combines quantitative computational and experimental approaches in the mechanistic investigation of hallucinogenic drug action of compounds in various structural classes including (1) indolealkylamines (eg, the hallucinogenic N,N-dimethyltryptamine); (2) ergolines (eg, D-LSD); and (3) phenylethylamines and phenylisopropylamines (eg, mescaline, DOI) (for reviews see Nichols,[1] Gresch et al,[2] and Aghajanian and Marek[3]) In the portion of this multifaceted work that is reviewed briefly below, we emphasize the information elicited from the computational modeling and simulations of mechanisms that can discriminate the actions of hallucinogens on the GPCRs in comparison to activation by nonhallucinogenic congeners. The aim of this quantitative modeling is to reveal the molecular details of the manner in which the hallucinogens trigger the mechanistically related subcellular elements that are responsible for their special properties. This type of information is tested, validated, and enhanced by the experimental component of the complete research program, and the insights are directed as well to the design of appropriate therapeutic measures.

The computational structure-function studies and simulation approaches use 3-dimensional (3-D) models of the receptor molecules and their interactions with ligands. Specific structure-based approaches have evolved for this purpose.[4,5] To enable the study of downstream signaling following ligand-receptor interaction, we have also elaborated larger scale models of GPCR functional entities, ranging from models of GPCR oligomerization,[6-8] to macromolecular interaction complexes with scaffolding proteins such as PDZ domains.[9-11] In addition, the newest type of investigation of hallucinogen mechanisms briefly described here aims to integrate the inferences and insights resulting from the studies at the discrete molecular level, into quantitative mechanistic models of signaling pathways in the cell.[12-15] Such an integrative approach is especially advantageous for the type of multi-disciplinary studies required to understand the mechanisms of drugs of abuse, because the computational studies must be combined with experimental efforts that are performed at several levels of organization (or "scales"). These scales cover the range from molecular and cellular aspects (eg, of signaling by hallucinogens and other ligands of the 5-HT receptors) to the integrated neurophysiological level, and whole animal behavior (eg, see range covered in[16-21]). The power of the integrative approach lies in the ability to address complete functional systems in which the effects of drugs of abuse are expressed. Examples of such whole systems that can now be modeled and understood quantitatively are the cellular signaling pathways and networks. This is made possible by new data management tools and computational approaches developed by us and others.[13-15] The quantitative modeling of signaling mechanisms can generate new mechanistic hypotheses that are suitable for experimental verification at the integrated system level (cell, tissue, organ) that is most pertinent to drug action. Our work discussed below provides specific illustrations of the success of such closely considered interactions and synergy between computational developments and experimental probing of the receptor systems (the combined approach).

The Synergy Between the Computational Modeling and Experimentation

Briefly summarized, the combined approach comprises the following stages:

1. 3-D constructs of molecular models are developed[4,22] and probed computationally in simulations of mutagenesis and structural perturbation,[23] in order to address characteristics of different states of the receptor molecules that relate to activation,[18] including oligomerization.[7,8]
2. The 3-D models serve in computational simulations of functional mechanisms involving structural rearrangements (eg, ligand-induced), or interactions in the signaling cascade, such as

   - dimerization,[7,8]
   - involvement in specific interactions with adaptor proteins such as PDZ-domains,[10,11] and
   - triggering of signaling pathways.[15]

These computational studies generate and/or probe mechanistic hypotheses regarding structural changes involved in the various states of the receptors and their signaling properties, for both wild type (WT) and mutant constructs. They are discussed in the subsequent section in light of the results from the cognate experimental studies in step (3) of the combined approach.

3. The activity of the corresponding constructs is measured in a variety of assays, including

- evaluation of pharmacological properties[23] and degrees of constitutive activity of the GPCRs defined by various measurable end points,[18,24]
- measurement of nature and extent of dimerization established in experiments ranging from co-IP to cross-linking, and including FRET/BRET, etc,[25-29]
- characterization of ligand-specific signaling pathways,[19] and
- creation of transgenic animals bearing the constructs to identify behavioral consequences.[20,30]

Recent progress in the development and application of the combined computational and experimental protocol is illustrated in the following sections for (1) intramolecular mechanisms triggering differential modes of ligand-dependent activation of GPCRs, and (2) the management of quantitative signaling data for modeling of cellular signaling pathways.

Intramolecular Mechanisms of Ligand-dependent Receptor Activation

Structural Motifs Acting as Functional Microdomains in G Protein-coupled Receptors

A key element in the development of a structure-based insight about the intramolecular mechanisms of ligand-dependent GPCR activation was our early observation that it is possible to parse the receptor structure into specific regions identified as structural motifs (SM) acting as (often conserved) functional microdomains (FM) (SM/FMs). Especially noteworthy here is that the crystal structure of rhodopsin confirmed the structural predictions regarding the key SM/FM that we obtained from the molecular models, and the functional properties of the SM/FMs we defined coincided with inferences from the crystal structure and were in agreement with the mechanisms suggested from molecular modeling and simulations of GPCRs in the rhodopsin-like family.[5,31]

The identification of conserved motifs in the structures of rhodopsin-like GPCRs that create microenvironments with special importance for the function of the receptor was an early consequence of the model-informed studies we undertook in the collaborative effort with several experimental laboratories. These motifs were shown to be sufficiently conserved in structure and function to merit a specific designation, and therefore we described them as SM/FMs in several different GPCRs.[5,17,18,24,32-34] The SM/FMs include, for example, the "ionic lock of the arginine cage", which we described in these publications and has subsequently been confirmed for many other GPCRs.[35-44]

The NPxxY motif conserved in TM7 of the rhodopsin-like GPCRs (including the 5-HT2 subtypes) is an SM/FM involved in receptor activation mechanisms, as demonstrated by our recent findings of the "locked-on" phenotype regulated through this motif.[18] Figure 17.1 summarizes some of the findings illustrating the effects of agonists and inverse agonists on the activity of the WT receptor, compared with one of the constitutively active constructs (Y7.53C) and the "locked-on" mutant Y7.53N. (Note the high basal activity of the mutants and the ability of the inverse agonists to reduce it for the Y7.53C, but not Y7.53N construct). Of importance, we showed through the identification of a "revertant" mutant phenotype[18] that this SM/FM connects to Helix 8 of the GPCRs. This connection through the direct interaction of residues at positions 7.53 and 7.60 is highlighted schematically in Fig.17.2 using representations of the rhodopsin structure.[45-49] The direct interaction of the NPxxY motif with Helix 8 is likely to be very significant in regulating the interactions of the C-terminal end of the GPCRs with various other cellular components involved in signaling (eg, the PDZ domains[10,22]). Like the other SM/FM we described, the functional properties of the NPxxY motif have been validated in other receptors as well,[50] including Rhodopsin.[49]

Another key SM/FM motif, which we were the first to identify as being involved in GPCR activation, triggers the regulation of the "ionic lock" through a series of specific structural rearrangements in the upper (more extracellular) end of the

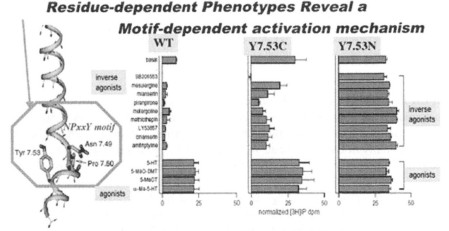

Conserved Helix 7 Tyrosine Acts as a Multistate Conformational Switch in the 5-HT2C Receptor: Identification of a Novel "Locked-on" Phenotype and Double Revertant Mutations"
C. Prioleau, I.Visiers, B.J. Ebersole, H. Weinstein and S.C. Sealfon-
JBC 2002, 277:36577-36584

Fig. 17.1 Data illustrating the functional role of Y7.53 in the NPxxY motif: Different activated states of the 5-HT2C receptors are produced by mutations at the 7.53 locus. The Y7.53C mutation produces a canonical constitutively activated phenotype, characterized by increased basal activity compared with WT, reduction of the basal activity by various inverse agonists, and activation by various agonists. In contrast, the constitutive activity of the Y7.53N mutant is shown to be irreversible (by any of the inverse agonists), and various agonists are unable to activate further the receptor, which appears locked in an "on" state.

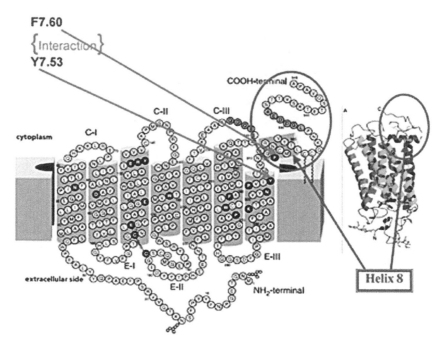

Fig. 17.2 The protein-protein interaction interface between a GPCR and its signaling environment is regulated by intramolecular interactions involving the NPxxY motif: The interaction between Y7.53 and the F7.60, which is in Hx8, controls the position of the helix and the C-terminal. This can regulate the interaction interface between the GPCRs and other proteins in the signaling cascade (eg, PDZ domains). The structural context is illustrated for the crystal structure of Rhodopsin.[45]

GPCR molecule. This SM/FM comprises the cluster of aromatic residues in TM6 surrounding the conserved Trp6.48, and straddling the conserved Pro6.50. [Note that we are using throughout the generic numbering system for GPCR residues defined initially in Ballesteros and Weinstein[51] and subsequently adopted widely in the relevant literature]. This motif, which in the 5-HT2A receptor comprises residues F6.44(332), W6.48(336), and F6.52(640) can vary somewhat in composition in different receptors, depending on the nature of the ligand. But these variations preserve the steric properties that can trigger the rearrangement of the other aromatic residues in the SM/FM in the manner of a "toggle switch"[4] that connects the ligand binding event to the rearrangements in the receptor structure leading to activation. The mechanism of activation, simulated in detail as reviewed by Visiers et al.[4] and Filizola et al.[5] explains the role of the central residue in the SM/FM W6.48, which was proposed much earlier by the Sakmar Lab (Lin and Sakmar[52]) to undergo a conformational rearrangement in the process of rhodopsin activation by light. The toggle switch mechanism of GPCR activation has now been incorporated in current accepted views of rhodopsin-like receptor function.[5,31,35-39,43,44,53-57]

Of importance, the modeling suggested that the ability to trigger this toggle switch determines the efficacy of a ligand. Since the position of a ligand in the binding site should affect its interaction with the aromatic cluster, the ligands will differ in the extent to which they can affect the toggle switch. As described in the following section, we had shown that even ligands differing little in chemical structure can adopt different positions in the receptor binding pocket, so that this detailed modeling identifies a structural mechanism for ligand-dependent mode of receptor activation. Notably, in the 5-HT2AR model, the compounds with hallucinogenic properties appear to adopt a very different position in the binding pocket compared with nonhallucinogenic congeners in the same family owing to the bulky substitutions of the cationic amine moiety in the hallucinogenic compounds, specifically 5-HT vs N,N-dimethyl congeners such as psylocin, or vs LSD.[23] While this is not likely to be the only source of difference in ligand-dependent conformations of the receptor produced by hallucinogens, it is a structurally explicit prototype for the concept of ligand-dependent functional selectivity.[58-61]

Hallucinogens and the Different Modes of G Protein-coupled Receptor Activation

The central working hypothesis that has emerged from our sustained investigation of the GPCR targets of hallucinogens attributes the hallucinogenic potential of certain compounds to the involvement of their structural elements in specific modes of interaction with the receptor, which produce distinct molecular mechanisms of receptor signaling. The hallucinogens are thus proposed to interact with the receptor molecules in a special manner that elicits, through these distinct interactions, a set of structural and dynamic receptor responses (including protein-protein interactions such as oligomerization, as well as selective PDZ-domain binding) that differ from those produced by other ligands, such as congeneric nonhallucinogens. This central hypothesis led to the investigation of discriminant factors responsible for the special properties underlying the effects of hallucinogenic drugs of abuse on the receptor molecules, and in particular those that result in triggering distinct signaling pathways. The discriminant actions of hallucinogens are of added interest because they can reveal generalizable concepts of ligand-specific receptor function,[60-62] and the inferences should be directly applicable to many other drugs of abuse mechanisms. The elements of these discriminant actions of the ligands on GPCRs include:

1. the modes of receptor response (conformational rearrangements and stabilization of activated states) responsible for protein-protein interactions ranging from oligomerization to interactions with scaffolding proteins (eg, PDZ domains), and
2. the relation to the selectivity and efficiency of signaling of (a) such conformational rearrangements, and (b) the resulting association/dissociation of protein-protein interactions (produced distinctively by the binding of this class of ligands).

Given the ability we developed to describe GPCR function in terms of SM/FMs, we sought first to reveal the distinct ligand-receptor interaction properties of such motifs. The involvement of the SM/FMs in giving rise to distinct receptor responses is emphasized by our findings discussed in the previous section, regarding the role of ligand orientation in the measurable receptor response. These insights emerged from modeling and computational simulations[16] involving the Ser3.36(159)Ala mutation in the 5-HT2AR. The results show that 5-HT2AR agonists that have unmodified cationic amine side chains interact with S3.36 in TM3, whereas those with substituted amines—such as the tryptamine-based hallucinogens Psylocin and N,N-dimethyl-tryptamine—are prevented from this interaction by steric repulsion. Surprisingly, this slight difference in mode of binding and orientation in the binding pocket was found experimentally (in the collaboration with the lab of Stuart Sealfon, Mount Sinai School of Medicine) to create significant differences in the pharmacological efficacy (relative to 5-HT). Similarly, alkyl substitution of the indole N1-amine in 5-HT and congeners (including LSD), which interacts with Ser5.46, reduced efficacy more markedly at the WT than at the Ser5.46Ala mutant receptor. Computational modeling of binding pocket interactions of ligands with WT and mutant-receptor constructs demonstrated how the Ser3.36 and Ser5.46 interactions serve to modify the agonist's favored position in the binding pocket. This provides a striking illustration of differential modes of binding leading to differential outcomes of receptor activation by ligands that exhibit only slight structural differences and constitutes a fundamental new realization in our understanding of GPCR function.

The definition of the SM/FMs provided a specific structural context for the functional implications of ligand-dependent modes of receptor activation. Thus, using the combined approach of experiment and simulation we showed how the differential ligand positioning by one of the binding pocket components, is "sensed" by yet another SM/FM—the aromatic cluster in TM6[63] that functions as the toggle switch described in the preceding section. The dynamics of the local rearrangements in the structure of the aromatic cluster, which can be triggered by ligand binding in the pocket and interaction with the F6.52 sensor, were probed with computational simulations in a 3-D model of the serotonin 5HT2AR.[4,5] The computed rearrangement of the aromatic cluster[64] in response to ligand binding, and the subsequent conformational change induced at the P6.50 kink, are the likely trigger for the transition from the inactive form to the active state of the receptor. The quantitative simulation details[4,65] support the hypothesis that the position of the agonist in the receptor is influenced by specific interactions in TMs3 and 5 and determines the degree of receptor activation by agonist through the conformational rearrangement mechanism involving the SM/FM in TM6. This coupling of SM/FM-mediated mechanism of ligand-specific receptor activation is central to understanding the manner in which drugs of abuse, such as the hallucinogens, acquire and express their special properties. Moreover, such mechanistic inferences have recently been shown to explain findings in other GPCRs[54,55,66] including those targeted by other drugs of abuse, such as the cannabinoids.[67]

Dynamic Elements of G Protein-coupled Receptor Signaling Mechanisms: New Insights and Methodological Imperatives for Their Investigation

Computational modeling studies seeking mechanistic insight into signaling components from quantitative simulations require reliable structural models of the receptors. For most, albeit not all, studies, these models must include responsibly constructed and appropriately modeled loops connecting the transmembrane (TM) segments. In a previous study,[68] we discussed the basis for this latter conclusion regarding the loops. The essential role for a rigorous representation of the loops was illustrated as well by results from our earlier work on the second intracellular loop (IL2) in the 5-HT2CR.[69] The study was performed to gain insight into the specific role of the intracellular loop segment following the conserved ArgAspTyr (DRY) motif and the "arginine cage" SM/FM in TM3 (see *Structural Motifs Acting as Functional Microdomains in GPCRs*). Specifically, we addressed the functional consequences of the surprising process of RNA editing discovered for the 5-HT2C receptor gene.[70,71] These adenosine-to-inosine RNA editing events for 5HT2C receptors were shown to result in sequence alterations at positions 156, 158, and 160 in the IL2 region. The edited receptor isoforms were shown to exhibit various extents of changes in their pharmacological and physiological phenotypes. To identify the molecular mechanism of these pharmacological effects of editing, we explored the conformational properties of the edited IL2 in comparison with the unedited construct, using an early form of our loop-structure-prediction methodology (we subsequently described an even more powerful and accurate version of the method[72,73]).

The calculations showed that a modification of a small element in the sequence (ie, a change from the unedited sequence **I[156]RN[158]PI[160]EHSRFN** [termed **INI**] to **VRGPVEHSRFN** [termed **VGV**]) causes a significant change in the preferred conformational orientation of the loop. A direct result is a significant change in the interaction surface of the 5-HT2C receptor with the cognate G-protein.[69] The quantitative analysis showed that parallel changes in the observed pharmacological properties of the modified (**VGV**) receptors are attributable directly to the effect that this change in the interaction surface has on the formation of the GPCR signaling complex with G-proteins.

The major lesson from these results was the high sensitivity of the signaling system to even relatively small changes in the interaction surface presented to other intracellular loops, and/or the G-protein. They highlight the relation between intramolecular rearrangements caused by ligand-induced activation of the GPCRs, and the manner in which the activation signal is propagated. Specifically, the structural consequences of ligand binding determine the mode of protein-protein interactions along the signaling cascade of the receptors. The regulation of such GPCR-signaling protein interaction surfaces by ligand-related structural changes in the receptor molecule, such as those illustrated above for the NPxxY motif (see Fig. 17.2), continues to be the subject of intensive studies in our laboratory.

The importance of the dynamic structural changes in the mechanisms of ligand-dependent GPCR activation points to important methodological conclusions concerning the appropriate approaches to modeling of detailed molecular mechanisms of GPCRs. In particular, the immediate environment of the receptor has emerged as an essential element in the representation and correct modeling of GPCRs for computational simulations (see Fig. 17.3). To achieve reliable results, the molecular models of the receptor structures used in computational simulations have to be complete and must include (1) the TM-connecting loops, constructed with appropriate structure-prediction methods and calculated explicitly,[65,68,72] and (2) the complex environment of the molecular system composed of protein/ligand/waters (ie, bulk water and the phospholipid bilayer).[68] Such molecular constructs (Fig. 17.3) are then suitable for the examination of interactions of various ligands from the results of extensive simulations of ligand-receptor complexes with the monomeric receptor structures, challenged by perturbations and control experiments. Clearly, any attempt to understand the mechanisms and effects of GPCR dimerization must take into account the environment. For discrete molecular representations of the membrane environment, it is necessary to carry out careful calibrations of the model.[74] Based on the evidence that rhodopsin reconstituted in artificial membranes is functional,[75] we use a hydrated patch of 1-Palmitoyl-2-oleoyl-*sn*-glycero-3-phosphocholine (POPC) lipid bilayer membrane to simulate the appropriate environment for receptor dimers. The size of a lipid unit cell that could accommodate a receptor dimer was calibrated with the dimer configuration with TM4 and TM5 at the interface recently proposed for rhodopsin,[76] which includes both TMs and loops regions. Our studies[74,77,78] have shown the appropriate distance between the solute protein

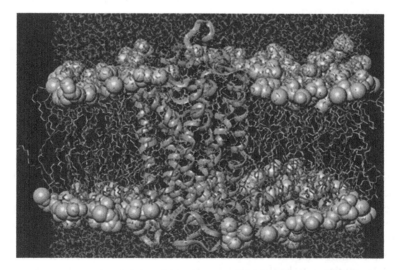

Fig. 17.3 Molecular model of the complete GPCR (rhodopsin) in an atomistic representation of its environment. (*See* also Color Insert).

and a simulation box boundary to correspond to ~4 to 5 layers of lipid molecules. According to this criterion, the unit cell was generated by duplicating and truncating a fully equilibrated POPC patch.[79] Based on the average size of a rhodopsin dimer (85 × 50 Å), as calculated from the oligomeric complex (PDB ID code: 1N3M), an orthorhombic lipid unit cell was selected for such studies, with a = 160 Å, b = 124 Å, and c = 98 Å. Pre-equilibrated water molecules were added at the edges of both lipid patches in the direction of the membrane normal, resulting in a system with 640 lipid molecules and 36 836 water molecules, for a total of 143 788 atoms (with the Rhodopsin dimer in this equilibrated POPC bilayer unit cell, the system size went up to 148 252 atoms).

The equilibration of the POPC bilayer unit cell using GROMACS with lipid parameters[80] and simple point charge (SPC) water model was performed after energy minimization in several cycles of steepest descent followed by conjugate gradient (converged at 100 kJ•mol^{-1}•nm^{-1}). These simulations are performed with semi-isotropic coupling, with the pressure, at 1.0 bar, coupled separately to the xy plane and z directions. Temperature is controlled with the weak coupling scheme of Berendsen, coupling each phase of lipid and water separately with a 310 K bath. The particle mesh Ewald (PME) summation algorithm is applied, with interpolation order set to 6 and maximum grid spacing for the fast Fourier transform (FFT) set to 0.12 nm. The Coulomb cut-off, and cut-off for the short-range neighbor list were both set to 0.9 nm, and a 1.2-nm Lennard-Jones cut-off was applied. The size of the system caused the potential energy of the system to reach a stable plateau only after 1-nanosecond simulation time; the converged area of the xy plane per lipid (61.8 Å^2), and the deuterium order parameter profile taken over the last 1 nanosecond of the trajectory were both close to the experimentally determined values.[81]

In view of the complexity of the intramolecular rearrangements produced by distinct effects of various ligands, and the delicate balance of protein-protein interactions involved in the signal transduction mechanism by GPCRs, there can no longer be any doubt that the modeling of such systems must reach a high level of physical realism in order to be useful for structure-function studies, as discussed and illustrated specifically in Mehler et al.[68] Unfortunately, such methodological imperatives are all too often neglected in computational attempts to describe structure-function relations of GPCRs. Not surprisingly, this neglect leads invariably to disappointingly wrongheaded inferences that are evident in publications on this subject. Unfortunately, it is not always recognized immediately how erroneous some of the inferences can be if they are reached from such flawed studies. Thus, GPCR models with loops attached to the TM region using methods other than careful structure prediction (eg, from the often used spurious homologies with short segments that are fished randomly from the Protein Data Bank, or from the generation of loop segment structures using weak methods such as energy minimization) produce misleading models, which lead to incorrect conclusions about important mechanisms such as the involvement of loops in ligand binding, or oligomerization. Similarly, bad approaches to structure-function modeling of GPCRs include energy-based minimization and/or dynamics simulations that are mistakenly performed in vacuum (using any variety of fixed-value "dielectric constants"). For these membrane proteins, the approach is flawed, because by neglecting the 3 different phases in which the loops and TM region are imbedded, the structures are subjected to artifacts (eg, the interaction of polar residues from the loops), with side chains in the TM regions. This type of spurious interaction in vacuum would have been prevented by a correct representation of the environment composed of the lipid, phospholipids head groups, and the surrounding aqueous medium. In the absence of appropriate modeling of the environment, the loops "collapse" toward the TM region and produce unacceptable artifacts.

Modeling G Protein-coupled Receptor Activity at the Systems Level

Signaling pathways, such as those triggered into action by ligands binding to the GPCRs, constitute the fundamental mechanisms underlying cell physiology and its connection to the environment. In turn, these signaling pathways interact, and they are interconnected in the cell's signaling networks that provide the mechanisms of regulation for most cellular functions. Not surprisingly, signaling pathways, networks, and the underlying molecular mechanisms are the focus of intense current research that encompasses both experimental and theoretical studies.[12,13,82-85] To integrate the results of our studies on the receptor mechanisms of hallucinogens, with the current understanding of such signaling pathways, we are developing specialized computational tools, and quantitative models of signaling cascades triggered by receptor activation.

The "models of signaling pathways" discussed in this section are distinct from the molecular models of receptors and protein-protein complexes that were the subject of the previous sections. A useful definition of the signaling models states: "A model, in this language, is simply a collection of hypotheses and facts brought together in an attempt to understand the [cellular] phenomenon...the facts and hypotheses are composed of the molecular species and the biochemical or electrophysiological transformations that are presumed to underlie the cellular events."[13] Therefore, these models provide a formal framework for understanding the mechanisms underlying a particular event in the cell. The models consist of the molecular species participating in the event, and the mechanisms (eg, protein-protein interactions, phosphorylation reactions) and diffusion fluxes in a particular compartment of the cell. The quantitative elements comprise the concentrations, locations, interaction rates and transport kinetics of the molecules involved in the event (eg, signaling), and they relate the hypothesized mechanisms to quantitative physicochemical details.[12] The models are used in simulations in which the equations are solved as a function of time and initial conditions (see below, section Systems—Level Modeling and Simulation in the Study of Hallucinogen Mechanisms). The quantitative information from these simulations contains the time-dependent changes in concentrations of cell components, and the results of their interactions.

We have been able to undertake this work with the support from the Program for Developing Computational and Theoretical Models in Drug Abuse and Addiction at National Institute on Drug Abuse (NIDA).

SigPath—A Comprehensive Information Management System

The large amount of data used in the modeling effort, as well as the resulting models, must be managed and maintained in a transparent and readily accessible database. The existing examples of bioinformatics databases offer large amounts of information about the parts that constitute an integrated system; they usually specialize in one type of biological entity (eg, gene, transcript, protein, specific classes of proteins). However, the modeling goals prompted us to design a new type of information management system (IMS), the SigPath project. This offers a new type of bioinformatics tool that integrates resources and scientific themes (see detailed description in Campagne et al,[15] and at the Institute for Computational Biomedicine website. Moreover, SigPath, which is freely available over the Internet (**http://www.sigpath.org**) both as a Web application and as source code released under the GNU General Public License, connects traditional bioinformatics databases with modeling environments (ie, mathematical modeling and simulation tools, such as Virtual Cell[12,86,87]) and acts as a bridge between bioinformatics and computational cell biology resources. The system differs from traditional bioinformatics databases in the following ways: (1) it stores the level of quantitative information needed to support the creation of quantitative models; (2) it organizes information as connected graphs of strongly typed elements of information; (3) it focuses on allowing end-users to manage information directly—see scheme in Fig. 17.4.

The development of SigPath enables us to seek the mechanistic details of hallucinogen activities through the integrative approach that combines findings from computational and modeling studies of interactions among cellular components, with those obtained experimentally. This integration makes it necessary to combine different types of data and information, including structural (eg, mutant constructs) as well as quantitative data (eg, on the concentrations of the components, and their kinetic interaction constants). The example of the activation of the MAPK1,2 pathway by 5-HT2AR ligands, described in the subsequent section illustrates as well the nature of criteria and choices in the development of the SigPath ontology. Thus, when considering the example of cellular compartments, one option is to define the representation of these compartments as contiguous subregions of space. Formally, this data representation choice calls for coding spatial geometries, for instance, as a combination of elementary volume elements (eg, through union and intersection), or as the space enclosed within a surface. However, there is a current paucity of spatial data about 3-D subcellular geometries, and the Virtual Cell tool we used (see below) was designed to work with 2-D geometries (eg, as acquired with various microscopy methods). We plan to extend the SigPath ontology, so that intracellular and extracellular compartments where biological entities have been experimentally observed will be represented by

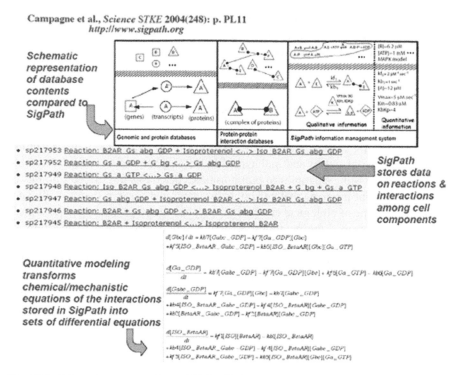

Fig. 17.4 Schematic representations of SigPath[15] characteristics: SigPath contents compared with traditional databases show the information management characteristics that include detailed reactions among the entries, as well as their quantitative parameters; the stored reaction information is illustrated, with specific identification numbers (sp-id of the form spxxxx, where x are running numbers) assigned by SigPath; the transformation of the reaction information into ODEs performed through transparent connections to mathematical modeling environments such as VirtualCell.[12]

the Compartment class (eg, membrane proteins that are produced in the ER, transfer to the Golgi and then to the plasma-membrane, can be described in this representation), and by the Localized Chemical class that positions the reagents in a specific cellular location (compartment or membrane). Reactions among molecules can then be represented in specific compartments or membranes, or across compartments in realistic 3-D representations that are based on experimental data from imaging at the appropriate level of detail.

Systems-level Modeling and Simulation in the Study of Hallucinogen Mechanisms

To reveal the discriminant features of the cellular mechanisms triggered by the hallucinogens' actions on the 5-HT2 receptors we studied, we must combine the mechanistic insights at the level of GPCR function, with the growing understanding of signal transduction pathways in the cells. In particular, the application of novel modeling approaches is needed to address the physiological consequences of the signal transduction processes as a series of intracellular interactions in the signal transduction pathways. To this end, we take advantage of bioinformatics tools[15] as described in the previous section, Sigpath—A Comprehensive Information Management System, and apply the accessible quantitative approaches for cell systems modeling (eg, see[12,13,86,88]) to study the structure-function relations of GPCRs in the context of their signaling pathways.

Understanding signal flow from the cell surface requires attention to the signaling events triggered at the receptors and propagated through protein-protein interactions. The schematic representation of a signaling pathway triggered by activation of the 5-HT2AR is shown in Fig. 17.5A. The involvement of the MAPK system in the signaling cascade linking the 5-HT2AR to PLA2 activation has been observed recently[89] and analyzed in comparison to other signaling modes.[90] As discussed in illuminating detail in a recent review by Nichols,[1] signaling of these receptors through Phospholypase C (PLC)[91-94] is complemented by apparently independent action in the PLA2 signaling cascade.[89,90,95] The importance of this pathway was emphasized in the review of hallucinogen mechanisms.[1] The exciting previous findings about the MAPK1,2 pathway from the Iyengar lab (Bhalla et al[96]) prompted a collaborative study focused on determining if simultaneous activation of the pathways activated through the 5HT1A and 5HT2A receptors leads to a switching of mitogen-activated protein kinase (MAPK 1,2). A schematic illustration of a possible way in which the signaling pathways triggered by activation of these 2 receptors could communicate in the activation of MAPK1,2 is given in Fig. 17.5B. As shown in the scheme, the putative interaction of the pathways to form a MAPK1,2 activation network triggered in combination by the 2 5-HT receptor subtypes is proposed to converge at phospholypaseC-bcta (PLCb). The possible intermediates involved in MAPK signaling are known to include PKC, Src and PI-3K, but the overall connectivity is strongly dependent on cell type, and the quantitative details of the signal flow through this pathway are not yet understood fully. In the collaborative studies with the Iyengar lab, Chiung-wen Chang has performed time course experiments of MAPK-1,2 phosphorylation in 2 cell lines, NIH3T3 and COS-7, transfected with 5-HT2A and 5-HT1A receptors individually and together. The preliminary results indicate that cotransfection of 5-HT2A and 5-HT1A receptors in COS-7 cells under stimulation of 5-MT (5-methyoxytryptamine), a general 5-HT1/5-HT2 agonist, produced prolonged activation of phospho-MAPK 1,2 compared with transfection with each of the receptors alone, but of a reduced magnitude. In NIH3T3 cells, prolonged activation of phospho-MAPK 1,2 was observed in cotransfected 5-HT2A and 5-HT1A receptors with treatment of a selective 5-HT2 agonist DOI ((+/−)-2,5-dimethoxy-4-iodoamphetamine), which has hallucinogenic properties and elicits the hallucinogen-specific transcriptome fingerprint.[19]

To simulate a detailed biochemical model of 5-HT2A receptor-mediated MAPK1,2 activation, biochemical parameters were obtained from the literature and computations were performed using Virtual Cell.[86,87] Briefly described, the quantitative modeling (simulation) procedure in Virtual Cell first converts the specified biochemical reaction steps into a system of ordinary differential equations (ODEs) and applies constraints related to mass conservation and pseudo steady-state

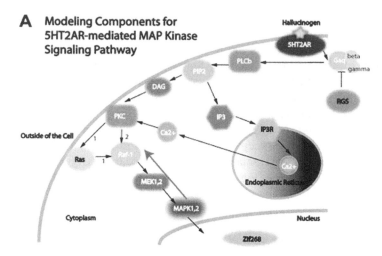

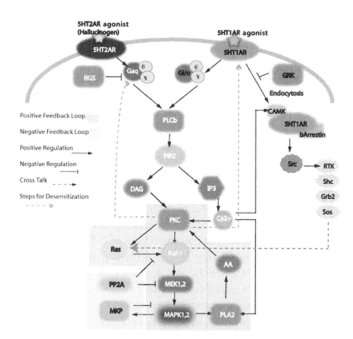

Fig. 17.5 Schematic representations of signaling pathways from 5-HT receptors to the MAPK system. (A) Signaling pathway triggered by activation of the 5-HT2A receptor coupled to Gαq; and (B) A putative combination of signaling pathways activated by ligand binding to both 5-HT2A and 5-HT1A receptors.

approximations, before applying numerical solvers to perform the simulations. The quantitative data stored in SigPath is converted automatically to systems of ODE, as illustrated schematically in Fig. 17.4, and conditions are imposed to solve these ODEs: (1) physical barriers are identified within the cellular system, such as the cell membrane, organelle membrane, etc; (2) the location of the reaction species is defined in each physical compartment; and (3) initial conditions are set for species concentrations and reactions, including the rate parameters. The results of the simulations are compared with data from measurements performed on control systems, or available in SigPath and the literature for cognate elements in other studied cell systems (cf[88,96-99]).

The main features of the results (not shown here) are in agreement with quantitative experimental data. Notably, the simulations serve to elucidate the role of the RGS proteins in regulating signaling from the agonist occupied receptor to downstream effectors. It is undoubtedly clear that such studies encounter major bottlenecks in the form of (1) the gathering and curation of the qualitative (pathway) data required for the models, and the quantitative data required for the simulations; and (2) the sheer paucity of such data. These have been considered in the development and population of the SigPath IMS, and in several responsible reviews in the current literature in systems biology.[12-14,82,83,88] Still, the value of modeling with the available levels of data for both hypothesis testing and experiment design have been considered to remain highly significant.[82] Ultimately, we expect increasingly more realistic representation of signaling in dynamic compartments within the cell, endowed with spatio-temporal characteristics obtained from experiment. Such models are likely to be increasingly necessary for development of an understanding of how the multiple functions of a cell are coordinated and regulated, and to evaluate the specifics of the perturbations caused by the hallucinogenic ligands of GPCRs.

Acknowledgments The research reviewed here is performed by a very talented group of current and past students and postdoctoral associates in the Weinstein lab, too numerous to thank individually, but worthy of very high praise. The longstanding collaboration in bioinformatics with Fabien Campagne at Weill Medical College, and with the experimental labs of Stuart Sealfon and Ravi Iyengar at Mount Sinai School of Medicine, New York, NY, and of Jonathan Javitch, Renee Hen, and Jay Gingrich at Columbia University, New York, NY, is acknowledged with pleasure and gratitude. The work was supported in part by National Institutes of Health (NIH) grants from the National Institute on Drug Abuse (K05–DA00060 and P01–DA12923), and by the Institute for Computational Biomedicine (ICB) at Weill Medical College of Cornell University. The computations were performed with the resources of the ICB and the Pittsburgh Supercomputer Center, Pittsburgh, PA, which are gratefully acknowledged.

References

1. Nichols DE. Hallucinogens. *Pharmacol Ther*. 2004; 101:131-181.
2. Gresch PJ, Strickland LV, Sanders-Bush E. Lysergic acid diethylamide-induced Fos expression in rat brain: role of serotonin-2A receptors. *Neuroscience*. 2002;114:707-713.
3. Aghajanian GK, Marek GJ. Serotonin and hallucinogens. *Neuropsychopharmacology*. 1999;21:16S-23S.

4. Visiers I, Ballesteros JA, Weinstein H. Three-dimensional representations of G protein-coupled receptor structures and mechanisms. *Methods Enzymol.* 2002;343:329-371.
5. Filizola M, Visiers I, Skrabanek L, Campagne F, Weinstein H. *Functional mechanisms of GPCRs in a structural context.* In: Schousboe A, Bräuner-Osborne H, eds. *Strategies in Molecular Neuropharmacology.* Totowa, NJ: Humana Press; 2003:235-266.
6. Filizola M, Weinstein H. The study of G-protein coupled receptor oligomerization with computational modeling and bioinformatics. *FEBS J.* In press.
7. Filizola M, Weinstein H. Structural models for dimerization of G-protein coupled receptors: the opioid receptor homodimers. *Biopolymers.* 2002;66:317-325.
8. Filizola M, Guo W, Javitch JA, Weinstein H. Oligomerization domains in G-protein coupled receptors: insights into the structural basis of GPCR association. In: Devi LA, ed. *The G-Protein Coupled Receptor Handbook.* Totowa, NJ: Humana Press Inc; 2005.
9. Beuming T, Skrabanek L, Niv MY, Mukherjee P, Weinstein H. PDZBase: a protein-protein interaction database for PDZ-domains. *Bioinformatics.* 2005;21:827-828.
10. Chang CW, Hassan SA, Weinstein H. Determinants for specificity in binding to the PDZ domain of PICK1. *Biophys J.* 2004;86:96a.
11. Madsen KL, Beuming T, Niv MY, et al. Molecular determinants for the complex binding specificity of the PDZ domain in pick 1. *J Biol Chem.* 2005;280:20539-20548.
12. Slepchenko BM, Schaff JC, Macara I, Loew LM. Quantitative cell biology with the Virtual Cell. *Trends Cell Biol.* 2003;13:570-576.
13. Slepchenko BM, Schaff JC, Carson JH, Loew LM. Computational cell biology: spatiotemporal simulation of cellular events. *Annu Rev Biophys Biomol Struct.* 2002;31:423-441.
14. Wachman ES, Poage RE, Stiles JR, Farkas DL, Meriney SD. Spatial distribution of calcium entry evoked by single action potentials within the presynaptic active zone. *J Neurosci.* 2004;24:2877-2885.
15. Campagne F, Neves S, Chang CW, et al. Quantitative information management for the biochemical computation of cellular networks. *Sci STKE.* 2004;2004:pl11.
16. Ebersole BJ, Visiers I, Weinstein H, Sealfon SC. Molecular basis of partial agonism: orientation of indoleamine ligands in the binding pocket of the human 5-HT2A serotonin receptor determines relative efficacy. *Mol Pharmacol.* 2003;63:36-43.
17. Visiers I, Ebersole BJ, Dracheva S, Ballesteros JA, Sealfon SC, Weinstein H. Structural motifs as functional microdomains in G-protein-coupled receptors: energetic considerations in the mechanism of activation of the serotonin 5-HT2A receptor by disruption of the ionic lock of the arginine cage. *Int J Quantum Chem.* 2002;88:65-75.
18. Prioleau C, Visiers I, Ebersole BJ, Weinstein H, Sealfon SC. Conserved helix 7 tyrosine acts as a multistate conformational switch in the 5HT2C receptor: identification of a novel "locked-on" phenotype and double revertant mutations. *J Biol Chem.* 2002;277:36577-36584.
19. Gonzalez-Maeso J, Yuen T, Ebersole BJ, et al. Transcriptome fingerprints distinguish hallucinogenic and nonhallucinogenic 5-hydroxytryptamine 2A receptor agonist effects in mouse somatosensory cortex. *J Neurosci.* 2003;23:8836-8843.
20. Gingrich JA, Ansorge MS, Merker R, Weisstaub N, Zhou M. New lessons from knockout mice: the role of serotonin during development and its possible contribution to the origins of neuropsychiatric disorders. *CNS Spectr.* 2003;8:572-577.
21. Ebersole BJ, Sealfon SC. Strategies for Mapping the Binding Site of the Serotonin 5HT2A Receptor. In: Iyengar R, Hildebrandt J, eds. *Methods in Enzymology.* San Diego, CA: Academic Press; 2001.
22. Beuming T, Weinstein H. A knowledge-based scale for the analysis and prediction of buried and exposed faces of transmembrane domain proteins. *Bioinformatics.* 2004;20:1822-1835. PubMed DOI: 10.1093/bioinformatics/bth143
23. Ebersole BJ, Visiers I, Weinstein H, Sealfon SC. Molecular basis of partial agonism: orientation of indoleamine ligands in the binding pocket of the human serotonin 5-HT2A receptor determines relative efficacy. *Mol Pharmacol.* 2003;63:36-43.

24. Ballesteros J, Kitanovic S, Guarnieri F, et al. Functional microdomains in G-protein-coupled receptors: the conserved arginine-cage motif in the gonadotropin-releasing hormone receptor. *J Biol Chem.* 1998;273:10445-10453.

25. Javitch JA. The ants go marching 2 by 2: oligomeric structure of G-protein-coupled receptors. *Mol Pharmacol.* 2004;66:1077-1082.

26. Filizola M, Olmea O, Weinstein H. Prediction of heterodimerization interfaces of G-protein coupled receptors with a new subtractive correlated mutation method. *Protein Eng.* 2002;15:881-885.

27. Filipek S, Teller DC, Palczewski K, Stenkamp R. The crystallographic model of rhodopsin and its use in studies of other G protein-coupled receptors. *Annu Rev Biophys Biomol Struct.* 2003;32:375-397.

28. Filipek S, Krzysko KA, Fotiadis D, et al. A concept for G protein activation by G protein-coupled receptor dimers: the transducin/rhodopsin interface. *Photochem Photobiol Sci.* 2004;3:628-638.

29. Hoffmann C, Gaietta G, Bunemann M, et al. A FlAsH-based FRET approach to determine G protein-coupled receptor activation in living cells. *Nat Methods.* 2005;2:171-176.

30. Zhuang X, Masson J, Gingrich JA, Rayport S, Hen R. Targeted gene expression in dopamine and serotonin neurons of the mouse brain. *J Neurosci Methods.* 2005;143:27-32.

31. Ballesteros JA, Shi L, Javitch JA. Structural mimicry in G protein-coupled receptors: implications of the high-resolution structure of rhodopsin for structure-function analysis of rhodopsin-like receptors. *Mol Pharmacol.* 2001;60:1-19.

32. Huang P, Li J, Chen C, Visiers I, Weinstein H, Liu-Chen LY. Functional role of a conserved motif in TM6 of the rat mu opioid receptor: constitutively active and inactive receptors result from substitutions of Thr6.34(279) with Lys and Asp. *Biochemistry.* 2001;40:13501-13509.

33. Flanagan CA, Zhou W, Chi L, et al. The functional microdomain in transmembrane helices 2 and 7 regulates expression, activation, and coupling pathways of the gonadotropin- releasing hormone receptor. *J Biol Chem.* 1999;274:28880-28886.

34. Xu W, Ozdener F, Li JG, et al. Functional role of the spatial proximity of Asp2.50(114) in TMH2 and Asn7.49(332) in TMH7 of the m opioid receptor. *FEBS Lett.* 1999;447:318-324.

35. Decaillot FM, Befort K, Filliol D, Yue S, Walker P, Kieffer BL. Opioid receptor random mutagenesis reveals a mechanism for G protein-coupled receptor activation. *Nat Struct Biol.* 2003;10:629-636.

36. Janz JM, Farrens DL. Rhodopsin activation exposes a key hydrophobic binding site for the transducin alpha-subunit C terminus. *J Biol Chem.* 2004;279:29767-29773.

37. Shapiro DA, Kristiansen K, Weiner DM, Kroeze WK, Roth BL. Evidence for a model of agonist-induced activation of 5-hydroxytryptamine 2A serotonin receptors that involves the disruption of a strong ionic interaction between helices 3 and 6. *J Biol Chem.* 2002;277:11441-11449.

38. Kroeze WK, Kristiansen K, Roth BL. Molecular biology of serotonin receptors structure and function at the molecular level. *Curr Top Med Chem.* 2002;2:507-528.

39. Meng EC, Bourne HR. Receptor activation: what does the rhodopsin structure tell us? *Trends Pharmacol Sci.* 2001;22:587-593.

40. Gerber BO, Meng EC, Dotsch V, Baranski TJ, Bourne HR. An activation switch in the ligand binding pocket of the C5a receptor. *J Biol Chem.* 2001;276:3394-3400.

41. Ghanouni P, Steenhuis JJ, Farrens DL, Kobilka BK. Agonist-induced conformational changes in the G-protein-coupling domain of the beta 2 adrenergic receptor. *Proc Natl Acad Sci USA.* 2001;98:5997-6002.

42. Ballesteros JA, Jensen AD, Liapakis G, et al. Activation of the beta 2-adrenergic receptor involves disruption of an ionic lock between the cytoplasmic ends of transmembrane segments 3 and 6. *J Biol Chem.* 2001;276:29171-29177.

43. Gether U. Uncovering molecular mechanisms involved in activation of G protein-coupled receptors. *Endocr Rev.* 2000;21:90-113.

44. Gether U, Asmar F, Meinild AK, Rasmussen SG. Structural basis for activation of G-protein-coupled receptors. *Pharmacol Toxicol.* 2002;91:304-312.

45. Palczewski K, Kumasaka T, Hori T, et al. Crystal structure of rhodopsin: a G-protein coupled receptor. *Science*. 2000;289:739-745.
46. Okada T, Ernst OP, Palczewski K, Hofmann KP. Activation of rhodopsin: new insights from structural and biochemical studies. *Trends Biochem Sci*. 2001;26:318-324.
47. Stenkamp RE, Teller DC, Palczewski K. Crystal structure of rhodopsin: a G-protein-coupled receptor. *ChemBioChem*. 2002;3:963-967.
48. Filipek S, Stenkamp RE, Teller DC, Palczewski K. G protein-coupled receptor rhodopsin: a prospectus. *Annu Rev Physiol*. 2003;65:851-879.
49. Fritze O, Filipek S, Kuksa V, Palczewski K, Hofmann KP, Ernst OP. Role of the conserved NPxxY(x)5,6F motif in the rhodopsin ground state and during activation. *Proc Natl Acad Sci USA*. 2003;100:2290-2295.
50. Kalatskaya I, Schussler S, Blaukat A, et al. Mutation of tyrosine in the conserved NPXXY sequence leads to constitutive phosphorylation and internalization, but not signaling, of the human B2 bradykinin receptor. *J Biol Chem*. 2004;279:31268-31276.
51. Ballesteros JA, Weinstein H. Integrated methods for the construction of three-dimensional models and computational probing of structure-function relations in G protein-coupled receptors. In: Sealfon SC, ed. *Receptor Molecular Biology*. San Diego, CA: Academic Press; 1995:366-428.
52. Lin SW, Sakmar TP. Specific tryptophan UV-absorbance changes are probes of the transition of rhodopsin to its active state. *Biochemistry*. 1996;35:11149-11159.
53. Shi L, Javitch JA. The second extracellular loop of the dopamine D2 receptor lines the binding-site crevice. *Proc Natl Acad Sci USA*. 2004;101:440-445.
54. Singh R, Hurst DP, Barnett-Norris J, Lynch DL, Reggio PH, Guarnieri F. Activation of the cannabinoid CB1 receptor may involve a W6 48/F3 36 rotamer toggle switch. *J Pept Res*. 2002;60:357-370.
55. Shi L, Liapakis G, Xu R, Guarnieri F, Ballesteros JA, Javitch JA. Beta2 adrenergic receptor activation: modulation of the proline kink in transmembrane 6 by a rotamer toggle switch. *J Biol Chem*. 2002;277:40989-40996.
56. McAllister SD, Hurst DP, Barnett-Norris J, Lynch D, Reggio PH, Abood ME. Structural mimicry in class A GPCR rotamer toggle switches: the importance of the F3.36(201)/W6.48(357) interaction in cannabinoid CB1 receptor activation. *J Biol Chem*. 2004;279:48024-48037.
57. McAllister SD, Rizvi G, Anavi-Goffer S, et al. An aromatic microdomain at the cannabinoid CB(1) receptor constitutes an agonist/inverse agonist binding region. *J Med Chem*. 2003;46:5139-5152.
58. Gay EA, Urban JD, Nichols DE, Oxford GS, Mailman RB. Functional selectivity of D2 receptor ligands in a Chinese hamster ovary hD2L cell line: evidence for induction of ligand-specific receptor states. *Mol Pharmacol*. 2004;66:97-105.
59. Mottola DM, Kilts JD, Lewis MM, et al. Functional selectivity of dopamine receptor agonists. 1. Selective activation of postsynaptic dopamine D2 receptors linked to adenylate cyclase. *J Pharmacol Exp Ther*. 2002;301:1166-1178.
60. Ghanouni P, Gryczynski Z, Steenhuis JJ, et al. Functionally different agonists induce distinct conformations in the G protein coupling domain of the beta 2 adrenergic receptor. *J Biol Chem*. 2001;276:24433-24436.
61. McLaughlin JN, Shen L, Holinstat M, Brooks JD, Dibenedetto E, Hamm HE. Functional selectivity of G protein signaling by agonist peptides and thrombin for the protease-activated receptor-1. *J Biol Chem*. 2005;280:25048-25059.
62. Vilardaga JP, Steinmeyer R, Harms GS, Lohse MJ. Molecular basis of inverse agonism in a G protein-coupled receptor. *Nature Chem Biol*. 2005;1:25-28.
63. Javitch JA, Ballesteros JA, Weinstein H, Chen J. A cluster of aromatic residues in the sixth membrane-spanning segment of the dopamine D2 receptor is accessible in the binding site crevice. *Biochemistry*. 1998;37:998-1006.

64. Javitch JA, Ballesteros JA, Weinstein H, Chen J. A cluster of aromatic residues in the sixth membrane-spanning segment of the dopamine D2 receptor is accessible in the binding-site crevice. *Biochemistry*. 1998;37:998-1006.
65. Filizola M, Hassan SA, Artoni A, Coller BS, Weinstein H. Mechanistic insights from a refined 3-dimensional model of integrin alphaIIbbeta3. *J Biol Chem*. 2004;279:24624-24630.
66. Liggett SB. Update on current concepts of the molecular basis of beta2-adrenergic receptor signaling. *J Allergy Clin Immunol*. 2002;110:S223-S227.
67. McAllister SD, Hurst DP, Barnett-Norris J, Lynch D, Reggio PH, Abood ME. Structural mimicry in class A G protein-coupled receptor rotamer toggle switches: the importance of the F3.36(201)/W6.48(357) interaction in cannabinoid CB1 receptor activation. *J Biol Chem*. 2004;279:48024-48037.
68. Mehler EL, Periole X, Hassan SA, Weinstein H. Key issues in the computational simulation of GPCR function: representation of loop domains. *J Comput Aided Mol Des*. 2002;16:841-853.
69. Visiers I, Hassan SA, Weinstein H. Differences in conformational properties of the second intracellular loop (IL2) in 5HT(2C) receptors modified by RNA editing can account for G protein coupling efficiency. *Protein Eng*. 2001;14:409-414.
70. McGrew L, Price RD, Hackler E, Chang MS, Sanders-Bush E. RNA editing of the human serotonin 5-HT2C receptor disrupts transactivation of the small G-protein RhoA. *Mol Pharmacol*. 2004;65:252-256.
71. Niswender CM, Copeland SC, Herrick-Davis K, Emeson RB, Sanders-Bush E. RNA editing of the human serotonin 5-hydroxytryptamine 2C receptor silences constitutive activity. *J Biol Chem*. 1999;274:9472-9478.
72. Hassan SA, Mehler EL, Zhang D, Weinstein H. Molecular dynamics simulations of peptides and proteins with a continuum electrostatic model based on screened Coulomb potentials. *Proteins*. 2003;51:109-125.
73. Hassan SA, Mehler EL, Weinstein H. Structure calculations of protein segments connecting domains with defined secondary structure: a simulated annealing monte carlo combined with biased scaled collective variables technique. In: Hark K, Schlick T, eds. *Lecture Notes in Computational Science and Engineering*. New York, NY: Springer Verlag, Ag; 2002:197-231.
74. Sankararamakrishnan R, Weinstein H. Surface tension parameterization in molecular dynamics simulations of a phospholipid-bilayer membrane: calibration and effects. *J Phys Chem B*. 2004;108:11802-11811.
75. Fong SL, Tsin AT, Bridges CD, Liou GI. Detergents for extraction of visual pigments: types, solubilization, and stability. *Methods Enzymol*. 1982;81:133-140.
76. Liang Y, Fotiadis D, Filipek S, Saperstein DA, Palczewski K, Engel A. Organization of the G protein-coupled receptors rhodopsin and opsin in native membranes. *J Biol Chem*. 2003;278:21655-21662.
77. Sankararamakrishnan R, Weinstein H. Molecular dynamics simulations predict a tilted orientation for the helical region of dynorphin A(1-17) in dimyristoylphosphatidylcholine bilayers. *Biophys J*. 2000;79:2331-2344.
78. Sankararamakrishnan R, Weinstein H. Positioning and stabilization of dynorphin peptides in membrane bilayers: the mechanistic role of aromatic and basic residues revealed from comparative MD simulations. *J Phys Chem B*. 2002;106:209-218.
79. Tieleman DP, Berendsen HJ, Sansom MS. An alamethicin channel in a lipid bilayer: molecular dynamics simulations. *Biophys J*. 1999;76:1757-1769.
80. Marrink SJ, Berger O, Tieleman P, Jahnig F. Adhesion forces of lipids in a phospholipid membrane studied by molecular dynamics simulations. *Biophys J*. 1998;74:931-943.
81. Petrache HI, Dodd SW, Brown MF. Area per lipid and acyl length distributions in fluid phosphatidylcholines determined by (2)H NMR spectroscopy. *Biophys J*. 2000;79:3172-3192.
82. Bock G, Goode JA, eds. In silico simulation of biological processes, Novartis Foundation Symposium 247. In: *Novartis Foundation Symposium. Vol 247*. Chichester, UK: John Wiley & Sons; 2002:262.
83. Fall C, Marland ES, Wagner JM, Tyson JJ. *Computational Cell Biology*. New York, NY: Springer Verlag; 2002.

84. Brown KS, Hill CC, Calero GA, et al. The statistical mechanics of complex signaling networks: nerve growth factor signaling. *Phys Biol.* 2004;1:184-195.
85. Barrios-Rodiles M, Brown KR, Ozdamar B, et al. High-throughput mapping of a dynamic signaling network in mammalian cells. *Science.* 2005;307:1621-1625.
86. Loew LM. The Virtual Cell project. *Novartis Found Symp.* 2002;247:151-160.Discussion 160-161, 198-206, 244-252.
87. Loew LM, Schaff JC. The Virtual Cell: a software environment for computational cell biology. *Trends Biotechnol.* 2001;19:401-406.
88. Sauro HM, Kholodenko BN. Quantitative analysis of signaling networks. *Prog Biophys Mol Biol.* 2004;86:5-43.
89. Kurrasch-Orbaugh DM, Parrish JC, Watts VJ, Nichols DE. A complex signaling cascade links the serotonin2A receptor to phospholipase A2 activation: the involvement of MAP kinases. *J Neurochem.* 2003;86:980-991.
90. Kurrasch-Orbaugh DM, Watts VJ, Barker EL, Nichols DE. Serotonin 5-hydroxytryptamine 2A receptor-coupled phospholipase C and phospholipase A2 signaling pathways have different receptor reserves. *J Pharmacol Exp Ther.* 2003;304:229-237.
91. Akin D, Manier DH, Sanders-Bush E, Shelton RC. Decreased serotonin 5-HT2A receptor-stimulated phosphoinositide signaling in fibroblasts from melancholic depressed patients. *Neuropsychopharmacology.* 2004;29:2081-2087.
92. Conn PJ, Sanders-Bush E. Selective 5HT-2 antagonists inhibit serotonin stimulated phosphatidylinositol metabolism in cerebral cortex. *Neuropharmacology.* 1984;23:993-996.
93. Roth BL, Nakaki T, Chuang DM, Costa E. Aortic recognition sites for serotonin (5HT) are coupled to phospholipase C and modulate phosphatidylinositol turnover. *Neuropharmacology.* 1984;23:1223-1225.
94. Sanders-Bush E, Tsutsumi M, Burris KD. Serotonin receptors and phosphatidylinositol turnover. *Ann N Y Acad Sci.* 1990;600:224-235.
95. Berg KA, Maayani S, Goldfarb J, Scaramellini C, Leff P, Clarke WP. Effector pathway-dependent relative efficacy at serotonin type 2A and 2C receptors: evidence for agonist-directed trafficking of receptor stimulus. *Mol Pharmacol.* 1998;54:94-104.
96. Bhalla US, Ram PT, Iyengar R. MAP kinase phosphatase as a locus of flexibility in a mitogen-activated protein kinase signaling network. *Science.* 2002;297:1018-1023.
97. Weng G, Bhalla US, Iyengar R. Complexity in biological signaling systems. *Science.* 1999;284:92-96.
98. Bruggeman FJ, Kholodenko BN. Modular interaction strengths in regulatory networks: an example. *Mol Biol Rep.* 2002;29:57-61.
99. Markevich NI, Hoek JB, Kholodenko BN. Signaling switches and bistability arising from multisite phosphorylation in protein kinase cascade. *J Cell Biol.* 2004;164:353-359.

Chapter 18
Recognition of Psychostimulants, Antidepressants, and Other Inhibitors of Synaptic Neurotransmitter Uptake by the Plasma Membrane Monoamine Transporters

Christopher K. Surratt,[1] Okechukwu T. Ukairo,[1] and Suneetha Ramanujapuram[1]

Abstract The plasma membrane monoamine transporters terminate neurotransmission by removing dopamine, norepinephrine, or serotonin from the synaptic cleft between neurons. Specific inhibitors for these transporters, including the abused psychostimulants cocaine and amphetamine and the tricyclic and SSRI classes of antidepressants, exert their physiological effects by interfering with synaptic uptake and thus prolonging the actions of the monoamine. Pharmacological, biochemical, and immunological characterization of the many site-directed, chimeric, and deletion mutants generated for the plasma membrane monoamine transporters have revealed much about the commonalities and dissimilarities between transporter substrate, ion, and inhibitor binding sites. Mutations that alter the binding affinity or substrate uptake inhibition potency of inhibitors by at least 3-fold are the focus of this review. These findings are clarifying the picture regarding substrate uptake inhibitor/transporter protein interactions at the level of the drug pharmacophore and the amino acid residue, information necessary for rational design of novel medications for substance abuse and a variety of psychiatric disorders.

Keywords transporter, neurotransmitter, antidepressant, addiction, cocaine

[1] Division of Pharmaceutical Sciences, Mylan School of Pharmacy, Duquesne University, Pittsburgh, PA 15282

Corresponding Author: Christopher K. Surratt, Duquesne University, Mellon Hall, Room 453, 600 Forbes Avenue, Pittsburg, PA 15282. Tel: (412) 396-5007; Fax: (412) 396-4660; E-mail: surratt@duq.edu

R.S. Rapaka and W. Sadée (eds.), *Drug Addiction.*
© American Association of Pharmaceutical Scientists 2008

Introduction

Plasma membrane transporters constitute the primary mechanism for synaptic clearance of neurotransmitter following Ca^{2+}-mediated exocytosis from synaptic vesicles. These proteins are responsible for translocating the cognate neurotransmitter from the extracellular space into the cytoplasm, at which point the neurotransmitter may be packaged into synaptic vesicles and recycled. The dopamine transporter (DAT), norepinephrine transporter (NET), and serotonin transporter (SERT) comprise the plasma membrane monoamine transporters, a subfamily that has been associated with psychostimulant actions and abuse, Parkinson's disease, attention deficit hyperactivity disorder, schizophrenia, narcolepsy, Lesch-Nyhan disease, postural hypotension, anxiety-related disorders, autism, and depression.[1-14] The plasma membrane monoamine transporters have been and will continue to be important therapeutic targets. Structure-function studies on the DAT, NET, and SERT can only increase the precision of rational drug design in treating the conditions mentioned above.

The plasma membrane monoamine transporters are members of the 12 transmembrane (TM) domain neurotransmitter:sodium symporter (NSS) family,[15] in which electrogenic transport of a neurotransmitter substrate across the cell membrane is driven by the naturally occurring neuronal Na^+ gradient. Cotransport of Cl^- is also required for the DAT, NET and SERT; the SERT additionally transports K^+, but in antiport fashion.[16] Aligning the amino acid sequences of the NSS family members guides delineation of monoamine transporter TM domain borders and other aspects of transporter secondary structure (Fig. 18.1, Table 18.1).[17] Such a sequence alignment can also yield clues as to which monoamine transporter amino acid residues probably contribute to the general protein infrastructure, which residues may play a role in substrate or ion recognition, and which residues are most likely to be responsible for a pharmacologic pattern unique to a given transporter. One problem in comparing pharmacologic findings between site-directed mutants of different transporters is that each residue of a given transporter is named according to its position in the polypeptide chain. Thus, only from the sequence alignment is the TM 1 aspartic acid residue D79 in the human DAT revealed to be at the position analogous to D75 in the human NET and D98 in the human SERT. Fortunately, a new nomenclature for identifying residues with respect to their relative position in a given NSS TM domain has been developed recently[17] and is employed here. The most conserved residue in a given TM domain is arbitrarily assigned Position 50; this number is preceded by the TM domain number. As an example, because W84 of hDAT TM 1 is the most conserved residue in this TM domain among the NSS proteins, this residue is termed $W_{1.50}$. V83, the hDAT residue immediately N-terminal to W84, is thus labeled $V_{1.49}$, and the immediately C-terminal R85 residue is labeled $R_{1.51}$. To facilitate the transition between the conventional and new nomenclatures, both numbering systems will be used (eg, $W84_{1.50}$), consistent with the suggestion of Weinstein, Javitch, and colleagues.[17]

Hundreds of plasma membrane monoamine transporter mutants have been constructed and characterized, but the large majority are not discussed here. This review

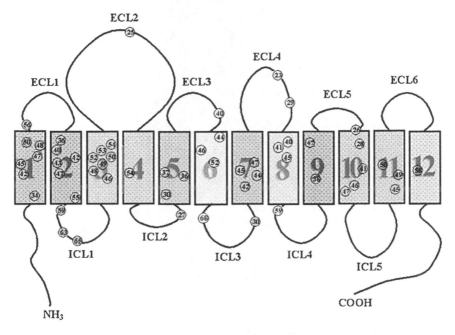

Fig. 18.1 Helical net topology scheme for discussed monoamine transporter mutations. The 12 TM domains are indicated by cylinders, color-coded to match the TM domain assignments of specific mutations listed in Table 18.1. Numbers inscribed in circles indicate specific positions of TM residues using the indexing system of Goldberg et al[17]; amino acid side chain assignments are listed in Table 18.1. Thus, the circled "34" in TM 1 refers to Position 1.34 in Table 18.1, in turn indicating that aspartic acid residues are found at this analogous position for the human DAT, NET, and SERT. Mutagenesis targets in the 6 extracellular loops (ECLs) and 5 intracellular loops (ICLs) are color-coded to indicate which of the flanking TM domains is used in the indexing system. Thus, the hDAT E218 residue in ECL 2 has been assigned Position 25 of TM 4 and is referred to as $E218_{4.25}$ in the text. (*See* also Color Insert).

focuses on discrete transporter residues that may contribute to recognition of inhibitors of substrate uptake. In this context, mutations of putative substrate binding site residues may also be discussed. NSS mutants for which the binding affinity or substrate uptake inhibition potency of uptake blockers is not altered by at least 3-fold are typically not discussed. Mutations that are believed to exert their effects via conformational changes or by altering the equilibrium between conformations are not emphasized but are discussed when the ≥ 3-fold pharmacologic shift was present. Mutants that displayed pronounced functional deficits and for which the extent of cell surface expression was ambiguous are not included. Regarding trafficking of mutants to the cell surface, wildtype-like B_{max} values for a ligand not expected to penetrate the plasma membrane (eg, the WIN 35,428 cocaine analog) were taken as proof of adequate cell surface expression.[18] Finally, findings from chimeric transporters are generally covered only when the study led to identification of specific residues critical for recognition of uptake inhibitors. To facilitate comparisons of specific mutations between monoamine transporters, the pharmacology of mutants in analogous positions are discussed one TM domain at a time.

Table 18.1 Discussed Amino Acid Residue Mutagenesis Targets and Their Counterparts at Analogous Positions in the DAT, NET, and SERT* (*See also* Color Insert).

	1.34	1.42	1.45	1.47	1.48	1.50	1.56	2.36	2.40	2.42	2.43	2.47	2.55	2.59
DAT	D68 (h)	F76 (r)	D79 (h)	A81 (h)	N82 (h)	W84 (h)	C90 (h)	F98 (r)	Y102 (h)	L104 (m)	F105 (m)	A109 (m)	E117 (h)	G121 (h)
SERT	D87 (h)	Y85 (h)	D98 (h)	G100 (h)	N101 (h)	W103 (h)	C109 (h)	F117 (h)	Y121 (h)	I123 (h)	M124 (r)	G128 (h)	E136 (h)	G140 (h)
NET	D64 (h)	F72 (h)	D75 (h)	A77 (h)	N78 (h)	W80 (h)	C86 (h)	F94 (h)	Y98 (h)	L100 (h)	F101 (h)	A105 (h)	E113 (h)	G117 (h)

	2.63	2.65	3.46	3.48	3.49	3.50	3.52	3.53	3.54	4.25	4.54	5.27	5.30	5.36
DAT	R125 (h)	G127 (h)	V152 (h)	F154 (r)	F155 (h)	Y156 (h)	V158 (h)	I159 (h)	I160 (h)	E218 (h)	V247 (h)	K264 (h)	W267 (h)	P272 (r)
SERT	R144 (h)	G146 (h)	I172 (r)	S174 (h)	Y175 (h)	Y176 (r)	T178 (h)	I179 (h)	M180 (h)	R234 (h)	F263 (h)	K279 (h)	W282 (h)	P288 (h)
NET	R121 (h)	G123 (h)	V148 (h)	F150 (h)	Y151 (h)	Y152 (h)	V154 (h)	I155 (h)	I158 (h)	E215 (h)	V244 (h)	K261 (h)	W264 (h)	P270 (h)

	5.37	6.40	6.44	6.46	6.52	6.68	7.30	7.42	7.44	7.45	7.47	8.23	8.29	8.40
DAT	Y274 (h)	E307 (h)	W311 (h)	D313 (h)	C319 (h)	Y335 (h)	D345 (h)	S356 (r)	S359 (h)	S359 (r)	F361 (r)	D385 (h)	F390 (r)	P402 (h)
SERT	Y289 (h)	E322 (h)	W326 (h)	D328 (h)	F334 (h)	Y350 (h)	D360 (h)	S372 (r)	S374 (h)	S375 (r)	F377 (h)	A401 (h)	F407 (h)	P418 (h)
NET	Y271 (h)	E304 (h)	W308 (h)	D310 (h)	F316 (h)	Y332 (h)	D342 (h)	S354 (h)	V356 (h)	S357 (h)	F359 (h)	E382 (h)	F388 (h)	S399 (h)

	8.41	8.45	8.59	9.38	9.47	10.26	10.28	10.41	10.46	10.47	11.45	11.49	11.50	12.58
DAT	L403 (h)	W406 (r)	D421 (h)	T455 (r)	T464 (r)	D476 (h)	F478 (h)	E490 (r)	F513 (b)	W496 (r)	W523 (h)	S528 (h)	P529 (h)	M569 (h)
SERT	A419 (h)	F423 (h)	D437 (h)	C473 (h)	T482 (h)	E493 (h)	F495 (b)	E508 (h)	S513 (h)	W514 (h)	W541 (h)	S545 (r)	P548 (h)	F586 (h)
NET	G400 (h)	W404 (h)	D418 (h)	T453 (h)	T462 (h)	D473 (h)	F475 (h)	E488 (h)	S493 (h)	W494 (h)	W521 (h)	S525 (h)	P526 (h)	M566 (h)

* DAT indicates dopamine transporter; NET, norepinephrine transporter; and SERT, serotonin transporter. Residues are grouped by TM domain and color-coded to match the transmembrane (TM) domain in Figure 1. Individual residues are named by their one-letter amino acid code and position in the polypeptide chain of that transporter, parenthetically followed by the species employed in mutagenesis studies (eg, "D68 (h)" refers to the aspartic acid residue of the human DAT). Residues at the analogous position in the neurotransmitter:sodium symporter (NSS) family sequence alignment are collectively named using the indexing system described in the Introduction (from Goldberg et al[17]). Thus, hDAT D68, hSERT D87, and hNET D64 are found at Position 34 in TM 1. In many cases, only one monoamine transporter was mutated at the indicated position; the analogous residues in the other 2 transporters are shown as points of reference.

Review

Transmembrane Domains

TM 1

A TM 1 aspartic acid residue common to the plasma membrane monoamine transporters but not shared by other NSS family members is the side chain perhaps most frequently postulated to directly contact cocaine and other nonsubstrate inhibitors, as well as substrates. This $D_{1.45}$ residue was the first to be mutated among NSS transporters,[19] an approach based on the G protein-coupled receptor model of a salt bridge between the positively charged agonist amino group and negatively charged TM domain carboxylate side chain.[20]

Consistent with the "salt bridge" premise, alanine, glycine, or glutamic acid substitution of rDAT $D79_{1.45}$ was reported to markedly decrease DAT affinities for dopamine and the cocaine analog WIN 35,428.[19] (The letters "h," "r," "m," "b," or "d" preceding the transporter name refer to the human, rat, mouse, bovine, or *Drosophila* species of that transporter, respectively.) On the other hand, recent findings with rDAT $D79_{1.45}E$ indicated no effect on dopamine affinity, only 3-fold losses in WIN 35,428, mazindol and methylphenidate affinities, and no effect on the dopamine uptake inhibition potency (DUIP) for these drugs.[21] Binding affinities and DUIPs for benztropine and its analogs were nevertheless typically altered substantially by this mutation.[22] The authors of the latter 2 studies question whether $D_{1.45}$ of the plasma membrane monoamine transporters is a logical counterion for the positively charged substrate amino group. A glycine side chain $(G_{1.45})$ is found in NSS family members including transporters for GABA, betaine, glycine, and proline, members whose cognate substrates share with the monoamines the positively charged amino group but lack aromatic groups.[21] The coincidence of an aspartic acid side chain at Position 1.45 in only those transporters recognizing aromatic substrates may indicate that $D_{1.45}$ serves as a strut supporting an aromatic binding site for the ligand.[22] Findings were inconsistent with, but did not rule out, formation of a salt bridge between $D_{1.45}$ and either dopamine, cocaine, or amphetamine.[21,22] $D75_{1.45}$ of the NET was intolerant to mutation, and like the DAT, only glutamate substitution of $D98_{1.45}$ yielded a functional SERT.[23] From experiments employing shortened tryptamine analogs, formation of a $D98_{1.45}$-serotonin salt bridge was judged to be probable.[23] Finally, the premise that a positively charged tropane nitrogen atom of cocaine or its analogs is critical for inhibition of dopamine uptake at the DAT[24] is in question,[25,26] as is formation of a $D_{1.45}$-cocaine salt bridge.[22]

Primarily to search for DAT TM residues capable of directly interacting with the positively charged moieties of substrates and inhibitors, conserved acidic and tryptophan hDAT residues were separately mutated and the mutant transporters characterized, including the TM 1 residues $D68_{1.34}$ and $W84_{1.50}$.[27] The conservative asparagine-for-aspartate mutant $D68_{1.34}N$, presumably positioned at the intracellular interface of TM 1[17,27] (Fig. 18.1), displayed 3- to 4-fold losses in affinity for the cocaine analog WIN 35,428 and in cocaine DUIP. The mutation did not appreciably affect recognition of the classic DAT inhibitor GBR-12909 or most of the hydroxy-piperidine GBR-like analogs tested; however, one such analog, (+)-R,R-D-84, sustained a 17-fold affinity loss. Of interest, this potential anticocaine therapeutic differs from one of the analogs unaffected by the mutation only in the position of a hydroxyl group, suggesting a direct interaction between D68$_{1.34}$ and the (+)-R,R-D-84 hydroxyl moiety.[28]

Human (W84$_{1.50}$L) and rat (W84$_{1.50}$A) DAT substitutions of the W$_{1.50}$ residue actually increased WIN 35,428 affinity and cocaine DUIP; dopamine K$_m$ (Michaelis constant) values were unaffected.[27,29] W84$_{1.50}$ may contribute to maintaining an intracellular-facing DAT conformation,[27] and Na$^+$-dependent conformational changes required for DAT function were impaired in hDAT W84$_{1.50}$L.[18] This mutant also displayed Na$^+$ sensitivity differences between cocaine and the diphenylmethoxy-bearing compounds benztropine and GBR-12,909. Taken with the aforementioned rDAT D79$_{1.45}$E results, the hDAT W84$_{1.50}$L findings suggest that TM 1 residues may provide discrimination between diphenylmethoxy-bearing compounds and classic inhibitors such as cocaine, WIN 35,428, and mazindol. Moreover, of several endogenous hDAT cysteine residues surveyed for accessibility to the methanethiosulfonate alkylating agent MTSET, the benztropine-induced DAT alkylation pattern diverged from those of cocaine, WIN 35,428, mazindol, and dopamine only at C90$_{1.56}$, a residue immediately extracellular to TM 1.[30] It is unclear whether these TM 1-associated inhibitor selectivities are solely due to DAT conformational differences or are indicative of TM 1 contributions to inhibitor binding sites.

SERT mutagenesis findings are consistent with direct interactions between TM 1 residues and uptake inhibitors or substrates. In addition to compensatory effects on serotonin analog affinities, the D98$_{1.45}$E mutant sustained serotonin uptake inhibition potency (SUIP) losses for cocaine, imipramine, and citalopram but not paroxetine or mazindol.[23] Human/*Drosophila* SERT chimera studies led to identification of hSERT Y95$_{1.42}$ (F90$_{1.42}$ in dSERT) as solely accounting for species differences in recognition of tryptamine analogs.[31] Using SERTs from the same 2 species, the hSERT Y95$_{1.42}$ side chain was previously postulated to sterically clash with the hydroxyl group of mazindol, while citalopram experienced no such hindrance.[32] The authors note that hSERT Y95$_{1.42}$ is one α-helical turn below D98$_{1.45}$ and therefore on the same face of TM 1, possibly facilitating coordination of the 2 residues in binding substrates and inhibitors.[31] Scanning cysteine accessibility mutagenesis (SCAM)[33] of all putative hSERT TM 1 residues revealed that D98$_{1.45}$C, G100$_{1.47}$C, and N101$_{1.48}$C were protected from MTSET inactivation by serotonin; G100$_{1.47}$C and N101$_{1.48}$C were similarly protected by cocaine.[34] The latter TM 1 residues are above (extracellular to) Y95$_{1.42}$ and D98$_{1.45}$ and may indeed be shielded from alkylation by the ligand; still, the ligand may have instead induced a conformational shift in SERT that in turn altered MTSET accessibility to the cysteine mutants. Nonsubstrates including cocaine are capable of altering DAT conformations in a manner sensitive to both the SCAM assay[30,35] and to changes in DAT vulnerability to proteases.[36]

Side chains at the position analogous to hSERT $Y95_{1.42}$ in other NSS members have been associated with substrate or inhibitor recognition. Alanine substitution of rDAT $F76_{1.42}$ decreased WIN 35,428 binding 4-fold without decreasing apparent surface expression. Dopamine potency in displacing [^{3}H]-WIN 35,428 at this mutant, however, increased ~300-fold, suggesting a significant perturbation in DAT structure or in available DAT conformations.[37] The hSERT tyrosine residue is conserved in only 1 of the 4 GABA transporters, with a glutamate side chain occupying the position in GAT-2, -3 and -4. Characterization of GAT-4 $E61_{1.42}$ mutants suggested that this side chain contributes to substrate binding.[38] Findings from TM 1 SCAM of GAT-1 were similar to hSERT in that the GAT-1 TM 1 also appears to contribute to the substrate permeation pathway.[34,39]

TM 2

Alanine replacement of rDAT $F98_{2.36}$, a residue putatively at the TM 2 extracellular interface, decreased WIN 35,428 binding 6-fold. The K_m value for dopamine uptake was unaffected, but dopamine turnover rate was greatly diminished.[37] $F98_{2.36}$ is largely conserved in the NSS family and perhaps less likely to directly contact specific uptake inhibitors. A mouse/*Drosophila* DAT chimera study led to identification of mDAT $F105_{2.43}$ as the residue chiefly responsible for the 10-fold higher DUIP of cocaine at the mDAT; this position is occupied by methionine in the dDAT. Of several mutations tested, only the presence of an aromatic side chain at mDAT position $105_{2.43}$ retained wildtype-like DUIPs for cocaine. It was not determined whether the effect of nonaromatic substitution of mDAT $F105_{2.43}$ on cocaine DUIP was direct or indirect.[40] Curiously, WIN 35,428 affinity at rDAT $F105_{2.43}$A decreased by only 2-fold relative to wildtype rDAT.[37] Methionine is also found at this position in some SERTs, but a phenylalanine residue one α-helical turn above, $F127_{2.40}$ in hSERT ($I108_{2.40}$ in mDAT), may play the role of mDAT $F105_{2.43}$ with respect to cocaine potency.[40] SCAM analysis of rSERT TM 2, however, did not identify residues that directly affected substrate binding or were accessible to alkylating agents.[41] Most recently, random mutagenesis of mDAT TM 2 residues in the vicinity of $F105_{2.43}$ generated the triple mutant $L104_{2.42}V/F105_{2.43}C/A109_{2.47}V$, which suffered 69- and 47-fold DUIP losses for cocaine and methylphenidate. The DUIPs for the substrates amphetamine and methamphetamine at the triple mutant were not significantly different from those at the wildtype mDAT.[42]

A glutamate residue at Position 2.55 ($E_{2.55}$) is absolutely conserved within the NSS family. This residue is thought to be at the cytoplasmic interface of TM 2 but could instead be the initial residue of ICL 1. If in the TM domain, $E_{2.55}$ would be only the third acidic TM residue and would likely be situated in a hydrophilic zone such as a ligand/ion pore. Human DAT and NET and rat GAT-1 proteins have been mutated at this position. The hDAT $E117_{2.55}Q$ mutation was not localized to the plasma membrane and was not characterized further.[27] Replacement of hNET $E113_{2.55}$ with alanine or aspartic acid compromised cell surface expression and eliminated norepinephrine uptake; substitution with glutamine was well tolerated. Affinity for the NET-selective inhibitor nisoxetine was reduced 10-fold at hNET $E113_{2.55}A$, with little or no change at $E113_{2.55}D$ and $E113_{2.55}Q$. Apparent affinities for substrates, measured by displacement of [^{3}H]-nisoxetine, were drastically reduced only at hNET $E113_{2.55}D$; cocaine and desipramine affinities were altered by less than 3-fold for all mutants. Thus, a 1-carbon shorter side chain at this position somehow profoundly disturbs substrate binding.[43] Glutamine substitution of the analogous rGAT-1 residue ($E101_{2.55}Q$) disrupted Na^+ binding, in turn disrupting GABA transport[44]; the hNET $E113_{2.55}Q$ mutant did not suffer the same functional consequences.[43]

TM 3

Human/bovine DAT chimeras identified a 54-residue segment encompassing TM 3 as especially critical for dopamine uptake and WIN 35,428 binding.[45] Remarkably, replacement of the bDAT TM 3 residue $I152_{3.46}$ with its conservative valine counterpart in the hDAT was found to almost single-handedly confer the superior substrate transport and WIN 35,428 binding characteristics of the hDAT.[46] Two positions away, $F154_{3.48}$ also appears to be relevant to cocaine recognition, as the rDAT $F154_{3.48}A$ mutation decreased cocaine affinity 10-fold without appreciably affecting substrate uptake.[47] $V152_{3.46}$ and $F154_{3.48}$ should be on opposite faces of DAT TM 3, meaning that both cannot directly contact the ligand. SCAM analysis of TM 3 of rSERT indicated that $I172_{3.46}$, the residue analogous to hDAT $V152_{3.46}$, is on the helical face accessible to ligands and external agents.[48] Moreover, $I172_{3.46}$ and $Y176_{3.50}$ of rSERT are in or near the binding sites for serotonin and cocaine.[48,49] Assuming that TM 3s of the DAT and SERT have similar orientations in the plasma membrane, $V152_{3.46}$ would be expected to face the ligand pore and $F154_{3.48}$ would face the lipid bilayer. $F155_{3.49}$ of DAT could still face the ligand pore, a residue conserved among DATs but replaced by tyrosine in SERTs and NETs. The rDAT $F155_{3.49}A$ mutant sustained a profound loss in apparent affinity for dopamine, but only a mild decrease in WIN 35,428 affinity.[37]

Two helical turns above $I172_{3.46}$, substrate transport but not cocaine binding by SERT $I179_{3.53}C$ was inactivated in the presence of MTSET. Neither substrate nor cocaine protected the mutant from the alkylating agent.[48] MTSET alkylation of the analogous NET mutant ($I155_{3.53}C$) was inhibited and enhanced by dopamine and cocaine, respectively. Substrate protection of this mutant was Na^+ and temperature dependent, suggesting a conformationally-sensitive protection mechanism as opposed to direct substrate occlusion of $I155_{3.53}C$ access.[49] In contrast to the SERT and NET, the analogous DAT mutant ($I159_{3.53}C$) was essentially insensitive to MTSET, in the presence or absence of dopamine or cocaine.[50] Thus, the $I_{3.53}$ residue in the monoamine transporters is less likely to directly contribute to ligand binding but has been proposed to contribute toward an external gate for the substrate permeation pathway.[49] Consistent with this idea, alanine mutation of the flanking $T178_{3.52}$ hSERT residue greatly accelerated serotonin translocation, apparently by modifying the equilibrium of SERT conformations.[51] Through human/bovine SERT species scanning and reverse mutations, $M180_{3.54}$, the other hSERT residue flanking $I179_{3.53}$, was found to substantially contribute to hSERT's higher SUIPs for the antidepressants citalopram, paroxetine, fluoxetine, and imipramine. A citalopram structure-activity series suggested that the heterocyclic nucleus of the drug interacts with $M180_{3.54}$.[52] This side chain also contributes to an allosteric citalopram binding site of the hSERT.[53]

TM 4

The pharmacologic profile of the hSERT $F263_{4.54}C$ mutant very closely resembles that of hSERT $T178_{3.52}A$ described above. Of 24 SERT mutants tested, only these 2 mutants displayed notable (~5-fold) K_m and V_{max} increases. The effect was amplified by combining the mutations, with K_m and V_{max} increases of 50- and 10-fold, respectively. A synergistic effect was also seen with respect to binding of the cocaine analog RTI-55, the double mutant sustaining a 60-fold affinity loss without a significant B_{max} change. Both individual mutants were insensitive to MTS reagent effects. The $F263_{4.54}$ residue alone appeared relatively unimportant with respect to the SUIPs of 5 inhibitors tested.[51]

TM 5

The $W267_{5.30}L$ hDAT mutation decreased cocaine DUIP by only 3-fold; uptake kinetics suggest that $W267_{5.30}$ contributes to an outward- (extracellular-) facing DAT conformation.[27] This residue is expected to border the cytoplasm. For hNET, the highly conserved $Y271_{5.37}$ residue was substituted with alanine, phenylalanine, or histidine; only the alanine mutant altered (decreased) the norepinephrine uptake inhibition potency (NUIP) of cocaine by 3-fold, with more modest effects on nisoxetine and desipramine NUIPs. Apparent affinities for norepinephrine and MPP^+ increased 3- to 4-fold at hNET $Y271_{5.37}A$.[54] Glycine replacement of rDAT $P272_{5.36}$ modestly reduced dopamine uptake but decreased WIN 35,428 binding affinity 10-fold without a reduction in B_{max} value. DUIPs for cocaine, mazindol, BTCP (1-[1-(2-benzo[b]thiopheneyl)cyclohexyl]piperidine hydrochloride), and trihexyphenidyl decreased by over 100-fold.[55] A subsequent study yielded very similar findings regarding dopamine uptake kinetics and WIN 35,428 binding with the same mutant and additionally characterized the rDAT $P272_{5.36}A$ mutation. The alanine mutant decreased WIN 35,428 affinity only 4-fold relative to wildtype rDAT.[56] Alanine replacement of the analogous hNET residue $P270_{5.36}$ yielded undetectable specific binding of nisoxetine and 11-, 3-, and 3-fold decreases in the NUIPs of nisoxetine, desipramine, and cocaine, respectively. Of 10 hNET proline residues mutated, only $P270_{5.36}A$ decreased recognition of uptake inhibitors by 3-fold or more.[57]

The number of TM proline residues is observed to be disproportionately large in transport proteins relative to other integral membrane proteins, yet it is unclear how such TM proline residues affect transporter protein structure and function.[58,59] In general, proline residues, and to a lesser extent glycine residues, disrupt α-helices, whereas alanine residues promote α-helix formation.[60] The extent of the α-helical "kink" induced by proline, however, is dependent on its environment,[61] and especially on neighboring residues.[62,63] Proline residues may serve a structural role, determining protein infrastructure by influencing helix-helix packing. Functional roles for TM proline residues include providing hinges that facilitate signal transduction, mediating conformational changes via *cis-trans* isomerization of the bond linking the proline to the preceding residue of the polypeptide, and providing a geometry that allows neighboring amide carbonyl oxygen atoms of the polypeptide to serve as cation binding sites.[64-66] The latter functional role is most likely for the monoamine transporters. Thus, $P272_{5.36}$ may provide a direct ligand binding site, a key Na^+ binding site that modulates transport or substrate or inhibitor recognition, or simply a kink necessary to the ligand or ion binding pocket.

TM 6

Leucine replacement of hDAT $W311_{6.44}$, putatively at the extracellular interface, decreased WIN 35,428 affinity 10-fold and cocaine DUIP over 3-fold; dopamine displacement of WIN 35,428 decreased by over 100-fold.[27] In contrast, alanine replacement of the rDAT counterpart ($W310_{6.44}A$) actually increased WIN 35,428 affinity 4-fold, and dopamine displacement of the cocaine analog was over 200 times more effective.[29] It should be noted that the rDAT binding was conducted at 4°C, compared with 37°C in the hDAT study.[27] Two residues away, the hDAT $D313_{6.46}N$ mutant did not notably affect WIN 35,428 or cocaine binding under normal assay conditions, and dopamine affinity was decreased.[27] While not believed to be part of the substrate or inhibitor binding sites, $D313_{6.46}$ may nevertheless regulate access to external dopamine in a Na^+-dependent fashion. This residue and $W84_{1.50}$ are involved in cation interactions, and control in part the ability of Na^+ to drive the DAT between inward- and outward-facing conformations, in turn influencing dopamine access and Na^+-dependent cocaine affinity.[67,68]

Searching for tricyclic antidepressant binding sites based on findings from chimeric studies,[69,70] nonconserved hNET residues from a region spanning TM 5 to TM 8 were replaced with the hDAT counterparts at each of 24 positions. The TM 6 residue $F316_{6.52}$ was the most important of the 24 for desipramine actions, as the hNET $F316_{6.52}C$ mutation reduced its DUIP 6-fold. Nortriptyline DUIP decreased 8-fold, but cocaine potency doubled. The reverse mutation in hDAT ($C319_{6.52}F$) increased DUIPs for these tricyclics, albeit less than 3-fold. $F316_{6.52}$ is conserved among all tricyclic-sensitive NSS members, mammalian or otherwise.[71] It remains to be elucidated if $F316_{6.52}$ directly interacts with tricyclic drugs.

TM 7

Simultaneous mutation of the rDAT $S356_{7.42}$ and $S359_{7.45}$ residues to glycine or alanine resulted in mild-to-insignificant reductions in WIN 35,428 binding affinity and significant but modest decreases in dopamine uptake. These residues are postulated to form hydrogen bonding interactions with the catechol hydroxyl groups of dopamine.[19] Again, this model was borrowed from that of Strader and colleagues, who demonstrated an association between β-adrenergic receptor TM serine residues and agonist hydroxyl groups.[72] The fact that a serine side chain is found at position 7.42 throughout the NSS family, including transporters for noncatechol substrates, argues against this model. In contrast, a serine is found at position 7.45 for the monoamine transporters and few other NSS members. The analogous hNET serine residues (S354$_{7.42}$ and S357$_{7.45}$) were singly and jointly switched to alanine. Affinity for nisoxetine was reduced 70-fold at hNET S354$_{7.42}$A, while affinity was unchanged at the S357$_{7.45}$A mutant. Affinities for dopamine and m- and p-tyramine, dopamine analogs lacking either of the catechol hydroxyl groups, were reduced at hNET S354$_{7.42}$A, but not in a manner that suggested a direct interaction with a catechol hydroxyl. Recognition of the 3 substrates by hNET S357$_{7.45}$A was indistinguishable from wildtype hNET. The authors concluded that formation of a hydrogen bond between these serine residues and substrates was unlikely.[73] Alanine mutation of either analogous rSERT serine residue (S372$_{7.42}$ and S375$_{7.45}$) only slightly diminished serotonin transport; inhibitor affinities were not investigated. Random mutagenesis of TM 7 revealed that most of the residues important to transporter function or Na$^+$ dependence were expected to share the same α-helical face, the face shared by S372$_{7.42}$ and S375$_{7.45}$.[74] TM 7 SCAM analysis indicated that this helical face is not directed toward a water-accessible pore. The TM 7 face containing S372$_{7.42}$ and S375$_{7.45}$ is probably involved in helix-helix interactions with another SERT TM domain, a role common to TM serine residues. In this way, TM 7 may transmit ion-driven conformational shifts in the protein.[75] There is no evidence that S372$_{7.42}$ and S375$_{7.45}$ contribute directly to inhibitor binding sites.

The presence of a third serine residue between S372$_{7.42}$ and S375$_{7.45}$ accounts in part for the lower tricyclic antidepressant DUIPs at the DAT relative to the hNET. Mutation of hNET V356$_{7.44}$ to the analogous hDAT serine residue decreased DUIPs for nortriptyline and desipramine by 10- and 4-fold, respectively. The DUIP for cocaine was not altered appreciably. The reverse mutation in hDAT (S359$_{7.44}$V) in turn increased DUIPs for nortriptyline and desipramine by 5- and 10-fold, respectively.[71]

Finally, alanine replacement of rDAT F361$_{7.47}$ decreased WIN 35,428 binding affinity by an order of magnitude without affecting dopamine uptake kinetics.[37] Positioned at the TM 7 midpoint, this side chain is largely conserved in the NSS family.

TM 8

DUIPs for desipramine and nortriptyline were respectively reduced 3- and 6-fold by substituting hNET G400$_{8.41}$ with leucine, the analogous hDAT residue. The reciprocal mutation in hDAT (L403$_{8.41}$G), however, did not affect the DUIPs for these drugs. The hNET triple mutant containing the aforementioned TM 6 and TM 7 substitutions (F316$_{6.52}$C/V356$_{7.44}$S/G400$_{8.41}$L) reduced desipramine and nortriptyline DUIPs 35- and 9-fold, with little change in dopamine uptake kinetics. Replacement of hNET $S399_{8.40}$ with the proline side chain found at hDAT position 8.40 did not affect inhibitor actions alone, but the double mutant $S399_{8.40}P/G400_{8.41}L$ decreased respective DUIPs for desipramine and nortriptyline by 1000- and 80-fold without altering cocaine DUIP or uptake kinetics. The dose-response curves for this double mutant were biphasic, and in fact correlate well with the high and low affinity IC_{50} values for tricyclics at hNET and hDAT, respectively.[71] Mutation of this region of TM 8 may alter the balance of inhibitor binding NET conformations.

For the rDAT, alanine substitution of $W406A_{8.45}$ decreased WIN 35,428 binding affinity by 3-fold; V_{max} and K_m values for dopamine uptake decreased 10-fold and 6-fold, respectively.[29] This residue is not far from the extracellular interface and is largely conserved in the NSS family, although a phenylalanine side chain is found at the same position in the SERT.

TM 9

TM 9 is underrepresented as a target for NSS structure-function studies on inhibitor recognition. Of the handful of mutants characterized with respect to uptake inhibitors, only 2 exhibited binding affinity or uptake inhibition potency shifts of 3-fold or more. WIN 35,428 binding affinities for the rDAT $T455_{9.38}A$ and $T464_{9.47}A$ mutants were, respectively, 20- and 7-fold lower than at the wildtype rDAT. Dopamine turnover was unchanged at rDAT $T455_{9.38}A$ and increased 5-fold at rDAT $T464_{9.47}A$.[76,77]

TM 10

TM 10 SERT residues at Positions 10.28 and 10.46 are reported to collaborate with the $M180_{3.54}$ side chain in accounting for the higher SUIPs of selected antidepressants at the hSERT compared with the bSERT. Gain-of-function bSERT mutants ($F495_{10.28}Y$ and $F513_{10.46}S$) and reverse hSERT mutants ($Y495_{10.28}F$ and $S513_{10.46}F$) confirmed that like hSERT $M180_{3.54}$, the presence of the hSERT side chain at each TM 10 position conferred higher SUIPs for citalopram and paroxetine. $S513_{10.46}$ and $M180_{3.54}$ were most important for fluoxetine and imipramine SUIPs. Because the SUIP gain-of-function was similar regardless of whether serine or alanine was substituted for bSERT $F513_{10.46}$, the phenylalanine side chain was postulated to confer steric hindrance in binding of these antidepressant uptake blockers. These TM 10 residues should lie on the same α-helical face and may line an antagonist binding pocket.[52]

For the rDAT, alanine mutation of $W496_{10.47}$ decreased WIN 35,428 binding affinity 6-fold, with minor effects on dopamine uptake kinetics.[29] This highly, but not absolutely, conserved residue should be within a helical turn of the cytoplasm. Finally, it should be noted that a glutamic acid residue is projected to be well within TM 10 ($E_{10.41}$), and a glutamic acid side chain is found at this position in over 50% of the NSS members, including the monoamine transporters. $E_{10.41}$ is one of only 2 monoamine transporter side chains with a full negative charge that almost certainly resides in the TM domains (the other being $D_{1.45}$); thus, $E_{10.41}$ would have to line a hydrophilic enclave such as a ligand or ion binding pore. Surprisingly, this residue has received little attention in structure-function studies. Other than a textual communication that the rDAT $E490_{10.41}A$ mutant was deficient in dopamine uptake and in registering an immunochemical signal[76]; no data are published on mutations at this position. A more conservative substitution (eg, $E_{10.41}Q$) may therefore be useful in searching for NSS protein contributors to ligand and ion recognition.

TM 11

Just as mutation of TM 10 residues compromised SUIPs of selected antidepressants, the rSERT $S545_{11.49}A$ mutant displayed a 7-fold SUIP decrease for citalopram, although high affinity binding of the drug was unchanged. Conversely, high affinity binding of imipramine was decreased 5-fold at the mutant, with a more subtle SUIP decrease. Of interest, this mutation allowed wildtype-like transport function when Li^+ was substituted for Na^+. An ion gating role for rSERT $S545_{11.49}$ may modulate conformational changes important for recognition of these antidepressants.[78] $S545_{11.49}$ is conserved among the monoamine transporters and highly conserved within the NSS family, occasionally replaced by threonine. Replacing the very highly conserved $P_{11.50}$ residue with alanine in the hNET actually increased (by 3-fold) NUIPs for nisoxetine, desipramine, and cocaine.[57]

TM 11 mutants displaying significant alterations in inhibitor affinities or uptake inhibition potencies are otherwise in short supply. WIN 35,428 affinity was decreased 4-fold at rDAT $W523_{11.45}A$. Dopamine uptake V_{max} was reduced 13-fold despite a wildtype-like B_{max} value.[29]

TM 12

Chimeric and point mutagenesis revealed that hSERT $F586_{12.58}$ almost solely accounts for the higher SUIPs of the tricyclic antidepressants imipramine, desipramine, and nortriptyline at hSERT relative to rSERT.[79,80] This hSERT phenylalanine residue is replaced by a valine side chain in other SERT species, and methionine in the DAT and NET. The relationship held for both gain-of-function (rSERT $V_{12.58}F$) and reverse (hSERT $F_{12.58}V$) mutants. SUIPs for cocaine, amphetamine, and nontricyclic antidepressants were not affected by this mutation. Curiously, the rSERT $V_{12.58}D$ mutation provided the same gain-of-function, but the rSERT $V_{12.58}Y$ mutation did not. Cocaine SUIP was also augmented by the $V_{12.58}D$ substitution.[80] That $V_{12.58}$ substitution with phenylalanine and aspartate side chains yields similar antidepressant potency increases suggests that different intramolecular interactions are formed that influence either the inhibitor binding sites or the prevalence of their preferred rSERT conformations. Introduction of a phenylalanine side chain at the analogous hNET position ($M566_{12.58}F$) did not alter DUIPs for the tricyclic compounds, suggesting a nonidentical antidepressant binding site for this transporter.[79,80]

Extratransmembranous Regions

Extracellular Loops

While it may be feasible to design a monoamine transporter-selective uptake inhibitor that reversibly binds to one or more extracellular loops (ECLs) and controls substrate access, binding sites for the classic, physiologically relevant inhibitors are believed to reside within the TM domains. Of the many ECL mutations created or found as polymorphisms within NSS family members, few have an appreciable effect on recognition of uptake inhibitors, and those that do are expected to alter transporter conformations as opposed to direct modification of inhibitor binding sites.[71,81]

Many mutations of putatively extracellular and intracellular residues have been generated for the purpose of detecting conformational shifts in, or mapping tertiary structure of, NSS family members. A few of these mutations were demonstrated to affect uptake inhibitor recognition. The hDAT $C90_{1.56}A$ mutant was prepared toward generating a DAT species lacking endogenous methanethiosulfonate-reactive cysteine residues.[35] This mutation did not alter affinity for WIN 35,428, but selectively compromised the DUIP of benztropine; DUIPs of cocaine, WIN 35,428, and mazindol were similar to wildtype hDAT. This very highly conserved ECL 1 residue is not expected to directly contact benztropine, but rather to differentially contribute toward stabilizing benztropine- versus cocaine-preferring DAT conformations.[30,35] Gether and colleagues have mutated many extratransmembranous hDAT residues in elucidating the endogenous Zn^{2+} binding site of the DAT, and in creating new Zn^{2+} sites toward mapping TM domain proximities.[50,82,83] In the course of this work, the extracellular hDAT mutants $E218_{4.25}Q$ (ECL 2), $E307_{6.40}Q$ (ECL 3), and $D385_{8.23}N$ (ECL 4) were found to sustain 4- to 5-fold losses in WIN 35,428 affinity.[83]

Regarding other ECL mutations, WIN 35,428 affinity decreased 5-fold as a result of the ECL 4 rDAT $F390_{8.29}A$ mutation; dopamine uptake was virtually eliminated.[37] Asparagine substitution of hDAT $D476_{10.26}$, a residue at the ECL 5/TM 10 interface, decreased WIN 35,428 affinity 4-fold, cocaine DUIP 3-fold, and apparent affinity (measured by K_m value) for dopamine 7-fold.[27] For the above ECL loop mutants, the inhibitor binding affinity and uptake inhibition potency losses are likely due to mutation-induced conformational changes; however, alterations in the actual inhibitor binding sites have not been ruled out.

Intracellular Segments

The N- and C-terminal tails of NSS family members do not appear to contain residues that directly contact inhibitors of substrate uptake. Nevertheless, mutagenesis studies indicate that selected N-terminal residues are physiologically relevant to the function of at least one inhibitor of monoamine uptake—amphetamine. As a structural analog of dopamine, the binding site for amphetamine, a monoamine transporter substrate, is expected to overlap with that of the neurotransmitter. The classical model posits that amphetamine uptake increases the percentage of inward-facing substrate binding sites of the transporter, facilitating reverse transport ("efflux") of cytoplasmic monoamine neurotransmitter into the synapse.[84] Recently, alanine substitution of the 5 hDAT N-terminal serine residues was found to almost eliminate amphetamine-mediated dopamine efflux without affecting dopamine uptake. Efflux was restored by substituting aspartic acid, a phosphorylation mimic, at 2 of the 5 positions.[85] The same N-terminal region is also required for PKC-mediated phosphorylation of the hDAT.[86] The necessity of phosphorylation for amphetamine-induced hDAT reverse transport but not for dopamine uptake suggests a problem with the classical "alternating access" model, and in fact, amphetamine actions at monoamine transporters may be better explained by an oligomeric DAT complex with separate moieties for forward and reverse transport.[87]

The remaining ICL mutants discussed below are not PKC substrates but are also not expected to make contact with the uptake inhibitor. In exploring the $G_{2.59}XXXR_{2.63}XG_{2.65}$ motif in the hNET ICL 1, the $G117_{2.59}A$ mutation decreased the NUIPs of desipramine and nisoxetine 5-fold without affecting that for cocaine. In contrast, alanine replacement of $G123_{2.65}$ did not alter the antidepressant NUIPs but decreased cocaine NUIP almost 3-fold. The results are consistent with the existence of nonidentical hNET binding sites for antidepressants and psychostimulants.[88] Mutation of these absolutely conserved residues probably disturbs inhibitor site infrastructure or the NET conformational equilibrium.

The intracellular hDAT mutations $K264_{5.27}A$ (ICL 2), $Y335_{6.68}A$ (ICL 3), $D345_{7.30}A$ (ICL 3), and $D421_{8.59}A$ (ICL 4) decreased WIN 35,428 affinity by 5-, 60-, 5-, and 9-fold, respectively. Cocaine DUIPs were reduced at the $K264_{5.27}A$, $Y335_{6.68}A$, and $D345_{7.30}A$ mutants by 5-, 70-, and 7-fold; for the same mutants, GBR-12,909 DUIPs were reduced 3-, 10-, and 3-fold.[50] A previous study of hDAT $Y335_{6.68}A$ revealed 10- to 150-fold DUIP decreases for WIN 35,428, cocaine, GBR-12,909, mazindol, and the cocaine analog RTI-55, but a 4-fold increase in amphetamine DUIP. Addition of micromolar Zn^{2+} concentrations substantially mitigated the DUIP losses.[89] As expected, the deficits appeared to be due to infrastructural changes; such changes may be shifting the equilibrium between DAT conformations.[50] The TM 3 $I159_{3.53}C$ mutation was introduced into these hDAT mutants, and resultant constructs were compared with hDAT $I159_{3.53}C$ for methanethiosulfonate reagent cross-linking in the presence or absence of Zn^{2+} or cocaine. The fact that cocaine decreased MTSET accessibility of the $I159_{3.53}C$ side chain in an otherwise wildtype hDAT protein but increased accessibility of this cysteine upon addition of the $K264_{5.27}A$, $Y335_{6.68}A$, or $D345_{7.30}A$ substitutions suggests that these 3 mutants employed a different cocaine-bound DAT conformation relative to wildtype hDAT.[50] Of interest, MTSET accessibility for hNET $I155_{3.53}C$ also increased upon addition of cocaine,[49] suggesting that the cocaine-bound state of hNET differs from that of hDAT.[50]

A recent in-depth study of hDAT $D345_{7.30}N$ indicated that like hDAT $Y335_{6.68}A$, $D345_{7.30}N$ is an ICL 3 mutation that increased DUIPs for amphetamine and other substrates. In addition, the usual uptake inhibition role of Zn^{2+} was actually reversed at these 2 mutants so that dopamine uptake was potentiated.[90] Unlike hDAT

Y335$_{6.68}$A, the D345$_{7.30}$N mutant did not affect inhibitor DUIPs, except for a 2-fold decrease in cocaine potency. The very low K$_m$ and V$_{max}$ values for dopamine uptake, the Zn^{2+} potentiation of uptake, and the lack of amphetamine-mediated dopamine efflux suggest that this mutation appears to render a preference for an inward-facing DAT conformation. A fascinating aspect of this mutant is that while most classical inhibitors potently block substrate uptake at hDAT D345$_{7.30}$N, high affinity specific binding of radiolabeled versions of the same inhibitors was undetectable under the same conditions. Detection of specific radioligand binding was also a function of whether the transfected cells were intact monolayers or membrane preparations at the time of assay.[90] This phenomenon is infrequently documented but has been reported in other DAT mutants.[21,91] One explanation for this curiosity is that the small percentage of remaining outward-facing DAT conformation(s) for hDAT D345$_{7.30}$N is insufficient for detection of binding of the inhibitor radiotracer, but adequate for higher levels of inhibitors and substrates to bind and drive the conformational cycling forward such that dopamine uptake (and its inhibition) is detected.[90] An alternative explanation is that DAT populations exist, possibly composed of multimeric DAT complexes[92-94] or DAT associated with intracellular factors,[95-98] and that the D345$_{7.30}$N mutation eliminates the population responsible for high affinity radioligand binding without affecting the population(s) most critical for substrate uptake and its inhibition.[21,22,91] Regardless of the explanation, a lack of correlation between an inhibitor's binding affinity and substrate uptake inhibition potency values at a given wildtype or mutant transporter protein is well documented.[21,22,88,90,99,100]

Conclusions

While elucidation of plasma membrane monoamine transporter inhibitor binding sites has progressed steadily, the lack of a crystal structure for any member of the NSS family has been a hindrance. Indeed, no high resolution structure is available for any mammalian transporter protein close to the NSS family on the phylogenetic tree, although recent DAT modeling based on the crystal structure of the bacterial 12 TM Na$^+$/H$^+$ transporter NhaA has yielded predictions largely consistent with the mutagenesis data regarding the role of specific DAT residues.[101-104] The very recently published crystal structure of a bacterial leucine transporter (LeuT$_{Aa}$), a protein with mild but definite amino acid sequence similarity to the NSS family, is also suggested to be a template for NSS protein modeling.[105] Binding pockets for the leucine substrate and one of 2 Na$^+$ atoms are created primarily by the middle portions of TM 1 and TM 6. Of interest, unwinding of the center of these 2 TM domains exposes main chain carbonyl oxygen and nitrogen atoms that H-bond to substrate and Na$^+$; no LeuT$_{Aa}$ side chains bearing a formal charge interact with the substrate. The unwound regions of TM 1 and TM 6 are also postulated to serve as hinges involved in interconversion of outward- and inward-facing transporter conformations. Still, it cannot be assumed at this point that the NSS proteins employ the same transport mechanism, or even that NSS TM domains are arrayed identically to LeuT$_{Aa}$ (eg, the significantly shorter ICL 1 segment for NSS proteins may preclude the TM 2-TM 3 spatial arrangement found in LeuT$_{Aa}$).

No direct contacts between a substrate uptake inhibitor and a specific amino acid residue side chain of a plasma membrane monoamine transporter protein have been unequivocally established, but findings for some of the above-discussed mutations make a compelling case for the proposed drug-protein association. The mutagenesis findings discussed here may serve to narrow the focus to specific TM domains in the search for inhibitor binding sites. TMs 1, 2, 3, 8, and 12 appear to be especially important contributors to inhibitor binding sites, but it should be noted that some of the remaining TM domains may not have been studied as rigorously in this respect. Monoamine transporter chimeras have implicated TMs 5 through 8 in inhibitor selectivity,[69,70,106] suggesting a closer inspection of TMs 5 through 7 is in order. Covalent cross-linking of radiolabeled photoaffinity ligands to the DAT followed by proteolytic and immunological peptide mapping revealed that GBR-12,909 and benztropine photoaffinity analogs labeled a fragment containing TMs 1 and 2, while the cocaine analog RTI-82 labeled a fragment containing TMs 4 through 7.[107-109] By expanding the arsenal of photoaffinity probes used and employing mass spectrometry of high-performance liquid chromatography (HPLC)-purified proteolysis fragments, this methodology should eventually identify the specific cross-linked amino acid side chains of the transporter protein.[110-112] Assuming that the alkyl chain tether of the photoaffinity probe is sufficiently short to ensure that the cross-linked transporter side chain lines the functional binding site of the uptake inhibitor, this approach may be the most promising in elucidating sites of action of cocaine, amphetamine, and antidepressants. Continuing refinement of structure-function methods and molecular modeling templates for the monoamine transporter proteins will likely yield superior medications in combating psychostimulant abuse and monoamine neurotransmitter-related psychiatric disorders.

Acknowledgments This work was supported by National Institutes of Health, Bethesda, MD, grants DA16604 and DA16604-S1.

References

1. Bannon MJ. The dopamine transporter: role in neurotoxicity and human disease. *Toxicol Appl Pharmacol*. 2005;204:355-360.
2. Rothman RB, Baumann MH. Monoamine transporters and psychostimulant drugs. *Eur J Pharmacol*. 2003;479:23-40.
3. Dougherty DD, Bonab AA, Spencer TJ, Rauch SL, Madras BK, Fischman AJ. Dopamine transporter density in patients with attention deficit hyperactivity disorder. *Lancet*. 1999;354:2132-2133.
4. Spencer TJ, Biederman J, Madras BK, et al. In vivo neuroreceptor imaging in attention-deficit/hyperactivity disorder: a focus on the dopamine transporter. *Biol Psychiatry*. 2005;57: 1293-1300.

5. Eriksen JL, Dawson TM, Dickson DW, Petrucelli L. Caught in the act: alpha-synuclein is the culprit in Parkinson's disease. *Neuron.* 2003;40:453-456.
6. Sidhu A, Wersinger C, Vernier P. Alpha-synuclein regulation of the dopaminergic transporter: a possible role in the pathogenesis of Parkinson's disease. *FEBS Lett.* 2004;565:1-5.
7. Dubertret C, Hanoun N, Ades J, Hamon M, Gorwood P. Family-based association study of the 5-HT transporter gene and schizophrenia. *Int J Neuropsychopharmacol.* 2005;8:87-92.
8. Keikhaee MR, Fadai F, Sargolzaee MR, Javanbakht A, Najmabadi H, Ohadi M. Association analysis of the dopamine transporter (DAT1)-67A/T polymorphism in bipolar disorder. *Am J Med Genet B Neuropsychiatr Genet.* 2005;135:47-49.
9. Wong DF, Harris JC, Naidu S, et al. Dopamine transporters are markedly reduced in Lesch-Nyhan disease in vivo. *Proc Natl Acad Sci USA.* 1996;93:5539-5543.
10. Hahn MK, Robertson D, Blakely RD. A mutation in the human norepinephrine transporter gene (SLC6A2) associated with orthostatic intolerance disrupts surface expression of mutant and wild-type transporters. *J Neurosci.* 2003;23:4470-4478.
11. Maron E, Kuikka JT, Shlik J, Vasar V, Vanninen E, Tiihonen J. Reduced brain serotonin transporter binding in patients with panic disorder. *Psychiatry Res.* 2004;132:173-181.
12. Sutcliffe JS, Delahanty RJ, Prasad HC, et al. Allelic heterogeneity at the serotonin transporter locus (SLC6A4) confers susceptibility to autism and rigid-compulsive behaviors. *Am J Hum Genet.* 2005;77:265-279.
13. Caspi A, Sugden K, Moffitt TE, et al. Influence of life stress on depression: moderation by a polymorphism in the 5-HTT gene. *Science.* 2003;301:386-389.
14. Inoue K, Itoh K, Yoshida K, Shimizu T, Suzuki T. Positive association between T-182C polymorphism in the norepinephrine transporter gene and susceptibility to major depressive disorder in a Japanese population. *Neuropsychobiology.* 2004;50:301-304.
15. Saier MH Jr. A functional-phylogenetic system for the classification of transport proteins. *J Cell Biochem.* 1999;75:84-94.
16. Rudnick G. Mechanisms of biogenic amine neurotransmitter transporters. In: Reith MEA, ed. *Neurotransmitter Transporters: Structure, Function, and Regulation.* Totowa, NJ: Humana Press Inc; 1997:73-100.
17. Goldberg NR, Beuming T, Soyer OS, Goldstein RA, Weinstein H, Javitch JA. Probing conformational changes in neurotransmitter transporters: a structural context. *Eur J Pharmacol.* 2003;479:3-12.
18. Chen N, Zhen J, Reith ME. Mutation of Trp84 and Asp313 of the dopamine transporter reveals similar mode of binding interaction for GBR12909 and benztropine as opposed to cocaine. *J Neurochem.* 2004;89:853-864.
19. Kitayama S, Shimada S, Xu H, Markham L, Donovan DM, Uhl GR. Dopamine transporter site-directed mutations differentially alter substrate transport and cocaine binding. *Proc Natl Acad Sci USA.* 1992;89:7782-7785.
20. Strader CD, Sigal IS, Candelore MR, Rands E, Hill WS, Dixon RAF. Conserved aspartic acid residues 79 and 113 of the β-adrenergic receptor have different roles in receptor function. *J Biol Chem.* 1988;263:10267-10271.
21. Wang W, Sonders MS, Ukairo OT, Scott H, Kloetzel MK, Surratt CK. Dissociation of high-affinity cocaine analog binding and dopamine uptake inhibition at the dopamine transporter. *Mol Pharmacol.* 2003;64:430-439.
22. Ukairo OT, Bondi CD, Newman AH, et al. Recognition of benztropine by the dopamine transporter (DAT) differs from that of the classical dopamine uptake inhibitors cocaine, methylphenidate and mazindol as a function of a DAT transmembrane 1 aspartic acid residue. *J Pharmacol Exp Ther.* 2005;314:575-583.
23. Barker EL, Moore KR, Rakhshan F, Blakely RD. Transmembrane domain I contributes to the permeation pathway for serotonin and ions in the serotonin transporter. *J Neurosci.* 1999;19:4705-4717.
24. Carroll FI, Lewin AH, Boja JW, Kuhar MJ. Cocaine receptor: biochemical characterization and structure-activity relationships of cocaine analogues at the dopamine transporter. *J Med Chem.* 1992;35:969-981.

25. Madras BK, Pristupa ZB, Niznik HB, et al. Nitrogen-based drugs are not essential for block-ade of monoamine transporters. *Synapse*. 1996;24:340-348.
26. Kozikowski AP, Simoni D, Roberti M, et al. Synthesis of 8-oxa analogues of norcocaine endowed with interesting cocaine-like activity. *Bioorg Med Chem Lett*. 1999;9:1831-1836.
27. Chen N, Vaughan RA, Reith ME. The role of conserved tryptophan and acidic residues in the human dopamine transporter as characterized by site-directed mutagenesis. *J Neurochem*. 2001;77:1116-1127.
28. Zhen J, Maiti S, Chen N, Dutta AK, Reith ME. Interaction between a hydroxypiperidine ana-logue of 4-(2-benzhydryloxy-ethyl)-1-(4-fluorobenzyl)piperidine and aspartate 68 in the human dopamine transporter. *Eur J Pharmacol*. 2004;506:17-26.
29. Lin Z, Wang W, Uhl GR. Dopamine transporter tryptophan mutants highlight candidate dopamine- and cocaine-selective domains. *Mol Pharmacol*. 2000;58:1581-1592.
30. Reith ME, Berfield JL, Wang LC, Ferrer JV, Javitch JA. The uptake inhibitors cocaine and benztropine differentially alter the conformation of the human dopamine transporter. *J Biol Chem*. 2001;276:29012-29018.
31. Adkins EM, Barker EL, Blakely RD. Interactions of tryptamine derivatives with serotonin transporter species variants implicate transmembrane domain I in substrate recognition. *Mol Pharmacol*. 2001;59:514-523.
32. Barker EL, Perlman MA, Adkins EM, et al. High affinity recognition of serotonin transporter antagonists defined by species-scanning mutagenesis. *J Biol Chem*. 1998;273:19459-19468.
33. Javitch JA, Shi L, Liapakis G. Use of the substituted cysteine accessibility method to study the structure and function of G protein-coupled receptors. *Methods Enzymol*. 2002;343:137-156.
34. Henry LK, Adkins EM, Han Q, Blakely RD. Serotonin and cocaine-sensitive inactivation of human serotonin transporters by methanethiosulfonates targeted to transmembrane domain I. *J Biol Chem*. 2003;278:37052-37063.
35. Ferrer JV, Javitch JA. Cocaine alters the accessibility of endogenous cysteines in putative extracellular and intracellular loops of the human dopamine transporter. *Proc Natl Acad Sci USA*. 1998;95:9238-9243.
36. Gaffaney JD, Vaughan RA. Uptake inhibitors but not substrates induce protease resistance in extracellular loop two of the dopamine transporter. *Mol Pharmacol*. 2004;65:692-701.
37. Lin Z, Wang W, Kopajtic T, Revay RS, Uhl GR. Dopamine transporter: transmembrane phe-nylalanine mutations can selectively influence dopamine uptake and cocaine analog recogni-tion. *Mol Pharmacol*. 1999;56:434-447.
38. Melamed N, Kanner BI. Transmembrane domains I and II of the gamma-aminobutyric acid transporter GAT-4 contain molecular determinants of substrate specificity. *Mol Pharmacol*. 2004;65:1452-1461.
39. Zhou Y, Bennett ER, Kanner BI. The aqueous accessibility in the external half of transmem-brane domain I of the GABA transporter GAT-1 is modulated by its ligands. *J Biol Chem*. 2004;279:13800-13808.
40. Wu X, Gu HH. Cocaine affinity decreased by mutations of aromatic residue phenylalanine 105 in the transmembrane domain 2 of dopamine transporter. *Mol Pharmacol*. 2003;63:653-658.
41. Sato Y, Zhang YW, Androutsellis-Theotokis A, Rudnick G. Analysis of transmembrane domain 2 of rat serotonin transporter by cysteine scanning mutagenesis. *J Biol Chem*. 2004;279:22926-22933.
42. Chen R, Han DD, Gu HH. A triple mutation in the second transmembrane domain of mouse dopamine transporter markedly decreases sensitivity to cocaine and methylphenidate. *J Neurochem*. 2005;94:352-359.
43. Sucic S, Paczkowski FA, Runkel F, Bonisch H, Bryan-Lluka LJ. Functional significance of a highly conserved glutamate residue of the human noradrenaline transporter. *J Neurochem*. 2002;81:344-354.
44. Keshet GI, Bendahan A, Su H, Mager S, Lester HA, Kanner BI. Glutamate-101 is critical for the function of the sodium and chloride-coupled GABA transporter GAT-1. *FEBS Lett*. 1995;371:39-42.

45. Lee SH, Kang SS, Son H, Lee YS. The region of dopamine transporter encompassing the 3rd transmembrane domain is crucial for function. *Biochem Biophys Res Commun.* 1998;246: 347-352.

46. Lee SH, Chang MY, Lee KH, Park BS, Lee YS, Chin HR. Importance of valine at position 152 for the substrate transport and 2beta-carbomethoxy-3beta-(4-fluorophenyl)tropane binding of dopamine transporter. *Mol Pharmacol.* 2000;57:883-889.

47. Lin Z, Uhl GR. Dopamine transporter mutants with cocaine resistance and normal dopamine uptake provide targets for cocaine antagonism. *Mol Pharmacol.* 2002;61:885-891.

48. Chen J-G, Sachpatzidis A, Rudnick G. The third transmembrane domain of the serotonin transporter contains residues associated with substrate and cocaine binding. *J Biol Chem.* 1997;272:28321-28327.

49. Chen J-G, Rudnick G. Permeation and gating residues in serotonin transporter. *Proc Natl Acad Sci USA.* 2000;97:1044-1049.

50. Loland CJ, Granas C, Javitch JA, Gether U. Identification of intracellular residues in the dopamine transporter critical for regulation of transporter conformation and cocaine binding. *J Biol Chem.* 2004;279:3228-3238.

51. Kristensen AS, Larsen MB, Johnsen LB, Wiborg O. Mutational scanning of the human serotonin transporter reveals fast translocating serotonin transporter mutants. *Eur J Neurosci.* 2004;19:1513-1523.

52. Mortensen OV, Kristensen AS, Wiborg O. Species-scanning mutagenesis of the serotonin transporter reveals residues essential in selective, high-affinity recognition of antidepressants. *J Neurochem.* 2001;79:237-247.

53. Chen F, Larsen MB, Neubauer HA, Sanchez C, Plenge P, Wiborg O. Characterization of an allosteric citalopram-binding site at the serotonin transporter. *J Neurochem.* 2005;92:21-28.

54. Paczkowski FA, Bryan-Lluka LJ. Tyrosine residue 271 of the norepinephrine transporter is an important determinant of its pharmacology. *Brain Res Mol Brain Res.* 2001;97:32-42.

55. Kopajtic T, Rucker C, Seidleck BK, Blaschak CJ, Surratt CK. Glycine substitution of selected dopamine transporter (DAT) proline residues predicted for transmembrane domains: effects on dopamine uptake and affinities for cocaine analogs and other DAT ligands. *Soc Neurosci Abs.* 1997;23:408.

56. Lin Z, Itokawa M, Uhl GR. Dopamine transporter proline mutations influence dopamine uptake, cocaine analog recognition, and expression. *FASEB J.* 2000;14:715-728.

57. Paczkowski FA, Bryan-Lluka LJ. Role of proline residues in the expression and function of the human noradrenaline transporter. *J Neurochem.* 2004;88:203-211.

58. Williams KA, Deber CM. Proline residues in transmembrane helices: structural or dynamic role? *Biochemistry.* 1991;30:8919-8923.

59. Brandl CJ, Deber CM. Hypothesis about the function of membrane-buried proline residues in transport proteins. *Proc Natl Acad Sci USA.* 1986;83:917-921.

60. Barlow DJ, Thornton JM. Helix geometry in proteins. *J Mol Biol.* 1988;201:601-619.

61. Li S-C, Goto NK, Williams KA, Deber CM. α-Helical, but not β-sheet, propensity of proline is determined by peptide environment. *Proc Natl Acad Sci USA.* 1996;93:6676-6681.

62. Ri Y, Ballesteros JA, Abrams CK, et al. The role of a conserved proline residue in mediating conformational changes associated with voltage gating of Cx32 gap junctions. *Biophys J.* 1999;76:2887-2898.

63. Visiers I, Weinstein H, Rudnick G, Stephan MM. A second site rescue mutation partially restores functional expression to the serotonin transporter mutant V382P. *Biochemistry.* 2003;42:6784-6793.

64. Sansom MS, Weinstein H. Hinges, swivels and switches: the role of prolines in signalling via transmembrane alpha-helices. *Trends Pharmacol Sci.* 2000;21:445-451.

65. Eisenman G, Dani JA. An introduction to molecular architecture and permeability of ion channels. *Annu Rev Biophys Biophys Chem.* 1987;16:205-226.

66. Sansom MSP. Proline residues in transmembrane helices of channel and transport proteins: a molecular modelling study. *Protein Eng.* 1992;5:53-60.

67. Chen N, Sun L, Reith ME. Cationic interactions at the human dopamine transporter reveal binding conformations for dopamine distinguishable from those for the cocaine analog 2 alpha-carbomethoxy-3 alpha-(4-fluorophenyl)tropane. *J Neurochem.* 2002;81:1383-1393.
68. Chen N, Reith ME. Na+ and the substrate permeation pathway in dopamine transporters. *Eur J Pharmacol.* 2003;479:213-221.
69. Buck KJ, Amara SG. Structural domains of catecholamine transporter chimeras involved in selective inhibition by antidepressants and psychomotor stimulants. *Mol Pharmacol.* 1995;48: 1030-1037.
70. Giros B, Wang Y, Suter S, Mestikawy SE, Pifl C, Caron MG. Delineation of discrete domains for substrate, cocaine, and tricyclic antidepressant interactions using chimeric dopamine-norepinephrine transporters. *J Biol Chem.* 1994;269:15985-15988.
71. Roubert C, Cox PJ, Bruss M, Hamon M, Bonisch H, Giros B. Determination of residues in the norepinephrine transporter that are critical for tricyclic antidepressant affinity. *J Biol Chem.* 2001;276:8254-8260.
72. Strader CD, Candelore MR, Hill WS, Sigal IS, Dixon RA. Identification of two serine residues involved in agonist activation of the beta-adrenergic receptor. *J Biol Chem.* 1989;264: 13572-13578.
73. Danek Burgess KS, Justice JB Jr. Effects of serine mutations in transmembrane domain 7 of the human norepinephrine transporter on substrate binding and transport. *J Neurochem.* 1999;73:656-664.
74. Penado KM, Rudnick G, Stephan MM. Critical amino acid residues in transmembrane span 7 of the serotonin transporter identified by random mutagenesis. *J Biol Chem.* 1998;273: 28098-28106.
75. Kamdar G, Penado KM, Rudnick G, Stephan MM. Functional role of critical stripe residues in transmembrane span 7 of the serotonin transporter: effects of Na+, Li+, and methanethio-sulfonate reagents. *J Biol Chem.* 2001;276:4038-4045.
76. Itokawa M, Lin Z, Cai NS, et al. Dopamine transporter transmembrane domain polar mutants: ΔG and ΔΔG values implicate regions important for transporter functions. *Mol Pharmacol.* 2000;57:1093-1103.
77. Uhl GR, Lin Z. The top 20 dopamine transporter mutants: structure-function relationships and cocaine actions. *Eur J Pharmacol.* 2003;479:71-82.
78. Sur C, Betz H, Schloss P. A single serine residue controls the cation dependence of substrate transport by the rat serotonin transporter. *Proc Natl Acad Sci USA.* 1997;94:7639-7644.
79. Barker EL, Kimmel HL, Blakely RD. Chimeric human and rat serotonin transporters reveal domains involved in recognition of transporter ligands. *Mol Pharmacol.* 1994;46:799-807.
80. Barker EL, Blakely RD. Identification of a single amino acid, Phenylalanine 586, that is responsible for high affinity interactions of tricyclic antidepressants with the human serotonin transporter. *Mol Pharmacol.* 1996;50:957-965.
81. Smicun Y, Campbell SD, Chen MA, Gu H, Rudnick G. The role of external loop regions in serotonin transport: loop scanning mutagenesis of the serotonin transporter external domain. *J Biol Chem.* 1999;274:36058-36064.
82. Norgaard-Nielsen K, Norregaard L, Hastrup H, Javitch JA, Gether U. Zn(2+) site engineering at the oligomeric interface of the dopamine transporter. *FEBS Lett.* 2002;524:87-91.
83. Loland CJ, Norregaard L, Gether U. Defining proximity relationships in the tertiary structure of the dopamine transporter: identification of a conserved glutamic acid as a third coordinate in the endogenous Zn(2+)-binding site. *J Biol Chem.* 1999;274:36928-36934.
84. Fischer JF, Cho AK. Chemical release of dopamine from striatal homogenates: evidence for an exchange diffusion model. *J Pharmacol Exp Ther.* 1979;208:203-209.
85. Khoshbouei H, Sen N, Guptaroy B, et al. N-terminal phosphorylation of the dopamine transporter is required for amphetamine-induced efflux. *PLoS Biol.* 2004;2:E78.
86. Granas C, Ferrer J, Loland CJ, Javitch JA, Gether U. N-terminal truncation of the dopamine transporter abolishes phorbol ester- and substance P receptor-stimulated phosphorylation without impairing transporter internalization. *J Biol Chem.* 2003;278:4990-5000.

87. Seidel S, Singer EA, Just H, et al. Amphetamines take two to tango: an oligomer-based counter-transport model of neurotransmitter transport explores the amphetamine action. *Mol Pharmacol*. 2005;67:140-151.
88. Sucic S, Bryan-Lluka LJ. The role of the conserved GXXXRXG motif in the expression and function of the human norepinephrine transporter. *Brain Res Mol Brain Res*. 2002;108:40-50.
89. Loland CJ, Norregaard L, Litman T, Gether U. Generation of an activating Zn(2+) switch in the dopamine transporter: mutation of an intracellular tyrosine constitutively alters the conformational equilibrium of the transport cycle. *Proc Natl Acad Sci USA*. 2002;99:1683-1688.
90. Chen N, Rickey J, Berfield JL, Reith ME. Aspartate 345 of the dopamine transporter is critical for conformational changes in substrate translocation and cocaine binding. *J Biol Chem*. 2004;279:5508-5519.
91. Lee FJ, Pristupa ZB, Ciliax BJ, Levey AI, Niznik HB. The dopamine transporter carboxyl-terminal tail: truncation/substitution mutants selectively confer high affinity dopamine uptake while attenuating recognition of the ligand binding domain. *J Biol Chem*. 1996;271:20885-20894.
92. Hastrup H, Karlin A, Javitch JA. Symmetrical dimer of the human dopamine transporter revealed by cross-linking Cys-306 at the extracellular end of the sixth transmembrane segment. *Proc Natl Acad Sci USA*. 2001;98:10055-10060.
93. Hastrup H, Sen N, Javitch JA. The human dopamine transporter forms a tetramer in the plasma membrane: cross-linking of a cysteine in the fourth transmembrane segment is sensitive to cocaine analogs. *J Biol Chem*. 2003;278:45045-45048.
94. Kilic F, Rudnick G. Oligomerization of serotonin transporter and its functional consequences. *Proc Natl Acad Sci USA*. 2000;97:3106-3111.
95. Torres GE, Yao WD, Mohn AR, et al. Functional interaction between monoamine plasma membrane transporters and the synaptic PDZ domain-containing protein PICK1. *Neuron*. 2001;30:121-134.
96. Lee KH, Kim MY, Kim DH, Lee YS. Syntaxin 1A and receptor for activated C kinase interact with the N-terminal region of human dopamine transporter. *Neurochem Res*. 2004;29: 1405-1409.
97. Sung U, Apparsundaram S, Galli A, et al. A regulated interaction of syntaxin 1A with the antidepressant-sensitive norepinephrine transporter establishes catecholamine clearance capacity. *J Neurosci*. 2003;23:1697-1709.
98. Deken SL, Beckman ML, Boos L, Quick MW. Transport rates of GABA transporters: regulation by the N-terminal domain and syntaxin 1A. *Nat Neurosci*. 2000;3:998-1003.
99. Pristupa ZB, Wilson JM, Hoffman BJ, Kish SJ, Niznik HB. Pharmacological heterogeneity of the cloned and native human dopamine transporter: disassociation of [^{3}H]WIN 35,428 and [^{3}H]GBR 12,935 binding. *Mol Pharmacol*. 1994;45:125-135.
100. Eshleman AJ, Carmolli M, Cumbay M, Martens CR, Neve KA, Janowsky A. Characteristics of drug interactions with recombinant biogenic amine transporters expressed in the same cell type. *J Pharmacol Exp Ther*. 1999;289:877-885.
101. Williams KA, Geldmacher-Kaufer U, Padan E, Schuldiner S, Kuhlbrandt W. Projection structure of NhaA, a secondary transporter from *Escherichia coli*, at 4.0 A resolution. *EMBO J*. 1999;18:3558-3563.
102. Williams KA. Three-dimensional structure of the ion-coupled transport protein NhaA. *Nature*. 2000;403:112-115.
103. Ravna AW, Sylte I, Dahl SG. Molecular model of the neural dopamine transporter. *J Comput Aided Mol Des*. 2003;17:367-382.
104. Ravna AW, Sylte I, Dahl SG. Molecular mechanism of citalopram and cocaine interactions with neurotransmitter transporters. *J Pharmacol Exp Ther*. 2003;307:34-41.
105. Yamashita A, Singh SK, Kawate T, Jin Y, Gouaux E. Crystal structure of a bacterial homologue of Na$^+$/Cl$^-$-dependent neurotransmitter transporters. *Nature*. 2005;437:215-223.
106. Lee SH, Chang MY, Jeon DJ, et al. The functional domains of dopamine transporter for cocaine analog, CFT binding. *Exp Mol Med*. 2002;34:90-94.

107. Vaughan RA. Photoaffinity-labeled ligand binding domains on dopamine transporters identified by peptide mapping. *Mol Pharmacol*. 1995;47:956-964.
108. Vaughan RA, Kuhar MJ. Dopamine transporter ligand binding domains: structural and functional properties revealed by limited proteolysis. *J Biol Chem*. 1996;271:21672-21680.
109. Vaughan RA, Agoston GE, Lever JR, Newman AH. Differential binding of tropane-based photoaffinity ligands on the dopamine transporter. *J Neurosci*. 1999;19:630-636.
110. Lever JR, Zou MF, Parnas ML, et al. Radioiodinated azide and isothiocyanate derivatives of cocaine for irreversible labeling of dopamine transporters: synthesis and covalent binding studies. *Bioconjug Chem*. 2005;16:644-649.
111. Vaughan RA, Parnas ML, Gaffaney JD, et al. Affinity labeling the dopamine transporter ligand binding site. *J Neurosci Methods*. 2005;143:33-40.
112. Wirtz SE, Parnas L, Jackson TV, et al. Identification of an MFZ 2-24 photoaffinity labeling site on the human dopamine transporter. *Soc Neurosci Abstr*. 2004;33:53-19.

Chapter 19
Dual Dopamine/Serotonin Releasers as Potential Medications for Stimulant and Alcohol Addictions

Richard B. Rothman,[1] Bruce E. Blough,[2] and Michael H. Baumann[1]

Abstract We have advocated the idea of agonist therapy for treating cocaine addiction. This strategy involves administration of stimulant-like medications (eg, monoamine releasers) to alleviate withdrawal symptoms and prevent relapse. A major limitation of this approach is that many candidate medicines possess significant abuse potential because of activation of mesolimbic dopamine (DA) neurons in central nervous system reward circuits. Previous data suggest that serotonin (5-HT) neurons can provide an inhibitory influence over mesolimbic DA neurons. Thus, it might be predicted that the balance between DA and 5-HT transmission is important to consider when developing medications with reduced stimulant side effects. In this article, we discuss several issues related to the development of dual DA/5-HT releasers for the treatment of substance use disorders. First, we discuss evidence supporting the existence of a dual deficit in DA and 5-HT function during withdrawal from chronic cocaine or alcohol abuse. Then we summarize studies that have tested the hypothesis that 5-HT neurons can dampen the effects mediated by mesolimbic DA. For example, it has been shown that pharmacological manipulations that increase extracellular 5-HT attenuate stimulant effects produced by DA release, such as locomotor stimulation and self-administration behavior. Finally, we discuss our recently published data about PAL-287 (naphthylisopropylamine), a novel non-amphetamine DA-/5-HT-releasing agent that suppresses cocaine self-administration but lacks positive reinforcing properties. It is concluded that DA/5-HT releasers might be useful therapeutic adjuncts for the treatment of cocaine and alcohol addiction, obesity, and even attention deficit disorder and depression.

[1] Clinical Psychopharmacology Section, Intramural Research Program, National Institute on Drug Abuse, National Institutes of Health, Department of Health and Human Services, Baltimore, MD

[2] Chemistry and Life Sciences Group, Research Triangle Institute International, Research Triangle Park, NC

Corresponding Author: Richard B. Rothman, Clinical Psychopharmacology Section, IRP, NIDA, NIH, PO Box 5180, 5500 Nathan Shock Drive, Baltimore, MD 21224. Tel: (410) 550-1598; Fax: (410) 550-2997; E-mail: rrothman@mail.nih.gov

R.S. Rapaka and W. Sadée (eds.), *Drug Addiction.*
© American Association of Pharmaceutical Scientists 2008

Keywords Alcohol, amphetamine, cocaine, dopamine, serotonin, treatment, transporter

Introduction

A major goal of this article is to review recent work from our lab that pertains to dual dopamine (DA)/serotonin (5-HT) releasers as potential medications for alcohol and psychostimulant addictions.[1-9] The term "psychostimulant" refers to drugs that produce a spectrum of effects in humans, including cardiovascular stimulation, mood elevation, and a decreased need for sleep. At higher doses, or after longer periods of use, stimulants can cause a range of disordered thought processes, including severe psychotic episodes. In laboratory animals, psychostimulants increase locomotor activity and are readily self-administered because of their powerful reinforcing properties. Psychostimulants are often described generally as "amphetamine-like," since amphetamine is the prototypical stimulant agent. Table 19.1 lists examples of stimulants, and Fig.19.1 depicts the chemical structures of drugs discussed in this article. It is noteworthy that many of these drugs are useful medications with long histories of efficacy and safety, whereas others are highly addictive substances[10-12] that are associated with considerable morbidity and mortality.[12,13] In some cases, such as amphetamine, the same drug can be a therapeutic entity or an abused substance, depending upon the context in which the drug is administered.

Most psychostimulants interact with monoamine neurons in the central nervous system (CNS). Neurons that synthesize, store, and release the monoamine transmitters norepinephrine (NE), DA, and 5-HT are widely distributed in the mammalian CNS. These neurons express specialized plasma membrane proteins that function to transport previously released transmitter molecules from the extracellular space

Table 19.1 Examples of Psychostimulants*

Drugs	Indication
Therapeutic	
Methylphenidate	Attention deficit disorder
Amphetamine	Attention deficit disorder/narcolepsy
Phentermine	Anorectic
Diethylpropion	Anorectic
Phendimetrazine	Anorectic
Benzphetamine	Anorectic
Abused	
Cocaine	
Methamphetamine	
3,4-Methylenedioxymethamphetamine	

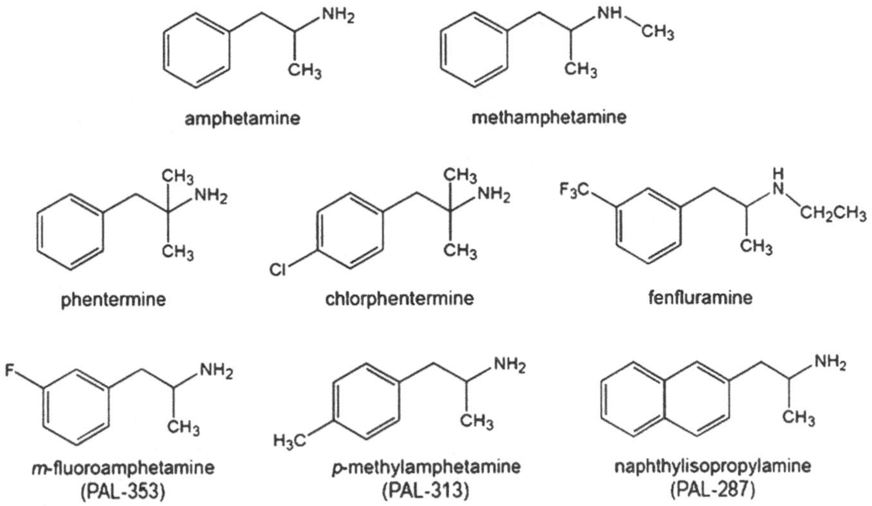

Fig. 19.1 Chemical structures of selected psychostimulants.

back into the cytoplasm.[14,15] Substantial evidence has shown that there are distinct transporter proteins expressed by NE neurons (NET), DA neurons (DAT), and 5-HT neurons (SERT). These proteins belong to a superfamily of Na^+/Cl^--dependent transporters that share genetic, structural, and functional homologies.[16,17] Under normal circumstances, the transporter-mediated uptake of monoamine transmitters is the principal mechanism for inactivation of monoaminergic signaling in the brain. The biogenic amine neurotransmitters and their receptors play a critical role in either the pathogenesis or the treatment of a wide range of psychiatric disorders.[18]

In general, drugs that target transporter proteins can be divided into 2 classes based on their precise mechanism of action: reuptake inhibitors and substrate-type releasers. Reuptake inhibitors bind to transporter proteins but are not themselves transported. These drugs elevate extracellular transmitter concentrations by blocking transporter-mediated recapture of transmitter molecules from the synapse. Substrate-type releasers bind to transporter proteins and are then transported into the cytoplasm of nerve terminals. "Releasers," a term used interchangeably with the term "substrates," elevate extracellular transmitter concentrations by a 2-pronged mechanism: (1) they promote efflux of transmitter by a process of transporter-mediated exchange, and (2) they increase cytoplasmic levels of transmitter by disrupting storage of transmitters in vesicles via interactions with vesicular monoamine transporter$_2$ (VMAT$_2$).[19,20] The exact mechanism underlying the transporter-mediated exchange mechanism is complex and still under intensive investigation.[21-23] The interaction with VMAT$_2$ can increase the pool of neurotransmitter available for release by transporter-mediated exchange. Because substrate-type releasing agents must be transported into nerve terminals to promote transmitter release, reuptake inhibitors can block the effects of releasers.

Dual-Deficit Model of Stimulant Addiction

The initial use of stimulants such as cocaine and methamphetamine produces a "high" or "rush" that is likely caused by elevations in extracellular DA levels in mesolimbic circuits, although some evidence indicates that elevations in extracellular NE may also contribute.[4,24] Similarly, alcohol-induced increases in mesolimbic DA are thought to underlie the positive reinforcing effects of this substance.[25] Episodic use of stimulants, especially when they are self-administered via smoking or the intravenous route, can lead to severe addiction in susceptible individuals. The persistent abuse of stimulants and alcohol causes long-term changes in neurochemistry and brain circuitry via processes of synaptic plasticity.[25-27] Both preclinical and human data suggest that withdrawal from drugs of abuse is associated with impairments in 5-HT neuronal function[28-30] in addition to the well-accepted deficits in DA function.[31] Compelling clinical evidence for 5-HT deficits in cocaine addiction is the occurrence of psychiatric symptoms resembling major depression following abstinence from binge cocaine use,[31,32] coupled with increased prevalence of suicidal ideation and suicide attempts among cocaine addicts.[33] A well-established role of 5-HT dysfunction in mediating depression and suicide[34] suggests that decreased synaptic 5-HT might play a role in cocaine and alcohol withdrawal states.[35] Indeed, the constellation of symptoms often reported by patients withdrawing from stimulant or alcohol use, such as depressed mood, suicidal ideations, obsessive thoughts of using drugs, intense drug craving, anhedonia, increased impulsivity, and susceptibility to drug-related cues presumably reflects long-term changes in brain function and structure. In particular, evidence points to deficits in DA and 5-HT neuronal function during withdrawal from alcohol and stimulant abuse.[30]

We have proposed a dual-deficit model of stimulant addiction in which drug-induced DA and 5-HT dysfunction contributes to withdrawal symptoms, drug craving, and relapse.[1,30,36,37] According to the dual-deficit model, depicted diagrammatically in Fig. 19.2, decreased synaptic DA during stimulant withdrawal underlies anhedonia and psychomotor retardation, whereas decreased synaptic 5-HT gives rise to depressed mood, obsessive thoughts, and lack of impulse control. Consistent with this model, rats receiving repeated injections of abused stimulants exhibit neurobiological changes similar to those observed in human patients with major depression.[30,38-40] If abstinent stimulant addicts exhibit DA and 5-HT deficits, a logical prediction of the dual-deficit model would be that pharmacotherapies capable of correcting abnormalities in DA and 5-HT function should be effective in treating stimulant and alcohol dependence.

In agreement with the dual-deficit hypothesis, drugs that release DA (phentermine, amphetamine) or 5-HT (fenfluramine) display properties consistent with the effective treatment of substance use disorders.[36,41-44] Indeed, administration of DA and 5-HT releasers alone, or in combination, decreases drug-seeking behavior in preclinical models of addiction. Acute and chronic administration of d-amphetamine, a DA-releasing agent, decreases cocaine self-administration behavior in rhesus monkeys.[45,46] As illustrated in Fig. 19.3, the DA-releasing agent phentermine suppresses

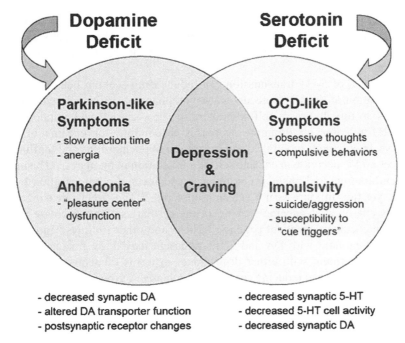

Fig. 19.2 The dual-deficit model of psychostimulant addiction. According to the model, withdrawal from chronic stimulant use leads to decreased synaptic availability of DA and 5-HT that, in turn, contributes to withdrawal symptoms, drug craving, and relapse. DA dysfunction underlies anhedonia and psychomotor disturbances, whereas 5-HT dysfunction causes depressed mood, obsessive thoughts, and lack of impulse control. Protracted withdrawal phenomena are postulated to contribute significantly to relapse. Taken from Rothman and Baumann.[5] OCD indicates obsessive-compulsive disorder; DA, dopamine; 5-HT, serotonin.

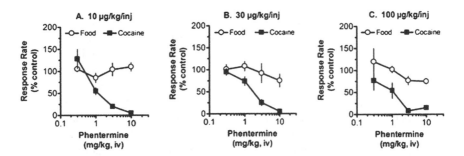

Fig. 19.3 Phentermine, administered intravenously, decreases cocaine self-administration. Taken from Wojnicki et al.[9] Acute effects of phentermine on rates of responding maintained under an FR 30 food (○), FR 30 cocaine (■) schedule with different unit doses (10–100 μg/kg/injection, left-right) of cocaine. Abscissa: dose of phentermine (mg/kg). Ordinate: effect, expressed as the mean (± SEM) percentage of individual control rates of responding (n = 3–4); control variability (filled symbols), expressed as the average of individual coefficients of variation. Inj indicates injection; IV, intravenous; FR, fixed ratio.

responding for cocaine without affecting food-reinforced behavior, and this effect is maintained by daily administration of phentermine.[9] These results provide a rationale for using DA-releasing agents as medications for treating cocaine addiction.[47,48]

Stimulation of 5-HT transmission can reduce drug-seeking behavior as well. Administration of the 5-HT precursor L-tryptophan, which increases brain 5-HT synthesis, to rats decreases self-administration of cocaine[49] and amphetamine.[50] The 5-HT releaser fenfluramine decreases responding for cocaine in rhesus monkeys. Interestingly, combined administration of phentermine and fenfluramine produces a 75% decrease in cocaine self-administration in monkeys.[51] The mixture of d-fenfluramine and phentermine reduces cocaine self-administration by 80% in rats, yet this mixture is not self-administered.[52] The 5-HT-releasing agents suppress cue-elicited cocaine-seeking behavior in rats[53] and decrease cocaine craving in cocaine-dependent patients.[54] These and other findings[36] indicate that combined treatment with DA and 5-HT releasers may have greater therapeutic value than treatment with either drug alone, in terms of decreasing stimulant self-administration and reducing cue-induced relapse. A growing body of evidence shows that DA-/5-HT-releasing agents may provide similar therapeutic benefits for alcohol dependence.[41,42,55]

Dual DA/5-HT Releasers as Agonist Treatments

The use of stimulant-like medications to treat stimulant addictions is known as agonist therapy. This strategy involves administering medications that are less potent and less addictive than cocaine or methamphetamine but decrease stimulant abuse because they share neurochemical properties with the illicit drugs.[56] Viewed from this perspective, agonist therapy is like neurochemical "normalization" therapy: by substituting for the abused drug, the treatment drug "normalizes" dysregulated neurochemistry.[5] Neurochemical normalization therapy has generated effective treatments for nicotine dependence[57] and opioid dependence[58,59] and has recently been explored for the treatment of cocaine dependence.[60-64] A major limitation of this approach as applied to stimulant addiction is that candidate medications often exhibit intrinsic abuse liability.[47] One possible advantage of treating stimulant and alcohol dependence with dual DA-/5-HT-releasing agents is that concurrent elevation of extracellular 5-HT can greatly reduce the typical psychomotor actions of DA releasers, including locomotor activity, reward, and self-administration behavior.

Several lines of evidence support the notion that elevations in synaptic 5-HT counteract the stimulant and reinforcing effects mediated by elevations in synaptic DA.[65,66] As noted above, L-tryptophan decreases cocaine[49] and amphetamine[50] self-administration in rats. Likewise, pretreatment with 5-HT reuptake inhibitors reduces intravenous cocaine self-administration in rats[67] and squirrel monkeys.[68] Cocaine analogs that have potent 5-HT transporter affinity[69] support less self-administration behavior than analogs with weak 5-HT transporter affinity. Moreover, as described

Table 19.2 Summary of Serotonergic and Dopaminergic Effects of Selected Releasing Agents*

Drug	[³H]5-HT Release EC$_{50}$ (nM)	[³H]DA Release EC$_{50}$ (nM)	Peak % Increase in Dialysate 5-HT (dose, mg/kg)	Peak % Increase in Dialysate DA (dose, mg/kg)	Self-Admini stered	Locomotor Activation
Amphet amine	1756	8.0	45 (0.3 mg/kg ip)	224 (0.3 mg/kg ip)	Yes	Strong
Phenter mine	3511	262	32 (1.0 mg/kg ip)	156 (1.0 mg/kg ip)	Yes	Strong
PAL-353	1937	24.2	170 (1.0 mg/kg IV)	432 (1.0 mg/kg IV)	Yes	Strong
Fenfluramine	79.3	>10 000	215 (1.0 mg/kg ip)	20 (1.0 mg/kg ip)	No	None
Chlorphe ntermine	30.9	2650	228 (1.0 mg/kg ip)	86 (1.0 mg/kg ip)	No	None
Phentermine + fenfluramine	NA	NA	222 (1.0 + 1.0 mg/kg, ip)	144 (1.0 + 1.0 mg/kg ip)	No	Weak
PAL-313	53.4	44.1	544 (1.0 mg/kg IV)	130 (1.0 mg/kg IV)	Weak	Weak
PAL-287	3.4	12.6	464 (1.0 mg/kg IV)	133 (1.0 mg/kg IV)	No	Weak

*A summary of data illustrating the tendency for increasing extracellular 5-HT to reduce reinforcing and locomotor effects mediated by increases in extracellular DA.[1-9] Microdialysis data for PAL-315 and PAL-353 are unpublished. 5-HT indicates serotonin; DA, dopamine; ip, intraperitoneally; PAL-353, *m*-fluoroamphetamine; IV, intravenously; PAL-313, *p*-methylamphetamine; PAL-287, naphthylisopropylamine.

in a recent review, agents that broadly activate brain 5-HT systems can reduce self-administration of stimulants and other drugs of abuse.[70] The "antistimulant" effect of increasing extracellular 5-HT is readily observed after combined administration of 5-HT releasers and DA releasers, or after administration of single agents that release both neurotransmitters. As summarized in Table 19.2, drugs that release [³H]DA more potently than [³H]5-HT in vitro (amphetamine, *m*-fluoroamphetamine, phentermine) increase endogenous extracellular DA much more than extracellular 5-HT in vivo. Such indirect DA agonists are strong locomotor stimulants and support self-administration behavior. Drugs that release [³H]5-HT more potently than [³H]DA (fenfluramine, chlorphentermine) increase endogenous extracellular 5-HT more than extracellular DA. Such indirect 5-HT agonists do not stimulate motor activity and do not support self-administration behavior.

Combining a DA releaser with a 5-HT releaser (phentermine plus fenfluramine), or a single molecule that has similar potencies for releasing DA and 5-HT, results in elevation of both extracellular 5-HT and DA. When the elevations in 5-HT are somewhat greater than the elevations in DA, there is minimal locomotor activation, coupled with minimal or no self-administration. The "antireward" effect of increasing extracellular 5-HT is also seen in the conditioned place preference (CPP) assay,

Fig. 19.4 FE (0.3 mg/kg) reduces PH (3 mg/kg) CPP. Ordinate: mean difference (sec) between time spent in the drug- and vehicle-paired sides of the test chamber. Abscissa: drug dose (mg/kg). Each column represents the mean conditioning score of 9 to 10 rats. Data taken from Rea et al.[3] *Significant place conditioning (Wilcoxon test, $P < .05$). FE indicates fenfluramine; PH, phentermine; CPP, conditioned place preference.

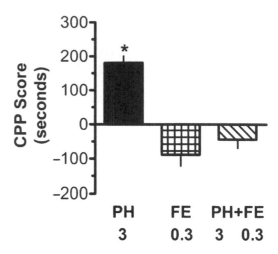

shown in Fig. 19.4, where a low dose of fenfluramine greatly reduces the positive CPP induced by phentermine. These considerations led us to predict that a single molecule that releases both 5-HT and DA would be able to decrease stimulant self-administration yet have minimal abuse liability. Such an agent would thereby provide the advantages of agonist therapy without the untoward side effects of a potential drug of abuse.

Potential Adverse Effects of 5-HT Releasers

Unfortunately, 5-HT-releasing agents are associated with several adverse effects of their own.[71] Based primarily on experience with fenfluramine, 3 potentially serious adverse effects need to be addressed when 5-HT releasers are developed as treatment agents: cardiac valvulopathy, serotonergic neurotoxicity, and primary pulmonary hypertension (PPH). The association of fenfluramine with an increased prevalence of cardiac valve disease led to its withdrawal from the marketplace in September 1997.[72] Recent investigations have demonstrated that norfenfluramine, the N-deethylated metabolite of fenfluramine, activates 5-HT$_{2B}$ receptors on heart valves to stimulate mitogenesis, and this action may represent the principal mechanism underlying cardiac valve disease.[73-75] The term "5-HT neurotoxicity," when used in the present context, refers to the fact that high-dose administration of selective 5-HT releasers (eg, fenfluramine) often causes persistent depletion of brain tissue 5-HT and SERT binding. A key observation is that not all 5-HT releasers deplete 5-HT.[2,76] As shown in Fig. 19.5, repeated administration of the 5-HT-releasing agent m-chlorophenylpiperazine (mCPP) fails to deplete brain 5-HT, despite producing elevations of extracellular 5-HT comparable to those produced by fenfluramine.[2] These data indicate that SERT-mediated release of 5-HT is necessary but not sufficient to produce long-term depletion of brain 5-HT.

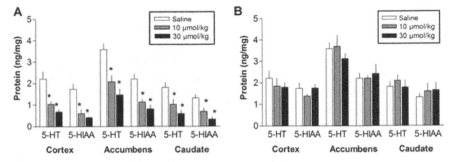

Fig. 19.5 Effects of dFEN and mCPP on brain tissue 5-HT and 5-HIAA. (A) Effects of high-dose dFEN or saline on postmortem tissue levels of 5-HT and 5-HIAA in cingulate cortex, nucleus accumbens, and caudate nucleus. dFEN was administered ip at 10 or 30 μmol/kg, every 2 hours, for 4 doses. Rats were killed 2 weeks after the dosing regimen. (B) Effects of high-dose mCPP or saline on postmortem tissue levels of 5-HT and 5-HIAA in cingulate cortex, nucleus accumbens, and caudate nucleus. mCPP was administered ip at 10 or 30 μmol/kg, every 2 hours, for 4 doses. Rats were killed 2 weeks after the dosing regimen. These doses of dFEN and mCPP produced comparable increases in extracellular 5-HT. Data are mean ± SEM expressed as ng/mg protein for 4 to 6 rats/group. *$P < .05$ compared with saline-treated group. Data taken from Baumann et al.[2] dFEN indicates d-fenfluramine; mCPP, m-chlorophenylpiperazine; 5-HT, serotonin; 5-HIAA, 5-hydroxyindoleacetic acid; ip, intraperitoneally.

Increasing evidence indicates that SERT sites are involved in the mechanism by which fenfluramine increases the risk of developing PPH (for review, see Rothman and Baumann[71] and references therein). For example, medications that increase the risk for PPH have in common the ability to release 5-HT by a SERT-mediated process. On the other hand, not all 5-HT releasers are associated with PPH. The antidepressant trazodone is not associated with PPH, yet its major metabolite, mCPP, is a potent SERT substrate, as noted above.[2] Experimental data from a mouse model of hypoxic pulmonary hypertension suggest that 5-HT$_{2B}$ receptors may also contribute to the pathogenesis of PPH.[77] The relevance of these findings to drug-induced PPH is not clear, since aminorex, a 5-HT releaser that caused an epidemic of PPH in the 1960s,[78] has minimal activity at 5-HT$_{2B}$ receptors. Viewed collectively, the available data suggest that it should be possible to develop dual DA/5-HT releasers devoid of fenfluramine-like adverse effects. In particular, we have suggested that a lead drug molecule should be chemically distinct from the phenylethylamine structure shared by amphetamine-like agents and should lack significant agonist activity at 5-HT$_{2B}$ receptors.[79]

PAL-287, a Non-Amphetamine DA/5-HT Releaser

Based in part on the above rationale, we sought to identify and characterize a non-amphetamine transporter substrate that would be a potent releaser of DA and 5-HT without affecting the release of NE. After an extensive evaluation of over 350 compounds, we found it virtually impossible to dissociate NE-and DA-releasing properties, perhaps because of phylogenetic similarities between NET and DAT. The first lead compound from our search was PAL-287 (naphthylisopropylamine; see structure in Fig. 19.1), a novel non-amphetamine monoamine releaser.[7] The in vitro potency of PAL-287 at releasing tritiated transmitter from DAT, NET, and SERT is 12.6 ± 0.4 nM, 11.1 ± 0.9 nM, and 3.4 ± 0.2 nM, respectively (Table 19.2). Figure 19.6 shows that administration of PAL-287 to rats increases extracellular 5-HT and DA in a dose-dependent manner, with larger effects on 5-HT than on DA. Functional studies with cloned human 5-HT_2 receptors reveal that PAL-287 is a full agonist at 5-HT_{2B} receptors ($EC_{50} = 40$ nM) and 5-HT_{2A} receptors ($EC_{50} = 466$ nM). The drug is a potent partial agonist at 5-HT_{2C} receptor sites ($EC_{50} = 2.3$ nM, $E_{MAX} = 20\%$), an effect that suggests possible anorectic actions of PAL-287.[80] The 5-HT_{2C} agonist activity may also contribute to the minimal reinforcing properties of PAL-287 despite the potent DA-releasing actions of the drug (see Czoty et al[81] for a review). The relatively weak potency at 5-HT_{2A} and 5-HT_{2B} receptors, as compared with its activity at SERT, suggests that PAL-287 may not activate 5-HT_{2A} and 5-HT_{2B} receptors in vivo.

As reported in Fig. 19.6, PAL-287 produces minimal ambulation and stereotypy (approximately one third of that produced by (+)-amphetamine) when administered to rats. Repeated high-dose administration of PAL-287 to rats (18 mg/kg intraperitoneally [ip] q 2 hours × 3 doses) fails to affect brain tissue 5-HT levels when assessed 2 weeks after injections, unlike (+)-methamphetamine (6.0 mg/kg ip q 2 hours × 3 doses) and (±)–3,4-methylenedioxymethamphetamine (MDMA)

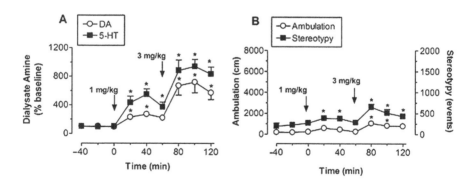

Fig. 19.6 Effects of PAL-287 on neurochemical and locomotor measures in rats. Taken from Rothman et al.[7] (A) Dose-response effects of PAL-287 on extracellular DA and 5-HT in rat prefrontal cortex, as determined by in vivo microdialysis. Rats received IV injection of 1 mg/kg PAL-287 at time 0, followed by 3 mg/kg 60 minutes later. Data are mean ± SEM for 7 rats/group, expressed as percentage of baseline. Baseline levels of DA and 5-HT were 0.43 ± 0.07 and 0.27 ± 0.06 pg/5 μL. (B) Dose-response effects of PAL-287 on ambulation and stereotypy in rats undergoing microdialysis sampling. Rats received IV injections of 1 mg/kg PAL-287 at time 0, followed by 3 mg/kg 60 minutes later. Data are mean ± SEM for 7 rats/group, expressed as distance traveled in cm (ambulation) and number of repetitive movements (stereotypy). $*P < .05$ compared with preinjection control, Duncan's post hoc test. DA indicates dopamine; 5-HT, serotonin; PAL-287, naphthylisopropylamine; IV, intravenous.

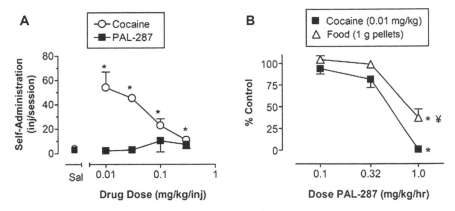

Fig. 19.7 Effects of PAL-287 in the monkey self-administration assay (taken from Rothman et al[7]). (A) Self-administration of cocaine and PAL-287 by rhesus monkeys. Drugs were available under an FR 25 schedule of reinforcement for 2 hours/day. Each point is the mean of 2 sessions of access to each dose of the drugs. Data are mean ± SEM for n = 4 monkeys. Symbols without bars have variability smaller than the points. *$P < .05$ compared with saline-injected control, Duncan's post hoc test. (B) Effects of chronic 7-day treatment with PAL-287 on cocaine- and food-maintained responding. Abscissa: Dose PAL-287 in mg/kg/hr (log scale). Ordinate: Percent control levels of cocaine- and food-maintained responding. Control values were defined as levels of cocaine- or food-maintained responding observed during 7 days of saline treatment. Each point shows mean data ± SEM for 3 monkeys collected during the last 3 days of each 7-day treatment. Two-way ANOVA indicated a significant effect of PAL-287 dose [$F(2,4) = 167$, $P = .0001$] but not a significant effect of reinforcer type [$F(2,2) = 7.26$, $P = 0.114$) or a significant interaction [$F(2,4) = 3.86$, $P = .116$]. Post hoc analysis was conducted with the Newman-Keuls test. *Indicates significant effect of PAL-287 dose in comparison to control for a given reinforcer, $P < .05$. ¥ Indicates that food-maintained responding was significantly greater than cocaine-maintained responding at that dose of PAL-287, $P < .05$. PAL-287 indicates naphthylisopropylamine; inj, injection; FR, fixed ratio.

(7.5 mg/kg ip q 2 hours × 3 doses), which cause significant 5-HT depletions. The data in Fig. 19.7 show that PAL-287 does not support self-administration behavior, and chronic administration of the drug decreases cocaine self-administration in rhesus monkeys. A dose of 1.0 mg/kg/hr PAL-287 significantly reduces both cocaine- and food-maintained responding; however, the suppression of cocaine self-administration is greater than the reduction in food-maintained responding.

Our results with PAL-287 confirm the hypothesis that a non-amphetamine substrate at DAT and SERT will release DA and 5-HT from neurons in vivo, be minimally reinforcing, and suppress ongoing cocaine self-administration. PAL-287 displays several desirable qualities for a candidate treatment medication, including minimal locomotor activation, lack of long-term 5-HT neurotoxicity, and low abuse potential. Future studies will be necessary to determine the potential of PAL-287 for increasing the risk for PPH, perhaps by determining its potency at human voltage-gated K[+] channels.[82] The present data with PAL-287 support the use of monoamine releasers as agonist medications for the treatment of stimulant addictions. A dose of 1.0 mg/kg/hr PAL-287 virtually eliminated cocaine self-administration in rhesus monkeys by the end of the 7-day treatment, although this effect was not entirely selective for cocaine vs food. We also note that the role of NE in the actions of PAL-287 is an important issue awaiting additional study.[4]

Conclusions

Our findings with PAL-287 in monkeys are similar to the suppression of cocaine self-administration produced by (+)-amphetamine, although amphetamine displays greater selectivity than PAL-287 in reducing cocaine self-administration as opposed to food-maintained responding.[83] Grabowski et al[61,84] showed that a slow-release formulation of (+)-amphetamine is effective in keeping cocaine addicts in treatment and reducing illicit cocaine use. We predict that agents with mixed DA-/5-HT-releasing activity, such as PAL-287, will possess the therapeutic effects of amphetamine-type monoamine releasers, while minimizing the adverse effects associated with the phenylethylamine structure. Based on observations that dual DA/5-HT releasers also suppress alcohol ingestion,[41,42,55] it is also likely that PAL-287 agents should also be tested as potential treatment agents for alcohol addiction, especially since dual DA/5-HT releasers suppress alcohol withdrawal seizures.[41] Although further work remains to refine PAL-287, in particular to reduce its potency at 5-HT_{2B} receptors, we believe that PAL-287 represents the prototype for a new generation of drugs that enhance biogenic amine release by acting as substrates at multiple biogenic amine transporters. It seems possible that drugs with a similar mode of action will provide neurochemical normalization therapy for the treatment of cocaine and alcohol addiction, and might be useful for treating depression, obsessive-compulsive disorder, attention deficit disorder, and obesity.

Acknowledgments This research was supported in part by the Intramural Research Program of the National Institutes of Health, National Institute on Drug Abuse; and grant number NIDA R01 DA12970 to Bruce Blough.

References

1. Baumann MH, Ayestas MA, Dersch CM, Brockington A, Rice KC, Rothman RB. Effects of phentermine and fenfluramine on extracellular dopamine and serotonin in rat nucleus accumbens: therapeutic implications. *Synapse*. 2000;36:102-113.
2. Baumann MH, Ayestas MA, Dersch CM, Rothman RB. 1-(m-Chlorophenyl)piperazine (mCPP) dissociates in vivo serotonin release from long-term serotonin depletion in rat brain. *Neuropsychopharmacology*. 2001;24:492-501.
3. Rea WP, Rothman RB, Shippenberg TS. Evaluation of the conditioned reinforcing effects of phentermine and fenfluramine in the rat: concordance with clinical studies. *Synapse*. 1998;30: 107-111.
4. Rothman RB, Baumann MH, Dersch CM, et al. Amphetamine-type central nervous system stimulants release norepinephrine more potently than they release dopamine and serotonin. *Synapse*. 2001;39:32-41.

5. Rothman RB, Baumann MH. Monoamine transporters and psychostimulant drugs. *Eur J Pharmacol*. 2003;479:23-40.
6. Rothman RB, Baumann MH. Serotonin releasing agents, Neurochemical, therapeutic and adverse effects. *Pharmacol Biochem Behav*. 2002;71:825-836.
7. Rothman RB, Blough BE, Woolverton WL, et al. Development of a rationally designed, low abuse potential, biogenic amine releaser that suppresses cocaine self-administration. *J Pharmacol Exp Ther*. 2005;313:1361-1369.
8. Wee S, Anderson KG, Baumann MH, Rothman RB, Blough BE, Woolverton WL. Relationship between the serotonergic activity and reinforcing effects of a series of amphetamine analogs. *J Pharmacol Exp Ther*. 2005;313:848-854.
9. Wojnicki FHE, Rothman RB, Rice KC, Glowa JR. Effects of phentermine on responding maintained under multiple fixed-ratio schedules of food and cocaine presentation in the rhesus monkey. *J Pharmacol Exp Ther*. 1999;288:550-560.
10. Castro FG, Barrington EH, Walton MA, Rawson RA. Cocaine and methamphetamine: differential addiction rates. *Psychol Addict Behav*. 2000;14:390-396.
11. Musto DF. Cocaine's history, especially the American experience. *Ciba Found Symp*. 1992;166:7-14. discussion 14-19.
12. Das G. Cocaine abuse in North America: a milestone in history. *J Clin Pharmacol*. 1993;33:296-310.
13. Centers for Disease Control and Prevention (CDC). Increasing morbidity and mortality associated with abuse of methamphetamine—United States, 1991-1994. *MMWR Morb Mortal Wkly Rep*. 1995;44:882-886.
14. Amara SG, Kuhar MJ. Neurotransmitter transporters: recent progress. *Annu Rev Neurosci*. 1993;16:73-93.
15. Masson J, Sagne C, Hamon M, el Mestikawy S. Neurotransmitter transporters in the central nervous system. *Pharmacol Rev*. 1999;51:439-464.
16. Blakely RD, De Felice LJ, Hartzell HC. Molecular physiology of norepinephrine and serotonin transporters. *J Exp Biol*. 1994;196:263-281.
17. Uhl GR, Johnson PS. Neurotransmitter transporters: three important gene families for neuronal function. *J Exp Biol*. 1994;196:229-236.
18. Amara SG, Sonders MS. Neurotransmitter transporters as molecular targets for addictive drugs. *Drug Alcohol Depend*. 1998;51:87-96.
19. Rudnick G, Clark J. From synapse to vesicle: the reuptake and storage of biogenic amine neurotransmitters. *Biochim Biophys Acta*. 1993;1144:249-263.
20. Rudnick G. Mechanisms of biogenic amine transporters. In: Reith MEA, ed. *Neurotransmitter Transporters: Structure, Function and Regulation*. Totowa, NJ: Humana Press; 1997:73-100.
21. Blakely RD, Defelice LJ, Galli A. Biogenic amine neurotransmitter transporters: just when you thought you knew them. *Physiology (Bethesda)*. 2005;20:225-231.
22. Sitte HH, Freissmuth M. Oligomer formation by Na+-Cl--coupled neurotransmitter transporters. *Eur J Pharmacol*. 2003;479:229-236.
23. Sulzer D, Sonders MS, Poulsen NW, Galli A. Mechanisms of neurotransmitter release by amphetamines: a review. *Prog Neurobiol*. 2005;75:406-433.
24. Alexander M, Rothman RB, Baumann MH, Endres CJ, Brasic JR, Wong DF. Noradrenergic and dopaminergic effects of (+)-amphetamine-like stimulants in the baboon Papio anubis. *Synapse*. 2005;56:94-99.
25. Koob GF. Alcoholism: allostasis and beyond. *Alcohol Clin Exp Res*. 2003;27:232-243.
26. Volkow ND, Li TK. Drug addiction: the neurobiology of behaviour gone awry. *Nat Rev Neurosci*. 2004;5:963-970.
27. Hyman SE. Addiction: a disease of learning and memory. *Am J Psychiatry*. 2005;162:1414-1422.
28. Weiss F, Parsons LH, Schulteis G, et al. Ethanol self-administration restores withdrawal-associated deficiencies in accumbal dopamine and 5-hydroxytryptamine release in dependent rats. *J Neurosci*. 1996;16:3474-3485.

29. Parsons LH, Koob GF, Weiss F. Serotonin dysfunction in the nucleus accumbens of rats during withdrawal after unlimited access to intravenous cocaine. *J Pharmacol Exp Ther.* 1995;274: 1182-1191.

30. Baumann MH, Rothman RB. Alterations in serotonergic responsiveness during cocaine withdrawal in rats: similarities to major depression in humans. *Biol Psychiatry.* 1998;44:578-591.

31. Dackis CA, Gold MS. New concepts in cocaine addiction: the dopamine depletion hypothesis. *Neurosci Biobehav Rev.* 1985;9:469-477.

32. Gawin FH, Kleber HD. Abstinence symptomatology and psychiatric diagnosis in cocaine abusers. *Arch Gen Psychiatry.* 1986;43:107-113.

33. Garlow SJ, Purselle D, D'Orio B. Cocaine use disorders and suicidal ideation. *Drug Alcohol Depend.* 2003;70:101-104.

34. Mann JJ. Neurobiology of suicidal behaviour. *Nat Rev Neurosci.* 2003;4:819-828.

35. Lesch KP. Alcohol dependence and gene x environment interaction in emotion regulation: is serotonin the link? *Eur J Pharmacol.* 2005;526:113-124.

36. Rothman RB, Elmer GI, Shippenberg TS, Rea W, Baumann MH. Phentermine and fenfluramine: preclinical studies in animal models of cocaine addiction. *Ann N Y Acad Sci.* 1998;844:59-74.

37. Baumann MH, Rothman RB. Serotonergic dysfunction during cocaine withdrawal: implications for cocaine-induced depression. In: Karch SB, ed. *Drug Abuse Handbook.* Boca Raton, FL: CRC Press; 1998:463-484.

38. Lin D, Koob GF, Markou A. Differential effects of withdrawal from chronic amphetamine or fluoxetine administration on brain stimulation reward in the rat—interactions between the two drugs. *Psychopharmacology (Berl).* 1999;145:283-294.

39. Markou A, Koob GF. Postcocaine anhedonia. An animal model of cocaine withdrawal. *Neuropsychopharmacology.* 1991;4:17-26.

40. Levy AD, Baumann MH, Van de Kar LD. Monoaminergic regulation of neuroendocrine function and its modification by cocaine. *Front Neuroendocrinol.* 1994;15:85-156.

41. Yu YL, Fisher H, Sekowski A, Wagner GC. Amphetamine and fenfluramine suppress ethanol intake in ethanol-dependent rats. *Alcohol.* 1997;14:45-48.

42. Halladay AK, Wagner GC, Hsu T, Sekowski A, Fisher H. Differential effects of monoaminergic agonists on alcohol intake in rats fed a tryptophan-enhanced diet. *Alcohol.* 1999;18: 55-64.

43. Hitzig P. Combined dopamine and serotonin agonists: a synergistic approach to alcoholism and other addictive behaviors. *Md Med J.* 1993;42:153-157.

44. Rothman RB, Gendron TM, Hitzig P. Combined use of fenfluramine and phentermine in the treatment of cocaine addiction: a pilot case series. *J Subst Abuse Treat.* 1994;11:273-275.

45. Glowa JR, Wojnicki FHE, Matecka D, Rice KC, Rothman RB. Effects of dopamine reuptake inhibitors on food- and cocaine-maintained responding, II: comparisons with other drugs and repeated administrations. *Exp Clin Psychopharmacol.* 1995;3:232-239.

46. Negus SS, Mello NK. Effects of chronic d-amphetamine treatment on cocaine- and food-maintained responding under a progressive-ratio schedule in rhesus monkeys. *Psychopharmacology (Berl).* 2003;167:324-332.

47. Grabowski J, Shearer J, Merrill J, Negus SS. Agonist-like, replacement pharmacotherapy for stimulant abuse and dependence. *Addict Behav.* 2004;29:1439-1464.

48. Rothman RB, Blough BE, Baumann MH. Appetite suppressants as agonist substitution therapies for stimulant dependence. *Ann N Y Acad Sci.* 2002;965:109-126.

49. McGregor A, Lacosta S, Roberts DC. L-tryptophan decreases the breaking point under a progressive ratio schedule of intravenous cocaine reinforcement in the rat. *Pharmacol Biochem Behav.* 1993;44:651-655.

50. Smith FL, Yu DS, Smith DG, Leccese AP, Lyness WH. Dietary tryptophan supplements attenuate amphetamine self-administration in the rat. *Pharmacol Biochem Behav.* 1986;25:849-855.

51. Glowa JR, Rice KC, Matecka D, Rothman RB. Phentermine/fenfluramine decreases cocaine self-administration in rhesus monkeys. *Neuroreport.* 1997;8:1347-1351.

52. Glatz AC, Ehrlich M, Bae RS, et al. Inhibition of cocaine self-administration by fluoxetine or D-fenfluramine combined with phentermine. *Pharmacol Biochem Behav.* 2002;71:197-204.

53. Burmeister JJ, Lungren EM, Neisewander JL. Effects of fluoxetine and d-fenfluramine on cocaine-seeking behavior in rats. *Psychopharmacology (Berl)*. 2003;168:146-154.
54. Buydens-Branchey L, Branchey M, Hudson J, Rothman M, Fergeson P, McKernin C. Effect of fenfluramine challenge on cocaine craving in addicted male users. *Am J Addict*. 1998;7: 142-155.
55. Halladay AK, Wagner GC, Sekowski A, Rothman RB, Baumann MH, Fisher H. Alterations in alcohol consumption, withdrawal seizures, and monoamine transmission in rats treated with phentermine and 5-hydroxy-L-tryptophan. *Synapse*. 2006;59:277-289.
56. Gorelick DA. The rate hypothesis and agonist substitution approaches to cocaine abuse treatment. *Adv Pharmacol*. 1998;42:995-997.
57. Henningfield JE. Nicotine medications for smoking cessation. *N Engl J Med*. 1995;333: 1196-1203.
58. Kreek MJ. Opiates, opioids and addiction. *Mol Psychiatry*. 1996;1:232-254.
59. Ling W, Rawson RA, Compton MA. Substitution pharmacotherapies for opioid addiction: from methadone to LAAM and buprenorphine. *J Psychoactive Drugs*. 1994;26:119-128.
60. Grabowski J, Roache JD, Schmitz JM, Rhoades H, Creson D, Korszun A. Replacement medication for cocaine dependence: methylphenidate. *J Clin Psychopharmacol*. 1997;17:485-488.
61. Grabowski J, Rhoades H, Schmitz J, et al. Dextroamphetamine for cocaine-dependence treatment: a double-blind randomized clinical trial. *J Clin Psychopharmacol*. 2001;21:522-526.
62. Kampman KM, Rukstalis M, Pettinati H, et al. The combination of phentermine and fenfluramine reduced cocaine withdrawal symptoms in an open trial. *J Subst Abuse Treat*. 2000;19: 77-79.
63. Walsh SL, Haberny KA, Bigelow GE. Modulation of intravenous cocaine effects by chronic oral cocaine in humans. *Psychopharmacology (Berl)*. 2000;150:361-373.
64. Alim TN, Jr, Rosse RB, Jr, Vocci FJ, Jr, Lindquist T, Deutsch SI. Diethylpropion pharmacotherapeutic adjuvant therapy for inpatient treatment of cocaine dependence: a test of the cocaine-agonist hypothesis. *Clin Neuropharmacol*. 1995;18:183-195.
65. Daw ND, Kakade S, Dayan P. Opponent interactions between serotonin and dopamine. *Neural Netw*. 2002;15:603-616.
66. Burmeister JJ, Lungren EM, Kirschner KF, Neisewander JL. Differential roles of 5-HT receptor subtypes in cue and cocaine reinstatement of cocaine-seeking behavior in rats. *Neuropsychopharmacology*. 2004;29:660-668.
67. Carroll ME, Lac ST, Asencio M, Kragh R. Fluoxetine reduces intravenous cocaine self-administration in rats. *Pharmacol Biochem Behav*. 1990;35:237-244.
68. Howell LL, Byrd LD. Serotonergic modulation of the behavioral effects of cocaine in the squirrel monkey. *J Pharmacol Exp Ther*. 1995;275:1551-1559.
69. Roberts DC, Phelan R, Hodges LM, et al. Self-administration of cocaine analogs by rats. *Psychopharmacology (Berl)*. 1999;144:389-397.
70. Higgins GA, Fletcher PJ. Serotonin and drug reward: focus on 5-HT2C receptors. *Eur J Pharmacol*. 2003;480:151-162.
71. Rothman RB, Baumann M. Therapeutic and adverse actions of serotonin transporter substrates. *Pharmacol Ther*. 2002;95:73-88.
72. Connolly HM, McGoon MD. Obesity drugs and the heart. *Curr Probl Cardiol*. 1999;24: 745-792.
73. Fitzgerald LW, Burn TC, Brown BS, et al. Possible role of valvular serotonin 5-HT$_{2B}$ receptors in the cardiopathy associated with fenfluramine. *Mol Pharmacol*. 2000;57:75-81.
74. Rothman RB, Baumann MH, Savage JE, et al. Evidence for possible involvement of 5-HT$_{2B}$ receptors in the cardiac valvulopathy associated with fenfluramine and other serotonergic medications. *Circulation*. 2000;102:2836-2841.
75. Setola V, Hufeisen SJ, Grande-Allen KJ, et al. 3,4-Methylenedioxymethamphetamine (MDMA, "ecstasy") induces fenfluramine-like proliferative actions on human cardiac valvular interstitial cells in vitro. *Mol Pharmacol*. 2003;63:1223-1229.

76. Nichols DE, Brewster WK, Johnson MP, Oberlender R, Riggs RM. Nonneurotoxic tetralin and indan analogues of 3,4-(methylenedioxy)amphetamine (MDA). *J Med Chem.* 1990;33: 703-710.
77. Launay JM, Herve P, Peoc'h K, et al. Function of the serotonin 5-hydroxytryptamine 2B receptor in pulmonary hypertension. *Nat Med.* 2002;8:1129-1135.
78. Gurtner HP. Aminorex and pulmonary hypertension. *Cor Vasa.* 1985;27:160-171.
79. Rothman RB, Baumann MH. Neurochemical mechanisms of phentermine and fenfluramine: therapeutic and adverse effects. *Drug Dev Res.* 2000;51:52-65.
80. Vickers SP, Clifton PG, Dourish CT, Tecott LH. Reduced satiating effect of d-fenfluramine in serotonin 5-HT(2C) receptor mutant mice. *Psychopharmacology (Berl).* 1999;143:309-314.
81. Czoty PW, Ginsburg BC, Howell LL. Serotonergic attenuation of the reinforcing and neuro-chemical effects of cocaine in squirrel monkeys. *J Pharmacol Exp Ther.* 2002;300:831-837.
82. Michelakis ED, Weir EK. Anorectic drugs and pulmonary hypertension from the bedside to the bench. *Am J Med Sci.* 2001;321:292-299.
83. Negus SS, Mello NK. Effects of chronic d-amphetamine treatment on cocaine- and food-maintained responding under a second-order schedule in rhesus monkeys. *Drug Alcohol Depend.* 2003;70:39-52.
84. Grabowski J, Rhoades H, Stotts A, et al. Agonist-like or antagonist-like treatment for cocaine dependence with methadone for heroin dependence: two double-blind randomized clinical trials. *Neuropsychopharmacology.* 2004;29:969-981.

Chapter 20
Receptors of Mammalian Trace Amines

Anita H. Lewin[1]

Abstract The discovery of a family of G-protein coupled receptors, some of which bind and are activated by biogenic trace amines, has prompted speculation as to the physiological role of these receptors. Observations associated with the distribution of these trace amine associated receptors (TAARs) suggest that they may be involved in depression, attention-deficit hyperactivity disorder, eating disorders, migraine headaches, and Parkinson's disease. Preliminary in vitro data, obtained using cloned receptors, also suggest a role for TAARs in the function of hallucinogens.

Keywords Trace amine associated receptor, TAAR, mammalian, G-protein coupled receptor, ADHD, hypothyroidism-associated depression, prepulse inhibition

Introduction

Endogenous amines such as tyramine, tryptamine, phenethylamine, and octopamine have long been known to be present in mammalian brain at potentially relevant physiological concentrations. In fact, some of these so-called trace amines have for over 25 years been thought to be associated with affective behavior,[1] paranoid chronic schizophrenia,[2] and depression.[3,4] Moreover, specific binding sites with unique pharmacology and localization for some tritium-labeled trace amines have been reported.[5-9] This mini-review provides a summary of the mammalian trace amine receptor literature up to the end of calendar year 2004.

[1] Chemistry and Life Sciences, Research Triangle Institute, Research Triangle Park, NC

Corresponding Author: Anita H. Lewin, Research Triangle Institute, PO Box 12194, Research Triangle Park, NC 27709-2194. Tel: (919) 541-6691; Fax: (919) 541-8868; E-mail: ahl@rti.org

Literature Review

Although trace amines have important functions in invertebrates, and particularly in insects, no role has been associated with these materials in mammals. The invertebrate receptors for trace amines, also referred to as octopamine receptors, are known to belong to the family of G-protein coupled receptors (GPCRs).[10] Four of them have been distinguished using pharmacological tools, and they have been found to show different coupling to second messenger systems, including activation and inhibition of adenylyl cyclase, activation of phospholipase C, and coupling to a chloride channel. Recently, octopamine receptors from mollusks and insects have been cloned. In humans and other mammals the existence of functional receptors for trace amines had, until recently, only been hypothesized.

A mammalian receptor for trace amines was identified with the discovery of a G-protein coupled receptor capable of binding both tyramine and phenethylamine and coupling to the stimulation of adenylate cyclase through Gαs G-protein, leading to accumulation of cAMP. In 2001, scientists[11] at Synaptic Corp (Paramus, NJ) reported the identification of a phylogenetic tree for the human, rat, and mouse trace amine receptors; human 5-HT receptors; human α1a receptor (AR-$_{\alpha 1a}$); GPR57; GPR58; putative neurotransmitter receptor (PNR); 5-HT$_{4\psi}$; Drosophila receptors for octopamine; 5-HT; and tyramine receptors from *Caenorhabditis elegans*, bee and locust, and a snail octopamine receptor. For rat, 14 trace amine receptors had been identified while 4 human trace amine receptors were found.[11] The abbreviation TA was used by these authors for these new receptors. Human and rat trace amine receptors were also described by Bunzow et al[12] who used the abbreviation TAR for the same receptors.

These newly discovered receptors have prompted multiple speculations regarding their physiological and pathological relevance. Trace amines have been hypothesized to act as neurotransmitters or neuromodulators,[13] as endogenous enhancer substances,[14] as monoamine releasers,[15] and even as vasoconstrictors.[16] A recent review has suggested that they may heterodimerize, for example, with dopamine (DA) receptors, which may increase the intrinsic activity of DA receptors by increasing their affinity to agonist ligands.[17] Indirect activation of dopamine autoreceptors by trace amines has also been proposed to be caused by an efflux of newly synthesized dopamine.[18]

Recently, a new nomenclature has been proposed for trace amine receptors.[19] Part of the rationale justifying the need for new nomenclature is because the terms TA and TAR are both used in other contexts. For example, *TA$_s$* has been used to refer to the human *GPR 102,* and *TAR* refers to *Escherichia coli* aspartate receptors. The new term trace amine associated receptor (TAAR) is proposed to avoid such ambiguity, as well as to include members of the trace amine receptor family that do not respond to trace amines (vide infra). Based on the sequential order of the receptor genes on the chromosomes as well as their phylogenetic relationships across species, a series of rules for the naming of TAARs has also been proposed. These rules stipulate that

- the term TAAR would be followed by a number identifying the specific ortholog;
- a letter suffix distinguishing genes that are paralogues would follow the number identifying the specific ortholog; and
- pseudogenes would be identified by the suffix P.

This mini-review will use this new nomenclature. Table 20.1 shows the new nomenclature and its relationship to terms used in previous publications. In addition, Table 20.1 demonstrates the identification of 19 individual TAARs for rat, 9 each for human and chimpanzee, and 16 for mouse.

Considerable homology had been reported between the human and rat TAARs: *hTAAR* 1 and *rTAAR* 1 share 79% identity; *hTAAR* 9 and *rTAA*R 9 share 87% identity; and *hTAAR* 6 and *rTAA*R 6 share 88% identity.[11] In fact, *hTAAR* 1 has been called the human ortholog of *rTAAR* 1.[12] For rhesus monkey, *TAAR* 1 and *TAAR* 9 were reported to be >96% homologous to the human orthologs, with only a single amino acid residue in the extracellular N terminus of monkey *TAAR* 1 differing from *hTAAR* 1.[20] Subsequent work revealed that although the chimpanzee *TAAR* 1 and *TAAR* 9P genes had 99.1% and 97.3% overall sequence identity, respectively, only 3 of the chimpanzee genes (*TAAR* 1, *TAAR* 5, and *TAAR* 6) had intact open reading frames, while the other 5 *TAAR* genes were pseudogenes.[19] Surprisingly, there are twice as many functional *TAAR* genes in human as in chimpanzee. An additional obvious interspecies difference is the absence of any functional counterpart of the rodent *TAAR* 7 orthologs in human.[19]

The reported phylogeny of the *TAAR* genes across species reveals the existence of 3 distinct subfamilies into which the orthologs can be grouped (Table 20.1).[19] All 4 species examined to date (human, chimpanzee, rat, and mouse) have at least one functional *TAAR* gene for each of the 3 subgroups, suggesting that each subgroup may have physiological relevance. At present putative, potential endogenous ligands for *TAAR* 1 and *TAAR* 4 have been identified. Specifically, in humans, *TAAR* 1 responds to tyramine,[11,21] β-phenethylamine,[11,21] octopamie,[11] and dopamine,[11] and the *TAAR* 4 is activated by tyramine[11] and β-phenethylamine.[11] No ligands are currently known to activate other TAARs. Overall, it has been concluded that TAARs represent a well-defined, coherent gene family, and not an extension of an established, closely related family, such as the 5-HT receptors.[19]

The discovery of the TAARs has prompted speculations as to their physiological role(s). Specifically, it has been pointed out[22] that although there do not appear to be any mammalian neurons using any of the trace amines, these molecules may function as traditional neuromodulators working through their own receptors. The fact that the mRNA for *rTAAR* 1 and *rTAAR* 4 receptor proteins is expressed in certain cells of the substantia nigra/ventral tegmental area, locus coeruleus, and dorsal raphe, which are all areas where cell bodies of the classic biogenic amines are found, further supports such a role for trace amines. Low levels of *hTAAR* 1, as well as *mTAAR* 1 mRNA, were found to be expressed in the amygdala. Only trace levels of *hTAAR* 1 were found in cerebellum, dorsal root ganglia, hippocampus, hypothalamus, medulla, and pituitary. *hTAAR* 6 mRNA at low level was also found to be expressed in amygdala, and *hTAAR* 8 mRNA was expressed in both amygdala and hippocampus.

Table 20.1 New Nomenclature and Classification for Trace Amine Associated Receptors*†

Sub-family	New Name	Old		Bp	Accession		Comments
		Name	Ref		Number	Reference	
Human							
1	TAAR 1	TA1	11,12	1020	AF200627 AF380185	15,16	Discrepancy: G864A
	TAAR 2	**GPR58**	11	921; 1056	AY702304 AF112460; AY703480‡	20	Discrepancies: C398T, C552T
	TAAR 3	**GPR57 P**	11	1030	AY702305 AF112461	20	Discrepancies: G57-, C134-
	TAAR 4	TA2 P, 5HT-4 P	11,12	1049	U88828	19	
2	TAAR 5	**PNR**	11	1014	AY702306 AF021818	21	Discrepancies: A118G, T770C
3	TAAR 6	TA4, TRAR4	11,22	1038	AF380192	15	
	TAAR 7	**Novel P**			AY803193§	15	
	TAAR 8	TA5, GPR102	11,20	1029	AF380193	15	
	TAAR 9	TA3	11,12	1047	AF380189 AL513524	15	Discrepancies: C9T, T181A
Chimpanzee							
1	TAAR 1	**Novel**		1020	AY702307		
	TAAR 2	**Novel P**		920; 1055	AY702308;∥		
	TAAR 3	**Novel P**		1030	AY702309		
	TAAR 4	**Novel P**		1049	AY702310		
2	TAAR 5	**Novel**		1014	AY702311		
3	TAAR 6	**Novel**		1038	AY702312		
	TAAR 7	**Novel P**			AY803194§		
	TAAR 8	**Novel P**		1027	AY702313		
	TAAR 9	**Novel P**		1048	AY702314		
Rat							
1	TAAR 1	**TA1**	11,12	999	AY702315 AF380186	15,16	Discrepancies: G72A, T509A, A660G, T867C; AF421352 discrepancy: A741G

	Receptor			Length	Accession		Notes
	TAAR 2	Novel		1020	AY702316 ¶		
	TAAR 3	Novel		1029	AY702317		
2	TAAR 4	TA2	11	1044	AF380188	15	
	TAAR 5	Novel	11	1014	AY702318	15	
3	TAAR 6	TA4	11	1038	AF380191	15	
	TAAR 7a	TA8	11	1077	AF380196	15	
	TAAR 7b	TA12	11	1077	AY702319 AF380200	15	Discrepancy: ATG is 75 bp downstream
	TAAR 7c	Novel		1077	AY702320		
	TAAR 7d	TA15	11	1077	AY702321 AF380203	15	Discrepancies: T198C, C199A, G282C, T292C, A373T, C459G
	TAAR 7e	TA14	11	1077	AY702322 AF380202	15	Discrepancies: C71T, G398C, C403A, C405A, C467T
	TAAR 7f	TA13P	11	1089	AY702323 AF380201	15	Discrepancies: C135A, T151C, G186A, T294G, T475G, A515G, G759A
	TAAR 7i	Novel P	11	1067	AY702324		
	TAAR 8a	TA11	11	1035; 1125	AF380199; AF380199	15	Using 2nd ATG
	TAAR 7g	TA9	11	1077	AF380197	15	
	TAAR 7h	TA6	11	1077	AF380194	15	
	TAAR 8b	TA7	11	1035; 1125	AF380195; AL513524	15	
	TAAR 8c	TA10	11	1035; 1125	AY702325 AF380198; AL513524	15	Discrepancy: G214A
	TAAR 9	TA3	11	1017	AF380190	15	
Mouse							
1	TAAR 1	TA1	11	999	AF380187	15	
	TAAR 2	Novel		1020	AY702326#		
	TAAR 3	Novel		1032	AY702327		
	TAAR 4	Novel		1044	AY702328		

(continued)

Table 20.1 (continued)

Sub-family	New Name	Old Name	Old Ref	Bp	Accession Reference	Accession Number	Accession Comments
2	TAAR 5	**Novel**		1014		AY702329	
3	TAAR 6	**Novel**		1038		AY702330	
	TAAR 7a	**Novel**		1077		AY702331	
	TAAR 7b	**Novel**		1077		AY702332	
	TAAR 7c	**Novel P**		1055		AY702333	
	TAAR 7d	**Novel**		1077		AY702334	
	TAAR 7e	**Novel**		1077		AY702335	
	TAAR 7f	**Novel**		1077		AY702336	
	TAAR 8a	**Novel**		1035		AY702337	
	TAAR 8b	**Novel**		1035		AY702338	
	TAAR 8c	**Novel**		1035		AY702339	
	TAAR 9	**Novel**		1047		AY702340	

*TAARs indicates trace amine associated receptors; ref, reference; bp, base pair; and PNR, putative neurotransmitter receptor. Genes that were resequenced are in bold. Data are adapted from Lindemann et al.[19]

†Genbank accession numbers or accession numbers referring to data from Roeder.[10]

‡Encoded by 2 exons. The presence of one transcript encompassing the coding sequence of both exons was proven on the level of cDNA.

§highly degenerated gene fragment (210bp), sharing 62.6% nucleotide sequence identity to the corresponding rat TAAR 7h sequence.

‖The intron/exon structure as well as coding sequences of human and chimpanzee are well conserved, suggesting that also chimpanzee TAAR 2 is encoded by 2 exons, which were amplified and sequenced separately from chimpanzee genomic DNA. However, the presence of transcripts encoding both exons has not been experimentally verified owing to unavailability of chimpanzee brain RNA.

¶Rat TAAR 2 is encoded by 2 exons. The presence of one transcript encompassing the coding sequence of both exons was proven on the level of cDNA.

#Mouse TAAR 2 is encoded by 2 exons. The presence of one transcript encompassing the coding sequence of both exons was proven on the level of cDNA.

It had been noted that *hTAAR* genes map to chromosome 6q23.2, close to SCDZ5, a susceptibility locus for schizophrenia, and it has been proposed that *hTAAR* 6 may be a susceptibility gene for schizophrenia.[23] Since the 6q chromosomal area has been linked to bipolar disorder, *hTAAR* 6 may be involved in both disorders. In addition, it has been suggested that[13] TAARs may be involved in depression, attention-deficit hyperactivity disorder (ADHD), eating disorders, migraine headaches, and Parkinson's disease.

Recently some specific data supporting the involvement of TAARs in attention-deficit hyperactivity disorder and in depression have been presented.[24] Specifically, it has been observed that phenethylamine levels may be deficient in ADHD brains, leading to the suggestion that ADHD may be associated with insufficient *TAAR* 1 activation. If this is the case, it would account for the effectiveness of inhibitors of the dopamine transporter as ADHD medications. Thus, these agents, which have been found to inhibit phenethylamine transport as well, will lead to increased phenethylamine levels, thereby ameliorating the symptoms of ADHD.

In support of the role of TAARs in depression, the observation that 3-iodothyronamine, an analog of tyramine and a metabolite of thyroid hormone, activates rat and mouse *TAAR* 1 heterologously expressed in HEK 293 cells in vitro has been interpreted to mean that *TAAR* 1 may play a role in depression associated with hypothyroidism.[25] Moreover, since synthetic 3-iodothyronamine injected intaperitoneally (mice) produces several physiological manifestations that are reminiscent of hypothyroidism-associated depression-like symptoms in humans (such as blocking the ability to thermoregulate and maintain normal cardiovascular tone at room temperature, depressing locomotor activity and metabolic rates, and elevating blood sugar levels),[25] *TAAR* 1 may be involved in these regulatory processes.

Only a very limited amount of information regarding activation of TAARs is available. Obtaining this information is difficult since the level of TAAR expression in both the central nervous system (CNS) and peripheral tissue is low. For *hTAAR* 1, only 15 to 100 copies/ng cDNA are expressed in amygdala, and <15 copies/ng cDNA are found in cerebellum, dorsal root ganglia, hippocampus, hypothalamus, medulla, and pituitary. The highest levels (100 copies/ng cDNA) are present in stomach.[11] Message from *hTAAR* 9, *hTAAR* 5, and *hTAAR* 6 was found in kidney; the first was also detected in the hippocampus and the latter 2 were also expressed in amygdala. All are expressed at low (<15 copies/ng cDNA) levels.[11] Countermanding these low receptor densities required the development of expression systems for screening purposes. This was accomplished by the cloning of rat, mouse, and human *TAAR* 1[11,12,19]; *rTAAR* 1 was stably expressed in HEK 293 cells,[12,19,26] as was *mTAAR* 1.[19] Transient transfection has been reported for *hTAAR* 1.[11] Stable expression of *hTAAR* 1 in HEK 293 cells was achieved by modification of the coding sequence by the addition of an influenza hemaglutinin viral leader sequence and by replacement of selected regions with the corresponding *rTAAR* 1 sequences.[19] A stable cell line expressing *hTAAR* 1 (no details given) has been reported.[21]

The rat clone was used to qualitatively screen several CNS-active compounds for activation of *rTAAR* 1. The results showed amphetamines and lysergic acid diethylamide (LSD)-related compounds to be agonists,[12] leading to the hope that

TAARs may provide insight into the molecular mode of action of these drugs of abuse. Evidence for the involvement of TAARs in psychostimulant activity has resulted from observations made in a line of mice lacking the *mTAAR* 1. These animals demonstrated reproducible deficits in prepulse inhibition, a condition that has been significantly correlated with abnormal functional interactions between the muscarinic, cholinergic, and dopaminergic systems,[27] with no difference in baseline startle response.[28] In addition, the mice lacking the *mTAAR* 1 displayed enhanced, dose-dependent sensitivity to the psychomotor stimulating effects of amphetamine, compared with the wild-type littermates, as well as a larger increase in the release of both dopamine and norepinephrine in the dorsal striatum. These observations have been interpreted to suggest that activation of *TAAR* 1 may serve to dampen the stimulatory effects of amphetamine.[28]

Use of the clones expressing *mTAAR* 1 and *rTAAR* 1 to screen thyronamine derivatives has demonstrated that both are activated by 3-iodothyronamine, a thyroid hormone derivative found in rodent brain.[26] Based on this observation, it has been suggested that a signaling pathway, stimulation of which leads to consequences opposite those associated with excess thyroid hormone, may exist. However, considering the significant differences in pharmacology observed[19] for rat and human *TAAR* 1 (see below and Table 20.2) such interpretations must be viewed with caution.

Table 20.2 Potency Values for Phenethylamine Analogs

		EC_{50} (µM)				
		rTAAR 1		*hTAAR* 1		*mTAAR* 1
Entry No.	Structure	Bunzow[12]	Lindeman[19]	Borowsky[11]	Lindemann[19]	Lindemann[19]
1	NH$_2$	0.24	0.9	0.324	0.3	0.66
2	NH$_2$ (HO)	0.069	0.21	0.214	1.07	1.37
3	NH$_2$ (HO)	5.4				
4	NH$_2$ (HO, HO)	5.9	5.14	6.7	15.78	11.76
5	OH, NH$_2$ (HO)	1.3	2.13	4.03	10.29	19.71
6	OH, NH$_2$ (HO, HO)		>50 000		>50 000	>50 000

(continued)

Table 20.2 (continued)

Entry No.	Structure	EC$_{50}$ (µM)				
		rTAAR 1		hTAAR 1		mTAAR 1
		Bunzow[12]	Lindeman[19]	Borowsky[11]	Lindemann[19]	Lindemann[19]
7	(phenethylamine, N–H N–CH$_3$)	0.3			0.16	0.15
8	(HO–phenyl, ethyl N–H N–CH$_3$)	0.14			2.05	1.02
9	(HO–phenyl, OH, N–H N–CH$_3$)	0.58				
10	(phenyl, NH$_2$)	0.21				
11	(phenyl, NH$_2$)	0.44				
12	(HO–phenyl, NH$_2$)	0.051				
13	(methylenedioxyphenyl, NH$_2$)	1.7				
14	(indole HN, NH$_2$)	0.3	5.24	>6	46.87	1.99
15	(indole OH, HN, NH$_2$)	>10	>50 000	>10	>50 000	>50 000

The potency of "trace amines" and their congeners to activate *TAAR* 1 are shown in Tables 20.2 and 20.3. The data in Table 20.2 emphasize the interspecies differences as well as the effects associated with expression systems. As pointed out in the literature[19] there appears to be greater correspondence between the assay data for mouse and human *TAAR* 1, than between mouse and rat *TAAR* 1. However, it needs to be understood that the number of data points is very small. Perhaps more meaningful is the difference observed between data obtained using stably and transiently expressed receptors, particularly for tryptamine (entry 14). It should also be

Table 20.3 Potency Values for Thyronamine Derivatives*

Substituents				EC$_{50}$ (µM)	
R$_1$	R$_2$	R$_3$	R$_4$	rTAAR 1	mTAAR 1
H	H	H	H	0.131	~1
I	H	H	H	0.014	0.112
H	H	I	H	~1	>1
I	H	I	H	0.041	~1
I	I	H	H	0.056	0.371
H	H	I	I	>1	>1
I	I	I	H	0.087	>1
I	H	I	I	>1	>1
I	I	I	I	>1	>1

* Data adapted from Grandy and Scanlon.[25]

noted that it is not known what effect the use of "modified" hTAAR 1 to prepare a stable expression system[19] has on potency to activate hTAAR 1. Despite these caveats, some trends are detectable. Thus, introduction of a p-hydroxy group provides for slightly increased potency (compare entries 1 and 2, 7 and 8, 10/11 and 12) whereas introduction of an m-hydroxy group decreases potency by about an order of magnitude (compare entries 1 and 3, 2 and 4, 5 and 6). Similarly, the replacement of one of the amine protons by a methyl group slightly enhances potency (compare entries 1 and 7, 2 and 8, 5 and 9). The effect of aromatic iodo substituents (Table 20.3) is intriguing. Again, interspecies differences are apparent. While a single m-iodo group increases potency by an order of magnitude in both mouse and rat receptors (compare entries 1 and 2), a second m-iodo group in the second aromatic ring (compare entries 2 and 4) has a modest effect in rTAAR 1, but a significantly larger effect in mTAAR 1.

In invertebrates lipophilicity, dipole moment, and molecular shape have been correlated to the agonist and antagonist efficacy of 49 trace amines in locust thoracic nerve cord.[29] Subsequent application of a 3-dimensional molecular field analysis to the same data set and to a larger set of 70 analogs, combined with a genetic algorithm/partial least squares statistical analysis, provided useful information in the characterization and differentiation of (insect) receptor types and subtypes.[30] Recently, a 3D quantitative structure activity relationship (QSAR) for a new series of 59 agonists provided a good correlation using a pharmacophore consisting of a positive charge center, aromatic ring, and 3 hydrophobic sites.[31] Clearly a significant amount of work remains to be done before any similar correlations can be performed for mammals and particularly humans.

At present the discovery of trace amine-associated receptors holds the promise of providing potentially important novel insights into the origins and treatments of CNS disorders. Although cloned membranes expressing hTAAR 1 have been prepared and used to screen a few compounds, the validity of these assays remains to be determined. In particular, the different results reported for the efficacy of ligands to activate *hTAAR* 1 must be resolved. Thus, the effects of modification of the coding sequence and replacement of certain segments with *rTAAR* 1 sequences to obtain a stable expression system for *hTAAR* 1, as well as the use of a transient expression system relative to stable expression system for *hTAAR* 1 must be ascertained before meaningful QSAR studies can be undertaken and before specific drug leads can be targeted for in vitro evaluation. Even more demanding will be the development of an animal model for in vivo testing. Homozygote *TAAR* 1 knockout mice are viable[13] and have been used to study the physiological role of *TAAR* 1 in the CNS.[28] However, considering the significant differences in pharmacology observed for rodent and human *hTAAR* 1 and in responses to trace amines and their analogs, it may be necessary to develop a *hTAAR* 1 transgenic rodent in order to get meaningful results.

Conclusions

Three distinct subfamilies of TAARs, comprising as many as 21 individual receptors, have been fully identified and characterized in human, chimpanzee, rat, and mouse. Significant interspecies differences have been found. Only 2 TAARs have had functional ligands, which are associated with them, identified. Owing to their low density in tissue, TAARs must be cloned and expressed for in vitro assays. At present very few stable expression systems have been generated. The scant data available suggest significant differences between results obtained in different expression systems and point to important species differences. The TAARs are an important new target for investigation in light of their likely involvement in neuropsychiatric and neurodegenerative disorders, as well as in drug abuse.

Acknowledgment The author is grateful to Dr David K. Grandy for discussions and review of the manuscript.

References

1. Sabelli HC, Mosnaim AD. Phenylethylamine hypothesis of affective behavior. *Am J Psychiatry*. 1974;131:695-699.
2. Potkin SG, Karoum F, Chuang LW, Cannon-Spoor HE, Phillips I, Wyatt RJ. Phenylethylamine in paranoid chronic schizophrenia. *Science*. 1979;206:470-471.
3. Davis BA, Boulton AA. The trace amines and their acidic metabolites in depression: an overview. *Prog Neuropsychopharmacol Biol Psychiatry*. 1994;18:17-45.
4. Sandler M, Ruthven CR, Goodwin BL, Coppen A. Decreased cerebrospinal fluid concentration of free phenylacetic acid in depressive illness. *Clin Chim Acta*. 1979;93:169-171.
5. Altar C, Wasley A, Martin L. Autoradiographic localization and pharmacology of unique 3Htryptamine binding sites in rat brain. *Neuroscience*. 1986;17:263-273.

6. Hauger R, Skolnick P, Paul S. Specific 3Hbeta-phenylethylamine binding sites in rat brain. *Eur J Pharmacol.* 1982;83:147-148.

7. Kellar KJ, Cascio CS. 3HTryptamine: high affinity binding sites in rat brain. *Eur J Pharmacol.* 1982;78:475-478.

8. Perry DC. 3Htryptamine autoradiography in rat brain and choroid plexus reveals two distinct sites. *J Pharmacol Exp Ther.* 1986;236:548-559.

9. Ungar F, Mosnaim A, Ungar B, Wolf M. Tyramine-binding by synaptosomes from rat brain: effect of centrally active drugs. *Biol Psychiatry.* 1977;12:661-668.

10. Roeder T. Octopamine in invertebrates. *Prog Neurobiol.* 1999;59:533-561.

11. Borowsky B, Adham N, Jones KA, et al. Trace amines: identification of a family of mammalian G protein-coupled receptors. *Proc Natl Acad Sci USA.* 2001;98:8966-8971.

12. Bunzow JR, Sonders MS, Arttmagangkul S, et al. Amphetamine, 3,4-methylenedioxymethamphetamine, lysergic acid diethylamide, and metabolites of the catecholamine neurotransmitters are agonists of a trace amine receptor. *Mol Pharmacol.* 2001;60:1181-1188.

13. Branchek TA, Blackburn TP. Trace amine receptors as targets for novel therapeutics: legend, myth and fact. *Curr Opin Pharmacol.* 2003;3:90-97.

14. Shimazu S, Miklya I. Pharmacological studies with endogenous enhancer substances: β-phenethylamine, tryptamine, and their synthetic derivatives. *Prog Neuropsychopharmacol Biol Psychiatry.* 2004;28:421-427.

15. Schmidt N, Ferger B. The biogenic trace amine tyramine induces pronounced hydroxyl radical production via monoamine oxidase dependent mechanism: an in vivo microdialysis study in mouse striatum. *Brain Res.* 2004;1012:101-107.

16. Davenport AP. Peptide and trace amine orphan receptors: prospects for new therapeutic targets. *Curr Opin Pharmacol.* 2003;3:127-134.

17. Berry MD. Mammalian central nervous system trace amines: pharmacologic amphetamines, physiologic neuromodulators. *J Neurochem.* 2004;90:257-271.

18. Geracitano R, Federici M, Prisco S, Bernardi G, Mercuri NB. Inhibitory effects of trace amines on rat midbrain dopaminergic neurons. *Neuropharmacology.* 2004;46:807-814.

19. Lindemann L, Ebeling M, Kratochwil NA, Bunzow JR, Grandy DK, Hoener MC. Trace amine associated receptors from structurally and functionally distinct subfamilies of novel G protein-coupled receptors. *Genomics.* 2005;85:372-385.

20. Miller GM, Madras BK. A trace amine receptor (TAR1) is a novel amphetamine receptor in primate brain poster. Paper presented at: Sixty-fifth Annual Meeting of the College on Problems of Drug Dependence (CPDD), June 15-19, 2003; Bal Harbour, FL.

21. Yin T, Tu Y, Johnstone EM, Little SP. A Characterization of the Trace Amine 1 Receptor (Program No. 961.5). Paper presented at: 2004 Abstract Viewer/Itinerary Planner, 2004 Online; Washington, DC: Society for Neuroscience.

22. Premont RT, Gainetdinov RR, Caron MG. Following the trace of elusive amines. *Proc Natl Acad Sci USA.* 2001;98:9474-9475.

23. Duan J, Martinez M, Sanders AR, et al. Polymorphisms in the trace amine receptor 4 (TRAR4) gene on chromosome 6q23.2 are associated with susceptibility to schizophrenia. *Am J Hum Genet.* 2004;75:624-638.

24. Madras BK, Verrico C, Jassen A, Miller GM. Attention Deficit Hyperactivity Disorder (ADHD): New Roles for Old Trace Amines and Monoamine Transporters poster. Paper presented at: The American College of Neuropsychopharmacology (ACNP) 43rd Annual Meeting, December 12-16, 2004; San Juan, Puerto Rico.

25. Grandy DK, Scanlan TS. Thyroid Hormone Metabolites and Depression: A New Twist on an Old Tale poster. Paper presented at: The American College of Neuropsychopharmacology (ACNP) 43rd Annual Meeting, December 12-16, 2004; San Juan, Puerto Rico.

26. Scanlan TS, Suchland KL, Hart ME, et al. 3-Iodothyronamine is an endogenous and rapid-acting derivative of thyroid hormone. *Nat Med.* 2004;10:638-642.

27. Jones CK, Eberle EL, Shaw DB, McKinzie DL, Shannon HE. Pharmacologic interactions between the muscarinic cholinergic and dopaminergic systems in the modulation of prepulse inhibition in rats. *J Pharmacol Exp Ther.* 2005;312:1055-1063.

28. Wolinsky TD, Swanson CJ, Zhong H, Smith KE, Branchek TA, Gerald CP. Deficit in Prepulse Inhibition and Enhanced Sensitivity to Amphetamine in Mice Lacking the Trace Amine-1 Receptor poster. Paper presented at: The American College of Neuropsychopharmacology (ACNP) 43rd Annual Meeting; December 12–16, 2004; San Juan, Puerto Rico.
29. Hirashima A, Pan C, Shinkai K, et al. Quantitative structure-activity studies of octopaminergic agonists and antagonists against nervous system of Locusta migratoria. *Bioorg Med Chem.* 1998;6:903-910.
30. Hirashima A, Nagata T, Pan C, Kuwano E, Taniguchi E, Eto M. Three-dimensional molecular field analyses of octopaminergic agonists and antagonists for the locust neuronal octopamine receptor class 3. *J Mol Graph Model.* 1999;17:198-218.
31. Hirashima A, Morimoto M, Kuwano E, Taniguchi E, Eto M. Three-dimensional common-feature hypotheses for octopamine agonist 2-(arylimino)imidazolidines. *Bioorg Med Chem.* 2002;10:117-123.

Part III
Drug Design: Nicotine, Opioids and Related Ligands

Chapter 21
The Role of Crystallography in Drug Design

Jeffrey R. Deschamps[1]

Abstract Structure and function are intimately related. Nowhere is this more important than the area of bioactive molecules. It has been shown that the enantioselectivity of an enzyme is directly related to its chirality. X-ray crystallography is the only method for determining the "absolute" configuration of a molecule and is the most comprehensive technique available to determine the structure of any molecule at atomic resolution. Results from crystallographic studies provide unambiguous, accurate, and reliable 3-dimensional structural parameters, which are prerequisites for rational drug design and structure-based functional studies.

Keywords structure, absolute configuration, opioid, pharmacophore, X-ray diffraction

Introduction

Structure and function are intimately related. X-ray crystallography is the most comprehensive technique available to determine the structure of any molecule at atomic resolution. "X-ray crystallography has become the sine qua non for elucidating the 3-dimensional structures of biologically interesting large and small molecules, providing the proverbial 'picture that is worth a thousand words'."[1] Accurate knowledge of molecular structures is a prerequisite for rational drug design and structure-based functional studies. Results from X-ray crystallographic studies provide unambiguous, accurate, and reliable 3-dimensional structural parameters at times even before complete chemical characterization is available. In addition, crystallography is the only method for determining the "absolute" configuration of a molecule. Absolute configuration is a critical property in biological systems as changes in this may alter the response of the biologic system.

---
[1] Laboratory for the Structure of Matter, Naval Research Laboratory, Washington, DC 20375

Corresponding Author: Jeffrey R. Deschamps, Research Chemist, Naval Research Laboratory, Code 6030, 4555 Overlook Avenue, Washington, DC 20375. Tel: (202) 767-0656; Fax: (202) 767-6874; E-mail: deschamps@nrl.navy.mil

R.S. Rapaka and W. Sadée (eds.), *Drug Addiction.*
© American Association of Pharmaceutical Scientists 2008

Conformation and Biologic Activity

The endogenous opioid peptides Leu- and Met-enkephalin (Try-Gly-Gly-Phe-Leu [Met]) were isolated from pig brain as a mixture.[2] These endogenous peptides are not receptor subtype specific and show binding affinity for both the μ and δ opioid receptors. Conformational studies indicate that small linear peptides, such as the enkephalins, can have many different conformations.[3] The lack of specificity may be related to the large number of conformations available to the peptides. However, in the crystalline state Leu-enkephalin has been shown to exist in only 3 conformations (Fig. 21.1), extended,[4] single β-bend,[5] and double β-bend,[6] while Met-enkephalin[7] has only been seen in an extended conformation. Thus the lack of specificity may be related to differential binding of these conformers at the various opioid receptors. Other investigators have speculated that the single-bend conformation, with its 2 intramolecular hydrogen bonds, provides the "rigid frame to which side chains are attached in a specific spatial relationship" required for activity.[5] Thus, systematic approaches for the design of potent and selective analogs of enkephalin have involved the application of both conformational and topographical constraints. Attempts to constrain the backbone to the single-bend conformation fall into 3 general categories: incorporation of residues that constrain the backbone conformation, cyclization of the peptide, or incorporation of constrained residues.

It is generally accepted that the most important pharmacophoric parameters in these opioids include the distance from the protonated amine to the tyrosine aromatic ring, the distance from the protonated amine to a second hydrophobic center (generally a second aromatic ring), and the distance between the tyrosine ring and hydrophobic center.[8] The pharmacophoric parameters for opioid peptides for which the X-ray crystallographic studies have been completed are summarized in Tables 21.1 and 21.2. Through examination of these parameters and the biologic activity we may begin

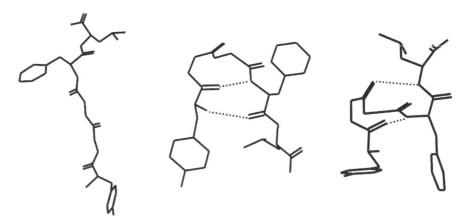

Fig. 21.1 Solid-state conformations of Leu-enkephalin: top—extended, middle—single-bend, bottom—double-bend.

to understand the relationship between structure and activity in this class of compounds.

Even though the cyclized peptide backbone is much more conformationally restricted than the linear enkephalin analogs, it still possesses significant residual flexibility due in part to the unsubstituted Gly residue at position 3. Attempts to

Table 21.1 Selected Pharmacophoric Parameters in Linear Opioid Peptides*

Compound	N -Tyr	N - Hydr	Ring-Ring	Angle	N - O	Tyr χ^1	Phe χ^1	CCDC	Ref
Extended									
LE-1	5.18	10.57	9.37	9.4	7.89	177	−63	BIXNIF10	4
	4.31	11.56	13.27	73.9	6.81	70	−55		
	4.10	11.58	13.90	62.4	6.60	53	−71		
	5.16	10.24	8.89	14.4	7.84	169	−68		
LE-2	5.13	14.26	13.21	67.3	7.83	175	−169	FABJEX	10
	4.10	10.52	11.80	42.1	6.55	62	−69		
ME-1	4.08	13.46	13.60	4.7	6.39	58	53	FABJIB	7
	4.00	13.13	13.63	6.3	6.42	68	65		
Metkephamide	5.10	10.05	12.76	36.6	7.88	176	−63	IDIHEI	11
	5.15	10.63	12.95	38.4	7.84	173	−55		
Range	3.8–5.2	7.5–13.4	8.9–13.9						
Single-bend									
LE-3	4.14	7.86	11.26	48.3	6.64	−80	−59	LENKPH11	5
	3.89	7.76	10.76	21.9	6.26	−53	−61		
	4.25	7.84	11.36	59.3	6.79	−87	−60		
	3.95	7.66	10.73	12.9	6.40	−52	−62		
LE-Br			11.34	54.5		−84	−69	NA	12
LE-Nle	5.19	7.71	9.58	26.0	7.89	−167	−73	CITXEI10	13
	5.13	5.00	8.15	41.3	7.81	−177	−74		
DTLET	5.16	8.84	10.83	70.3	7.88	169	−73	HICJUY	14
DADLE	5.13	7.18	9.34	41.7	7.80	−166	−71	HIHYAY	15
TGGP	3.03	6.14	9.07	46.0	6.34	−63	−168	TGGPDH10	16
Biphalin (1:4)†	5.20	7.20	8.57	84.6	7.90	176	−56	NA	17
Range	4.1–5.2	5.0–8.9	8.1–11.4						
Double-bend									
LE-4	5.18	6.70	4.99	79.1	7.89	177	−67	GEWWAG	6
RTI02	5.15	7.45	4.87	83.4	7.84	−150	−61	SUPBOU	18
Biphalin (8:5)†	5.10	6.70	5.95	67.4	7.80	175	−58	NA	17
Range	5.1–5.2	6.7–7.5	4.8–5.0						

*CCDC indicates Cambridge Crystallographic Data Center; Ref, reference; and NA, not applicable. In all cases except the Tic peptides the second aromatic ring is part of a Phe residue and there are 2 amino acids between the Try and Phe residues (except for JOM-13, which has only 1). For the Tic peptides the distances quoted for N-Hydrophobic and Ring-Ring refer to the relationship between Tyr[1] and Tic[2] (1–3) or Phe[3] (1–3), where possible values were determined from the X-ray coordinates using SHELXTL[9]; all distances are reported in Å.

† Biphalin is a mixed agonist, which binds to both μ and δ opioid receptors. Because of these "mixed" properties, the pharmacophoric parameters have been split into the single- and double-bend sections based on the similarity of the 1 to 4 and 5 to 8 regions to other entries.

Table 21.2 Selected Pharmacophoric Parameters in Cyclic and Tic Containing Opioid Peptides*

Compound	N -Tyr	N - Hydr	Ring-Ring	Angle	N - O	Tyr χ^1	Phe χ^1	CCDC	Ref
Cyclic									
DPDPE	4.04	13.35	14.95	47.5	6.49	−68	−67	HESFUG	[19]
	4.14	12.28	15.91	59.6	6.55	−70	−67		
	2.99	12.82	13.18	41.3	6.36	−61	−69		
[D-Ala]- DPDPE	5.13	12.69	13.98	62.9	7.76	174	− 64	WIPYEZ	[20]
[L-Ala]- DPDPE	5.16	8.00	12.06	20.0	7.82	−174	−66	WIPYAY	[20]
	5.13	7.54	11.56	35.0	7.83	179	−62		
	3.80	7.74	10.23	53.1	7.83	−174	−56		
	3.83	7.93	10.58	32.9	7.81	−179	−46		
DPMPT	5.17	12.10	13.69	60.2	7.88	171	63	WIPXUD	[21]
[Nle,Gly]- DPLPE	5.12	12.59	12.93	73.0	7.77	−165	−76	NA	unpub†
	5.23	13.05	14.67	59.0	7.95	174	−86		
[Ser³]- DPDPE	4.01	11.24	14.20	31.0	6.43	57	177	NA	unpub†
	3.98	9.08	12.45	88.6	6.38	57	−69		
Range	3.0–5.3	7.5–13.35	10.2–15.9						
JOM-13	4.34	8.03	10.95	60.9	6.84	71	−83	YECDUF	[22]
	5.17	4.57	9.57	78.4	7.86	−171	−70		
Range	4.3–5.2	4.6–8.0	9.6–11.0						
Tic									
TIPP (1–2)	5.16	7.37	5.93	51.5	7.86	168	57	SUPBUA	[18]
TIPP (1–3)	5.16	8.30	9.21	43.1	7.86	168	−62		
D-TIPP (1–2)	4.18	6.78	6.74	50.0	6.61	−74	47	CALFEB	[23]
	5.17	6.53	6.27	76.0	7.86	−174	−48		
D-TIPP (1–3)	4.18	9.97	12.67	89.8	6.61	−74	−67		[23]
	5.17	9.43	9.55	55.0	7.86	−174	−59		
cyclo- [Tyr-Tic]	3.95	6.00	5.35	21.1	6.37	−60	54		[24]
boc-Tyr-Tic	3.92	6.84	8.45	13.9	6.28	−62	49	QAMWEG	[25]
Tyr-D-Tic	5.15	6.77	3.90	4.0	7.83	−172	−47	ROHFEZ	[26]
	5.15	6.90	3.93	1.3	7.84	−178	−55		
Tyr-D-Tic- NH₂	5.15	6.93	4.12	5.8	7.81	−169	−49	ROHFID	[26]
DmDmT*	5.24	7.30	5.07	13.3	7.94	−170	43	TUSMOJ	[27]
DmTA*	5.15	7.28	6.27	64.8	7.86	−178	64	TUSMUP	[27]
DmDmTA*	5.22	7.19	6.54	57.4	7.91	−168	62	TUSNAW	[27]
Range	3.9–5.2	6.0–10.0	3.9–12.7						

*CCDC indicates Cambridge Crystallographic Data Center; ref, reference; NA, not applicable; DmDmT, N,N-dimethyl-(2,6-dimethyl-Try)-Tic; DmTA, dimethyl-Tyr-Tic-NH-adamantain; and DmDmTA, N,N-dimethyl-(2,6-dimethyl-Try)-Tic-NH-adamantain.

† Deschamps JR, George C, Flippen-Anderson JL, Hruby V. Unpublished data. March 1998.

reduce this flexibility have included replacing Gly[3] with bulkier residues (eg, l- and d-Ala[20]), replacing one of the bridging residues with a more conformationally restricted moiety such as mercaptoproline,[21] or removing the Gly[3] residue altogether to form a more rigid cyclic tetrapeptide.[22]

The rationally designed linear peptides in Fig. 21.1 and 21.2 exhibit only folded conformations in the solid state with the single-bend peptides being agonists and a double-bend peptide acting as an antagonist. The tighter winding in the double bend brings the 2 aromatic rings to within 5 Å of one another, much closer than what is observed for this approach in any of the other phenylalanine (Phe)-containing peptides. For the tetra-hydroisoquinoline carboxylic acid (Tic) peptides, which show activity as μ agonists and δ antagonists, the distances fall in the range observed for the folded peptides. Despite difficulties in predicting which modifications increase selectivity or potency, the constraints applied to the peptide ligands have produced compounds with higher selectivity and potency.

Nonpeptide Ligands

Petsko[28] noted, "Chirality is fundamental in biology. The building blocks of proteins, the naturally occurring amino acids, are chiral." Milton and coworkers[29] showed that inverting the chirality of an entire enzyme also inverts its enantioselectivity. Thus absolute configuration is critical to proper function in biological systems. Nonbiological systems can also have a handedness. Inequivalence observed in crystallographic data of zinc sulfide was related to the absolute configuration of the crystal.[30] This effect was later shown to be general and applied to a variety of chiral structures to determine their absolute configuration.[31] In general determination of absolute configuration requires a heavy atom in the structure. Alternatively, inclusion of a salt of known chirality can be used to set the hand of the complex. With the advent of area detectors, crystallographers are now collecting more "redundant" data. Small differences in certain data pairs can be exploited to determine the absolute configuration.[32]

The naturally occurring opioid peptides are chiral, as are all proteins. A change in the configuration at a single chiral center can alter the pharmacological properties of a molecule.[33,34] Nonpeptide ligands bind to the same receptors as the endogenous opioid peptides and must mimic the arrangement of binding groups present in the opioid peptides. It is therefore no surprise that the nonpeptide ligands are chiral and that crystallography is used to track chiral syntheses and confirm, or determine, the absolute configuration of products.

The opioid alkaloid, morphine, has been around for almost 200 years,[35] and it is still widely used as an analgesic despite its undesirable side effects that include respiratory depression, reduced heart rate, nausea, vomiting, dizziness, sluggishness, sweating, and with repeated use addiction. Thus, the search for a better analgesic has been the search for a substance with morphine's beneficial properties without its undesirable side effects. There is some evidence of topologic similarity between

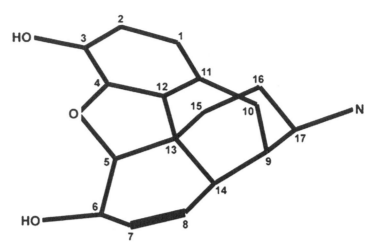

Fig. 21.2 Structure of morphine[37] showing the numbering of the heterocyclic atoms.

morphine and the endogenous opioid peptides.[36] Building on this, many nonpeptide opioids are based on the morphine skeleton (Fig. 21.2). Structural elements are modified or eliminated in efforts to circumvent unwanted effects. This often results in simplification that serves another function as it is not economic to synthesize a complex structure, such as morphine, on a large scale.[38,39] Extensive studies on morphine have shown that it requires the 3-hydroxyl group of the phenol ring for maximum activity, and that the hydroxyl group on C-6 be omitted or modified without losing activity.[34]

Further studies showed that the opioid pharmacophore could be simplified by eliminating the tetrahydrofuran ring and one cyclohexyl ring (ie, the bridging O, C6, C7, and C8) from morphine to produce the benzomorphans (Fig. 21.3). Other simplifications of the opioid pharmacophore lead to the development of the phenylmorphans. Like benzomorphans, phenylmorphans are formed by eliminating the tetrahydrofuran ring and one cyclohexyl ring, but only C10 and the bridging O are removed (Fig. 21.4). This progression has continued with newer ligands being either more potent, more selective, or both. Thomas et al showed that potent antagonists could be produced from phenylmorphans,[41] while Hashimoto and his coworkers found that (-)-(1R,5S,1'R)-3-[2-(1'-methyl-2'-phenylethyl)-2-azabicyclo[3,3,1]non-5-yl]-phenol is a moderately potent opioid antagonist.[42]

Other modifications can convert an agonist to an antagonist. The structurally related family of etorphine, buprenorphine, and diprenorphine (Fig. 21.5) are produced by altering the substituent on N17. Etorphine, with only a methyl substituent on the nitrogen, is an agonist, while buprenorphine and diprenorphine, which both have a methylcyclopropyl substituent on the nitrogen, are partial or complete antagonists. The differences in overall activity of buprenorphine and diprenorphine

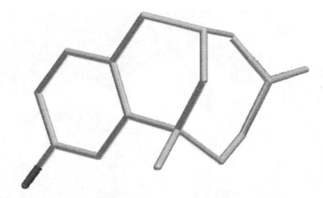

Fig. 21.3 Benzomorphans lack the fourth 6-membered ring and the bridging ether linkage, which forms the 5-membered ring. Shown is 4-methylhomobenzomorphan.[40]

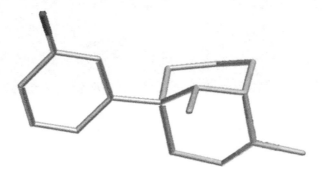

Fig. 21.4 Phenylmorphans are formed by eliminating the tetrahydrofuran ring and one cyclohexyl ring by removing C10 and the bridging O in morphine. Shown is 2,9beta-gimethyl-5-(3-hydroxyphenyl)-2-azabicyclo(3.3.1)nonan-2-ium.[41]

are attributable to the substitution of a methyl group for a t-butyl group (off C7 of the morphine skeleton) converting a mixed agonist-antagonist (buprenorphine) to a pure antagonist (diprenorphine).

Discussion

Despite overlaps in the range of distances separating the pharmacophores in the opioid peptides, some useful insights can be gained from a plot of the separation between the aromatic rings and the distance from the protonated amine to the second hydrophobic center (ie, aromatic ring) (Fig. 21.6). For the purpose of comparison

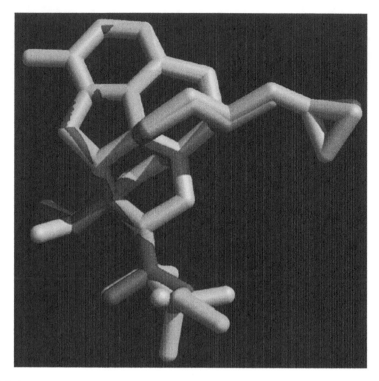

Fig. 21.5 Superimposition of etorphine (green), buprenorphine (yellow), and diprenorphine (red) shows the structural similarity of these compounds despite their divergent activities (ie, agonist, mixed agonist-antagonist, and antagonist, respectively).[43]

only, structures of potent highly selective ligands were initially used (filled symbols). Examining only these entries, it would appear that the δ-agonists (black squares) cluster along a diagonal, while the μ-agonists (black circles) and δ-antagonists (black triangles) form tight nonoverlapping clusters. Addition of some weak δ-agonists (open symbols) continues to show the same trend as was seen for the strong δ-agonists. The range of separations observed for weak μ-agonists (open circles) overlaps with that of the δ-antagonists in this simplistic 2-dimensional plot.

A large number of poorly selective agonists (denoted by the + symbols in (Fig. 21.6) were added in an attempt to classify these compounds. The majority of these "mixed agonists" are enkephalins, thus it is not surprising that they plot in the same general area as the δ-agonists. Enkephalin is considered a δ-agonist, although it has rather poor selectivity.[44] Only one of these mixed agonists plotted in the region of the μ-agonists. It lies between the strong and weak μ-agonists. This is the double-bend conformation of Leu-enkephalin. The presence of the δ-antagonists in this same region confuses the picture, but it is interesting to note that a protected derivative of the δ-antagonist N,N-diallyl-Tyr-Aib-Aib-Phe-Leu-OH[18] shares this double-bend conformation.

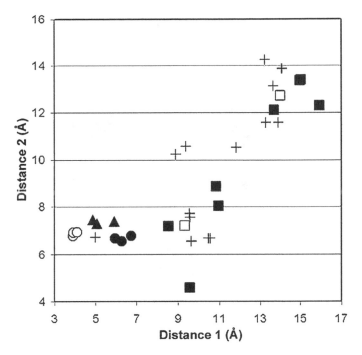

Fig. 21.6 Separation of pharmacophoric elements in opioid peptides. Distance 1 is the distance between the 2 hydrophobic regions (ie, rings); distance 2 is the separation between the amine (ie, N-terminal amino group) and the second hydrophobic region (ie, Phe[4]). Included are strong (■) and weak (□) δ-agonists, strong (●) and weak (○) μ-agonists, δ-antagonists (▲), and poorly selective compounds (+).

Part of the difficulty in quantifying the optimal separation of the pharmacophores may be due to conformational flexibility remaining even in the conformationally constrained peptides (Fig. 21.7). This problem was previously noted by Lomize and his colleagues.[22] Although nonpeptide ligands eliminate many of these problems, small structural changes may result in large changes in activity. Our ability to design highly potent and highly specific ligands is limited by our poor understanding of the molecular recognition necessary for proper receptor binding and activation. The final answers may not be available until structural information is obtained for the receptors themselves, both with and without bound ligands.

Highly potent and selective peptide agonists and antagonists have been synthesized. The utility of these compounds as drugs is limited mainly by their nature—they are peptides. In general, the peptide drugs are not given orally but are administered by the parenteral route. This requirement complicates their use and thus limits their utility. The nonpeptide ligands can be administered orally and thus have found their way into widespread use. Nonpeptide ligands also eliminate the problems associated with flexibility found even in highly constrained peptide ligands. The endogenous opioid peptides are somewhat effective in relieving pain and do not exhibit the undesirable side effects associated with the nonpeptide ligands. If problems with

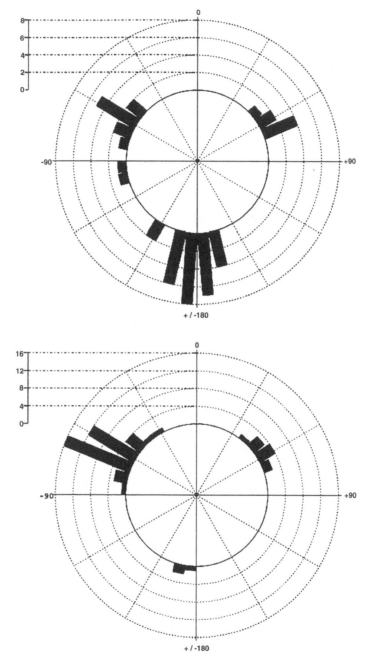

Fig. 21.7 Side chain conformers in the opioid peptides: top—tyrosine (residue 1) x^1 torsion angle, bottom—phenylalanine (residue 4) x^1 torsion angle.

drug delivery could be overcome, peptide-based drugs may offer the best of both worlds, effective analgesia and little or no side effects.

Conclusions

Crystallographic studies play a vital role on drug design. The results from X-ray crystallographic studies provide accurate and reliable 3-dimensional structural parameters. In addition, crystallography is the only method for determining the "absolute" configuration of a molecule, a critical property in biological systems as changes in this may alter the response of the biologic system. Medicinal chemists have made considerable progress in producing more potent and selective opioid peptides by constraining the peptide conformation. Further progress requires translating the linear modifications made to the peptide ligands into the 3-dimensional framework of the receptor. The results of crystallographic studies allow pharmacophoric parameters to be calculated from the 3-dimensional coordinates. These can then be used along with data on biologic activity to guide future development. The use of 3-dimensional data allows comparison of the relative position of groups thought to be important in binding to the receptor even in structurally dissimilar compounds.

Acknowledgments This research was supported in part by the National Institute for Drug Abuse (NIDA), Bethesda, MD, and the Office of Naval Research (ONR), Arlington, VA.

References

1. Griffin JF, Duax WL, eds. *Molecular Structure and Biological Activity*. New York, NY: Elsevier Biomedical; 1982.
2. Hughes J, Smith TW, Kosterlitz HW, Fothergill LA, Morgan BA, Morris HR. Identification of 2 related pentapeptides from brain with potent opiate agonist activity. *Nature*. 1975;258:577-579.
3. Temussi PA, Picone D, Castiglione-Morelli MA, Motta A, Tancredi T. Bioactive conformation of linear peptides in solution: an elusive goal. *Biopolymers*. 1989;28:91-107.
4. Karle IL, Karle J, Mastropaolo D, Camerman A, Camerman N. [Leu-5]enkepalin - 4 co-crystallizing conformers with extended backbones that form an anti-parallel beta-sheet. *Acta Crystallogr*. 1983;B39:625-637.
5. Smith D, Griffin JF. Conformation of [Leu-5]enkephalin rrom X-ray-diffraction: features important for recognition at opiate receptor. *Science*. 1978;199:1214-1216.
6. Aubry A, Birlirakis N, Sakarellos-Daitsiotis M, Sakarellos C, Marraud M. A crystal molecular-conformation of leucine-enkephalin related to the morphine molecule. *Biopolymers*. 1989;28:27-40.
7. Doi M, Tanaka M, Ishida T, et al. Crystal-structures of [Met⁵] and [(4-bromo)Phe⁴,Met⁵]e nkephalins: formation of a dimeric antiparallel beta-structure. *J Biochem (Tokyo)*. 1987;101:485-490.
8. Loew GH. Molecular modeling of opioid analgesics. *Mod Drug Discovery*. 1999;2:24-30.
9. *SHELXTL [Computer program]. Version 6.10*. Madison, Wisconsin: Bruker AXS Inc. 2000.
10. Griffin JF, Langs DA, Smith GD, Blundell TL, Tickle IJ, Bedarkar S. The crystal-structures of [Met⁵] enkephalin and a third form of [Leu⁵] enkephalin: observations of a novel pleated β-sheet. *Proc Natl Acad Sci USA*. 1986;83:3272-3276.

11. Deschamps JR, Flippen-Anderson JL, Brine GA, Hayes JP, George C. Boc-tyrosyl-D-alanyl-glycyl-N-methyl-pnenylalanyl-O-methyl-methionine hydrate: a protected analog of metkeph-amid. *Acta Crystallogr.* 2002;58E:o13-o15.

12. Ishida T, Kenmotsu M, Mino Y, et al. X-Ray diffraction studies of enkephalins: crystal-structure of [(4'-bromo)Phe⁴,Leu⁵] enkephalin. *Biochem J.* 1984;218:677-689.

13. Stezowski JJ, Eckle E, Bajusz SA. Crystal-structure determination for Tyr-d-Nle-Gly-Phe-Nles [Nles=MetCH₂CH₂CH₂CH(NH₂)SO₃H]: an active synthetic enkephalin analog. *J Chem Soc Chem Comm.* 1985;11:681-682.

14. Deschamps JR, George C, Flippen-Anderson JL. [D-Ala²,D-Leu⁵]-enkephalin (DADLE). *Acta Crystallogr.* 1996;52:1583-1585.

15. Flippen-Anderson JL, Deschamps JR, Ward KB, George C, Houghten R. The crystal structure of deltakephalin: a δ-selective opioid peptide with a novel β-bend-like conformation. *Int J Pept Protein Res.* 1994;44:97-104.

16. Fournie-Zaluski M, Prange T, Pascard C, Roques BP. Enkephalin related fragments: conforma-tional studies of the tetrapeptides Tyr-Gly-Gly-Phe and Gly-Gly-Phe-X (X = Leu, Met) by X-ray and ¹H NMR spectroscopy. *Biochem Biophys Res Commun.* 1977;79:1199-1206.

17. Flippen-Anderson JL, Deschamps JR, George C, Hruby VJ, Misicka A, Lipkowski AW. Crystal structure of biphalin - multireceptor opioid peptide. *J Pept Res.* 2002;59:123-133.

18. Flippen-Anderson JL, George C, Deschamps JR, Reddy PA, Lewin AH, Brine GA. X-ray structures of a potent δ-receptor selective opioid antagonist and a protected form of the δ-receptor antagonist ICI 174,864. *Lett Pept Sci.* 1994;1:107-115.

19. Flippen-Anderson JL, Hruby VJ, Collins N, George C, Cudney B. X-ray structure of [D-Pen²,D-Pen⁵]enkephalin, a highly potent, delta-opioid receptor-selective compound: com-parisons with proposed solution conformations. *J Am Chem Soc.* 1994;116:7523-7531.

20. Collins N, Flippen-Anderson JL, Haaseth R, et al. Conformational determinants of agonist versus antagonist properties of [D-Pen²,D-Pen⁵]-enkephalin (DPDPE) analogs at opioid recep-tors: comparison of x-ray crystallographic structure, solution ¹H NMR data, and molecular dynamic simulations of [L-Ala³]DPDPE and [D-Ala³]DPDPE. *J Am Chem Soc.* 1996;118:2143-2152.

21. Nikiforovich GV, Kover KE, Kolodziej SA, et al. Design and comprehensive conformational studies of Tyr¹-cyclo(D-Pen²-Gly³-Phe⁵-l-3-Mpt⁵) and Tyr(1)-cyclo(Pen²-Gly³-Phe⁵-d-3-Mpt⁵): novel conformationally constrained opioid peptides. *J Am Chem Soc.* 1996;118:959-969.

22. Lomize AL, Flippen-Anderson JL, George C, Mosberg HI. Conformational-analysis of the delta-receptor-selective, cyclic opioid peptide, Tyr-cyclo[D-Cys-Phe-D-Pen]OH (JOM-13): comparison of X-ray crystallographic structures, molecular mechanics simulation, and ¹H-NMR data. *J Am Chem Soc.* 1994;116:429-436.

23. Flippen-Anderson JL, Deschamps JR, George C, et al. X-ray structure of Tyr-D-Tic-Phe-Phe-NH₂ (D-TIPP-NH₂), a highly potent μ-receptor selective opioid agonist: comparisons with proposed model structures. *J Pept Res.* 1997;49:384-393.

24. Ciajolo MR, Balboni G, Picone D, et al. A solution and solid-state structure of the diketopi-perazine of tyrosyl-tetrahydroisoquinoline-3-carboxylic acid. *Int J Pept Protein Res.* 1995;46:134-138.

25. Deschamps JR, Flippen-Anderson JL, George C. 2-[N-(*t*-Butoxycarbonyl)tyrosyl]-1,2,3,4-tetrahydroisoquinoline-3-carboxylic acid nitromethane solvate. *Acta Crystallogr.* 2001;57E:o87-o90.

26. Deschamps JR, Flippen-Anderson JL, Moore C, Cudney R, George C. Tyrosyl-D-tetrahydroi-soquinoline-3-carboxylic acid and tyrosyl-D-tetrahydroisoquinoline-3-carboxamide. *Acta Crystallogr.* 1997;C53:1478-1482.

27. Bryant SD, George C, Flippen-Anderson JL, et al. Crystal structures of dipeptides containing the DMT-TIC pharmacophore. *J Med Chem.* 2002;45:5506-5513.

28. Petsko GA. On the other hand.... *Science.* 1992;256:1403-1404.

29. Milton RC, Milton SCF, Kent BBH. Total chemical synthesis of a D-enzyme: the enantiomers of HIV-1 protease show demonstration of reciprocal chiral substrate specificity. *Science.* 1992;256:1445-1448.

30. Coster D, Knol KS, Prins JA. Unterschiede in der intensität der röntgenstrahlen-feflexion an den beiden 111-flächen der zinkblende. *Z Phys*. 1930;63:345-369.
31. Bijvoet JM, Peerdeman AF, van Bommel AJ. Determination of the absolute configuration of optically active compounds by means of X-rays. *Nature*. 1951;168:271-272.
32. Flack HD. On enantiomorph-polarity estimation. *Acta Crystallogr*. 1983;A39:876-881.
33. Schiller PW, Nguyen TMD, Weltrowska G, et al. Differential stereochemical requirments of μ vs δ opioid receptors for ligand binding and signal transduction: development of a class of potent and highly δ-selective peptide antagonists. *Proc Natl Acad Sci USA*. 1992;89:11871-11875.
34. Balboni G, Guerrini R, Salvadori S, et al. Evaluation of the Dmt-Tic pharmacophore: conversion of a potent delta-opioid receptor antagonist into a potent delta agonist and ligands with mixed properties. *J Med Chem*. 2002;45:713-720.
35. Eddy NB, May EL. The search for a better analgesic. *Science*. 1973;181:407-414.
36. Schiller PW, Yam CF, Lis M. Evidence of topographical analogy between methionine-enkephalin and morphine derivatives. *Biochemistry*. 1977;16:1831-1838.
37. Gylbert L. The crystal and molecule structure of morphine hydrochloride trihydrate. *Acta Crystallogr*. 1973;B29:1630-1635.
38. Thomas G. *Medicinal Chemistry: An Introduction*. Chichester, UK: John Wiley & Sons; 2000.
39. Foye WO, Lemke TL, Williams DA. *Principles of Medicinal Chemistry*. Baltimore, MD: Williams & Wilkins; 1995.
40. Michel AG, Evrard G, Norberg B, Milchert E. Molecular-Structure of Opiate Alkaloids. 2. Crystal-Structures of 4-Methylhomobenzomorphan Hydrobromide (I) and 4,12-beta-Dimethylhomobenzomorphan (II). *Can J Chem*. 1988;66:1763-1769.
41. Thomas JB, Zheng XL, Mascarella SW, et al. N-substituted 9β-methyl-5-(3-hyroxyphenyl)morphans are opioid receptor pure antagonists. *J Med Chem*. 1998;41:4143-4149.
42. Hashimoto A, Jabobson AE, Rothman RB, et al. Probes for narcotic receptor mediated phenomena. 28. New opioid antagonists from enantiomeric analogues of *m*-hydroxyphenyl-N-phenylethylmorphan. *Bioorg Med Chem*. 2002;10:3319-3329.
43. Flippen-Anderson JL, George C, Bertha CM, Rice KC. X-ray crystal structures of potent opioid receptor ligands: etonitazene, *cis*-(+)-3-methylfentanyl, etorphine, diprenorphine, and buprenorphine. *Heterocycles*. 1994;39:751-766.
44. Hruby VJ, Gehrig CA. Recent developments in the design of receptor specifico-peptides. *Med Res Rev*. 1989;9:343-401.

Chapter 22
Opioid Peptide-Derived Analgesics

Peter W. Schiller[1]

Abstract Two recent developments of opioid peptide-based analgesics are reviewed. The first part of the review discusses the dermorphin-derived, cationic-aromatic tetrapeptide H-Dmt-D-Arg-Phe-Lys-NH$_2$ ([Dmt^1]DALDA, where Dmt indicates 2',6'-dimethyltyrosine), which showed subnanomolar μ receptor binding affinity, extraordinary μ receptor selectivity, and high μ agonist potency in vitro. In vivo, [Dmt^1]DALDA looked promising as a spinal analgesic because of its extraordinary antinociceptive effect (3000 times more potent than morphine) in the mouse tail-flick assay, long duration of action (4 times longer than morphine), and lack of effect on respiration. Unexpectedly, [Dmt^1]DALDA also turned out to be a potent and long-acting analgesic in the tail-flick test when given subcutaneously (s.c.), indicating that it is capable of crossing the blood-brain barrier. Furthermore, little or no cross-tolerance was observed with s.c. [Dmt^1]DALDA in morphine-tolerant mice. The second part of the review concerns the development of mixed μ agonist/δ antagonists that, on the basis of much evidence, are expected to be analgesics with a low propensity to produce tolerance and physical dependence. The prototype pseudopeptide H-Dmt-TicΨ[CH$_2$NH]Phe-Phe-NH$_2$ (DIPP-NH$_2$[Ψ], where Tic indicates 1,2,3,4-tetrahydroisoquinoline-3-carboxylic acid) showed subnanomolar μ and δ receptor binding affinities and the desired μ agonist/δ antagonist profile in vitro. DIPP-NH$_2$[Ψ] produced a potent analgesic effect after intracerebroventricular administration in the rat tail-flick assay, no physical dependence, and less tolerance than morphine. The results obtained with DIPP-NH$_2$[Ψ] indicate that mixed μ agonist/δ antagonists look promising as analgesic drug candidates, but compounds with this profile that are systemically active still need to be developed.

[1] Laboratory of Chemical Biology and Peptide Research, Clinical Research Institute of Montreal, 110 Pine Avenue West, Montreal, Quebec, Canada H2W 1R7

Corresponding Author: Peter W. Schiller, 110 Pine Avenue West, Montreal, Quebec, Canada H2W 1R7. Tel: (514) 987-5576; Fax: (514) 987-5513; E-mail: schillp@ircm.qc.ca

Introduction

The clinical treatment of severe pain relies heavily upon opioid analgesics, most of which act via μ opioid receptors. Morphine and other centrally acting μ opioid analgesics produce, in addition to the analgesic effect, several side effects—including inhibition of gastrointestinal motility, respiratory depression, tolerance, and physical dependence—that limit their use in pain treatment. Kappa opioid agonists have also been shown to be potent analgesics; however, it has long been recognized that centrally acting κ agonists have limited usefulness in humans because of their psychotomimetic and dysphoric effects.[1,2] Delta opioid agonists are known to produce analgesic effects when given intrathecally (i.th)[3,4] or intracerebroventricularly (i.c.v.).[4] There is evidence to indicate that they induce less tolerance and physical dependence than μ analgesics, no respiratory depression, and few or no adverse gastrointestinal effects.[5-7] Among the peptide δ opioid agonists, [D-Pen^2, D-Pen^5]enkephalin (DPDPE) produced only a weak, centrally mediated analgesic effect after systemic administration, indicating that it does not cross the blood-brain barrier (BBB) to a significant extent.[8] Interestingly, the δ-selective and highly stable cyclic lanthionine enkephalin analog H-Tyr-c[D-Val$_L$-Gly-Phe-D-Ala$_L$]-OH was as active as morphine in producing centrally mediated analgesia when given intraperitoneally.[9] Several nonpeptide compounds showing potent and selective δ agonist activity in vitro were developed. These include TAN-67,[10] the racemic compound BW373U86,[11] and its chemically modified enantiomer SNC80.[12] These compounds produced analgesic effects when administered i.th. or i.c.v. but showed very low or no analgesic activity when given systemically. Furthermore, both BW373U86 and SNC80 produced convulsions in mice. Numerous compounds structurally derived from SNC80 were synthesized, and some were shown to be potent and selective δ agonists in in vitro assays.[13] However, analgesic data for these compounds have not yet been published. It remains to be seen whether δ opioid agonists that are efficacious enough to produce strong centrally mediated analgesic effects when given systemically or orally can indeed be developed.

Progress has been made in the development of peripherally acting κ and μ opioid agonists (for a review, see DeHaven-Hudkins and Dolle).[14] Since such compounds have no or very low ability to cross the BBB, they are expected not to produce the typical side effects mediated by central κ and μ opioid receptors (vide supra). There is evidence to indicate that peripherally restricted opioid analgesics produce antinociceptive effects under inflammatory conditions through local interaction with opioid receptors present on peripheral nerve terminals. Peripherally acting κ and μ opioid agonists may be effective as analgesics in various inflammatory pain states, for the treatment of visceral and postoperative pain, and as antipruritic agents. Most of the peripherally restricted opioids developed so far are still in the preclinical phase, and their promise as therapeutic agents needs to be confirmed in clinical trials.

In this paper, we review 2 recent developments of opioid peptide-based analgesics with novel activity profiles or with distinct physicochemical properties. The first part discusses the pharmacological characteristics of the μ opioid agonist tetrapeptide

H-Dmt-D-Arg-Phe-Lys-NH$_2$ ([Dmt^1]DALDA, where Dmt indicates 2′,6′-dimethyl-tyrosine), which has therapeutic potential for use in spinal analgesia and is capable of crossing the BBB. The second part discusses the development of opioid peptides that act as agonists at the μ opioid receptor and as antagonists at the δ receptor. Opioid compounds with such a mixed μ agonist/δ antagonist profile look promising as analgesics with a low propensity to produce tolerance and dependence.

[Dmt^1]DALDA

The dermorphin-derived tetrapeptide H-Tyr-D-Arg-Phe-Lys-NH$_2$ (DALDA)[15] carries a net positive charge of 3+. In vitro it displayed μ agonist activity in the guinea pig ileum (GPI) assay, low nanomolar μ receptor binding affinity, and extraordinary μ receptor selectivity (Table 22.1). Replacement of the Tyr^1 residue in this peptide with 2′,6′-dimethyltyrosine (Dmt) led to a compound, [Dmt^1]DALDA, which showed 180-fold increased μ agonist potency in the GPI assay, subnano-molar μ receptor binding affinity, and still excellent μ receptor selectivity.[16] The high μ receptor binding affinity and excellent μ selectivity of this peptide were confirmed in another binding study that, furthermore, indicated some preference for μ$_1$ receptors (K$_i$ = 0.05 ± 0.02 nM) over μ$_2$ receptors (K$_i$ = 0.27 ± 0.13 nM).[17] When a calf striatal membrane binding assay was used, [^{3}H][Dmt^1]DALDA binding was shown to be far less sensitive than [^{3}H]H-Tyr-D-Ala-Gly-N^{2}MePhe-Gly-ol ([^{3}H]DAMGO) binding to the effects of divalent and sodium cations, and guanine nucleotides.[18] The observation that [Dmt^1]DALDA showed plateaus suggestive of a partial agonist in [^{35}S]GTPγS binding assays using brain and spinal cord membranes was in agreement with the demonstrated ability of [^{3}H][Dmt^1]DALDA to label agonist and antagonist conformations of μ receptors expressed in Chinese hamster ovary (CHO) cells. In the [^{35}S]GTPγS binding assay using CHO cells, [Dmt^1]DALDA showed high efficacy with the μ receptor and with several of its splice variants, but its potency (EC$_{50}$) varied markedly among some of the splice variants despite similar affinities in the receptor binding assays. In general,

Table 22.1 In Vitro Opioid Activity Profiles of DALDA Peptides*[16]

Compound	GPI IC$_{50}$, nM†	MVD IC$_{50}$, nM†	Receptor Binding	
			K$_i$^{μ}, nM†	K$_i$ Ratio (μ/δ/κ)
H-Tyr-D-Arg-Phe-Lys-NH$_2$ (DALDA)	254 ± 27	781 ± 146	1.69 ± 0.25	1/11 400/2500
H-Dmt-D-Arg-Phe-Lys-NH$_2$ ([Dmt^1] DALDA)	1.41 ± 0.29	23.1 ± 2.0	0.143 ± 0.015	1/14 700/156
Morphine	29.3 ± 2.2	155 ± 31	1.00 ± 0.04	1/33/217

*Dmt indicates 2′,6′-dimethyltyrosine; GPI, guinea pig ileum; MVD, mouse vas deferens.
†Mean of 3–6 determinations ± standard error of the mean.

[Dmt^1]DALDA activated GTPγS binding more potently than did DAMGO. Taken together, these observations indicate that [Dmt^1]DALDA and DAMGO differ in the way they activate these receptors.

As expected on the basis of its structural characteristics, [Dmt^1]DALDA was found to be highly stable against enzymatic degradation when incubated in sheep blood.[19] When given i.th. to rats, [Dmt^1]DALDA was extremely active in producing an analgesic effect in the tail-flick assay: it was 3000 times more potent than morphine.[20] The same extraordinary antinociceptive potency of i.th. [Dmt^1]DALDA was also observed in the mouse tail-flick assay.[19] The observation that [Dmt^1]DALDA had only 7-fold higher μ receptor binding affinity than morphine (Table 22.1) suggested that this peptide may produce its extraordinarily potent antinociceptive effect via additional mechanisms. Interestingly, it was found that [Dmt^1]DALDA inhibited norepinephrine uptake in rat spinal cord synaptosomes with an IC$_{50}$ of 4.1 μM.[20] Thus, i.th. administration of [Dmt^1]DALDA results in activation of both μ opioid receptors and α$_2$-adrenergic receptors in a synergistic manner known to potentiate the antinociceptive effect of μ opioid agonists.[21] This interpretation is in tune with the observation that the antinociceptive response to [Dmt^1]DALDA was attenuated by i.th. yohimbine, an α$_2$-adrenergic antagonist.[20] Furthermore, it was shown that i.th. [Dmt^1]DALDA in mice caused the release of dynorphin-like and met-enkephalin-like peptides in the spinal cord that then acted on κ and μ receptors, respectively, to potentiate the potency of i.th. [Dmt^1]DALDA.[22] Thus, [Dmt^1]DALDA may be regarded as a spinal analgesic with triple action. The duration of the antinociceptive effect of [Dmt^1]DALDA (13 hours) in the rat tail-flick assay was 4 times longer than that of morphine (3 hours) when the 2 drugs were given i.th. at equipotent doses ($3 \times$ ED$_{50}$).[20] The long duration of action of [Dmt^1]DALDA may be due to not only its enzyme resistance but also the slow clearance from the spinal cord due to the peptide's high positive charge. Unlike morphine, [Dmt^1]DALDA produced no respiratory depression after i.th. administration at a dose of $30 \times$ ED$_{50}$, most likely because at the very low dose level required for producing the analgesic effect, significant rostral distribution of the drug to the medullary respiratory centers does not occur.[20] Because [Dmt^1]DALDA has low propensity to produce respiratory depression after i.th. administration, it may be a candidate for a safe spinal opioid in patients. However, this peptide did produce quite profound tolerance after chronic i.th. administration.[23,24] When given i.c.v. to mice, [Dmt^1]DALDA was 119 times more potent than morphine in the tail-flick test in one study[17] and 217 times more potent in another.[23]

Unexpectedly, [Dmt^1]DALDA also produced a potent antinociceptive effect in the mouse tail-flick test when given subcutaneously (s.c.), being 218 times more potent than morphine in one study[17] and 36 times more potent in another.[23] These results indicate that this peptide is capable of crossing the BBB. The duration of the analgesic effect produced by s.c. [Dmt^1]DALDA (12 hours) was again much longer than that determined for s.c. morphine (3 hours) at equipotent doses ($5 \times$ ED$_{50}$). A pharmacokinetic study performed with sheep (intravenous infusion) revealed that the elimination half-life of [Dmt^1]DALDA (118 minutes) was 4 times longer than that of morphine (30 minutes).[19] Both the metabolic stability and the long elimination half-life of this peptide may be responsible for its prolonged analgesic effect after systemic administration. In contrast to morphine-induced analgesia, [Dmt[1]]DALDA (s.c.) supraspinal analgesia was insensitive to several antisense probes targeting the different exons of MOR-1[17] and, unlike morphine, retained its analgesic actions in MOR-1 knockout mice.[25] Furthermore, various strains of mice showed differential sensitivities to morphine and [Dmt[1]]DALDA analgesia. These observations indicate that [Dmt[1]]DALDA is a μ opioid analgesic showing significant pharmacological differences in comparison with morphine. [Dmt[1]]DALDA did produce tolerance when chronically administered s.c. to mice[23]; however, little or no cross-tolerance was observed with this peptide given s.c. in morphine-tolerant mice.[17,26] The latter observation raises the interesting possibility that morphine-tolerant patients could be switched over to [Dmt[1]]DALDA for better pain relief.

The demonstrated ability of [Dmt[1]]DALDA to cross the BBB prompted studies examining whether this peptide could penetrate into Caco-2 cells.[27] Cellular uptake could be demonstrated using tritiated [Dmt[1]]DALDA in an incubation experiment, as well as the dansylated analog H-Dmt-Arg-Phe-Dap(dns)[28] in a confocal laser scanning microscopy study. Furthermore, it was demonstrated that [Dmt[1]]DALDA could translocate across Caco-2 cell monolayers.[27] These observations provide an explanation for this peptide's ability to penetrate into the central nervous system (CNS) after systemic administration and suggest that it may even have reasonable oral bioavailability. The mechanism of the cellular uptake of [Dmt[1]]DALDA remains to be elucidated; however, it has been established that it is not receptor mediated and does not involve a transporter or endocytosis.[27] [Dmt[1]]DALDA is a cationic-aromatic peptide consisting of alternating aromatic and basic amino acids, and it may enter cells via a local destabilization of the plasma membrane. Taken together, the results obtained with [Dmt[1]]DALDA demonstrate that potent and stable peptide drugs showing slow clearance and ability to cross the BBB can be developed.

Mixed μ Agonist/δ Antagonists

Two studies have indicated that selective δ receptor blockade with a δ antagonist greatly reduced the development of morphine tolerance and dependence.[29,30] Several interesting observations in relation to this phenomenon have been made. Chronic morphine treatment was shown to result in an upregulation of δ binding sites in rats.[31] A study using different strains of mice demonstrated that the intensity of the withdrawal syndrome after chronic morphine treatment correlated with the level of δ binding sites.[32] Furthermore, the development of morphine tolerance and dependence following chronic morphine administration was blocked by an antisense oligodeoxynucleotide to the δ opioid receptor.[33] Finally, morphine was shown to retain its μ receptor mediated analgesic activity in δ opioid receptor knockout mice without producing tolerance upon chronic administration.[34] Very recently, δ receptor antagonists were shown to enhance morphine-mediated i.th. analgesia, possibly as a consequence of μ-δ receptor heterodimerization.[35] These various observations clearly indicate that δ opioid receptors play a major role in the development of morphine tolerance and dependence and provide a rationale for the development of an opioid compound acting as an agonist at the μ receptor and as an antagonist at the δ receptor. Such a mixed μ agonist/δ antagonist would be expected to be an analgesic with low propensity to produce analgesic tolerance and physical dependence, and might be of benefit in the management of chronic pain. Furthermore, it has been shown that the δ antagonist naltrindole reversed alfentanil (a μ agonist) induced respiratory depression[36] and enhanced colonic propulsion.[37] These results suggest that a mixed μ agonist/δ antagonist might also cause less respiratory depression and less inhibition of gastrointestinal transit than a μ agonist like morphine.

The first known compound with a mixed μ agonist/δ antagonist profile was the tetrapeptide amide H-Tyr-Tic-Phe-Phe-NH$_2$ (TIPP-NH$_2$).[38] This compound showed modest μ agonist potency in the GPI assay (IC$_{50}$ = 1.70 ± 0.22 μM) and quite high δ antagonist potency in the mouse vas deferens (MVD) assay against the δ agonist DPDPE (K$_e$ = 18.0 ± 2.2 nM). In agreement with the bioassay data, TIPP-NH$_2$ displayed relatively low affinity for μ receptors (K$_i^\mu$ = 78.8 ± 7.1 nM) and high affinity for δ receptors (K$_i^\delta$ = 3.0 ± 1.5 nM) in the rat brain membrane binding assays, indicating that it was quite δ-selective (K$_i^\mu$/K$_i^\delta$ = 26.3). In an effort to strengthen the μ agonist component of TIPP-NH$_2$ without compromising its δ antagonist properties, the Tyr[1] residue was replaced with Dmt. The resulting compound, H-Dmt-Tic-Phe-Phe-NH$_2$ (DIPP-NH$_2$), showed much improved μ agonist potency in the GPI assay (IC$_{50}$ = 18.2 ± 1.8 nM) and retained very high δ antagonist activity in the MVD assay (K$_e$ = 0.209 ± 0.037 nM)[39] (Table 22.2). The receptor binding data were in agreement with these results and indicated that DIPP-NH$_2$ was still somewhat δ receptor-selective, as indicated by the ratio of the binding inhibition constants (K$_i^\mu$/K$_i^\delta$ = 10.1). Reduction of the peptide bond between Tic[2] and Phe[3] of DIPP-NH$_2$

Table 22.2 In Vitro Opioid Activity Profiles of Mixed μ Agonist/δ Antagonists and Related Compounds*

Compound	GPI IC$_{50}$, nM	MVD K$_e$, nM[‡]	Receptor Binding K$_i^\mu$, nM	K$_i^\delta$, nM
H-Dmt-Tic-Phe-Phe-NH$_2$	18.2 ± 1.8	0.209 ± 0.037	1.19 ± 0.11	0.118 ± 0.016
H-Dmt-TicΨ[CH$_2$NH]Phe-Phe-NH$_2$ (DIPP-NH$_2$[Ψ])	7.71 ± 0.31	0.537 ± 0.026	0.943 ± 0.052	0.447 ± 0.007
[Dmt¹]DALDA→CH$_2$CH$_2$NH←TICP[Ψ]	66.5 ± 5.4	2.40 ± 0.58	14.0 ± 1.5	4.79 ± 0.50
[Dmt¹]DALDA	1.41 ± 0.29	—	0.143 ± 0.015	2100 ± 310
TICP[Ψ]	Inactive	0.175 ± 0.025	1050 ± 10	0.259 ± 0.047

*DALDA indicates H-Dmt-D-Arg-Phe-Lys-NH$_2$; Dmt, 2',6'-dimethyltyrosine; GPI, guinea pig ileum; MVD, mouse vas deferens; TICP[Ψ], H-Tyr-TicΨ[CH$_2$NH]Cha-Phe-OH, where Cha indicates cyclohexylalanine. Mean of 3–6 determinations ± standard error of the mean.

[†]Displacement of [³H]DAMGO (μ-selective) and [³H]DSLET (δ-selective) from rat brain membrane binding sites.

[‡]Determined against DPDPE.

resulted in the highly stable pseudopeptide H-Dmt-TicΨ[CH$_2$NH]Phe-Phe-NH$_2$ (DIPP-NH$_2$[Ψ]), which displayed further increased μ agonist potency in the GPI assay (IC$_{50}$ = 7.71 nM) and retained very high δ antagonist activity (K$_e$ = 0.537 nM) in the MVD assay.[39] DIPP-NH$_2$[Ψ] showed subnanomolar binding affinities for both μ and δ receptors and thus turned out to be a "balanced" μ agonist/δ antagonist (K$_i^\mu$/K$_i^\delta$ = 2.11). In the rat tail-flick test, DIPP-NH$_2$[Ψ] given i.c.v. produced a potent analgesic effect (ED$_{50}$ = 0.04 μg), being ~3 times more potent than morphine (ED$_{50}$ = 0.11 μg).[39] At high doses (i.c.v.) it produced less acute analgesic tolerance than morphine but still a certain level of chronic tolerance. Unlike morphine, DIPP-NH$_2$[Ψ] produced no physical dependence upon chronic i.c.v. infusion at high dose levels (up to 4.5 μg/h) over a 7-day period.[39] Thus, the in vivo pharmacological behavior of DIPP-NH$_2$[Ψ] with regard to analgesic activity and the development of tolerance and dependence was, to a large extent, as expected for a mixed μ agonist/δ antagonist. However, DIPP-NH$_2$[Ψ] showed a limited ability to cross the BBB, and mixed μ agonist/δ antagonists capable of penetrating into the CNS and showing improved bioavailability in general have yet to be developed.

In DIPP-NH$_2$[Ψ] no clear distinction can be made between structural moieties that confer μ agonist properties to the molecule and moieties that are responsible for δ antagonist behavior. An alternative approach to the development of mixed μ agonist/δ antagonists is the design of compounds containing a known μ agonist and a known δ antagonist as distinct moieties. In an effort to develop a mixed μ agonist/δ antagonist capable of crossing the BBB, we recently synthesized a chimeric peptide containing [Dmt^1]DALDA and the potent and selective δ antagonist (inverse agonist) H-Tyr-TicΨ[CH$_2$NH]Cha-Phe-OH (TICP[Ψ]), where Cha indicates cyclohexylalanine[40] connected "tail-to-tail" via a short linker.[41] This peptide, H-Dmt→D-Arg→Phe→Lys-NH-CH$_2$-CH$_2$-NH-Phe←Cha[NHCH$_2$]ΨTic←Tyr←H ([Dmt^1]DALDA→CH$_2$CH$_2$NH←TICP[Ψ]) is expected to cross the BBB because it contains [Dmt^1]DALDA, which by itself effectively penetrates into the CNS (*vide supra*) and which likely will confer BBB crossing ability to the entire chimeric peptide construct. [Dmt^1]DALDA→CH$_2$CH$_2$NH←TICP[Ψ] showed high μ and δ receptor binding affinities in the opioid receptor binding assays (K$_i^\mu$ = 14 nM; K$_i^\delta$ = 4.8 nM) and the expected μ agonist/δ antagonist profile [IC$_{50}$(GPI) = 66 nM; K$_e^\delta$(MVD) = 2.40 nM] (Table 22.2). In comparison with [Dmt^1]DALDA, the chimeric peptide has 47-fold lower μ agonist potency in the GPI assay and 98-fold lower μ receptor binding affinity. It has 14-fold lower δ antagonist potency than TICP[Ψ] in the MVD assay and 18-fold lower δ receptor binding affinity. Despite these reductions in potency, the chimeric peptide still has quite high μ agonist and δ antagonist potencies because of the extraordinarily high potencies of its 2 constituents. It is possible that the reduced potency of [Dmt^1]DALDA→CH$_2$CH$_2$NH←TICP[Ψ] is due to some interference between the 2 components caused specifically by their "tail-to-tail" coupling. This chimeric peptide is currently being examined for its ability to produce a centrally mediated antinociceptive effect after administration by various routes.

Pyridomorphinans with a partial μ agonist/δ antagonist profile in vitro have been reported to produce a partial or full agonist effect in the warm-water tail-withdrawal assay after i.c.v. administration and a reduced level of tolerance.[42,43] The best compound of this class was 10-fold less potent than morphine. Taken together, the results obtained with DIPP-NH$_2$[Ψ] and with the pyridomorphinans indicate that mixed μ agonist/δ antagonists look promising as analgesic drug candidates; however, compounds with this profile that have higher μ agonist potency and higher efficacy and that are systemically active still need to be developed.

Acknowledgments This work was supported by grants from the Canadian Institutes of Health Research (MOP-5655) and the National Institute on Drug Abuse (DA-08924).

References

1. Pfeiffer A, Brantl V, Herz A, Emrich HM. Psychotomimesis mediated by kappa opiate receptors. *Science*. 1986;233:774-776.
2. Walsh SL, Strain EC, Abreu ME, Bigelow GE. Enadoline, a selective kappa opioid agonist: comparison with butorphanol and hydromorphone in humans. *Psychopharmacology (Berl)*. 2001;157:151-162.
3. Yaksh TL. In vivo studies on spinal opiate receptor systems mediating antinociception, I: mu and delta receptor profiles in the primate. *J Pharmacol Exp Ther*. 1983;226:303-316.
4. Porreca F, Mosberg HI, Hurst R, Hruby VJ, Burks TF. Roles of mu, delta and kappa opioid receptors in spinal and supraspinal mediation of gastrointestinal transit effects and hot-plate analgesia in the mouse. *J Pharmacol Exp Ther*. 1984;230:341-348.
5. Cowan A, Zhu XZ, Mosberg HI, Omnaas JR, Porreca F. Direct dependence studies in rats with agents selective for different types of opioid receptor. *J Pharmacol Exp Ther*. 1988;246:950-955.
6. Cheng PY, Wu D, Decena J, Soong Y, McCabe S, Szeto HH. Opioid-induced stimulation of fetal respiratory activity by [D-Ala^2]deltorphin, I. *Eur J Pharmacol*. 1993;230:85-88.
7. Galligan JJ, Mosberg HI, Hurst R, Hruby VJ, Burks TF. Cerebral delta opioid receptors mediate analgesia but not the intestinal motility effects of intracerebroventricularly administered opioids. *J Pharmacol Exp Ther*. 1984;229:641-648.
8. Weber SJ, Greene DL, Sharma SD, et al. Distribution and analgesia of [^{3}H][D-Pen^2, D-Pen^5]enkephalin and two halogenated analogs after intravenous administration. *J Pharmacol Exp Ther*. 1991;259:1109-1117.
9. Svensson CI, Rew Y, Malkmus S, et al. Systemic and spinal analgesic activity of a δ-opioid-selective lanthionine enkephalin analog. *J Pharmacol Exp Ther*. 2003;304:827-832.
10. Kamei J, Saitoh A, Ohsawa M, et al. Antinociceptive effects of the selective non-peptidic δ-opioid receptor antagonist TAN-67 in diabetic mice. *Eur J Pharmacol*. 1995;276: 131-135.
11. Chang K-J, Rigdon GC, Howard JL, McNutt RW. A novel, potent and selective nonpeptidic delta opioid receptor agonist BW373U86. *J Pharmacol Exp Ther*. 1993;267:852-857.
12. Calderon SN, Rothman RB, Porreca F, et al. Probes for narcotic receptor mediated phenomena, 19: synthesis of (+)-4-(αR)-α-((2S,5R)-4-allyl-2,5-dimethyl-1-piperazinyl)-3-methoxybenzyl]-N,N-diethylbenzamide (SNC80): a highly selective, nonpeptide delta opioid receptor agonist. *J Med Chem*. 1994;37:2125-2128.
13. Plobeck N, Delorme D, Wei Z-Y, et al. New diarylmethylpiperazines as potent and selective nonpeptidic δ opioid receptor agonists with increased in vitro metabolic stability. *J Med Chem*. 2000;43:3878-3894.
14. DeHaven-Hudkins DL, Dolle RE. Peripherally restricted opioid agonists as novel analgesic agents. *Curr Pharm Des*. 2004;10:743-757.

15. Schiller PW, Nguyen TM-D, Chung NN, Lemieux C. Dermorphin analogues carrying an increased positive net charge in their "message" domain display extremely high μ-opioid receptor selectivity. *J Med Chem.* 1989;32:698-703.
16. Schiller PW, Nguyen TM-D, Berezowska I, et al. Synthesis and in vitro opioid activity profiles of DALDA analogues. *Eur J Med Chem.* 2000;35:895-901.
17. Neilan CL, Nguyen TM-D, Schiller PW, Pasternak GW. Pharmacological characterization of the dermorphin analog [Dmt¹]DALDA, a highly potent and selective μ-opioid peptide. *Eur J Pharmacol.* 2001;419:15-23.
18. Neilan CL, Janvey AJ, Bolan E, et al. Characterization of the binding of [³H][Dmt¹]H-Dmt-D-Arg-Phe-Lys-NH₂, a highly potent opioid peptide. *J Pharmacol Exp Ther.* 2003;306:430-436.
19. Szeto HH, Lovelace JL, Fridland G, et al. In vivo pharmacokinetics of selective μ-opioid peptide agonists. *J Pharmacol Exp Ther.* 2001;298:57-61.
20. Shimoyama M, Shimoyama N, Zhao G-M, Schiller PW, Szeto HH. Antinociceptive and respiratory effects of intrathecal H-Tyr-D-Arg-Phe-Lys-NH₂ (DALDA) and [Dmt¹]DALDA. *J Pharmacol Exp Ther.* 2001;297:364-371.
21. Reimann W, Schlutz H, Selve N. The antinociceptive effects of morphine, desipramine, and serotonin and their combinations after intrathecal injection in the rat. *Anesth Analg.* 1999;88:141-145.
22. Szeto HH, Soong Y, Wu D, Qian X, Zhao G-M. Endogenous opioid peptides contribute to antinociceptive potency of intrathecal [Dmt¹]DALDA. *J Pharmacol Exp Ther.* 2003;305: 696-702.
23. Zhao GM, Wu D, Soong Y, et al. Profound spinal tolerance after repeated exposure to a highly selective μ-opioid peptide agonist: role of δ-opioid receptors. *J Pharmacol Exp Ther.* 2002;302:188-196.
24. Ben Y, Smith AP, Schiller PW, Lee NM. Tolerance develops in spinal cord, but not in brain with chronic [Dmt¹]DALDA treatment. *Br J Pharmacol.* 2004;143:987-993.
25. Neilan CL, King MA, Rossi G, et al. Differential sensitivities of mouse strains to morphine and [Dmt¹]DALDA analgesia. *Brain Res.* 2003;974:254-257.
26. Riba P, Ben Y, Nguyen TM-D, Furst S, Schiller PW, Lee NM. [Dmt¹]DALDA is highly selective and potent at μ opioid receptors, but is not cross-tolerant with systemic morphine. *Curr Med Chem.* 2002;9:31-39.
27. Zhao K, Luo G, Zhao G-M, Schiller PW, Szeto HH. Transcellular transport of a highly polar 3+ net charge opioid tetrapeptide. *J Pharmacol Exp Ther.* 2003;304:425-432.
28. Berezowska I, Chung NN, Lemieux C, Zelent B, Szeto HH, Schiller PW. Highly potent fluorescent analogues of the opioid peptide [Dmt¹]DALDA. *Peptides.* 2003;24:1195-1200.
29. Abdelhamid EE, Sultana M, Portoghese PS, Takemori AE. Selective blockage of delta opioid receptors prevents the development of morphine tolerance and dependence in mice. *J Pharmacol Exp Ther.* 1991;258:299-303.
30. Fundytus ME, Schiller PW, Shapiro M, Weltrowska G, Coderre TJ. The highly selective δ-opioid antagonist H-Tyr-TicΨ[CH₂-NH]Phe-Phe-OH (TIPP[Ψ]) attenuates morphine tolerance and dependence. *Eur J Pharmacol.* 1995;286:105-108.
31. Rothman RB, Danks JA, Jacobson AE, Burke TR, Jr, Rice KE, Holaday JW. Morphine tolerance increases mu-noncompetitive delta binding sites. *Eur J Pharmacol.* 1986;124:113-119.
32. Yukhananov RY, Klodt PM, Riva AD, Zeitsev SV, Masky AI. Opiate withdrawal correlates with the presence of DSLET high-affinity binding. *Pharmacol Biochem Behav.* 1994;49: 1109-1112.
33. Kest B, Lee CY, McLemore GL, Inturrisi CE. An antisense oligodeoxynucleotide to the delta opioid receptor (DOR-1) inhibits morphine tolerance and acute dependence in mice. *Brain Res Bull.* 1996;39:185-188.
34. Zhu Y, King MA, Schuller AG, et al. Retention of supraspinal delta-like analgesia and loss of morphine tolerance in delta opioid receptor knock-out mice. *Neuron.* 1999;24:243-252.
35. Gomes I, Gupta A, Filipovska J, Szeto HH, Pintar JE, Devi LA. A role for heterodimerization of μ and δ opiate receptors in enhancing morphine analgesia. *Proc Natl Acad Sci USA.* 2004;101:5135-5139.

36. Freye E, Latasch L, Portoghese PS. The delta receptor is involved in sufentanil-induced respiratory depression—opioid subreceptors mediate different effects. *Eur J Anaesthesiol.* 1992;9:457-462.
37. Foxx-Orenstein AE, Jin JG, Grider JR. 5HT4 receptor agonists and delta opioid receptor antagonists act synergistically to stimulate colonic propulsion. *Am J Physiol.* 1998;275: G979-G983.
38. Schiller PW, Nguyen TM-D, Weltrowska G, et al. Differential stereochemical requirements of μ vs δ opioid receptors for ligand binding and signal transduction: development of a class of potent and highly δ-selective peptide antagonists. *Proc Natl Acad Sci USA.* 1992;89: 11871-11875.
39. Schiller PW, Fundytus ME, Merovitz L, et al. The opioid μ agonist/δ antagonist DIPP-NH$_2$[Ψ] produces a potent analgesic effect, no physical dependence, and less tolerance than morphine in rats. *J Med Chem.* 1999;42:3520-3526.
40. Schiller PW, Weltrowska G, Berezowska I, et al. The TIPP opioid peptide family: development of δ antagonists, δ agonists and mixed μ agonist/δ antagonists. *Biopolymers (Peptide Science).* 1999;51:411-425.
41. Weltrowska G, Lemieux C, Chung NN, Schiller PW. A chimeric opioid peptide with mixed μ agonist/δ antagonist properties. *J Pept Res.* 2004;63:63-68.
42. Ananthan S, Kezar HS, III, Carter RL, et al. Synthesis, opioid receptor binding, and biological activities of naltrexone-derived pyrido- and pyrimidomorphinans. *J Med Chem.* 1999;42: 3527-3538.
43. Ananthan S, Khare NK, Saini SK, et al. Identification of opioid ligands possessing mixed μ agonist/δ antagonist activity among pyridomorphinans derived from naloxone, oxymorphone, and hydromorphone. *J Med Chem.* 2004;47:1400-1412.

Chapter 23
Opioid Ligands with Mixed μ/δ Opioid Receptor Interactions: An Emerging Approach to Novel Analgesics

Subramaniam Ananthan[1]

Abstract Opioids are widely used in the treatment of severe pain. The clinical use of the opioids is limited by serious side effects such as respiratory depression, constipation, development of tolerance, and physical dependence and addiction liabilities. Most of the currently available opioid analgesics exert their analgesic and adverse effects primarily through the opioid μ receptors. A large number of biochemical and pharmacological studies and studies using genetically modified animals have provided convincing evidence regarding the existence of modulatory interactions between opioid μ and δ receptors. Several studies indicate that δ receptor agonists as well as δ receptor antagonists can provide beneficial modulation to the pharmacological effects of μ agonists. For example, δ agonists can enhance the analgesic potency and efficacy of μ agonists, and δ antagonists can prevent or diminish the development of tolerance and physical dependence by μ agonists. On the basis of these observations, the development of new opioid ligands possessing mixed μ agonist/δ agonist profile and mixed μ agonist/δ antagonist profile has emerged as a promising new approach to analgesic drug development. A brief overview of μ-δ interactions and recent developments in identification of ligands possessing mixed μ agonist/δ agonist and μ agonist/δ antagonist activities is provided in this report.

Keywords Analgesics, Opioid Ligands, Mixed Mu/Delta agonists, Mixed Mu agonist/Delta antagonists, Peptides, Nonpeptides

Introduction

Opioid analgesics are the standard therapeutic agents for the treatment of moderate-to-severe pain. These drugs exert their analgesic activity through their interaction with the opioid μ, δ, or κ receptors as agonists. The clinical usefulness of μ opioid

---

[1] Organic Chemistry Department, Southern Research Institute, Birmingham, AL

Corresponding Author: Subramaniam Ananthan, Organic Chemistry Department, Southern Research Institute, Birmingham, AL 35255. Tel: (205) 581-2822; Fax: (205) 581-2726; E-mail: ananthan@sri.org

R.S. Rapaka and W. Sadée (eds.), *Drug Addiction*.
© American Association of Pharmaceutical Scientists 2008

agonists such as morphine, however, is limited by significant side effects such as respiratory depression, constipation, development of tolerance and physical dependence, and addiction potential. One approach to limit μ-receptor-mediated side effects is to selectively target δ and κ opioid receptors. This approach has been explored using agonist ligands selective for δ and κ opioid receptors but has seen only limited success. The δ agonists generally display limited analgesic efficacy and κ receptor agonists are limited to their use as peripheral analgesics owing to their psychotomimetic and dysphoric central effects. An alternative approach that is gaining considerable interest is the development of compounds that possess mixed opioid activity at the different opioid receptors.[1,2]

Several lines of evidence indicate the existence of physical and functional interactions between the opioid receptors, particularly between the μ and δ receptors. Several biochemical and pharmacological studies using μ and δ receptor ligands gave an early indication of such interactions between the μ and δ receptors.[3-6] The μ and δ opioid receptors exist on overlapping populations of neurons in pain-modulating regions of the central nervous system, and the presence of both μ and δ receptors within the same neuron has been demonstrated.[7] In recent years, several studies have shown that μ and δ receptors form functionally distinct heterodimeric or hetero-oligomeric complexes.[8-11] The physiological and pharmacological significance of μ-δ interactions have been substantiated by recent studies using opioid receptor gene knockout animals.[12] The existence of intermodulatory effects between μ and δ receptors has spawned a new interest in the pursuit of ligands with a mixed interaction profile at the μ and δ receptors as a novel therapeutic approach for the treatment of pain. Presented herein is a brief overview of ligands that possess a mixed μ agonist/δ agonist or μ agonist/δ antagonist profile of activity.

Mixed μ Agonists/δ Agonists

Several early studies using coadministration of μ and δ agonist ligands demonstrated that both the potency and efficacy of μ agonists can be increased by δ agonists. Vaught and Takemori found that Leu[5]-enkephalin given at subantinociceptive doses could potentiate the analgesic actions of morphine.[13] Several other studies extended these observations to synergistic antinociceptive effects between other μ agonists and δ agonists.[14-16] The activation of δ opioid receptors has been reported to have synergistic effect on μ opioid functional activities in cells transfected with μ and δ receptors.[7,8,17] Treatment of rats or mice for several days with μ agonists leads to translocation of δ opioid receptors to neuronal plasma membranes and enhances δ-receptor-mediated antinociception.[18] These observations imply that addition of a δ agonist may allow for the treatment of pain with lower doses of μ agonists, and ligands possessing dual agonist activities at the δ and μ receptors may allow for the effective treatment of pain with lessened μ-receptor-mediated side effects.[19,20]

Peptide ligands possessing μ and δ agonist activity

There have been several reports on peptide ligands that display high-affinity binding and agonist actions at both μ and δ receptors. Of particular interest among peptide ligands possessing dual agonist actions at μ and δ receptors are biphalin and biphalin analogs. Biphalin, (Tyr-D-Ala-Gly-Phe-NH)$_2$, binds to both μ and δ receptors with high affinity. It is a highly potent analgesic and is as potent as etorphine in the tail-flick test when it is administered by intracerebroventricular (icv) injection.[21,22] This peptide also produces antinociceptive effects comparable to morphine after systemic injection and has been shown to produce less dependence than morphine on chronic use.[23,24] Several explanations have been proposed for biphalin's high potency. Most of these focused on the presence of 2 pharmacophores in one molecule and on the possible synergistic interactions between the μ and δ receptors. Although a definitive explanation for the extraordinary potency of biphalin is still not available, it has been suggested that its high agonist activity at both μ and δ receptor may be a contributing factor.[25] Several biphalin analogs have been synthesized to understand the structural elements responsible for its high activity and to identify ligands with enhanced antinociceptive activity, blood brain barrier (BBB) penetration, and stability toward enkephalinases. Simplified fragment analogs of biphalin such as Tyr-D-Ala-Gly-Phe-NHNH←Phe and analogs with nonhydrazine linkers such the piperazine **1** (Fig. 23.1) also display μ and δ bioactivity comparable to biphalin. Two cyclic biphalin analogs, **2** and **3**, have recently been synthesized through replacing

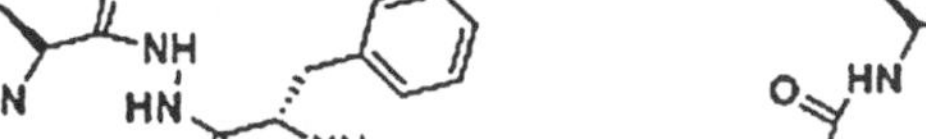

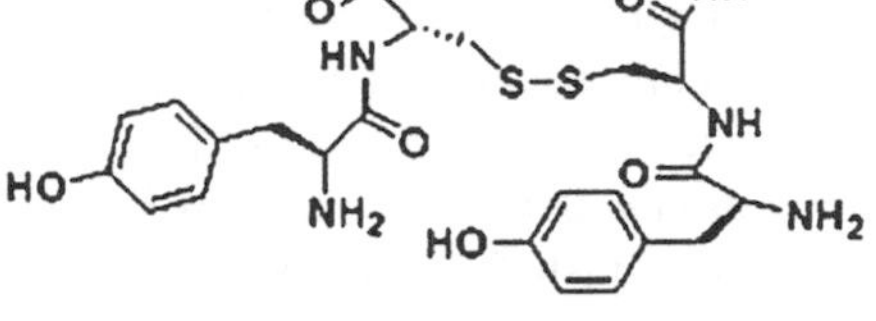

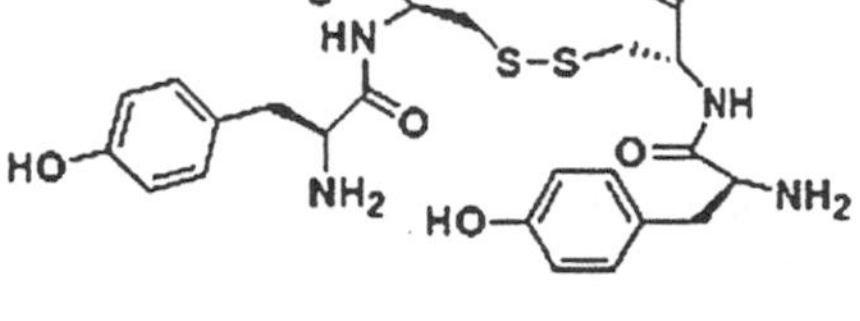

Fig. 23.1 Chemical Structures of Compounds 1-3.

the D-alanine residues in the 2,2′ positions of biphalin with L- and D-cysteine and formation of intramolecular disulfide bond between the cysteine thiol groups. While the cyclic peptide **2** containing L-cysteine residues displayed reduced potencies, the cyclic peptide **3** containing the D-cysteine residues displayed potencies similar to that of biphalin in binding and functional bioassays in mouse vas deferens (MVD) and guinea pig ileum (GPI) smooth muscle preparations. In agonist efficacy determinations using [^{35}S]GTPγS binding in cells expressing human δ opioid receptor and rat μ opioid receptor, compound **3** displayed δ and μ receptor activation capacities (E_{max} at δ = 100%; E_{max} at μ = 47%) higher than the activation levels displayed by biphalin (E_{max} at δ = 27%; E_{max} at μ = 25%).[26]

Structural manipulations on peptides containing the Dmt-Tic (Dmt = 2′,6′-dimethyltyrosine, -Tic = tetrahydroisoquinoline-3-carboxylic acid) pharmacophore have produced compounds possessing varying intrinsic activities including those that display agonist activity at both μ and δ receptors.[27] The tripeptide amide, H-Dmt-Tic-Gly-NHPh was one such compound that displayed mixed μ/δ agonist activity. It was found to be nearly equipotent as an agonist at δ (pEC$_{50}$ = 8.52) and μ (pEC$_{50}$ = 8.59) receptors in functional assays in smooth muscles.[28] Endomorphin-2 (Tyr-Pro-Phe-NH$_2$) is a peptide possessing μ agonist activity coupled with weak δ agonist activity. The replacement of the Tyr residue in this peptide with Dmt residue yielded a compound (Dmt-Pro-Phe-NH$_2$) endowed with high agonist activity at both μ (IC$_{50}$ in GPI = 0.07 nM) and δ (IC$_{50}$ in MVD = 1.87 nM) sites owing to simultaneous increase in agonist potency at both the receptors.[29] Some of the C-terminal arylamide analogs such as Dmt-Pro-Phe-NH-1-naphthyl also displayed mixed μ/δ agonist activities.[30] Another Dmt containing peptide that has recently been shown to possess mixed μ/δ agonist activity is the tetrapeptide H-Dmt-D-Arg(NO$_2$)-Phe-Lys-(Z)-NH$_2$. This compound displayed potent agonist activity in the GPI (IC$_{50}$ = 0.509 nM) and MVD (IC$_{50}$ = 1.69 nM) bioassays.[31]

Nonpeptide ligands possessing μ and δ agonist activity

The therapeutic potential of nonpeptide ligands with dual agonist activity at μ and δ receptors has also attracted attention in recent years. Since the identification of nonpeptide agonist ligands such as BW373U86 (**4**) and SNC80 (**5**) (Fig. 23.2), a significant amount of research effort has been expended on the discovery and development of nonpeptide agonists of the δ receptors.[32,33] Some of the studies using a combination of these nonpeptide δ agonists with μ agonists gave evidence supporting potential clinical advantages of a compound with combined μ and δ receptor agonist activities.[34] In studies with rats, additive analgesic effects were observed when the μ agonist fentanyl was administered in combination with the δ agonist BW373U86. Moreover, the coadministration was shown to diminish fentanyl-induced muscle rigidity (straub tail) and attenuate BW373U86-mediated seizures. In other studies it has been found that prolonged coadministration of morphine and BW373U86 attenuated the development and expression of morphine-induced dependence and

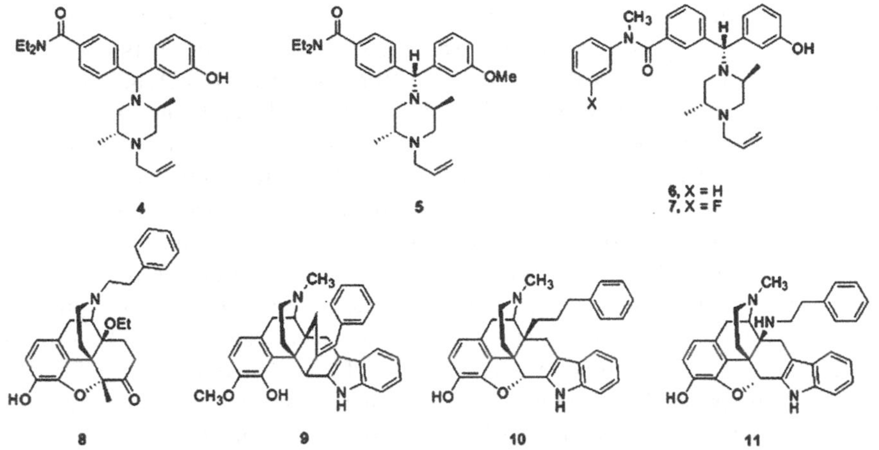

Fig. 23.2 Structures of δ agonists BN373U86(**4**), SNC 80(**5**), and nonpeptide ligands possessing mixed μ and δ agonist activity.

tolerance in rats.[35] Coadministration of BW373U86 with alfentanil led to significant attenuation of alfentanil-induced respiratory depression.[36] On the basis of these results, suggesting that compounds with mixed μ and δ receptor agonist activity may be useful in producing analgesic effects with fewer adverse effects, nonpeptide ligands possessing a mixed agonist profile of activity have been pursued. Structural changes involving the placement of the diethylamide function of BW373U86 at the meta position and conversion of the diethylamide to *N*-methylanilide yielded compound **6** possessing mixed δ/μ agonist activity. A series of aryl ring-substituted analogs of **6** also displayed mixed μ/δ agonist activity similar to that of the parent compound.[20] From this series of compounds, the *m*-fluorophenyl compound **7** (DPI-3290) has undergone extended evaluations. DPI-3290 displayed nonselective high-affinity binding to all 3 opioid receptors. In MVD it decreased electrically induced tension in a concentration-dependent manner with IC_{50} values of 1.0, 6.2, and 25 nM at δ, μ, and κ receptors, respectively. When administered intravenously to rats, it displayed potent dose-dependent antinociceptive activity with an ED_{50} value of 0.05 mg/kg in tail-pinch latency assay. The antinociceptive activity of this compound was partially blocked by the δ opioid receptor antagonist naltrindole and completely blocked by naloxone. It has been suggested that the antinociceptive actions of this compound result from its combined action at both δ and μ receptors.[37] In further studies it has been demonstrated that the respiratory depression profile of DPI-3290 was distinct from those observed with morphine and fentanyl, and DPI-3290 improved rather than added to the respiratory depression caused by alfentanil.[38]

Among epoxymorphinan ligands investigated by Schmidhammer and coworkers, several 14-alkoxy derivatives were found to display high affinity binding to all 3 opioid receptors with potent agonist activity in vitro and in vivo. Among these, the 14-ethoxymetopon derivative **8** possessing a phenylethyl group on N-17 retained high affinity binding at the μ (K_i = 0.16 nM) and δ (K_i = 3.14 nM) receptors with diminished binding affinity at the κ (K_i = 83.2 nM) receptor. This compound displayed agonist activity in the GPI (IC_{50} = 1.9 nM) and in the MVD (IC_{50} = 9.7 nM) bioassays. In antinociceptive evaluations, this compound was found to be 60-fold more potent than morphine in the hot-plate test. In its ability to induce constipation, however, its potency was equal to that of morphine.[39] Several morphinan compounds reported by Grundt and coworkers have displayed mixed μ/δ agonist profile of activity. For example, among a series of 3-hydroxy-4-methoxyindolomorphinans, compound **9** was found to display full or nearly full agonist activity at all 3 receptors in the [^{35}S]GTPγS binding assay using Chinese hamster ovary (CHO) cells expressing the individual human opioid receptors. Its agonist potency at μ (EC_{50} = 44.7 nM) and δ (EC_{50} = 42.6 nM) receptors was higher than at κ receptors (EC_{50} = 323 nM).[40] The indolomorphinan **10** and **11** were also found to possess mixed μ/δ agonist activity. The 14-phenethylamino compound **11** was a potent μ agonist (EC_{50} = 5.33 nM, % stimulation = 91%) and partial δ agonist (EC_{50} = 0.95 nM, % stimulation = 33%). It has been suggested that the high potency and low efficacy of this compound at the δ receptors could translate into δ antagonist activity in vivo and might therefore display properties of a μ agonist/δ antagonist in vivo.[41]

Mixed μ Agonists/δ Antagonists

A large body of evidence indicates that δ receptor antagonists suppress tolerance, physical dependence, and related side effects of μ agonists without affecting their analgesic activity. In studies using the δ receptor antagonist naltrindole, it was demonstrated that the δ antagonist greatly reduced the development of morphine tolerance and dependence in both the acute and chronic models without affecting the analgesic actions of morphine.[42,43] Continuous infusion of the δ selective antagonist TIPP[ψ] by the icv route in parallel with continuous administration of morphine by the subcutaneous (sc) route to rats attenuated the development of morphine tolerance and dependence to a large extent.[44] The development of morphine tolerance and dependence following chronic morphine administration was blocked by antisense oligonucleotides to the δ opioid receptors.[45-47] Furthermore, studies with δ receptor knockout mice have documented the critical role of δ receptors in the development of opioid tolerance. In contrast to wild-type mice, in which the analgesic response to a fixed morphine dose was lost within 5 days, the δ opioid knockout mice failed to develop tolerance following daily administration of 5 mg/kg of morphine, sc, for 8 days. After 10 days of chronic morphine dosing, cumulative dose-response curves revealed a significant 2.8-fold shift to the right of the morphine ED_{50} in wild-type mice, whereas the potency of morphine in the δ receptor knockout mice remained unchanged following chronic morphine administration.[48] Recently, compelling evidence for the involvement of δ opioid receptors in the development of morphine-induced tolerance has been obtained through studies using knock-in mice in which the native μ receptors were replaced by mutant μ receptors (S196A), which confers μ agonism to the antagonist ligand naltrexone. In these animals, an analgesic response was observed with acute administration of naltrexone, and chronic administration of naltrexone did not result in tolerance to naltrexone itself or to morphine. This lack of tolerance in these animals was attributed to concurrent blockade of δ opioid receptors with activation of μ receptors. Further studies using wild-type and knock-in mice revealed that inhibition of δ opioid receptor must occur at the time of μ activation to prevent tolerance development. Tolerance development could therefore be prevented by δ receptor blockade but cannot be reversed once it has occurred.[49] These observations clearly indicate that δ opioid receptors play a major role in the development of morphine tolerance and dependence and provide a rationale for the development of opioid ligands that act as an agonist at the μ receptor and as an antagonist at the δ receptor. Such a mixed μ agonist/δ antagonist would be expected to be an analgesic with low propensity to produce analgesic tolerance and physical dependence and might be of benefit in the management of chronic pain. Moreover, studies indicating that the δ antagonist naltrindole reversed alfentanil-induced respiratory depression[50] and enhanced colonic propulsion[51] suggest that a mixed μ agonist/δ antagonist may be less prone to cause respiratory depression and gastrointestinal side effects.

Peptide ligands possessing mixed μ agonist/δ antagonist activity

The first peptide ligand with μ agonist/δ antagonist properties was reported by Schiller and coworkers.[52] Among the analogs of the moderately μ selective β-casomorphin-5, H-Tyr-c[D-Orn-Phe-D-Pro-Gly-], replacement of the Phe[3] residue by 2-naphthylalanine (2-Nal) gave the peptide H-Tyr-c[D-Orn-2-Nal-D-Pro-Gly-], which displayed high affinity for both μ and δ receptors. This compound was an agonist in GPI smooth muscle assay and a moderately potent antagonist against various δ agonists in the MVD assay.[52] Ligands with a more balanced μ agonist/δ antagonist profile of activity were discovered among analogs of the tetrapeptide amide H-Tyr-Tic-Phe-Phe-NH$_2$ (TIPP-NH$_2$). Substitution of Dmt for Tyr[1] in TIPP-NH$_2$ and reduction of the peptide bond between Tic[2] and Phe[3] led to a compound, H-Dmt-Ticψ[CH$_2$-NH]Phe-Phe-NH$_2$ (DIPP-NH$_2$[ψ]), which showed high μ agonist potency and very high δ antagonist activity in the GPI and MVD bioassays. When administered icv, DIPP-NH$_2$[ψ] produced a potent antinociceptive effect in the rat tail-flick test and produced less tolerance than morphine and no physical dependence on chronic administration at high dose levels, thus fulfilling to a large extent the expectations based on the mixed μ agonist/δ antagonist concept with regard to analgesic activity and development of tolerance and dependence.[53] Recently, chimeric peptides containing a μ agonist fragment and δ antagonist fragment have also been synthesized and evaluated. The chimeric peptide resulting from linking the μ agonist H-Dmt-D-Arg-Phe-Lys-NH$_2$ ([Dmt[1]]DALDA) and the δ antagonist H-Tyr-Ticψ[CH$_2$-NH]Cha-Phe-OH (TICP[ψ]) (Cha = cyclohexylalanine) tail-to-tail using H$_2$N-CH$_2$-CH$_2$-NH$_2$ as the linker has been shown to display the expected μ agonist/δ antagonist profile in the GPI and MVD bioassays. The δ antagonist and μ agonist potencies of this chimeric peptide, however, were lower than the potencies of DIPP-NH$_2$[ψ].[54]

Ligands possessing mixed μ agonist/δ antagonist profile have been found among several analogs containing the Dmt-Tic pharmacophore.[27] For example, the Dmt-Tic analog lacking the COOH function in the Tic moiety displayed relatively nonselective binding to the δ and μ receptors with high δ antagonism (pA2 = 7.41) and modest μ agonism (pEC$_{50}$ = 6.31) with an E_{max} of 52% in smooth muscle bioassays.[55] Among N- and C-modified Dmt-Tic analogs, the N,N-dimethylated adamantyl-amide, N,N-(Me$_2$)Dmt-Tic-NH-1-adamantane, was found to display high affinity binding to δ and μ receptors (K_i at δ = 0.16 nM, K_i at μ = 1.12 nM) with potent δ antagonist (pA$_2$ = 9.06 in MVD) and μ agonist (IC$_{50}$ = 16 nM in GPI) activities.[56] The benzylamide peptide, H-Dmt-Tic-Gly-NH-CH$_2$-Ph, was also found to be a potent μ agonist (pEC$_{50}$ = 8.57) and δ antagonist (pA2 = 9.25) in the smooth muscle assays.[28] The heteroaryl analog, H-Dmt-Tic-NH-CH$_2$-Bid (Bid = 1H-benzimidazole-2-yl) similarly displayed potent δ antagonist activity coupled with weak μ agonist activity.[57]

Nonpeptide ligands possessing mixed μ agonist/δ antagonist activity

In a series of naltrindole analogs possessing phenyl-, phenoxy-, and benzyloxy substituents that were synthesized and evaluated for potential selective binding at the putative δ receptor subtypes, one of the compounds, the 7'-phenoxynaltrindole (12, Fig. 23.3) was found to display potent δ antagonist activity with a K_e of 0.25 nM in the MVD and weak μ agonist activity with an IC$_{50}$ of 450 nM in the GPI.[58] The first nonpeptide ligand with a mixed δ antagonist/μ agonist profile that was examined in some detail came from another series of compounds possessing the pyridomorphinan framework. The naltrexone-derived 4-chlorophenyl substituted pyridomorphinan 13 (SoRI 9409), displayed potent δ antagonist (K_e = 0.66 nM in the MVD) and moderate μ agonist (IC$_{50}$ = 163 nM in the GPI) activities in the smooth muscle preparations. In antinociceptive evaluations, this compound displayed partial agonist activity in the warm-water tail-withdrawal assay and full agonist activity in the acetic acid writhing assay after icv or intraperitoneal (ip) injections. Studies in mice with selective antagonists characterized this compound as a partial μ agonist/δ antagonist. Significantly, in contrast to morphine, repeated icv injection of an A$_{90}$ dose of this compound did not produce any significant antinociceptive tolerance.[59,60] Paradoxically, however, when the profile of this compound was determined using [^{35}S]GTPγS binding assays, it failed to display μ agonist activity in guinea pig caudate membranes as well as in cloned cells expressing human μ opioid receptors.[61] In an effort to identify compounds with μ agonist/δ antagonist activity in vitro and in vivo, an expanded series of pyridomorphinans

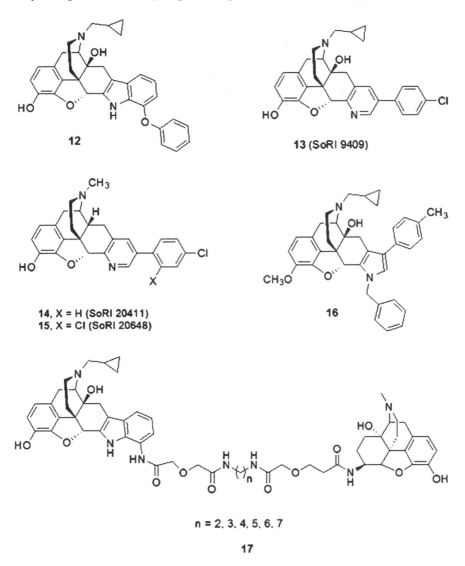

Fig. 23.3 Structures of nonpeptide ligands possessing mixed μ agonist/δ antagonist activity (**12–16**) and bivalent ligands possessing μ agonist and δ antagonist pharmacopores (**17**).

derived from naloxone, oxymorphone, and hydromorphone framework were synthesized and evaluated. These efforts led to the identification of hydromorphone-derived pyridomorphinans **14** (SoRI 20411) and **15** (SoRI 20648) as compounds possessing μ agonist/δ antagonist activity in both the [^{35}S]GTPγS binding and smooth muscle functional assays. In analgesic activity evaluations, **14** was found to be the more efficacious compound with an A_{50} potency value of 42.8 nmol in the warm-water tail-withdrawal assay in mice. The antinociceptive activity of this compound was completely blocked by the μ selective antagonist β-FNA, confirming that the analgesic activity of this compound was indeed mediated through the μ receptors. In conformity with the expectations, this mixed μ agonist/δ antagonist ligand did not produce any significant tolerance on repeated administration.[62] Compounds possessing δ antagonist and weak μ agonist activity have been found in other C-ring annulated morphinans such as the pyrrolomorphinans. Among a limited number of such pyrrolomorphinans synthesized and evaluated, it was found that compound **16** possessing a 4-methylphenyl substituent on the pyrrole ring displayed δ antagonist activity with a K_e of 14.1 nM and partial μ agonist activity with and EC_{50} of 1360 nM and E_{max} of 34% in $[^{35}S]GTP\gamma S$ binding assays in CHO cells expressing human δ and μ opioid receptors.[63]

Portoghese and coworkers have, for a long time, pursued the design of bivalent ligands to probe opioid receptor complexes.[64-67] The recent demonstration of the existence of μ-δ receptor hetero-oligomeric complexes has spurred further interest in the design of such bivalent ligands that could potentially interact with these receptor complexes. Of particular interest among such series of bivalent ligands are the bivalent ligands **17,** which possess a μ agonist and a δ antagonist pharmacophore. These bivalent ligands possess the oxymorphamine unit as the μ agonist pharmacophore and 7'-aminonaltrindole as the δ antagonist pharmacophore connected by spacers of length ranging from 19 to 25 Å. These compounds were evaluated in mice for acute antinociception in tail-flick test and were found to be more potent than morphine and fully efficacious. These were also evaluated for their ability to induce tolerance and dependence. Morphine and the bivalent ligand with the shortest spacer (**17,** n = 2) promoted the development of tolerance and dependence. The bivalent ligands with slightly longer spacers (**17,** n = 3 and n = 4) produced tolerance but not dependence. Ligands with the longest spacers (**17,** n = 5, 6, and 7) did not produce tolerance or physical dependence.[68,69]

Conclusions

The development of potent opioid analgesics devoid of the limiting side effects has been the goal of considerable research efforts. Accumulating evidence strongly support the existence of physical and functional interactions between the opioid μ and δ receptors. Recent studies using μ agonists along with δ agonists or δ antagonists have provided convincing evidence that there could be clear therapeutic advantages in combining the actions of μ agonists with that of a δ agonist or a δ antagonist. Recent successes in the identification of peptide and nonpeptide ligands possessing mixed μ agonist/δ agonist and μ agonist/δ antagonist profiles, and the encouraging results obtained in studies with these ligands is an exciting development in opioid drug discovery. It is likely that the pursuit of this new approach will lead to novel analgesics superior to those currently available for the treatment of pain.

Acknowledgments The author would like to acknowledge the financial support of the National Institute on Drug Abuse (Grant No. DA08883), National Institutes of Health, Bethesda, MD.

References

1. Aldrich JV, Vigil-Cruz SC. Narcotic analgesics. In: Abraham DJ, ed. *Burger's Medicinal Chemistry and Drug Discovery. Vol 6.* New York, NY: John Wiley & Sons; 2003:329-481.
2. Friderichs E. Opioids. In: Buschmann H, Christoph T, Friderichs E, Maul C, Sundermann B, eds. *Analgesics, From Chemistry and Pharmacology to Clinical Application.* Weinheim, Germany: Wiley-VCH; 2002:127-150.
3. Rapaka RS, Porreca F. Development of delta opioid peptides as nonaddicting analgesics. *Pharm Res.* 1991;8:1-8.
4. Traynor JR, Elliott J. δ-Opioid receptor subtypes and cross-talk with μ-receptors. *Trends Pharmacol Sci.* 1993;14:84-86.
5. Rothman RB, Holaday JW, Porreca F. Allosteric coupling among opioid receptors: evidence for an opioid receptor complex. In: Herz A, Akil H, Simon EJ, eds. *Handbook of Experimental Pharmacology: Opioids I. Vol 104.* Berlin, Germany: Springer-Verlag; 1993:217-237.
6. Jordan BA, Cvejic S, Devi LA. Opioids and their complicated receptor complexes. *Neuropsychopharmacology.* 2000;23:S5-S18.
7. Egan TM, North RA. Both mu and delta opiate receptors exist on the same neuron. *Science.* 1981;214:923-924.
8. Gomes I, Jordan BA, Gupta A, Trapaidze N, Nagy V, Devi LA. Heterodimerization of mu and delta opioid receptors: a role in opiate synergy. *J Neurosci.* 2000;20:RC110.
9. George SR, Fan T, Xie Z, et al. Oligomerization of mu- and delta-opioid receptors. Generation of novel functional properties. *J Biol Chem.* 2000;275:26128-26135.
10. Levac BA, O'Dowd BF, George SR. Oligomerization of opioid receptors: generation of novel signaling units. *Curr Opin Pharmacol.* 2002;2:76-81.
11. Fan T, Varghese G, Nguyen T, Tse R, O'Dowd BF, George SR. A role for the distal carboxyl tails in generating the novel pharmacology and G protein activation profile of mu and delta opioid receptor hetero-oligomers. *J Biol Chem.* 2005;280:38478-38488.
12. Kieffer BL. Opioids: first lessons from knockout mice. *Trends Pharmacol Sci.* 1999;20:19-26.
13. Vaught JL, Takemori AE. Differential effects of leucine and methionine enkephalin on morphine-induced analgesia, acute tolerance and dependence. *J Pharmacol Exp Ther.* 1979;208:86-90.
14. Horan P, Tallarida RJ, Haaseth RC, Matsunaga TO, Hruby VJ, Porreca F. Antinociceptive interactions of opioid delta receptor agonists with morphine in mice: supra- and sub-additivity. *Life Sci.* 1992;50:1535-1541.
15. He L, Lee NM. Delta opioid receptor enhancement of mu opioid receptor-induced antinociception in spinal cord. *J Pharmacol Exp Ther.* 1998;285:1181-1186.
16. Porreca F, Takemori AE, Sultana M, Portoghese PS, Bowen WD, Mosberg HI. Modulation of mu-mediated antinociception in the mouse involves opioid delta-2 receptors. *J Pharmacol Exp Ther.* 1992;263:147-152.
17. Martin NA, Prather PL. Interaction of co-expressed mu- and delta-opioid receptors in transfected rat pituitary GH(3) cells. *Mol Pharmacol.* 2001;59:774-783.
18. Cahill CM, Morinville A, Lee MC, Vincent JP, Collier B, Beaudet A. Prolonged morphine treatment targets delta opioid receptors to neuronal plasma membranes and enhances delta-mediated antinociception. *J Neurosci.* 2001;21:7598-7607.
19. Coop A, Rice KC. Role of delta-opioid receptors in biological processes. *Drug News Perspect.* 2000;13:481-487.
20. Bishop MJ, Garrido DM, Boswell GE, et al. 3-(alphaR)-alpha-((2S,5R)-4-allyl-2,5-dimethyl-1-piperazinyl)-3-hydroxyben zyl)-N-alkyl-N-arylbenzamides: potent, non-peptidic agonists of both the mu and delta opioid receptors. *J Med Chem.* 2003;46:623-633.

21. Lipkowski AW, Konecka AM, Sroczynska I. Double-enkephalins-synthesis, activity on guinea-pig ileum, and analgesic effect. *Peptides*. 1982;3:697-700.
22. Horan PJ, Mattia A, Bilsky EJ, et al. Antinociceptive profile of biphalin, a dimeric enkephalin analog. *J Pharmacol Exp Ther*. 1993;265:1446-1454.
23. Silbert BS, Lipkowski AW, Cepeda MS, Szyfelbein SK, Osgood PF, Carr DB. Analgesic activity of a novel bivalent opioid peptide compared to morphine via different routes of administration. *Agents Actions*. 1991;33:382-387.
24. Yamazaki M, Suzuki T, Narita M, Lipkowski AW. The opioid peptide analogue biphalin induces less physical dependence than morphine. *Life Sci*. 2001;69:1023-1028.
25. Abbruscato TJ, Thomas SA, Hruby VJ, Davis TP. Brain and spinal cord distribution of biphalin: correlation with opioid receptor density and mechanism of CNS entry. *J Neurochem*. 1997;69:1236-1245.
26. Mollica A, Davis P, Ma SW, Porreca F, Lai J, Hruby VJ. Synthesis and biological activity of the first cyclic biphalin analogues. *Bioorg Med Chem Lett*. 2006;16:367-372.
27. Bryant SD, Jinsmaa Y, Salvadori S, Okada Y, Lazarus LH. Dmt and opioid peptides: a potent alliance. *Biopolymers*. 2003;71:86-102.
28. Balboni G, Guerrini R, Salvadori S, et al. Evaluation of the Dmt-Tic pharmacophore: conversion of a potent delta-opioid receptor antagonist into a potent delta agonist and ligands with mixed properties. *J Med Chem*. 2002;45:713-720.
29. Okada Y, Fujita Y, Motoyama T, et al. Structural studies of [2′,6′-dimethyl-L-tyrosine1] endomorphin-2 analogues: enhanced activity and cis orientation of the Dmt-Pro amide bond. *Bioorg Med Chem*. 2003;11:1983-1994.
30. Fujita Y, Tsuda Y, Li T, et al. Development of potent bifunctional endomorphin-2 analogues with mixed mu-/delta-opioid agonist and delta-opioid antagonist properties. *J Med Chem*. 2004;47:3591-3599.
31. Balboni G, Cocco MT, Salvadori S, et al. From the potent and selective mu opioid receptor agonist H-Dmt-D-Arg-Phe-Lys-NH(2) to the potent delta antagonist H-Dmt-Tic-Phe-Lys(Z)-OH. *J Med Chem*. 2005;48:5608-5611.
32. Calderon SN, Coop A. SNC 80 and related delta opioid agonists. *Curr Pharm Des*. 2004;10:733-742.
33. Eguchi M. Recent advances in selective opioid receptor agonists and antagonists. *Med Res Rev*. 2004;24:182-212.
34. O'Neill SJ, Collins MA, Pettit HO, McNutt RW, Chang KJ. Antagonistic modulation between the delta opioid agonist BW373U86 and the mu opioid agonist fentanyl in mice. *J Pharmacol Exp Ther*. 1997;282:271-277.
35. Lee PH, McNutt RW, Chang KJ. A nonpeptidic delta opioid receptor agonist, BW373U86, attenuates the development and expression of morphine abstinence precipitated by naloxone in rat. *J Pharmacol Exp Ther*. 1993;267:883-887.
36. Su YF, McNutt RW, Chang KJ. Delta-opioid ligands reverse alfentanil-induced respiratory depression but not antinociception. *J Pharmacol Exp Ther*. 1998;287:815-823.
37. Gengo PJ, Pettit HO, O'Neill SJ, et al. DPI-3290 [(+)-3-((alpha-R)-alpha-((2S,5R)-4-allyl-2,5-dimethyl-1-piperazinyl)-3-hydroxybenzyl)-N-(3-fluorophenyl)-N-methylbenzamide]. I. A mixed opioid agonist with potent antinociceptive activity. *J Pharmacol Exp Ther*. 2003;307:1221-1226.
38. Gengo PJ, Pettit HO, O'Neill SJ, Su YF, McNutt R, Chang KJ. DPI-3290 [(+)-3-((alpha-R)-alpha-((2S,5R)-4-Allyl-2,5-dimethyl-1-piperazinyl)-3-hydroxybenzyl)-N-(3-fluorophenyl)-N-methylbenzamide]. II. A mixed opioid agonist with potent antinociceptive activity and limited effects on respiratory function. *J Pharmacol Exp Ther*. 2003;307:1227-1233.
39. Lattanzi R, Spetea M, Schullner F, et al. Synthesis and biological evaluation of 14-alkoxymorphinans. 22.(1) Influence of the 14-alkoxy group and the substitution in position 5 in 14-alkoxymorphinan-6-ones on in vitro and in vivo activities. *J Med Chem*. 2005;48:3372-3378.
40. Grundt P, Martinez-Bermejo F, Lewis JW, Husbands SM. Opioid binding and in vitro profiles of a series of 4-hydroxy-3-methoxyindolomorphinans. Transformation of a delta-selective

ligand into a high affinity kappa-selective ligand by introduction of a 5,14-substituted bridge. *J Med Chem.* 2003;46:3174-3177.

41. Grundt P, Jales AR, Traynor JR, Lewis JW, Husbands SM. 14-amino, 14-alkylamino, and 14-acylamino analogs of oxymorphindole. Differential effects on opioid receptor binding and functional profiles. *J Med Chem.* 2003;46:1563-1566.

42. Abdelhamid EE, Sultana M, Portoghese PS, Takemori AE. Selective blockage of delta opioid receptors prevents the development of morphine tolerance and dependence in mice. *J Pharmacol Exp Ther.* 1991;258:299-303.

43. Hepburn MJ, Little PJ, Gingras J, Kuhn CM. Differential effects of naltrindole on morphine-induced tolerance and physical dependence in rats. *J Pharmacol Exp Ther.* 1997;281: 1350-1356.

44. Fundytus ME, Schiller PW, Shapiro M, Weltrowska G, Coderre TJ. Attenuation of morphine tolerance and dependence with the highly selective delta-opioid receptor antagonist TIPP[psi]. *Eur J Pharmacol.* 1995;286:105-108.

45. Kest B, Lee CE, McLemore GL, Inturrisi CE. An antisense oligodeoxynucleotide to the delta opioid receptor (DOR-1) inhibits morphine tolerance and acute dependence in mice. *Brain Res Bull.* 1996;39:185-188.

46. Suzuki T, Ikeda H, Tsuji M, Misawa M, Narita M, Tseng LF. Antisense oligodeoxynucleotide to delta opioid receptors attenuates morphine dependence in mice. *Life Sci.* 1997;61: PL165-PL170.

47. Sanchez-Blazquez P, Garcia-Espana A, Garzon J. Antisense oligodeoxynucleotides to opioid mu and delta receptors reduced morphine dependence in mice: role of delta-2 opioid receptors. *J Pharmacol Exp Ther.* 1997;280:1423-1431.

48. Zhu Y, King MA, Schuller AG, et al. Retention of supraspinal delta-like analgesia and loss of morphine tolerance in delta opioid receptor knockout mice. *Neuron.* 1999;24:243-252.

49. Roy S, Guo X, Kelschenbach J, Liu Y, Loh HH. In vivo activation of a mutant mu-opioid receptor by naltrexone produces a potent analgesic effect but no tolerance: role of mu-receptor activation and delta-receptor blockade in morphine tolerance. *J Neurosci.* 2005;25:3229-3233.

50. Freye E, Latasch L, Portoghese PS. The delta receptor is involved in sufentanil-induced respiratory depression-opioid subreceptors mediate different effects. *Eur J Anaesthesiol.* 1992;9:457-462.

51. Foxx-Orenstein AE, Jin JG, Grider JR. 5-HT4 receptor agonists and delta-opioid receptor antagonists act synergistically to stimulate colonic propulsion. *Am J Physiol.* 1998;275:G979-G983.

52. Schmidt R, Vogel D, Mrestani-Klaus C, et al. Cyclic beta-casomorphin analogues with mixed mu agonist/delta antagonist properties: synthesis, pharmacological characterization, and conformational aspects. *J Med Chem.* 1994;37:1136-1144.

53. Schiller PW, Fundytus ME, Merovitz L, et al. The opioid mu agonist/delta antagonist DIPP-NH(2)[Psi] produces a potent analgesic effect, no physical dependence, and less tolerance than morphine in rats. *J Med Chem.* 1999;42:3520-3526.

54. Weltrowska G, Lemieux C, Chung NN, Schiller PW. A chimeric opioid peptide with mixed mu agonist/delta antagonist properties. *J Pept Res.* 2004;63:63-68.

55. Santagada V, Balboni G, Caliendo G, et al. Assessment of substitution in the second pharmacophore of Dmt-Tic analogues. *Bioorg Med Chem Lett.* 2000;10:2745-2748.

56. Salvadori S, Guerrini R, Balboni G, et al. Further studies on the Dmt-Tic pharmacophore: hydrophobic substituents at the C-terminus endow delta antagonists to manifest mu agonism or mu antagonism. *J Med Chem.* 1999;42:5010-5019.

57. Balboni G, Salvadori S, Guerrini R, et al. Potent delta-opioid receptor agonists containing the Dmt-Tic pharmacophore. *J Med Chem.* 2002;45:5556-5563.

58. Ananthan S, Johnson CA, Carter RL, et al. Synthesis, opioid receptor binding, and bioassay of naltrindole analogues substituted in the indolic benzene moiety. *J Med Chem.* 1998;41: 2872-2881.

59. Ananthan S, 3rd, Kezar HS, 3rd, Carter RL, et al. Synthesis, opioid receptor binding, and biological activities of naltrexone-derived pyrido- and pyrimidomorphinans. *J Med Chem.* 1999;42:3527-3538.

60. Wells JL, Bartlett JL, Ananthan S, Bilsky EJ. In vivo pharmacological characterization of SoRI 9409, a nonpeptidic opioid mu-agonist/delta-antagonist that produces limited antinociceptive tolerance and attenuates morphine physical dependence. *J Pharmacol Exp Ther.* 2001;297:597-605.

61. Xu H, Lu YF, Rice KC, Ananthan S, Rothman RB. SoRI 9409, a nonpeptide opioid mu receptor agonist/delta receptor antagonist, fails to stimulate [35S]-GTP-gamma-S binding at cloned opioid receptors. *Brain Res Bull.* 2001;55:507-511.

62. Ananthan S, Khare NK, Saini SK, et al. Identification of opioid ligands possessing mixed mu agonist/delta antagonist activity among pyridomorphinans derived from naloxone, oxymorphone, and hydromorphone. *J Med Chem.* 2004;47:1400-1412.

63. Srivastava SK, Husbands SM, Aceto MD, Miller CN, Traynor JR, Lewis JW. 4'-Arylpyrrolomorphinans: effect of a pyrrolo-N-benzyl substituent in enhancing delta-opioid antagonist activity. *J Med Chem.* 2002;45:537-540.

64. Portoghese PS. Bivalent ligands and the message-address concept in the design of selective opioid receptor antagonists. *Trends Pharmacol Sci.* 1989;10:230-235.

65. Portoghese PS, Edward E. Smissman-Bristol-Myers Squibb Award Address. The role of concepts in structure-activity relationship studies of opioid ligands. *J Med Chem.* 1992;35:1927-1937.

66. Portoghese PS. From models to molecules: opioid receptor dimers, bivalent ligands, and selective opioid receptor probes. *J Med Chem.* 2001;44:2259-2269.

67. Daniels DJ, Kulkarni A, Xie Z, Bhushan RG, Portoghese PS. A bivalent ligand (KDAN-18) containing delta-antagonist and kappa-agonist pharmacophores bridges delta2 and kappa1 opioid receptor phenotypes. *J Med Chem.* 2005;48:1713-1716.

68. Lenard NR, Moore JB, Daniels DJ, Portoghese PS, Roerig SC. Bivalent Ligands With Mu Agonist and Delta Antagonist Pharmacophores: Spacer Length Dependence of Tolerance and Physical Dependence Suggests Associated Mu and Delta Receptors [abstract]. *Neuroscience* [Society for Neuroscience, Abstract Viewer and Itinerary Planner]. 2004: Abstract 406.10.

69. Daniels DJ, Lenard NR, Etienne CL, et al. Opioid-induced tolerance and dependence in mice is modulated by the distance between pharmacopores in a bivalent ligand series. *Proc Natl Acad Sci USA.* 2005;102:19208-19213.

Chapter 24
Small-Molecule Agonists and Antagonists of the Opioid Receptor-Like Receptor (ORL1, NOP): Ligand-Based Analysis of Structural Factors Influencing Intrinsic Activity at NOP

Nurulain Zaveri,[1] Faming Jiang,[1] Cris Olsen,[1] Willma Polgar,[1] and Lawrence Toll[1]

Abstract The recently discovered fourth member of the opioid receptor family, the nociceptin receptor (NOP) and its endogenous ligand, the heptadecapeptide nociceptin, are involved in several central nervous system pathways, such as nociception, reward, tolerance, and feeding. The discovery of small-molecule ligands for NOP is being actively pursued for several therapeutic applications. This review presents a brief overview of the several recently reported NOP ligands, classified as NOP agonists and antagonists, with an emphasis on the analysis of the structural features that may be important for modulating the agonist/antagonist profile (intrinsic activity) of these ligands. Structure-activity relationships in our own series of dihydroindolinone-based NOP ligands and those of the various reported ligands indicate that the lipophilic substituent on the common basic nitrogen present in all NOP ligands plays a role in determining the agonist/antagonist profile of the NOP ligand. This analysis provides a basis for the rational drug design of NOP ligands of desired intrinsic activity and provides a framework for developing pharmacophore models for high affinity binding and intrinsic activity at the NOP receptor. Since NOP agonists and antagonists both have therapeutic value, rational approaches for obtaining both within a high-affinity binding class of compounds are very useful for designing potent and selective NOP ligands with the desired profile of intrinsic efficacy.

Keywords nociceptin, opioid receptor-like, ORL1, NOP, agonist, antagonist, intrinsic activity

Introduction

Since its discovery in 1994, the opioid receptor-like receptor (ORL1, NOP), the fourth member of the opioid receptor family, has been shown to be widely distributed in the brain and periphery.[1,2] The endogenous ligand for this receptor is a 17–amino acid peptide, nociceptin or orphanin FQ (N/OFQ). The functional roles of the

[1] Biosciences Division, SRI International, Menlo Park, CA 94025

Corresponding Author: Nurulain Zaveri, Drug Discovery Program Director, Biosciences Division, SRI International, 333 Ravenswood Ave, Menlo Park, CA 94025. Tel: 650-859-6041; Fax: 650-859-3153; E-mail: nurulain.zaveri@sri.com

R.S. Rapaka and W. Sadée (eds.), *Drug Addiction.*
© American Association of Pharmaceutical Scientists 2008

NOP-N/OFQ system are still under active investigation, and the system's involvement in pain, tolerance and withdrawal, and other pathways is still not completely understood. It is clear, though, that this new member of the opioid receptor family plays a significant role in pathways of pain, anxiety, learning and memory, reward and tolerance, feeding, renal systems and circadian rhythms (see Mogil and Pasternak and Calo et al for excellent reviews on the pharmacology of the NOP-N/OFQ system).[3,4]

Despite significant sequence homology of this G-protein-coupled receptor with the classical opioid receptors, opioids do not bind the NOP receptor. However, several known small-molecule central nervous system (CNS)–active drugs show appreciable affinity for the NOP receptor. Neuroleptics such as pimozide and spiroxatrine and clinically used opiates such as buprenorphine have significant affinity for NOP,[5] which perhaps plays a role in the overall systemic effects of these drugs. Indeed, Lutfy et al[6] recently showed that the ceiling effect of the antinociceptive action of the mu partial agonist buprenorphine is in fact due to its activation of the ORL1 receptor. Determining structural features of small-molecule drugs that may lead to recognition at the NOP receptor is important for understanding the profiles of the systemic action of CNS drugs. On the other hand, small-molecule nonpeptide ligands for the NOP receptor are valuable as tools and broaden the armamentarium of CNS therapeutics that can be employed to treat several neurological disorders.

Several small-molecule NOP ligands have now been reported both in public and patent literature.[7,8] NOP agonists are being pursued as potential therapeutics for anxiety, analgesia, cough, and drug abuse. NOP antagonists have been considered for their utility in treating obesity and learning deficits.

Although many different classes of NOP ligands have been reported, no pharmacophore models have been defined for NOP binding, selectivity compared with opioid receptors, or intrinsic activity (agonist vs antagonist activity) at the receptor. In this review, we describe a preliminary 2-D pharmacophore that can be used as a starting point for understanding the structural parameters that play a role in determining the binding and selectivity as well as the intrinsic activity of small-molecule NOP ligands. This analysis is based on the structure-activity relationships (SAR) observed in our own series of NOP ligands[9] and is confirmed by activities reported for other classes of NOP ligands. Our analysis provides a basis for the rational drug design of NOP ligands and will be particularly useful for designing NOP agonists or antagonists as desired.

Factors that need to be considered while designing high-affinity NOP ligands are (1) binding affinity for the NOP receptor, (2) selectivity for NOP vs opioid and other receptors, and (3) intrinsic activity (agonist/antagonist activity). From the analysis presented below for NOP ligands, it appears that the first 2 factors, binding affinity and selectivity, can usually be modulated together, whereas intrinsic activity can be modulated through a distinct set of structural features.

With a few notable exceptions, almost all reported NOP ligands, agonists as well as antagonists, exhibit similar structural features that fall into a 2-D pharmacophoric pattern. Most ligands have a central alicyclic core ring containing the protonatable

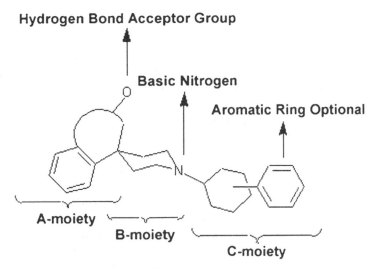

Fig. 24.1 Preliminary 2-D pharmacophore depicting the 3 common elements present in most NOP ligands reported thus far.

basic nitrogen, a heterocyclic moiety distal to the protonatable nitrogen by at least 3 carbons, and a lipophilic moiety on the basic nitrogen. This pharmacophore is shown in Fig. 24.1. For the ease of discussion, we name the 3 pharmacophoric elements: (1) the heterocyclic A moiety, (2) the basic nitrogen-containing B moiety, and (3) the lipophilic C moiety on the basic nitrogen. From the results of our own studies and observations with other reported classes, we propose the hypothesis that the heterocyclic A portion is an important determinant of binding affinity and selectivity vs the opioid receptors, whereas the lipophilic C moiety plays a role in the intrinsic activity of the ligand at the receptor. From our analysis presented below, we propose that within the same class of NOP ligands, classified according to the heterocyclic A scaffold, it is possible to modulate the intrinsic activity of the ligand, to generate agonists and antagonists as desired, by the appropriate choice of the lipophilic C moiety. This analysis provides a rational approach to the design of potent and selective NOP agonists and antagonists, which can be further exploited for their therapeutic potential. Needless to say, optimization of all 3 pharmacophoric features will lead to an increase in binding affinity and selectivity, but only modifications in the C moiety appear to predict agonist-antagonist activity. This is similar to the effect of the nitrogen substituent in opiate ligands, where a change from N-Me in the agonists morphine and oxymorphone, to an N-allyl or N-cyclopropylmethyl, results in switching intrinsic activity to that of the antagonists nalorphine and naloxone, respectively.

NOP Receptor Agonists

The nonpeptide NOP agonist ligand that has been studied most extensively is the triazaspirodecanone **Ro 64–6198**, reported by the Roche group (Fig. 24.2).[10] The Roche series of spiropiperidines were obtained by optimization of a high-throughput screening lead, **1**, containing the triazaspirodecanone (comprising the A and B moiety of the proposed pharmacophore) and a substituted 2-tetralinyl moiety as the lipophilic C moiety directly linked to the basic piperidine nitrogen.[11] This lead compound, which lacked selectivity over the other opioid receptors and was an agonist at NOP, was optimized to improve selectivity, mainly through modifications of the lipophilic C moiety of the piperidine nitrogen. Most of the C moieties examined contained some aromatic character, eg, **2**, **3**, **Ro 65–6570**, and **Ro 64–6198** (Fig. 24.2). Modest 10-fold selectivity was obtained with **3** and **Ro 65–6570** (Table 24.1), and notably, all these compounds were still agonists in functional assays at NOP. The Roche group also examined alicyclic C moieties at the piperidine nitrogen on the same triazaspirodecanone A-moiety scaffold, to improve selectivity.[12] Substituents such as cyclooctyl (**4**), cyclononyl (**5**), and 4-isopropylcyclohexyl (**6**)

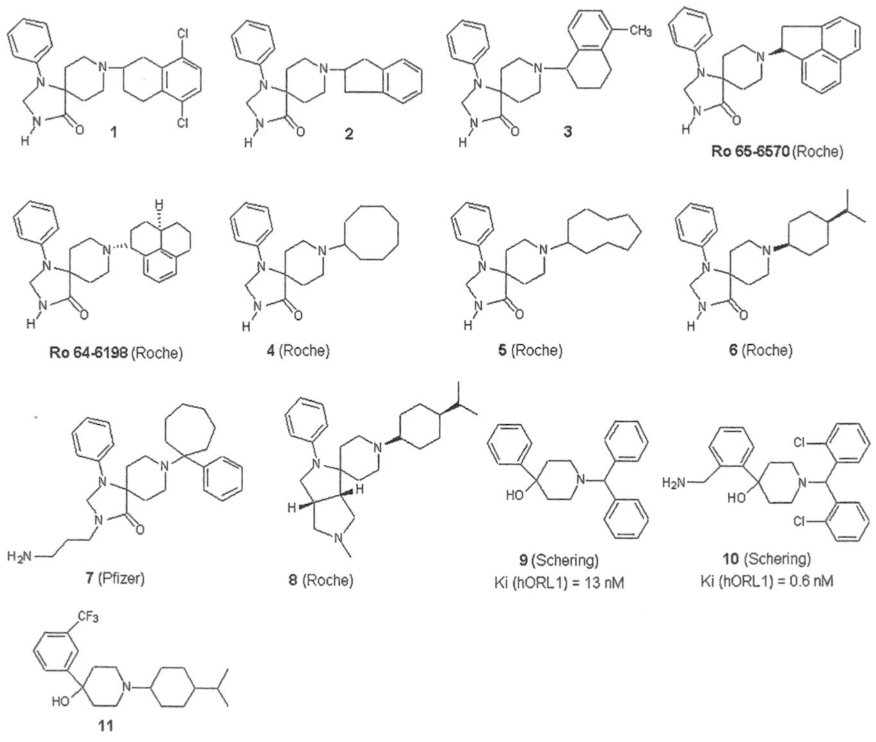

Fig. 24.2 Structures of reported NOP agonists. NOP, nociceptin.

Table 24.1 Binding Affinities of Reported NOP Ligands From Fig. 24.2 at the NOP and Opioid Receptors*

| | Receptor Binding | | | | Functional Activity | |
| | K_i (nM) | | | | GTPγS | |
	ORL	μ	κ	δ	EC_{50} (nM)	% Stim
1	5.6	7.2	44.2	680	1500	100
2	2.5	26.0	161	710		
3	1.4	31.7	44	460		
Ro 65–6570	0.52	5.9	26	250	40	100
Ro 64–6198	0.39	46	89	1380	38	100
4	1.9	13	9.1	>200		
5	0.24	3.2	3.9	>200		
6	0.079	3.2	26	242		
7	NA					
8	0.49	537	309	2138		100
9	13					
10	0.6					
11	12	36	4153	5674		

*The binding affinity values in the above table have been taken from the publications describing the respective ligands and are for discussion only. These represent values from different experiments conducted in different laboratories and, as such, cannot to be used to compare ligands reported by different research groups.

afforded a 10-fold increase in binding affinity and a 40-fold selectivity vs mu opioid receptors (Table 24.1). All these ligands were agonists at NOP. Pfizer also patented a series of triazaspirodecanones exemplified by **7**, as agonists at the NOP receptor.[13]

In an effort to further improve selectivity, the Roche group reported a series of hexahydropyrrolopyrroles as highly selective NOP agonists.[14] The most potent and selective compound resulting from this series was **8**, containing the cis-4-isopropyl-cyclohexyl as the lipophilic C moiety. This compound had a binding affinity K_i of 0.49 nM, and more important, was over 1000-fold more selective at NOP than the opioid receptors. It is worth noting that the same lipophilic C substituent, cis-4-isopropylcyclohexyl, on the triazaspirodecanone A moiety as in **6** afforded selectivities of only 10-fold (Fig. 24.1). This indicates that the A moiety plays a greater role in the selectivity for NOP vs the other opioid receptors. This trend is further confirmed by our own results with the indolinone series of NOP ligands (see below).

Schering reported a series of phenylpiperidines (eg, **9** and **10**) as NOP agonists in a broad patent.[15] The phenylpiperidine class of NOP ligands represents a deviation from the usual A-moiety pharmacophore, in which most A moieties of reported ligands are heterocyclic rings. Nevertheless, the phenylpiperidines do possess the aromatic ring that is present in all A moieties. Notable, however, are the C moieties reported for the Schering agonists **9** and **10**. These agonists contain the bulky diphenylmethane as the C moiety. Although the selectivities of these compounds vs the opioid receptors were not reported, these C moieties were a departure from the usual alicyclic or cycloaromatic C moieties in the Roche and Pfizer agonists. Recently, another research group from Purdue Pharma also reported a series of phenylpiperidines, among which compound **11**, containing the 4-isopropylcyclohexyl ring as the C moiety directly linked to the basic piperidine nitrogen, was the most potent agonist but with only 3-fold selectivity vs mu receptors.[16] This further confirms the trend that the A moiety plays a significant role in the binding affinity and selectivity vs the opioid receptors.

Analysis of the C moieties of all the agonists from different classes of NOP ligands indicates that the C portion (Fig. 24.1) of piperidine-based agonists can either contain significant aromatic character, as in **Ro 65–6570**, **Ro 64–6198**, and phenylpiperidines **9/10**, or contain lipophilic alicyclic rings like the cyclononyl and isopropylcyclohexyl. Assuming that these ligands bind at the same site on the NOP receptor, with the protonated basic piperidine nitrogen as an anchoring point, the binding site must be able to accommodate both these types of C moieties, such that binding of these ligands will result in transduction of a signaling event, leading to agonist action (intrinsic activity).

NOP Receptor Antagonists

The first nonpeptide NOP antagonist to be reported was **J-113397**, belonging to a class of benzimidazolinones, patented by Banyu Pharmaceutical Co.[17,18] **J-113397** was obtained through optimization of a high-throughput screening lead, **12** (Fig. 24.3), which contained an N-benzyl C moiety and was a nonselective NOP agonist. Selectivity

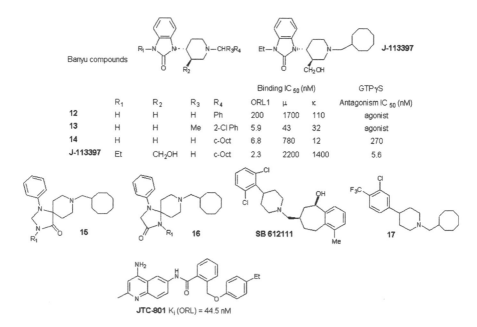

Fig. 24.3 Structures of reported NOP antagonists. NOP, nociceptin.

increased 30-fold when an α-methyl substituent was introduced onto the N-benzyl group and a 2-chloro substituent was added on the pendant phenyl ring as in **13** (Fig. 24.3), likely because of restrictive conformational freedom of the substituted N-benzyl group. However, this compound was still an agonist at NOP. When the piperidine nitrogen substituent (C moiety) was changed to cyclooctylmethyl, the resulting compound **14** retained the affinity and selectivity but was now an antagonist at NOP. Further optimization of binding affinity was achieved through modifications of the benzimidazolinone A moiety and the piperidine ring, resulting in the potent antagonist **J-113397**.

Another series of antagonists reported by Banyu were the isomeric triazaspirodecanones **15** and **16**, identical in the A and B moieties to the Roche and Pfizer agonist ligands **2** to **7** but containing lipophilic C moieties attached to the piperidine nitrogen by a 1-carbon linker, similar to the cyclooctylmethyl substituent of **J-113397**.[19] This indicates that with the same heterocyclic A moiety, the triazaspirodecanone, it was possible to obtain antagonists by a subtle 1-carbon homologation of the lipophilic C moiety on the piperidine nitrogen. This trend was also observed in our series of indolinones, as described in detail below.

Among the phenylpiperidine class of compounds, **SB-612111** (Fig. 24.3) was recently reported as an NOP antagonist that had a 174-fold selectivity over the mu opioid receptor.[20] It contains a cycloaromatic C moiety attached to the piperidine nitrogen by a 1-carbon linker, a feature that is commonly noted with NOP antagonists. Phenylpiperidines such as **17** reported by Purdue Pharma,[16] containing the same cyclooctylmethyl C moiety as **J-113397**, were also NOP antagonists. These observations and the results from our SAR on the indolinone series of NOP ligands, described below, indicate that the cyclooctylmethyl group could be a preferred C moiety for obtaining NOP antagonists in any heterocyclic class of NOP ligands.

One notable exception to the preliminary pharmacophore described in Fig. 24.1 is the NOP antagonist, JTC-801, a 4-aminoquinoline, reported by Japan Tobacco Inc.[21] Furthermore, JTC-801 is the only small-molecule NOP antagonist that has demonstrated analgesic activity in vivo, in models of both acute and neuropathic pain, not reversed by naloxone.[22-24] The flat planar structure of JTC-801 is clearly distinct from that of almost all reported NOP ligands. It is likely that JTC-801 binds to the NOP receptor at a site partially overlapping the active site where most piperidine-based ligands anchor, via the electrostatic interaction of the protonated basic nitrogen of the ligand, and the Asp-130 at the active site.[25] Studies with photoaffinity ligands could confirm these observations.

As discussed above, although several extensive series of NOP ligands have been reported, only agonists or antagonists have been reported within the same structural class. The Banyu series of benzimidazolinones that resulted in the antagonist **J-113397** did contain agonists such as **13** (Fig. 24.3); however, no rational design of NOP agonists or antagonists within the same structural class had been reported until we reported our series of indolinone-based NOP ligands, discussing the modulation of agonist/antagonist activity by subtle changes in the C moiety in this structural class.[9] Our results, discussed below, provide new insights into the rational design of selective ligands for the NOP receptor and shed light on the pharmacophoric requirements for intrinsic activity at the receptor.

NOP Receptor Agonists and Antagonists From the Dihydroindol-2-one Structural Class Give Insights Into the Modulation of Intrinsic Activity by Structural Manipulation of the C Moiety

We recently reported a new structural class of NOP ligands based on the dihydroindol-2-one A moiety.[9] This series was particularly interesting because, unlike with previously reported classes of NOP ligands, modifications of the piperidine N-substituent (C moiety) afforded potent agonists as well as antagonists. Our SAR studies show that there are specific structural characteristics of the C moiety (size, shape, lipophilic volume, distance from the protonated nitrogen) that are responsible for transduction of intrinsic activity at the NOP receptor. This information can be used for designing potent agonists or antagonists of any class of NOP ligands containing appropriately selective A moieties.

We obtained this indolinone class of NOP ligands through a random screening hit, **18**, containing the N-benzyl group as the C moiety (Table 24.2). Replacement of the C moiety with a cyclooctylmethyl group, as in **19** (Table 24.2), provided a significant increase in binding affinity at NOP and reduced affinity at the opioid receptors, resulting in a ligand that was 38-fold more selective than κ receptors. In GTPγS assays for functional activity, **19** was found to be an antagonist ($K_e = 15\,nM$). We continued our structural modifications of the C moiety and introduced other alicyclic lipophilic groups based on our results with the cyclooctylmethyl group. When the C moiety was a cyclooctyl group, compound **20**, it improved binding affinity and selectivity for the receptor, but importantly, converted the compound into an agonist, with an EC_{50} of $20\,nM$. This subtle structural change in the C moiety, therefore, changed the intrinsic activity of the molecule without affecting the binding affinity. Our results with different C moieties showed several interesting trends. C moieties such as the decahydronaphthyl (**21**, **22**) and 4-isopropylcyclohexyl (**23**) gave potent agonist ligands with good binding affinities. Although the decahydronaphthyl and 4-isopropylcyclohexyl groups appear to be optimally sized lipophilic groups for the C moiety and have afforded potent ligands on various scaffolds, discussed earlier, these groups on the indolinone scaffold did not afford the same selectivity (only 40-fold vs kappa) vs the opioid receptors as seen when the same C moieties were on the hexahydropyrrolopyrrole scaffold (~1000-fold) reported by Roche (**8**, Fig. 24.2). This finding indicates that the heterocyclic A moiety at the 4-position of the piperidine ring of NOP ligands is an important determinant of selectivity of that structural class over the opioid receptors.

However, when these lipophilic substituents of the C moiety were placed 1 methylene carbon away from the piperidine nitrogen (compounds **24** and **25**), it resulted not only in decreased binding but also in complete loss of agonist activity. There appears to be a volume constraint of the size of the lipophilic group around the piperidine nitrogen. Compounds **26** to **28**, which contain more compacted bicyclic lipophilic groups and are 1 carbon removed from the basic nitrogen, have higher affinity and are antagonists at the receptor. This finding is also illustrated by the increase in binding affinity observed when the extended 4-isopropyl group of **24** is

Table 24.2 Binding Affinities and Functional Activities of the New Piperidin-4-yl-1,3-dihydroindol-2-ones at the NOP and Opioid Receptors[*]

| R | Receptor Binding[a] | | | | Functional Activity[a] | | |
| | K_i (nM) | | | | NOP [^{35}S] GTPγS | | |
	NOP	μ	κ	δ	EC_{50} (nM)	% Stim	K_e^{b} (nM)
18	201 ± 51	91.1 ± 16	84.5 ± 0.8	ND[c]	174 ± 51	18 ± 2	
19	6.04 ± 0.42	14.4 ± 1.1	229 ± 33	>10 K	>10 K	—	15.3 ± 1.6
20	1.39 ± 0.42	29.9 ± 2.1	42.7 ± 1.0	ND	19.9 ± 3.4	59.1 ± 7.1	
21	4.67 ± 1.96	16.4 ± 3.3	137 ± 2	ND	74.9 ± 2	78 ± 14	
22	5.64 ± 2.89	10.6 ± 1.2	52.1 ± 31.5	ND	16 ± 3	62 ± 6	
23	3.96 ± 1.55	8.0 ± 0.97	148 ± 9	ND	26.3 ± 8	100	
24	183 ± 29	117 ± 4	1146 ± 392	ND	>10 K		
25	366 ± 100	1190 ± 514	454 ± 127	ND	>10 K		
26	15.5 ± 7.1	27.8 ± 5.4	175 ± 3	ND	>10 K		67.1 ± 7.8

(continued)

Table 24.2 (continued)

27		22.0 ± 8.9	115 ± 0.9	372 ± 0.2	>10K	>10K	ND
28		27.9 ± 8.7	118 ± 1.2	318 ± 27	>10K	>10K	ND
29		7.49 ± 0.78	2.70 ± 0.5	31.7 ± 4.82	>10K	28.7 ± 0.6	45 ± 5
30		9.98 ± 2.8	3.44 ± 0.46	43.9 ± 9.2	ND	82.3 ± 16	60 ± 10
31		27.8 ± 4.7	14.2 ± 1.4	61.4 ± 21.2	ND	63 ± 15	74 ± 14
32		71.1 ± 25	81 ± 13	10.96 ± 2	ND	406 ± 2	56 ± 1
33		>10K	227 ± 80	343 ± 92	>10K	>10K	

*NOP indicates nociceptin; GTP - guanidine triphosphate; EC$_{50}$ - Concentration at which 50% effect is observed; Stim - Stimulation; ND - Not Determined. Receptor binding and [^{35}S]GTPγS binding were conducted as described previously, in Zaveri et al.[9]

[a] - Receptor binding and [^{35}S] GTPgammaS binding were conducted as described previously.

[b] - K_e = [A]/(dose ration-1); [A] = antagonist concentration

[c] - Not Determined

conformationally constrained into the bicyclo ring of **26**, resulting in a significant increase in binding affinity but not intrinsic activity. Our results show that when the piperidyl N-1 is directly linked to the cyclic C moiety (as in **20–23** and **29**), the compounds are potent NOP agonists, whereas those ligands that are linked via a methylene (**19**, **22–24**) are antagonists at the NOP receptor. However, when alkyl groups are added back on the methylene linker, as in **30** to **32**, agonist activity is regained. The complete loss of binding affinity of the biscyclohexylmethyl-containing compound **33** confirms that there is a size constraint on the volume of the lipophilic region around the basic piperidine nitrogen.

Our results suggest that (1) there is a lipophilic binding site in the vicinity of the protonated nitrogen binding site, which must be occupied (by the C moiety) for optimum binding affinity, for both agonist as well as antagonist ligands; (2) there may be a specific binding area of limited size, close to where the protonated nitrogen binds, that triggers an agonist response when the lipophilic binding site is occupied by an appropriately sized and placed C moiety; and (3) the 1-carbon homologation of the C moiety allows binding to the lipophilic site for good affinity but does not allow binding to the agonist trigger site. Such compounds do not trigger an agonist response and are antagonists. This analysis can be visualized in Fig. 24.4, in which the agonists and antagonists from the dihydroindolinone class are superimposed in their low-energy conformations. The agonists (**20**, **23**, and **30**) and antagonists (**19** and **26**) possess C moieties that occupy the lipophilic binding pocket proximal to the protonated nitrogen binding site. In addition, the agonist groups interact with the putative agonist trigger site. The 1-carbon homologation of the

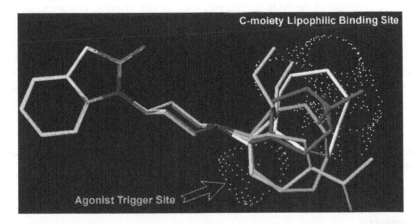

Fig. 24.4 Overlay of the dihydroindolinone-based agonists **20** (green), **23** (cyan), and **30** (yellow) with the antagonists **19** (white) and **26** (magenta). The lipophilic site that must be occupied by the C-moiety for good binding affinity is depicted by the white van der Waals surface. The green van der Waals surface represents the agonist trigger site, which when occupied by the agonists (eg **20**, **23**, **30**), triggers signal transduction leading to intrinsic activity. Antagonists **19** and **20** bind to the lipophilic site and have good affinity but do not interact with the agonist trigger site and therefore lack intrinsic activity. (*See* also Color Insert).

lipophilic group in the antagonist ligands places the C moiety in the lipophilic binding pocket but does not allow interaction with the agonist trigger site (Fig. 24.4). These analyses can be further confirmed with site-directed mutagenesis studies of residues lining the NOP active site close to where the protonated nitrogen binds. An alternate explanation for these observations is that the optimally sized lipophilic C moieties directly linked to the protonated nitrogen bind to and stabilize an agonist receptor conformation that can transduce the agonist signal. C moieties 1 carbon away can still bind the receptor with high affinity but do not induce the agonist conformational change and therefore lack intrinsic activity. It appears very likely that the shape and volume of the lipophilic C moiety play a role in the transduction of intrinsic activity at the receptor, as illustrated by comparing the lead antagonist **19** and compound **29** (Table 24.2). Compound **29**, in which the cyclooctyl ring is linked to the methylene carbon linker of the cyclooctylmethyl group, can be considered a conformationally restricted analog of antagonist **19**. This structural modification retains the binding affinity in **29** but converts the antagonist profile of **19** to a partial agonist profile of **29**, suggesting that the extended nature of the cyclooctylmethyl and other groups linked via a methylene linker stabilize an antagonist conformation or, conversely, that compacted lipophilic groups stabilize an agonist conformation or interact with an agonist trigger site.

Conclusions

The ligand-based analysis presented can be confirmed by complementary studies with the 3-D model of the NOP receptor as well as site-directed mutagenesis of the NOP receptor. Our analysis provides the first basis for the rational design of high-affinity NOP agonists and antagonists and for understanding the structural factors that influence intrinsic activity at the NOP receptor. Future studies will address the issue of selectivity vs the opioid and other receptors. Such analyses are important for effective drug design of NOP ligands that can be developed as therapeutics to harness the potential of this receptor in pain, tolerance, withdrawal, and other important CNS pathways.

Acknowledgment The work presented in this review was supported by a grant from the National Institute on Drug Abuse (DA 14026).

References

1. Bigoni R, Giuliani S, Calo' G, et al. Characterization of nociceptin receptors in the periphery: in vitro and in vivo studies. *Naunyn Schmiedebergs Arch Pharmacol.* 1999;359:160-167.
2. Mollereau C, Mouledous L. Tissue distribution of the opioid receptor-like (ORL1) receptor. *Peptides.* 2000;21:907-917.

3. Mogil JS, Pasternak GW. The molecular and behavioral pharmacology of the orphanin FQ/ nociceptin peptide and receptor family. *Pharmacol Rev.* 2001;53:381-415.
4. Calo' G, Guerrini R, Rizzi A, Salvadori S, Regoli D. Pharmacology of nociceptin and its receptor: a novel therapeutic target. *Br J Pharmacol.* 2000;129:1261-1283.
5. Zaveri N, Polgar WE, Olsen CM, et al. Characterization of opiates, neuroleptics, and synthetic analogs at ORL1 and opioid receptors. *Eur J Pharmacol.* 2001;428:29-36.
6. Lutfy K, Eitan S, Bryant C, et al. Buprenorphine-induced antinociception is mediated by mu-opioid receptors and compromised by concomitant activation of opioid receptor-like receptors. *J Neurosci.* 2003;23:10331-10337.
7. Zaveri N. Peptide and nonpeptide ligands for the nociceptin/orphanin FQ receptor ORL1: research tools and potential therapeutic agents. *Life Sci.* 2003;73:663-678.
8. Ronzoni S, Peretto I, Giardina GA. Lead generation and lead optimization approaches in the discovery of selective, nonpeptide ORL-1 receptor agonists and antagonists. *Expert Opin Ther Patents.* 2001;11:525-546.
9. Zaveri NT, Jiang F, Olsen CM, et al. A novel series of piperidin-4-yl-1,3-dihydroindol-2-ones as agonist and antagonist ligands at the nociceptin receptor. *J Med Chem.* 2004;47:2973-2976.
10. Wichmann J, Adam G, Rover S, et al. Synthesis of (1S,3aS)-8-(2,3,3a,4,5, 6-hexahydro-1H-phenalen-1-yl)-1-phenyl-1,3,8-triaza-spiro[4. 5]decan-4-one, a potent and selective orphanin FQ (OFQ) receptor agonist with anxiolytic-like properties. *Eur J Med Chem.* 2000;35:839-851.
11. Rover S, Adam G, Cesura AM, et al. High-affinity, non-peptide agonists for the ORL1 (orphanin FQ/nociceptin) receptor. *J Med Chem.* 2000;43:1329-1338.
12. Rover S, Wichmann J, Jenck F, Adam G, Cesura AM. ORL1 receptor ligands: structure-activity relationships of 8-cycloalkyl-1-phenyl-1,3,8-triaza-spiro[4.5]decan-4-ones. *Bioorg Med Chem Lett.* 2000;10:831-834.
13. Ito F, Ohashi Y, inventors. Pfizer, Inc., assignee. 1,3,8-Triazaspiro[4,5]decanone compounds as ORL1-receptor agonists. European patent application, European patent 0 997 464 A1. July 10, 1999.
14. Kolczewski S, Adam G, Cesura AM, et al. Novel hexahydrospiro[piperidine-4,1 [3,4-c]pyrroles]: highly selective small-molecule nociceptin/orphanin FQ receptor agonists. *J Med Chem.* 2003;46:255-264.
15. Tulshian D, Ho G, Silverman L, et al, inventors. Schering Corporation, assignee. High affinity ligands for nociceptin receptor ORL-1. US patent 6 262 066 B1. July 17, 2001.
16. Chen Z, Miller WS, Shan S, Valenzano KJ. Design and parallel synthesis of piperidine libraries targeting the nociceptin (N/OFQ) receptor. *Bioorg Med Chem Lett.* 2003;13:3247-3252.
17. Kawamoto H, Ozaki S, Itoh Y, et al. Discovery of the first potent and selective small molecule opioid receptor-like (ORL1) antagonist: 1-[(3R,4R)-1-cyclooctylmethyl-3-hydroxymethyl-4-piperidyl]-3-ethyl-1, 3-dihydro-2H-benzimidazol-2-one (J-113397). *J Med Chem.* 1999;42:5061-5063.
18. Ozaki S, Kawamoto H, Ito Y, Hayashi K, Hirano K, Iwasawa Y, inventors. Banyu Pharmaceutical Co., assignee. New 2-oxoimidazole derivatives. US patent 6 258 825. July 10, 2001.
19. Kawamoto H, Ozaki S, Ito Y, Iwazawa Z, inventors. Banyu Pharmaceutical Co, assignee. 4-Oxoimidazolidine-5-spiro-nitrogen-containing heterocyclic compound. Japan patent application 20001169476. June 20, 2000.
20. Zaratin PF, Petrone G, Sbacchi M, et al. Modification of nociceptin and morphine tolerance by the selective ORL-1 antagonist (-)-cis-1-methyl-7-[[4-(2,6-dichlorophenyl)piperidin-1-yl]methyl]-6,7,8,9-tetrahydro-5H-benzocyclohepten-5-ol (SB-612111). *J Pharmacol Exp Ther.* 2004;308:454-461.
21. Shinkai H, Ito T, Iida T, Kitao Y, Yamada H, Uchida I. 4-Aminoquinolines: novel nociceptin antagonists with analgesic activity. *J Med Chem.* 2000;43:4667-4677.
22. Yamada H, Nakamoto H, Suzuki Y, Ito T, Aisaka K. Pharmacological profiles of a novel opioid receptor-like1 (ORL1) receptor antagonist, JTC-801. *Br J Pharmacol.* 2002;135:323-332.
23. Muratani T, Minami T, Enomoto U, et al. Characterization of nociceptin/orphanin FQ-induced pain responses by the novel receptor antagonist N-(4-amino-2-methylquinolin-6-yl)-

2-(4-ethylphenoxymethyl)benzamide monohydrochloride. In: *J Pharmacol Exp Ther.* vol. 303. 2002:424-430.

24. Mabuchi T, Matsumura S, Okuda-Ashitaka E, et al. Attenuation of neuropathic pain by the nociceptin/orphanin FQ antagonist JTC-801 is mediated by inhibition of nitric oxide production. *Eur J Neurosci.* 2003;17:1384-1392.

25. Mouledous L, Topham CM, Moisand C, Mollereau C, Meunier JC. Functional inactivation of the nociceptin receptor by alanine substitution of glutamine 286 at the C terminus of transmembrane segment VI: evidence from a site-directed mutagenesis study of the ORL1 receptor transmembrane-binding domain. *Mol Pharmacol.* 2000;57:495-502.

Chapter 25
Kappa Opioid Antagonists: Past Successes and Future Prospects

Matthew D. Metcalf[1] and Andrew Coop[1]

Abstract Antagonists of the kappa opioid receptor were initially investigated as pharmacological tools that would reverse the effects of kappa opioid receptor agonists. In the years following the discovery of the first selective kappa opioid antagonists, much information about their chemistry and pharmacology has been elicited and their potential therapeutic uses have been investigated. The review presents the current chemistry, ligand-based structure activity relationships, and pharmacology of the known nonpeptidic selective kappa opioid receptor antagonists. This manuscript endeavors to provide the reader with a useful reference of the investigations made to define the structure-activity relationships and pharmacology of selective kappa opioid receptor antagonists and their potential uses as pharmacological tools and as therapeutic agents in the treatment of disease states.

Keywords Opioid, Opiate, Receptor, Kappa, Antagonist

Introduction

The opioid receptor system consists of 3 types of heterogeneous, G-protein–coupled, opioid receptors mu (μ), delta (δ), and kappa (κ), which have been pharmacologically characterized and cloned.[1-4] Each opioid receptor type has selective agonists and antagonists that bind to and produce effects unique to that individual receptor type. The prototypical agonist acting through opioid receptors is morphine (**1**) (Fig. 25.1), though not selective, it functions as a mu opioid agonist. Mu opioid agonists produce the classic opioid effects: analgesia, euphoria, respiratory depression, constipation, nausea, cough suppression, and the development of tolerance and dependence.[5]

[1] Department of Pharmaceutical Sciences, University of Maryland School of Pharmacy, 20 Penn Street, Baltimore, MD 21201

Corresponding Author: Andrew Coop, Department of Pharmaceutical Sciences, University of Maryland School of Pharmacy, 20 Penn Street, Baltimore, MD 21201. Tel: (410)-706-2209; Fax: (410)-706-5017; E-mail: acoop@rx.umaryland.edu

R.S. Rapaka and W. Sadée (eds.), *Drug Addiction.*
© American Association of Pharmaceutical Scientists 2008

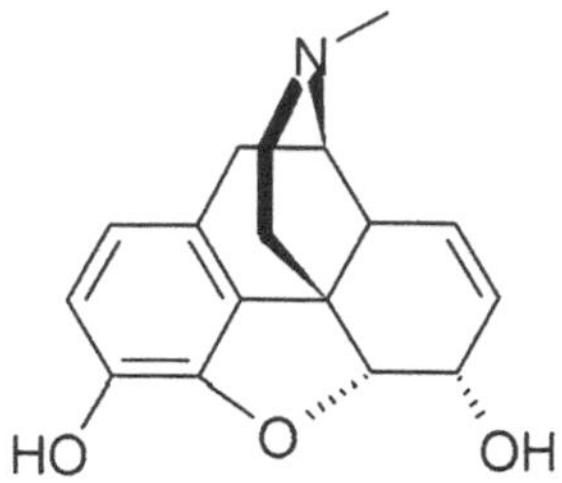

(1) Morphine

Fig. 25.1 Structure of morphine.

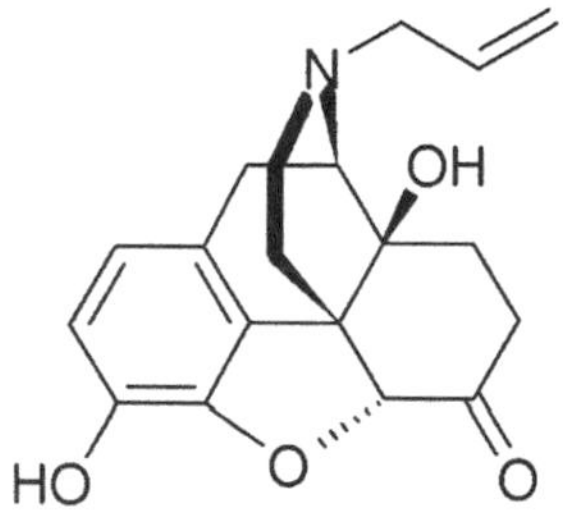

(2) Naloxone

Fig. 25.2 Structure of naloxone.

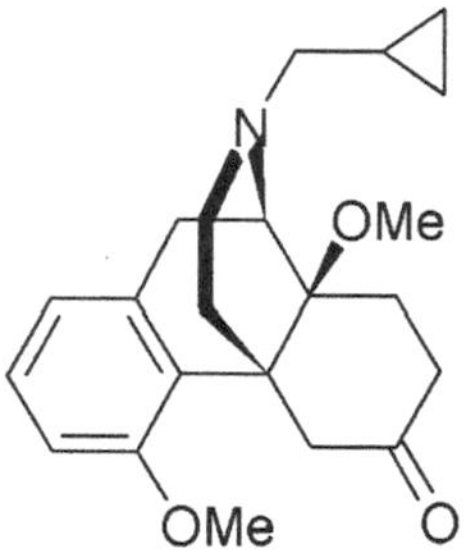

(3) Cyprodime

Fig. 25.3 Structure of cyprodime.

The prototypical opioid antagonist naloxone (**2**) (Fig. 25.2) functions as a mu opioid antagonist, though it is also not selective for mu opioid receptors. Selective mu opioid antagonists such as cyprodime (**3**) (Fig. 25.3) reverse the effects of mu opioid agonists only and are used as tools in pharmacological assays.[5,6] Selective delta opioid agonists such as SNC 80 (**4**) (Fig. 25.4) produce weak analgesia, mild convulsions, and immunostimulation.[7] Selective delta antagonists such as naltrindole (**5**) (Fig. 25.5) are being investigated for their potential use as immunosuppressants and modulation of the tolerance effect of mu opioid agonists.[7]

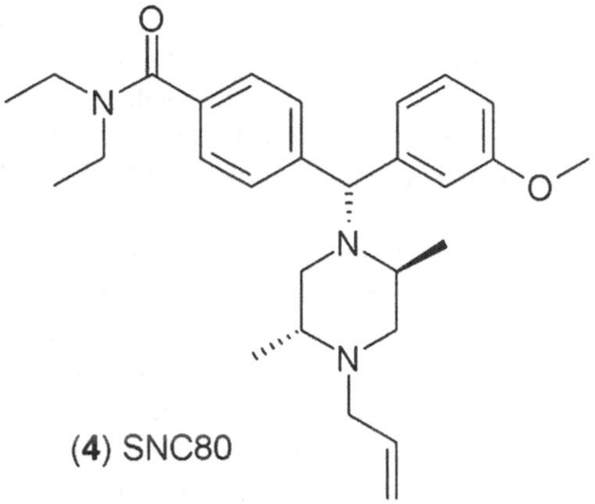

Fig. 25.4 Structure of SNC80.

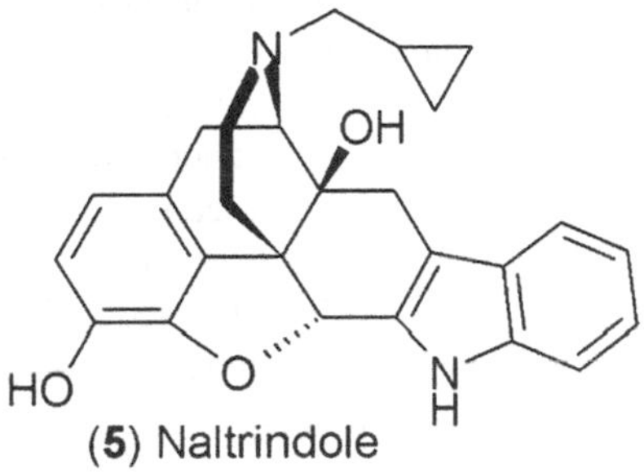

Fig. 25.5 Structure of naltrindole.

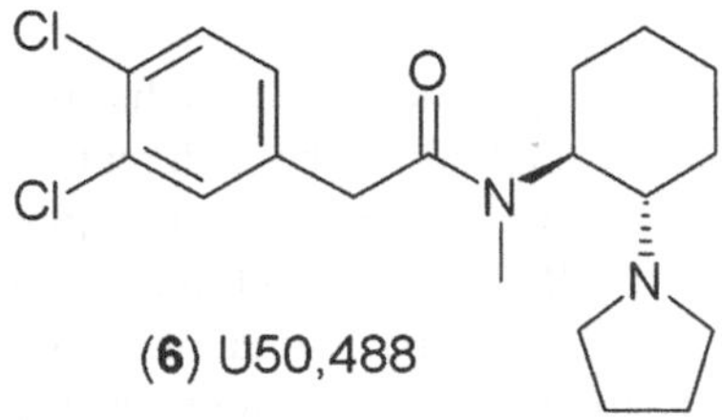

Fig. 25.6 Structure of U50,488.

Selective agonists and antagonists for kappa opioid receptors have also been investigated. Selective kappa opioid agonists such as U50,488 (**6**) (Fig. 25.6) produce analgesia, diuresis, dysphoria, and show antipruritic activity,[8] whereas selective kappa opioid antagonists are being explored for their effects in the treatment of a wide variety of areas including cocaine addiction,[9] depression,[10] and feeding behavior,[11] and have been proposed as a treatment for psychosis and schizophrenia.[12] In this manuscript we present currently known chemical classes of selective kappa opioid antagonists, their pharmacology, and ligand-based structure-activity relationships (SAR).

While this manuscript focuses on nonpeptidic selective kappa opioid receptor antagonists, several related issues with peptidic opioids will briefly be addressed. Four different types of endogenous mammalian peptides[13] have been identified that act upon opioid receptors: endorphins, enkephalins, endomorphins, and dynorphins. The dynorphin family of peptides acts predominantly as kappa opioid receptor agonists and peptidic antagonists for the kappa receptor are known.[14,15] Those interested in an excellent discussion of peptidic kappa opioid antagonists should refer to the analgesics chapter in Burger's Medicinal Chemistry.[16] Further, the nonselective kappa opioid antagonist buprenorphine will not be covered due to its mu opioid agonist actions. Those seeking information on buprenorphine should seek John Lewis' excellent book of the same title (Cowan and Lewis[17]). Subtypes of kappa opioid receptors have been proposed through the results of pharmacological assays, but only one type of kappa opioid receptor has been cloned so far.[2] Further, it has been shown that receptor dimerization between the kappa and delta opioid receptors produces a dimer that possesses the pharmacological profile of the kappa-2 subtype,[18] and that the kappa-1 and kappa-2 receptor subtypes may be different affinity states of the same receptor,[19] which may explain the pharmacological findings of subtypes of kappa opioid receptors.[20] Therefore, this article will not differentiate between subtypes of kappa opioid receptors. Target-based modeling of kappa opioid antagonists has been performed[21-27] and an excellent review is available,[28] however this review will focus on ligand-based SAR. We endeavor herein to cover nonpeptidic, selective kappa opioid antagonists including the most recent chemical and pharmacological developments.

Competitive Kappa Opioid Antagonists

Antagonist selectivity for the kappa opioid receptor has been a goal of chemists and pharmacologists since the recognition of the different subtypes of opioid receptors.[20] Early accomplishments in developing kappa opioid antagonists produced Mr 2266 (7a) (Fig. 25.7) and WIN 44,441 (quadazocine) (7b).[29] While occasionally used[30] for their historical value as kappa opioid antagonists, these compounds are not selective[20] antagonists for the kappa opioid receptor. The first nonpeptide selective kappa opioid antagonist, triethyleneglycolnaltrexamine (TENA) (8) (Fig. 25.8), was developed by Erez et al.[31] TENA (8), a derivative of β-naltrexamine (8a), contains 2 naltrexone (9) (Fig. 25.9) pharmacophores linked by a spacer. While superior to Mr 2266 (7a) and quadazocine (7b), TENA (8) possesses only a modest selectivity for kappa receptors over mu and delta opioid receptors[32] (Table 25. 1). Although TENA (8) was not an ideal selective kappa opioid antagonist, it was very useful as a lead compound in the development of selective kappa opioid antagonists. Numerous structural modifications of the spacing linker[33-35] involving the substituents, length, flexibility, and conformation led to a short, rigid, pyrrole ring

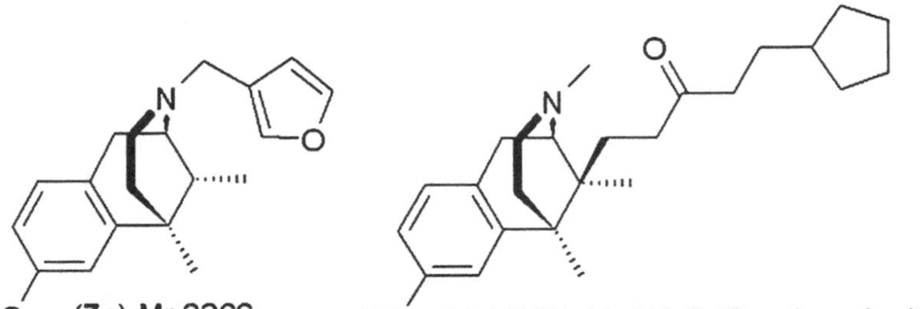

(7a) Mr 2266 (7b) WIN 44,441-3 (Quadazocine)

Fig. 25.7 Structures of Mr 2266 and WIN 44,441–3.

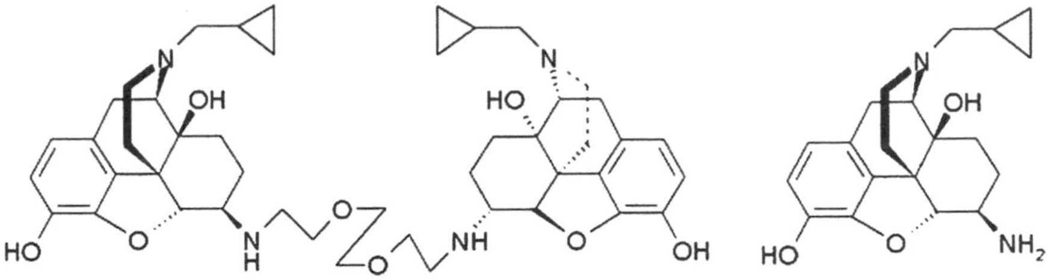

(8) TENA (8a) ß-naltrexamine

Fig. 25.8 Structures of TENA and β-naltrexamine.

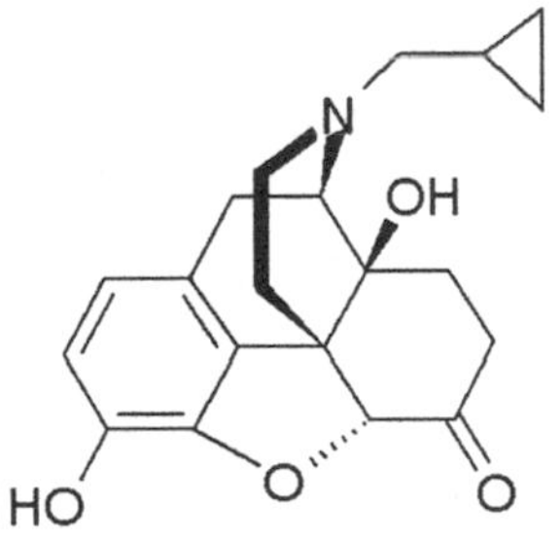

(9) Naltrexone

Fig. 25.9 Structure of naltrexone.

Table 25.1 Opioid Antagonist Activities of TENA (**8**) in the GPI and MVD[*,32]

	IC_{50} ratio				
Antagonist	Ethylketozocine (κ)	U50,488 (κ)	Morphine (μ)	DADLE (δ)	κ/μ
Naloxone (**2**)	7.2	-	46.8		0.2
TENA (**8**)	19.6	111.5	4.2	1.2	4.7 (26.6)
Mr 2266 (**7a**)	9.6	9.9	7.9	1.5	1.2 (1.3)
quadazocine (**7b**)	4.6	-	16	-	0.3

*GPI indicates guinea pig ileum assay; MVD, mouse vas deferens assay.

between the 2 pharmacophores as the optimal spacer. This spacing linker produced the selective kappa opioid receptor antagonists[36] binaltorphimine (BNI) (**10**) (Fig. 25.10) and norbinaltorphimine (norBNI) (**11**).

While developing these compounds, Takemori and Portoghese[37,38] used the "message-address" concept,[39] originally applied to proteins, and his "bivalent-ligand" approach (2 pharmacophores covalently attached to one another) in the development of kappa opioid antagonists TENA (**8**) and norBNI (**11**).[21,40] Later, the message address concept was used in the development of other kappa opioid antagonists.[22,41,42] The "message-address" concept is used to explain the selective binding of ligands to different subtypes of receptors within a general receptor class (here the mu [μ], delta [δ], and kappa [κ] subtypes of the general class of opioid receptors). Briefly, the "message" portion (scaffold) of the ligand provides the affinity for the general class of receptor, and the "address" portion, a chemically specific function, confers specificity for the individual receptor subtype (Fig. 25.11).

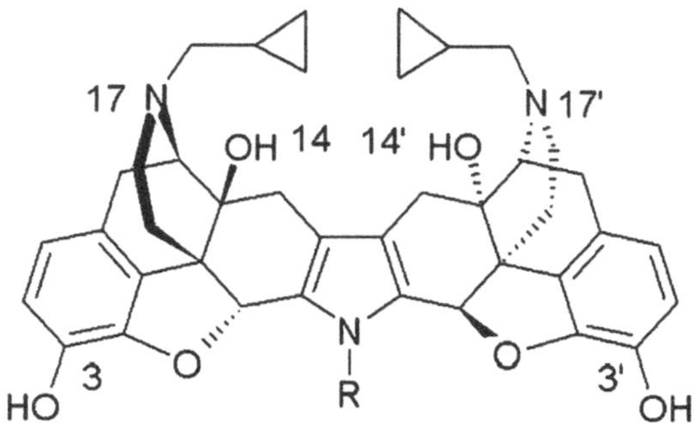

(**10**) R = methyl = BNI
(**11**) R = H = norBNI

Fig. 25.10 Structures of Binaltorphimine and norBinaltorphimine.

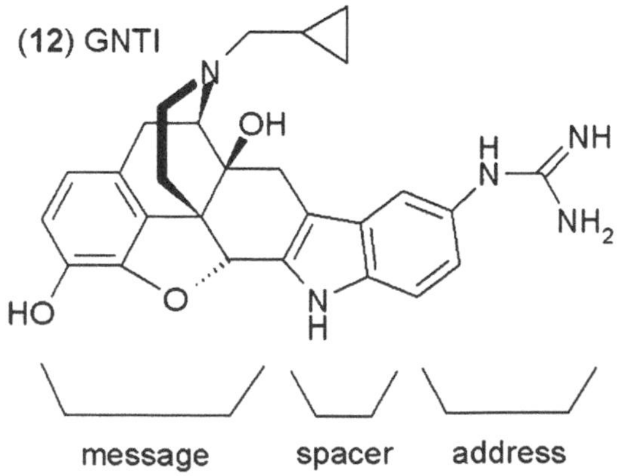

Fig. 25.11 Structure of guanidinenaltrindole detailing the message-address concept.

Examples include the transformation of the nonselective opioid antagonist naltrexone (**9**) to the selective delta opioid antagonist naltrindole (**5**),[37,38] and the transformation of naltrindole (**5**) to the kappa specific antagonist 5'-guanidinonaltrindole (GNTI) (**12**).[22] For an in an in-depth discussion of the "message-address concept" please refer to the eloquently presented argument and discussion in Takemori and Portoghese,[37] Portoghese,[38] and more current, though condensed, discussions by Sharma et al[23] and Thomas et al.[41]

NorBNI and Analogs

In 1987, Portoghese et al[29,36] reported the selective kappa opioid receptor antagonists binaltorphimine (BNI) (**10**) and norbinaltorphimine (norBNI) (**11**); the latter has become the prototype kappa opioid antagonist ligand. Both ligands displayed high selectivity and potency for kappa opioid receptors (Table 25. 2). A subsequent paper[43] describes (−) norBNI (**11**) compared with its "unnatural" (+) enantiomer (**13**) (Fig. 25.12) and its (±) diasterisomer (**14**) (Fig. 25.13). The difference in the molecules is best appreciated by the perspective drawings in Fig. 25.14 and 25.15. This series showed that (+)-norBNI (**13**) was inactive while (±)-norBNI (**14**) displayed increased potency, but decreased specificity as a kappa opioid antagonist (Table 25. 2). A series of analogs (**15–23**) (Fig. 25.16) of norBNI (**11**) was synthesized to test replacements of the 3, 14, 3', and 14' hydroxyls, and the N-17 and N-17' substituents[44] (Table 25. 3). Additionally, Schmidhammer's group reported 2 norBNI (**11**) analogs[45] (**24, 25**) (Fig. 25.17) and 2 BNI (**10**) analogs[46] (**26, 27**) (Fig. 25.18) with the 14 and 14' positions occupied by methoxy groups (Table 25. 4). Another study[47] presented data on replacements of the nitrogen in the pyrrole ring with the thiophene (**28**) (Fig. 25.19) and pyran (**29**) (Fig. 25.20) analogs of norBNI (Table 25. 5). Also, 2 octahydroisoquinoline BNI (**10**) analogs[40] (**30, 31**) (Fig. 25.21) have been synthesized and tested (Table 25. 6). Another study[48] of norBNI analogs analyzed the results of sequential replacements (**32–42**) (Fig. 25.22) of the N-17' substituent (Table 25. 7) and 2 more (**43, 44**) with only binding data.[21] A 3'-dehydroxy analog[49] of norBNI (**45**) (Fig. 25.23) has also been prepared (Table 25. 8). A radio ligand form of norBNI (**46**) (Fig. 25.24) has also been synthesized[50] and possesses high binding affinity and selectivity for kappa receptors.

Table 25.2 Opioid Antagonist Activities of BNI (2), norBNI (3) and Stereoisomers in the GPI and MVD[*,36,43]

Antagonist	K_e in nM			K_e ratio	
	(κ)	(μ)	(δ)	μ/κ	δ/κ
BNI (**10**)	0.14	11	5.7	79	41
(−)-norBNI (**11**)	0.41	13	20	32	49
(±)-norBNI (**14**)	0.08	1.1	1.3	14	16
naltrexone (**9**)	5.5	1.0	24	0.2	4.4

*GPI indicates guinea pig ileum assay; MVD, mouse vas deferens assay; norBNI, norbinaltorphimine.

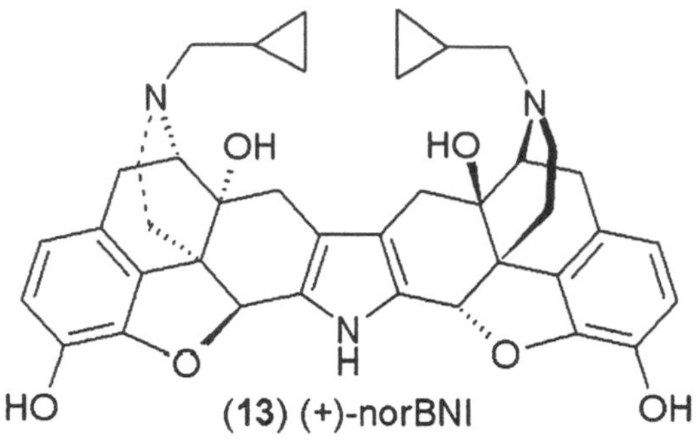

Fig. 25.12 Structure of (+)-norBinaltorphimine.

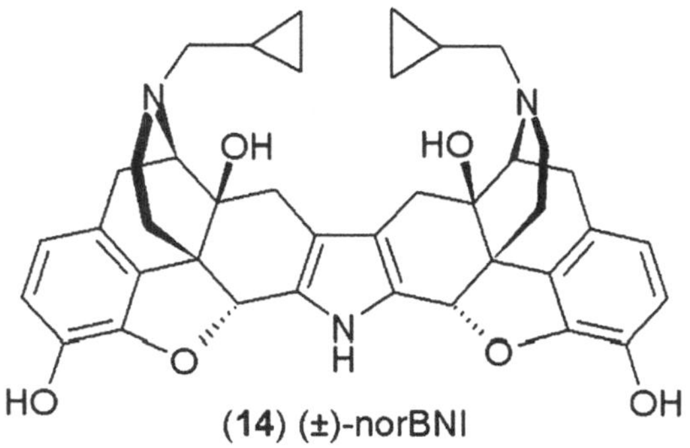

Fig. 25.13 Structure of (±)-norBinaltorphimine.

Perspective drawing of (11) (-)-norBNI

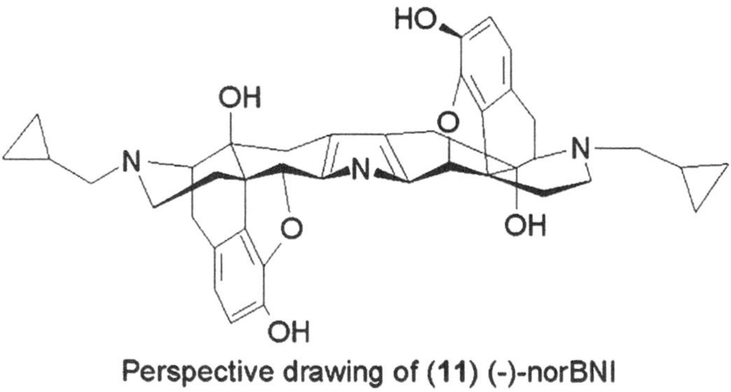

Fig. 25.14 Perspective model of (–)-norBinaltorphimine.

The overall conclusions that can be drawn from these analogs suggest a structure activity relationship as follows. Only one antagonist pharmacophore is necessary for kappa antagonist activity, as suggested by data on compounds **11, 14, 15–18,** and **31**. A second basic nitrogen is necessary for kappa opioid antagonist activity,

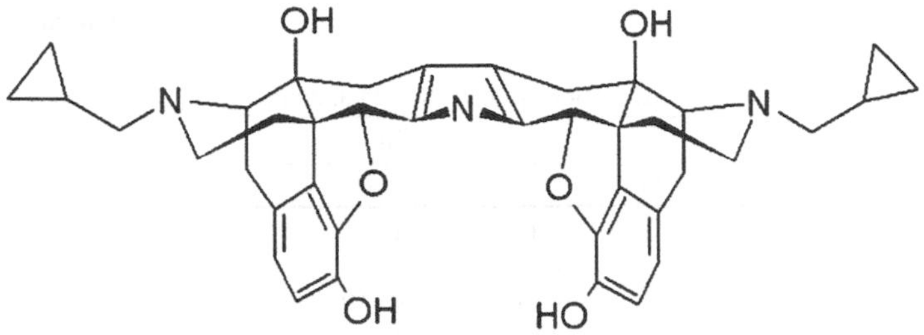

Perspective drawing of (14) (±)-norBNI

Fig. 25.15 Perspective model of (±)-norBinaltorphimine.

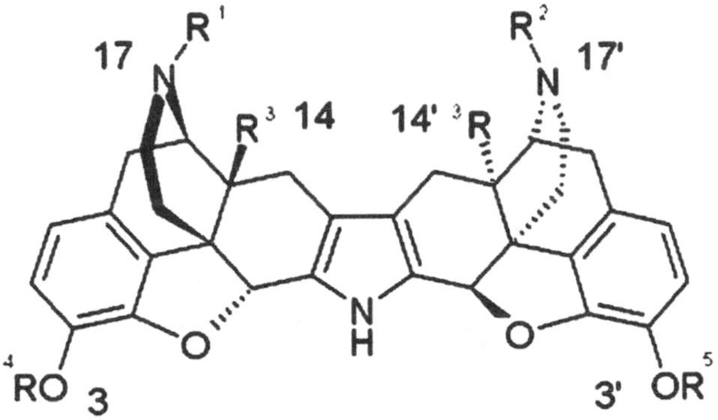

	R¹	R²	R³	R⁴	R⁵
15	allyl	allyl	OH	H	H
16	Methyl	Methyl	OH	H	H
17	Methyl	Methyl	H	H	H
18	Methyl	Methyl	H	Methyl	Methyl
19	CPM	CPM	OAc	Ac	Ac
20	CPM	CPM	OAc	H	H
21	CPM	CPM	OH	Methyl	Methyl
22	CPM	CPM	OH	H	Methyl
23	CPM	Methyl	OH	H	H

CPM = cyclopropyl methyl, OAc = acetate, Ac = acetyl

Fig. 25.16 Structures of norBinaltorphimine analogs.

Table 25.3 Opioid Antagonist Activities of norBNI (**11**) and analogs in the GPI and MVD[*,44]

Antagonist	Conc. nM	K_e in nM			K_e ratio	
		(κ)	(μ)	(δ)	μ/κ	δ/κ
BNI (**10**)	20	0.14	11	5.7	79	41
norBNI (**11**)	20	0.41	13	20	32	49
15	100	0.91	≥250	≥143 (pa)	≥275	≥157
16	20	a	a			
17	10	a	a			
18	100	a	a			
19	100					
20	100	0.38	42	12	111	32
21	20	7.1				
22	200	1.3	38	45	29	35
23	200	1.9	21	41	11	22
naltrexone (**9**)	100	5.5	1.0	24	0.2	4.4

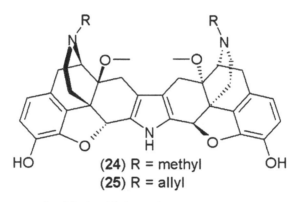

(24) R = methyl
(25) R = allyl

Fig. 25.17 Structures of norBinaltorphimine analogs.

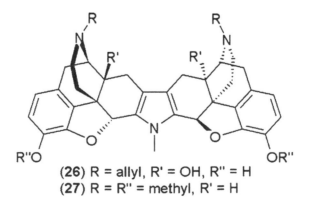

(26) R = allyl, R' = OH, R'' = H
(27) R = R'' = methyl, R' = H

Fig. 25.18 Structures of Binaltorphimine analogs.

Table 25.4 Opioid Antagonist Activities of norBNI and two analogs in the GPI and MVD*,45,46

Antagonist	K_e in nM			Selectivity ratio	
	(κ)	(μ)	(δ)	μ/κ	δ/κ
norBNI (11)	0.02	27	22	1350	1100
24	0.6	88	4.6	147	8
25	0.03	0.36	2.3	12	77
26	0.11	5.7	6.1	52	6

*GPI indicates guinea pig ileum assay; MVD, mouse vas deferens assay; norBNI, norbinaltorphimine, a = agonist; pa = partial agonist.
*GPI indicates guinea pig ileum assay; MVD, mouse vas deferens assay; norBNI, norbinaltorphimine.

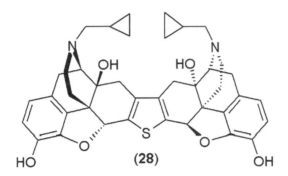

Fig. 25.19 Structure of Pyran analog of norBinaltorphimine.

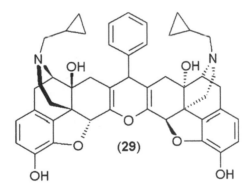

Fig. 25.20 Structure of Furan analog of norBinaltorphimine.

Table 25.5 Opioid Antagonist Activities in the GPI and MVD*,47

Antagonist	K_e in nM			μ/κ	δ/κ
	(κ)	(μ)	(δ)		
norBNI (11)	0.55	14	10.6	25	19
naltrexone (9)	5.5	1.0	24	0.2	4.4
28	2.6	41	33	16	13
29	2.6	39	36	15	14

*GPI indicates guinea pig ileum assay; MVD, mouse vas deferens assay; norBNI, norbinaltorphimine.

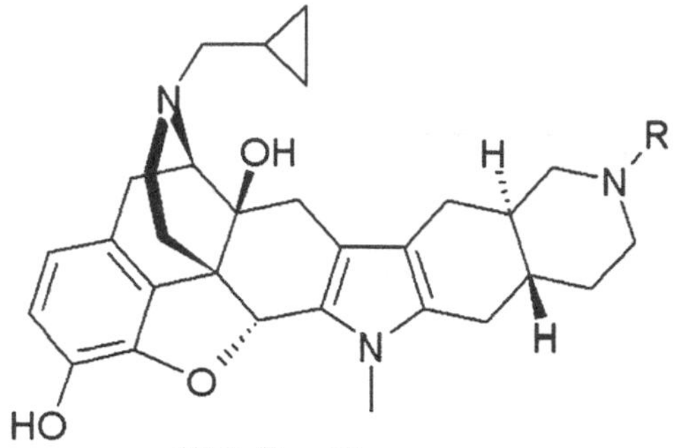

(30) R = Cbz
(31) R = H

Fig. 25.21 Structures of Octahydroisoquinoline analogs of norBinaltorphimine.

Table 25.6 Opioid Antagonist Activities in GPI and MVD[*,40]

Antagonist	IC$_{50}$ ratio			Selectivity ratio	
	(κ)	(μ)	(δ)	κ/μ	κ/δ
norBNI (**11**)	181	8.3	10.4	22	17
30	1.6	1.7	9.2	0.9	0.2
31	40	1	1.1	40	36

*GPI indicates guinea pig ileum assay; MVD, mouse vas deferens assay; norBNI, norbinaltorphimine.

although the functionality of the nitrogen may vary, suggested by data on compounds **11, 14, 23, 30–44**. One phenolic hydroxyl is necessary for activity (although there is loss of potency when the second hydroxyl is masked or eliminated), as suggested by data on compounds **11, 18, 19, 22, 23, 27, 31, 45**. The 14 and 14′ hydroxyls can be methylated or acetylated and still retain activity suggested by data on compounds **19, 20, 24, 25**. The pyrrole spacer can have increased size (sulfur) and be functionalized (methylated) and retain activity, as suggested by data on compounds **10, 11, 26, 28, 29**.

Indolomorphinan Kappa Opioid Antagonists

In 1993, Portoghese's group (Olmstead et al[51]) presented a series of 3 amidines (**47–49**) (Fig. 25.25), based on the naltrindole (NTI) (**5**) pharmacophore, which converted the selective delta opioid antagonist naltrindole (**5**) into selective kappa opioid antagonists (Table 25. 9). Subsequently, the same group reported the preparation of guanidinonaltrindole[22] (GNTI) (**12**); the 5′-guanidinyl derivative of naltrindole. GNTI (**12**) (Fig. 25.11) showed increased affinity, selectivity, and potency over norBNI (**11**); with pA$_2$ values of 10.40, 8.49, and 7.81, respectively, for kappa, mu,

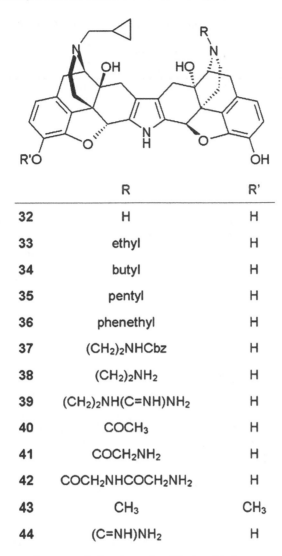

	R	R'
32	H	H
33	ethyl	H
34	butyl	H
35	pentyl	H
36	phenethyl	H
37	(CH$_2$)$_2$NHCbz	H
38	(CH$_2$)$_2$NH$_2$	H
39	(CH$_2$)$_2$NH(C=NH)NH$_2$	H
40	COCH$_3$	H
41	COCH$_2$NH$_2$	H
42	COCH$_2$NHCOCH$_2$NH$_2$	H
43	CH$_3$	CH$_3$
44	(C=NH)NH$_2$	H

Fig. 25.22 Structures of asymmetrical analogs of norBinaltorphimine.

and delta cloned human opioid receptors in Chinese hamster ovary (CHO) cells.[52] A series of GNTI analogs[24] (**12, 50–71**) (Fig. 25.26) were synthesized with GNTI being the most potent and selective of the series (Table 25. 10). ANTI (**58**) would eventually be tested[10] as a peripherally active GNTI (**12**) derivative. Lewis' group published data (Jales et al[53]) on a butyl amidine (**72**); similar but less potent than norBNI (**11**), in the [^{35}S]GTPγS assay (kappa K$_i$ (nM) = 0.12, 0.17, and 0.039 for compounds **55**, **72**, and **11**, respectively) (Fig. 25.27). Portoghese also presented

Table 25.7 Opioid Antagonist Activities of norBNI and N-17' substituted analogs in the GPI and MVD[*,48]

Antagonist	IC$_{50}$ ratio			Selectivity ratio	
	(κ)	(μ)	(δ)	κ/μ	κ/δ
norBNI (11)	181	8.3	10.4	22	17
32	41	1.9	8.5	22	4.8
33	22	1.6	6.3	14	3.5
34	61	1.8	1.9	34	32
35	27	3.1	3.1	8.7	8.7
36	44	1.8	2.4	24	18
37	26	4.5	4.6	5.7	5.7
38	20	1.6	1.9	12.5	10
39	27	1.7	1.0	15	27
40	4.3	1.8	2.8	2.4	1.5
41	11.8	1.4	2.2	8.4	5.4
42	9.6	2.0	0.67	4.8	

*GPI indicates guinea pig ileum assay; MVD, mouse vas deferens assay; norBNI, norbinaltorphimine.

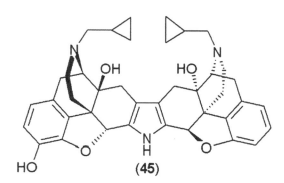

Fig. 25.23 Structure of 14'-Desoxy analog of norBinaltorphimine.

Table 25.8 Antagonist Potency in the [^{35}S]GTPγS assay in Guinea Pig Caudate Membranes[*,49]

Antagonist	K$_i$ (nM)			μ/κ	δ/κ
	(κ)	(μ)	(δ)		
norBNI (11)	0.038	16.7	10.2	439	268
45	0.13	5.55	>300	43	>2307

*NorBNI indicates norbinaltorphimine.

(Sharma et al[23]) a sequential substitution of the guanidine moiety (**73–75**) (Fig. 25.28) at each position of the naltrindole (**5**) scaffold. The results showed the 4' GNTI (**73**) was inactive (K$_e$ >1000nM at all opioid receptors), 6'-GNTI (**74**) showed selective kappa opioid agonist activity (51-fold greater potency than

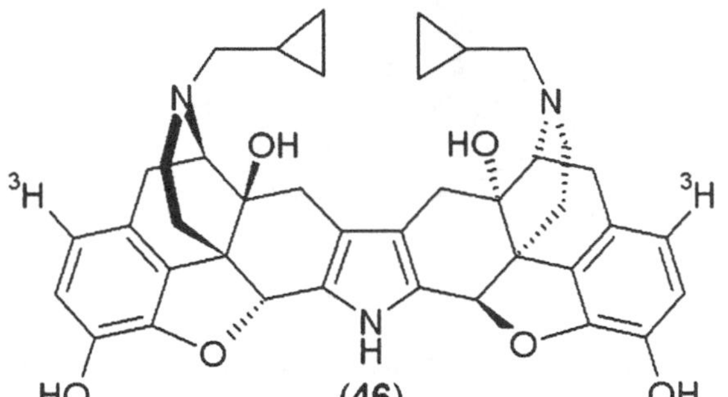

Fig. 25.24 Structure of tritiated analog of norBinaltorphimine.

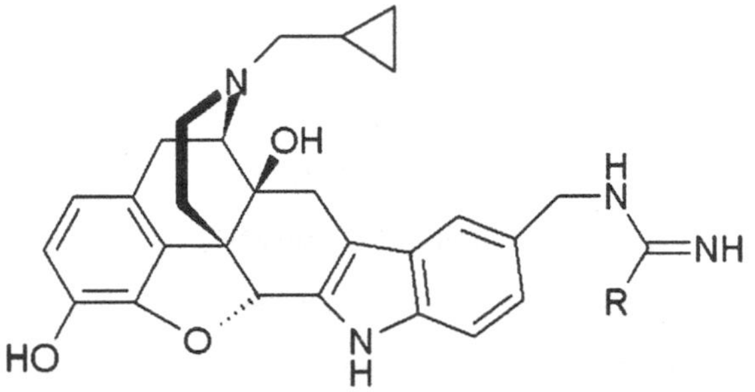

(47) R = ethyl
(48) R = propyl
(49) R = butyl

Fig. 25.25 Structures of amidine kappa opioid antagonists.

Table 25.9 Opioid Antagonist Activities of NTI and 5' substituted analogs in the GPI and MVD*, 51

Antagonist	IC50 ratio			Selectivity ratio	
	(κ)	(μ)	(δ)	κ/μ	κ/δ
NTI (5)	1.3	11.2	459		
norBNI (11)	181	8.3	10.4	22	17
47	159	11.3	2.28	14	69
48	185	19.3	3.00	10	62
49	439	15.7	4.71	28	93

*NTI indicates naltrindole; GPI, guinea pig ileum assay; MVD, mouse vas deferens assay; norBNI, norbinaltorphimine.

morphine in the guinea pig ileum assay (GPI) and reversed by norBNI (11), and 7'-GNTI (75) showed selective delta antagonist activity (K_e = 0.96 in the mouse vas deferens assay [MVD]). Husbands' group presented a series of amides, amidines, and urea analogs of GNTI (Black et al[54]) (76–94) (Fig. 25.29, 25.30, 25.31 and 25.32)

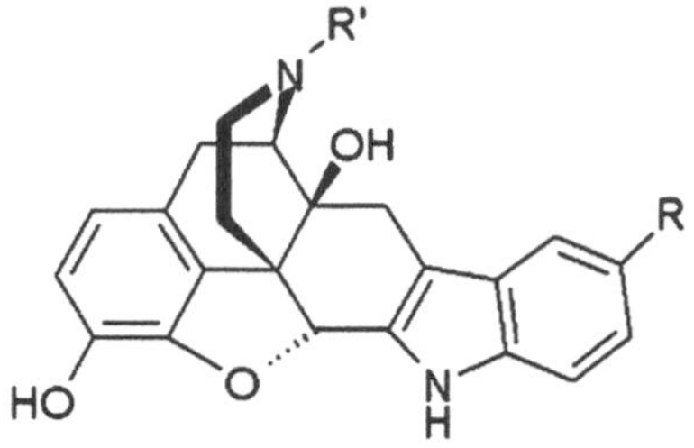

	R	R'
50	-NH(C=NH)NH$_2$	Methyl
51	-(C=NH)NH$_2$	CPM
52	-CH$_2$(C=NH)NH$_2$	CPM
53	-NH$_2$	CPM
54	-CH$_2$NH$_2$	CPM
55	-CH$_2$CH$_2$NH$_2$	CPM
56	-NH(C=NH)CH$_3$	CPM
57	-CH$_2$NH(C=NH)CH$_3$	CPM
ANTI (58)	-CH$_2$CH$_2$NH(C=NH)CH$_3$	CPM
GNTI (12)	-NH(C=NH)NH$_2$	CPM
59	-CH$_2$NH(C=NH)NH$_2$	CPM
60	-CH$_2$CH$_2$NH(C=NH)NH$_2$	CPM
61	-NH(C=NH)NH(C=NH)NH$_2$	CPM
62	-N(CH$_3$)$_2$	CPM
63	-CH$_2$N(CH$_3$)$_2$	CPM
64	-CH$_2$CH$_2$N(CH$_3$)$_2$	CPM
65	-N$^+$(CH$_3$)$_3$I$^-$	CPM
66	-CH$_2$N$^+$(CH$_3$)$_3$I$^-$	CPM
67	-CH$_2$CH$_2$N$^+$(CH$_3$)$_3$I$^-$	CPM
68	-NH(C=N-CN)NH$_2$	CPM
69	-CH$_2$NH(C=N-CN)NH$_2$	CPM
70	-NH(C=S)NH$_2$	CPM
71	-NH(C=NH)SCH$_3$	CPM

CPM = cyclopropyl methyl

Fig. 25.26 Structures of guanidinenaltrindole analogs.

Table 25.10 Opioid Antagonist Activities of GNTI and analogs in the GPI and MVD*.[24]

Antagonist	K_e in nM			K_e ratio	
	(κ)	(μ)	(δ)	μ/κ	δ/κ
norBNI (**11**)	0.4[a]	13	11	31	33 κ/δ
50	17			6.3 κ/μ	41 κ/δ
51	0.7	16		22	142 κ/δ
52	2.2			22 κ/μ	26[i]
53		57		1.5 κ/μ	0.4 κ/δ
54	34	61	18	1.8	0.5
55	2.1			15 κ/μ	21 κ/δ
56	1.0	16		15	52 κ/δ
57	6.1	8.8		1.4	17.3 κ/δ
ANTI (**58**)	0.3[a]	7.6	18	27	65
GNTI (**12**)	0.2[a]	30		193	366 κ/δ
59	0.6	11		19	172 κ/δ
60	1.7	12	3.4	7.3	2.0
61	0.2	14		74	512 κ/δ
62	6.8	36		5.3	6.6 κ/δ
63	0.8	9.8		12	87 κ/δ
64	3.2			13 κ/μ	18 κ/δ
65	3.1			13 κ/μ	9.1 κ/δ
66	0.7	4.0		6.2	154 κ/δ
67	0.4[a]	5.7		13	96 κ/δ
68	3.1	16	9.1	5.1	2.9
69	2.9	18	5.9	6.2	2.0
70	7.2	38		5.3	12 κ/δ
71	0.5[a]	16		33	115 κ/δ

All compounds tested at 100 nM except [a]Tested at 20 nM.
*GNTI indicates guanidinonaltrindole; GPI, guinea pig ileum assay; MVD, mouse vas deferens assay; norBNI, norbinaltorphimine; ANTI, 5'-acetamidinoethylnaltrindole.

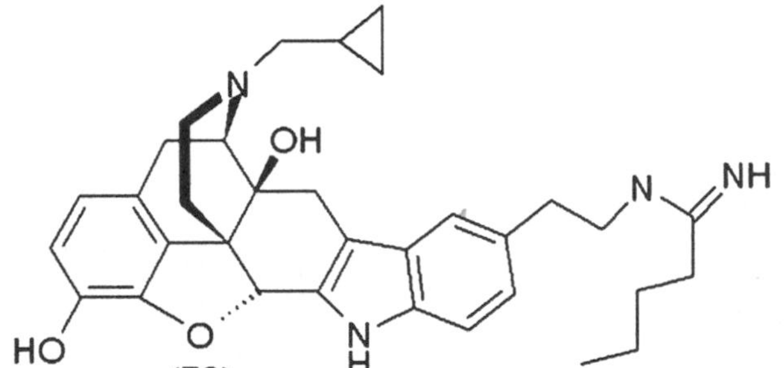

Fig. 25.27 Structure of amidine guanidinenaltrindole analog.

(Table 25. 11). These compounds, especially the ureas, showed less selectivity and potency than norBNI in the [^{35}S]GTPγS assay. Following this work, this group presented a series of guanidine-substituted analogs of GNTI[55] (**95–109**) (Figs. 25.33, 25.34, 25.35 and 25.36) (Table 25. 12). In 2003, Ananthan et al[56] published a pyrido-morphinan kappa opioid antagonist (**110**) (Fig. 25.37); while only slightly preferring

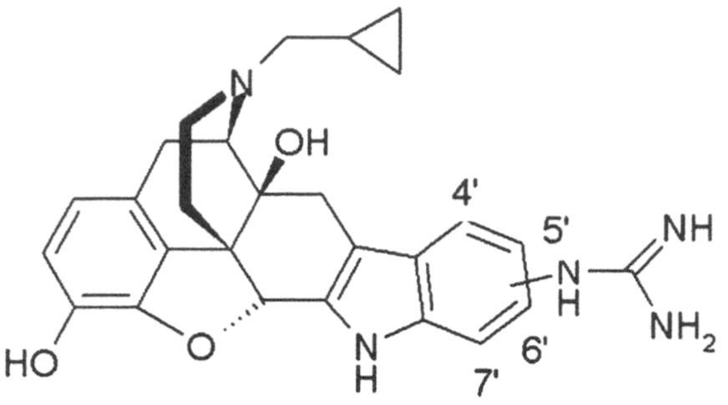

(12) 5'-guanidine = 5'-GNTI = GNTI
(73) 4'-guanidine = 4'-GNTI
(74) 6'-guanidine = 6'-GNTI
(75) 7'-guanidine = 7'-GNTI

Fig. 25.28 Structures of guanidinenaltrindole positional isomers.

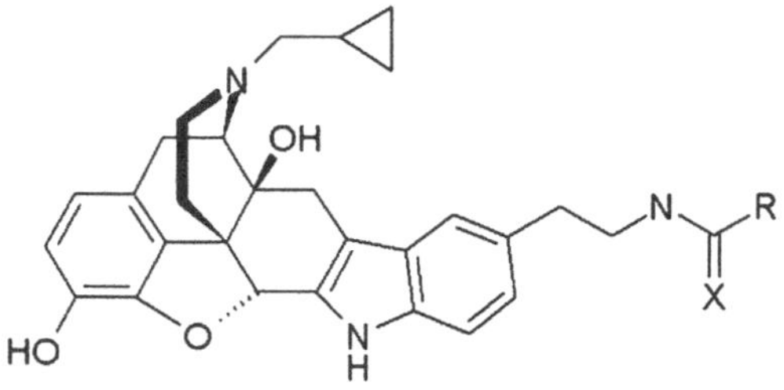

(76) X = O, R = Ethyl
(77) X = O, R = Propyl
(78) X = O, R = Butyl
(79) X = NH, R = Methyl
(80) X = NH, R =Ethyl
(81) X = NH, R =Propyl
(82) X = NH, R =n-butyl
(83) X = NH, R =iso-butyl

Fig. 25.29 Structures of amide and amidine guanidinenaltrindole analogs.

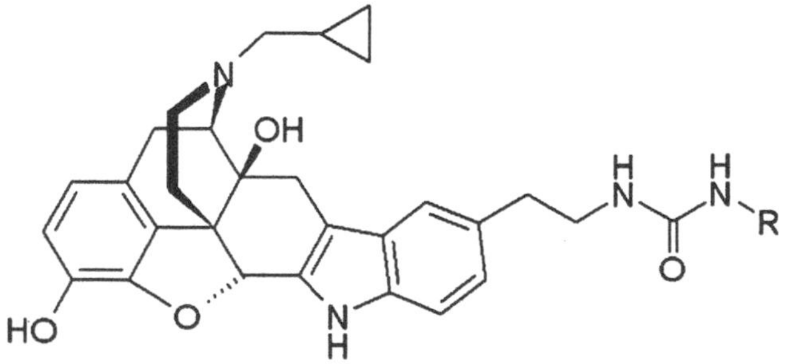

(84) R = ethyl
(85) R = n-butyl
(86) R = n-hexyl

Fig. 25.30 Structures of urea guanidinenaltrindole analogs.

[^{35}S]GTPγS (K_i = 1.0, 6.1, and 6.5 nM for kappa, mu, and delta, respectively), this compound (**110**) serves as another lead compound in the development of future kappa opioid antagonists.

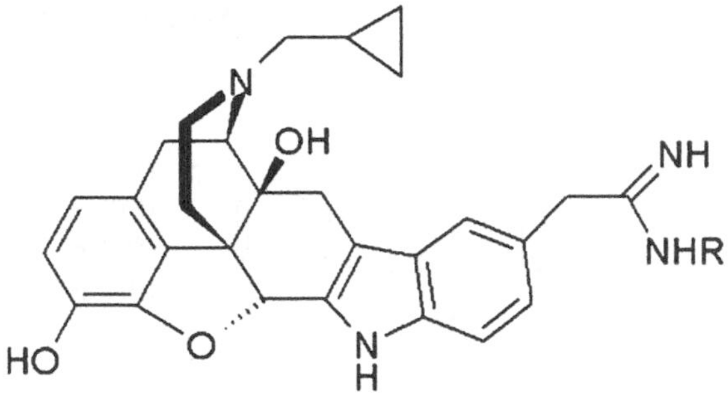

(87) R = *n*-propyl
(88) R = *n*-pentyl
(89) R = *n*-heptyl

Fig. 25.31 Structures of amidine guanidinenaltrindole analogs.

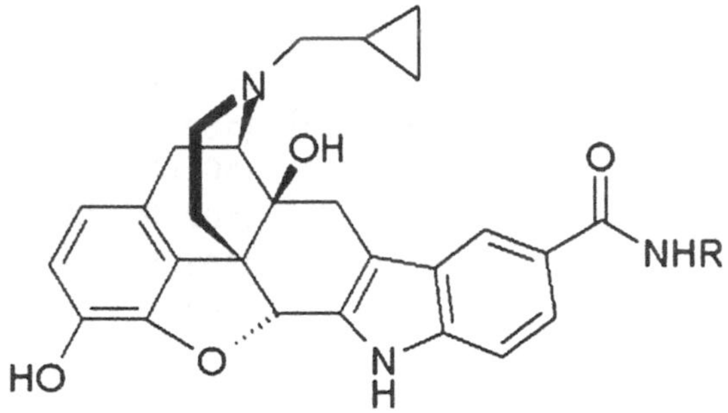

(90) R = *n*-heptyl
(91) R = Benzyl
(92) R = Phenethyl
(93) R = (CH₂)₄Ph
(94) R = *p*-MeO-Benzyl

Fig. 25.32 Structures of amide guanidinenaltrindole analogs.

Table 25.11 Antagonist Activities in the [^{35}S]GTPγS assay in Human Recombinant Receptors in CHO cells[*,54]

| Antagonist | K_i (nM) | | | μ/κ | δ/κ |
	(κ)	(μ)	(δ)		
norBNI (11)	0.04	18.9	4.42	484	113
76	0.48	4.94	0.38	10	1
77	0.35	3.17	0.30	9	1
78	0.46	3.37	0.23	7	0.5
79	0.21	3.78	1.79	18	9
80	0.24	4.70	1.77	20	7
81	0.18	4.21	1.89	23	11
82	0.17	5.33	3.31	31	20
83	0.32	14.73	5.23	46	16
84	2.47	1.60	0.65	0.6	0.3
85	1.52	1.63	0.53	1	0.3
86	1.71	1.79	1.04	1	0.6
87	0.05	3.19	4.41	64	88
88	0.21	5.61	3.83	27	18
89	0.37	2.04	5.83	6	16
90	0.29	6.86	6.95	24	24
91	0.73	4.40	2.99	6	4
92	0.17	2.70	1.21	16	7
93	0.26	2.78	5.15	10	20
94	0.28	0.94	6.20	3	22

[*]CHO indicates Chinese hamster ovary; norBNI, norbinaltorphimine.

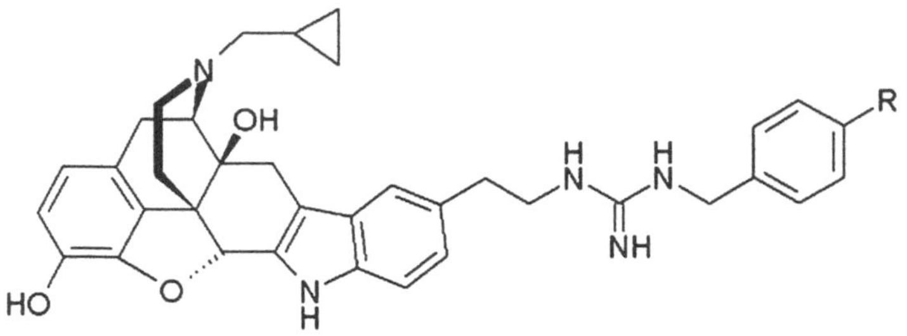

R (95) R = H
   (96) R = Cl
   (97) R = NO$_2$
   (98) R = NH$_2$

Fig. 25.33 Structures of substituted guanidinenaltrindole analogs.

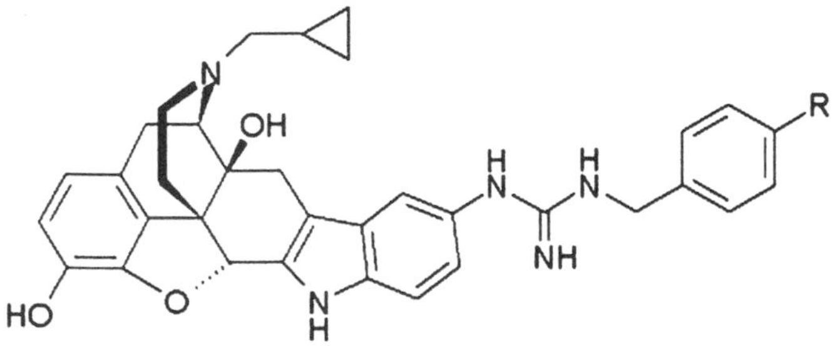

(99) R = H
(100) R = Cl
(101) R = NO$_2$
(102) R = NH$_2$
(103) R = OH
(104) R = m OH

Fig. 25.34 Structures of substituted guanidinenaltrindole analogs.

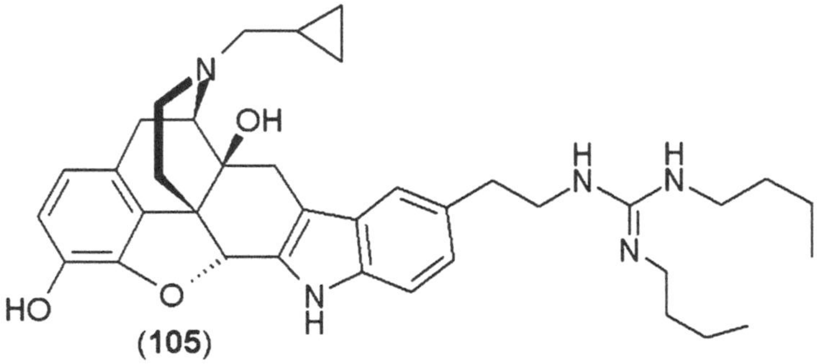

(105)

Fig. 25.35 Structures of di-substituted guanidinenaltrindole analogs.

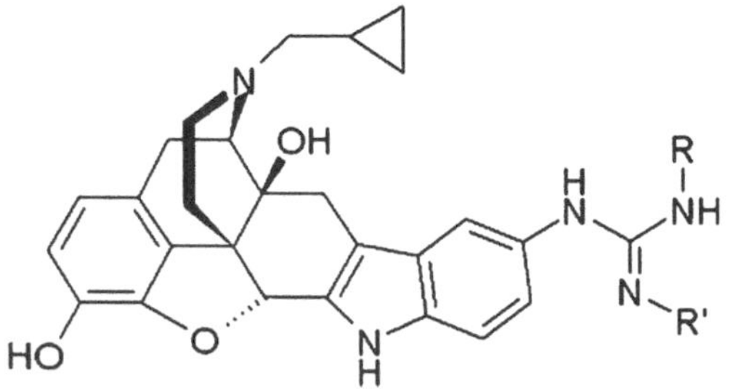

(106) R = R' = n-butylH
(107) R = R' = n-propyl
(108) R = n-propyl, R' = CPM
(109) R = benzyl, R' = CPM

Fig. 25.36 Structures of di-substituted guanidinenaltrindole analogs.

Table 25.12 Antagonist Potency in the [^{35}S]GTPγS assay in Cloned Human Opioid Receptors[*,55]

Antagonist	K_i (nM)			μ/κ	δ/κ
	(κ)	(μ)	(δ)		
norBNI (11)	0.04	18.9	4.42	484	113
GNTI (12)	0.04	3.23	15.49	81	389
60	0.40	1.25	0.88	3	2
95	0.13	2.94	1.36	23	10
96	0.23	2.61	1.48	11	6
97	0.17	2.20	1.34	13	8
98	0.25	1.57	0.95	6	4
99	0.06	1.41	4.09	24	68
100	0.14	5.24	7.67	37	55
101	0.18	3.71	16.66	21	93
102	0.09	1.22	10.80	14	120
103	0.10	12.66	18.31	127	183
104	0.13	4.28	4.35	33	33
105	0.39	4.62	1.05	12	3
106	0.44	5.66	5.24	13	12
107	0.26	4.59	2.43	18	9
108	0.08	3.26	6.31	41	79
109	0.17	2.75	3.28	16	19

* norBNI indicates norbinaltorphimine; GNTI, guanidinonaltrindole.

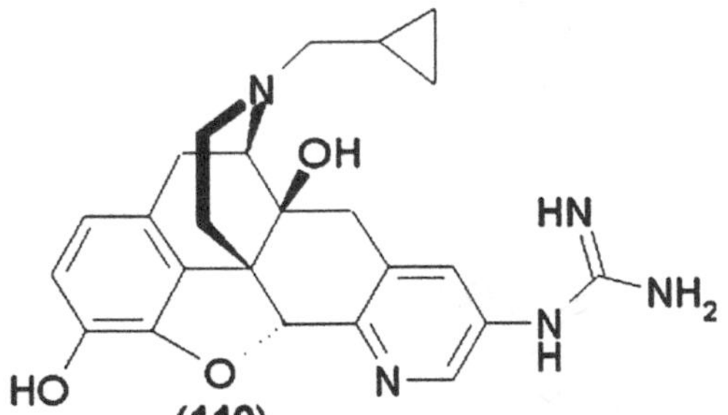

Fig. 25.37 Structure of pyridomorphinan guanidinenaltrindole analog.

The results from the indolomorphinan analogs seem to confirm the SAR found in the norBNI analogs (single pharmacophore, 2 basic nitrogens, spacing ring[s], phenolic hydroxyl), also adding, perhaps, that increasing the basicity of the second basic nitrogen leads to increased potency, as suggested by compounds **12, 58, 67**.

Non-Epoxymorphinans

In 2001 Carroll's group presented the phenylpiperidine-based, selective kappa opioid antagonist JDTic (**111**) (Fig. 25.38), a trans-(3R,4R)-dimethyl-4-(3-hydroxyphenyl)piperidine (Thomas et al[57]). While many 4-phenylpiperidine N-substituted derivatives have been previously prepared,[58,59] none were selective kappa opioid receptor antagonists until JDTic (**111**). JDTic (**111**) was based on a previous nonselective compound (**112**) that was kappa preferring (Table 25.13). The same group followed this discovery with the publication of a series of phenyl-morphan kappa opioid antagonists[60] (**113–117**) (Fig. 25.39); the best (**113**) was similar, but less potent than norBNI (kappa antagonist K_e = 0.24 and 0.04 nM, respectively, in the [^{35}S]GTPγS assay with cloned human opioid receptors). In a follow-up SAR study of the JDTic pharmacophore, a series of compounds[41] (**118– 126**) (Figs. 25.40 and 25.41) (Table 25. 14) was presented that highlighted the necessity for 2 basic nitrogens, similar to norBNI (**11**) and GNTI (**12**), and for and 2 phenolic hydroxyls for kappa opioid antagonist activity in the [^{35}S]GTPγS assay. In another study, Carroll presented a comparison of the dehydroxy analogs of norBNI (**45**) and JDTic (**111**) (Thomas et al[49]) (Table 25. 15). This analysis showed both compounds lose potency when the second hydroxyl group is deleted from their structure. Husbands recently presented a series of amino tetralin derivatives (Grundt et al[61]) (**127–141**) (Fig. 25.42) that produced a nonselective kappa opioid antagonist (**141**) (Table 25. 16). This work is similar to that of Thomas et al,[59] which produced the kappa opioid antagonist (**112**) and led to the development of the selective kappa opioid antagonist JDTic (**111**). These results likely indicate the amino tetralin pharmacophore is poised for development of selective kappa opioid antagonists.

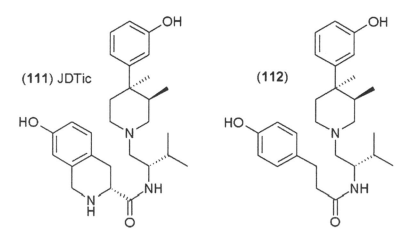

Fig. 25.38 Structures of JDTic and its lead compound.

Table 25.13 Antagonist Potency in the [^{35}S]GTPγS assay in Guinea Pig Caudate Membranes[57]

	K_i (nM)				
Antagonist	(κ)	(μ)	(δ)	μ/κ	δ/κ
norBNI (**11**)	0.038	16.7	10.2	439	268
JDTic (**111**)	0.02	2.16	>300	108	>15000
112	4.7	7.25	450	1.5	96

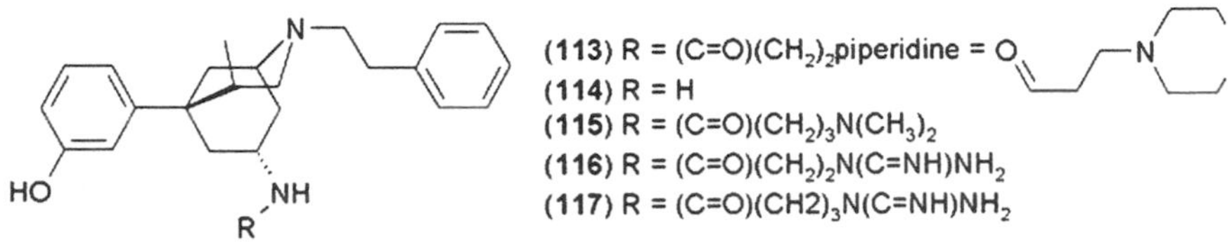
HO
NH
R
N
(113) R = (C=O)(CH$_2$)$_2$piperidine = O
N
(114) R = H
(115) R = (C=O)(CH$_2$)$_3$N(CH$_3$)$_2$
(116) R = (C=O)(CH$_2$)$_2$N(C=NH)NH$_2$
(117) R = (C=O)(CH2)$_3$N(C=NH)NH$_2$

Fig. 25.39 Structures of phenylmorphan JDTic analogs.

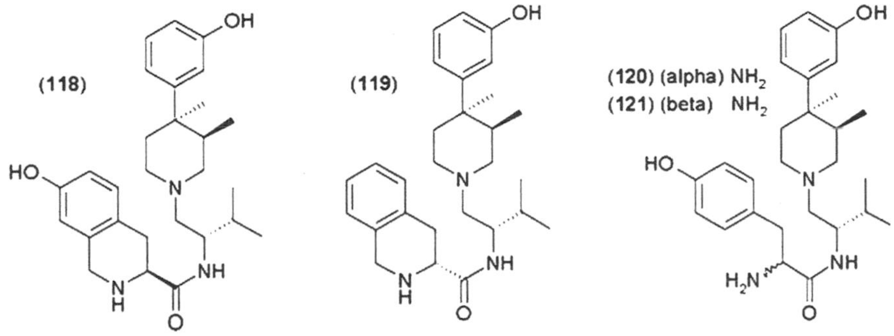
(118)
(119)
(120) (alpha) NH$_2$
(121) (beta) NH$_2$
OH
HO
N
NH
H
O
H$_2$N

Fig. 25.40 Structures of JDTic analogs.

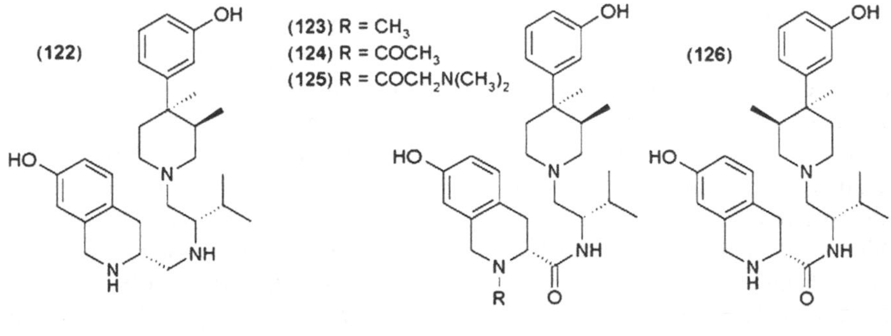
(122)
(123) R = CH$_3$
(124) R = COCH$_3$
(125) R = COCH$_2$N(CH$_3$)$_2$
(126)
OH
HO
N
NH
H
R
O

Fig. 25.41 Structures of JDTic analogs.

Table 25.14 Antagonist Potency in the [^{35}S]GTPγS assay in Guinea Pig Caudate Membranes[*,29]

Antagonist	K_e (nM)			μ/κ	δ/κ
	(κ)	(μ)	(δ)		
norBNI (**11**)	0.038	16.7	10.2	440	268
JDTic (**111**)	0.02	2.16	>300	108	>15000
112	4.7	7.25	450	1.5	96
118	4.2	11	327	2.6	78
119	11.5	68.6	147	5.9	12.8
120	44.6	12	334	0.3	7.5
121	30	16.5	452	0.55	15
122	0.20	12.8	>300	64	>15000
123	0.37	12.7	>300	34	810
124	19.6	17.4	>300	0.9	15
125	0.16	29	628	181	3925
126	16.7	178	>300	10.7	>18

*norBNI indicates norbinaltorphimine.

Table 25.15 Antagonist Potency in the [^{35}S]GTPγS assay in Guinea Pig Caudate Membranes[*,49]

Antagonist	K_i (nM)			μ/κ	δ/κ
	(κ)	(μ)	(δ)		
norBNI (**11**)	0.038	16.7	10.2	439	268
45	0.13	5.55	>300 nM	43	>2307
JDTic (**111**)	0.02	2.16	>300	108	>15000
110	11.5	68.6	213	6	18
119	4.7	7.25	450	1.5	96

*norBNI indicates norbinaltorphimine.

Irreversible Kappa Opioid Antagonists, UPHIT and DIPPA

In an effort to develop site-directed affinity labels of the kappa opioid receptor, the Rice group (de Costa et al[62]) discovered UPHIT (**142**) (Fig. 25.43). UPHIT (**142**) was based on their previous compound[63] (**143**) that was able to irreversibly inhibit [^{3}H]U69,593 binding to kappa opioid receptors with an IC$_{50}$ of 100 nM, but was unable to irreversibly inhibit kappa opioid receptors when administered intracerebroventricularly (i.c.v.). Based on the design of U50,488 (**144**), a potent selective kappa opioid agonist, UPHIT contains an isothiocyanate acetylating group and was able to irreversibly inhibit 98% specific binding of [^{3}H]U69,593 to guinea pig kappa opioid receptors compared with control when 100 μg was administered i.c.v.[62] Portoghese's group followed UPHIT (**142**) with DIPPA (**145**) (Fig. 25.44) (Chang et al[64,65]), which also contained an isothiocyanate acetylating group, though located on a different portion of the molecule. DIPPA (**145**) displayed irreversible kappa opioid antagonism in vitro, B_{max} (fmol/mg) [^{3}H]U69,593 of 3.55 (87% decrease in number of [^{3}H]U69,593 binding sites) and kappa opioid agonism in the GPI and MVD (IC$_{50}$ = 23.8 and 14.9 nM, respectively). DIPPA (**145**) also displayed kappa opioid agonism in vivo with an ED$_{50}$ ratio of 16.7 at

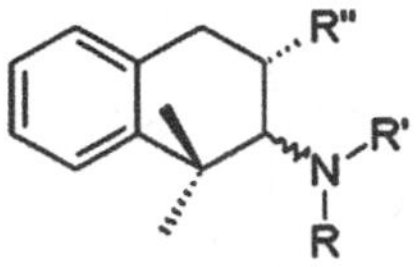

	R	R'	R"
127	CH₃	CH₃	H
128	n-propyl	H	H
129	n-propyl	CH₃	H
130	n-propyl	n-propyl	H
131	cyclopropylmethyl (CPM)	H	H
132	CPM	CH₃	H
133	CPM	CPM	H
134	allyl	H	H
135	allyl	CH₃	H
136	allyl	allyl	H
137	Cinnamyl	H	H
138	Cinnamyl	CH₃	H
139	Cinnamyl	Cinnamyl	H
140	(N is β) H	(N is β) H	OCH₃
141	(N is β) H	(N is β) Cinnamyl	OCH₃

CPM = cyclopropyl methyl

Fig. 25.42 Structures of aminotetralins.

Table 25.16 Antagonist Potency in the [^{35}S]GTPγS assay in Human Cloned Opioid Receptors*,[61]

Antagonist	K$_i$ (nM)		
	(κ)	(μ)	(δ)
norBNI (11)	0.039	18.9	4.42
NTX (9)	1.86	0.59	5.44
NTI (5)	4.95	4.26	0.11
137	42.7	67.7	NT
140	49.3	agonist	NT
141	2.12	2.62	26.3

*norBNI indicates norbinaltorphimine; NTI, naltrindole; NTX, naltrexone.

kappa opioid receptors [(ED$_{50}$ of DIPPA [1.53 μmol] in norBNI [11] treated mice [norBNI dose of 12.25 μmol/kg s.c. 3.5 hours before DIPPA] divided by the control ED$_{50}$) (ED$_{50}$ ratio 1.25 and 3.03 for mu [β-FNA] and delta [NTI] receptors)] in the mouse abdominal stretch assay.[65] However DIPPA (**145**) also displayed

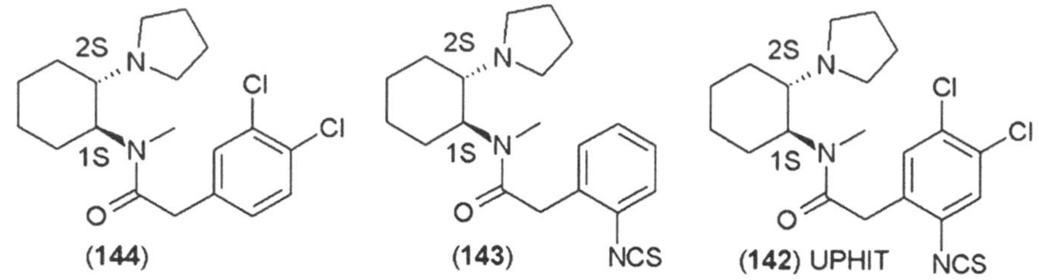

Fig. 25.43 Structures of UPHIT and analogs.

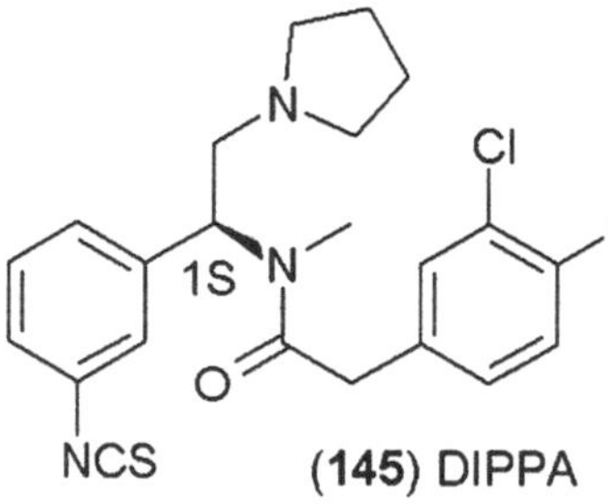

Fig. 25.44 Structure of DIPPA.

kappa opioid antagonism in the tail flick assay with an ED_{50} ratio of 9.1 (U50,488) at kappa receptors compared with 1.8 for mu (morphine) and 1.3 for delta (DPDPE) receptors.[65] The in vivo kappa opioid effects appeared to be short-term agonism (peak at one-half hour, duration less than 4 hours), followed by long-term antagonism (peak at 4 hours, duration of 48 hours).[65] Portoghese notes (Change et al[64]) that β-chlornaltrexamine (β-CNA) (another affinity label, for mu opioid receptors) also displays short-term agonism followed by long-term antagonism.

Additional Information

While in review, an article was published by the Husbands group detailing additional information about the norBNI pharmacophore (Chauvignac et al[66]). This work showed that benzylation of the pyrrole nitrogen in norBNI (**11**) and its 17, 17 -diNmethyl analog (**16**) produced compounds with mu opioid partial agonism. This was a change in efficacy for the benzylated norBNI (**146**) (Fig. 25.45), which displayed mu opioid partial agonism in the [^{35}S]GTPγS assay (EC_{50} 187 nM, 38% stimulation) and also some kappa opioid partial agonism (EC_{50} 1906 nM, 29% stimulation). The 17, 17 -diNmethyl analog (**147**) had increase potency in the [^{35}S]GTPγS assay EC_{50} 526 nM, compared with EC_{50} 1388 nM for compound **16**.

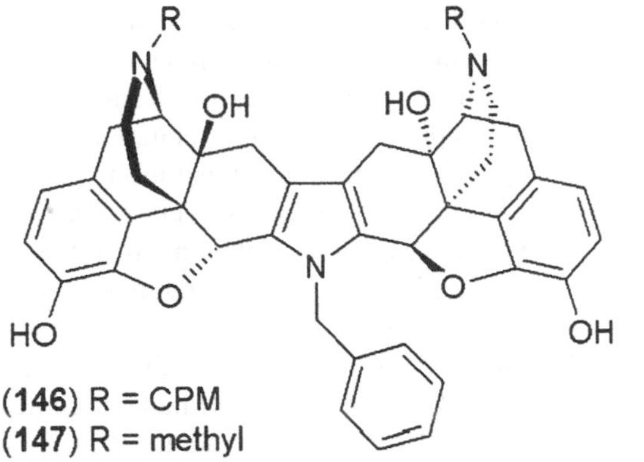

(146) R = CPM
(147) R = methyl

Fig. 25.45 Structures of benzylated norBinaltorphimine analogs.

These findings represent a significant addition to the pharmacophore of norBNI-based analogs.

Time Course of Kappa Opioid Receptor Antagonists

Two interesting characteristics of currently described kappa opioid receptor antagonists are their delay in onset of action and their long duration of action. Both norBNI and GNTI display these characteristics, and recently JDTic has been confirmed as having a similarly long duration of action and delayed onset of action.

All 3 kappa opioid antagonists (norBNI, GNTI, JDTic) show a delay in the onset of their effects as kappa opioid antagonists. The slow onset of kappa opioid antagonists is discussed by Negus et al[67] as "unusual among opioid antagonists … For comparison, the mu-[and kappa] selective opioid antagonist quadazocine and the delta-selective opioid antagonist naltrindole produce their peak effects in less than one hour, and these antagonist effects lasted less than one day." Citing other articles,[68,69] GNTI,[67] JDTic,[70] and norBNI[71] all produce their peak effects after 24 hours. GNTI did not alter the ED_{50} of morphine after 1 hour or 1 day[67] and norBNI is not selective for kappa antagonism over mu opioid antagonism until after 24 hours.[72,73]

NorBNI has been reported to have various long durations of action when administered peripherally and centrally in several different species. In peripheral administration, norBNI produced the following results. In one study[72] male ddY mice were administered norBNI subcutaneously (s.c.) and retained kappa antagonistic actions in the tail pinch test for as long as 4 and 8 days (no end time limit reported). In another study,[71] rhesus monkeys were administered norBNI s.c. and experienced kappa opioid antagonism as long as 14 and 21 days in the tail withdrawal assay. A third study[73] reports after administration of norBNI s.c., male NIH mice experienced kappa opioid antagonism for at least 4 weeks in the writhing assay, but did not retain kappa opioid antagonist effects at 8 weeks. In a fourth study, administration of norBNI s.c. to rhesus monkeys significantly blocked U-50,488 (kappa opioid agonist) attenuation of morphine-induced scratching through 21 days after norBNI administration.[74] Upon central administration, norBNI also displays a long duration of action. One study[75] showed that Sprague-Dawley rats experienced kappa antagonism, after intracisternal (i.c.) administration of norBNI, at 1, 7, and 21 days in the paw-lick and hot-plate tests. Another study[76] reports kappa opioid antagonism after i.c.v. administration of nor-BNI in male ICR mice for up to 28 days in the tail flick test. A study in Sprague-Dawley rats[10] showed that i.c.v. norBNI had antidepressant-like activity in the forced swim test at 48 and 72 hours after administration, which was similar to and directly compared with GNTI. A third study[77] reports that rhesus monkeys administered norBNI i.c. experienced kappa opioid antagonism 49 days after administration in the tail withdrawal assay. In a study conducted with pigeons, norBNI was ineffective at 1 hour, displayed a 3-fold reduction in kappa agonist potency at 8 days, a 10-fold reduction in agonist potency between 2 and 3 weeks, with control sensitivity returning only at 112 days.[78] These studies show that the duration of a single, smallest effective dose of norBNI is on the order of weeks in rats, mice, and monkeys, and months in pigeons.

GNTI and JDTic also demonstrate long durations of action. A study[67] showed rhesus monkeys receiving intramuscular (i.m.) GNTI experienced significant kappa antagonism at 2 days, lasted as long as 10 days in some of the monkeys, and returned to control in 14 days in the schedule controlled behavior assay. GNTI also displays a long duration of action when administered centrally. A study in Sprague-Dawley rats[10] showed that i.c.v. GNTI had antidepressant like activity in the forced swim test at 48 and 72 hours after administration, which was similar to and directly compared with nor-BNI. JDTic (Fig. 25.2) was reported to have a long duration of action, which is comparable with GNTI.[67] This initial report[67] was confirmed in a recent study[70] that showed JDTic (p.o. or s.c.) had kappa opioid antagonist effects at 24 hours, 7 days, and 28 days in male ICR mice in the tail flick test. In the same study, JDTic showed that when given to squirrel monkeys i.m., they displayed a right shift in the antinociceptive (shock titration) ED_{50} of U50,488 (a kappa opioid agonist) up to 10 days after administration. Also in this same paper, JDTic and norBNI both showed significant reduction of U50,488-induced diuresis in Sprague-Dawley rats up to 3 weeks.

In Vivo Effects

NorBNI has demonstrated selective kappa opioid antagonism of antinociceptive responses in the tail flick assay in mice i.c.v.[76,79] and s.c.,[79] in the mouse antiwrithing assay i.c.v[72,79] and s.c.,[73] in the tail withdraw assay in rhesus monkeys i.c.[77] and s.c[71], in the hot plate test in rats i.c.,[75] and in the tail pinch assay in mice s.c.[72] NorBNI has also suppressed kappa opioid agonist–induced diuresis in the rat s.c.[80] and i.c.[81] BNI demonstrated selective kappa opioid antagonist activity in the mouse writing assay 90 minutes pretreatment time.[29]

JDTic has demonstrated[70] selective kappa opioid antagonism of antinociceptive responses in the mouse tail flick test p.o. or s.c., shock titration assay in squirrel monkeys i.m., and also suppressed kappa opioid agonist–induced diuresis s.c. in rats.

Potentially the most exciting work with kappa opioid antagonists has been their effects on the behaviors induced by the administration of cocaine. Experimentally naive rats pretreated (48 hours) with s.c. norBNI had decreased intake of cocaine when offered at reinforcement threshold level, but not when cocaine was presented at higher, double-threshold level, doses.[9] In one study, the aversive effects of cocaine-conditioned place preference were blocked in rats pretreated with norBNI, which had also been given herpes simplex virus vector delivering cAMP response element binding protein (HSV-CREB).[82] In a following study,[83] rats given HSV-CREB and treated with norBNI displayed increased latencies to become immobile in the forced swim test, which were similar to rats given HSV-mCREB, which downregulates dynorphin production, and sham surgery (indicating an antidepressant effect of norBNI). Another study presented data that demonstrated mice pretreated with norBNI and exposed to stress via the forced swim test did not develop increased sensitivity to cocaine-conditioned place preference testing, which non-norBNI–treated mice developed,[84] again indicating an antidepressant-like effect of norBNI.

Another exciting area where kappa opioid antagonists are being explored as therapeutic agent is their potential use in the treatment of depression. The kappa opioid antagonists norBNI i.c.v., GNTI i.c.v., and ANTI intraperitoneal (i.p.) all displayed antidepressant-like activity in the forced swim test.[10] A recent study[85] of norBNI, administered s.c. in male CD1 mice, showed no effect in the forced swim test, however, it must be noted that norBNI was administered only 30 minutes before the test, a time when norBNI is not effective as a selective kappa opioid antagonist.[71-73] A study of norBNI in Sprague-Dawley rats showed an antidepressant-like effect in the learned helplessness model when norBNI was injected i.c.v., and intra-accumbens, but not when injected into the hippocampus (all trials conducted 3 days after injection).[86] Another study of norBNI showed an antidepressant effect in the learned helplessness model when injected into the hippocampus and the nucleus accumbens of male Sprague-Dawley rats.[87]

Scratching behavior has also been attributed to administration of kappa opioid antagonists. In one study,[88] norBNI administered s.c. produced dose-dependant scratching behavior (at the injection site) in IRC mice beginning within 5 minutes of injection and disappeared within 2 hours. This effect was dose-dependently reversed with both a histamine antagonist (chlorpheniramine) and a kappa agonist (U-50,488).[88] In another study,[89] GNTI administered s.c. to male Swiss mice precipitated frenzied scratching (at the site of injection) within 5 minutes, which tapered off between 40 and 80 minutes. This behavior was decreased by pretreatment with both centrally active (enadoline) and peripherally active (ICI 204448) kappa opioid agonists. Additionally the study indicated that i.c.v. and intrathecal (i.t.) administration of GNTI did not produce the scratching behavior. Other studies indicate that norBNI did not affect scratching behavior. When norBNI was administered s.c. to male ICR mice there was no scratching effect noted after 24 hours,[90] but no description was given for the prior 24-hour time period immediately following the injection of norBNI. When norBNI was administered to rhesus monkeys s.c. there were no scratching responses detected in the 3 hours following injection and also none 24 hours after administration.[91] This administration of s.c. norBNI significantly blocked U-50,488 attenuation of morphine-induced scratching for a period 21 days after norBNI administration.[91] Another study in which norBNI was administered i.c.v. to male ddY mice, notes that norBNI treatment did not affect scratching behavior.[92] Taken together, these studies suggest that administration of a s.c. dose of kappa opioid antagonist may produce scratching behavior, however this behavior occurs during a time period (immediately following injection) when kappa opioid antagonist effects are inconsistent. After a time period of 24 hours or more after administration, when kappa opioid antagonists display kappa opioid antagonistic effects, there has been no induction of scratching behavior reported.

Feeding behavior is another area where kappa opioid antagonists have been studied for their impact. NorBNI has produced the following: reduction of butorphanol-induced feeding in male Sprague-Dawley rats,[93] reduction in weight and food intake in lean and obese Zucker rats,[94] reduction of deprivation-induced food intake in rats,[95] reduction of sucrose intake in sham-fed rats,[96] reduction of GABA agonist–induced feeding in male Sprague-Dawley rats,[97] reduction of NPY-induced feeding in male Sprague-Dawley rats,[98] reduction of glucose solution intake in female Long-Evans rats.[99] GNTI has been shown to reduce U50,488-, DAMGO-, and deprivation-induced feeding behavior in rats.[11]

Both norBNI and GNTI have been explored in various other pharmacological models. NorBNI has also been studied for various other effects on systems including enhancement of morphine-induced sensitization in the rat,[100] the hypothalamic pituitary-axis,[101] modulation of morphine-induced reward,[102] instrumental learning in the spinal cord,[103] decrease of THC-induced place aversion,[104] reversal of kappa opioid agonist–induced increases of [^{35}S]GTPγS binding,[105] enhanced binding in butorphanol-dependent rats,[106] enhancement of noradrenalin release,[107] kappa opioid inhibitory tone,[108] the enhancement of allodynia,[109] antagonism of kappa opioid agonist induced hypothermia,[110] antagonism of the effects of kappa agonist anticonvulsant effects in the maximum electroshock seizure model,[111] increases in the activity of tuberohypophysial dopamine neurons in male Long-Evans rats,[112] effects on the heart,[113-115] attenuation of the discriminative stimulus effects of kappa agonists in squirrel monkeys,[116] and attenuation of kappa agonist–induced food-reinforced responding in pigeons[78,117] and rats.[118]

GNTI has been studied for its effects on systems including: the enhancement of allodynia,[109] antagonism of the effects of kappa opioid agonists in schedule controlled behavior in rhesus monkeys,[67] and antagonism of the discriminative stimulus effects of salvinorin A (a kappa opioid agonist) in rhesus monkeys.[30]

Conclusions

Selective kappa opioid antagonists have been sought since the discovery of multiple opioid receptor types in the 1970s. Several compounds with kappa opioid selective pharmacology are now available for further research and numerous lead compounds have been presented that provide excellent candidates for future development. The structure activity relationships of the currently known selective kappa opioid antagonists indicate the need for a traditional antagonist pharmacophore that contains a second basic nitrogen. The pharmacology of the selective kappa opioid antagonists shows a delay in onset of action, a very long duration of action, and presents various possibilities for the treatment of human disease states.

Acknowledgments We wish to thank the National Institute on Drug Abuse for providing funds for our opioid studies (DA-13583). We also wish to thank Christopher Cunningham and Susan Gillenberger for their kind reading and commentary on this manuscript.

References

1. Wang JB, Johnson PS, Persico AM, Hawkins AL, Griffin CA, Uhl GR. Human mu opiate receptor – cDNA and genomic clones, pharmacologic characterization and chromosomal assignment. *FEBS Lett.* 1994;338:217-222.
2. Mansson E, Bare L, Yang D. Isolation of a human kappa opioid receptor cDNA from placenta. *Biochem Biophys Res Commun.* 1994;202:1431-1434.
3. Kieffer BL, Befort K, Gavriaux-Ruff C, Hirth CG. The opioid receptor: isolation of a cDNA by expression cloning and pharmacological characterization. *Proc Natl Acad Sci USA.* 1992;89:12048-12052.
4. Peters GR, Gaylor S. Human central nervous system (CNS) effects of a selective kappa opioid agonist [abstract] *Clin Pharmacol Ther.* 1989;45:130.
5. Casy AF, Parfitt RT. *Opioid Analgesics.* New York and London: Plenum Press; 1986.
6. Schmidhammer H. Opioid receptor antagonists. *Prog Med Chem.* 1998;35:83-132.
7. Coop A, Rice KC. Role of delta-opioid receptors in biological processes. *Drug News Perspect.* 2000;13:481-487.
8. Rees DC. Chemical structures and biological activities of non-peptide selective kappa opioid ligands. *Prog Med Chem.* 1992;29:109-139.
9. Kuzmin AV, Gerrits MAFM, Van Ree JM. Kappa-opioid receptor blockade with nor-binaltorphimine modulates cocaine self-administration in drug-naïve rats. *Eur J Pharmacol.* 1998;358:197-202.
10. Mague SD, Pliakas AM, Todtenkopf MS, et al. Antidepressant-like effects of kappa-opioid receptor antagonists in the forced swim test in rats. *J Pharmacol Exp Ther.* 2003;305:323-330.
11. Jewett DC, Grace MK, Jones RM, Billington CJ, Portoghese PS, Levine AS. The kappa-opioid antagonist GNTI reduces U50,488-, DAMGO-, and deprivation-induced feeding, but not butorphanol- and neuropeptide-Y-induced feeding in rats. *Brain Res.* 2001;909:75-80.
12. Roth BL, Baner K, Westkaemper R, et al. Salvinorin A: a potent naturally occurring nonnitrogenous kappa opioid selective agonist. *Proc Natl Acad Sci USA.* 2002;99:11934-11939.
13. Schmidhammer H. Opioid receptor antagonists. *Prog Med Chem.* 1998;35:83-132.
14. Bennett MA, Murray TF, Aldrich JV. Identification of arodyn, a novel acetylated dynorphin A-(1–11) analogue, as a κ opioid receptor antagonist. *J Med Chem.* 2002;45:5617-5619.

15. Weltrowska G, Lu Y, Lemieux C, Chung NN, Schiller PW. A novel cyclic enkephalin analogue with potent opioid antagonist activity. *Bioorg Med Chem Lett.* 2004;14:4731-4733.
16. Aldrich JV. Analgesics. In: Abraham DJ, ed. *Burger's Medicinal Chemistry and Drug Discovery, Volume 6, Nervous System Agents.* 6th ed. New York: John Wiley and Sons; 2003:329-482.
17. Cowan A, Lewis JW. *Buprenorphine: Combatting Drug Abuse with a Unique Opioid.* New York: John Wiley and Sons; 1995.
18. Devi LA. Heterodimerization of G-protein-coupled receptors: pharmacology, signaling, and trafficking. *Trends Pharmacol Sci.* 2001;22:532-537.
19. Rusovici DE, Negus SS, Mello NK, Bidlack JM. κ-opioid receptors are differentially labeled by arylacetamides and benzomorphans. *Eur J Pharmacol.* 2004;485:119-125.
20. Zimmerman DM, Leander JD. Selective opioid receptor agonists and antagonists: research tools and potential therapeutic agents. *J Med Chem.* 1990;33:895-902.
21. Larson DL, Jones RM, Hjorth SA, Schwartz TW, Portoghese PS. Binding of norbinaltorphimine (norBNI) congeners to wild-type and mutant mu and kappa opioid receptors: molecular recognition loci for the pharmacophore and address components of kappa antagonists. *J Med Chem.* 2000;43:1573-1576.
22. Jones RM, Hjorth SA, Schwartz TW, Portoghese PS. Mutational evidence for a common κ antagonist binding pocket in the wild-type κ and mutant μ[K303E] opioid receptors. *J Med Chem.* 1998;41:4911-4914.
23. Sharma SK, Jones RM, Metzger TG, Ferguson DM, Portoghese PS. Transformation of a κ–opioid receptor antagonist to a κ–agonist by transfer of a guanidinium group form the 5'- to the 6'-position of naltrindole. *J Med Chem.* 2001;44:2073-2079.
24. Stevens WC, Jones RM, Subramanian G, Metzger TG, Ferguson DM, Portoghese PS. Potent and selective indolomorphinan antagonists of the kappa-opioid receptor. *J Med Chem.* 2000;43:2759-2769.
25. Metzger TG, Paterlini MG, Ferguson DM, Portoghese PS. Investigation of the selectivity of oxymorphone- and naltrexone-derived ligands via site directed mutagenesis of opioid receptors: exploring the 'address' recognition locus. *J Med Chem.* 2001;44:857-862.
26. Kong H, Raynor K, Yano H, Takeda J, Bell GI, Reisine T. Agonists and antagonists bind to different domanins of the cloned κ opioid receptor. *Proc Natl Acad Sci USA.* 1994;91:8042-8046.
27. Hjorth SA, Thirstrup K, Grandy DK, Schwartz TW. Analysis of selective binding epitopes for the κ-opioids receptor antagonist nor-binaltorphimine. *Mol Pharmacol.* 1995;47:1089-1094.
28. Eguchi M. Recent Advances in selective opioid receptor agonists and antagonists. *Med Res Rev.* 2004;24:182-212.
29. Portoghese PS, Lipkowski AW, Takemori AE. Binaltorphimine and nor-binaltorphimine, potent and selective κ-opioid receptor antagonists. *Life Sci.* 1987;40:1287-1292.
30. Butelman ER, Harris TJ, Kreek MJ. The plant-derived hallucinogen, salvinorin A, produces kappa-opioid agonist-like discriminative effects in rhesus monkeys. *Psychopharmacology (Berl).* 2004;172:220-224.
31. Erez M, Takemori AE, Portoghese PS. Narcotic antagonistic potency of bivalent ligands which contain β-naltrexamine. Evidence for bridging between proximal recognition sites. *J Med Chem.* 1982;25:847-849.
32. Portoghese PS, Takemori AE. TENA, a selective kappa opioid receptor antagonist. *Life Sci.* 1985;36:801-805.
33. Botros S, Lipkowski AW, Takemori AE, Portoghese PS. Investigation of the structural requirements for the κ-selective opioid receptor antagonist, 6β,6β-[ethlenebis(oxyethyleneimino)]bis[17-(cyclopropylmethyl)-4,5α-epoxymorphinan-3,14-diol] (TENA). *J Med Chem.* 1986;29:874-876.
34. Portoghese PS, Ronsisvalle G, Larson DL, Takemori AE. Synthesis and opioid antagonist potencies of naltrexamine bivalent ligands with conformationally restricted spacers. *J Med Chem.* 1986;29:1650-1653.

35. Portoghese PS, Larson DL, Sayre LM, et al. Opioid agonist and antagonist bivalent ligands. The relationship between spacer length and selectivity at multiple opioid receptors. *J Med Chem.* 1986;29:1855-1861.

36. Portoghese AS, Lipkowski AW, Takemori AE. Bimorphinans as highly selective, potent κ opioid receptor antagonists. *J Med Chem.* 1987;30:238-239.

37. Takemori AE, Portoghese PS. Selective naltrexone-derived opioid receptor antagonists. *Annu Rev Pharmacol Toxicol.* 1992;32:239-269.

38. Portoghese PS. Bivalent ligands and the message-address concept in the design of selective opioid receptor antagonists. *Trends Pharmacol Sci.* 1989;10:230-235.

39. Schwyzer R. ACTH: a short introductory review. *Ann N Y Acad Sci.* 1977;297:3-26.

40. Lin C, Takemori AE, Portoghese PS. Synthesis and κ-opioid antagonist selectivity of a nor-binaltorphimine congener. Identification of the address moiety reqired for κ-antagonist activity. *J Med Chem.* 1993;36:2412-2415.

41. Thomas JB, Atkinson RN, Vinson A, et al. Identification of (3R)-7-Hydroxy-*N*-((1S)-1-{[(3R,4R)-4-(3-hydroxyphenyl)-3,4-dimethyl-1-piperidinyl]methyl}-2-methylpropyl)-1,2,3,4-tetrahydro-3-isoquinolinecarboxamide as a novel potent and selective opioid κ receptor antagonist. *J Med Chem.* 2003;46:3127-3137.

42. Grundt P, Williams IA, Lewis JW, Husbands SM. Identification of a new scaffold for κ opioid receptor antagonism based on the 2-amino-1,1-dimethyl-7-hydroxytetralin pharmacophore. *J Med Chem.* 2004;47:5069-5075.

43. Portoghese PS, Nagase H, Takemori AE. Only one pharmacophore is required for the κ opioid antagonist selectivity of norbinaltorphimine. *J Med Chem.* 1988;31:1344-1347.

44. Portoghese PS, Nagase H, Lipkowski AW, Larson DL, Takemori AE. Binaltorphimine-related bivalent ligands and their κ opioid receptor antagonist selectivity. *J Med Chem.* 1988;31:836-841.

45. Schmidhammer H, Ganglbauer E, Mitterdorfer J, Rollinger JM, Smith CFC. Synthesis and biological evaluation of 14-alkoxymorphinans 14,14′-dimethoxy analogues of norbinaltorphimine: synthesis and determination of their κ opioid antagonist selectivity. *Helv Chim Acta.* 1990;73:1779-1783.

46. Schmidhammer H, Smith CFC. A simple and efficient method for the preparation of binaltorphimine and derivatives and determination of their κ opioid antagonist selectivity. *Helv Chim Acta.* 1989;72:675-677.

47. Portoghese PS, Garzon-Aburbeh A, Nagase H, Lin C, Takemori AE. Role of the spacer in conferring κ opioid receptor selectivity to bivalent ligands related to norbinaltorphimine. *J Med Chem.* 1991;34:1292-1296.

48. Portoghese PS, Lin C, Farouz-Grant R, Takemori AE. Structure-activity relationship of N17′substituted norbinaltorphimine congeners. Role of the N17′ basic group in the interaction with a putative address subsite on the κ opioid receptor. *J Med Chem.* 1994;37: 1495-1500.

49. Thomas JB, Fix SE, Rothman RB, et al. Importance of phenolic address groups in opioid kappa receptor selective antagonists. *J Med Chem.* 2004;47:1070-1073.

50. Marki A, Otvos F, Toth G, Hosztafi S, Borsodi A. Tritiated kappa receptor antagonist norbinaltorphimine: synthesis and in vitro binding in three different tissues. *Life Sci.* 2000;66:43-49.

51. Olmsted SL, Takemori AE, Portoghese PS. A remarkable change of opioid receptor selectivity on the attachment of a peptidomimetic κ address element to the δ antagonist, naltrindole: 5′-[(N²-alkylamidino)methyl]naltrindole derivatives as a novel class of κ opioid receptor antagonists. *J Med Chem.* 1993;36:179-180.

52. Jones RM, Portoghese PS. 5′-Guanidinonaltrindole, a highly selective and potent κ-opioid receptor antagonist. *Eur J Pharmacol.* 2000;396:49-52.

53. Jales AR, Husbands SM, Lewis JW. Selective κ-opioid antagonists related to naltrindole. Effect of side-chain spacer in the 5′-amidinoalkyl series. *Bioorg Med Chem Lett.* 2000;10:2259-2261.

54. Black SL, Jales AR, Brandt W, Lewis JW, Husbands SM. The role of the side chain in determining relative δ- and κ-affinity in C5'-substituted analogues of naltrindole. *J Med Chem.* 2003;46:314-317.
55. Black SL, Chauvignac C, Grundt P, et al. Guanidino N-substituted and N,N-disubstituted derivatives of the κ-opioid antagonist GNTI. *J Med Chem.* 2003;46:5505-5511.
56. Ananthan S, Kezar HS, Saini SK, et al. Synthesis, opioid receptor binding, and functional activity of 5'-subsitituted 17-cyclopropylmethylpyrido[2',3',:6,7]morphinans. *Bioorg Med Chem Lett.* 2003;13:529-532.
57. Thomas JB, Atkinson RN, Rothman RB, et al. Identification of the first *trans*-(3R,4R)-dimethyl-4-(3-hydroxyphenyl)piperidine derivative to possess highly potent and selective opioid κ receptor antagonist activity. *J Med Chem.* 2001;44:2687-2690.
58. Zimmerman DM, Leander JD, Cantrell BE, et al. Structure-activity relationships of *trans*-3, 4-dimethyl-4-(3-hydroxyphenyl)piperidine antagonists for μ- and κ-opioid receptors. *J Med Chem.* 1993;36:2833-2841.
59. Thomas JB, Fall MJ, Cooper JB, et al. Identification of an opioid κ receptor subtype-selective N-substituent for (+)-(3R,4R)-dimethyl-4-(3-hydroxyphenyl)piperidine. *J Med Chem.* 1998;41:5188-5197.
60. Thomas JB, Atkinson RN, Namdev N, et al. Discovery of an opioid κ receptor selective pure antagonist from a library of N-substituted 4β-methyl-5-(3-hydroxyphenyl)morphans. *J Med Chem.* 2002;45:3524-3530.
61. Grundt P, Williams IA, Lewis JW, Husbands SM. Identification of a new scaffold for opioid receptor antagonism based on the 2-amino-1,1-dimethyl-7-hydroxytetralin pharmacophore. *J Med Chem.* 2004;47:5069-5075.
62. de Costa BR, Band L, Rothman RB, et al. Synthesis of an affinity ligand ('UPHIT') for in vivo acylation of the κ-opioid receptor. *FEBS Lett.* 1989;249:178-182.
63. de Costa BR, Rothman RB, Bykov V, Jacobson AE, Rice KC. Selective and enantiospecific acylation of κ opioid receptors by (1S,2S)-*trans*-2-isothiocyanato-N-methyl-N-[2-(1-pyrrolidi nyl)cyclohecyl]benzeneacetamide. Demonstration of κ receptor heterogeneity. *J Med Chem.* 1989;32:281-283.
64. Chang AC, Takemori AE, Portoghese PS. 2-(3,4-dichlorophenyl)-N-methyl-N-[(1S)-1-(3-isothiocyanatophenyl)-2-(1-pyrrolidinyl)ethyl]acetamide: an opioid receptor affinity label that produces selective and long-lasting κ antagonism in mice. *J Med Chem.* 1994;37:1547-1549.
65. Chang AC, Takemori AE, Ojala WH, Gleason WB, Portoghese PS. κ opioid receptor selective affinity labels: electrophilic benzeneacetamides as κ-selective opioid antagonists. *J Med Chem.* 1994;37:4490-4498.
66. Chauvignac C, Miller CN, Srivastava SK, Lewis JW, Husbands SM, Traynor JR. Major effect of pyrrolic N-benzylation in norbinaltorphiminie, the selective κ-opioid receptor antagonist. *J Med Chem.* 2005;48:1676-1679.
67. Negus SS, Mello NK, Linsenmayer DC, Jones RM, Portoghese PS. Kappa opioid antagonist effects of the novel kappa antagonist 5'-guanidinonaltrindole (GNTI) in an assay of schedule-controlled behavior in rhesus monkeys. *Psychopharmacology (Berlin).* 2002;163:412-419.
68. Bertalmio AJ, Woods JH. Differentiation between *mu* and *kappa* receptor-mediated effects in opioid drug discrimination: apparent pA_2 analysis. *J Pharmacol Exp Ther.* 1987;243: 591-597.
69. Negus SS, Butelman ER, Chang KJ, DeCosta B, Winger G, Woods JH. Behavioral effects of the systemically active *delta* opioid agonist BW373U86 in rhesus monkeys. *J Pharmacol Exp Ther.* 1994;270:1025-1034.
70. Carroll I, Thomas JB, Dykstra LA, et al. Pharmacological properties of JDTic: a novel κ-opioid receptor antagonist. *Eur J Pharmacol.* 2004;501:111-119.
71. Butelman ER, Negus SS, Ai Y, deCosta BR, Woods JH. Kappa opioid antagonist effects of systemically administered nor-binaltorphimine in a thermal antinociception assay in rhesus monkeys. *J Pharmacol Exp Ther.* 1993;267:1269-1276.

72. Endoh T, Matsuura H, Tanaka C, Nagase H. Nor-binaltorphimine: a potent and selective kappa-opioid receptor antagonist with long-lasting activity in vivo. *Arch Int Pharmacodyn Ther*. 1992;316:30-42.

73. Broadbear JH, Negus SS, Butelman ER, de Costa BR, Woods JH. Differential effects of systemically administered nor-binaltorphimine (nor-BNI) on kappa-opioid agonists in the mouse writhing assay. *Psychopharmacology (Berlin)*. 1994;115:311-319.

74. Ko MCH, Lee H, Song MS, et al. Activation of κ-opioid receptors inhibits pruritus evoked by subcutaneous or intrathecal administration of morphine in monkeys. *J Pharmacol Exp Ther*. 2003;305:173-179.

75. Jones DNC, Holtzman SG. Long term kappa opioid receptor blockade following nor-binaltorphimine. *Eur J Pharmacol*. 1992;215:345-348.

76. Horan P, Taylor J, Yamamura HI, Porreca F. Extremely long-lasting antagonistic actions of nor-binaltorphimine (nor-BNI) in the mouse tail-flick test. *J Pharmacol Exp Ther*. 1992;260:1237-1243.

77. Ko MCH, Johnson MD, Butelman ER, Willmont KJ, Mosberg HI, Woods JH. Intracisternal nor-binaltorphimine distinguishes central and peripheral kappa-opioid antinociception in rhesus monkeys. *J Pharmacol Exp Ther*. 1999;291:1113-1120.

78. Jewett DC, Woods JH. Nor-binaltorphimine: a very, very long acting kappa opioid antagonist in pigeons. *Behav Pharmacol*. 1995;6:815-820.

79. Takemori AE, Ho BY, Naeseth JS, Portoghese PS. Nor-binaltorphimine, a highly selective kappa-opioid antagonist in analgesic and receptor binding assays. *J Pharmacol Exp Ther*. 1988;246:255-258.

80. Takemori AE, Schwartz MM, Portoghese PS. Suppression by nor-binaltorphimine of *kappa* opioid-mediated diuresis in rats. *J Pharmacol Exp Ther*. 1988;247:971-974.

81. Ko MCH, Willmont KJ, Lee H, Flory GS, Woods JH. Ultra-long antagonism of kappa opioid agonist-induced diuresis by intracisternal nor-binaltorphimine in monkeys. *Brain Res*. 2003;982:38-44.

82. Carlezon WA Jr, Thome J, Olson VG, et al. Regulation of cocaine reward by CREB. *Science*. 1998;282:2272-2275.

83. Pliakas AM, Carlson RR, Neve RL, Konradi C, Nestler EJ, Carlexon WA. Altered responsiveness to cocaine and increased immobility in the forced swim test associated with elevated cAMP response element-binding protein expression in nucleus accumbens. *J Neurosci*. 2001;21:7397-7403.

84. McLaughlin JP, Marton-Popovici M, Chavkin C. κ opioid receptor antagonism and prodynorphin gene disruption block stress-induced behavioral responses. *J Neurosci*. 2003;23:5674-5683.

85. Berrocoso E, Rojas-Corrales MO, Mico JA. Non-selective opioid receptor antagonism of the antidepressant-like effect of venlafaxine in the forced swimming test in mice. *Neurosci Lett*. 2004;363:25-28.

86. Newton SS, Thome J, Wallace TL, et al. Inhibition of cAMP response element-binding protein or dynorphin in the nucleus accumbens produces an antidepressant-like effect. *J Neurosci*. 2002;22:10883-10890.

87. Shirayama Y, Ishida H, Iwata M, Hazama G, Kawahara R, Duman RS. Stress increases dynorphin immunoreactivity in limbic brain regions and dynorphin antagonism produces antidepressant-like effects. *J Neurochem*. 2004;90:1258-1268.

88. Kamei J, Nagase H. Norbinaltorphimine, a selective κ opioid receptor antagonist, induces an itch-associated response in mice. *Eur J Pharmacol*. 2001;418:141-145.

89. Cowan A, Inan S, Kehner GB. GNTI, a kappa receptor antagonist, causes compulsive scratching in mice. *The Pharmacologist*. 2002;44:A51.

90. Togashi Y, Umeuchi H, Okano K, et al. Antipruritic activity of the κ-opioid receptor agonist, TRK-820. *Eur J Pharmacol*. 2002;435:259-264.

91. Ko MCH, Lee H, Song MS, et al. Activation of κ-opioid receptors inhibits pruritus evoked by subcutaneous of intrathecal administration of morphine in monkeys. *J Pharmacol Exp Ther*. 2003;305:173-179.

92. Umeuchi H, Togashi Y, Honda T, et al. Involvement of central μ-opioid system in the scratching behavior in mice, and the suppression of it by the activation of κ-opioid system. *Eur J Pharmacol*. 2003;477:29-35.

93. Levine AS, Grace M, Portoghese PS, Billington CJ. The effect of selective opioid antagonists on butorphanol-induced feeding. *Brain Res*. 1994;637:242-248.

94. Cole JL, Berman N, Bodnar RJ. Evaluation of chronic opioid receptor antagonist effects upon weight and intake measures in lean and obese zucker rats. *Peptides*. 1997;18:1201-1207.

95. Bodnar RJ, Glass MJ, Ragnauth A, Cooper ML. General, μ and κ opioid antagonists in the nucleus accumbens alter food intake under deprivation, glucoprivic and palatable conditions. *Brain Res*. 1995;700:205-212.

96. Leventhal L, Kirkham TC, Cole JL, Bodnar RJ. Selective actions of central μ and κ opioid antagonists upon sucrose intake in sham-fed rats. *Brain Res*. 1995;685:205-210.

97. Khaimova E, Kandov Y, Israel Y, Cataldo G, Hadjimarkou MM, Bodnar RJ. Opioid receptor subtype antagonists differentially alter GABA agonist-induced feeding elicited from either the nucleus accumbens shell or ventral tegmental area regions in rats. *Brain Res*. 2004;1026:284-294.

98. Kotz CM, Grace MK, Billington CJ, Levine AS. The effect of norbinaltorphimine, β-funaltrexamine and naltrindole on NPY-induced feeding. *Brain Res*. 1993;631:325-328.

99. Calcagnetti DJ, Calcagnetti RL, Fanselow MS. Centrally administered opioid antagonists, nor-binaltorphimine, 16-methyl cyprenorphine, and Mr2266, suppress intake of a sweet solution. *Pharmacol Biochem Behav*. 1990;35:69-73.

100. Spanagel R, Shippenberg TS. Modulation of morphine-induced sensitization by endogenous κ opioid systems in the rat. *Neurosci Lett*. 1993;153:232-236.

101. Williams KL, Ko MHC, Rice KC, Woods JH. Effect of opioid receptor antagonists on hypothalamic-pituitary-adrenal activity in rhesus monkeys. *Psychoneuroendocrinology*. 2003;28:513-528.

102. Narita M, Kishimoto Y, Ise Y, Yajima Y, Misawa K, Suzuki T. Direct evidence for the involvement of the mesolimbic κ-opioid system in the morphine-induced rewarding effect under an inflammatory pain-like state. *Neuropsychopharmacology*. 2005;30:111-118.

103. Joynes RL, Grau JW. Instrumental learning within the spinal cord: III. Prior exposure to noncontingent shock induces a behavioral deficit that is blocked by an opioid antagonist. *Neurobiol Learn Mem*. 2004;82:35-51.

104. Cheng HY, Laviolette SR, van der Kooy D, Penninger JM. DREAM ablation selectively alters THC place aversion and analgesia but leaves intact the motivational and analgesic effects of morphine. *Eur J Neurosci*. 2004;19:3033-3041.

105. Mizoguchi H, Leitermann RJ, Narita M, Nagase H, Suzuki T, Tseng LF. Region-dependant G-protein activation by κ-opioid receptor agonists in the mouse brain. *Neurosci Lett*. 2004;356:145-147.

106. Fan L, Tien L, Tanaka S, et al. Enhanced binding of nor-binaltorphimine to κ-opioid receptors in rats dependent on butorphanol. *J Neurosci Res*. 2003;72:781-789.

107. Cosentino M, Marino F, DePonti F, et al. Tonic modulation of neurotransmitter release in the guinea-pig myenteric plexus: effect of μ and κ opioid receptor blockade and of chronic sympathetic denervation. *Neurosci Lett*. 1995;194:185-188.

108. Ossipov MH, Kovelowski CJ, Wheeler-Aceto H, et al. Opioid antagonists and antisera to endogenous opioids increase the nociceptive response to formalin: demonstration of an opioid *kappa* and *delta* inhibitory tone. *J Pharmacol Exp Ther*. 1996;277:784-788.

109. Obara I, Mika J, Schafer MK-H, Przewlocka B. Antagonists of the κ-opioid receptor enhance allodynia in rats and mice after sciatic nerve ligation. *Br J Pharmacol*. 2003;140:538-546.

110. Baker AK, Meert TF. Functional effects of systemically administered agonists and antagonists of μ, δ, and κ opioid receptor subtypes on body temperature in mice. *J Pharmacol Exp Ther*. 2002;302:1253-1264.

111. Tortella FC, Echevarria E, Lipkowski AW, Takemori AE, Portoghese PS, Holaday JW. Selective kappa antagonist properties of nor-binaltrophimine in the rat seizure model. *Life Sci*. 1989;44:661-665.

112. Manzanares J, Lookingland KJ, LaVigne SD, Moore KE. Activation of tuberohypophysial dopamine neurons following intracerebroventricular administration of the selective kappa opioid receptor antagonist nor-binaltorphimine. *Life Sci.* 1991;48:1143-1149.
113. McIntosh M, Kane K, Parratt J. Effects of selective opioid receptor agonists and antagonists during myocardial ischaemia. *Eur J Pharmacol.* 1992;210:37-44.
114. Llobel F, Laorden ML. Effects of μ-, δ-, and κ-opioid antagonists in atrial preparations from failing human hearts. *Gen Pharmacol.* 1997;28:371-374.
115. Cao Z, Liu L, VanWinkle DM. Activation of δ- and κ-opioid receptors by opioid peptides protects cardiomyocytes via K_{ATP} channels. *Am J Physiol Heart Circ Physiol.* 2003;285: H1032-H1039.
116. Carey GJ, Bergman J. Enadoline discrimination in squirrel monkeys: effects of opioid agonists and antagonists. *J Pharmacol Exp Ther.* 2001;297:215-223.
117. Jewett DC, Woods JH. Nor-binaltorphimine: an ultra-long acting kappa-opioid antagonist in pigeons. *Behav Pharmacol.* 1995;6:815-820.
118. Picker MJ, Mathewson C, Allen RM. Opioids and rate of positively reinforced behavior: III. Antagonism by the long-lasting kappa antagonist norbinaltorphimine. *Behav Pharmacol.* 1996;7:495-504.

Chapter 26
In Vitro and Direct In Vivo Testing of Mixture-Based Combinatorial Libraries for the Identification of Highly Active and Specific Opiate Ligands

Richard A. Houghten,[1] Colette T. Dooley,[1] and Jon R. Appel[1]

Abstract The use of combinatorial libraries for the identification of novel opiate and related ligands in opioid receptor assays is reviewed. Case studies involving opioid assays used to demonstrate the viability of combinatorial libraries are described. The identification of new opioid peptides composed of L-amino acids, D-amino acids, or L-, D-, and unnatural amino acids is reviewed. New opioid compounds have also been identified from peptidomimetic libraries, such as peptoids and alkylated dipeptides, and those identified from acyclic (eg, polyamine, urea) and heterocyclic (eg, bicyclic guanidine) libraries are reviewed.

Keywords positional scanning libraries, opioid receptor, in vivo screening, mixtures, peptides, peptidomimetics

Introduction

Binding to opioid receptors was first demonstrated in 1973[1-3]; the endogenous peptides were first discovered in 1975.[4] Since then, the search for new opioid ligands with better selectivity has continued. The search for the "holy grail" of opiates—that is, an opiate ligand without the traditional side effects (addiction, tolerance, respiratory depression, etc)—is ongoing, though with diminished expectations. Thousands of analogs of the natural opioid peptides enkephalin, dynorphin, endorphin, dermenkephalin, and dermorphin have been synthesized over the past 20 years and used to determine the workings of the opioid receptor family. More recently, highly selective compounds (in most cases structurally related to the classic opiates, eg, morphine) have been identified and used as research tools. Why then would one want to identify additional compounds that interact with opioid receptors? First, the question

---

[1]Torrey Pines Institute for Molecular Studies, San Diego, CA

Corresponding Author: Richard A. Houghten, Torrey Pines Institute for Molecular Studies, 3550 General Atomics Court, San Diego, CA 92121. Tel: (858) 455-3803; Fax: (858) 455-3804; E-mail: houghten@tpims.org

R.S. Rapaka and W. Sadée (eds.), *Drug Addiction.*
© American Association of Pharmaceutical Scientists 2008

of the existence, number, and nature of subtypes of the 3 receptors remains unanswered. Two subtypes have been proposed for the mu receptor (μ_1, μ_2); delta receptor subtypes have been classified by 2 different schools of thought, into δ_1 and δ_2 by one school and δ_{cx} and δ_{ncx} by another; and subtypes reported for the kappa receptor include κ_1, κ_2, κ_3, κ_{1a}, κ_{1b}, κ_{2a}, and κ_{2b}.[5] To date, only a single gene has been identified for each of the 3 opioid receptors, mu,[6,7] delta,[8,9] and kappa.[10] While alternate splicing and posttranslational modifications may prove to be responsible for receptor subtype expression, they have yet to be verified with pharmacological data. New ligands specific for, rather than selective for, the receptor subtypes would greatly facilitate binding studies. Structurally distinct new ligands may cover the binding spectrum of a particular receptor more completely and indicate whether ligands are binding to slightly different positions on the same receptor, thus giving rise to different inhibition profiles. The inability to determine specific ligands for the receptor subtypes may indicate that the differences observed in vivo are due to postbinding events (signaling). Second, new ligands may prove more useful as tools for in vivo study. Structurally diverse ligands will aid in the study of analgesic efficacy, addiction, and tolerance and will delineate central and peripheral antinociception, thus leading to effective new analgesics or treatments for drug abuse.

This review covers the use of combinatorial libraries in opioid binding assays, from an early demonstration of the concept to recently identified peptide and nonpeptide ligands. In our own research we have used combinatorial libraries to study opioids and, conversely, have used opioid receptors to study combinatorial libraries. This approach has demonstrated that mixture-based libraries can be used with a wide range of compound classes. It has also led to the development of a more rapid means of deconvolution for the identification of a wide variety of new ligands for the opioid receptors, and as first reported herein, a proof of concept illustration of its direct use in selected in vivo assays for the identification of inherently more advanced "hits" than those identified via traditional target-based in vitro assays.

Synthetic Combinatorial Libraries

Synthetic combinatorial libraries were originally described for peptides but are now used with a wide variety of compound types; such libraries are responsible for the remarkable transformation of the manner in which new therapeutics and diagnostics are identified. The term *combinatorial* was originally applied to describe collections of compounds containing all possible combinations of the building blocks used in their preparation. "Combinatorial library" is a term now more generally used to describe collections of compounds ranging in number from a few dozen to more than 10^{12}. The first libraries described truly were combinatorial, since they represented a complete set of the compounds possible with the building blocks used and were generated either biologically (using molecular biology techniques) or synthetically. In the former, the peptide or protein diversity was presented on the surface of filamentous phage particles or plasmids.[11-13] In the latter, synthetic chemistry was used to generate a diversity of peptides attached to a solid support. The first synthetic combinatorial library described in the literature was composed of mixtures of tens to hundreds of thousands of octapeptides on plastic pins.[14] This was followed by 2 simultaneous reports in 1991, the first of which described a second immobilized method, referred to as the one bead/one peptide approach.[15] Immobilized libraries can be assayed for binding to soluble receptors (eg, antibodies). However, the vast majority of receptors are membrane-bound and cannot be readily screened with libraries attached to a support. Chemical synthesis of libraries on a solid support, which are subsequently cleaved and screened in solution, allows for a wider range of assays to be screened. This approach was first presented in the second of the 2 reports from 1991.[16,17] The ability to screen mixtures that are free in solution confers decided advantages, in that a broad spectrum of assays can be used without alteration, and the concentration of the library mixtures being screened can be varied to adjust to the needs of the particular assay.

There remain 2 schools of thought regarding the screening of combinatorial libraries: (1) screen the greatest diversity possible, primarily through the use of mixtures, or (2) screen smaller diversities, primarily through the use of parallel arrays in conjunction with high-throughput screening. Although the successful use of mixture-based libraries was presented more than a decade ago, until recently the trend in the pharmaceutical industry has been to synthesize libraries as large parallel arrays of individual compounds, which are then screened individually or in small pools. Studies performed by our own and other laboratories, however, have shown that mixture-based libraries are a rapid, cost-effective means for the identification of extremely active, highly specific individual compounds.[18]

Combinatorial libraries are synthesized using solid-phase chemistry involving the consecutive incorporation of multifunctional building blocks with orthogonal protecting groups[19,20] and contain a varied number of diversity positions. The solid support is typically polystyrene, but libraries have also been synthesized on plastic pins[14] paper,[21] cotton,[22] and silicon chips.[23] Since amide bond formation on the solid phase has been optimized through 30 years of solid-phase peptide synthesis, it has been used extensively in combinatorial synthesis.

One of 2 methods is used to generate the approximate equimolarity required for mixture-based libraries. In the first, equimolarity is achieved by mixing precoupled resins (a process termed divide-couple-recombine,[16] split synthesis,[15] or portioning-mixing[24]). In the second, mixtures of incoming reagents are used during coupling.[25] The latter method also enables incorporation of mixture positions after the defined position has been incorporated, which is critical for most positional scanning libraries.

The initial combinatorial libraries described were all peptide libraries. Because of well-developed synthetic methods, amino acids and short peptides can be used as starting materials for the synthesis of low-molecular-weight heterocyclic libraries. The ability to exhaustively transform whole libraries of compounds to libraries of entirely different pharmacophores has been developed in our laboratory.[26-31] With this approach (termed libraries from libraries), the original diversity in a library may be expanded via chemical modification of the entire library. For example, peptide libraries may be modified by exhaustive methylation of their amide bonds to yield peptidomimetics,[31] by complete reduction of the backbone amide carbonyl groups to yield polyamines,[32] or by a combination of both to obtain alkylated polyamines.

Unlike parallel array libraries, mixture-based libraries must be deconvoluted to identify active compounds. While several mixture deconvolution methods have been described, including direct sequencing, encoded tags, high-performance liquid chromatography, mass spectrometry, and orthogonal synthesis, they have not been applied to the identification of opioid ligands and thus will not be discussed further in this review. The 2 most widely used deconvolution strategies for soluble combinatorial libraries are iterative[16,17] and positional scanning.[33,34] The iterative deconvolution approach uses a step-by-step selection and enhancement process to identify individual compounds. The most active sequence in this process is thus identified by the systematic reduction in the number of compounds in the most active mixture. The positional scanning deconvolution approach is a more rapid means to gather information about all possible variable positions in a soluble mixture library and was first presented by our laboratory in 1992.[33] As an illustration of the method for a simple tetrapeptide combinatorial library, envision 4 different amino acids (D, F, I, N) incorporated at each of 4 different variable positions, resulting in 256 (4^4) possible peptides. When this diversity is arranged as a positional scanning synthetic combinatorial library (PS-SCL), 16 peptide mixtures (4 separate mixtures for each of the 4 positions) are synthesized. The 4 positional sublibraries, namely O_1XXX-NH_2, XO_2XX-NH_2, XXO_3X-NH_2, and XXXO_4-NH_2, contain all 256 peptides but differ in the arrangement of peptides within the mixtures and hence the location of the position defined. Thus, the 4 mixtures in O_1XXX-NH_2 are DXXX-NH_2, FXXX-NH_2, IXXX-NH_2, and NXXX-NH_2. Mixture DXXX-NH_2 contains the 64 peptides containing D at position 1. In sublibrary XO_2XX-NH_2 mixture XDXX-NH_2 contains the 64 peptides with D at position 2. The only peptides that mixtures DXXX-NH_2 and XDXX-NH_2 share are the 16 that have D in both positions (DDXX-NH_2). In this example, assume that the sequence FIND-NH_2 is the sole tetrapeptide having activity, with the other 255 being completely inactive. Since each positional sublibrary contains all 256 peptides, the individual tetrapeptide is present in only 1 mixture in each of the 4 positional sublibraries. Thus, the mixtures having activity will be FXXX-NH_2, XIXX-NH_2, XXNX-NH_2, and XXXD-NH_2 because of activity of FIND-NH_2. These 4 amino acids in their respective positions yield the sequence FIND in the initial screening. The corresponding peptide is then synthesized and tested for activity. It should be noted that the activity observed for each of the 4 mixtures is due to the presence of the tetrapeptide FIND-NH_2 in each mixture and is not due to the individual amino acids (F, I, N, and D) that occupy the defined positions. Often, more than 1 mixture is found to have activity at each position. Building block selection for the synthesis of individual compounds is based first on the activity of the mixture, but if there are too many possibilities, then similarities in chemical character may be used to reduce the number of individual compounds to be made. Freier and coworkers have provided an excellent discussion of the theoretical and experimental aspects of iterative and positional scanning deconvolution.[35,36]

Identification of Opioid Ligands: Case Studies Using Combinatorial Libraries

The monoclonal antibody (mAb) 3E7 raised against β-endorphin was used in many of the first screens of combinatorial libraries as a receptor of convenience. The antigenic determinant recognized by this antibody is well understood and represents the 6 residues of the N-terminal of β-endorphin, YGGFMT. This antibody is also known to bind to a variety of other related endogenous opioid ligands having similar N-terminal residues. This antigen/antibody system proved to be a good model for the early testing of library feasibility.[37] mAb 3E7 was first used in conjunction with the molecular biology approach, in which a library of peptide sequences was expressed on the N terminus of pIII, a fusion protein.[11] When a process of affinity purification termed *biopanning* was used, the enkephalin sequences YGGFM and YGGFL were not initially found, but peptides that bound with high affinity to mAb 3E7 (YGAFMQ, 13 nM) were reported. Using a related approach with mAb 3E7, McLafferty et al[38] tested a phage display library. Five of the 6 clones derived from the library contained sequences related to YGGF boarded by cysteine residues. mAb 3E7 was also used to demonstrate the principle of an approach in which thousands of individual peptides were synthesized on the silica surfaces of microchips using light-directed synthesis.[23] In this study, 1024 individual peptides were synthesized and screened to determine their binding to mAb 3E7. Active sequences (15 peptides) were found after visualization using a fluorescein-labeled antibody. The one bead/one peptide approach[15] was also examined using mAb 3E7, in which binding was monitored by an alkaline phosphatase assay to produce a blue color in active beads. Specific peptides were identified by Edman degradation microsequencing. Six sequences were identified, the most active of which was found to be YGGFQ ($Ki = 15$ nM). Kassarjian et al[39] used a similar process with I^{125}-labeled anti-β-endorphin mAb 3E7. Salmon et al[40] used an improved version of this approach, in which small quantities of peptide were released into and tested in solution. mAb 3E7 was again employed to verify the use of this library approach—3 peptide sequences were identified, 1 of which corresponded with the first 4 positions of methionine- and leucine-enkephalin. Although screening membrane-bound receptors is now possible, one bead/one peptide libraries have not been screened in membrane-bound opioid receptor assays.

Use of libraries with membrane-bound receptors has so far been limited to those that can be screened with compounds free in solution. Such a library was used in a case study our laboratory performed employing a μ opioid receptor binding assay and a hexapeptide synthetic combinatorial library composed of 400 different mixtures, each of which contained an equimolar mixture of 130 321 hexapeptides, for a library total of 52 128 400 L-amino acid hexapeptides. Two of the 6 positions were specifically defined using 20 naturally occurring L-amino acids (O); the remaining 4 positions were made up of mixtures of 19 amino acids (X; cysteine excluded). In the initial screening all 400 mixtures were tested at a single concentration for their ability to inhibit binding of tritiated DAMGO. IC_{50} values were subsequently determined for the most effective peptide mixtures. YGXXXX-NH$_2$ was found to be the most effective inhibiting mixture. An iterative process was performed in which the subsequent X positions of YGXXXX-NH$_2$ were successively defined. For each of the 4 iterations, 20 peptide mixtures were synthesized. The final deconvolution yielded sequences in which the first 5 residues corresponded to the naturally occurring opioid peptide sequences of methionine and leucine enkephalin (YGGFMA-NH$_2$ IC$_{50}$ = 28 nM and YGGFLG-NH$_2$ IC$_{50}$ = 59 nM[41]).

Positional scanning deconvolution was also demonstrated using the mu opioid receptor binding assay as a case study.[34] A hexapeptide PS-SCL consisting of 6 separate sublibraries, each having a single position defined with the remaining 5 positions as mixtures (O$_1$XXXXX-NH$_2$, XO$_2$XXXX-NH$_2$, XXO$_3$XXX-NH$_2$, XXXO$_4$XX-NH$_2$, XXXXO$_5$X-NH$_2$, and XXXXXO$_6$-NH$_2$; 108 separate peptide mixtures), was screened. Each mixture was composed of ~18^5 = 1 889 568 hexapeptides (cysteine and tryptophan were omitted). The 18 mixtures making up each of the 6 separate sublibraries addressed a single position in the hexapeptide. Each of the 6 positional sublibraries were different arrangements of the same 34 012 224 hexapeptides (18 × 18^5 = 34 012 224). Used in concert, the data derived from the 108 mixtures yielded information about the most important amino acids for every position in the hexapeptide. This library was tested to determine the most active amino acids at each position. Peptides comprising all possible combinations of the amino acids active at each position were synthesized (position 1: tyrosine; position 2: glycine; position 3: glycine and phenylalanine; position 4-phenylalanine; position 5: phenylalanine, tyrosine, methionine, and leucine; and position 6: phenylalanine, arginine, and tyrosine). This generated 1 × 1 × 2 × 1 × 4 × 3 = 24 individual hexapeptides. The IC$_{50}$ values obtained for these peptides ranged from 17 nM to 3276 nM. Nine peptides had activities below 200 nM, 5 of which possessed the sequences of methionine- or leucine-enkephalin within the first 5 residues.

Identification of Novel Opioid Peptides

L-Amino Acid Libraries

Screening of an N-acetylated library, Ac-OOXXXX-NH$_2$, in a μ binding assay yielded new opioid antagonists with no homology to known opioid peptides.[42,43] The individual peptides derived from this library have been termed acetalins. Three peptides, Ac-RFMWMR-NH$_2$, Ac-RFMWMK-NH$_2$, and Ac-RFMWMT-NH$_2$, were tested for their selectivity among opioid receptors in μ, δ, κ$_1$, κ$_2$, and κ$_3$ receptor binding assays. These peptides showed high affinity for μ and κ$_3$ opioid receptors, somewhat lower affinity for δ receptors, weak affinity for κ$_1$ receptors, and no affinity for κ$_2$ receptors. They were found to be potent μ receptor antagonists in the guinea pig ileum assay and relatively weak antagonists in the mouse vas deferens assay. These peptides represent a new class of opioid receptor ligands. This study exemplifies the power of mixture-based combinatorial libraries for the identification of new ligands; such ligands would not have been found using classical structure-activity relationship (SAR) techniques.

Iterations were completed for additional mixtures found to have activity in the initial screening of the nonacetylated and acetylated hexapeptide libraries OOXXXX-NH$_2$ and Ac-OOXXXX-NH$_2$.[44] Two new series of nonacetylated hexapeptides not related to the enkephalins were identified, YPFGFO-NH$_2$ and WWPKHO-NH$_2$ (where O = 1 of 20 L-amino acids). Both possessed high affinity (IC$_{50}$ values of the most active peptides were 10–15 nM) and selectivity for the μ receptor, individuals of which were found to be μ agonists. Two additional series were identified from the acetylated library, Ac-FRWWYO-NH$_2$ and Ac-RWIGWO-NH$_2$ (IC$_{50}$ values of the most active peptides were 5–10 nM). The peptide Ac-FRWWYM-NH$_2$ was determined to be an agonist for the μ receptor, whereas the peptide Ac-RWIGWR-NH$_2$ was found to be an antagonist at this receptor. In total, 6 different families of sequences were identified from the 2 libraries (Table 26.1).

A positional scanning format of the hexapeptide library, in which 2 positions are defined for each sublibrary, was used to identify ligands for the delta receptor. The 3 related L-amino acid sublibraries (composed of identical hexapeptides but differing in the location of their defined positions, OOXXXX-NH$_2$, XXOOXX-NH$_2$, and XXXXOO-NH$_2$) were used to identify a new ligand for the delta receptor, YGFDLV-NH$_2$ (IC$_{50}$ =15 nM). This peptide is similar to the sequences found when a single-position-defined positional scanning library was used in an earlier study, YHGWLV-NH$_2$ and YGMHLV-NH$_2$.[47] YGFDLV-NH$_2$ was found to be an agonist at the delta receptor.

An N-acetylated positional scanning decapeptide library was screened in binding assays specific for the kappa receptor. The library was made up of ~3 trillion decapeptides, with each of the 200 mixtures of these 2 separate libraries composed of ~200 billion decapeptides per mixture. From this extremely large pool of compounds, 2 peptide sequences having high affinities for the kappa receptor were identified from the N-acetylated library: Ac-YRTRYRYRRR-NH2 (IC$_{50}$ = 28 nM) and Ac-RGWFHYKPKR-NH2 (IC$_{50}$ = 30 nM).

Burgess et al synthesized a library made up of a total of 96 peptides based on the sequences YGGFL-NH$_2$ and YGGFLRF-NH$_2$ to explore the effects of incorporating 2,3 methanoamino acids, in particular stereoisomers of 2,3 methanoleucine.[52] None of the compounds, however, were found to show improved activity over the native peptides. The authors concluded that binding in mu and delta receptors is governed by amino acids other than the leu[5] residue.

D-Amino Acid Libraries

A mixture-based combinatorial library containing all D-amino acid hexapeptides (Ac-ooxxxx-NH$_2$) was used to identify a novel ligand for the μ opioid receptor, Ac-rfwink-NH$_2$ (IC$_{50}$ = 18 nM).[49] While the first 2 amino acid side chains (Arg and Phe) and the presence of the N-terminal acetyl is similar to that found in the acetalins,

Table 26.1 Opioid Ligands Identified From Combinatorial Libraries

Library	Receptor	Total No. of Compounds	Deconvolution	Individual Compound	Activity (nM)	Agonist/ Antagonist	Ref
Tetrapeptide OXXX-NH$_2$	Mu	6 × 10^6	Iterative	YmFA-NH$_2$	IC$_{50}$ = 2	Agonist	45
Tetrapeptide OXXX-NH$_2$	Mu	6 × 10^6	PosScan	Y(DNve)G(L-Nal)-NH$_2$	K$_i$ = 0.4	Agonist	46
Tetrapeptide OXXX-NH$_2$	Mu	6 × 10^6	PosScan	YrAW-NH$_2$	K$_i$ = 1.8	Agonist	46
	Delta	6 × 10^6	PosScan	Wy(aAba)R-NH$_2$	K$_i$ = 7	Agonist	46
	Kappa	6 × 10^6	PosScan	ff(DNle)r-NH$_2$	K$_i$ = 1	Agonist	46
Hexapeptide OOXXXX-NH$_2$	Mu	52 × 10^6	Iterative	YGGFMA-NH$_2$	IC$_{50}$ = 28	Agonist	41
	Mu	52 × 10^6	Iterative	YPFGFR-NH$_2$	IC$_{50}$ = 13	Agonist	44
	Mu	52 × 10^6	Iterative	WWPR-NH$_2$	IC$_{50}$ = 10	Agonist	44
	Delta	52 × 10^6	Iterative	YGGFLV-NH$_2$	IC$_{50}$ = 10	Agonist	
Hexapeptide Ac-OOXXXX-NH$_2$	Mu	52 × 10^6	Iterative	Ac-RFMWMK-NH$_2$	IC$_{50}$ = 5	Antagonist	42
	Mu	52 × 10^6	Iterative	Ac-RWIGWR-NH$_2$	IC$_{50}$ = 5	Antagonist	44
	Mu	52 × 10^6	Iterative	Ac-FRWWYM-NH$_2$	IC$_{50}$ = 33	Agonist	44
Hexapeptide OXXXXX-NH$_2$	Mu	34 × 10^6	PosScan	YGGFMY-NH$_2$	IC$_{50}$ = 17	Agonist	34
	Delta	34 × 10^6	PosScan	YHGWLV-NH$_2$	IC$_{50}$ = 61	Not reported	47
	Delta	34 × 10^6	Pos Scan	YGMHLV-NH$_2$	IC$_{50}$ = 45	Not reported	47
Hexapeptide OOXXXX -NH$_2$	Delta	52 × 10^6	PosScan	YGFDLV-NH$_2$	IC$_{50}$ = 15	Agonist	47
Decapeptide Ac-OXXXXXXXXX-NH$_2$	Kappa	3.2 × 10^{12}	PosScan	Ac-YRTRYRRYRR-NH$_2$	IC$_{50}$ = 28	none	
Hexapeptide Ac-OOXXXX-NH$_2$	Orphanin	52 × 10^6	PosScan	Ac-RYYRWK-NH$_2$	IC$_{50}$ = 23	Agonist	48

Hexapeptide D-amino acids Ac-OOXXXX-NH$_2$	Mu	52×10^6	Iterative	Ac-rfwink-NH$_2$	IC$_{50}$ = 18	Agonist	49
Hexapeptide D-amino acids OOXXXX-NH$_2$	Mu	52×10^6	Iterative	Iftwyr-NH$_2$ Rh-aOrn-R-7Aha-r-	IC$_{50}$ = 5	Not reported	
Rhodamine-OXXX-NH$_2$	Kappa	7.3×10^6	PosScan	NH$_2$	K$_i$ = 5.7	Agonist	50
Trimer peptoid	Mu	3672	Iterative	CHIR 4531	K$_i$ = 6	Not reported	51
Peptide/ peptidomimetic	Mu and delta	96	Parallel	YGGF(2,3 methanoleucine) -NH$_2$	Not reported	Not reported	52
N-alkylated dipeptide	Mu	57 500	Iterative	TPI 418-1	IC$_{50}$ = 3	Agonist	53
Heptamine	Mu	37 791 360	PosScan	TPI 27-11	IC$_{50}$ = 14	Antagonist	54
Urea	Mu	126 000	Iterative	TPI 632-4	IC$_{50}$ = 100	Not reported	28
Hydantoins	Sigma	38 880	PosScan	TPI 610-2	IC$_{50}$ = 62	Not reported	29
Tetrahydroisoquinoline	Sigma	43 472	Iterative	TPI 462-4	IC$_{50}$ = 56	Not reported	55
Bicyclic guanidine	Kappa	102 459	PosScan	TPI 614-1	IC$_{50}$ = 37	Not reported	18
Piperidine	Kappa	288	Parallel	RTI 5989-29	Ki = 6.9	Antagonist	56

the D form of the amino acids was found to be essential. The systematic replacement of each of the 6 positions with each of the 20 L-amino acids yielded inactive peptides. The all-D-amino acid peptide exhibits high selectivity for μ receptors (K_i values: $\mu_1 = 16 \pm 0.5$ nM, $\mu_2 = 41 \pm 4.8$ nM). Ac-rfwink-NH$_2$ had a K_i value of greater than 1500 nM for delta receptors, had very low affinity in assays for the κ_1 ($K_i > 2000$ nM) and κ_2 ($K_i > 5000$ nM) receptor subtypes, and had only modest affinity in assays for κ_3 receptors ($K_i = 288 \pm 71$ nM). Ac-rfwink-NH$_2$ was shown to be a full agonist in the guinea pig ileum assay ($EC_{50} = 433 \pm 43$ nM). This activity was antagonized by naloxone at a low concentration ($K_e = 3.80$ nM), indicating that it was an opioid effect mediated through interaction with μ opioid receptors. Ac-rfwink-NH$_2$ is a potent agonist at the μ receptor and induces long-lasting analgesia in mice. The in vivo potency of Ac-rfwink-NH$_2$ ($ED_{50} = 0.6$ nmol, intracerebroventricular) was found to be approximately twice that obtained for morphine ($ED_{50} = 1.29$ nmol, icv). Ac-rfwink-NH$_2$ produced antinociception equal to that of morphine following intraperitoneal (ip) administration. Since analgesia produced by ip-administered Ac-rfwink-NH$_2$ is blocked by icv administration of naloxone, this peptide is most likely able to cross the blood-brain barrier.

A nonacetylated library made up entirely of D-amino acid hexapeptides (ooxxxx-NH$_2$) was also found to have activity at the mu receptor. Four iterative syntheses (20 mixtures for each iteration) were performed on each of the 2 mixtures found to be most active: imxxxx-NH$_2$ and itxxxx-NH$_2$. Upon completion of the iterative deconvolution process, the 2 peptides found to bind with the highest affinity to the mu receptor were iftwyr-NH$_2$ ($IC_{50} = 5$ nM) and imswwg-NH$_2$ ($IC_{50} = 10$ nM) (Table 26.1). These peptides are yet another class of opioid peptide, in that they do not have the typical N-terminal free tyrosine of endogenous ligands or the N-terminal arginine of the acetalins or Ac-rfwink-NH$_2$.

Mixed L- and D-Amino Acid Libraries

A synthetic peptide combinatorial library composed of mixtures of 50 different L-, D-, and unnatural amino acids (OXXX-NH$_2$) was screened in the 3 opioid binding assays. The tetrapeptide library contained 6.5 million peptides and required iterative deconvolution. Iterations were completed for the most active mixture at the mu receptor. After 3 iterative syntheses (50 mixtures each), the most active individual peptide found was YmFA-NH$_2$ ($IC_{50} = 2$ nM). This compound was found to be a highly mu-specific receptor agonist.[45] A tetrapeptide positional scanning library that differed slightly in the amino acid making up the library was also synthesized and screened. Following an extensive study,[46] individual compounds were identified for all 3 opioid receptors, mu, delta, and kappa. The most active peptide for the mu receptor was Y(D-Nve-)G(L-Nal)-NH$_2$ ($Ki = 0.4$ nM), while the most mu-selective peptide found was YrAW-NH$_2$, with μ:δ and μ:κ ratios of greater than 1000 (Table 26.1). The most selective peptide identified for the delta receptor was Wy(aAba)R-NH$_2$ ($Ki = 7$ nM). The most active peptide identified for the kappa receptor was ff(D-Nle)r-NH$_2$ (Ki = 1 nM). The tetrapeptides identified for the kappa receptor were highly selective for this receptor, with κ:μ and κ:δ ratios of greater than 10 000.[46] The kappa-selective peptide kaffiralin (ffir-NH$_2$) is a full agonist in the GTPγS binding assay (EC$_{50}$ = 10 nM hKOR-CHO cells). Kaffiralin generated a full dose-response curve in the mouse 55°C warm water tail flick assay and in the acetic acid writhing test after icv administration. It was ~10-fold more potent in the writhing test than in the tail flick test. After ip administration, kaffiralin did not produce a full dose-response curve in the tail flick assay, but it did in the writhing test. It was antagonized by an ip injection of nor-binaltorphimine (nor-BNI) but not an icv injection of nor-BNI. When given by ip administration, ffir-NH$_2$ may produce antinociception at spinal or peripheral receptors instead of supraspinal receptors. There was no evidence of the peptide crossing the blood-brain barrier (J. Bidlack and B. Urban, oral communication, 1999).

Fluorescent-Labeled Libraries

In a recent study, kappa-selective peptides having intrinsic fluorescent properties were identified from a rhodamine-labeled tetrapeptide PS-SCL.[50] From a library of ~7.3 million rhodamine-labeled tetrapeptides, more than 250 individual peptides were synthesized from the most active mixtures. Eight individual rhodamine-labeled peptides were identified that were specific for the kappa opioid receptor, having binding affinities ranging from 5 to 20 nM (Table 26.1). The majority of the most active peptides identified contained at least 2 positively charged residues. Such strongly positively charged compounds have the potential for nonspecific binding to the receptor through ionic interactions. This was found not to be the case since the same peptides lacking a rhodamine label did not inhibit binding of the radioligand to the kappa receptor (K$_i$ >10 μM). As rhodamine and rhodamine sulfonyl amide had no inhibitory activity, the peptide sequence together with the rhodamine moiety were necessary components of a single molecule responsible for receptor binding. We are currently pursuing a range of other fluorescent groups in a similar manner with both peptide and nonpeptide libraries for the identification of opioid receptor–specific ligands.

Orphanin FQ/Nociceptin

In October and November 1995, 2 separate reports were published[57,58] on the identification of the endogenous ligand for the orphan receptor ORL1, a potential member of the opioid family of receptors. After establishing a binding assay in rat brain using tritiated orphanin FQ,[48] a hexapeptide positional scanning library containing 2 defined positions (1200 mixtures) was used to identify hexapeptide ligands for this receptor. The most active peptide found was Ac-RYYRWK-NH$_2$. The 5 most active compounds were found to be agonists using 3 separate biochemical bioassays: inhibition of cyclic adenosine monophosphate (cAMP) accumulation, stimulation of [^{35}S]GTPγS binding, and inhibition of electrically induced contractions in the mouse vas deferens.[59]

Peptidomimetic Libraries

The first use of a peptidomimetic library for the identification of opioids was described by Zuckermann et al,[51] who screened a library of 5000 peptoids (oligo-N-substituted glycines). The library, composed of 3 sets of monomers (22 different monomers) from commercially available amines, and with the amino terminus either as a free amine, N-acetylated or capped with cyclohexylurea, contained 204 peptoid trimers in 18 different mixtures. This library was screened in a μ-specific radioreceptor assay with ^{3}H-DAMGO as the radioligand. Through use of an iterative process in which the most active mixture from the first screening was deconvoluted by individually defining the first, second, and third positions in sequential order, 3 highly active compounds were found. The most active compound, CHIR 4531, had a K_i value of 6 nM.

A dipeptidomimetic library based on a dipeptide scaffold with the C-terminal and middle amide hydrogens replaced separately with 5 different alkyl groups (methyl, ethyl, allyl, benzyl, or naphthylmethyl) was also used to identify opioid ligands.[53] The 2 variable amino acid positions of this library were made up of 50 different L-, D-, and nonproteinogenic amino acids. The library, which contained 57 500 different compounds and was screened against all 3 opioid receptors, required 2 iterative syntheses to identify individual compounds. Highly active individual compounds were identified for each of the 3 receptors: mu (TPI 418-1 Ki = 6 nM), delta (TPI 452-19 Ki = 39 nM), and kappa (TPI 419-19 Ki = 1 nM) (Fig. 26.1). All 3 were found to be agonists at their particular receptors. The selectivity of the mu and kappa compounds was high, while that of the delta ligand was poor, with the compound binding equally to kappa receptors.

Nonpeptide Libraries

In contrast to the stepwise synthesis of peptidomimetics mentioned above, the transformation of peptide libraries to libraries of entirely different pharmacophores has been reported.[31] The approach, termed libraries from libraries, extends the diversity obtained with peptide libraries via chemical modification. Peptide libraries have been successfully modified by exhaustive methylation of their amide bonds to yield peptidomimetics[31] and/or by reduction of the backbone amide carbonyl groups to yield polyamines.[32]

A chemically modified peptide library in which all of the peptide amide carbonyls were reduced to methylenes was screened for opioid ligands. Mu-selective opioid

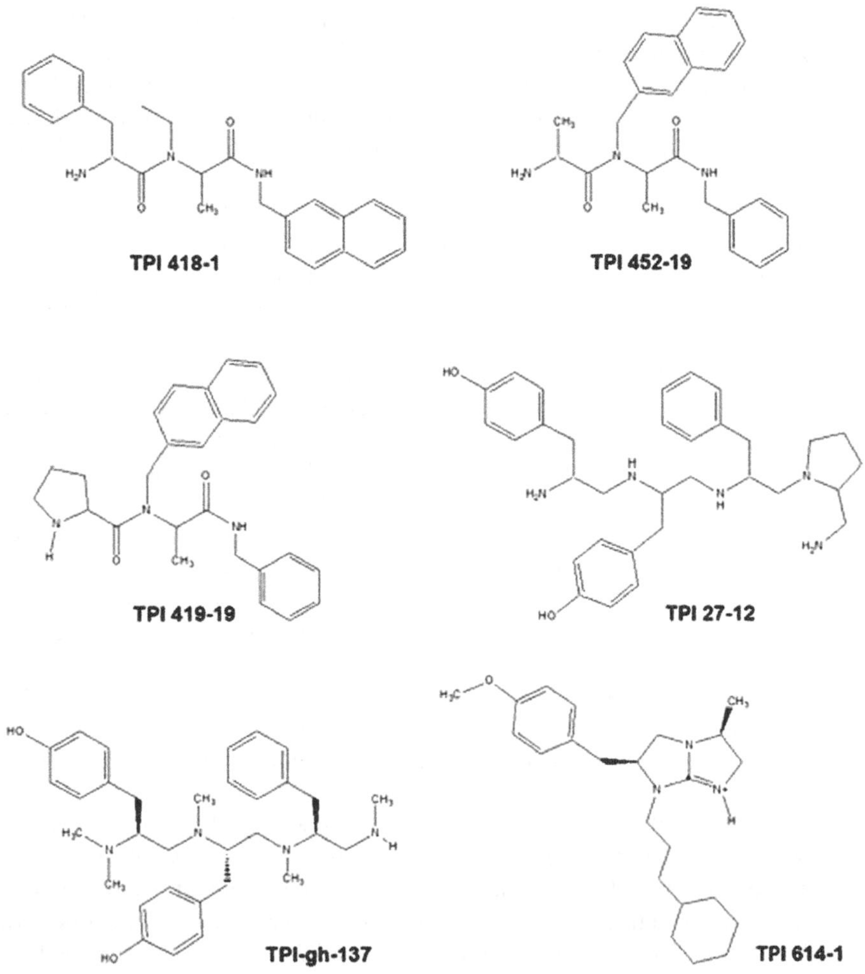

Fig. 26.1 Structures of nonpeptide compounds identified for opioid receptors.

compounds were identified from a library made up of 52 million different heptamines.[54] The library was obtained from the chemical transformation of a C-terminal amide hexapeptide positional scanning library. Combinations of the most active residues found at each position were synthesized as peptides, then reduced, and the activities of the resulting heptamines were determined. The activities of the individual compounds identified ranged from 14 to 345 nM. A truncation analog of the most active individual heptamine, red[YYFPTM-NH$_2$], was found to be equally active (red[YYFP-NH$_2$] IC$_{50}$ = 16 nM, Fig. 26.1). It was found to be a selective mu antagonist in the guinea pig ileum assay. Preliminary results indicated that this compound was toxic to mice at high doses. A series of derivatives were then synthesized in which the backbone nitrogens of the compounds red[YYFP] and red[YYF] were per-alkylated with methyl, ethyl, allyl, benzyl, or naphthylmethyl. The most active compound found was TPI-gh-137 (IC_{50} = 0.5 nM, Fig. 26.1), which was found to be a highly specific, pure antagonist at the mu receptor. It was also found to be much less toxic than the unmodified pentamine from which it was derived. This example illustrates how compounds may be further refined after initial identification from a library.

A bicyclic guanidine library containing more than 100 000 different heterocyclic compounds was screened in the opiate assays. Twenty-four (3 × 4 × 2) individual bicyclic guanidines were then synthesized and tested for activity; they were found to range from 37 to 10 000 nM. The most active compound found was TPI 614-1 (IC_{50} = 37 nM, Fig. 26.1).

Even when libraries are not derived from peptide precursors, diversity in many libraries is achieved through the use of amino acid side chains. A library of over 125 000 linear N,N'-di-substituted ureas was used to identify ligands for mu and sigma receptors. The 276 separate mixtures in this library were each made up of 452 different linear ureas. Two separate iterative deconvolutions were performed for the most active mixtures found for the mu and sigma receptors. The most active compound found for the mu receptor was TPI 632-4 (IC_{50} = 100 nM). Two active compounds were identified having activity at the sigma receptor, TPI 634-6 (IC_{50} = 5 nM) and TPI 632-9 (IC_{50} = 30 nM).[28] Similarly, individual compounds were identified for the sigma receptor from a dialkylated hydantoin library. The 2 most active compounds found were TPI 610-2 (IC_{50} = 62 nM) and TPI 610-4 (IC_{50} = 64 nM).[29] A library of 43 472 isoquinolines was also used to identify new sigma receptor ligands. The most active compound identified from this library was TPI 462-4 (IC_{50} = 56 nM).[55]

A parallel synthetic strategy of 288 compounds was used by Thomas et al to identify kappa antagonists. The library was designed around N-substituted (+)-(3R,4R)-dimethyl-4-(-3-hydroxyphenyl)piperidine, a compound known to have nonselective opioid antagonist activity.[56] The most active compound identified was RTI 5989-29 (Fig. 26.1), which was found to have a Ki of 7 nM. The compound was found to have antagonist activity at both the kappa and mu receptors (Table 26.1).

In Vivo Screening of Mixture-Based Libraries

Our laboratory has more than 15 years of experience in the synthesis and screening of mixture-based combinatorial libraries in target-based in vitro assays. It is now imperative to explore the enormous potential of the direct in vivo testing of the many mixture-based chemically diverse libraries as a superior approach to drug discovery. Our future studies will seek to demonstrate that the direct in vivo screening and deconvolution of mixture-based combinatorial libraries is a better approach to the identification of fundamentally more "advanced" therapeutic candidates. This new approach should prove faster and cheaper than the typical target-based drug discovery process.

A series of preliminary experiments have been conducted as proof of concept studies to validate the use of mixture-based libraries reported to exhibit opioid activity in an in vivo model. In this study we compared the activity of mixtures of tetrapeptides each containing 125 000 tetrapeptides. These peptide mixtures were based on the known active dermorphin analog 2,6-dimethyltyrosine-DALDA ([Dmt]-DALDA = H-Dmt-D-Arg-Phe-Lys-NH$_2$). Dmt-DALDA was identified through the outstanding classical synthetic medicinal chemistry effort by Schiller's group.[60] These compounds have high mu opioid receptor affinity[60,61] with proven in vivo antinociceptive properties in mice.[62] The Dmt-tyrosine group of [Dmt]-DALDA has been shown to be an essential component, as demonstrated by both in vitro and in vivo data. We therefore synthesized a positively biased mixture of 125 000 tetrapeptide compounds in which Dmt-tyrosine was fixed at the first position (Dmt-XXX). This mixture was examined for its activity and compared with the antinociceptive effect of the known active individual Dmt-DALDA and 2 negatively biased tetrapeptide mixtures (F-XXX and k-XXX, which are 800 and 3580 times less active in vitro, respectively; Table 26.2).

To assess the antinociceptive effects of these mixtures, we used the mouse tail flick assay since it is well established, yields clear and reproducible end points, and can differentiate between mu and kappa activity. Dmt-XXX, at a dose of 100 mg/kg, was active and had duration of action comparable to the individual compound [Dmt]-DALDA at 10 mg/kg (Fig. 26.2). This effect appears to be specific since F-XXX-NH$_2$ was inactive at comparable doses. It was also observed that Dmt-XXX was longer acting than morphine (ie, 5 hours vs 1 hour), a property already reported for [Dmt]-DALDA,[62] and was maintained for the mixtures containing Dmt on the N-terminal. As anticipated, the mixtures required greater absolute doses than the individual compounds.

After achieving these results, we performed a single iteration by synthesizing the anticipated next Dmt-r-XX mixture; the second position was defined with D-arginine,

Table 26.2 Mu Binding (K$_i$) and cAMP (IC$_{50}$) Data for Selected Individual and Tetrapeptide Mixtures*

				Binding K$_i$ (nM)	cAMP IC-50 (µM)	No of Compounds
L-(Dmt)-Tyr	X	X	X	16.2	6.8	125 000
L-Tyr	X	X	X	592.2	651.2	125 000
L-Phe	X	X	X	13 000	1027	125 000
D-Pro	X	X	X	41 238	ND	125 000
L-Lys	X	X	X	55 920	ND	125 000
D-Lys	X	X	X	58 030	ND	125 000
D-Asp	X	X	X	84 380	ND	125 000
L-(Dmt)-Tyr	D-Arg	X	X	4.5	0.4	2500
L-Tyr	D-Arg	X	X	136.0	91.3	2500
Dmt-DALDA: L-(Dmt)-Tyr	D-Arg	L-Phe	L-Lys	0.2	0.002	1
DALDA: L-Tyr	D-Arg	L-Phe	L-Lys	5.5	0.8	1

*cAMP, cyclic adenosine monophosphate; ND, not determined.

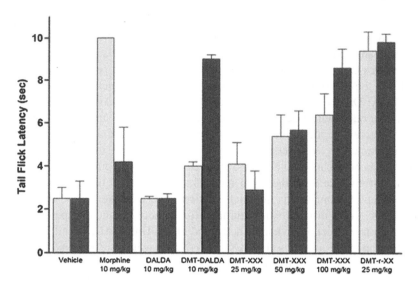

Fig. 26.2 Comparison of in vivo activity of tetrapeptide mixtures and individual compounds using tail flick assay. Tail flick latency is the average of 2 readings per animal, 10 animals per compound. Vehicle is 10% Trappsol. Light bars = 30 minutes postinjection, dark bars = 5 hours postinjection.

which is the amino acid found in DALDA. This iteration decreases the complexity of the mixtures from 125 000 compounds (OXXX) to 2500 compounds (OOXX). The antinociceptive effects of these mixtures were tested in the tail flick assay as before. As the tetrapeptide mixture becomes more defined, one would expect an increase in activity when testing at the same concentration. It is of note that when decreasing the mixture size from 125 000 for Dmt-XXX to 2500 for Dmt-r-XX the increase in activity was modest (4-fold in vitro) while the decrease in mixture size was 50-fold. This discrepancy can be explained by several different mechanisms. Clearly, more than 1 substitution at the second position can be accepted and activity retained (lysine may be an acceptable replacement for arginine). Additionally, it is important to point out that we fixed D-arginine at the second position simply as a test study to expand this proof of concept for the use of mixture-based combinatorial libraries directly in vivo. There is in fact no reason to assume that D-arginine is the most functionally useful amino acid at the second position, especially in vivo. At 5 hours postinjection at a dose of 25 mg/kg this peptide mixture of 2500 tetrapeptides was clearly more active than morphine (Fig. 26.2). Six others were tested in vivo (Y-XXX, F-XXX, p-XXX, K-XXX, k-XXX, and D-XXX, data not shown), and the activities of these mixtures in binding and cAMP assays are shown in Table 26.2. This expected correlation between the in vitro and in vivo activities was found for all except k-XXX, which had significant tail flick activity from 30 minutes all the way through the 5-hour cutoff point. Of clear significance in this study was that k-XXX, while having very poor activity in vitro, was clearly active in the tail flick test. This may be due to several factors, including the interaction at an unknown nonopiate receptor, the inhibition or stimulation of an enzyme, or a translational factor or signaling event. This result illustrates perhaps the central most exciting aspect of the proposed studies, namely the direct in vivo identification of mixtures that may be active as pain-modulating agents at sites other than the expected 3 opiate receptors. These preliminary results are encouraging, and testing will be continued to determine individual compounds.

Conclusions

A wide range of combinatorial libraries, from peptides to low-molecular-weight heterocyclic compounds, have been successfully screened in assays specific for the opioid receptors and have enabled the identification of new ligands for these receptors. New opioid peptides found from combinatorial libraries range in length from tetramers to decamers. The compounds described in this review are the most active found and represent only a fraction of the number of individual peptides and non-peptidic compounds synthesized and tested. All the peptides found have an amide at the carboxyl terminus, as all libraries screened were in this format. Some of the peptides resemble the classical opioids—they possess a tyrosine at position 1 and a tertiary amino group on the N terminus. The peptide YPWFPO-NH$_2$ is a hexapeptide analog of the recently described tetrapeptide endomorphin-1 (YPWF-NH$_2$), thought to be the endogenous ligand for the mu receptor.[63] The delta-selective hexapeptides identified possess both Tyr[1] and Leu[5] but differ from each other and the enkephalins at the remaining positions. YHGWLV-NH$_2$ has a conservative replacement of Phe[4] by Trp[4]; thus, it differs from the enkephalin mainly at the His[2]. It is assumed that Val[6] is redundant, although this has not yet been tested. The 2 remaining delta peptides have replacements at the fourth and fifth positions (YGMHLV-NH$_2$ and YGFDLV-NH$_2$). Novel peptides identified for the opioid receptors were found to contain basic residues (arginine and lysine), and many also contain tryptophan. Basic residues are found in position 1 in the acetalins and in the all D-amino acid peptide, Ac-rfwink-NH$_2$. They are also found on the C-terminal residue in peptides selective for mu, delta, or kappa (WWPR-NH$_2$, Wy(Nve)R-NH$_2$, and f(D-nal)(D-nle) r-NH$_2$, respectively). The highly active and receptor-specific tetrapeptide ligands have been fully developed and are now in phase I human trials.

It is still unclear what is required for a compound to bind to opioid receptors and what the effect of binding will be. It was assumed that compounds identified from very large mixture-based libraries would in virtually all instances be identified as antagonists since it was reasoned that there must be many more ways to block a binding interaction with one of many thousands of compounds than to bind and affect a secondary signaling event. Antagonists need only bind to a receptor in order to block another ligand from binding, whereas an agonist must not only bind but also induce a conformational change in the receptor in order to achieve signal transduction. Thus, the mu agonist activity of Ac-rfwink-NH$_2$ was unexpected. Furthermore, the acetalins

(Ac-RFMWMK-NH$_2$), which have sequence similarities to Ac-rfwink-NH$_2$ although they are composed entirely of L-amino acids, were found to be antagonists. Certainly the identification of the opioid peptide Ac-rfwink-NH$_2$, which does not require a phenolic hydroxyl or a tertiary amino group to be an agonist, challenges the preconception that these pharmocophores are required for agonist activity. Since then we have found that greater than 80% of the new sequences identified are agonists at the opioid receptors. Whether the high percentage of agonists found is due to a bias resulting from the specific radioligand used in the initial library screen has yet to be determined.

The high numbers of different compounds identified raises the question of the plasticity of the opioid receptors. Why are new ligands of widely varying structures so readily identified for the opioid receptors, particularly the mu receptor? This is not the case for other G-coupled receptors, even for the orphanin FQ/nociceptin receptor, at which few libraries are found to have activity. The plasticity of the mu receptor may account for the high numbers of novel agonists identified. The data obtained from in vivo studies on these new opioid ligands should generate interesting insights into this question.

Finally, the use of mixture-based libraries for direct in vivo testing for the identification of inherently more advanced "hits" was demonstrated here in a proof of concept illustration. This process, found to work well in preliminary studies with peptides and classic low molecular weight heterocyclic mixtures, will make the drug discovery process much faster than it has been with traditional target-based in vitro assays. Future studies will explore the enormous potential of the direct in vivo testing of the many mixture-based chemical of diverse libraries in an effort to reduce the time and resources required for drug discovery. This new approach is expected to lead to the identification of novel pain-modulating agents for the 3 opiate receptors and the identification of ligands to a variety of other orphan receptors that may play a role in pain regulation.

Acknowledgments This work was funded by National Institute on Drug Abuse Grant No DA09410 and the Arthritis and Cancer Pain Research Institute. The in vivo studies were performed in collaboration with Mixture Sciences Inc, San Diego, CA, and PsychoGenics Inc, Tarrytown, NY.

References

1. Pert CB, Snyder SH. Properties of opiate-receptor binding in rat brain. *Proc Natl Acad Sci USA*. 1973;70:2243-2247.
2. Simon EJ, Hiller JM, Edelman I. Stereospecific binding of the potent narcotic analgesic (3H) etorphine to rat-brain homogenate. *Proc Natl Acad Sci USA*. 1973;70:1947-1949.
3. Terenius L. Characteristics of the "receptor" for narcotic analgesics in synaptic plasma fraction from rat brain. *Acta Pharmacol Toxicol (Copenh)*. 1973;33:377-384.
4. Hughes J, Smith TW, Kosterlitz HW, Fothergill LA, Morgan BA, Morris HR. Identification of two related pentapeptides from the brain with potent opiate agonist activity. *Nature*. 1975;258:577-579.
5. Fowler CJ, Fraser GL. Mu-, delta-, and kappa-opioid receptors and their subtypes. A critical review with emphasis on radioligand binding experiments. *Neurochem Int*. 1994;24: 401-426.

6. Chen Y, Mestek A, Liu J, Hurley JA, Yu L. Molecular cloning and functional expression of a mu opioid receptor from rat brain. *Mol Pharmacol.* 1993;44:8-12.
7. Fukuda K, Kato S, Mori K, Nishi M, Takeshima H. Primary structures and expression from cDNAs of rat opioid receptor delta and mu subtypes. *FEBS Lett.* 1993;327:311-314.
8. Kieffer BL, Befort K, Gaveriaux-Ruff C, Hirth CG. The delta opioid receptor: isolation of a cDNA by expression cloning and pharmacological characterization. *Proc Natl Acad Sci USA.* 1992;89:12048-12052.
9. Evans CJ, Jr, Keith DE, Jr, Morrison H, Magendzo K, Edwards RH. Cloning of delta opioid receptor by functional expression. *Science.* 1992;258:1952-1955.
10. Yasuda K, Raynor K, Kong H, et al. Cloning and functional comparison of kappa and delta opioid receptors from mouse brain. *Proc Natl Acad Sci USA.* 1993;90:6736-6740.
11. Cwirla SE, Peters EA, Barrett RW, Dower WJ. Peptides on phage: a vast library of peptides for identifying ligands. *Proc Natl Acad Sci USA.* 1990;87:6378-6382.
12. Devlin JJ, Panganiban LC, Devlin PE. Random peptide libraries: a source of specific protein binding molecules. *Science.* 1990;249:404-406.
13. Scott JK, Smith GP. Searching for peptide ligands with an epitope library. *Science.* 1990;249: 386-390.
14. Geysen HM, Rodda SJ, Mason TJ. A priori delineation of a peptide which mimics a discontinuous antigenic determinant. *Mol Immunol.* 1986;23:709-715.
15. Lam KS, Salmon SE, Hersh EM, Hruby VJ, Kazmierski WM, Knapp RJ. A new type of synthetic peptide library for identifying ligand-binding activity. *Nature.* 1991;354:82-84.
16. Houghten RA, Pinilla C, Blondelle SE, Appel JR, Dooley CT, Cuervo JH. Generation and use of synthetic peptide combinatorial libraries for basic research and drug discovery. *Nature.* 1991;354:84-86.
17. Houghten RA, Appel JR, Blondelle SE, Cuervo JH, Dooley CT, Pinilla C. The use of synthetic peptide combinatorial libraries for the identification of bioactive peptides. *Biotechniques.* 1992;13:412-421.
18. Houghten RA, Pinilla C, Appel JR, et al. Mixture-based synthetic combinatorial libraries. *J Med Chem.* 1999;42:3743-3778.
19. Merrifield RBJ. Solid phase peptide synthesis, I: the synthesis of a tetrapeptide. *J Am Chem Soc.* 1963;85:2149-2154.
20. Merrifield B. Solid phase synthesis. *Science.* 1986;232:341-347.
21. Frank R. Spot-synthesis: an easy and flexible tool to study molecular recognition. In: Epton R, ed. *Innovation and Perspectives in Solid Phase Synthesis: Peptides, Proteins and Nucleic Acids.* Birmingham, UK: Mayflower Worldwide; 1994:509-512.
22. Eichler J, Houghten RA. Identification of substrate-analog trypsin inhibitors through the screening of synthetic peptide combinatorial libraries. *Biochemistry.* 1993;32:11035-11041.
23. Fodor SPA, Read JL, Pirrung MC, Stryer L, Lu AT, Solas D. Light-directed, spatially addressable parallel chemical synthesis. *Science.* 1991;251:767-773.
24. Furka A, Sebestyen F, Asgedom M, Dibo G. General method for rapid synthesis of multicomponent peptide mixtures. *Int J Pept Protein Res.* 1991;37:487-493.
25. Ostresh JM, Winkle JH, Hamashin VT, Houghten RA. Peptide libraries: determination of relative reaction rates of protected amino acids in competitive couplings. *Biopolymers.* 1994;34:1681-1689.
26. Ostresh JM, Schoner CC, Hamashin VT, Nefzi A, Meyer J-P, Houghten RA. Solid phase synthesis of trisubstituted bicyclic guanidines via cyclization of reduced N-acylated dipeptides. *J Org Chem.* 1998;63:8622-8623.
27. Nefzi A, Ostresh JM, Houghten RA. Solid phase synthesis of 1, 3, 4, 7-tetrasubstituted perhydro-1,4-diazepine-2,5-diones. *Tetrahedron Lett.* 1997;38:4943-4946.
28. Nefzi A, Ostresh JM, Meyer J-P, Houghten RA. Solid phase synthesis of heterocyclic compounds from linear peptides: cyclic ureas and thioureas. *Tetrahedron Lett.* 1997;38:931-934.
29. Nefzi A, Dooley CT, Ostresh JM, Houghten RA. Combinatorial chemistry: from peptides and peptidomimetics to small organic and heterocyclic compounds. *Bioorg Med Chem Lett.* 1998;8:2273-2278.

30. Nefzi A, Giulianotti M, Houghten RA. Solid phase synthesis of 2, 4, 5-trisubstituted thiomorpholin-3-ones. *Tetrahedron Lett.* 1998;39:3671-3674.

31. Ostresh JM, Husar GM, Blondelle SE, Dörner B, Weber PA, Houghten RA. "Libraries from libraries": chemical transformation of combinatorial libraries to extend the range and repertoire of chemical diversity. *Proc Natl Acad Sci USA.* 1994;91:11138-11142.

32. Cuervo JH, Weitl F, Ostresh JM, Hamashin VT, Hannah AL, Houghten RA. Polyalkylamine chemical combinatorial libraries. In: Maia HLS, ed. *Peptides 94: Proceedings of the 23rd European Peptide Symposium.* Leiden, The Netherlands: ESCOM; 1995:465-466.

33. Pinilla C, Appel JR, Blanc P, Houghten RA. Rapid identification of high affinity peptide ligands using positional scanning synthetic peptide combinatorial libraries. *Biotechniques.* 1992;13:901-905.

34. Dooley CT, Houghten RA. The use of positional scanning synthetic combinatorial libraries for the rapid determination of opioid receptor ligands. *Life Sci.* 1993;52:1509-1517.

35. Konings DAM, Wyatt JR, Ecker DJ, Freier SM. Deconvolution of combinatorial libraries for drug discovery: theoretical comparison of pooling strategies. *J Med Chem.* 1996;39:2710-2719.

36. Wilson-Lingardo L, Davis PW, Ecker DJ, et al. Deconvolution of combinatorial libraries for drug discovery: experimental comparison of pooling strategies. *J Med Chem.* 1996;39:2720-2726.

37. Dooley CT, Houghten RA. A comparison of combinatorial library approaches for the study of opioid compounds. *Perspect Drug Disc Design.* 1995;2:287-304.

38. McLafferty MA, Kent RB, Ladner RC, Markland W. M13 bacteriophage displaying disulfide-constrained microproteins. *Gene.* 1993;128:29-36.

39. Kassarjian A, Schellenberger V, Turck CW. Screening of synthetic peptide libraries with radiolabeled acceptor molecules. *Pept Res.* 1993;6:129-133.

40. Salmon SE, Lam KS, Lebl M, et al. Discovery of biologically active peptides in random libraries: solution-phase testing after staged orthogonal release from resin beads. *Proc Natl Acad Sci USA.* 1993;90:11708-11712.

41. Houghten RA, Dooley CT. The use of synthetic peptide combinatorial libraries for the determination of peptide ligands in radioreceptor assays: opioid peptides. *Bioorg Med Chem Lett.* 1993;3:405-412.

42. Dooley CT, Chung NN, Schiller PW, Houghten RA. Acetalins: opioid receptor antagonists determined through the use of synthetic peptide combinatorial libraries. *Proc Natl Acad Sci USA.* 1993;90:10811-10815.

43. Dooley CT, Hope S, Houghten RA. Rapid identification of novel opioid peptides from an N-acetylated synthetic combinatorial library. *Regul Pept.* 1994;54:87-88.

44. Dooley CT, Kaplan RA, Chung NN, Schiller PW, Bidlack JM, Houghten RA. Six highly active mu-selective opioid peptides identified from two synthetic combinatorial libraries. *Pept Res.* 1995;8:124-137.

45. Dooley CT, Hope SK, Houghten RA. Identification of tetrameric opioid peptides from a combinatorial library of L-, D- and nonproteinogenic amino acids. In: Maia HLS, ed. *Peptides 94: Proceedings of the 23rd European Peptide Symposium.* Leiden, The Netherlands: ESCOM; 1995:805-806.

46. Dooley CT, Ny P, Bidlack JM, Houghten RAJ. Selective ligands for the mu, delta, and kappa opioid receptors from a single mixture-based tetrapeptide positional scanning combinatorial library. *Biol Chem.* 1998;273:18848-18856.

47. Pinilla C, Appel JR, Blondelle SE, et al. Versatility of positional scanning synthetic combinatorial libraries for the identification of individual compounds. *Drug Dev Res.* 1994;33:133-145.

48. Dooley CT, Houghten RA. Orphanin FQ: receptor binding and analog structure activity relationships in rat brain. *Life Sci.* 1996;59:PL23-PL29.

49. Dooley CT, Chung NN, Wilkes BC, et al. An all D-amino acid opioid peptide with central analgesic activity from a combinatorial library. *Science.* 1994;266:2019-2022.

50. Houghten RA, Dooley CT, Appel JR. De novo identification of highly active fluorescent kappa opioid ligands from a rhodamine labeled tetrapeptide positional scanning library. *Bioorg Med Chem Lett.* 2004;14:1947-1951.
51. Zuckermann RN, Martin EJ, Spellmeyer DC, et al. Discovery of nanomolar ligands for 7-transmembrane G-protein-coupled receptors from a diverse N-(substituted)glycine peptoid library. *J Med Chem.* 1994;37:2678-2685.
52. Burgess K, Li W, Linthicum DS, et al. Libraries of opiate and anti-opiate peptidomimetics containing 2,3 methanoleucine. *Bioorg Med Chem.* 1997;5:1867-1871.
53. Dorner B, Ostresh JM, Blondelle SE, Dooley CT, Houghten RA. Peptidomimetic synthetic combinatorial libraries. *Adv Amino Acid Mimetics Peptidomimetics.* 1997;1:109-125.
54. Dooley CT, Houghten RA. Identification of mu-selective polyamine antagonists from a synthetic combinatorial library. *Analgesia.* 1995;1:400-404.
55. Griffith MC, Dooley CT, Houghten RA, Kiely JS. Solid-phase synthesis, characterization, and screening of a 43,000 compound tetrahydroisoquinoline combinatorial library. In: Chaiken IM, Janda KD, eds. *Molecular Diversity and Combinatorial Chemistry: Libraries and Drug Discovery.* Washington, DC: American Chemical Society; 1996:50-57.
56. Thomas JB, Fall MJ, Cooper JB, et al. Identification of an opioid kappa receptor subtype-selective N-substituent for (+)-(3R,4R)-dimethyl-4-(3-hydroxyphenyl)piperidine. *J Med Chem.* 1998;41:5188-5197.
57. Meunier JC, Mollereau C, Toll L, et al. Isolation and structure of the endogenous agonist of the opioid receptor-like ORL1 receptor. *Nature.* 1995;377:532-535.
58. Reinscheid RK, Nothacker HP, Bourson A, et al. Orphanin FQ: a neuropeptide that activates opioidlike G protein-coupled receptor. *Science.* 1995;270:792-794.
59. Dooley CT, Spaeth CG, Berzetei-Gurske IP, et al. Binding and in vitro activities of peptides with high affinity for the nociceptin/orphanin FQ receptor, ORL1. *J Pharmacol Exp Ther.* 1997;283:735-741.
60. Schiller PW, Nguyen TM, Berezowska I, et al. Synthesis and in vitro opioid activity profiles of DALDA analogues. *Eur J Med Chem.* 2000;35:895-901.
61. Zhao GM, Qian X, Schiller PW, Szeto HH. Comparison of [Dmt1] DALDA and DAMGO in binding and G protein activation at mu, delta, and kappa opioid receptors. *J Pharmacol Exp Ther.* 2003;307:947-954.
62. Shimoyama M, Shimoyama N, Zhao GM, Schiller PW, Szeto HH. Antinociceptive and respiratory effects of intrathecal H-Tyr-D-Arg-Phe-Lys-NH2 (DALDA) and [Dmt1] DALDA. *J Pharmacol Exp Ther.* 2001;297:364-371.
63. Zadina JE, Hackler L, Ge L-J, Kastin AJ. A potent and selective endogenous agonist for the mu opiate receptor. *Nature.* 1997;386:499-502.

Chapter 27
Current Status of Immunologic Approaches to Treating Tobacco Dependence: Vaccines and Nicotine-Specific Antibodies

Mark G. LeSage,[1] Daniel E. Keyler,[1] and Paul R. Pentel[1]

Abstract In contrast to current pharmacotherapies, immunologic approaches to treating tobacco dependence target the drug itself rather than the brain. This approach involves the use of nicotine-specific antibodies that bind nicotine in serum, resulting in a decrease in nicotine distribution to the brain and an increase in nicotine's elimination half-life. This review summarizes the literature examining the effects of immunologic interventions on the pharmacokinetics and behavioral effects of nicotine in animal models, as well as recent phase I and II clinical trials in humans. Studies using various vaccines and nicotine-specific antibodies in rodents have shown that immunization can significantly reduce the behavioral effects of nicotine that are relevant to tobacco dependence (eg, nicotine self-administration). These findings provide proof of principle that immunologic interventions could have utility in the treatment of tobacco dependence. Thus far, phase I clinical trials of nicotine vaccines have not produced any serious adverse events in humans and have produced dose-dependent increases in serum antibody levels. Although preliminary data from these small trials suggest that vaccination can facilitate abstinence from tobacco use, more advance trials are needed. By acting outside the nervous system, immunologic approaches are less likely to produce the adverse side effects associated with current medications. In addition, the unique mechanism of action of immunotherapy makes it particularly suitable for combination with other pharmacological approaches. Taken together, the work completed to date provides substantial evidence that immunologic interventions could play an important role in future treatment strategies for tobacco dependence.

Keywords tobacco, nicotine, vaccination, passive immunization, antibodies, pharmacokinetics

[1] Minneapolis Medical Research Foundation, Department of Medicine, University of Minnesota Medical School, Minneapolis, MN

Corresponding Author: Mark G. LeSage, Minneapolis Medical Research Foundation, 914 South 8th Street, D3-850, Minneapolis, MN 55404. Tel: (612) 347-5118; Fax: (612) 337-7372; E-mail: lesag002@umn.edu

R.S. Rapaka and W. Sadée (eds.), *Drug Addiction.*
© American Association of Pharmaceutical Scientists 2008

455

Introduction

Tobacco dependence is the most common form of drug abuse. There are an estimated 71.5 million adult cigarette smokers, and smoking is associated with over 400 000 deaths per year in the United States.[1] Thus, treatment of tobacco dependence continues to be a major public health priority.[2] Nicotine is considered the primary chemical in tobacco that is responsible for engendering tobacco use and dependence.[3,4] Although it is clear that other compounds in tobacco and nonpharmacologic variables can play a role in the development and maintenance of tobacco dependence, the primary role of nicotine has broad empirical support providing a strong rationale for targeting its effects in the development of interventions for tobacco dependence. Nicotine produces its addictive effects by altering neuropharmacological processes in the brain. For example, nicotine produces an increase in extracellular dopamine in the nucleus accumbens,[5] an effect common with other drugs of abuse (eg, heroin, cocaine[6,7]). Currently available pharmacotherapies for tobacco dependence involve administration of a medication that substitutes for or modifies some aspect of these neuropharmacological effects of nicotine. For example, the most commonly used medication for smoking cessation is nicotine replacement therapy (NRT), which involves delivery of pure nicotine via transdermal patches or other routes as a substitute for the nicotine otherwise derived from using tobacco. The atypical antidepressant bupropion, which primarily inhibits dopamine and norepinephrine transporters, is another first-line medication used for tobacco dependence.[8] Both NRT and bupropion significantly increase quit rates over placebo.[9-11] However, despite their efficacy in promoting cessation, the vast majority of smokers that use NRT or bupropion fail to quit.[8,10] There is a clear need for improved pharmacotherapies for nicotine dependence.

The approach of targeting the neuropharmacological actions of nicotine in the brain poses 2 significant challenges. First, the neuropharmacological mechanisms involved in nicotine's effects are also important in mediating normal functioning of the nervous system. Thus, medications targeting nicotine's neuropharmacological effects may alter normal functioning and produce undesired side effects. Second, nicotine acts through multiple neuropharmacological mechanisms to produce its addictive effects. Finding one receptor-based medication or a combination of such medications that targets more than one these critical mechanisms is difficult. Development of alternative strategies that circumvent these challenges is of interest. One alternative is an immunologic approach, which targets nicotine itself rather than the brain. This approach involves the production of nicotine-specific antibodies in serum that bind nicotine in blood and reduce nicotine distribution to brain. As a result, vaccination can reduce the addictive effects of nicotine, and thereby facilitate treatment of tobacco dependence. By acting outside the brain, immunologic approaches should lack the central nervous system (CNS) sides effects associated with other types of medications. By preventing nicotine distribution to brain, all of nicotine's neuropharmacological effects in brain are attenuated.

An immunologic approach to treating drug dependence was first suggested over 30 years ago, when it was reported that immunization against heroin could reduce the likelihood that monkeys would self-administer the drug. Since then, vaccines and drug-specific antibodies have been developed that are effective in modifying the pharmacokinetics and behavioral effects of a range of drugs of abuse in animals, including cocaine, phencyclidine, and methamphetamine.[12,13] The purpose of the present article is to review the literature examining immunologic approaches against nicotine. Focus will be primarily on studies employing preclinical animal models, but brief coverage of recent early-phase clinical trials in humans will also be provided. Finally, several issues regarding the clinical application of immunologic interventions will be discussed.

Mechanism of Action

Nicotine, or any other drug of abuse, serves as a positive reinforcer. That is, it increases the frequency of behaviors, such as smoking tobacco, that lead to its delivery to the brain. This positive reinforcing effect of nicotine then leads to high sustained rates of smoking that are a hallmark of tobacco dependence and associated with many adverse health consequences (eg, lung cancer, cardiovascular disease). Thus, the positive reinforcing effect of nicotine on behavior is a cornerstone of tobacco dependence, and a primary behavioral target for medication development. Medications that attenuate nicotine's reinforcing effects should be useful in facilitating cessation of tobacco use.

The pharmacokinetic properties of drugs (ie, absorption, distribution, metabolism, elimination) are key determinants of their reinforcing effects. The dose of nicotine reaching the brain determines whether it has no effect, reinforcing effects, or punishing effects on behavior.[5,14] The speed with which nicotine is absorbed and reaches the brain also determines the strength of its reinforcing effects. Smoking, which produces peak blood levels within 10 to 20 seconds, is more reinforcing than chewing nicotine gum, which produces peak blood levels within 15 to 30 minutes. Conversely, slower metabolism and elimination of nicotine has been associated with lower rates of smoking needed to maintain a desired blood level and rate of reinforcement.[15-17] Because of their key role in determining the reinforcing effects of nicotine, these pharmacokinetic processes represent a potential pharmacological target for developing medications that attenuate nicotine's reinforcing effects and thereby facilitate smoking cessation. This is the primary goal of an immunologic approach to treating tobacco dependence.

Immunization against nicotine involves using nicotine-specific antibodies that bind nicotine in serum. In an immunized subject, nicotine-specific antibody is present in the bloodstream and extracellular fluid. The antibody is excluded from the brain because it is too large to cross the blood-brain barrier. When an immunized subject receives nicotine, a substantial fraction of the drug is bound to antibody, sequestered in blood, and prevented from entering the brain to thereby produce its reinforcing effects on tobacco use. In addition, the binding of nicotine by antibody makes it less available for metabolism. Thus, vaccination markedly slows nicotine's elimination half-life. Consequently, the rate of smoking could be reduced by prolonging the effect of nicotine from each cigarette and delaying the nicotine deprivation that leads to smoking the next cigarette. It is important to note that, although immunization against nicotine reduces the ability of the drug to bind to nicotinic cholinergic receptors, it should not be considered analogous to a nicotinic acetylcholinergic receptor antagonist such as mecamylamine. Receptor antagonists block the binding of endogenous compounds (eg, acetylcholine) to receptors, while antibodies do not. Moreover, nicotine-specific antibodies have the additional effect of increasing the elimination half-life of nicotine, while receptor antagonists do not.

Immunological Methods

Active Versus Passive Immunization

Immunization against nicotine can be achieved by 2 methods. Active immunization (hereafter referred to as vaccination) involves repeated administration of an immunogen to the subjects being studied in order to stimulate the immune system to produce nicotine-specific antibodies. Passive immunization involves the production of antibodies in some other species (eg, rabbits) or in vitro, which are then purified and administered to the subjects being studied. Each method has advantages and disadvantages. Vaccination requires relatively few administrations (eg, 1 injection per month for 3 to 4 months) to produce a high serum level of antibody that persists for several months. It is also relatively inexpensive. The primary disadvantages of vaccination are the delay to achieving required antibody levels and the inability to control those levels. Passive immunization also offers several advantages, including the ability to (a) achieve the required serum level of antibody virtually immediately, compared with the 1 to 2 months needed for vaccination, (b) control the antibody dose to study dose-response relationships, and (c) examine the effects of high antibody doses that cannot be achieved with vaccination alone. The primary disadvantages of passive immunization are that it requires more frequent injections to maintain required antibody levels and is more expensive than vaccination.

Vaccine Formulation and Administration

Nicotine is too small (molecular weight [MW] 167 kD) to elicit an immune response (ie, it is not immunogenic). Thus, regular tobacco users do not have antibodies against it. Nicotine is rendered immunogenic by conjugating (ie, linking) the drug itself or a structurally related compound (ie, hapten) to an immunogenic carrier protein to form a complete immunogen, referred to as a conjugate vaccine. Various types of carrier proteins have been employed, including keyhole limpet hemocyanin (KLH),[18-20] a 19-residue peptide,[21] recombinant cholera toxin B subunit,[22] and recombinant pseudomonas exoprotein A.[23] The latter 2 have the advantage of being used previously in vaccines administered to humans. The conjugation of nicotine to a carrier protein has typically been accomplished using a linker, such as succinic acid. One vaccine in development uses virus-like particles formed from the bacteriophage Qb instead of a carrier protein.[24] Most vaccines are prepared for administration by mixing the complete immunogen with an adjuvant (eg, Freund's in animals, alum in humans), which enhances the immune response. The peptide-based vaccine mentioned above does not use additional adjuvant.

After the initial injection of vaccine, periodic booster doses are needed to maintain satisfactory antibody levels, since exposure to nicotine by itself does not elicit an anamnestic (ie, booster response). Vaccination schedules in rats typically involve 2 to 4 injections at 2 to 4 week intervals. No studies have been published directly comparing different schedules to suggest an optimal one. Vaccination schedules during early clinical trials in humans have involved 2 to 6 injections also at 2 to 4 week intervals.

Specific Vaccines and Antibodies

The effects of 9 different nicotine vaccines have been reported in rodents,[18-22,24-27] 3 of which have been tested in phase I and II clinical trials.[24,28,29] The effects of passive immunization using various forms of nicotine-specific antibody have also been examined in several studies in rodents.[20,23,30,31] Although the formulation varies between these vaccines and antibodies, their mechanism of action is the same and their pharmacokinetic and behavioral effects in animals and humans are generally similar.

Antibody Characteristics

Three characteristics of vaccines that are relevant to treating drug abuse include its immunogenicity, and the affinity and specificity of the elicited antibodies. Immunogenicity refers to the serum concentration of antibody that is achieved. In order to be maximally effective, a vaccine must elicit and maintain a high serum concentration of antibody throughout the period of interest, because higher ratios of antibody to nicotine result in greater binding of nicotine in serum. Affinity refers to the strength with which the elicited antibodies bind the drug. Specificity refers to the extent to which the antibodies bind nicotine in preference to other compounds. Greater specificity reduces competition from other compounds for binding capacity, improves safety, and reduces the likelihood of adverse side effects. Vaccine formulation can influence these 3 properties. For example, specificity is influenced by linker position. Linkers that are distant from prime sites of metabolism help to elicit antibodies that preferentially bind nicotine over its metabolites.[18,23] In addition, immunogenicity appears to be influenced by the design of the hapten.[26]

All of the vaccines studied to date in animals have been sufficiently immuno-genic to elicit significant concentrations of nicotine-specific antibody in serum (eg, 0.1–0.29 mg/mL[18,32,33]) that bind nicotine with high affinity (eg, K_d 37–50 nM[23,24]). These antibodies also generally show high specificity for nicotine, as binding of other compounds is very low (cross-reactivity with other compounds such as nico-tine metabolites, acetylcholine, or other neurotransmitters is typically less than 5%[18,19,22,24]).

Preclinical Studies in Nonhumans

Pharmacokinetic Studies

The effects of vaccination or passive immunization on nicotine pharmacokinetics have been studied using both acute and chronic nicotine dosing protocols. Acute protocols have typically involved rapid delivery of a single intravenous (IV) dose of 0.01 to 0.03 mg/kg nicotine (equivalent on a weight basis to the nicotine absorbed from two thirds to 2 cigarettes by a smoker), with serum and brain nicotine levels measured 1 to 60 minutes postinfusion. Chronic protocols have involved either repeated bolus doses (0.003–0.03 mg/kg IV) or continuous infusion of nicotine via subcutaneous (sc) osmotic mini-pump (eg, 1.0 mg/kg/d). These protocols have been designed to achieve serum nicotine concentrations approximating that of moderate to heavy smokers (10–40 ng/mL).

Nicotine binding in serum

The binding of nicotine to serum proteins is normally quite low (<10%). However, in rats immunized against nicotine, 80% to 99% of nicotine in serum is bound to nicotine-specific antibody.[18,23,30] Consequently, studies have shown that total serum nicotine concentrations in immunized subjects are 300% to 850% higher than that in controls (Fig. 27.1).[22,23,32] This increase in nicotine binding results in up to a 92% decrease in the concentration of nicotine that is unbound in serum and capable of entering the brain.[33] In passively immunized rats, this effect has been shown to be directly related to antibody dose and affinity.[30]

Nicotine distribution to brain

The significant decrease in unbound serum nicotine concentrations in immunized subjects results in an associated decrease in nicotine distribution to brain. Across various animal studies, brain nicotine concentrations are 40% to 92% lower in vac-cinated subjects compared with controls within the first few minutes after a single nicotine dose.[22,32] Similar results have been obtained with passive immunization

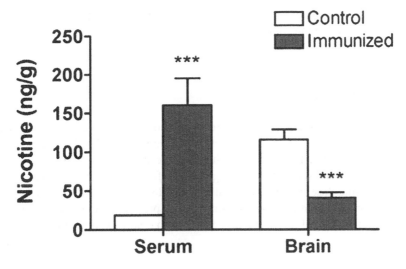

Fig. 27.1 Mean (± SEM) serum and brain nicotine concentrations in vaccinated and control rats. Three minutes after a single IV nicotine dose (0.03 mg/kg), the serum nicotine concentration was higher in vaccinated rats, and brain nicotine concentration was 64% lower than control rats. ***Significantly different from control, $P < .001$ (from Pentel et al, 2000[23] with permission from Elsevier).

(30%–90% reduction,[20,23,30] Fig. 27.1). This attenuation of the early distribution of nicotine to brain is particularly important because the positive subjective and reinforcing effects of nicotine are apparent within minutes after the first few puffs of a cigarette.[34] Several variables have been shown to influence the efficacy of immunization in reducing nicotine distribution to brain. First, effects are greatest in subjects with the highest serum concentration of antibody and, thus, the greatest capacity to bind nicotine.[35] Second, when higher single nicotine doses are administered, the degree of reduction in nicotine distribution to brain can be somewhat less (58%).[20] Third, when nicotine is administered chronically via repeated bolus doses or a continuous infusion, immunization has relatively little effect on the chronic accumulation of nicotine in brain (23%–29% reduction[35,36]). However, immunization still substantially reduces the peak level of nicotine produced by each individual dose. Finally, the efficacy in reducing nicotine distribution to brain has been shown to be directly related to antibody dose and affinity in passively immunized rats.[23,30]

One clinical concern is that a smoker could overcome the reduced distribution of nicotine to brain by increasing nicotine intake (ie, compensating) and overwhelming the binding capacity of the antibody. As a result, the desired CNS effects of nicotine could still be achieved. However, studies in animals have shown that both the cumulative distribution of nicotine to brain and distribution of a single dose are significantly decreased even when the nicotine dosing protocol provides a total nicotine dose exceeding the estimated binding capacity of antibody by up to 33-fold.[36] This finding suggests that the immediate rewarding and reinforcing effects of nicotine could still be suppressed in the context of increased nicotine exposure (eg, compensatory smoking).

Nicotine elimination

Because bound nicotine is protected from metabolism and excretion, vaccination restricts metabolism to the unbound fraction of nicotine, thereby slowing the overall elimination of nicotine from the body. Studies have shown that nicotine clearance is reduced by 90%, and serum half-life is prolonged from 0.8 hours up to 6 hours after a single nicotine dose in immunized rats.[35,37] As discussed above, this finding suggests that immunization could reduce smoking by prolonging the effects of nicotine and reducing the rate of nicotine intake required to obtain desired effects.

Behavioral Studies

The studies discussed above clearly demonstrate that immunization against nicotine can have profound effects on nicotine pharmacokinetics by reducing nicotine distribution to brain and slowing nicotine elimination. However, it is also clear that nicotine distribution to brain is not completely prevented, especially under some conditions of chronic nicotine exposure. Therefore, the question of whether these pharmacokinetic effects are large enough to alter the dependence-related behavioral effects of nicotine must be addressed. Significant progress has been made over the past 5 years addressing this question, as the effects of nicotine-specific antibodies have been characterized in a wide range of animal behavioral models. Some of these models (eg, locomotor behavior, seizures), although not particularly germane to the behavioral features of tobacco dependence, are useful for demonstrating that nicotine-specific antibodies can attenuate the behavioral effects of nicotine. The other models that have been used (eg, nicotine withdrawal, self-administration) are more relevant to tobacco dependence in that they model more closely the type of nicotine exposure and specific diagnostic criteria associated with tobacco dependence.

Locomotor behavior

As with other psychomotor stimulant drugs (eg, cocaine), nicotine induces an increase in locomotor activity when administered to rodents in a familiar environment.[38] To demonstrate this effect, rats are initially habituated to (ie, familiarized with) an activity test chamber for 3 sessions. Nicotine or saline is then administered prior to a test session and an activity score is obtained. Rats exposed to nicotine exhibit significantly higher levels of locomotor activity compared with saline-treated rats (Fig. 27.2). Passive immunization against nicotine has been shown to block this locomotor-stimulant effect of a single dose of nicotine, while cocaine-induced locomotor activity is unaffected.[23] Thus, the effects of passive immunization are specific to nicotine's locomotor stimulant effects as opposed to drug-induced locomotor stimulation in general.

With repeated administration of the same dose, the locomotor-stimulating effect of nicotine progressively increases (ie, locomotor sensitization is observed).[38] The putative neural substrate that mediates this effect is the mesolimbic dopamine system, the same system involved in the reinforcing effects of nicotine. The neuroadaptations that result from repeated exposure to nicotine may render this system more sensitive to the drug. As such, immunization may be less effective in attenuating the locomotor stimulant effects of nicotine in sensitized rats. However, both vaccination and passive immunization have been shown to attenuate the locomotor-stimulant effects of nicotine in rats after repeated exposure to nicotine, with passive immunization doing so in dose-dependent fashion.[20]

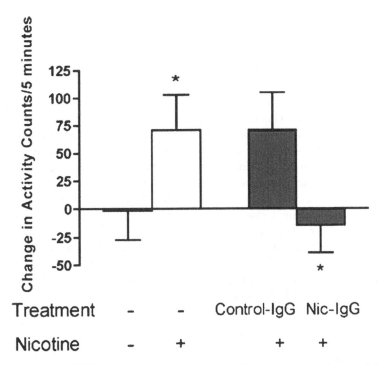

Fig. 27.2 Mean (± SEM) change in locomotor activity in rats after nicotine administration (0.28 mg, sc). In rats that were not vaccinated (open bars), nicotine-induced a significant increase in locomotor activity. However, nicotine-specific antibody (Nic-IgG) completely blocked the nicotine-induced increase in activity observed in control rats. *Significantly different from control IgG + nicotine, $P < .05$ (from Pentel et al, 2000[23] with permission from Elsevier).

Nicotine-induced seizures

At toxic doses, nicotine can induce seizures in both humans and animals. The large doses required to induce seizures in rats provide a rigorous test of an antibody's ability to reduce nicotine distribution to brain and nicotine-induced behavioral effects. In one study, vaccination was shown to reduce the incidence of seizures and distribution of nicotine to brain following a dose (2 mg/kg) that was 28-fold higher than the estimated binding capacity of the antibody.[39] The serum nicotine concentration produced by this dose in control rats (1050 ng/mL) was 25 to 50 times that of a regular smoker (10 to 40 mg/kg). This finding correlates well with pharmacokinetic studies showing continued efficacy despite a high degree of saturation of antibody and demonstrates that vaccination can effectively reduce the behavioral effects of nicotine even when such large nicotine doses are administered.

Nicotine relief of nicotine withdrawal syndrome

Part of the diagnostic criteria for tobacco dependence is the presence of a withdrawal syndrome upon termination of tobacco use. This withdrawal syndrome is characterized by several somatic and affective signs and symptoms, including gastrointestinal discomfort, depressed mood, irritability, anxiety, difficulty concentrating, and craving for tobacco. Tobacco withdrawal is important because many studies have shown it is one factor that can motivate relapse and undermine cessation success.[40] For example, smokers who experience withdrawal upon quitting may relapse because the nicotine obtained from smoking terminates the aversive withdrawal symptoms. This relief of withdrawal serves as another source of reinforcement that can maintain tobacco use. Consistent with this notion is that nicotine replacement products promote cessation in part because they relieve withdrawal symptoms. The ability of nicotine to relieve withdrawal can be modeled in animals. Rats are first made dependent on nicotine by administering a continuous sc nicotine infusion for 1 week. Termination of the infusion then results in a withdrawal syndrome characterized by a range of behavioral signs (eg, writhing, body shakes, tremors). If nicotine is administered again, the frequency of behavioral signs of withdrawal significantly decreases. However, in passively immunized rats, nicotine fails to reduce signs of withdrawal (Fig. 27.3).[31] Thus, to the extent that withdrawal motivates tobacco use, this finding suggests that immunization against nicotine could reduce the likelihood of relapse by rendering tobacco use less effective in relieving withdrawal.

Subjective effects

When humans use tobacco, they report various sensations or subjective effects. To the extent that these effects play a role in facilitating the development and maintenance

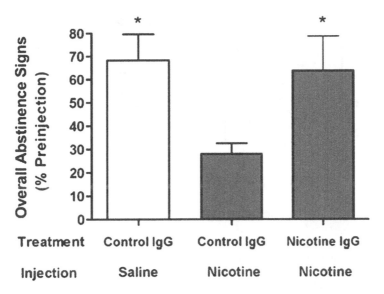

Fig. 27.3 Mean (± SEM) overall abstinence signs following sc injection of either nicotine (0.12 mg/kg) or saline during nicotine withdrawal in rats. Values are expressed as a percentage of signs observed prior to injection. Rats were passively immunized 25 hours earlier with either nicotine-specific antibody (Nicotine IgG) or control immunogen (Control IgG). Nic-IgG completely reversed the decrease in abstinence signs produced by nicotine that was observed in rats administered control IgG. *Significantly different from control IgG + nicotine, $P < .05$ (from Malin et al, 2001[31] with permission from Elsevier).

of tobacco dependence, blocking these effects may promote cessation of tobacco use. Animals can be taught to distinguish between the subjective effects of nicotine and other compounds using a drug discrimination procedure. This technique involves training rats to press one lever (nicotine lever) in a test chamber after administration of a dose of nicotine, and a different lever (saline lever) after administration of saline. In well-trained rats, nicotine comes to serve as a discriminative stimulus, such that the majority of lever presses will occur on the nicotine lever when nicotine is administered. Moreover, when the dose of nicotine is decreased, lever pressing decreases on the nicotine lever and increases on the saline lever, demonstrating that the subjective effects of nicotine are dose related. In one study using this paradigm, rats that were passively immunized against nicotine emitted fewer responses on the nicotine lever after a nicotine injection than control rats (Fig. 27.4).[41] Another study using a related paradigm showed that the rate of acquisition of a nicotine discrimination was slower in vaccinated rats.[21] Thus, both vaccination and passive immunization can attenuate the subjective effects of nicotine. This finding suggests that immunization against nicotine might reduce the pleasurable subjective effects of tobacco use and thereby facilitate cessation.

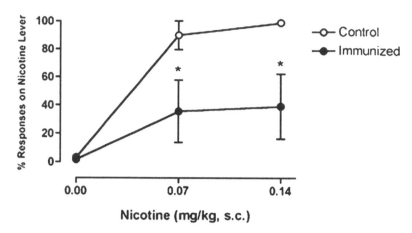

Fig. 27.4 Mean (±SEM) percentage of total responses made on the nicotine lever as a function of nicotine dose in immunized and control rats. Immunized rats exhibited a significantly lower percentage of responses on the nicotine lever following nicotine administration than control rats. *Significantly different from control, $P < .05$ (from Malin et al, 2002[41] with permission from Elsevier).

Reinforcing Effects

As discussed above, a hallmark of drug dependence is the high rate with which the drug is self-administered. Most drugs that are abused by humans, including nicotine, are also self-administered by animals. As such, nicotine self-administration in animals is considered a preclinical model of tobacco dependence, and studies of such behavior are thought to be relevant to the analysis and treatment of this disorder.[5] In a nicotine self-administration (NSA) procedure, IV nicotine infusions are administered contingent upon the animal emitting a specified response (eg, lever press). Both rodents and primates will exhibit robust levels of responding for nicotine infusions, and medications that reduce NSA in animals are thought to have potential utility in facilitating cessation of tobacco use in humans. Three phases of NSA often examined are acquisition, maintenance, and reinstatement. These 3 phases are considered relevant to similar phases of tobacco use in humans, such as initiation of use, continuation of use, and relapse after a quit attempt, respectively. The effects of nicotine vaccines on each of these phases of NSA have been examined.

In a recent study examining acquisition of NSA,[25] rats were vaccinated with nicotine or control immunogen prior to being given access to nicotine for 3 weeks. NSA was significantly lower in vaccinated rats compared with controls during the acquisition period, with vaccinated rats earning 38% fewer infusions during the last week of training (Fig. 27.5A) The percentage of rats meeting acquisition criteria in the vaccinated group was lower (36%) than that in the control group (70%), but this difference was not statistically significant. In the subgroup of rats that acquired NSA, infusion rates were similar to those in control rats (Fig. 27.5B), indicating

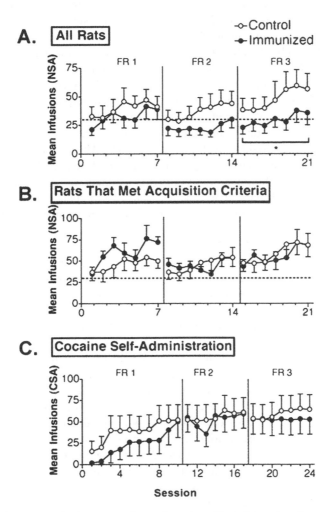

Fig. 27.5 Effects of vaccination on nicotine and cocaine self-administration. One week after their fourth and final vaccine dose, rats were placed in operant chambers where they had access to IV drug infusions 23 h/d. For the first week each response on an active lever (FR 1) produced an infusion of drug (0.01 mg/kg nicotine or 0.2 mg/kg cocaine). In the second and third weeks, 2 (FR 2) or 3 (FR 3) responses respectively were required for each infusion. (A) Number of nicotine infusions earned in immunized and control rats during the acquisition period. The dotted line indicates the minimum number of infusions required to meet acquisition criteria. At the end of week 3, responding was significantly lower in immunized rats compared with controls ($^*P < .05$). (B) Data for 5 vaccinated rats, which did meet acquisition criteria are shown. Their rates of NSA were similar to those of controls, suggesting that compensation did not occur. (C) Number of cocaine infusions in immunized and control rats during acquisition. No significant effect of vaccination on acquisition of cocaine self-administration was observed (from LeSage et al, in press, with permission from Springer Science and Business Media).

that this subgroup did not compensate by increasing their infusion rate to surmount the effects of vaccination on nicotine pharmacokinetics. In a parallel experiment, vaccination did not affect acquisition of cocaine self-administration, demonstrating its specificity for nicotine (Fig. 27.5C). These findings suggest a potential role for vaccination in the prevention of tobacco dependence.

In the same study, the effects of vaccination on the maintenance of NSA were also examined. Rats were initially trained to self-administer nicotine, and then vaccinated with nicotine or control immunogen, while NSA continued to be monitored. The effects of vaccination on food-maintained responding were similarly examined to determine the specificity of vaccination effects. NSA was significantly reduced in vaccinated rats compared with controls after the final (4th) vaccine injection, with a mean reduction of 57% (Fig. 27.6A). The slow onset of effect may have been owing to the slow development of antibody levels (and thus reduction of the nicotine dose reaching the brain) or that some nicotine still reaches the brain. Moreover, NSA has been shown to be less sensitive to changes in dose than self-administration of other drugs of abuse,[5] and this may have also contributed to the slow onset of effect. No effect on food-maintained responding was observed (unpublished data, 2005, Fig. 27.6B). There was no evidence that vaccinated rats attempted to compensate for altered nicotine distribution, as no significant increase in NSA was observed at any point during the vaccination period. These findings suggest a potential role for vaccination in facilitating cessation or reduction of tobacco use.

The effects of vaccination on reinstatement of NSA have also been examined. In this model, after rats are trained to self-administer nicotine, saline is substituted for nicotine to extinguish responding to low levels. Once extinction is achieved, a single priming dose of nicotine is administered prior to an extinction session. Reinstatement is evident when the priming infusion of nicotine produces a significant increase in responding on the lever that produced nicotine infusions during training. In one study,[42] rats were vaccinated with nicotine or control immunogen during the extinction period prior to the reinstatement test. While control rats exhibited a significant increase in responding following a low priming dose of nicotine, vaccinated rats did not. Thus, vaccination blocked the ability of a low dose of nicotine to reinstate NSA. This finding suggests a role for vaccination in preventing relapse to tobacco use.

Although the findings from animal studies are encouraging and suggest a potential role for immunologic approaches to treating or preventing tobacco dependence, they should be interpreted with some caution. In some studies employing passive immunization, the antibody affinity and dose used was higher than that which has been achieved by vaccination, which could possibly exaggerate efficacy. However, the nicotine dose used in some of these studies was much higher than those in smokers, thus providing a rigorous test of immunization. Although some of the animal models discussed above are somewhat relevant to essential features of tobacco dependence (nicotine withdrawal, NSA), their relevance to tobacco use in humans is not entirely clear. These models differ from tobacco use in humans along

A. Nicotine Self-Administration

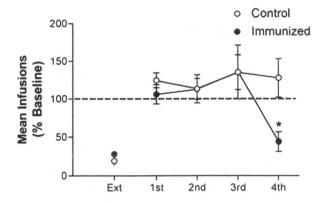

B. Food-Maintained Responding

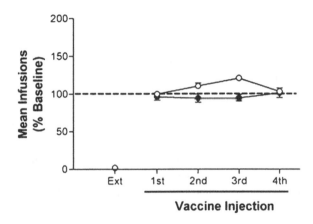

Fig. 27.6 Effects of vaccination on the maintenance of nicotine self-administration and responding for food pellets. Rats were initially trained to lever press for nicotine infusions (0.03 mg/kg/infusion) or food pellets. Responding was then extinguished and reacquired. After reacquisition of responding, rats received 4 doses of nicotine or control vaccine, while continuing to have access to nicotine (A) or food (B). Nicotine self-administration was reduced after the fourth vaccine dose in immunized rats compared with controls ($P < .05$). Immunization had no significant effect on food-maintained responding (unpublished data). *Significantly different from control, $P < .05$. (from LeSage et al, 2005, with permission from Springer Science and Business Media).[25]

several dimensions, including the route of nicotine administration, nicotine dose, and patterns of administration. In addition, the potential influence of nonpharmacological variables (sensory effects of smoke, social factors) that are known to promote tobacco use in humans on the efficacy of immunization remains to be determined. Development of better animal models may be helpful, but ultimately clinical trials in humans are needed to address some of these issues.

Studies in Humans

Immugenicity and Adverse Effects

The results of phase I and II clinical trials have been reported for 3 nicotine vaccines: NicVAX,[28] NicQb,[24] and TA-NIC.[29] The vaccination schedule in these clinical trials consisted of 2 to 6 doses of vaccine at an interval of 2 to 4 weeks, and a later booster dose was administered in 2 trials.[27,28] As in animal studies, serum antibody levels were low after the first dose and increased significantly after each subsequent dose. Marked variability in antibody levels between subjects has been observed. Antibody levels decreased by 50% over 6 to 8 weeks after the last vaccine injection of the initial immunization period but increased again when a booster dose was administered.[28] Thus, periodic booster doses would be needed to maintain antibody levels above some minimally acceptable value. In one trial, antibody levels in some subjects were in the range of that found to be effective in animal studies.[28] However, it is not yet clear what level of antibody will be necessary for efficacy in humans (see Clinical Issues).

No adverse events have been reported other than local reactions (eg, soreness or redness at the injection site) and mild systemic reactions (eg, flu-like symptoms such as fever, headache, malaise). Occurrence of these symptoms in placebo and vaccine groups was not significantly different, suggesting that they were the result of the adjuvant used rather than the immunogen. All symptoms resolved within 1 to 4 days without medical intervention. The lack of adverse effects is consistent with animal studies, demonstrating the specificity of antibodies for binding nicotine rather than endogenous compounds such as acetylcholine. These findings suggest that nicotine vaccines are well tolerated in humans and support the notion that immunotherapy may lack the side effects associated with other types of medication.

Potential Efficacy

Although these phase I and II clinical trials were not designed to examine the efficacy of vaccination in facilitating reduction or cessation of tobacco use, smoking status was nonetheless a secondary end point, thus providing a preliminary indication of efficacy.

In the TA-NIC trial,[27] participants were instructed to quit after receiving 6 vaccine injections at 1 of 3 doses over 12 weeks and were then boosted at 32 weeks. Quit rates were greater in the group receiving the highest vaccine dose than in the control group (38% vs 8%), but group size was small and statistical analysis was not reported. In the NicQb trial, participants who were motivated to quit were instructed to do so after the second monthly vaccine injection and received 3 additional monthly injections thereafter. Only a single vaccine dose was tested. Smoking cessation counseling was provided to all participants at each visit during the first 3 months. Although abstinence rates confirmed by self-report and expired air CO did not differ between the vaccine and control groups, a subgroup of vaccinated participants with the highest antibody levels exhibited significantly higher abstinence rates than controls (57% vs 31%, n = 30/53 vs 25/80). In the NicVax trial,[28] participants were neither motivated to quit nor instructed to do so. Participants received 3 monthly vaccine injections at 1 of 3 doses followed by a booster dose at 6 months. A greater percentage of subjects achieved 30 days of continuous abstinence (confirmed by self-report and expired air CO) in the high-dose vaccine group (40%) compared with the control group (8%). There was no evidence of increased smoking according to self-report, expired air CO, and urinary NNAL (a tobacco carcinogen nicotine metabolite). Thus, smokers did not try to compensate for possible reductions in nicotine distribution to brain.

It is important to stress that these initial clinical findings are preliminary, owing to small sample sizes and the necessity to stratify vaccinated participants based on antibody level to observe differences between groups. However, it is encouraging to see that despite the marked differences between these studies (ie, the motivation of participants to quit, whether they were instructed to do so, and whether they received concurrent counseling), they all showed a similar trend toward efficacy. Moreover, the fact that efficacy was only achieved in participants receiving the highest vaccine dose or achieving the highest antibody levels is consistent with animal studies showing that the greatest effect of vaccination in altering nicotine pharmacokinetics is observed in rats with the highest antibody levels.[33,35] Thus, development of improved vaccine formulations or vaccination schedules that elicit higher antibody levels may be necessary to improve efficacy.

Clinical Issues

Advantages of Immunologic Approaches

As discussed above, immunologic approaches to treating tobacco dependence have 3 key advantages. First, immunization appears to be safe because of its low cross-reactivity with compounds other than nicotine. Second, immunization only requires a brief series of monthly injections to produce effects that can endure for months. The lack of major side effects and relatively minimal dosing requirements could be associated with improved patient compliance. Third, its unique mechanism of action makes it well suited for combination with other pharmacotherapies. Both the animal and human data thus far show that the efficacy of vaccination is limited. Despite best efforts to improve on immunologic methods in their own right, combining immunization with other medications may be necessary to maximize efficacy.

Potential Concerns

The lack of control over antibody levels and large variability between subjects is the primary limitation of vaccination. Both the animal and human studies discussed in this review show that achieving the highest antibody levels possible will be essential to maximizing the efficacy of vaccination. In addition, the slow development of antibody levels and onset of effect could discourage tobacco users who are eager to quit from trying vaccination, as treatment would need to be initiated months before the quit attempt. Methods of boosting immunogenicity need to be explored in order to address these issues. Passive immunization with a high-affinity antibody could be combined with vaccination to provide any desired antibody level and an immediate onset of effect. However, passive immunization is much more expensive and requires more frequent dosing, and potential side effects could occur (eg, allergic reactions).

To the extent that nicotine plays a role in the adverse effects of maternal smoking on fetal outcomes, immunization against nicotine could play a role in protecting the fetus from some of these adverse effects. Studies are needed to assess the safety of immunizing pregnant smokers and the efficacy of immunization in reducing fetal exposure to nicotine. Animal studies have shown that immunization reduces nicotine distribution to maternal brain in pregnant female rats to a similar extent as in male rats.[37,43] In addition, immunization reduces nicotine distribution to fetal brain by up to 63% after a single nicotine dose. Although nicotine distribution to whole fetus is not reduced, immunization reduces the concentration of unbound nicotine in fetal serum. These findings suggest that immunization should not exacerbate the adverse effects of prenatal nicotine exposure and comment on the safety of immunizing pregnant smokers against nicotine.

There is concern that compensatory increases in smoking could occur to surmount the effects of immunization, possibly leading to increases in exposure to other harmful constituents in tobacco. However, there has been no evidence of compensation in either animals self-administering nicotine or smoking in humans. It is also possible that immunization could precipitate withdrawal. Although this has not been examined in animal models of nicotine withdrawal, one clinical trial found no evidence of vaccination precipitating withdrawal.[28]

Vaccination would not address the effects of nicotine withdrawal, such as craving or negative affect, that would likely occur upon cessation of tobacco use. As discussed above, withdrawal can be a strong motivator for relapse and dropping out of treatment. Although immunization may attenuate the ability of a smoking lapse to relieve withdrawal, the withdrawal may be severe enough for a smoker to abandon continuing treatment. Thus, combining vaccination with therapies directed against withdrawal processes may be helpful or even necessary for vaccination to be effective in treating tobacco dependence. Fortunately, this should be feasible owing to the unique mechanism of action of immunization and the low probability of adverse interactions that can be associated with combining other forms of pharmacotherapy.

Immunologic interventions target the role of nicotine in tobacco addiction. However, nonpharmacologic factors such as the environmental context and the sensory aspects of smoking also clearly play a role in tobacco dependence. These stimuli come to serve as powerful conditioned reinforcers that help to maintain tobacco use. Although immunization does not target these factors directly, it can help to alter the control of these stimuli. Whenever tobacco use occurs in a vaccinated user and nicotine cannot produce its reinforcing effects, then the association between nicotine at these nonpharmacological stimuli is broken and the stimuli should eventually lose their conditioned reinforcing strength.

Finally, other compounds in tobacco, such as acetaldehyde or nornicotine, may also play a role in the reinforcing effects of tobacco use. Although vaccination against nicotine will not impact these factors, it could be combined with other pharmacotherapies that do.

Conclusion

Immunization against nicotine can significantly attenuate several behavioral effects of nicotine in animals that are considered relevant to tobacco dependence in humans. These findings suggest that immunologic interventions could have use in the treatment of tobacco dependence. Initial clinical trials have demonstrated that nicotine vaccines are safe and produce substantial serum levels of nicotine-specific antibody in humans. Although preliminary data from these small trials suggest that vaccination may facilitate abstinence from tobacco use, more advance trials are needed to validate this finding. Taken together, the research to date suggests that immunological interventions could play an important role in future treatments for tobacco dependence. The primary role of such interventions will likely be in preventing relapse in smokers who are motivated to quit. By preventing a lapse from producing positive subjective and reinforcing effects, vaccination might prevent progression to full relapse. Another potential role for immunologic interventions is in facilitating reduction of tobacco use in people who are unwilling or unable to quit. It is generally accepted that the most effective approach to treating tobacco dependence is concurrent use of medications and behavioral therapy. Despite the significant therapeutic potential of immunological interventions, they do not target the nonpharmacological factors that maintain tobacco dependence and will likely be maximally effective when combined with behavioral interventions that motivate abstinence from tobacco use.

Acknowledgments Supported by National Institutes of Health grants DA10714, P50-DA013333, and DA15668.

References

1. Centers for Disease Control and Prevention (CDC). Annual smoking-attributable mortality, years of potential life lost, and economic costs–United States, 1995–1999. *MMWR Morb Mortal Wkly Rep*. 2002;51:300-303.

2. U. S. Department of Health and Human Services. *Healthy People 2010. With understanding and improving health and objectives for improving health.* Washington, DC: US Department of Health and Human Services; 2000.

3. Harvey DM, Yasar S, Heishman SJ, Panlilio LV, Henningfield JE, Goldberg SR. Nicotine serves as an effective reinforcer of intravenous drug-taking behavior in human cigarette smokers. *Psychopharmacology (Berl).* 2004;175:134-142.

4. Stolerman IP, Jarvis MJ. The scientific case that nicotine is addictive. *Psychopharmacology (Berl).* 1995;117:2–10. Discussion 14-20.

5. Corrigall WA. Nicotine self-administration in animals as a dependence model. *Nicotine Tob Res.* 1999;1:11-20.

6. Gerrits MA, Petromilli P, Westenberg HG, Di Chiara G, van Ree JM. Decrease in basal dopamine levels in the nucleus accumbens shell during daily drug-seeking behaviour in rats. *Brain Res.* 2002;924:141-150.

7. Wonnacott S, Sidhpura N, Balfour DJ. Nicotine: from molecular mechanisms to behaviour. *Curr Opin Pharmacol.* 2005;5:53-59.

8. Fiore MC. US public health service clinical practice guideline: treating tobacco use and dependence. *Respir Care.* 2000;45:1200-1262.

9. Ferry L, Johnston JA. Efficacy and safety of bupropion SR for smoking cessation: data from clinical trials and five years of postmarketing experience. *Int J Clin Pract.* 2003;57:224-230.

10. Fiore MC, Smith SS, Jorenby DE, Baker TB. The effectiveness of the nicotine patch for smoking cessation: a meta-analysis. *JAMA.* 1994;271:1940-1947.

11. Hurt RD, Sachs DP, Glover ED, et al. A comparison of sustained-release bupropion and placebo for smoking cessation. *N Engl J Med.* 1997;337:1195-1202.

12. Haney M, Kosten TR. Therapeutic vaccines for substance dependence. *Expert Rev Vaccines.* 2004;3:11-18.

13. Pentel PR, Keyler DE. Vaccines to treat drug addiction. In: Levine MM, Kaper JB, Rappuoli R, Liu MA, Good MF, eds. *New Generation Vaccines.* New York, NY: Marcel Dekker; 2004.

14. Goldberg SR, Spealman RD. Suppression of behavior by intravenous injections of nicotine or by electric shocks in squirrel monkeys: effects of chlordiazepoxide and mecamylamine. *J Pharmacol Exp Ther.* 1983;224:334-340.

15. Benowitz NL, Perez-Stable EJ, Herrera B. Jacob Pr. Slower metabolism and reduced intake of nicotine from cigarette smoking in Chinese-Americans. *J Natl Cancer Inst.* 2002;94:108-115.

16. Malaiyandi V, Sellers EM, Tyndale RF. Implications of CYP2A6 genetic variation for smoking behaviors and nicotine dependence. *Clin Pharmacol Ther.* 2005;77:145-158.

17. Schoedel KA, Hoffmann EB, Rao Y, Sellers EM, Tyndale RF. Ethnic variation in CYP2A6 and association of genetically slow nicotine metabolism and smoking in adult Caucasians. *Pharmacogenetics.* 2004;14:615-626.

18. Hieda Y, Keyler DE, Vandevoort JT, et al. Active immunization alters the plasma nicotine concentration in rats. *J Pharmacol Exp Ther.* 1997;283:1076-1081.

19. de Villiers SH, Lindblom N, Kalayanov G, et al. Active immunization against nicotine suppresses nicotine-induced dopamine release in the rat nucleus accumbens shell. *Respiration.* 2002;69:247-253.

20. Carrera MR, Ashley JA, Hoffman TZ, et al. Investigations using immunization to attenuate the psychoactive effects of nicotine. *Bioorg Med Chem.* 2004;12:563-570.

21. Sanderson SD, Cheruku SR, Padmanilayam MP, et al. Immunization to nicotine with a peptide-based vaccine composed of a conformationally biased agonist of C5a as a molecular adjuvant. *Int Immunopharmacol.* 2003;3:137-146.

22. Cerny EH, Levy R, Mauel J, et al. Preclinical development of a vaccine "against smoking." *Onkologie.* 2002;25:406-411.

23. Pentel PR, Malin DH, Ennifar S, et al. A nicotine conjugate vaccine reduces nicotine distribution to brain and attenuates its behavioral and cardiovascular effects in rats. *Pharmacol Biochem Behav.* 2000;65:191-198.

24. Maurer P, Jennings GT, Willers J, et al. A therapeutic vaccine for nicotine dependence: preclinical efficacy, and Phase I safety and immunogenicity. *Eur J Immunol.* 2005;35:2031-2040.

25. LeSage MG, Keyler DE, Hieda Y. Effects of a nicotine conjugate vaccine on the acquisition and maintenance of nicotine self-administration in rats. *Psychopharmacology (Berl).* 2005;1-8.

26. Meijler MM, Jr, Matsushita M, Jr, Altobell L, Jr, Wirsching P, Janda KD. A new strategy for improved nicotine vaccines using conformationally constrained haptens. *J Am Chem Soc.* 2003;125:7164-7165.

27. St Clair Roberts J, Akers CVR, Vanhinsbergh L, McKenna KA, Wood DM, Jack L. Longitudinal safety and immunogenicity data of TA-NIC, a novel nicotine vaccine. Proceedings of the Ninth Annual Meeting of the Society for Research on Nicotine and Tobacco Ninth Annual Meeting of the Society for Research on Nicotine and Tobacco; February 19–22, 2003; New Orleans, LA. Middletown, WI: Society for Research on Nicotine and Tobacco; 2003.

28. Hatsukami D, Rennard S, Jorenby DE, et al. Safety and immunogenicity of a nicotine conjugate vaccine in current smokers. *Clin Pharmacol Ther.* 2005;78:456-467.

29. St Clair Roberts J, Dobson J, Wood D, Settles M. Safety and immunogenicity of a human nicotine conjugate vaccine. *Drug Alcohol Depend.* 2002;66:S148.

30. Keyler DE, Roiko SA, Benlhabib E, et al. Monoclonal nicotine-specific antibodies reduce nicotine distribution to brain in rats: dose- and affinity-response relationships. *Drug Metab Dispos.* 2005;33:1056-1061.

31. Malin DH, Lake JR, Lin A, et al. Passive immunization against nicotine prevents nicotine alleviation of nicotine abstinence syndrome. *Pharmacol Biochem Behav.* 2001;68:87-92.

32. de Villiers SH, Lindblom N, Kalayanov G, Gordon S, Johansson AM, Svensson TH. Active immunization against nicotine alters the distribution of nicotine but not the metabolism to cotinine in the rat. *Naunyn Schmiedebergs Arch Pharmacol.* 2004;370:299-304.

33. Satoskar SD, Keyler DE, LeSage MG, Raphael DE, Ross CA, Pentel PR. Tissue-dependent effects of immunization with a nicotine conjugate vaccine on the distribution of nicotine in rats. *Int Immunopharmacol.* 2003;3:957-970.

34. Perkins KA, Jacobs L, Sanders M, Caggiula AR. Sex differences in the subjective and reinforcing effects of cigarette nicotine dose. *Psychopharmacology (Berl).* 2002;163:194-201.

35. Keyler DE, Hieda Y, St Peter J, Pentel PR. Altered disposition of repeated nicotine doses in rats immunized against nicotine. *Nicotine Tob Res.* 1999;1:241-249.

36. Hieda Y, Keyler DE, Ennifar S, Fattom A, Pentel PR. Vaccination against nicotine during continued nicotine administration in rats: immunogenicity of the vaccine and effects on nicotine distribution to brain. *Int J Immunopharmacol.* 2000;22:809-819.

37. Keyler DE, Dufek MB, Calvin AD, et al. Reduced nicotine distribution from mother to fetal brain in rats vaccinated against nicotine: time course and influence of nicotine dosing regimen. *Biochem Pharmacol.* 2005;69:1385-1395.

38. Stolerman IP. Interspecies consistency in the behavioural pharmacology of nicotine dependence. *Behav Pharmacol.* 1999;10:559-580.

39. Tuncok Y, Hieda Y, Keyler DE, et al. Inhibition of nicotine-induced seizures in rats by combining vaccination against nicotine with chronic nicotine infusion. *Exp Clin Psychopharmacol.* 2001;9:228-234.

40. Shiffman S, West R, Gilbert D. Recommendation for the assessment of tobacco craving and withdrawal in smoking cessation trials. *Nicotine Tob Res.* 2004;6:599-614.

41. Malin DH, Alvarado CL, Woodhouse KS, et al. Passive immunization against nicotine attenuates nicotine discrimination. *Life Sci.* 2002;70:2793-2798.

42. Lindblom N, de Villiers SH, Kalayanov G, Gordon S, Johansson AM, Svensson TH. Active immunization against nicotine prevents reinstatement of nicotine-seeking behavior in rats. *Respiration.* 2002;69:254-260.

43. Keyler DE, Shoeman D, LeSage MG, Calvin AD, Pentel PR. Maternal vaccination against nicotine reduces nicotine distribution to fetal brain in rats. *J Pharmacol Exp Ther.* 2003;305:587-592.

Chapter 28
New Paradigms and Tools in Drug Design for Pain and Addiction

Victor J. Hruby,[1,3] Frank Porreca,[2] Henry I. Yamamura,[2] Gordon Tollin,[1,3]
Richard S. Agnes,[1] Yeon Sun Lee,[1] Minying Cai,[1] Isabel Alves,[1,3]
Scott Cowell,[1] Eva Varga,[2] Peg Davis,[2] Zdzislaw Salamon,[3] William Roeske,[2]
Todd Vanderah,[2] and Josephine Lai[2]

Abstract New modalities providing safe and effective treatment of pain, especially prolonged pathological pain, have not appeared despite much effort. In this mini-review/overview we suggest that new paradigms of drug design are required to counter the underlying changes that occur in the nervous system that may elicit chronic pain states. We illustrate this approach with the example of designing, in a single ligand, molecules that have agonist activity at μ and δ opioid receptors and antagonist activities at cholecystokinin (CCK) receptors. Our findings thus far provide evidence in support of this new approach to drug design. We also report on a new biophysical method, plasmon waveguide resonance (PWR) spectroscopy, which can provide new insights into information transduction in G-protein coupled receptors (GPCRs) as illustrated by the δ opioid receptor.

Keywords drug design, neuropathic pain, bifunctional ligands, plasmon waveguide resonance spectroscopy, GPCRs, opioid receptors, cholecystokinin receptors

Introduction

Despite much effort, medications providing effective and tolerable treatment of chronic abnormal pains such as neuropathic pain have not appeared in the past 2 decades. The reasons for this are multifaceted and involve cultural, political, economic, social, and scientific considerations. From a scientific perspective it has become increasingly clear that current methods of drug design[1] are inadequate and require revision when considering the nonphysiological state of the nervous system, which is associated with chronic pain.[2]

[1] Department of Chemistry, University of Arizona, Tucson, AZ

[2] Department of Pharmacology, University of Arizona, Tucson, AZ

[3] Departments of Biochemistry and Molecular Biophysics, University of Arizona, Tucson, AZ

Corresponding Author: Victor J. Hruby, Regents Professor, Department of Chemistry, University of Arizona, Tucson, AZ 85721. Tel: (520) 621-6332; Fax: (520) 621-8407; E-mail: hruby@u.arizona.edu

Many recent studies[3-5] have suggested that in neuropathic pain states adaptations occur in the central and peripheral nervous systems that may change the expected pain-relieving actions of analgesics such as morphine. An additional complication is the recent understanding that in addition to their pain-relieving actions, opioids can elicit unexpected development of hyperalgesia, or an increase in sensitivity to normally noxious and also to nonnoxious stimuli, resulting in enhancement of pain.[6,7] Adaptations that can occur in the nervous system in conditions of chronic pain include increases in the expression and activity of endogenous neurotransmitters, such as cholecystokinin (CCK), which may act both as pronociceptive substances and produce "anti-opioid" effects as well.[8] Both of these actions will diminish the analgesic actions of opioids, reducing the expected therapeutic benefit of these drugs. In this article, we outline a new approach for designing drugs that will be effective in these pain states and illustrate this approach by designing single ligands that can act as both agonists at opioid receptors and antagonists at CCK receptors. Additionally, the possibility that opiate use may produce increased sensitivity to pain is an aspect of pain management that is now receiving considerable attention, as indicated by the spate of recent blinded clinical studies. Investigations performed with patients undergoing surgery showed that intraoperative opiate administration resulted in increased postoperative pain and increased the dose required for postoperative analgesics in order to achieve analgesia.[9]

Finally, we discuss a new biophysical method, plasmon waveguide resonance (PWR) spectroscopy that allows, for the first time, direct examination, in real time, of the structural changes that occur to G-protein coupled receptors (GPCRs) in model membrane bilayers when the receptor interacts with agonists, antagonists, and inverse agonists, and the effects on G-protein-receptor interactions on these different receptor-occupied conformational states. These studies can be done without any spectroscopic labels, radioactive moieties, or other structure modifications that often can interfere with or change the nature of the interactions. Surprising results are obtained that suggest a major revision of current models of GPCR-mediated effects.

Materials and Methods

Peptide Synthesis

Peptide synthesis of the ligands discussed here was accomplished by standard methods of solid phase peptide synthesis using the N^{α}-Fmoc strategy.[10] The synthesized peptides were purified by gel filtration and preparative reverse-phase high-performance liquid chromatography (HPLC) generally using a gradient system composed of acetonitrile and 0.1% aqueous trifluoroacetic acid. Purity was assessed by thin layer chromatography in 3 solvent systems and by analytic HPLC. Further analysis of the structure was determined using high-resolution mass spectrometry and amino acid analysis, and by nuclear magnetic resonance spectroscopy in selected samples. The peptides generally were greater than 98% pure.

Binding Assays

Receptor binding affinities to the δ- and μ-opioid receptors were performed with membrane preparations using methods previously reported.[11] Binding affinities to the CCK receptors (CCK-1 and CCK-2) were made using stably transfected cell lines that express the human CCK-1 or CCK-2 receptors (the cDNA were gifts from Dr. Alan Kopin) using published methods that were recently published. Radiolabeled ligands used were [³H]c[DPen,²DPen⁵]-enkephalin (DPDPE) or [³H]-deltorphin II for the δ opioid receptor, D-Phe-c[Cys-Tyr-D-Trp-Arg-Thr-Pen]-Thr-NH$_2$ ([³H]CTAP) or [D-Ala², Gly-OH⁵]-enkephalin ([³H]DAMGO) for the μ-opioid receptor, and [³H]CCK-8 (sulfated) for the CCK-1 and CCK-2 receptors. Multiple assays were performed for each ligand reported, and the results were analyzed statistically.

Bioassay

In vitro functional bioassays were determined using the guinea pig ileum (GPI, μ), mouse vas deferens (MVD, δ), and the unstimulated GPI/LMMP (CCK receptor) (versus the sulfated CCK-8 for antagonist activity) as described previously.[12] Multiple assays were performed for each ligand, and the results were analyzed statistically.

Plasmon-Waveguide Resonance Spectroscopy

PWR spectra were obtained by resonance excitation of conduction electron oscillations (plasmons) by polarized light from a CW laser at wavelengths of 632.8 or 543.5 nm incident on the back surface of a thin metal film (Ag) coated by a layer of SiO$_2$ deposited on a glass prism,[13,14] using a Proterion Corp (Piscataway, NJ) instrument that had a spectral resolution of 1 millidegree (mdeg). The sample to be analyzed (a solid-supported lipid bilayer membrane) was immobilized on the resonator SiO$_2$ surface and placed in contact with an aqueous medium to which proteins and ligands could be introduced. The deposited molecules (eg, bilayer, GPCRs, G-proteins) change the resonance characteristics and thereby influence the plasmon spectra. The PWR spectra, which are plots of reflected light intensity versus the incident angle, can be obtained with light whose electric vector is either parallel or perpendicular to the plane of the resonator surface (s- or p-polarization, respectively). From these spectra 2 refractive index values (n_s and n_p) as well as the sample thickness (t) can be determined. This provides information about changes in the mass density, structural asymmetry, and molecular orientation that results from the molecular interactions occurring at the resonator surface.[15,16]

Receptor Purification and Characterization; Incorporation of hDOR Into a Lipid Bilayer by Detergent Dilution Followed by Ligand or G-Protein Addition

A fully functional human δ opioid receptor (hDOR) with a Myc and His tag was stably transfected into a Chinese hamster ovary cell line (CHO-K1) and was solubilized and purified as previously reported.[16,17] For studies in which the receptors were prebound with ligand (to study G-protein interactions with the liganded receptor), the solubilized purified receptors were incubated with saturating amounts of a peptide agonist (DPDPE), a nonpeptide agonist (SNC80), or an antagonist (Naltrindole, NTI) for 1 to 2 hours at 4°C prior to introduction into the PWR cell that contained a previously prepared lipid bilayer, which was assembled as previously reported.[16] This bilayer is formed within the orifice of a Teflon sheet on the PWR cell surface that separates the resonator from the aqueous medium. This provides a lipid bilayer with an annulus of lipid at the borders of the orifice, which allows lipid molecules to move into and out of the bilayer in response to protein insertion and/or changes in the protein conformation. In general, the lipid bilayers consisted of egg phosphatidylcholine (PC) and 1-palmitoyl2-oleyl-*sn*-glycero-3-phosphoglycerol (Avanti Polar Lipids, Alabaster, AL) (75/25 mol/mol) prepared as previously reported.[17] The receptors (either unoccupied or ligand occupied) were incorporated into the lipid bilayer by introducing the purified detergent-solubilized hDOR receptor in 30 mM octyl glucoside-containing buffer into the aqueous compartment of the resonator prism under conditions that dilute the detergent to below the critical micelle concentration (CMC), which allows the receptor protein to spontaneously insert into the lipid bilayer. Based on a variety of control experiments, the evidence suggests that the receptor molecules insert bidirectionally into the lipid bilayer; that is, with the extracellular side facing both the silica surface (this allows examination of G-protein interactions with the receptor) and the aqueous compartment (this allows examination of ligand-receptor interactions). G-proteins examined include mixtures of $G_{\alpha o}$, $G_{\alpha i1}$, $G_{\alpha i2}$, and $G_{\alpha i3}$ (or pure single G_α subunits) and a βγ subunit complex (a mixture of the different βγ subtypes present in the brain—both obtained from Calbiochem, EMD Biosciences, La Jolla, CA). Aliquots of ligand or G-protein solutions were incrementally added to increase their concentration so as to effectively examine the dose-response of these molecules. For the GTPγS (Sigma, St Louis, MO.) binding studies, the G-protein-receptor complex formation was at full saturation before GTPγS was added (again incrementally). In these experiments, the changes in the spectra were monitored using both *s*- and *p*-polarized light. From these experiments, hyperbolic saturation curves corresponding to a plot of the concentration of the ligand (or G-protein) added versus the resonance position angle (in mdeg) can be obtained to provide K_D values using standard curve fitting procedures.

Results and Discussion

As discussed above, our analysis of the changes in the expression of neurotransmitters and their receptors that accompany the development of neuropathic pain and prolonged pain of various origins suggested to us that the design of a single ligand that had agonist activities at both δ and μ opioid receptors, and antagonist activity at CCK-1 and especially CCK-2 receptors, would provide a ligand that could directly address the changes in gene expression in the brain and spinal cord that accompany these pain states. Two specific approaches to the design of such ligands were considered: (1) development of a single ligand with overlapping pharmacophores for the opioid receptors and the CCK receptors, and (2) development of a single ligand that possessed the agonist pharmacophore for the μ and δ opioid receptors, and the antagonist pharmacophore for the CCK-1 and CCK-2 receptors joined together by a spacer. This latter approach, though successfully pursued, will not be further discussed here. The idea of developing a peptide or peptidomimetic ligand, which possesses affinity for both opioid and CCK receptors in a single molecule rather than in 2 separate molecules, was chosen for several reasons: (1) economy of structure especially when using the concept of overlapping pharmacophores in design, (2) development of a single moiety that would have a single mode of delivery, transport, metabolism, and biodistribution and a single toxicity (such a molecule would more easily obtain approval as a new drug by the Food and Drug Administration [FDA]), and (3) an opportunity to evaluate a new approach to drug design for disease states in which changes in gene expression are believed to have occurred and are important components of the disease state. If successful, we believe this approach can be applied to many other diseases such as cancer and diabetes.

In previous research directed to obtaining analogs of CCK-8 with selectivity for the CCK-2 (or CCK-1) receptor, we obtained a ligand we designated as SNF-9007 (H-Asp-Tyr-D-Phe-Gly-Trp-NMeNle-Asp-Phe-NH$_2$, Fig. 28.1), which was highly potent and selective for the CCK-2 receptor[18] but which had weak agonist activity at the δ and μ opioid receptors.[18] Furthermore, we noticed, based on our modeling studies of the highly δ opioid selective cyclic enkephalin analog DPDPE[19] and of the CCK-8 structure, that they possessed similar topographical 3-dimensional

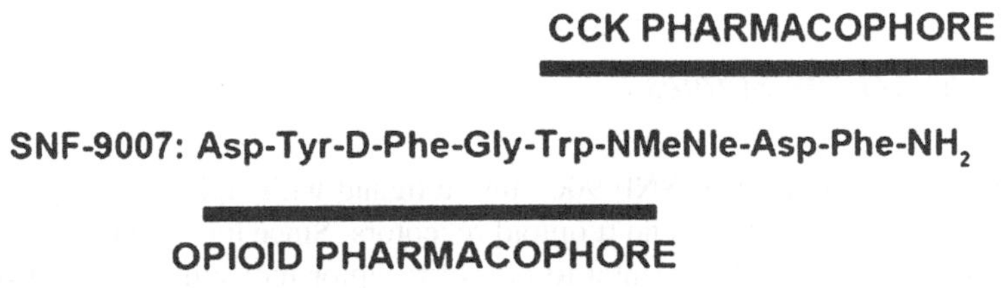

CCK PHARMACOPHORE
▬▬▬▬▬▬▬▬▬▬▬▬▬▬▬

SNF-9007: Asp-Tyr-D-Phe-Gly-Trp-NMeNle-Asp-Phe-NH$_2$
▬▬▬▬▬▬▬▬▬▬▬

OPIOID PHARMACOPHORE

Fig. 28.1 Design of a single molecule with overlapping pharmacophores for opioid and CCK receptors.

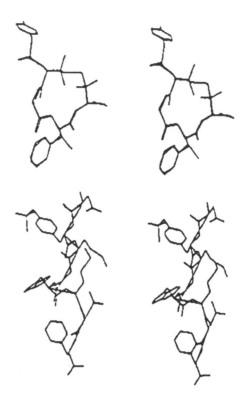

Fig. 28.2 Similarities between the conformations of DPDPE (top) and CCK$_8$ (bottom) shown in stereoview.

structures, especially in the placement of critical aromatic residues important to both pharmacophores (Fig. 28.2).[20,21] Further modeling suggested that the 2 pharmacophores (DPDPE and CCK-8) could be overlapped in a single structure such as SNF-9007 (Fig. 28.1). As outlined below we felt that further modification in such a structure could provide a single ligand with the desired biological activity profile.

Structure-Activity Studies

Our first goal was to convert SNF-9007 into a ligand with higher binding affinities and agonist activities at the δ and μ opioid receptors. Since the amino terminal Asp residue in SNF-9007 is detrimental to opioid receptor molecular recognition, and not essential for CCK receptor binding, we removed it and obtained compound **1** (Table 28.1), which had much improved affinity (~40-fold) for both the δ ($K_i = 6.8$ nM) and μ ($K_i = 136$ nM) receptors. We then further improved the opioid binding affinity of **1** by replacing the D-Phe² residue with other D-amino acid residues known to

Table 28.1 Increasing the Binding Affinity at Opioid Receptors by Modifying SNF-9007*

Compound	Opioid, K_i (nM)		CCK, K_i (nM)	
	$\delta^\dagger$	$\mu^\ddagger$	CCK-1§	CCK-2§
H-Asp-Tyr-D-Phe-Gly-Trp-NMeNle-Asp-Phe-NH$_2$ (SNF-9007)	250	5200	3300	2.1
1. H-Tyr-D-Phe-Gly-Trp-NMeNle-Asp-Phe-NH$_2$	6.8	136	10 000	2.1
2. H-Tyr-D-Ala-Gly-Trp-NMeNle-Asp-Phe-NH$_2$	14	46	5700	2.1
3. H-Tyr-D-Nle-Gly-Trp-NMeNle-Asp-Phe-NH$_2$	1.6	25	3900	0.60
4. H-Tyr-Gly-Gly-Trp-NMeNle-Asp-Phe-NH$_2$	2010	610	870	1.3

*CCK indicates cholecystokinin.
[†] Competitive binding assay versus [³H]DPDPE.
[‡] Competitive binding assay versus DAMGO.
[§] Competitive binding assay versus [³H]CCK-8.

Table 28.2 SAR Studies to Balance the Selectivity for CCK-1 and CCK-2 Receptors*

Compound	K_i (nM)		K_i (nM)	
	$\delta^\dagger$	$\mu^\ddagger$	CCK-1§	CCK-2§
1. H-Tyr-D-Phe-Gly-Trp-NMeNle-Asp-Phe-NH$_2$	6.8	136	10 000	2.1
5. H-Tyr-D-Phe-Gly-Trp-Nle-Asp-Phe-NH$_2$	0.42	80	116	8.1
6. H-Tyr-D-Ala-Gly-Trp-Nle-Asp-Phe-NH$_2$	39.1	3.3	5700	146
7. H-Tyr-D-Nle-Gly-Trp-Nle-Asp-Phe-NH$_2$	2.9	27	11.2	15.8

*CCK indicates cholecystokinin.
[†] Competitive binding assay versus [³H]DPDPE.
[‡] Competitive binding assay versus DAMGO.
[§] Competitive binding assay versus [³H]CCK-8.

produce potent opioid ligands: (A) D-Ala in **2**; (B) D-Nle in **3**; and (C) Gly in **4**. Significant improvements in binding affinity were seen for both **2** and **3** (Table 28.1), but surprisingly **4** had considerably reduced potency. Since enkephalin itself has a Gly in position 2, the reason for the large loss in binding affinity of **4** for opioid receptors is not clear.

It should be noted that the binding affinities of analogs **1** to **4** for the CCK-1 and CCK-2 receptors were largely unchanged by these modifications to the N-terminal dipeptide residues of SNF-9007. Thus, we next sought to improve the binding of SNF-9007 for the CCK-1 receptor in particular to obtain a ligand with more balanced binding affinities for the 2 CCK receptors. As shown in Table 28.2, this was accomplished by using **1** (Table 28.1) as the starting ligand, and substituting the N-MeNle^5 residue with a Nle residue, which was known from our previous studies of CCK[22] to give ligands with more balanced CCK-1 and CCK-2 binding affinities. In addition we put a D-Phe (**5**) or a D-Ala (**6**) or a D-Nle^2 residue in position 2 (Table 28.2). In general, these modifications led to increased binding affinities for the CCK-1 receptor (90-fold for **5**, 2-fold for **6**, and 900-fold for **7**), although with some decrease in binding affinities for the CCK-2 receptor. Most important, **7** was found

Table 28.3 Conversion to High-Affinity CCK Antagonist Activity*

[D-Trp[4]]Analogues	Opioid, K_i (nM)		CCK, K_i (nM)	
	δ[†]	μ[‡]	CCK-1[§]	CCK-2[§]
1. H-Tyr-D-Phe-Gly-Trp-NMeNle-Asp-Phe-NH₂	22	2.5	10 000	2.1
8. H-Tyr-D-Phe-Gly-D-Trp-NMeNle-Asp-Phe-NH₂	0.55	5.7	1080	1.6
9. H-Tyr-D-Ala-Gly-D-Trp-NMeNle-Asp-Phe-NH₂	1.9	20	32	1.3

*CCK indicates cholecystokinin.

[†] Competitive binding assay versus [³H]DPDPE.

[‡] Competitive binding assay versus DAMGO.

[§] Competitive binding assay versus [³H]CCK-8.

to have very balanced binding affinity for both the CCK-1 and CCK-2 receptors. High affinity binding was retained for the μ and δ receptors as well.

Finally, we converted the analogs to ligands, which would be expected to have antagonist activity at CCK receptors (Table 28.3). It is well known from previous structure-activity relationships (SAR) studies with both CCK peptides and peptidomimetics that conversion of the L-Trp in CCK analogs to a D-Trp leads to compounds that are antagonists at CCK receptors. Hence, starting with **1** we replaced the L-Trp residue with a D-Trp residue to give **8** (Table 28.3), and we also made an analog with a D-Ala² residue (**9**, Table 28.3). In both cases, analogs with potent binding affinities for the δ, μ, and CCK-2 receptors were obtained, and for **9** at the CCK-1 receptor as well. Of surprise, **8** still had weak affinity for the CCK-1 receptor, presumably because of the presence of a N-MeNle⁵ residue (although **9** also had this residue, it had high affinity for the CCK-1 receptor). As expected, **8** and **9** were antagonists at the CCK receptors (data not shown).

Finally, we examined the design of cyclic ligands related to the linear ligands discussed above. The linear analogs were converted to cyclic analogs using a rational approach for making cyclic analogs from linear analogs by topographical modification and cyclization.[23,24] In this case, we cyclized using structural modifications at positions 2 and 5 of the linear analogs discussed above. Both cyclic disulfide and cyclic lactam analogs were examined. Here we will report on our work with cyclic disulfides. In this approach we substituted position 2 with either D-Cys or D-Pen, whereas in position 5 we substituted with either D-Cys, Cys, or Pen (Table 28.4). Based on previous studies of cyclic opioid ligands based on DPDPE, which were extended at the C-terminal,[25,26] it was anticipated that an L-Cys or L-Pen residue in the analogs would lead to higher affinity analogs on opioid receptors. As shown in Table 28.4 this turned out to be the case at the δ receptor (**13** and **14** versus **15**, **16**, and **17**) but not at the μ receptor, although **15** had the highest affinity at both the δ and μ receptors as expected. All of the cyclic disulfides had good to very good antagonist activities at the CCK receptors (Table 28.4).

In preliminary studies we have examined whether these ligands have binding affinity and, most important, in vivo activity in animal models of neuropathic pain and anti-allodynic effects. Using the linear analog RSA 601 (H-Tyr-D-Phe-Glu-D-Trp-NMeNle-Asp-Phe-NH₂) we have found that these compounds demonstrate

Table 28.4 Conformational Constraint With Disulfide Cyclization*

Cyclic Disulfide Analogues	Opioid Agonist (nM) MVD(δ)[†]		CCK Antagonist[§] (nM) GPI(μ)[‡]
7. H-Tyr-D-Nle-Gly-Trp-Nle-Asp-Phe-NH$_2$	22.7	206	192
13. H-Tyr-D-Cys-Gly-Trp-D-Cys-Asp-Phe-NH$_2$	84	182	37.8
14. H-Tyr-c[D-Cys-Gly-Trp-D-Cys]-Asp-Phe-NH$_2$	119	282	23
15. H-Tyr-c[D-Cys-Gly-Trp-Cys]-Asp-Phe-NH$_2$	0.45	63	7.6
16. H-Tyr-c[D-Pen-Gly-Trp-Cys]-Asp-Phe-NH$_2$	9.5	151	19
17. H-Tyr-c[D-Cys-Gly-Trp-Pen]-Asp-Phe-NH$_2$	15	290	24

*CCK indicates cholecystokinin.
[†]Functional assay at mouse vas deferens (δ).
[‡]Functional assay at guinea pig ileum (μ).
[§]Competitive binding assay at the guinea pig ileum, longitudinal muscle with myeuteric plexus (GPI/LMMP).

dose-dependent activity using a descending facilitation animal pain model for neuropathic pain and in an in vivo anti-allodynic assay. Further studies are in progress to confirm these findings. However, it does appear that as predicted by our basic working hypothesis, ligands with the novel biological activities profiles of our new ligands can indeed provide for the first time ligands that are actually effective for neuropathic pain and allodynia. Studies are continuing to further expand on this model.

Use of a Novel Biophysical Method to Directly Examine Structural Changes of GPCRs in Membrane Bilayers

Efforts to examine directly the structural properties of integral membrane proteins such as GPCRs have been hampered by their intrinsic properties in the bilayers in which they are located in vivo, including (1) their relatively low abundance, (2) the difficulties in solubilizing them in a biologically active state, (3) their anisotropic properties in the bilayers, (4) the difficulty in crystallizing them so as to obtain high resolution structures, (5) the complexity of their molecular interactions (ligands, the trimeric G-proteins), and (6) the need to use radiolabels or even more problematic fluorescent probes to examine these interactions.

Here we report on a new method, PWR spectroscopy, which can overcome all of these difficulties. The method uses resonant excitation by light of plasmons, which are electronic oscillations, in a thin metal film (eg, silver) coated with a thicker dielectric layer (in our case silica), which is deposited on the surface of a prism. This setup generates a surface-localized evanescent electromagnetic field at the interface of the coated prism and the external aqueous medium. In this way, the optical properties of materials immobilized at this surface including lipid bilayers, GPCRs in the bilayers, the interactions of the GPCRs with their cognate ligands, and interactions with their G-proteins can be probed. This allows for the characterization

of thermodynamic, kinetic, and structural properties and features of a wide variety
of biomembrane systems (see references 12–16 for details of the instrumentation
and its applications to anisotropic structural analysis). Most important, this method
can be done with a very high degree of sensitivity (femtomole quantities of immobilized receptor, for example) and without the need for any labels or other structural
modifications. For example, the kinetics and thermodynamics of ligand binding can
be examined directly, and insights into the conformational/structural changes that
result from ligand-receptor interactions can be obtained. This is possible because,
in contrast to surface plasmon resonance (SPR) spectra, PWR spectra can be
excited with both parallel and perpendicular polarized light, allowing characterization of molecular orientation within the membrane and evaluation of the anisotropy
inherent in this system rather than simple changes in mass. Furthermore, PWR is
much more sensitive than SPR owing to the much narrower line widths of PWR
spectra, which allows quantitative measurement with a single proteolipid bilayer
and nanomolar amounts of protein in the sample cell.

For our initial studies with GPCRs we chose the cloned hDOR, which had been
modified at the C-terminus with Myc and His tags. This GPCR mediates pain
response in acute pain. CHO cells containing the hDOR were harvested and
homogenized, and the membrane fraction was solubilized in an octylglucoside-
containing buffer and purified by column chromatography and affinity chromatography and evaluated for purity and the ability to bind δ opioid ligands. A lipid
bilayer containing 75 mol% egg PC and 25 mol% palmitoyl-oleoyl-phosphatidyl-
glycerol (POPG) was used to form a bilayer (Fig. 28.3A) within an orifice in a
Teflon spacer on the prism. The bilayer formed is quite stable and is anchored to
the orifice by an annulus of lipid solution. This bilayer readily incorporates the
hDOR by introducing the detergent solubilized hDOR into the aqueous compartment under conditions that dilute the detergent to below the CMC (Fig. 28.3A).
Once the receptor is inserted into the bilayer, solutions of ligands or soluble proteins such as G proteins, or other molecules or ions can be added to the aqueous
compartment of the PWR instrument. Insertion of the hDOR can be performed with
the receptor either unoccupied or occupied by an agonist, antagonist, or inverse
agonist (Fig. 28.3A). The ligand occupied receptor (agonist, antagonist, or inverse
agonist occupied) can subsequently be used to interrogate the G-protein binding
processes (Fig. 28.3B, C) and in turn guanosine 5'-diphosphate/guanosine
5'-triphosphate (GPD/GTP) exchange (GTPγ-S binding) can be monitored in real
time for changes in the PWR spectra (Fig. 3B, C) using both s-polarized and
p-polarized light. Fitting of the changes in spectra as a result of, for example,
changes in agonist ligand concentration to a hyperbolic binding isotherm can be
done to determine K_D values for binding of the ligand to the hDOR. Similar studies
can be made with prebound antagonist and inverse agonists, peptides, and nonpeptides.
The plasmon resonance spectra depend on 3 properties of the proteolipid bilayers:
the refractive index (n), the absorption coefficient (k), and the thickness (t) of the immobilized layer. Both s-polarized and p-polarized light can be used to examine the
anisotropic behavior of the system. From this process information can be obtained
about the changes in structure that accompany interaction of the receptor with ligands

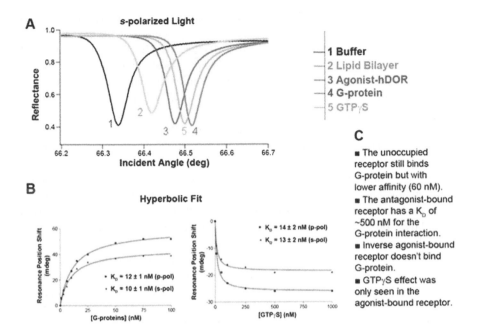

Fig. 28.3 PWR equilibrium spectra following the changes of reflectance for study of G-protein receptors in lipid bilayers: (A) PWR equilibrium spectra for various experimental situations, (B) PWR binding isotherm for G-protein binding to agonist-bound DPDPE-hDOR complex (left) and subsequent measurement of GTPγS binding (right), and (C) Other observations made using PWR spectroscopy with other unoccupied or ligand-occupied hDORs.

and G-protein. For example, we have shown that incorporation of hDOR into a bilayer follows a hyperbolic curve consistent with single uniform site in the bilayers and allows calculation of mass density for closely packed molecules from which the surface area occupied per molecule can be determined.[16] The value obtained ($1200\,Å^2$) is consistent with the expected molecular structure of the receptor. Furthermore, as expected, n_p values are greater than n_s values again consistent with insertion of a cylindrically shaped receptor protein (an asymmetric structure) into a rod-shaped lipid bilayer. Finally, the thickness of the proteolipid membrane increases from $53\,Å$ before receptor insertion, to $68\,Å$ after hDOR addition. These values are consistent with known structural features of the lipid bilayer and the receptor.

Following insertion of the receptors into the bilayer, ligand binding to the receptor can be examined in detail by adding increasing concentrations of agonist (Fig. 28.3B), antagonist, or inverse agonist ligands (Fig. 28.3C). We have examined these binding interactions in detail using PWR spectroscopy by monitoring the changes in the PWR spectra that occur on adding increasing concentrations of the ligand to the receptor.[27] In these studies we have found that the binding of the ligand to the receptor leads to different changes in the spectra for s-polarized and p-polarized light consistent with an anisotropic change in structure in the binding process.

Furthermore, these changes are quite different when agonists, antagonists, and an inverse agonist bind to the receptor, completely in agreement with the interpretation that each of these receptor-occupied states has a different conformation. Of interest, some peptide agonists and nonpeptide agonists show different anisotropic spectral changes suggesting a different conformation for each of these agonist-occupied-receptor states. This observation is consistent with previous observations we have made using μDORs modified by site-specific mutagenesis.[28]

Fitting the changes in PWR spectra that occur as the concentration of ligand is increased to saturation to a hyperbolic binding isotherm can directly provide the K_D values for ligand binding to the receptor. We have examined several agonists and antagonists of the hDOR and a known inverse agonist and have shown that the K_D values obtained are very similar to those reported in the literature, generally using brain membrane preparations.[27] We thus conclude that our receptor preparations in lipid bilayers provide a good approximation to the structural and functional properties of the receptors in living systems.

With this in mind, we extended our studies to examine the binding of G-proteins to the incorporated hDOR and examined the PWR spectral changes that accompany the addition of the G-proteins (Fig. 28.3B). In these experiments, the hDOR receptor was inserted into the membrane bilayers either unoccupied by a binding ligand, or occupied by an agonist, an antagonist, or an inverse agonist. We found that prebinding of a ligand to the receptor results in changes in G-protein interaction with the occupied receptor that varies with the ligand type (agonist, antagonist, or inverse agonist). This finding demonstrates that the receptor inserts into the membrane bi-directionally and thus permits exploration of processes that occur on both extracellular and intracellular membrane surfaces. This fortunate situation has allowed us to examine the consequences of the interaction of G-proteins with variously occupied receptors to provide novel insights that may provide a completely new way to do structure-biological activity relationships in drug design. We briefly discuss some of these findings below.

The δ opioid agonist (DPDPE)[19]-occupied receptor was inserted in the lipid bilayer and then was interrogated with a purified mixture of the predominant forms of the pertussis toxin-sensitive G-proteins from bovine brain (Calbiochem, EMD Biosciences) associated with the DOR containing $G_{\alpha o}$, $G_{\alpha i1}$, $G_{\alpha i2}$, and $G_{\alpha i3}$ and the βγ subunit complex.[29] When these were incrementally added, changes in PWR spectra were observed (Fig. 28.3B). As shown in Fig. 28.3, saturation was obtained at higher concentrations, and again the K_D value of the binding of the G-protein to the agonist occupied hDOR could be determined by fitting the data to a hyperbolic binding isotherm. As can be seen, both s-polarized and p-polarized light gave the same K_D value as expected. After saturation of the receptor with the G-protein was reached, GTPγS was added and, as before, the changes in the PWR spectra were monitored as shown in Fig. 28.3C. The K_D value for GTPγS binding was found to be ~14 nM. Note that the anisotropic spectral changes seen with GTPγS binding were in the opposite direction as those seen for G-protein binding to the DPDPE-occupied receptor. We interpret this result to be caused by the release of the alpha subunit of the G-protein after GTP/GDP exchange. Note that the G-protein binding to the agonist-occupied receptor and the GTPγS binding to the G-protein have K_D values of similar magnitude. Similar experiments with the antagonist (naltrindole)-occupied hDOR showed that the G-protein was only weakly bound to the receptor (K_D ~500 nM), and that the GTPγS apparently does not bind to the G-protein in this case (data not shown). This finding is consistent with expectation, showing that these interactions reflect receptor biology. By directly monitoring these effects, PWR allows them to be quantified, which is very difficult to do by other methods. This has important implications for drug discovery protocols.

Of interest, unoccupied hDOR still binds the G-protein but with an intermediate affinity (~60 nM) but no GTPγS binding was detected. Again, as expected, the inverse agonist-occupied receptor does not bind the G-protein nor is any GTPγS binding detected. These results further validate as previously discussed (*vide supra*) that the hDOR assumes different structures depending on the nature of the ligand bound to it (agonist, antagonist, inverse agonist, and unoccupied receptor). This picture is quite different from that usually depicted in biochemistry or pharmacology textbooks and reviews. These 4 different conformational states appear to be essential for the proper functioning of information transduction that is used for biological function in response to changes in the environment of the cell.

If one uses the purified Gα-protein subtypes ($G_{\alpha o}$, $G_{\alpha i1}$, $G_{\alpha i2}$, and $G_{\alpha i3}$) in combination with the βγ subunits and then interrogates them with either ligand-occupied hDORs or the unliganded state, a remarkably diverse set of transduction pathways emerges (Table 28.5).[30] Examining first the DPDPE-bound hDOR, there is a 40-fold difference in binding of the different G-protein subtypes. Moreover there no longer is a uniformly close 1:1 correspondence between G-protein binding to the

Table 28.5 K_D Values (nM) for Binding of the Different G-Protein Subtypes to the Different Liganded States of the Human δ Opioid Receptor

Agonist (DPDPE)-bound				
G-Protein subtype	$G_{\alpha o}$	$G_{\alpha i1}$	$G_{\alpha i2}$	$G_{\alpha i3}$
$K_D^{\text{G-protein}}$ (nM)	10 ± 1	300 ± 30	7 ± 1	43 ± 5
$K_D^{\text{GTPγS}}$ (nM)	400 ± 50	4.2 ± 0.5	9.9 ± 0.7	82 ± 10

Unliganded Receptor				
G-Protein subtype	$G_{\alpha o}$	$G_{\alpha i1}$	$G_{i\alpha i2}$	$G_{\alpha i3}$
$K_D^{\text{G-protein}}$ (nM)	21 ± 1.8	80 ± 9	585 ± 70	95 ± 10
$K_D^{\text{GTPγS}}$ (nM)	1900 ± 200	*	*	*

Partial Agonist (morphine)-bound				
G-Protein subtype	$G_{\alpha o}$	$G_{\alpha i1}$	$G_{\alpha i2}$	$G_{\alpha i3}$
$K_D^{\text{G-protein}}$ (nM)	43 ± 5	33 ± 8	310 ± 27	17 ± 3
$K_D^{\text{GTPγS}}$ (nM)	925 ± 125	93 ± 11	1650 ± 130	910 ± 142

Agonist (SNC 80)-bound				
G-Protein subtype	$G_{\alpha o}$	$G_{\alpha i1}$		$G_{\alpha i2}$	$G_{\alpha i3}$
$K_D^{\text{G-protein}}$ (nM)	5 ± 0.5	215 ± 33	209 ± 33	14 ± 1.1	19 ± 2
$K_D^{\text{GTPγS}}$ (nM)	10 ± 1.8	2.2 ± 0.4	2.4 ± 0.3	97 ± 14	24 ± 3

* No G-protein activation up to 5 μM of GTPγS

agonist-occupied receptor and GTPγS binding. Thus, in the case of the $G_{\alpha i2}$ protein, there is essentially 1 to 1 correspondence, but for the other high-affinity G-protein $G_{\alpha o}$ there is up to a 40-fold difference in G-protein binding to the agonist-occupied receptor and GTPγS binding. Since transduction requires both the G-protein binding event and GDP/GTP exchange, clearly the most likely transduction pathway in this case will be via the $G_{\alpha i2}$ protein. Remarkably, a completely different picture emerges when examining these binding events with a nonpeptide-hDOR complex, namely, the SNC80-hDOR complex (Table 28.5). In this case, the G-protein, which binds most strongly to the hDOR is the $G_{\alpha o}$ protein and this also has potent GTPγS binding. On the other hand, although the $G_{\alpha i2}$ protein binds strongly to the agonist-occupied DOR, a 7-fold decrease in GTPγS binding occurs.

Also of interest is the observation that the partial agonist for the hDOR (morphine) chooses yet another G-protein, $G_{\alpha i1}$ (Table 28.5), and all of the other G-proteins bind GTPγS very weakly and thus are unlikely to transduce any message very well. By enabling a quantitative measure of the affinity between the receptor and G-protein subtypes, PWR spectroscopy offers a unique approach and new insights into the molecular mechanisms that may govern the efficacy of opioids. Conventional analyses by and large evaluate the influence of receptor/G-protein complexes on the affinity of ligands for the receptors; the analyses make the assumption that some predominant conformation(s) of the receptor or receptor/G-protein complexes dictate the affinity of the agonist for the receptor and, by assumption, the ensuing efficacy for a particular signaling pathway. The PWR analysis instead evaluates the dynamic interactions between the receptor and G-proteins as a result of agonist occupancy. The data presented here show that the full agonists, DPDPE and SNC80, and the partial agonist, morphine, confer very different profiles on the hDOR for G-protein binding and subsequent GTP exchange. One interpretation of the current data is that the more efficiently an agonist can induce G-protein binding and GTP exchange, and furthermore coupling to multiple G-protein subtypes, the more efficacious the agonist would be at that receptor. The affinity of hDOR for $G_{\alpha o}$, $G_{\alpha i2}$, and $G_{\alpha i3}$ upon SNC80 occupancy versus the affinity of hDOR for $G_{\alpha i3}$ only and low affinity for GTP when occupied by morphine is a case in point.

The above observations may explain the often-suggested idea of apparent "subtypes" of δ opioid receptors. Rather, our studies suggest that these different "subtypes" may result from the different transduction pathways induced by the ligand as defined by relative efficacy of the ligands in different tissues. Actually, since different pathological pain disease states may be a result of different phenotypes, the nature of the ligand for the GPCR may result in the emergence of a specific phenotypic response depending on the nature of the ligand. If this is the case, then PWR spectroscopy provides a unique and powerful assay system for developing drug ligands that can address specific pathological pain conditions.

We also have examined whether the interactions of the ligands with the receptor are modulated or different when individual G-proteins are present. That is, is there a reciprocal effect of the G-protein binding to the receptor on the affinity of the ligand for the receptor? In general we have found that the G-proteins have no effect on antagonist and inverse-agonist binding, which is consistent with current conclusions from classical binding and second messenger studies. On the other hand, in the presence of G-proteins, agonists such as DPDPE and SNC80 bind with 6- to 8-fold higher affinity to the hDOR than when no G-proteins are present, demonstrating that in the absence of G-proteins the hDOR is in a lower affinity state than when in their presence. This observation is in agreement with a model in which G-protein promotes a high affinity state of the receptor for agonists.

Finally, we have examined the binding of the α and $\beta\gamma$ subunits of the hDOR when it is occupied with agonists such as DPDPE and SNC80 and the partial agonist morphine. Surprisingly, we found in all cases that the highest affinity α subunit ($G_{\alpha i2}$ for DPDPE-occupied receptor, $G_{\alpha o}$ for the SNC80-occupied receptor, and $G_{\alpha i1}$ for the morphine-occupied receptor) bound less tightly by a factor of 5 to 7 than the $\beta\gamma$ subunit. These data suggest that both the G_{α} and the $\beta\gamma$ subunits consist of intrinsic structures that allow them to interact with the hDOR independently of each other. The affinity of the $\beta\gamma$ subunit for the hDOR is consistent with the proposed function of this subunit complex whose association with the receptor is essential for initiating receptor internalization. The current model proposes that the G-protein trimeric complexes have the best structural characteristics for interacting with a G-protein coupled receptor. Thus, the $\beta\gamma$ subunit is critical, by complexing with the alpha subunits to form the trimeric G-protein complex, to facilitate the G-protein's affinity for hDOR. Experimental evidence in the literature suggests that the beta/gamma subunits serve as a GTPase activating protein (GAP) whose function is to promote the formation of the functional G-protein trimers. The data from the PWR analysis support this hypothesis and suggest further that the $\beta\gamma$ subunits contribute significantly to the G protein's binding to the agonist-occupied receptor.

These and others studies demonstrate that PWR spectroscopy provides a powerful new tool for investigating proteolipid structural changes involving GPCRs in various aspects of transmembrane signaling including binding of ligands to the receptor, the interactions of G-proteins and G-protein subunits with the receptor in various receptor states, and GTPγS binding to the G-proteins when the GPCRs are unoccupied or occupied with agonists, antagonists, or inverse-agonists. Of note, all these experiments can be done without the need for radiolabels, fluorescent labels, or structural modifications of the receptor by mutagenesis, all of which can lead to artifacts that are difficult to determine. On the other hand, it might be argued that our studies do not correspond to the actual biological system, which is much more complicated. Whereas there is certainly some validity in such arguments and caution must be exercised in interpreting such "model studies" in terms of actual biological processes, our studies thus far have indicated that in terms of binding K_D values and other parameters that can be examined by PWR spectroscopy, and compared with other biochemical and biophysical methods that are more traditionally considered as "biological systems" (membrane preparation and whole cells), we have obtained very good agreement between the latter studies and those obtained with our reconstitution methods and using PWR spectroscopy. Furthermore, there is a long and successful history of reconstitution of membrane proteins into lipid bilayer vesicles. There is no reason to think that reconstitution into a solid-supported planar bilayer would be any less successful. We conclude that it is reasonable to suggest that PWR spectroscopy should be useful for examining further aspects of transmembrane signaling such as the effects of other modulatory proteins that are involved in GPCR signaling, including clathrins, β-arrestins, kinases, phosphatases, and ion channels. In addition we hope to be able to address directly the significance (or not) of homomeric and heteromeric GPCR dimerization in signal transduction as well as the role of lipid structure, lipid rafts, and other structural modulators of the lipid bilayer that might be important in modulation of GPCR signal transduction pathways.

Conclusions

Clearly the developments stemming from genomics and proteomics for examining systemic changes that occur during the development of diseases such as neuropathic pain, cancer, and diabetes is demanding a reevaluation of our past approaches to drug development. In this context, new biophysics methods such as PWR spectroscopy are providing important physical tools for examining more carefully the mechanisms involved in such critical biological activities as transmembrane signaling, protein-ligand interactions, and protein-protein interactions.

In terms of optimized drug discovery for disease, clearly the application of current strategies of parallel or combinatorial synthesis and high throughput assays, have not provided many new insights into how best to address drug design and discovery. It is very clear that nervous system changes and cellular changes that occur in the setting of injury and disease need to be examined from the viewpoint of how therapy can address these changes directly and not simply modulate or ameliorate symptoms of the disease state. It is critical to realize that the target for treatment has changed from the "normal" state, and hence these system level adaptations must be considered in drug design and treatment strategies. Drugs need to be designed for optimal activity in the disease states, so that they can overcome and/or ameliorate adaptations of the cellular and or nervous system. Of interest, as we have shown here, design will often involve ligands with activities at more than one "biological" target. The development of concepts of overlapping pharmacophores, multivalent ligands, and systems-based design are critical new approaches that are in need of new ideas and new paradigms.

Acknowledgments This study was supported by grants from the United States Public Health Service, GM 59630 (GT and ZS), and National Institute of Drug Abuse, DA 06284 (VJH), DA 1339 (VJH), and DA 12394 (FP), which are gratefully acknowledged.

References

1. Hruby VJ. Designing peptide receptor agonists and antagonists. *Nat Rev Drug Discov.* 2002;1:847-858.
2. Ossipov MH, Lai J, Porreca F. Mechanisms of experimental neuropathic pain: Integration from animal models. In: McMahon S, Koltzenburg M, eds. *Wall and Melzack's Textbook of Pain.* 5th ed. New York, NY: Elsevier; 2005:929-946.

3. Ossipov MH, Porreca F. Challenges in the development of novel treatment strategies for neuropathic pain. *NeuroRx.* 2005;2:650-661.
4. Vera-Portocarrero LP, Zhang ET, Ossipov MH, et al. Descending facilitation from the rostral ventromedial medulla maintains nerve injury-induced central sensitization. *Neuroscience.* In press.
5. Ossipov MH, Porreca F. Descending modulation of pain. In: Merskey H, Loeser JD, Dubner R, eds. *The Paths of Pain 1975-2005.* Seattle, WA: IASP Press; 2005:117-130.
6. Xie JY, Herman SD, Stiller CO, et al. Cholecystokinin in the rostral ventromedial medulla mediates opioid-induced hyperalgesia and antinociceptive tolerance. *J Neurosci.* 2005;25:409-416.
7. King T, Ossipov MH, Vanderah TW, Porreca F, Lai J. Is paradoxical pain induced by sustained opioid exposure an underlying mechanism of opioid antinociceptive tolerance? *Neurosignals.* 2005;14:194-205.
8. Heinricher MM, Neubert MJ. Neural basis for the hyperalgesic action of cholecystokinin in the rostral ventromedial medulla. *J Neurophysiol.* 2004;92:1982-1989.
9. Wilcox GL, Stone LS, Ossipov MH, Lai J, Porreca F. Pharmacology of pain and analgesia. In: Pappagallo M, ed. *The Neurologic Basis of Pain.* New York, NY: McGraw-Hill; 2004:31-52.
10. Hruby VJ, Meyer J-P. Chemical synthesis of peptides. In: Hecht SM, ed. *Bioorganic Chemistry: Peptides and Proteins.* New York, NY: Oxford University Press; 1998:27-64.
11. Misicka A, Lipkowski AW, Horvath R, et al. Topographical requirements for δ opioid ligands: common structural features of dermenkephalin and deltorphin. *Life Sci.* 1992;51:1025-1032.
12. Kramer TH, Davis P, Hruby VJ, Burks TF, Porreca F. In vitro potency, affinity and agonist efficacy of highly selective δ opioid receptor ligands. *J Pharmacol Exp Ther.* 1993;266:577-584.
13. Salamon Z, Macleod HA, Tollin G. Coupled plasmon-waveguide resonators: a new spectroscopic tool for probing proteolipid film structure and properties. *Biophys J.* 1997;73:2791-2797.
14. Salamon Z, Tollin G. Plasmon resonance spectroscopy: probing molecular interactions at surfaces and interfaces. *Spectroscopy.* 2005;15:161-175.
15. Tollin G, Salamon Z, Hruby VJ. Techniques: plasmon-waveguide resonance (PWR) spectroscopy as a tool to study ligand-GPCR interactions. *Trends Pharmacol Sci.* 2003;24:655-659.
16. Salamon Z, Cowell S, Varga E, Yamamura HI, Hruby VJ, Tollin G. Plasmon resonance studies of agonist/antagonist binding to the human δ-opioid receptor: new structural insights into receptor-ligand interactions. *Biophys J.* 2000;79:2463-2474.
17. Alves ID, Salamon Z, Varga E, Yamamura HI, Tollin G, Hruby VJ. Direct observation of G-protein binding to the human δ-opioid receptor using plasmon-waveguide resonance spectroscopy. *J Biol Chem.* 2003;278:48890-48897.
18. Slaninová J, Knapp RJ, Wu J, et al. Opioid receptor binding properties of analgesic analogues of cholecystokinin octapeptide. *Eur J Pharmacol.* 1991;200:195-198.
19. Mosberg HI, Hurst R, Hruby VJ, et al. Bis-penicillamine enkephalins possess highly improved specificity toward δ opioid receptors. *Proc Natl Acad Sci USA.* 1983;80:5871-5874.
20. Hruby VJ, Fang SN, Kramer TH. Analogues of cholecystokinin$_{26-33}$ selective for B-type CCK receptors possess δ opioid receptor agonist activity in vitro and in vivo: Evidence for similarities in CCK-B and δ opioid receptor requirements. In: Hodges RS, Smith JA, eds. Peptides: Chemistry, Structure and Biology. Proceedings of the 13th American Peptide Symposium; June 20-25, 1993; Alberta, Canada. Leiden, The Netherlands: ESCOM Publishers; 1994: 669-671.
21. Nikiforovich GV, Hruby VJ, Prakash O, Gehrig CA. Topographical requirements for δ-selective opioid peptides. *Biopolymers.* 1991;31:941-955.
22. Hruby VJ, Fang SN, Knapp R, Kazmierski WM, Lui GK, Yamamura HI. Cholecystokinin analogues with high affinity and selectivity for brain membrane receptors. *Int J Pept Protein Res.* 1990;35:566-573.
23. Hruby VJ. Conformational restrictions of biologically active peptides via amino acid side chain groups. *Life Sci.* 1982;31:189-199.

24. Hruby VJ, Al-Obeidi F, Kazmierski WM. Emerging approaches in the molecular design of receptor selective peptide ligands: conformational, topographical and dynamic considerations. *Biochem J.* 1990;268:249-262.
25. Bartosz-Bechowski H, Davis P, Slaninova J, et al. Cyclic enkephalin analogues that are hybrids of DPDPE-related peptides and Met-enkephalin-Arg-Gly-Leu: prohormone analogues that retain good potency and selectivity for δ opioid receptors. *J Pept Res.* 1999;53:329-336.
26. Hruby VJ, Bartosz-Bechowski H, Davis P, et al. Cyclic enkephalin analogues with exceptional potency and selectivity for δ-opioid receptors. *J Med Chem.* 1997;40:3957-3962.
27. Alves ID, Cowell SM, Salamon Z, Devanathan S, Tollin G, Hruby VJ. Different structural states of the proteolipid membrane are produced by ligand binding to the human δ-opioid receptor as shown by plasmon-waveguide resonance spectroscopy. *Mol Pharmacol.* 2004;65:1248-1257.
28. Hosohata Y, Varga EV, Stropova D, et al. Mutation W284L of the human δ opioid receptor reveals agonist specific conformational mechanisms of G-protein activation. *Life Sci.* 2001;68:2233-2242.
29. Alves ID, Salamon Z, Varga E, Yamamura HI, Tollin G, Hruby VJ. Direct observation of G-protein binding to the human δ-opioid receptor using plasmon-waveguide resonance spectroscopy. *J Biol Chem.* 2003;278:48890-48897.
30. Alves ID, Ciano KA, Boguslavsky V, et al. Selectivity, cooperativity, and reciprocity in the interactions between the δ-opioid receptor, its ligands, and G-proteins. *J Biol Chem.* 2004;279:44673-44682.

Part IV
Opioids: General

Chapter 29
Neuropeptide-Processing Enzymes: Applications for Drug Discovery

Lloyd D. Fricker[1]

Abstract Neuropeptides serve many important roles in communication between cells and are an attractive target for drug discovery. Neuropeptides are produced from precursor proteins by selective cleavages at specific sites, and are then broken down by further cleavages. In general, the biosynthetic cleavages occur within the cell and the degradative cleavages occur postsecretion, although there are exceptions where intracellular processing leads to inactivation, or extracellular processing leads to activation of a particular neuropeptide. A relatively small number of peptidases are responsible for processing the majority of neuropeptides, both inside and outside of the cell. Thus, inhibition of any one enzyme will lead to a broad effect on several different neuropeptides and this makes it unlikely that such inhibitors would be useful therapeutics. However, studies with mutant animals that lack functional peptide-processing enzymes have facilitated the discovery of novel neuropeptides, many of which may be appropriate targets for therapeutics.

Keywords carboxypeptidase, peptidomics, prohormone convertase, peptide biosynthesis

Neuropeptides and Their Biosynthetic Pathways

Neuroendocrine peptides function in a large number of physiological processes including feeding and body weight regulation, fluid intake and retention, pain, anxiety, memory, circadian rhythms and sleep/wake cycles, and reward pathways.[1,2] Altogether, there are hundreds of peptides that have been detected in brain and

[1] Department of Molecular Pharmacology, Albert Einstein College of Medicine, 1300 Morris Park Avenue, Bronx, NY 10461

Corresponding Author: Lloyd D. Fricker, Department of Molecular Pharmacology, Albert Einstein College of Medicine, 1300 Morris Park Avenue, Bronx, NY 10461. Tel: (718) 430-4225; Fax: (718) 430-8954; E-mail: fricker@aecom.yu.edu

R.S. Rapaka and W. Sadée (eds.), *Drug Addiction.*   497
© American Association of Pharmaceutical Scientists 2008

other tissues, although only a fraction has known biological functions. The biological activity of peptides is usually mediated by G-protein coupled receptors, or in some cases, by enzyme-linked receptors (such as the insulin receptor). Because there are a large number of orphan G-protein coupled receptors, it is likely that there are peptides with undiscovered functions.[2,3] One approach to identifying novel neuropeptides makes use of a mutant animal lacking a peptide-processing enzyme, discussed in more detail after an overview of the peptide-processing enzymes.

When the amino acid sequences of peptide precursors were first discovered in the 1970s, it was immediately clear that generation of the active forms of the peptides required processing of the precursor at sites containing 2 or more basic amino acids.[4] In most cases, the sites were either Lys-Arg or Arg-Arg. Analysis of hundreds of peptide precursor cleavage sites in a variety of organisms has extended these earlier observations and confirmed that Lys-Arg and Arg-Arg constitute the vast majority of all cleavage sites, while Arg-Lys and Lys-Lys are found with much less frequency.[5] In addition to these sites, some cleavages occur at sites containing pairs of basic amino acids separated by 2, 4, or 6 other residues.[6] For many years, these sites were described as "monobasic" and the enzymes responsible for cleavage were thought to be distinct from the "dibasic" site enzymes. However, in the past decade it has become clear that the enzymes capable of processing precursors at Arg-Arg sites can also cleave at Arg-X-X-Arg sites, and the general consensus has recently been described as Arg-X_n-Arg, where n is either 0, 2, 4, or 6.[7,8] Several different peptide precursors are also cleaved at sites containing a single basic residue, with no upstream Arg in the appropriate position.[9] Often, these single basic sites are Pro-Arg sequences, and it is not yet clear if any of the identified prohormone convertases can cleave at these sites.

In addition to the classical pathway that involves cleavage at basic amino acids, several peptides have been detected that arise from cleavage at nonbasic residues or at basic residues that don't fit the typical consensus site.[9-16] In some cases, these peptides may be formed after secretion when the peptides are exposed to extracellular peptidases. However, several peptides that are formed from cleavage at nontypical sites appear to be present within purified secretory vesicles.[10] The enzymes responsible for these nontraditional cleavages are not currently known, although there are candidates (described below).

Peptide-Processing Enzymes

The finding that peptide precursors contain basic amino acids separating the various bioactive and/or spacer regions led to the prediction that a trypsin-like endopeptidase initially cleaved the precursors, thereby generating intermediates with C-terminal basic residues.[4] These basic residues would then be removed by a carboxypeptidase B-like enzyme, in many cases producing the final peptide (Fig. 29.1). In some cases, additional posttranslational processing steps are required such as C-terminal amidation, N-terminal acetylation, or other modifications (glycosylation, sulfation, and phosphorylation).

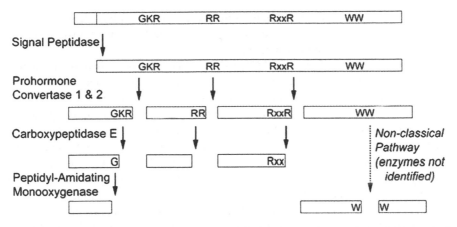

Fig. 29.1 Classical and nonclassical neuropeptide processing scheme. First, the N-terminal sequence that drives translocation of the protein into the lumen of the endoplasmic reticulum is co-translationally removed by a signal peptidase. Then, in the classical scheme, the prohormone is typically processed at sites containing Lys-Arg (KR), Arg-Arg (RR), or Arg-Xaa$_n$-Arg, where n is 2, 4, or 6 (RxxR shown in figure). Processing at these basic amino acids involves endopeptidase action by an enzyme such as prohormone convertase 1 or 2 followed by the removal of the C-terminal basic residue(s) primarily by carboxypeptidase E, although an additional enzyme (carboxypeptidase D) is also able to contribute to processing. An amidating enzyme that is broadly expressed in the neuroendocrine system converts C-terminal Gly residues into a C-terminal amide. In addition to this classical pathway, a large number of peptides have been found that result from cleavage at nonbasic residues. An example of this nonclassical pathway for the generation of a peptide previously found in brain is indicated; this fragment of chromogranin B involves cleavage between 2 adjacent Trp residues (WW). Many other nonbasic cleavage sites have been reported, including other hydrophobic residues, short chain aliphatic residues, and acidic residues. The enzymes responsible for the nonclassical pathway are not clear. Some of these nonclassical processing events may occur after secretion and be mediated by extracellular peptidases, although some of the nonbasic mediated cleavages appear to occur within the secretory pathway.

Two "trypsin-like" endopeptidases appear to be involved in the production of neuropeptides.[7,8] These enzymes, designated prohormone convertase 1 (PC1, also known as PC3) and prohormone convertase 2 (PC2), are broadly expressed in the neuroendocrine system.[17-20] Although some cell types express only 1 of the 2 enzymes, many neuroendocrine cells express both. Within the cell, PC1 and PC2 are enriched in peptide-containing secretory vesicles.[7,8] The pH optima of these enzymes are in the 5 to 6 range, corresponding to the moderately acidic pH of the interior of the secretory vesicles. These enzymes are serine proteases of the subtilisin family and are strongly activated by Ca^{2+}.[7,8] The combination of decreasing pH and increasing calcium levels activates PC1 and PC2 once they leave the Golgi apparatus. In addition, there are specific inhibitors of PC1 (named proSAAS) and PC2 (named 7B2) that also function to block enzyme activation early in the secretory pathway.[21,22] Both proSAAS and 7B2 bind tightly to their respective enzymes and are slowly cleaved by them. Interestingly, the products of this cleavage remain potent inhibitors until a carboxypeptidase removes the C-terminal basic residues, thereby rendering the inhibitor inactive.[23,24]

The substrate specificities of PC1 and PC2 have been studied with purified enzymes, in cell culture, and in mice with disruptions of either one of the 2 genes.[15,25-27] Based on these studies, it appears that both PC1 and PC2 are able to cleave many of the same substrates although there are some sites cleaved preferentially by each. For example, PC2 cleaves the Lys-Lys sites in proopiomelanocortin (necessary to generate α-melanocyte-stimulating hormone, corticotrophin-like intermediate lobe peptide, and β-endorphin 1–27), whereas PC1 has negligible activity toward these sites in proopiomelanocortin but cleaves Lys-Lys sites in proenkephalin.[28-30] As predicted from the early studies on prohormone processing, PC1 and PC2 cleave on the C-terminal side of the basic residue(s); these residues often need to be removed by a carboxypeptidase before the peptide has biological activity.

The major peptide-processing carboxypeptidase was discovered in 1982 and named enkephalin convertase as well as carboxypeptidase E (CPE).[31,32] Because the enzyme is broadly expressed in the neuroendocrine system and processes many peptides in addition to enkephalin, the latter name is more appropriate. Subsequently, the name carboxypeptidase H was used for this enzyme, although this is rarely used in recent publications. CPE is a member of the metallocarboxypeptidase family, requiring Zn^{2+} in the active site for catalysis.[32,33] Unlike most other metallocarboxypeptidases, CPE also binds Ca^{2+} and this causes a slight activation and increase in stability.[34] CPE cleaves C-terminal Lys, Arg, and His residues from the C-terminus of a large number of peptides including those ending with Pro-Arg, although these bonds are cleaved orders of magnitude more slowly than peptides with penultimate amino acids other than Pro.[35-37]

For many years, CPE was thought to be the only carboxypeptidase involved in neuropeptide processing because it was the sole activity detected in purified secretory vesicles. However, studies on the $Cpe^{fat/fat}$ mice challenged this assumption: these mice lack functional CPE due to a point mutation in the Cpe gene that changes a Ser into a Pro and destabilizes the protein structure.[38,39] Despite the absence of CPE activity in these mice, detectable levels of the mature forms of peptides are produced, albeit at reduced levels.[14,38,40-43] This result suggested that an additional carboxypeptidase was involved in peptide processing. A search for CPE-like enzymes led to the discovery of carboxypeptidase D (CPD).[44] However, CPD is primarily localized to the *trans* Golgi network and although some CPD can enter the immature secretory vesicles, no CPD is detectable in the mature secretory vesicle.[45,46] Thus, only the processing reactions that are initiated in the *trans* Golgi network and immature vesicles can be completed by CPD to produce the mature peptide. Because the majority of peptide processing occurs later in the secretory pathway, CPD is only able to play a moderate role and CPE is the major peptide-processing carboxypeptidase.

In addition to the endopeptidase and carboxypeptidase processing steps, some peptides require further processing reactions. It has been estimated that ~50% of all known bioactive peptides have a C-terminal amide residue.[47] However, if one considers all peptides that have been detected in brain, pituitary, and other tissues, and not just those peptides with known biological activities, the fraction of amidated peptides is considerably smaller. Still, this is an important modification that is essential for the biological activity of many peptides. In order for a peptide to get amidated it must have a C-terminal Gly residue. This Gly is converted to an amide residue by 2 distinct enzyme activities that are contained within a single multifunctional protein, peptidyl-glycine-α-amidatingmonooxygenase (PAM).[48] The N-terminal domain is a hydroxylating monooxygenase that oxidizes the alpha carbon of the Gly in a reaction that uses copper, oxygen, and ascorbate.[49] Then, the C-terminal lyase domain releases glyoxylate, leaving behind the nitrogen of the Gly as the C-terminal amide residue.[50] PAM is broadly distributed throughout the neuroendocrine system and appears to be the only amidating activity present in tissues.

Other posttranslational processing events include acetylation, sulfation, phosphorylation, glycosylation, and additional proteolytic cleavages.[51] There are also rare modifications such as n-octanoylation of a Ser residue within the peptide ghrelin.[52] Except for sulfation, the enzymes responsible for these modifications haven't been well characterized.[53,54] The additional proteolytic cleavages are intriguing, and a large number have been found in recent studies using mass spectrometry to characterize the precise form of peptides present in extracts of brain and pituitary.[9,13-16,55] In some cases the peptides may be processed after secretion by extracellular peptidases such as endopeptidase 25.11 (also known as neprilysin, enkephalinase, and other names), angiotensin-converting enzyme, and several amino peptidases.[56,57] The extracellular processing does not always lead to inactivation of the peptide; in some cases, the product of the processing reaction has a distinct profile of receptor binding compared with the original peptide.[58,59] In these cases, the extracellular reaction serves more of a modulatory role than an inhibitory one. While some of the nonbasic residue-directed cleavages are likely to occur outside the cell, others happen within the secretory pathway based on analyses of purified secretory vesicles[10,60] or on posttranslational modifications. For example, fragments of α-melanocyte-stimulating hormone (α-MSH) are found in pituitary extracts that lack 1 or 2 N-terminal residues normally present on α-MSH, but containing an N-terminal acetyl group.[14] Because the acetylation reaction is only known to occur within the secretory pathway, and not following secretion, the presence of an acetyl group on the N terminus indicates that the cleavage occurred within the secretory pathway. The enzymes that cleave peptides within the secretory pathway at nonbasic sites are not known, but candidates include endothelin-converting enzyme-2 (ECE2) and the recently discovered carboxypeptidases A5 and A6. These latter 2 enzymes are detected in certain brain and/or pituitary cell types, and are predicted to be present within the secretory pathway and to cleave peptides at C-terminal aliphatic or aromatic residues.[61,62] ECE2 was originally described as a member of the endothelin-converting enzyme family, although ECE2 only has ~50% amino acid sequence identity to other members of this gene family and also has a neuroendocrine distribution.[63] Furthermore, ECE2 has been reported to be present in the secretory pathway and to be maximally active at pH 5 to 6, coinciding with the intravesicular pH range. Finally, ECE2 was tested with several peptides and found to cleave quite selectively.[64] Further studies are needed to examine the precise role of ECE2 and other enzymes in the intracellular processing of neuropeptides.

Peptide-Processing Enzymes and Drug Discovery

Typically, enzymes are considered to be potential drug targets if inhibition of the enzyme would produce a useful therapeutic effect. In this sense, most of the peptide-processing enzymes are poor targets for drugs for 2 reasons. First, many of these enzymes have too broad a role, and it is unlikely that inhibition would achieve a selective beneficial effect. For example, mice lacking PAM activity are not viable (John Pintar, oral communication, July 2001). While mice lacking CPE activity are viable, the phenotype is not considered to be desirable in a drug: obesity,[38] increased anxiety (Reeta Biswas and Lloyd Fricker, unpublished data, July 2001), and abnormal sexual behavior.[65] Secondly, the intracellular peptide-processing enzymes present a difficult target for drug development due to pharmacokinetic issues. Inhibitors of the enzymes that target basic amino acids (ie, the PCs and CPE) tend to contain multiple charges and therefore do not readily penetrate the cell. However, to be effective as inhibitors in vivo, the compound would need to enter not only the cell but also the secretory vesicles. Although the extracellular peptide-processing enzymes do not have this problem with pharmacokinetic issues, they generally share the problem of nonspecificity.

An alternative approach to drug discovery is to use the peptide-processing enzymes to identify novel peptides, some of which are likely to bind to orphan receptors. Knowledge of the ligands for these orphan receptors is important for the development of drugs that target these receptors. This peptidomics approach was originally described as a method to isolate CPE substrates from mice lacking CPE activity (ie, *Cpe^fat/fat* mice) although it should work for any organism that has a reduced level of a peptide-processing enzyme and which subsequently has elevated levels of the enzyme's substrates.[9] The basic approach is to use an affinity column that binds the peptide precursors to isolate these precursors from tissue extracts (Fig. 29.2). To reduce the number of false positives, it is useful to compare the results with control organisms that have normal levels of the processing enzyme with the results from the organisms with reduced enzyme levels; those peptides present at different levels in the 2 extracts are likely to be substrates for the enzyme in vivo. Then, once the peptides have been affinity purified, they can be easily detected and identified using mass spectrometry (Fig. 29.2).

In the case of the *Cpe^fat/fat* mice, the Lys- and Arg-extended processing intermediates that accumulate in the absence of CPE activity can be readily purified with anhydrotrypsin agarose (Fig. 29.2). This protein binds peptides with C-terminal basic residues (ie, trypsin products), but unexpectedly, doesn't bind peptides with

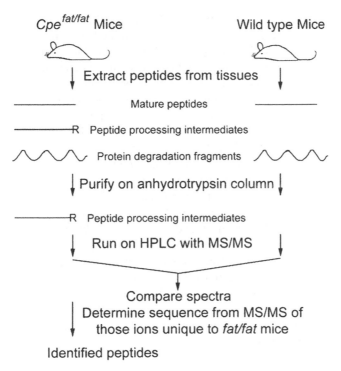

Fig. 29.2 Purification of neuropeptide-processing intermediates from *Cpe^fat/fat* mouse tissues. Peptides extracted from brain or other tissues of *Cpe^fat/fat* mice fall into 1 of 3 categories. One group includes the mature forms of neuropeptides. These are generally present in *Cpe^fat/fat* mice at lower levels than in wild-type mice. Another group of peptides is the peptide-processing intermediates that are C-terminally extended with basic residues (ie, the immediate substrates of CPE). These are greatly increased in the *Cpe^fat/fat* mice, relative to wild-type mice, which show undetectable levels of most of these peptides. The third group of "peptides" represents protein degradation fragments that are either normally present in the tissue due to protein turnover or which may be induced by postmortem changes during the dissection and/or extraction. Some of these protein degradation fragments may contain C-terminal basic residues. The anhydrotrypsin column is used to purify peptides containing C-terminal basic residues from the other peptides. Then, the peptides are analyzed on HPLC with on-line tandem mass spectrometry (MS/MS) so that peptide sequence information can be obtained. The spectra from analysis of *Cpe^fat/fat* and wild-type mice is compared; those peptides common to the 2 spectra typically represent protein breakdown fragments that contain C-terminal basic residues while those peptides unique to the *Cpe^fat/fat* mice represent CPE substrates (ie, neuropeptide processing intermediates or other proteins that are normally processed by PCs and CPE within the secretory pathway).

internal basic residues (ie, trypsin substrates). It is not known why the conversion of trypsin into anhydrotrypsin eliminates its ability to bind substrates and enhances its ability to bind products. After purification of *Cpe^fat/fat* mouse brain or pituitary extracts on the anhydrotrypsin column, hundreds of peptides were detected that were not present in the extracts from wild-type mice.[9] A large number of known neuropeptide-processing intermediates were identified, which both validates the approach and confirms the importance of CPE for the biosynthesis of numerous peptides. The known peptides or peptide-processing intermediates identified in *Cpe^{fat/fat}* brain and pituitary include fragments of proopiomelanocortin, proenkephalin, prodynorphin, preprotachykinin A and B, provasopressin, prooxytocin, promelanin concentrate hormone, proneurotensin, chromogranin A and B, and secretogranin II.[9,12-16] Fragments of other proteins that are processed by CPE in the secretory pathway were also identified, such as N- and/or C-terminal pieces of the peptide-processing enzymes PC1, PC2, and PAM (above references,[9,12-16] and Fa-Yun Che and Lloyd Fricker, unpublished data, August 2005). Some of the identified peptides represent novel cleavages or posttranslational modifications such as acetylation, glycosylation, phosphorylation, and oxidation. In addition, novel peptides were identified that were subsequently found to be encoded by a novel protein, which was subsequently named proSAAS.[22] One function of proSAAS is to inhibit PC1 early in the secretory pathway. Because mice overexpressing proSAAS are slightly overweight even though PC1 activity does not appear to be affected, it is likely that the proSAAS-derived peptides serve other functions, possibly as neuropeptides.[22,66,67] Many more peptides have been found with partial amino acid sequences that do not match the database of known peptide precursors; these may represent additional novel peptides.

Future Directions

The overall goal of the peptidomic studies is to identify the biological activity of each peptide, and this knowledge could be then used for drug discovery. Because peptides are involved in so many physiological processes, practically any disorder, from addiction to anxiety, would be a potential area that could benefit from drugs based on neuropeptide receptors. The experimentally difficult part of this concept is the determination of the function of each peptide. The peptidomics approach described in Fig. 29.2 provides a simple and elegant method to isolate a large number of peptide-processing intermediates, and mass spectrometry provides an efficient and sensitive approach to identify these peptides. However, the determination of function remains an extremely low-throughput venture. For example, a typical approach to determine the function of a protein is to generate transgenic and/or knockout mice, which can take several years to produce and characterize. Another approach is to determine which physiological states regulate the levels of each peptide, and then to use this knowledge to predict the function of the peptide. Although one would still need to directly test the peptide(s) for the proposed function, this approach would reduce the number of tests. For example, the peptides present in hypothalamus that are regulated by food deprivation are potentially involved in the control of body weight/energy balance. Similarly, peptides upregulated or downregulated by the chronic administration of drugs of abuse may be important mediators of the reward mechanisms and/or may contribute to the underlying neurochemical changes that lead to addiction. While this approach is not without false positives, it can at least reduce the number of candidate functions for a particular peptide. For example, the peptide hypocretin/orexin was found in one study to be upregulated by food deprivation, although subsequent studies suggested that this peptide was more involved in arousal states than in food intake.[68-70] However, it makes sense that in times of food deprivation an animal would spend more time awake and foraging for food, so the regulation of hypocretin/orexin by food deprivation is consistent with a function in both arousal and feeding.

It is possible to obtain accurate quantitative data from mass spectrometry if differential isotopic labels are incorporated into 2 samples that are then combined and analyzed.[71,72] The relative abundance of the material in the 2 samples can be readily determined by comparing the peak height of the heavy and light isotopic labels.[12,13,73] Using this approach, a large number of hypothalamic peptides were found to be altered by food deprivation.[16] Further refinement of the technique, both by improved extraction methods and by analysis on capillary columns with nanospray mass spectrometry will allow for the detection of even more peptides in each sample. Subsequent studies need to be performed to test the proposed function for each peptide, and to identify the receptors through which these peptides function. The peptidomics approach to identify and quantify neuropeptides provides a powerful method to rapidly screen for peptides, both known and novel, that contribute to a variety of physiological processes and it is likely that this information will be useful for drug development.

Acknowledgments This work was supported in part by National Institutes of Health grants DA-04494, DK-51271, DA-17665, and DK-67350. Thanks to Dr Hui Pan for helpful discussions.

References

1. Clynen E, De Loof A, Schoofs L. The use of peptidomics in endocrine research. *Gen Comp Endocrinol*. 2003;132:1-9.
2. Strand FL. Neuropeptides: general characteristics and neuropharmaceutical potential in treating CNS disorders. *Prog Drug Res*. 2003;61:1-37.
3. Tanaka H, Yoshida T, Miyamoto N, et al. Characterization of a family of endogenous neuropeptide ligands for the G protein-coupled receptors GPR7 and GPR8. *Proc Natl Acad Sci USA*. 2003;100:6251-6256.
4. Docherty K, Steiner DF. Post-translational proteolysis in polypeptide hormone biosynthesis. *Annu Rev Physiol*. 1982;44:625-638.
5. Lindberg I, Hutton JC. Peptide processing proteinases with selectivity for paired basic residues. In: Fricker LD, ed. *Peptide Biosynthesis and Processing*. Boca Raton, FL: CRC Press; 1991:141-174.
6. Devi L. Peptide processing at monobasic sites. In: Fricker LD, ed. *Peptide Biosynthesis and Processing*. Boca Raton, FL: CRC Press; 1991:175-198.

7. Zhou A, Webb G, Zhu X, Steiner DF. Proteolytic processing in the secretory pathway. *J Biol Chem.* 1999;274:20745-20748.

8. Seidah NG, Prat A. Precursor convertases in the secretory pathway, cytosol and extracellular milieu. *Essays Biochem.* 2002;38:79-94.

9. Che F-Y, Yan L, Li H, Mzhavia N, Devi L, Fricker LD. Identification of peptides from brain and pituitary of Cpe^{fat}/Cpe^{fat} mice. *Proc Natl Acad Sci USA.* 2001;98:9971-9976.

10. Sigafoos J, Chestnut WG, Merrill BM, Taylor LCE, Diliberto EJ, Viveros OH. Novel peptides from adrenomedullary chromaffin vesicles. *J Anat.* 1993;183:253-264.

11. Vilim FS, Aarnisalo AA, Nieminen M, et al. Gene for pain modulatory neuropeptide NPFF: induction in spinal cord by noxious stimuli. *Mol Pharmacol.* 1999;55:804-811.

12. Che F-Y, Fricker LD. Quantitation of neuropeptides in Cpe^{fat}/Cpe^{fat} mice using differential isotopic tags and mass spectrometry. *Anal Chem.* 2002;74:3190-3198.

13. Che F-Y, Fricker LD. Quantitative peptidomics of mouse pituitary: comparison of different stable isotopic tags. *J Mass Spectrom.* 2005;40:238-249.

14. Che F-Y, Biswas R, Fricker LD. Relative quantitation of peptides in wild type and $Cpe^{fat/fat}$ mouse pituitary using stable isotopic tags and mass spectrometry. *J Mass Spectrom.* 2005;40:227-237.

15. Pan H, Nanno D, Che FY, et al. Neuropeptide processing profile in mice lacking prohormone Convertase-1. *Biochemistry.* 2005;44:4939-4948.

16. Che FY, Yuan Q, Kalinina E, Fricker LD. Peptidomics of $Cpe^{fat/fat}$ mouse hypothalamus: effect of food deprivation and exercise on peptide levels. *J Biol Chem.* 2005;280: 4451-4461.

17. Smeekens SP, Steiner DF. Identification of a human insulinoma cDNA encoding a novel mammalian protein structurally related to the yeast dibasic processing protease Kex2. *J Biol Chem.* 1990;265:2997-3000.

18. Seidah NG, Marcinkiewicz M, Benjannet S, et al. Cloning and primary sequence of a mouse candidate prohormone convertase PC1 homologous to PC2, furin, and Kex2: distinct chromosomal localization and messenger RNA distribution in brain and pituitary compared to PC2. *Mol Endocrinol.* 1991;5:111-122.

19. Smeekens SP, Avruch AS, LaMendola J, Chan SJ, Steiner DF. Identification of a cDNA encoding a second putative prohormone convertase related to PC2 in AtT-20 cells and islets of Langerhans. *Proc Natl Acad Sci USA.* 1991;88:340-344.

20. Schafer MKH, Day R, Cullinan WE, Chretien M, Seidah NG, Watson SJ. Gene expression of prohormone and proprotein convertases in the rat CNS: a comparative in situ hybridization analysis. *J Neurosci.* 1993;13:1258-1279.

21. Braks JAM, Martens GJM. 7B2 is a neuroendocrine chaperone that transiently interacts with prohormone convertase PC2 in the secretory pathway. *Cell.* 1994;78:263-273.

22. Fricker LD, McKinzie AA, Sun J, et al. Identification and characterization of proSAAS, a granin-like neuroendocrine peptide precursor that inhibits prohormone processing. *J Neurosci.* 2000;20:639-648.

23. Zhu X, Rouille Y, Lamango NS, Steiner DF, Lindberg I. Internal cleavage of the inhibitory 7B2 CT peptide by PC2: a potential mechanism for its inactivation. *Proc Natl Acad Sci USA.* 1996;93:4919-4924.

24. Cameron A, Fortenberry Y, Lindberg I. The SAAS granin exhibits structural and functional homology to 7B2 and contains a highly potent hexapeptide inhibitor of PC1. *FEBS Lett.* 2000;473:135-138.

25. Furuta M, Yano H, Zhou A, et al. Defective prohormone processing and altered pancreatic islet morphology in mice lacking active SPC2. *Proc Natl Acad Sci USA.* 1997;94:6646-6651.

26. Furuta M, Zhou A, Webb G, et al. Severe defect in proglucagon processing in islet A-cells of prohormone convertase 2 null mice. *J Biol Chem.* 2001;276:27197-27202.

27. Zhu X, Orci L, Carroll R, Norrbom C, Ravazzola M, Steiner DF. Severe block in processing of proinsulin to insulin accompanied by elevation of des-64,65 proinsulin intermediates in islets of mice lacking prohormone convertase 1/3. *Proc Natl Acad Sci USA.* 2002;99: 10299-10304.

28. Zhou A, Bloomquist BT, Mains RE. The prohormone convertases PC1 and PC2 mediate distinct endoproteolytic cleavages in a strict temporal order during proopiomelanocortin biosynthetic processing. *J Biol Chem.* 1993;268:1763-1769.
29. Breslin MB, Lindberg I, Benjannet S, Mathis JP, Lazure C, Seidah NG. Differential processing of proenkephalin by prohormone convertases 1(3) and 2 and furin. *J Biol Chem.* 1993;268:27084-27093.
30. Zhou A, Mains RE. Endoproteolytic processing of proopiomelanocortin and prohormone convertases 1 and 2 in neuroendocrine cells overexpressing prohormone convertases 1 or 2. *J Biol Chem.* 1994;269:17440-17447.
31. Fricker LD, Snyder SH. Enkephalin convertase: purification and characterization of a specific enkephalin-synthesizing carboxypeptidase localized to adrenal chromaffin granules. *Proc Natl Acad Sci USA.* 1982;79:3886-3890.
32. Fricker LD. Carboxypeptidase E. *Annu Rev Physiol.* 1988;50:309-321.
33. Aloy P, Companys V, Vendrell J, et al. The crystal structure of the inhibitor-complexed carboxypeptidase D domain II as a basis for the modelling of regulatory carboxypeptidases. *J Biol Chem.* 2001;276:16177-16184.
34. Nalamachu SR, Song L, Fricker LD. Regulation of carboxypeptidase E: effect of Ca2+ on enzyme activity and stability. *J Biol Chem.* 1994;269:11192-11195.
35. Fricker LD, Snyder SH. Purification and characterization of enkephalin convertase, an enkephalin-synthesizing carboxypeptidase. *J Biol Chem.* 1983;258:10950-10955.
36. Smyth DG, Maruthainar K, Darby NJ, Fricker LD. C-terminal processing of neuropeptides: involvement of carboxypeptidase H. *J Neurochem.* 1989;53:489-493.
37. Chen H, Jawahar S, Qian Y, et al. A missense polymorphism in the human carboxypeptidase E gene alters its enzymatic activity: possible implications in type 2 diabetes mellitus. *Hum Mutat.* 2001;18:120-131.
38. Naggert JK, Fricker LD, Varlamov O, et al. Hyperproinsulinemia in obese *fat/fat* mice associated with a point mutation in the carboxypeptidase E gene and reduced carboxypeptidase E activity in the pancreatic islets. *Nat Genet.* 1995;10:135-142.
39. Varlamov O, Leiter EH, Fricker LD. Induced and spontaneous mutations at Ser202 of carboxypeptidase E: effect on enzyme expression, activity, and intracellular routing. *J Biol Chem.* 1996;271:13981-13986.
40. Fricker LD, Berman YL, Leiter EH, Devi LA. Carboxypeptidase E activity is deficient in mice with the fat mutation: effect on peptide processing. *J Biol Chem.* 1996;271:30619-30624.
41. Rovere C, Viale A, Nahon J, Kitabgi P. Impaired processing of brain proneurotensin and promelanin-concentrating hormone in obese *fat/fat* mice. *Endocrinology.* 1996;137:2954-2958.
42. Udupi V, Gomez P, Song L, et al. Effect of carboxypeptidase E deficiency on progastrin processing and gastrin mRNA expression in mice with the fat mutation. *Endocrinology.* 1997;138:1959-1963.
43. Cain BM, Wang W, Beinfeld MC. Cholecystokinin (CCK) levels are greatly reduced in the brains but not the duodenums of *Cpe^fat/Cpe^fat* mice: a regional difference in the involvement of carboxypeptidase E (Cpe) in pro-CCK processing. *Endocrinology.* 1997;138:4034-4037.
44. Song L, Fricker LD. Purification and characterization of carboxypeptidase D, a novel carboxypeptidase E-like enzyme, from bovine pituitary. *J Biol Chem.* 1995;270:25007-25013.
45. Varlamov O, Fricker LD. Intracellular trafficking of metallocarboxypeptidase D in AtT-20 cells: localization to the trans-Golgi network and recycling from the cell surface. *J Cell Sci.* 1998;111:877-885.
46. Varlamov O, Eng FJ, Novikova EG, Fricker LD. Localization of metallocarboxypeptidase D in AtT-20 cells: potential role in prohormone processing. *J Biol Chem.* 1999;274:14759-14767.
47. Eipper BA, Milgram SL, Husten EJ, Yun HY, Mains RE. Peptidylglycine alpha-amidating monooxygenase: a multifunctional protein with catalytic, processing, and routing domains. *Protein Sci.* 1993;2:489-497.

48. Ouafik LH, Stoffers DA, Campbell TA, et al. The multifunctional peptidylglycine alpha-amidating monooxygenase gene: exon/intron organization of catalytic, processing, and routing domains. *Mol Endocrinol.* 1992;6:1571-1584.
49. Prigge ST, Mains RE, Eipper BA, Amzel LM. New insights into copper monooxygenase and peptide amidation: structure, mechanism, and function. *Cell Mol Life Sci.* 2000;57:1236-1259.
50. Kolhekar AS, Mains RE, Eipper BA. Peptidylglycine alpha-amidating monooxygenase: an ascorbate-requiring enzyme. *Meth Enzymol.* 1997;279:35-43.
51. Bradbury AF, Smyth DG. Modification of the N- and C-termini of bioactive peptides: amidation and acetylation. In: Fricker LD, ed. *Peptide Biosynthesis and Processing* Boca Raton, FL: CRC Press; 1991:231-250.
52. Kojima M, Hosoda H, Date Y, Nakazato M, Matsuo H, Kangawa K. Ghrelin is a growth-hormone-releasing acylated peptide from stomach. *Nature.* 1999;402:656-660.
53. Lee RWH, Huttner WB. Tyrosine O-sulfated proteins of PC1 pheochromocytoma cells and their sulfation by tyrosylprotein sulfotransferase. *J Biol Chem.* 1983;258:11326-11332.
54. Bennett HPJ. Glycosylation, phosphorylation, and sulfation of peptide hormones and their precursors. In: Fricker LD, ed. *Peptide Biosynthesis and Processing.* Boca Raton, FL: CRC Press; 1991:111-140.
55. Svensson M, Skold K, Svenningsson P, Andren PE. Peptidomics-based discovery of novel neuropeptides. *J Proteome Res.* 2003;2:213-219.
56. Turner AJ. Exploring the structure and function of zinc metallopeptidases: old enzymes and new discoveries. *Biochem Soc Trans.* 2003;31:723-727.
57. Albiston AL, Ye S, Chai SY. Membrane bound members of the M1 family: more than aminopeptidases. *Protein Pept Lett.* 2004;11:491-500.
58. Kim SI, Grum-Tokars V, Swanson TA, et al. Novel roles of neuropeptide processing enzymes: EC3.4.24.15 in the neurome. *J Neurosci Res.* 2003;74:456-467.
59. Smith AI, Clarke IJ, Lew RA. Post-secretory processing of peptide signals: a novel mechanism for the regulation of peptide hormone receptors. *Biochem Soc Trans.* 1997;25:1011-1014.
60. Goumon Y, Lugardon K, Gadroy P, et al. Processing of proenkephalin-A in bovine chromaffin cells. Identification of natural derived fragments by N-terminal sequencing and matrix-assisted laser desorption ionization-time of flight mass spectrometry. *J Biol Chem.* 2000;275:38355-38362.
61. Wei S, Segura S, Vendrell J, et al. Identification and characterization of three members of the human metallocarboxypeptidase gene family. *J Biol Chem.* 2002;277:14954-14964.
62. Fontenele-Neto JD, Kalinina E, Feng Y, Fricker LD. Identification and distribution of mouse carboxypeptidase A-6. *Brain Res Mol Brain Res.*
63. Emoto N, Yanagisawa M. Endothelin-converting enzyme-2 is a membrane-bound, phosphoramidon-sensitive metalloprotease with acidic pH optimum. *J Biol Chem.* 1995;270:15262-15268.
64. Mzhavia N, Pan H, Che F-Y, Fricker LD, Devi LA. Characterization of endothelin-converting enzyme-2. Implication for a role in the nonclassical processing of regulatory peptides. *J Biol Chem.* 2003;278:14704-14711.
65. Srinivasan S, Bunch DO, Feng Y, et al. Deficits in reproduction and pro-gonadotropin-releasing hormone processing in male Cpefat mice. *Endocrinology.* 2004;145:2023-2034.
66. Qian Y, Devi LA, Mzhavia N, Munzer S, Seidah NG, Fricker LD. The C-terminal region of proSAAS is a potent inhibitor of prohormone convertase 1. *J Biol Chem.* 2000;275:23596-23601.
67. Wei S, Feng Y, Che F-Y, et al. Obesity and diabetes in transgenic mice expressing proSAAS. *J Endocrinol.* 2004;180:357-368.
68. Sakurai T, Amemiya A, Ishii M, et al. Orexins and orexin receptors: a family of hypothalamic neuropeptides and G-protein-coupled receptors that regulate feeding behavior. *Cell.* 1998;92:573-585.
69. Preti A. Orexins (hypocretins): their role in appetite and arousal. *Curr Opin Investig Drugs.* 2002;3:1199-1206.
70. Rodgers RJ, Ishii Y, Halford JC, Blundell JE. Orexins and appetite regulation. *Neuropeptides.* 2002;36:303-325.

71. Tao WA, Aebersold R. Advances in quantitative proteomics via stable isotope tagging and mass spectrometry. *Curr Opin Biotechnol*. 2003;14:110-118.
72. Goshe MB, Smith RD. Stable isotope-coded proteomic mass spectrometry. *Curr Opin Biotechnol*. 2003;14:101-109.
73. Che F-Y, Eipper BA, Mains RE, Fricker LD. Quantitative peptidomics of pituitary glands from mice deficient in copper transport. *Cell Mol Biol*. 2003;49:713-722.

Chapter 30
CNS Drug Delivery: Opioid Peptides and the Blood-Brain Barrier

Ken A. Witt[1] and Thomas P. Davis[2]

Abstract Peptides are key regulators in cellular and intercellular physiological responses and possess enormous promise for the treatment of pathological conditions. Opioid peptide activity within the central nervous system (CNS) is of particular interest for the treatment of pain owing to the elevated potency of peptides and the centrally mediated actions of pain processes. Despite this potential, peptides have seen limited use as clinically viable drugs for the treatment of pain. Reasons for the limited use are primarily based in the physiochemical and biochemical nature of peptides. Numerous approaches have been devised in an attempt to improve peptide drug delivery to the brain, with variable results. This review describes different approaches to peptide design/modification and provides examples of the value of these strategies to CNS delivery of peptide drugs. The various modes of modification of therapeutic peptides may be amalgamated, creating more efficacious "hybrid" peptides, with synergistic delivery to the CNS. The ongoing development of these strategies provides promise that peptide drugs may be useful for the treatment of pain and other neurologically-based disease states in the future.

Keywords DPDPE, biphalin, transport, delivery strategies

Introduction

In recent years, there have been several important advancements in the development of peptide therapeutics. Nevertheless, the targeting of peptide drugs to the central nervous system (CNS) remains a formidable undertaking. Delivery of efficacious

[1] Pharmaceutical Sciences, School of Pharmacy, Southern Illinois University, Edwardsville, 200 University Park Drive, Edwardsville, IL., 62026, USA

[2] Department of Medical Pharmacology, College of Medicine, The University of Arizona, LSN 542, 1501 N. Campbell Avenue, Tucson, Arizona 85724

Corresponding Author: Thomas P. Davis, Department of Pharmacology, P.O. Box 245050, The University of Arizona, Tucson, AZ 85724. Tel: (520) 626-7643; Fax: (520) 626-4053; E-mail: davistp@u.arizona.edu

R.S. Rapaka and W. Sadée (eds.), *Drug Addiction.*
© American Association of Pharmaceutical Scientists 2008

peptide drugs is limited by their poor bioavailability due to low metabolic stability and high clearance by the liver. In addition, peptides are generally water-soluble compounds that will not enter the CNS readily, via passive diffusion, due to the existence of the blood-brain barrier (BBB). The aim of this review is to assess many of the chemical modifications developed to date and to discuss the various delivery-enhancing strategies necessary to produce viable CNS acting opioid peptide drugs.

Peptide Characterization

The capacity of a peptide to cross the BBB and enter the brain is dependent upon several compositional factors, including size, flexibility, conformation, biochemical properties of amino acids, and amino acid arrangement. Peptide composition also determines, in part, the degree of protein binding, enzymatic stability, cellular sequestration, uptake into nontarget tissue, clearance rate, and affinity for protein carriers. Other aspects independent of peptide composition must also be considered, such as cerebral blood flow, diet, age, sex, species (for experimental studies), dosing route, and effects of existing pathological conditions. Each of these factors must be considered for an appropriated study design strategy.

In this review we focus on opioid peptides with emphasis on 2 unique and well characterized enkephalin analogs, DPDPE and biphalin. Each of these peptides has been the focus of numerous studies to examine novel mechanisms in which to enhance delivery of peptides into the CNS. An additional advantage of using opioid peptides in the examination of new technologies and structural/chemical modifications is the definitive CNS-mediated end point (ie, analgesia) and the well-characterized biochemical nature of the opioid receptors.

Role of the Blood-Brain Barrier in CNS Drug Delivery

The brain is one of the least accessible organs for the delivery of active pharmacological compounds. Despite its relatively high nutrient support and exchange requirements, the uptake of any compound is strictly regulated by the BBB. The surface area of the human BBB is estimated to be 5000 times greater than that of the blood-cerebrospinal fluid barrier, and therefore the BBB is considered to be the primary barrier controlling the uptake of drugs into the brain parenchyma.[1] To understand why the BBB is such a significant impediment to peptide drug delivery, its characteristics must first be assessed. The BBB is a unique physical and enzymatic barrier that segregates the brain from the systemic circulation. BBB capillary endothelia lack fenestrations and are sealed by tight junctions, which inhibit any significant paracellular transport.[2-4] Specific transporters exist at the BBB that permit nutrients to enter the brain and toxicants/waste products to exit.[5] The BBB further functions as a diffusional restraint, with selective discrimination of substance transcytosis based on lipid solubility, molecular size, and charge.[6] In addition, the BBB has a high concentration of drug-efflux-transporters (ie, P-glycoprotein, multi-drug resistant protein, breast cancer resistant protein) in the luminal membranes of the cerebral capillary endothelium. These efflux transporters actively remove a broad range of drug molecules from the endothelial cell cytoplasm before they cross into the brain parenchyma. Last, the "enzymatic barrier" component of the BBB, capable of rapidly metabolizing peptide drugs and nutrients,[7-10] is also of great significance in regard to peptide viability. As amino acids and their associated linkage are highly susceptible to enzymatic degradation, the nature and concentration of specific enzymes at the BBB can greatly affect the efficacy of a given peptide-based drug.[11,12]

The influence of brain pathology on the functioning of the BBB must also be integrated into the development of the peptide delivery strategies. The development of new drugs and drug-vectors must also contend with potential pathological conditions of the patient. Several disease states result in enhanced BBB permeability to fluid and/or solutes[13] including hypoxia-ischemia and inflammatory mechanisms involving the BBB in septic encephalopathy, HIV-induced dementia, multiple sclerosis, and Alzheimer disease. The list of factors that may contribute to changes in drug bioavailability (eg, changes in BBB cytoarchitecture, protein binding, receptor site, enzymes) during a pathological state is extensive and must be taken into account for appropriate drug design. Specific changes at the BBB, such as opening/disruption of tight junctions, increased pinocytosis, changes in nutrient transport, and pore formation may enhance/reduce drug uptake. Table 30.1 lists several potential conditions and factors shown to induce changes at the BBB.

Table 30.1 Potential causes of blood-brain barrier alteration*

Paracellular opening:	hyperosmolarity[14]; acidic pH[15]; burn encephalopathy[16]; experimental autoimmune encephalitis[17,18]; multiple sclerosis[19,20]; chemical mediators associated with inflammation: (TNFα,[21] IL-1β,[22] histamine,[23] serotonin,[24] bradykinin,[25] Thrombin,[26] and reactive oxygen species[27]); ischemia[28-30]; lead[31]; aluminum[32]; post-ischemia reperfusion[33,34]; electromagnetic fields[35]; systemic lupus erythematosus[36]
Increased Pinocytosis:	acute hypertension[37,38]; microwave irradiation[39]; ischemia[40,41]; seizures[42]; heat stroke[16]; brain injury[43]; tumors[44]; development[45,46]; hypervolemia[47]; immobilization stress[48]; hypothermia (<16°C)[49]; post-radiation[39,50]; hyperbaric conditions[51]; lead encephalopathy[52]; mercury[53]; Tricyclic antidepressants[54]; meningitis[55,56]; multiple sclerosis[57,58]; lymphostatic encephalopathy[59]
Pore Formation:	Tricyclic antidepressants (chlorpromazine, nortriptyline)[60]; Ischemia[61]

(continued)

Table 30.1 (continued)

Disease / toxicant transport changes:	Diabetes (GLUT-1)[62,63]; Alzheimer's disease (β-amyloid, RAGE, LRP receptor)[64-66]; Wernickes-Korsakoff syndrome (thiamine)[67,68]; Eating / weight disorders (insulin and leptin)[69-71]; hypertension (choline)[72]

TNFα: tissue necrosis factor-α; IL-1β: interleukin-1β; GLUT-1: glucose transporter type-1; RAGE: receptor for advanced glycation end products; LRP: lipoprotein receptor-related protein (Adapted from Pardridge 1991[11])

Delivery Strategies to Enhance Peptide Delivery to the CNS

Peptide drug delivery to the brain may be divided into 3 general categories:

1. Invasive procedures, which include transient osmotic opening of the BBB,[73,74] shunts,[75] and biodegradable implants.[76,77] These procedures can be highly traumatic and often have low therapeutic efficiency with substantial side effects.
2. Pharmacologically-based approaches to increase the passage through the BBB by increasing specific biochemical attributes of a compound. This may be accomplished either by chemical modification of the peptide molecule itself, or by the attachment or encapsulation of the peptide in a substance that increases permeability, stability, bioavailability, and/or receptor affinity. In addition, modification of drug structure and/or addition of constituents (eg, lipophilicity enhancers, polymers, antibodies) may enhance drug concentration within the CNS, with a reduced toxic profile.
3. Physiologic-based strategies exploit the various carrier mechanisms at the BBB, which have been characterized in recent years for nutrients, peptide and nonpeptide hormones, and transport proteins. These strategies can be combined, dependent of the nature of a given peptide, creating "hybrid" peptides, resulting in synergistic CNS delivery and end-effect.

Peptide drug modification can be broadly divided into several categories: lipidization, structural modification to enhance stability, glycosylation, increasing affinity for nutrient transporters, prodrugs, vector-based, cationization, and polymer conjugation/encapsulation. Table 30.2 provides a listing of these strategies to increase peptide uptake into the brain, with associated advantages and limitations.

Lipidization

Lipid solubility is a key factor in determining the rate at which a drug passively crosses the BBB. The presence of hydroxyl groups on peptides tends to promote hydrogen bonding with water leading to a concomitant decrease in the partition

Table 30.2 Modes of Peptide Modification to Enhance CNS Delivery*

Strategy	Advantages	Limitations
Lipidization	Increases membrane permeability	Increases plasma protein binding
		Intracellular sequestration
		Increased hepato-biliary elimination
		Non-specific targeting
		Receptor interference
		Increase size of molecule may counter membrane permeability enhancement
Structural modification to enhance stability	Increases stability	Potential decrease in membrane transport
	Potential increase in membrane transport	Potential decrease in receptor affinity
	Potential increase in receptor affinity	
Glycosylation	Increases membrane permeability	Nonspecific targeting
	Increases stability	Receptor interference
	Increases serum half-life	
Nutrient Transport	Drug entry not dependent upon passive diffusion	Limited capacity of carriers
	Potentially specific targeting	Potential interference with endogenous substrate of carrier
		Specificity of carrier
		Similarity of carrier mechanisms throughout body may reduce specificity of targeting
Prodrug	Increases membrane permeability and/or pharmacokinetics	Kinetics of drug release must be precise
	Potential target specificity based on design of cleavable linker and/or enhancer moiety	Requires optimization of linker and drug attachment
	"Redox" prodrugs lock drug in tissue	Charged "Redox" prodrugs are rapidly eliminated from body
Vector-based	Specific membrane targeting	Delivery to brain is directly limited to the transporter concentration
	Linker strategies may be incorporated to enhance stability and detachment of vector portion	

(continued)

Table 30.2 (continued)

Strategy	Advantages	Limitations
		Potential downregulation of transporters with continual dosing
		Potential interference with endogenous substrate of carrier/ transporter
		Requires optimization of linker and drug attachment
		Altered pharmacokinetic profile
		Significant cost in design and production
Cationization	Increases membrane permeability	Increases plasma protein binding
	Increases serum half-life	Immune complex formation
		Non-specific targeting
		Rapid elimination of charged moiety
Polymer conjugation	Increases stability	Hydrophobic polymers reduce membrane permeability
	Increases serum-half life	
	Decreases elimination rate	Decrease receptor binding with improper selection or placement of polymer
	Decreases immunogenicity/ toxicity	
	Decreases protein binding	
	Potential for control-release design	Nonspecific targeting

* Adapted for Witt et al, 2001[12]

coefficient (ie, lipophilicity) and resultant decrease in membrane permeability.[78] Peptide drugs generally contain polar functional groups that impart a degree of dipolarity and hydrogen bonding. The amino acids that compose a peptide determine the respective polarity. The overall balance of polar to nonpolar groups within a drug molecule can be reduced either by removal of a polar group or addition of a nonpolar group.[6] In addition, the relative positioning of polar to nonpolar amino acids (ie, whether polar/nonpolar groups are at the center or ends of a given peptide) will also determine the capability of a peptide to transport across a biological membrane.[6]

Methylation has been shown to reduce the overall hydrogen bond potential. Dimethylation of the tyrosine on the synthetic opioid peptide DPDPE has been shown to significantly enhance analgesia with a concomitant enhancement of bioavailability.[79] This structural modification resulted in a 10-fold increase in the potency over the nonmethylated DPDPE at the delta opioid receptor and a 35-fold increase in potency at the μ-opioid receptor, while substantial delta receptor selectivity was maintained. In another study, the placement of 3 methyl groups on the phenylalanine of DPDPE induced changes in lipophilicity and BBB permeability.[80] These alterations were contingent upon the specific conformation of the respective methyl groups on the phenylalanine. The trimethylated DPDPE was also shown to alter efflux (ie, reduced P-glycoprotein affinity), metabolism, and analgesia, based on the diastereoisomer configuration of the nonaromatic methyl group.[80] Thus, during formulation, the stereoselectivity of the peptide drug must be assessed with preservation of optimal bioavailability and receptor binding affinity.

Halogenation of peptides can also enhance lipophilicity and BBB permeability. Halogenation of peptides such as DPDPE,[81,82] DPLPE,[83] and biphalin[84] have shown to significantly enhance BBB permeability in a manner dependent upon the conjugated halogen (Cl, Br, F, I). Addition of chlorine on the Phe4 residue of DPDPE led to a significant increase in permeability in both in vivo[81] and in vitro studies.[82] Addition of 2 chlorine atoms onto DPDPE further increased BBB permeability, beyond that of the single chlorine. An identical trend was observed for chlorinated biphalin, with an increased BBB permeability both in situ and in vitro.[84] However, when fluorine was added to DPDPE, permeability did not increase, while fluorine addition to biphalin greatly diminished BBB permeability. Another method to increase lipophilicity is through acylation or alkylation of the N-terminal amino acid.[85] Acylation of peptides and proteins has consistently proven to be an effective means to increase membrane permeability with limited interference in receptor binding. Acyl derivatives of DADLE,[86,87] DPDPE,[88] thyrotropin-releasing hormone (TRH),[88,89] and insulin[90] have also shown improved absorption through artificial and biological membranes and enhanced enzymatic stability, while retaining pharmacological activity.

There are many strategies designed to enhance lipid solubility of drugs, but lipidization does have several limitations. Since highly lipid-soluble drugs may be extensively plasma protein bound, there is the potential for a reduction in the amount of free or exchangeable drug in the plasma, thereby compromising brain uptake.[91] The site of modification or attachment of substances/molecules to increase lipophilicity must also be taken into account, as receptor binding affinity may be diminished if alterations are within the pharmacophore region, thus reducing biological activity. Last, enhancement of lipophilicity alone may not necessarily improve BBB transport. Factors such as size, stability, intracellular sequestration, nontarget organ uptake, efflux rates, and P-glycoprotein (P-gp) efflux affinity must also be considered.

Structural modification to enhance stability

Structural design to reduce enzymatic degradation is another approach used to enhance peptide bioavailability to the CNS. These modifications require extensive analytical investigation to define the site of enzymatic cleavage and the proteolytic enzymes that act upon a specific peptide.[11] Enzyme masking strategies include modification of the amino acid terminus, with N-acylation or pyroglutamyl residues, to reduce aminopeptidase M activity.[85,92] However, such modifications may result in reduced biological activity; for example, opioid peptides require the amino terminus to be free for effective receptor binding.[93,94] An alternative modification for opioids, to reduce aminopeptidase activity, is to substitute the Glycine[2] (Gly[2]) residue with a D-Alanine[2] (D-Ala[2]) residue. Substitution of D-Ala[2] for L-Gly[2] at the N-terminal of met-enkephalin, and amidation of its C-terminus, produce greater enzymatic stability.[95] In addition, the substitution of D-Ala[2] and D-Leucine[5] (D-Leu[5]) DADLE has been shown to significantly increase half-life by reducing enzymatic proteolysis.[96] Modifications of amino acids or attachment of secondary structures onto peptides within these regions may also reduce enzyme degradation.

Other modes to reduce enzymatic degradation and increase membrane permeability of peptides include the introduction of conformational constraints and altering chirality of amino acids. Cyclization of peptides may reduce hydrogen bonding, increase lipophilicity, and reduce the hydrodynamic radius in solution, thereby enhancing membrane permeability.[97-100] This conversion of linear peptides into cyclic conformationally constrained peptides, via a disulfide-bridge, has met with considerable success. The use of disulfide-bridge constrained peptide analogs has been shown to significantly reduce enzymatic degradation,[81,101] with the potential advantage of enhanced specificity for receptor subtypes.[102] In the case of linear met-enkephalin, the conversion into the cyclic analog (DPDPE) (Fig. 30.1) resulted in a δ-opioid-specific peptide[103] with

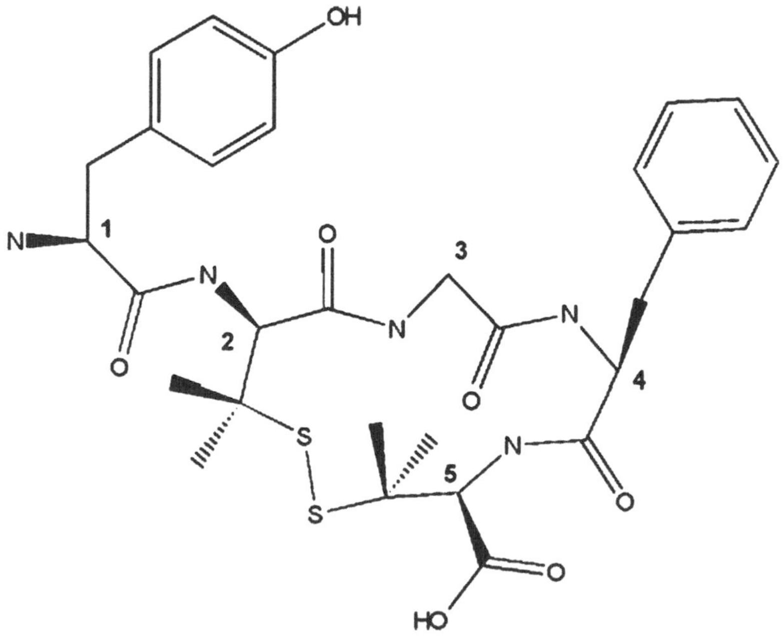

Fig. 30.1 Structure of DPDPE[106] NH2-Tyr1-D-Pen2-Gly3-Phe4-D-Pen5-OH.

a saturable mode of transport at the BBB.[104-106] Due to the incorporation of 2 D-penicillamine residues and conformational restriction by a disulfide bridge, DPDPE is enzymatically stable.[101,107] Another variation on conformational bridging is shown with the opioid peptide biphalin (Fig. 30.2), a unique analog containing 2 enkephalin sequences linked by a hydrazide bridge. Thus, biphalin has 2 biologically active pharmacophores, with affinity for both µ- and δ-opioid receptors.[108-110]

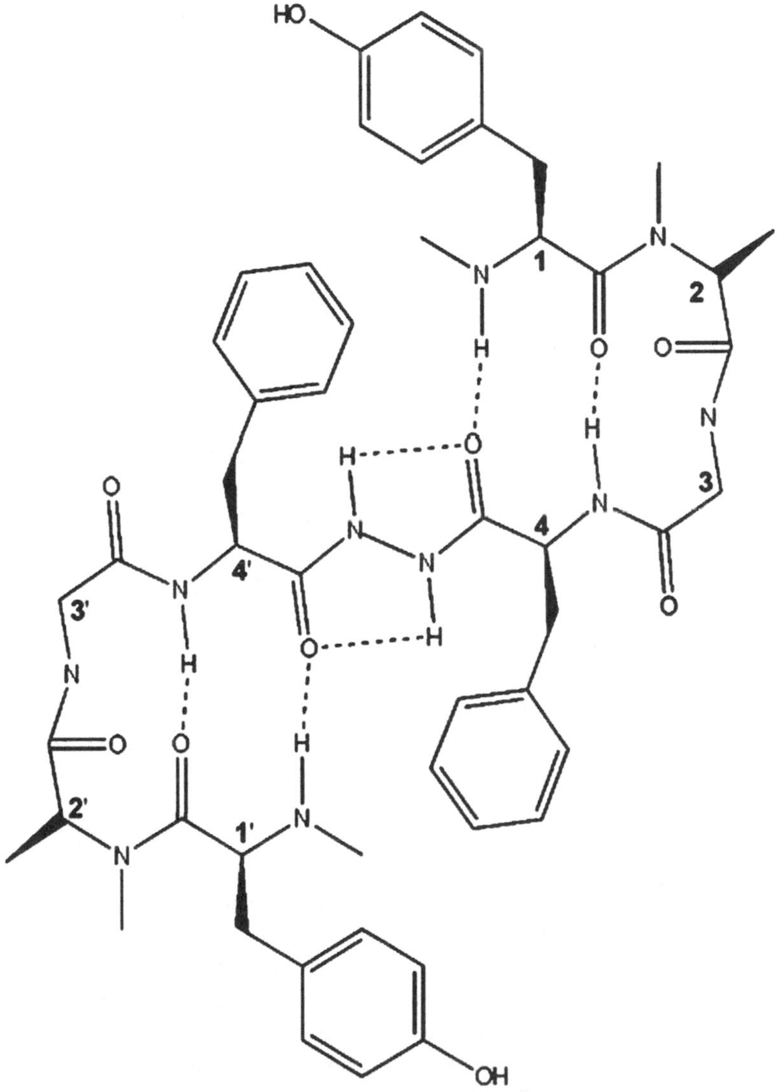

Fig. 30.2 Structure of Biphalin[106] NH_2-Tyr[1]-D-Ala[2]-Gly[3]-Phe[4]-NH-NH-Phe[4']-Gly[3']-D-Ala[2']-Tyr[1'].

Administered intracerebroventricularly in mice, biphalin was 6.7- and 257-fold more potent than etorphine or morphine, respectively, in eliciting analgesia.[111] Biphalin is protected from aminopeptidase activity by D-Ala residues in the 2 and 2′ positions and is protected from carboxy peptidase activity by the hydrazide bridge.

Glycosylation

The addition of carbohydrate moieties to a peptide (glycopeptide) produces changes in the molecular structure that, in turn, can have dramatic effects on the pharmaco-dynamic and/or pharmacokinetic properties.[112] Glycosylation has proven to enhance biodistribution of multiple substances to the brain.[113,114] Attachment of simple sugars to enkephalins increases their penetration of the BBB and allows the resulting glycopeptide analogs to function effectively as drugs. Several different sugar moieties have been investigated, including glucose and xylose, with respective sugars exhibiting variations in BBB permeability.[115] The improved analgesia exhibited by glycosylated opioids may be due to increased bioavailability of glycopeptides via higher metabolic stability,[116] reduced clearance,[117] and improved BBB transport.[115] Improved analgesia has also been reported for glycosylated deltorphin,[118,119] cyclized methionine enkephalin analogs,[115,120] and linear leucine enkephalin analogs.[121] The δ-selective glycosylated leu-enkephalin amide, H_2N-Tyr-D-Thr-Gly-Phe-Leu-Ser(βD-Glc)-$CONH_2$, produces analgesic effects similar to morphine, even when administered peripherally, yet possesses reduced dependence liability as indicated by naloxone-precipitated withdrawal studies.[115] Although the mode of enhanced transport at the BBB has yet to be fully elucidated for glycosylated peptides, the improved BBB transport is not related to increased lipophilicity, given that octanol/saline distribution studies of glycosylated peptides indicate that the addition of glucose significantly reduced lipophilicity, thereby reducing passive diffusion.[115] In addition, endocytotic mechanisms have been shown to transport glyc-osylated peptides.[122-125] Of interest, recent studies indicate that transport through the BBB may hinge on the amphipathic nature of the glycopeptides.[126] That is, the amphipathic glycopeptides possess 2 conflicting solubility states: one state that is completely water soluble, and another at water-membrane phase boundaries. However, simply producing highly amphipathic sequences is not enough to promote systemic delivery and penetration of the BBB. The glycopeptide sequence must be capable of assuming a water-soluble random coil conformation (ie, "biousian" activity), comparable to micelle formation, and the barrier between the 2 states must be low enough for rapid interconversion between the 2 states.[127] In addition, it was proposed that some glycopeptides promote a negative membrane curvature at the endothelial cell wall, with the negative curvature leading to increased rates of endocytosis, which in turn result in enhanced BBB transport.[127]

A caveat in regard to opioid peptide glycosylation is that a reduction in affinity for the μ-opioid receptor occurs upon glycosylation. Yet, there is virtually no effect on δ binding or efficacy.[128] This finding is consistent with Schwyzer's membrane compartment theory,[129] which suggests that the μ-receptor binding site resides in a more hydrophilic environment than the binding site for the δ-opioid receptor. This is important because, the primary analgesic action of opioid-based drugs is theorized to be regulated through the μ-opioid receptor.

Nutrient Transporters

Peptide drug design may also incorporate specific molecular characteristics that enable the drug to be transported by one or more of the inwardly directed nutrient carriers. The BBB expresses several transport systems for nutrients and endogenous compounds.[130,131] Utilization of these transport systems is a potential strategy for controlling the delivery of drugs into the brain. These drugs must have a molecular structure mimicking the endogenous nutrient. The prototypical example is levo-dopa, a lipid-insoluble precursor of dopamine that has been used for the treatment of Parkinson's disease because it contains the carboxyl and α-amino groups that allow it to compete for transport across the BBB by the large neutral amino acid carrier.[132] Biphalin, a potent opioid analgesic,[111,133] is a peptide drug that has been shown to use the neutral amino acid carrier system to gain entry into the brain.[134] Chemical groups could be designed with the ability to attach to specific drugs rendering them substrates for carriers, or drugs specifically designed for a carrier mechanism. The hexose and large neutral amino acid carriers have the highest capacity and presently are the best candidates for delivery of substrates to the brain. Lower capacity carriers may also be utilized for highly potent peptide drugs. Peptides, which generally require low concentrations to induce effect, are most appropriate for this type of targeting design. Yet, the complexity in designing a peptide to target specific nutrient transporters requires a great deal of knowledge of both peptide and transporter. Nevertheless, these transport mechanisms may also be advantageous targets for prodrug and vector-mediated approaches to enhance peptide delivery to the brain.

Prodrugs

Prodrugs contain a pharmacologically active moiety that is either conjugated to a molecule with a known transporter or to a lipophilicity enhancer, which is cleaved at or near the site of action, allowing drug to induce its effect. The rationale for prodrug design is that the structural requirements necessary to elicit a desired pharmacological action and those necessary to provide optimal delivery to the target receptor site may not be the same. The ideal prodrug is enzymatically stable in the blood, but rapidly degraded to the active parent compound once it is within the target tissue. Esters have shown particular promise in the area of prodrug design for brain delivery, owing to the abundance of endogenous esterases in the CNS.

Esterification or amidation of amino, hydroxyl, or carboxylic acid-containing drugs may greatly enhance lipid solubility, and thus brain entry.[135,136] Once in the CNS, hydrolysis of the modifying group releases the active compound. Both aromatic benzoyl esters[135] and branched chain tertiary butyl esters[137] have shown stability in plasma, while still remaining adequately cleaved within the CNS. Lipophilic amino acids, such as phenylalanine (Phe), can be used as the cleavable unit. The addition of a Phe group to DPDPE at the amino terminal resulted in enhanced permeability at the BBB.[138] Chains of nonpolar amino acids could further enhance lipophilicity, albeit the balance between molecular size and degree of lipophilic enhancement must be assessed individually.

Another prodrug design focuses on the redox system,[139,140] in which a lipophilic attachment (eg, 1,4-dihydro) is converted to the hydrophilic quaternary form, effectively "locking" the drug in the tissue.[141] When a drug is conjugated to a methyldihydropyridine carrier and subsequently oxidized by NADH-linked dehydrogenases in the brain, it results in a quaternary ammonium salt, which does not cross back through the BBB endothelium.[142] Similar design has been explored with a wide variety of drugs, such as steroids, antivirals, neurotransmitters, anticonvulsants, and peptides (leucine enkephalin analog and TRH analog).[141,143] The primary difficulties with the redox design are that any tissue may take up the lipophilic moiety, and rapid elimination of the charged salt form occurs.

Prodrug design is presently at the forefront of pharmaceutical exploration in terms of CNS targeting. The difficulty with prodrugs lies primarily within the pharmacokinetics. Precise placement and choice of cleavable moiety must be optimized to obtain the most efficacious pharmacokinetic profile.

Vector-based

Physiologic vector-based strategies involve the use of existing BBB transport properties to enhance brain entry of a specific drug, much the same as prodrugs. The principle of the vector-mediated or chimeric delivery strategy lies in the coupling of a moderately impermeable peptide to a substance that increases the affinity to and transport across a biological membrane via receptor-mediated or absorptive-mediated endocytosis. After entry into the brain, these chimeric drugs release via enzymatic cleavage, allowing the drug to initiate a pharmacological action in the brain. This technology may be adapted for use with peptide pharmaceuticals, nucleic acid therapeutics, and small molecules. Important design considerations of such chimeric peptides include vector specificity for the brain, pharmacokinetics of the vector, and placement and cleavability of the linker between the drug and vector. Multiple concepts for such systems exist,[144-147] with present focus on antibody attachment and chemical linker strategies.

Receptor-mediated vectors for brain delivery must be specific. There are several potential receptors at the BBB that may serve this purpose. The plasma protein transferrin is able to bind and undergo endothelial endocytosis in brain capillaries and has proven to be a suitable vector. A murine monoclonal antibody (OX26) to the transferrin receptor has been successfully used to increase brain uptake of proteins and peptides. An analog of the opioid peptide dermorphin ([Lys7]dermorphin) was conjugated to the OX26 vector, demonstrating analgesia, which was reversed by naloxone.[148] Cationized albumin has also been used as a vector to enhance peptide uptake, via adsorptive-mediated endocytosis. When cationized albumin was conjugated to β-endorphin, it yielded increased uptake into isolated brain endothelial cells, as compared with β-endorphin alone.[149]

Several additional caveats should be considered with use of a receptor-mediated vector design. There exists the potential competition between the vector-drug and the endogenous ligand for the receptor as such endocytotic mechanisms tend to have low capacity in the brain. This phenomenon would result in decreased vector transport and/or decreased concentration of a required nutrient to the brain, resulting in a subsequent pathology. Last, the quantity of drug delivered to the brain is directly limited by transporter concentration. Transporter capacity may become saturated or downregulated over time, decreasing the ability to deliver an adequate and consistent dosage of drug to elicit a pharmacological effect. This possibility is important if the use of a drug requires consistent and repeated doses. Therefore, this approach would likely require extremely potent therapeutic peptides, which may be most effective for acute disease states.

Cationization

Cationization of peptides is a manner of increasing membrane entry via absorptive-mediated endocytosis (AME).[145,150-153] Presence of anionic sites on BBB endothelium brings about attraction of cationized substances to the membrane surface.[154] The dynorphin-like analgesic peptide E-2078, and the adrenocorticotropic hormone (ACTH) analog, ebiratide, are polycationic peptides at physiologic pH shown to internalize into brain capillaries by AME.[155-158] The μ-opioid receptor-selective [D-Arg²]-dermorphin tetrapeptide analogs H-Tyr-D-Arg-Phe-Sar-OH, and H-Tyr-D-Arg-Phe-β-Ala-OH (TAPA) were developed,[159] showing potent analgesic activity with low physical and psychological dependence.[160] It was reported that TAPA crosses the BBB via AME, which is triggered by binding of the peptides to negatively charged sites on the surface of brain capillary endothelial cells.[152] Yet, when 2 additional [D-Arg²]-dermorphin analogs were designed (Nαamidino-Tyr-D-Arg-Phe-β-Ala-OH (ADAB) and Nα-amidino-Tyr-D-Arg-Phe-MeβAla-OH (ADAMB), the peptides exhibited a slower degree of analgesic onset, attributed to the parallel decrease in AME across the BBB.[153]

Cationized albumin attached to beta-endorphin, in a vector-based manner, showed significant increases in membrane uptake by AME.[161] Cationized albumin displayed longer serum half-life and a general selectivity to the brain.[147] In addition, avidin-cationized albumin conjugates have been proposed to affect the delivery of biotinylated, phosphodiesterase, antisense oligodeoxynucleotides to the brain.

These conjugates retain function (ie, inactivation of target mRNAs) and impart a degree of stability to serum and cellular enzymes.[162]

Unfortunately the potential toxicity of this strategy limits its clinical use as a therapeutic. Cationized proteins have been shown to induce immune complex formation with membranous nephropathy,[163,164] and increased cerebral and peripheral vascular permeability.[150,151,165] Cationized albumin has been shown to be significantly cleared by the kidney and liver, posing a potential toxicological threat as well.[147,166,167] This approach is also nonspecific as to tissue uptake, unless additionally coupled to a selective vector.

Polymer conjugation/encapsulation

Structural modifications can be obtained by the covalent conjugation of peptides to polymers. Polymer conjugations are used to increase peptide stability, reduce elimination, and reduce immunogenicity.[168-172] Chemical modification of peptides with macromolecular polymers, such as poly(ethylene glycol) (PEG),[170,172] and poly(styrene maleic acid),[173,174] shows significant promise.

Pegylation is a procedure of growing interest for enhancing the therapeutic and biotechnological potential of peptides and proteins. When PEG is correctly linked to a peptide it will modify many of the pharmacokinetic features, while theoretically maintaining the primary biological activity (ie, enzymatic activity or receptor recognition). PEG chains may contain linear and branched structures, which can be conjugated directly to the peptide drug or linked in a prodrug manner. PEG conjugation masks the peptide's surface and increases the molecular size, thereby reducing immune response, enzymatic degradation, toxicity, and renal ultrafiltration.[171] PEGs may also produce improved physical and thermal stability, as well as increased solubility.[175] The principal disadvantage of pegylation is the potential loss of activity with improper choice of PEG (ie, length, branching, chemical design) or unfavorable choice of attachment site. Another considerable disadvantage to pegylation, in regard to CNS focused drug delivery, is the enhanced hydrophilicity and molecular size that can bring about significant reductions in passive diffusion across the BBB.

When the opioid peptide DPDPE was pegylated, decreased clearance, reduced plasma protein binding, and first-pass elimination was shown, while increases in the analgesic effect following intravenous administration was demonstrated.[176] BBB permeability of the pegylated form was not significantly different when compared with the native form, despite enhanced hydrophilicity. This finding was possibly owing to an association with the saturable mechanism observed at the BBB[104] or a reversal of P-gp affinity[177] of the native compound.

Encapsulation, via nanoparticles and liposomes, may also be an effective manner by which to increase delivery to the brain. Nanoparticles are polymeric particles ranging in size between 10 and 1000 nm, which have a polysorbate overcoating. Drugs can be bound in the form of a solid solution or dispersion, or they can be absorbed to the surface of the particle or chemically attached. Polysorbate-80 nanoparticles have been shown to enhance delivery of the leu-enkephalin analog dalargin.[178] The particles are thought to mimic low density lipoproteins (LDL) and could therefore be taken up into the endothelium of the BBB via the LDL receptor. Enhanced transport of these nanoparticles may also involve tight junction modulation[179] or P-gp inhibition.[180] Liposomes are composed of a phospholipids bilayer that may act as a carrier for both hydrophilic and hydrophobic drugs. The beneficial attributes of liposomes are enhanced plasma half-life, decreased clearance, and decreased toxicity of associated drug.[181] One such liposome formulation is the pluronic copolymer P85, a self-forming micelle preparation that encapsulates a drug. The P85 formulation has been shown to enhance the delivery of digoxin into the brain,[182] and to enhance the analgesic profile of biphalin, DPDPE, and morphine,[183] with the mechanism of action theorized to be the inhibition of P-gp. One of the negatives of the P85 micellular formulations is the observation that P85 may function via depletion of ATP, which would reduce P-gp activity, yet may also result in undesired responses within the endothelium.[184]

Conclusion

Despite significant impediments of brain-directed peptide therapeutics, several delivery strategies show considerable promise for enhancement of CNS uptake. The specific biochemical modifications and delivery enhancers addressed in this review can be combined to create "hybrid" peptides, able to take advantage of multiple components of BBB passage. With this understanding, opioid peptide hybrids, specifically designed for increased brain entry, may provide highly potent treatment for CNS-mediated pain.

References

1. Crone C. The blood-brain barrier -facts and questions. In: Siesjo B, Sorensen S, eds. *Ion Homeostasis of the Brain.* Copenhagen: Munksgaard; 1971:52-62.
2. Brightman MW, Reese TS. Junctions between intimately apposed cell membranes in the vertebrate brain. *J Cell Biol.* 1969;40:648-677.
3. Rubin LL, Staddon JM. The cell biology of the blood-brain barrier. *Annu Rev Neurosci.* 1999;22:11-28.
4. Kniesel U, Wolburg H. Tight junctions of the blood-brain barrier. *Cell Mol Neurobiol.* 2000;20:57-76.
5. Tamai I, Tsuji A. Transporter-mediated permeation of drugs across the blood-brain barrier. *J Pharm Sci.* 2000;89:1371-1388.
6. Habgood MD, Begley DJ, Abbott NJ. Determinants of passive drug entry into the central nervous system. *Cell Mol Neurobiol.* 2000;20:231-253.
7. Vorbrodt AW. Ultrastructural cytochemistry of blood-brain barrier endothelia. *Prog Histochem Cytochem.* 1988;18:1-99.

8. Minn A, Ghersi-Egea JF, Perrin R, Leininger B, Siest G. Drug metabolizing enzymes in the brain and cerebral microvessels. *Brain Res Brain Res Rev.* 1991;16:65-82.
9. Brownlees J, Williams CH. Peptidases, peptides, and the mammalian blood-brain barrier. *J Neurochem.* 1993;60:793-803.
10. el-Bacha RS, Minn A. Drug metabolizing enzymes in cerebrovascular endothelial cells afford a metabolic protection to the brain. *Cell Mol Biol.* 1999;45:15-23.
11. Pardridge WM. *Peptide Drug Delivery to the Brain.* New York: Raven Press Ltd; 1991.
12. Witt KA, Gillespie TJ, Huber JD, Egleton RD, Davis TP. Peptide drug modifications to enhance bioavailability and blood-brain barrier permeability. *Peptides.* 2001;22:2329-2343.
13. Banks WA, Kastin AJ. Passage of peptides across the blood-brain barrier: pathophysiological perspectives. *Life Sci.* 1996;59:1923-1943.
14. Brightman MW, Hori M, Rapoport SI, Reese TS, Westergaard E. Osmotic opening of tight junctions in cerebral endothelium. *J Comp Neurol.* 1973;152:317-325.
15. Nagy Z, Szabo M, Huttner I. Blood-brain barrier impairment by low pH buffer perfusion via the internal carotid artery in rat. *Acta Neuropathol (Berl).* 1985;68:160-163.
16. Basch A, Fazekas IG. Increased permeability of the blood-brain barrier following experimental thermal injury of the skin. A fluorescent and electron microscopic study. *Angiologica.* 1970;7:357-364.
17. Hirano A, Dembitzer HM, Becker NH, Levine S, Zimmerman HM. Fine structural alterations of the blood-brain barrier in experimental allergic encephalomyelitis. *J Neuropathol Exp Neurol.* 1970;29:432-440.
18. Muller DM, Pender MP, Greer JM. Blood-brain barrier disruption and lesion localisation in experimental autoimmune encephalomyelitis with predominant cerebellar and brainstem involvement. *J Neuroimmunol.* 2005;160:162-169.
19. Kirk J, Plumb J, Mirakhur M, McQuaid S. Tight junctional abnormality in multiple sclerosis white matter affects all calibres of vessel and is associated with blood-brain barrier leakage and active demyelination. *J Pathol.* 2003;201:319-327.
20. Plumb J, McQuaid S, Mirakhur M, Kirk J. Abnormal endothelial tight junctions in active lesions and normal-appearing white matter in multiple sclerosis. *Brain Pathol.* 2002;12:154-169.
21. Yang GY, Gong C, Qin Z, Liu XH, Lorris Betz A. Tumor necrosis factor alpha expression produces increased blood-brain barrier permeability following temporary focal cerebral ischemia in mice. *Brain Res Mol Brain Res.* 1999;69:135-143.
22. Blamire AM, Anthony DC, Rajagopalan B, Sibson NR, Perry VH, Styles P. Interleukin-1beta-induced changes in blood-brain barrier permeability, apparent diffusion coefficient, and cerebral blood volume in the rat brain: a magnetic resonance study. *J Neurosci.* 2000;20:8153-8159.
23. Gulati A, Dhawan KN, Shukla R, Srimal RC, Dhawan BN. Evidence for the involvement of histamine in the regulation of blood-brain barrier permeability. *Pharmacol Res Commun.* 1985;17:395-404.
24. Sharma HS, Dey PK. Probable involvement of 5-hydroxytryptamine in increased permeability of blood-brain barrier under heat stress in young rats. *Neuropharmacology.* 1986;25:161-167.
25. Schurer L, Temesvari P, Wahl M, Unterberg A, Baethmann A. Blood-brain barrier permeability and vascular reactivity to bradykinin after pretreatment with dexamethasone. *Acta Neuropathol (Berl).* 1989;77:576-581.
26. Guan JX, Sun SG, Cao XB, Chen ZB, Tong ET. Effect of thrombin on blood brain barrier permeability and its mechanism. *Chin Med J (Engl).* 2004;117:1677-1681.
27. Lee HS, Namkoong K, Kim DH, et al. Hydrogen peroxide-induced alterations of tight junction proteins in bovine brain microvascular endothelial cells. *Microvasc Res.* 2004;68:231-238.
28. Lo EH, Pan Y, Matsumoto K, Kowall NW. Blood-brain barrier disruption in experimental focal ischemia: comparison between in vivo MRI and immunocytochemistry. *Magn Reson Imaging.* 1994;12:403-411.
29. Fischer S, Wiesnet M, Marti HH, Renz D, Schaper W. Simultaneous activation of several second messengers in hypoxia-induced hyperpermeability of brain derived endothelial cells. *J Cell Physiol.* 2004;198:359-369.

30. Brown RC, Davis TP. Hypoxia/aglycemia alters expression of occludin and actin in brain endothelial cells. *Biochem Biophys Res Commun.* 2005;327:1114-1123.
31. Struzynska L, Walski M, Gadamski R, Dabrowska-Bouta B, Rafalowska U. Lead-induced abnormalities in blood-brain barrier permeability in experimental chronic toxicity. *Mol Chem Neuropathol.* 1997;31:207-224.
32. Kim YS, Lee MH, Wisniewski HM. Aluminum induced reversible change in permeability of the blood-brain barrier to [14C]sucrose. *Brain Res.* 1986;377:286-291.
33. Yang CS, Chang CH, Tsai PJ, Chen WY, Tseng FG, Lo LW. Nanoparticle-based in vivo investigation on blood-brain barrier permeability following ischemia and reperfusion. *Anal Chem.* 2004;76:4465-4471.
34. Dobbin J, Crockard HA, Ross-Russell R. Transient blood-brain barrier permeability following profound temporary global ischaemia: an experimental study using 14C-AIB. *J Cereb Blood Flow Metab.* 1989;9:71-78.
35. Schirmacher A, Winters S, Fischer S, et al. Electromagnetic fields (1.8 GHz) increase the permeability to sucrose of the blood-brain barrier in vitro. *Bioelectromagnetics.* 2000;21:338-345.
36. Abbott NJ, Mendonca LL, Dolman DE. The blood-brain barrier in systemic lupus erythematosus. *Lupus.* 2003;12:908-915.
37. Hansson HA, Johansson BB. Induction of pinocytosis in cerebral vessels by acute hypertension and by hyperosmolar solutions. *J Neurosci Res.* 1980;5:183-190.
38. Nag S, Robertson DM, Dinsdale HB. Quantitative estimate of pinocytosis in experimental acute hypertension. *Acta Neuropathol (Berl).* 1979;46:107-116.
39. Neubauer C, Phelan AM, Kues H, Lange DG. Microwave irradiation of rats at 2.45 GHz activates pinocytotic-like uptake of tracer by capillary endothelial cells of cerebral cortex. *Bioelectromagnetics.* 1990;11:261-268.
40. Petito CK. Early and late mechanisms of increased vascular permeability following experimental cerebral infarction. *J Neuropathol Exp Neurol.* 1979;38:222-234.
41. Cipolla MJ, Crete R, Vitullo L, Rix RD. Transcellular transport as a mechanism of blood-brain barrier disruption during stroke. *Front Biosci.* 2004;9:777-785.
42. Nitsch C, Goping G, Klatzo I. Pathophysiological aspects of blood-brain barrier permeability in epileptic seizures. *Adv Exp Med Biol.* 1986;203:175-189.
43. Lossinsky AS, Vorbrodt AW, Wisniewski HM. Ultracytochemical studies of vesicular and canalicular transport structures in the injured mammalian blood-brain barrier. *Acta Neuropathol (Berl).* 1983;61:239-245.
44. Long DM. Capillary ultrastructure and the blood-brain barrier in human malignant brain tumors. *J Neurosurg.* 1970;32:127-144.
45. Lossinsky AS, Vorbrodt AW, Wisniewski HM. Characterization of endothelial cell transport in the developing mouse blood-brain barrier. *Dev Neurosci.* 1986;8:61-75.
46. Engelhardt B. Development of the blood-brain barrier. *Cell Tissue Res.* 2003;314:119-129.
47. Horton JC, Hedley-Whyte ET. Protein movement across the blood-brain barrier in hypervolemia. *Brain Res.* 1979;169:610-614.
48. Sharma HS, Dey PK. Impairment of blood-brain barrier (BBB) in rat by immobilization stress: role of serotonin (5-HT). *Indian J Physiol Pharmacol.* 1981;25:111-122.
49. Wells LA. Alteration of the blood-brain barrier system by hypothermia: critical time period vs. critical temperature. *Comp Biochem Physiol A.* 1973;44:293-296.
50. Albert EN, Kerns JM. Reversible microwave effects on the blood-brain barrier. *Brain Res.* 1981;230:153-164.
51. Lanse SB, Lee JC, Jacobs EA, Brody H. Changes in the permeability of the blood-brain barrier under hyperbaric conditions. *Aviat Space Environ Med.* 1978;49:890-894.
52. Sundstrom R, Muntzing K, Kalimo H, Sourander P. Changes in the integrity of the blood-brain barrier in suckling rats with low dose lead encephalopathy. *Acta Neuropathol (Berl).* 1985;68:1-9.
53. Kuwabara T, Yuasa T, Hidaka K, Igarashi H, Kaneko K, Miyatake T. The observation of blood-brain barrier of organic mercury poisoned rat: a Gd-DTPA enhanced magnetic resonance study. *No To Shinkei.* 1989;41:681-685.

54. Sarmento A, Albino-Teixeira A, Azevedo I. Amitriptyline-induced morphological alterations of the rat blood-brain barrier. *Eur J Pharmacol*. 1990;176:69-74.
55. Quagliarello VJ, Long WJ, Scheld WM. Morphologic alterations of the blood-brain barrier with experimental meningitis in the rat. Temporal sequence and role of encapsulation. *J Clin Invest*. 1986;77:1084-1095.
56. Tunkel AR, Rosser SW, Hansen EJ, Scheld WM. Blood-brain barrier alterations in bacterial meningitis: development of an in vitro model and observations on the effects of lipopolysaccharide. *In Vitro Cell Dev Biol*. 1991;27A:113-120.
57. Pozzilli C, Bernardi S, Mansi L, et al. Quantitative assessment of blood-brain barrier permeability in multiple sclerosis using 68-Ga-EDTA and positron emission tomography. *J Neurol Neurosurg Psychiatry*. 1988;51:1058-1062.
58. Wuerfel J, Bellmann-Strobl J, Brunecker P, et al. Changes in cerebral perfusion precede plaque formation in multiple sclerosis: a longitudinal perfusion MRI study. *Brain*. 2004;127:111-119.
59. Joo F, Zoltan OT, Csillik B, Foldi M. Increased permeability of the blood-brain barrier in lymphostatic encephalopathy. An electron microscopic study. *Angiologica*. 1969;6:318-325.
60. Pardridge WM, Crawford IL, Connor JD. Permeability changes in the blood-brain barrier induced by nortriptyline and chlorpromazine. *Toxicol Appl Pharmacol*. 1973;26:49-57.
61. Preston E, Foster DO. Evidence for pore-like opening of the blood-brain barrier following forebrain ischemia in rats. *Brain Res*. 1997;761:4-10.
62. Simpson IA, Appel NM, Hokari M, et al. Blood-brain barrier glucose transporter: effects of hypo- and hyperglycemia revisited. *J Neurochem*. 1999;72:238-247.
63. Pardridge WM, Triguero D, Farrell CR. Downregulation of blood-brain barrier glucose transporter in experimental diabetes. *Diabetes*. 1990;39:1040-1044.
64. Deane R, Du Yan S, Submamaryan RK, et al. RAGE mediates amyloid-beta peptide transport across the blood-brain barrier and accumulation in brain. *Nat Med*. 2003;9:907-913.
65. Deane R, Wu Z, Sagare A, et al. LRP/amyloid beta-peptide interaction mediates differential brain efflux of Abeta isoforms. *Neuron*. 2004;43:333-344.
66. Zlokovic BV. Neurovascular mechanisms of Alzheimer's neurodegeneration. *Trends Neurosci*. 2005;28:202-208.
67. Harata N, Iwasaki Y. The blood-brain barrier and selective vulnerability in experimental thiamine-deficiency encephalopathy in the mouse. *Metab Brain Dis*. 1996;11:55-69.
68. Gibson GE, Calingasan NY, Baker H, Gandy S, Sheu KF. Importance of vascular changes in selective neurodegeneration with thiamine deficiency. *Ann N Y Acad Sci*. 1997;826:516-519.
69. Banks WA. Leptin transport across the blood-brain barrier: implications for the cause and treatment of obesity. *Curr Pharm Des*. 2001;7:125-133.
70. Kastin AJ, Akerstrom V. Glucose and insulin increase the transport of leptin through the blood-brain barrier in normal mice but not in streptozotocin-diabetic mice. *Neuroendocrinology*. 2001;73:237-242.
71. Pan W, Akerstrom V, Zhang J, Pejovic V, Kastin AJ. Modulation of feeding-related peptide/protein signals by the blood-brain barrier. *J Neurochem*. 2004;90:455-461.
72. Kang YS, Terasaki T, Tsuji A. Dysfunction of choline transport system through blood-brain barrier in stroke-prone spontaneously hypertensive rats. *J Pharmacobiodyn*. 1990;13:10-19.
73. Kroll RA, Neuwelt EA. Outwitting the blood-brain barrier for therapeutic purposes: osmotic opening and other means. *Neurosurgery*. 1998;42:1083-1099.
74. Rapoport SI. Osmotic opening of the blood-brain barrier: principles, mechanism, and therapeutic applications. *Cell Mol Neurobiol*. 2000;20:217-230.
75. Alexander B, Li X, Benjamin IS, Segal MB, Sherwood R, Preston JE. A quantitative evaluation of the permeability of the blood brain barrier of portacaval shunted rats. *Metab Brain Dis*. 2000;15:93-103.
76. Emerich DF, Tracy MA, Ward KL, et al. Biocompatibility of poly (DL-lactide-co-glycolide) microspheres implanted into the brain. *Cell Transplant*. 1999;8:47-58.
77. Benoit JP, Faisant N, Venier-Julienne MC, Menei P. Development of microspheres for neurological disorders: from basics to clinical applications. *J Control Release*. 2000;65:285-296.

78. Chikhale EG, Ng KY, Burton PS, Borchardt RT. Hydrogen bonding potential as a determinant of the in vitro and in situ blood-brain barrier permeability of peptides. *Pharm Res.* 1994;11: 412-419.
79. Hansen DW, Jr, Stapelfeld A, Savage MA, et al. Systemic analgesic activity and delta-opioid selectivity in [2,6- dimethyl-Tyr1,D-Pen2,D-Pen5]enkephalin. *J Med Chem.* 1992;35:684-687.
80. Witt KA, Slate CA, Egleton RD, et al. Assessment of stereoselectivity of trimethylphenyla-lanine analogues of delta-opioid [D-Pen(2),D-Pen(5)]-enkephalin. *J Neurochem.* 2000;75:424-435.
81. Weber SJ, Greene DL, Sharma SD, et al. Distribution and analgesia of [3H][D-Pen2, D-Pen5]enkephalin and two halogenated analogs after intravenous administration. *J Pharmacol Exp Ther.* 1991;259:1109-1117.
82. Weber SJ, Abbruscato TJ, Brownson EA, et al. Assessment of an in vitro blood-brain barrier model using several [Met5]enkephalin opioid analogs. *J Pharmacol Exp Ther.* 1993;266: 1649-1655.
83. Gentry CL, Egleton RD, Gillespie T, et al. The effect of halogenation on blood-brain barrier permeability of a novel peptide drug. *Peptides.* 1999;20:1229-1238.
84. Abbruscato TJ, Williams SA, Misicka A, Lipkowski AW, Hruby VJ, Davis TP. Blood-to-central nervous system entry and stability of biphalin, a unique double-enkephalin analog, and its halogenated derivatives. *J Pharmacol Exp Ther.* 1996;276:1049-1057.
85. Bradbury AF, Smyth DG. Modification of the N- and C- termini of bioactive peptides: amida-tion and acetylaion. In: Fricker LD, ed. *Peptide Biosysthesis and Processing.* Boca Raton: CRC Press; 1991:231-242.
86. Bak A, Gudmundsson OS, Friis GJ, Siahaan TJ, Borchardt RT. Acyloxyalkoxy-based cyclic prodrugs of opioid peptides: evaluation of the chemical and enzymatic stability as well as their transport properties across Caco-2 cell monolayers. *Pharm Res.* 1999;16:24-29.
87. Uchiyama T, Kotani A, Tatsumi H, et al. Development of novel lipophilic derivatives of DADLE (leucine enkephalin analogue): intestinal permeability characateristics of DADLE derivatives in rats. *Pharm Res.* 2000;17:1461-1467.
88. Bundgaard H, Moss J. Prodrugs of peptides. 6. Bioreversible derivatives of thyrotropin- releas-ing hormone (TRH) with increased lipophilicity and resistance to cleavage by the TRH-specific serum enzyme. *Pharm Res.* 1990;7:885-892.
89. Yamamoto A. Improvement of intestinal absorption of peptide and protein drugs by chemical modification with fatty acids. *Nippon Rinsho.* 1998;56:601-607.
90. Asada H, Douen T, Waki M, et al. Absorption characteristics of chemically modified-insulin derivatives with various fatty acids in the small and large intestine. *J Pharm Sci.* 1995;84:682-687.
91. Audus KL, Chikhale PJ, Miller DW, Thompson SE, Borchardt RT. Brain uptake of drugs: The influence of chemical and biological factors. *Advance in Drug Research.* 1992;23:3-64.
92. Veber DF, Freidinger RM. The design of metabolically-stable peptide analogs. *Trends Neurosci.* 1985;8:392-396.
93. Bewley TA, Li CH. Evidence for tertiary structure in aqueous solutions of human beta- endor-phin as shown by difference absorption spectroscopy. *Biochemistry.* 1983;22:2671-2675.
94. Chaturvedi K, Shahrestanifar M, Howells RD. mu Opioid receptor: role for the amino terminus as a determinant of ligand binding affinity. *Brain Res Mol Brain Res.* 2000;76:64-72.
95. Roemer D, Pless J. Structure activity relationship of orally active enkephalin analogues as analgesics. *Life Sci.* 1979;24:621-624.
96. Uchiyama T, Kotani A, Kishida T, et al. Effects of various protease inhibitors on the stability and permeability of [D-Ala2,D-Leu5]enkephalin in the rat intestine: comparison with leucine enkephalin. *J Pharm Sci.* 1998;87:448-452.
97. Knipp GT, Vander Velde DG, Siahaan TJ, Borchardt RT. The effect of beta-turn structure on the passive diffusion of peptides across Caco-2 cell monolayers. *Pharm Res.* 1997;14:1332-1340.
98. Wang B, Nimkar K, Wang W, et al. Synthesis and evaluation of the physicochemical properties of esterase- sensitive cyclic prodrugs of opioid peptides using coumarinic acid and phenylpropionic acid linkers. *J Pept Res.* 1999;53:370-382.

99. Borchardt RT. Optimizing oral absorption of peptides using prodrug strategies. *J Control Release*. 1999;62:231-238.

100. Gudmundsson OS, Jois SD, Vander Velde DG, Siahaan TJ, Wang B, Borchardt RT. The effect of conformation on the membrane permeation of coumarinic acid- and phenylpropionic acid-based cyclic prodrugs of opioid peptides. *J Pept Res*. 1999;53:383-392.

101. Weber SJ, Greene DL, Hruby VJ, Yamamura HI, Porreca F, Davis TP. Whole body and brain distribution of [3H]cyclic [D-Pen2,D-Pen5] enkephalin after intraperitoneal, intravenous, oral and subcutaneous administration. *J Pharmacol Exp Ther*. 1992;263:1308-1316.

102. Mosberg HI, Hurst R, Hruby VJ, et al. Cyclic penicillamine containing enkephalin analogs display profound delta receptor selectivities. *Life Sci*. 1983;33:447-450.

103. Knapp RJ, Sharma SD, Toth G, et al. [D-Pen2,4'-125I-Phe4,D-Pen5]enkephalin: a selective high affinity radioligand for delta opioid receptors with exceptional specific activity. *J Pharmacol Exp Ther*. 1991;258:1077-1083.

104. Thomas SA, Abbruscato TJ, Hruby VJ, Davis TP. The entry of [D-penicillamine2,5]enkeph alin into the central nervous system: saturation kinetics and specificity. *J Pharmacol Exp Ther*. 1997;280:1235-1240.

105. Egleton RD, Davis TP. Transport of the delta-opioid receptor agonist [D-penicillamine2,5] enkephalin across the blood-brain barrier involves transcytosis1. *J Pharm Sci*. 1999;88:392-397.

106. Liao S, Alfaro-Lopez J, Shenderovich MD, et al. De novo design, synthesis, and biological activities of high-affinity and selective non-peptide agonists of the delta-opioid receptor. *J Med Chem*. 1998;41:4767-4776.

107. Brownson EA, Abbruscato TJ, Gillespie TJ, Hruby VJ, Davis TP. Effect of peptidases at the blood brain barrier on the permeability of enkephalin. *J Pharmacol Exp Ther*. 1994;270:675-680.

108. Lipkowski AW, Konecka AM, Sadowski B. Double enkephalins. *Pol J Pharmacol Pharm*. 1982;34:69-71.

109. Lipkowski AW, Konecka AM, Sroczynska I. Double-enkephalins–synthesis, activity on guinea-pig ileum, and analgesic effect. *Peptides*. 1982;3:697-700.

110. Romanowski M, Zhu X, Ramaswami V, et al. Interaction of a highly potent dimeric enkephalin analog, biphalin, with model membranes. *Biochim Biophys Acta*. 1997;1329:245-258.

111. Horan PJ, Mattia A, Bilsky EJ, et al. Antinociceptive profile of biphalin, a dimeric enkephalin analog. *J Pharmacol Exp Ther*. 1993;265:1446-1454.

112. Lis H, Sharon N. Protein glycosylation. Structural and functional aspects. *Eur J Biochem*. 1993;218:1-27.

113. Poduslo JF, Curran GL. Glycation increases the permeability of proteins across the blood-nerve and blood-brain barriers. *Brain Res Mol Brain Res*. 1994;23:157-162.

114. Jakas A, Horvat S. The effect of glycation on the chemical and enzymatic stability of the endogenous opioid peptide, leucine-enkephalin, and related fragments. *Bioorg Chem*. 2004;32:516-526.

115. Egleton RD, Mitchell SA, Huber JD, et al. Improved bioavailability to the brain of glycosylated Met-enkephalin analogs. *Brain Res*. 2000;881:37-46.

116. Powell MF, Jr, Stewart T, Jr, Otvos L, Jr, et al. Peptide stability in drug development. II. Effect of single amino acid substitution and glycosylation on peptide reactivity in human serum. *Pharm Res*. 1993;10:1268-1273.

117. Fisher JF, Harrison AW, Bundy GL, Wilkinson KF, Rush BD, Ruwart MJ. Peptide to glycopeptide: glycosylated oligopeptide renin inhibitors with attenuated in vivo clearance properties. *J Med Chem*. 1991;34:3140-3143.

118. Tomatis R, Marastoni M, Balboni G, et al. Synthesis and pharmacological activity of deltorphin and dermorphin- related glycopeptides. *J Med Chem*. 1997;40:2948-2952.

119. Negri L, Lattanzi R, Tabacco F, et al. Dermorphin and deltorphin glycosylated analogues: synthesis and antinociceptive activity after systemic administration. *J Med Chem*. 1999;42:400-404.

120. Polt R, Porreca F, Szabo LZ, et al. Glycopeptide enkephalin analogues produce analgesia in mice: evidence for penetration of the blood-brain barrier. *Proc Natl Acad Sci USA*. 1994;91:7114-7118.

121. Bilsky EJ, Egleton RD, Mitchell SA, et al. Enkephalin glycopeptide analogues produce analgesia with reduced dependence liability. *J Med Chem.* 2000;43:2586-2590.
122. Banks WA, Kastin AJ, Akerstrom V. HIV-1 protein gp120 crosses the blood-brain barrier: role of adsorptive endocytosis. *Life Sci.* 1997;61:PL119-PL125.
123. Broadwell RD, Balin BJ, Salcman M. Transcytotic pathway for blood-borne protein through the blood-brain barrier. *Proc Natl Acad Sci USA.* 1988;85:632-636.
124. Mackic JB, Stins M, McComb JG, et al. Human blood-brain barrier receptors for Alzheimer's amyloid-beta 1-40. Asymmetrical binding, endocytosis, and transcytosis at the apical side of brain microvascular endothelial cell monolayer. *J Clin Invest.* 1998;102:734-743.
125. Fillebeen C, Descamps L, Dehouck MP, et al. Receptor-mediated transcytosis of lactoferrin through the blood-brain barrier. *J Biol Chem.* 1999;274:7011-7017.
126. Palian MM, Boguslavsky VI, O'Brien DF, Polt R. Glycopeptide-membrane interactions: glycosyl enkephalin analogues adopt turn conformations by NMR and CD in amphipathic media. *J Am Chem Soc.* 2003;125:5823-5831.
127. Egleton RD, Bilsky EJ, Tollin G, et al. Biousian glycopeptides penetrate the blood-brain barrier. *Tetrahedron Asymmetry.* 2005;16:65-75.
128. Elmagbari NO, Egleton RD, Palian MM, et al. Antinociceptive structure-activity studies with enkephalin-based opioid glycopeptides. *J Pharmacol Exp Ther.* 2004;311:290-297.
129. Sargent DF, Schwyzer R. Membrane lipid phase as catalyst for peptide-receptor interactions. *Proc Natl Acad Sci USA.* 1986;83:5774-5778.
130. Begley DJ. The blood-brain barrier: principles for targeting peptides and drugs to the central nervous system. *J Pharm Pharmacol.* 1996;48:136-146.
131. Tsuji A, Tamai II. Carrier-mediated or specialized transport of drugs across the blood- brain barrier. *Adv Drug Deliv Rev.* 1999;36:277-290.
132. Wade LA, Katzman R. Synthetic amino acids and the nature of L-DOPA transport at the blood- brain barrier. *J Neurochem.* 1975;25:837-842.
133. Silbert BS, Lipkowski AW, Cepeda MS, Szyfelbein SK, Osgood PF, Carr DB. Analgesic activity of a novel bivalent opioid peptide compared to morphine via different routes of administration. *Agents Actions.* 1991;33:382-387.
134. Abbruscato TJ, Thomas SA, Hruby VJ, Davis TP. Brain and spinal cord distribution of biphalin: correlation with opioid receptor density and mechanism of CNS entry. *J Neurochem.* 1997;69:1236-1245.
135. Ghosh MK, Mitra AK. Enhanced delivery of 5-iodo-2'-deoxyuridine to the brain paren-chyma. *Pharm Res.* 1992;9:1173-1176.
136. Lambert DM, Geurts M, Scriba GK, Poupaert JH, Dumont P. Simple derivatives of amino acid neurotransmitters. Anticonvulsant evaluation of derived amides, carbamates and esters of glycine and beta-alanine. *J Pharm Belg.* 1995;50:194-203.
137. Greig NH, Stahle PL, Shetty HU, et al. High-performance liquid chromatographic analysis of chlorambucil tert.-butyl ester and its active metabolites chlorambucil and phenylacetic mustard in plasma and tissue. *J Chromatogr.* 1990;534:279-286.
138. Greene DL, Hau VS, Abbruscato TJ, et al. Enkephalin analog prodrugs: assessment of in vitro conversion, enzyme cleavage characterization and blood-brain barrier permeability. *J Pharmacol Exp Ther.* 1996;277:1366-1375.
139. Bodor N, Shek E, Higuchi T. Delivery of a quaternary pyridinium salt across the blood-brain barrier by its dihydropyridine derivative. *Science.* 1975;190:155-156.
140. Prokai L, Prokai-Tatrai K, Bodor N. Targeting drugs to the brain by redox chemical delivery systems. *Med Res Rev.* 2000;20:367-416
141. Bodor N, Buchwald P. Recent advances in the brain targeting of neuropharmaceuticals by chemical delivery systems. *Adv Drug Deliv Rev.* 1999;36:229-254.
142. Brewster ME, Estes KS, Bodor N. Improved delivery through biological membranes. 32. Synthesis and biological activity of brain-targeted delivery systems for various estradiol derivatives. *J Med Chem.* 1988;31:244-249.
143. Prokai-Tatrai K, Prokai L, Bodor N. Brain-targeted delivery of a leucine-enkephalin analogue by retrometabolic design. *J Med Chem.* 1996;39:4775-4782.

144. Zlokovic BV. Cerebrovascular permeability to peptides: manipulations of transport systems at the blood-brain barrier. *Pharm Res.* 1995;12:1395-1406.

145. Pardridge WM, Boado RJ, Kang YS. Vector-mediated delivery of a polyamide ("peptide") nucleic acid analogue through the blood-brain barrier in vivo. *Proc Natl Acad Sci USA.* 1995;92:5592-5596.

146. Pardridge WM. Vector-mediated drug delivery to the brain. *Adv Drug Deliv Rev.* 1999;36:299-321.

147. Bickel U, Yoshikawa T, Pardridge WM. Delivery of peptides and proteins through the blood-brain barrier. *Adv Drug Deliv Rev.* 2001;46:247-279.

148. Bickel U, Kang YS, Pardridge WM. In vivo cleavability of a disulfide-based chimeric opioid peptide in rat brain. *Bioconjug Chem.* 1995;6:211-218.

149. Pardridge WM, Triguero D, Buciak JL. Beta-endorphin chimeric peptides: transport through the blood-brain barrier in vivo and cleavage of disulfide linkage by brain. *Endocrinology.* 1990;126:977-984.

150. Vehaskari VM, Chang CT, Stevens JK, Robson AM. The effects of polycations on vascular permeability in the rat. A proposed role for charge sites. *J Clin Invest.* 1984;73:1053-1061.

151. Hardebo JE, Kahrstrom J. Endothelial negative surface charge areas and blood-brain barrier function. *Acta Physiol Scand.* 1985;125:495-499.

152. Deguchi Y, Miyakawa Y, Sakurada S, et al. Blood-brain barrier transport of a novel micro 1-specific opioid peptide, H-Tyr-D-Arg-Phe-beta-Ala-OH (TAPA). *J Neurochem.* 2003;84:1154-1161.

153. Deguchi Y, Naito Y, Ohtsuki S, et al. Blood-brain barrier permeability of novel [D-arg2]dermorphin (1–4) analogs: transport property is related to the slow onset of antinociceptive activity in the central nervous system. *J Pharmacol Exp Ther.* 2004;310:177-184.

154. Chakrabarti S, Sima AA. The presence of anionic sites in basement membranes of cerebral capillaries. *Microvasc Res.* 1990;39:123-127.

155. Terasaki T, Hirai K, Sato H, Kang YS, Tsuji A. Absorptive-mediated endocytosis of a dynorphin-like analgesic peptide, E-2078 into the blood-brain barrier. *J Pharmacol Exp Ther.* 1989;251:351-357.

156. Terasaki T, Takakuwa S, Saheki A, et al. Absorptive-mediated endocytosis of an adrenocorticotropic hormone (ACTH) analogue, ebiratide, into the blood-brain barrier: studies with monolayers of primary cultured bovine brain capillary endothelial cells. *Pharm Res.* 1992;9:529-534.

157. Shimura T, Tabata S, Terasaki T, Deguchi Y, Tsuji A. In-vivo blood-brain barrier transport of a novel adrenocorticotropic hormone analogue, ebiratide, demonstrated by brain microdialysis and capillary depletion methods. *J Pharm Pharmacol.* 1992;44:583-588.

158. Yu J, Butelman ER, Woods JH, Chait BT, Kreek MJ. Dynorphin A (1–8) analog, E-2078, crosses the blood-brain barrier in rhesus monkeys. *J Pharmacol Exp Ther.* 1997;282:633-638.

159. Ukai M, Kobayashi T, Mori K, Shinkai N, Sasaki Y, Kameyama T. Attenuation of memory with Tyr-D-Arg-Phe-beta-Ala-NH2, a novel dermorphin analog with high affinity for mu-opioid receptors. *Eur J Pharmacol.* 1995;287:245-249.

160. Paakkari P, Paakkari I, Vonhof S, Feuerstein G, Siren AL. Dermorphin analog Tyr-D-Arg2-Phe-sarcosine-induced opioid analgesia and respiratory stimulation: the role of mu 1-receptors? *J Pharmacol Exp Ther.* 1993;266:544-550.

161. Kumagai AK, Eisenberg JB, Pardridge WM. Absorptive-mediated endocytosis of cationized albumin and a beta- endorphin-cationized albumin chimeric peptide by isolated brain capillaries. Model system of blood-brain barrier transport. *J Biol Chem.* 1987;262:15214-15219.

162. Boado RJ, Pardridge WM. Complete inactivation of target mRNA by biotinylated antisense oligodeoxynucleotide-avidin conjugates. *Bioconjug Chem.* 1994;5:406-410.

163. Adler SG, Wang H, Ward HJ, Cohen AH, Border WA. Electrical charge. Its role in the pathogenesis and prevention of experimental membranous nephropathy in the rabbit. *J Clin Invest.* 1983;71:487-499.

164. Huang JT, Mannik M, Gleisner J. In situ formation of immune complexes in the choroid plexus of rats by sequential injection of a cationized antigen and unaltered antibodies. *J Neuropathol Exp Neurol.* 1984;43:489-499.

165. Nagy Z, Peters H, Huttner I. Charge-related alterations of the cerebral endothelium. *Lab Invest.* 1983;49:662-671.
166. Bergmann P, Kacenelenbogen R, Vizet A. Plasma clearance, tissue distribution and catabolism of cationized albumins with increasing isoelectric points in the rat. *Clin Sci (Lond).* 1984;67:35-43.
167. Pardridge WM, Triguero D, Buciak J. Transport of histone through the blood-brain barrier. *J Pharmacol Exp Ther.* 1989;251:821-826.
168. Mumtaz S, Bachhawat BK. Conjugation of proteins and enzymes with hydrophilic polymers and their applications. *Indian J Biochem Biophys.* 1991;28:346-351.
169. Francis GE, Fisher D, Delgado C, Malik F, Gardiner A, Neale D. PEGylation of cytokines and other therapeutic proteins and peptides: the importance of biological optimisation of coupling techniques. *Int J Hematol.* 1998;68:1-18.
170. So T, Ito HO, Hirata M, Ueda T, Imoto T. Extended blood half-life of monomethoxypolyethylene glycol-conjugated hen lysozyme is a key parameter controlling immunological tolerogenicity. *Cell Mol Life Sci.* 1999;55:1187-1194.
171. Reddy KR. Controlled-release, pegylation, liposomal formulations: new mechanisms in the delivery of injectable drugs. *Ann Pharmacother.* 2000;34:915-923.
172. Tsutsumi Y, Onda M, Nagata S, Lee B, Kreitman RJ, Pastan I. Site-specific chemical modification with polyethylene glycol of recombinant immunotoxin anti-Tac(Fv)-PE38 (LMB-2) improves antitumor activity and reduces animal toxicity and immunogenicity. *Proc Natl Acad Sci USA.* 2000;97:8548-8553.
173. Duncan R. Drug-polymer conjugates: potential for improved chemotherapy. *Anticancer Drugs.* 1992;3:175-210.
174. Mu Y, Kamada H, Kaneda Y, et al. Bioconjugation of laminin peptide YIGSR with poly(styrene co-maleic acid) increases its antimetastatic effect on lung metastasis of B16-BL6 melanoma cells. *Biochem Biophys Res Commun.* 1999;255:75-79.
175. Veronese FM. Peptide and protein PEGylation: a review of problems and solutions. *Biomaterials.* 2001;22:405-417.
176. Witt KA, Huber JD, Egleton RD, et al. Pharmacodynamic and pharmacokinetic characterization of poly(ethylene glycol) conjugation to met-enkephalin analog [D-Pen2, D-Pen5]-enkephalin (DPDPE). *J Pharmacol Exp Ther.* 2001;298:848-856.
177. Chen C, Pollack GM. Altered disposition and antinociception of [D-penicillamine(2,5)] enkephalin in mdr1a-gene-deficient mice. *J Pharmacol Exp Ther.* 1998;287:545-552.
178. Kreuter J, Alyautdin RN, Kharkevich DA, Ivanov AA. Passage of peptides through the blood-brain barrier with colloidal polymer particles (nanoparticles). *Brain Res.* 1995;674:171-174.
179. Kreuter J. Nanoparticulate systems for brain delivery of drugs. *Adv Drug Deliv Rev.* 2001;47:65-81.
180. Woodcock DM, Linsenmeyer ME, Chojnowski G, et al. Reversal of multidrug resistance by surfactants. *Br J Cancer.* 1992;66:62-68.
181. Reddy KR. Controlled-release, pegylation, liposomal formulations: new mechanisms in the delivery of injectable drugs. *Ann Pharmacother.* 2000;34:915-923.
182. Batrakova EV, Miller DW, Li S, Alakhov VY, Kabanov AV, Elmquist WF. Pluronic P85 enhances the delivery of digoxin to the brain: in vitro and in vivo studies. *J Pharmacol Exp Ther.* 2001;296:551-557.
183. Witt KA, Huber JD, Egleton RD, Davis TP. Pluronic p85 block copolymer enhances opioid peptide analgesia. *J Pharmacol Exp Ther.* 2002;303:760-767.
184. Batrakova EV, Li S, Li Y, Alakhov VY, Kabanov AV. Effect of pluronic P85 on ATPase activity of drug efflux transporters. *Pharm Res.* 2004;21:2226-2233.

Chapter 31
Cell-Permeable, Mitochondrial-Targeted, Peptide Antioxidants

Hazel H. Szeto[1]

Abstract Cellular oxidative injury has been implicated in aging and a wide array of clinical disorders including ischemia-reperfusion injury; neurodegenerative diseases; diabetes; inflammatory diseases such as atherosclerosis, arthritis, and hepatitis; and drug-induced toxicity. However, available antioxidants have not proven to be particularly effective against many of these disorders. A possibility is that some of the antioxidants do not reach the relevant sites of free radical generation, especially if mitochondria are the primary source of reactive oxygen species (ROS). The SS (Szeto-Schiller) peptide antioxidants represent a novel approach with targeted delivery of antioxidants to the inner mitochondrial membrane. The structural motif of these SS peptides centers on alternating aromatic residues and basic amino acids (aromatic-cationic peptides). These SS peptides can scavenge hydrogen peroxide and peroxynitrite and inhibit lipid peroxidation. Their antioxidant action can be attributed to the tyrosine or dimethyltyrosine residue. By reducing mitochondrial ROS, these peptides inhibit mitochondrial permeability transition and cytochrome c release, thus preventing oxidant-induced cell death. Because these peptides concentrate >1000-fold in the inner mitochondrial membrane, they prevent oxidative cell death with EC_{50} in the nM range. Preclinical studies support their potential use for ischemia-reperfusion injury and neurodegenerative disorders. Although peptides have often been considered to be poor drug candidates, these small peptides have excellent "druggable" properties, making them promising agents for many diseases with unmet needs.

Keywords reactive oxygen species, free radicals, mitochondrial permeability transition, apoptosis, ischemia-reperfusion injury

[1] Department of Pharmacology, Joan and Sanford I. Weill Medical College of Cornell University, New York, NY

Corresponding Author: Hazel H. Szeto, Department of Pharmacology, Weill Medical College of Cornell University, 1300 York Avenue, New York, NY, 10021. Tel: (212) 746-6232; Fax: (212) 746-8835; E-mail: hhszeto@med.cornell.edu

R.S. Rapaka and W. Sadée (eds.), *Drug Addiction.*
© American Association of Pharmaceutical Scientists 2008

Introduction

Reactive oxygen species (ROS) can damage cells by oxidizing membrane phospho lipids, proteins, and nucleic acids. These damaging effects of ROS are normally kept under control by endogenous antioxidant systems including glutathione, ascorbic acid, and enzymes such as superoxide dismutase (SOD), glutathione peroxidase, and catalase. Oxidative stress occurs when antioxidant systems are overwhelmed by ROS, and the resulting oxidative damage can lead to cell death.

Sources of ROS

NADPH oxidase on the plasma membrane, and cytoplasmic enzymes such as xanthine oxidase and nitric oxide synthase, can all generate superoxide anion ($O_2^{\bullet-}$). In addition, mitochondria are a major source of ROS[1] (see Fig. 31.1). Superoxide anion is produced by the electron transport chain on the inner mitochondrial membrane, and the rate of production is dependent on mitochondrial potential. In the presence of mitochondrial SOD, $O_2^{\bullet-}$ can be converted to hydrogen peroxide (H_2O_2), which can then diffuse out of mitochondria into the cytoplasm. In the presence of high iron concentrations, H_2O_2 can form the highly reactive hydroxyl radical ($OH^{\bullet}$) via the Fenton reaction. $O_2^{\bullet-}$ can also react with nitric oxide to form the highly reactive peroxynitrite ($ONOO^-$).

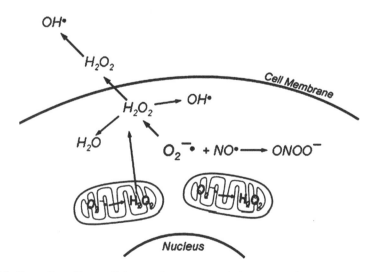

Fig. 31.1 Formation of intracellular reactive oxygen and nitrogen species.

Consequences of Reactive Oxygen and Reactive Nitrogen Species

Reactive oxygen and reactive nitrogen species can cause damage to all cellular macromolecules, including nucleic acids, proteins, carbohydrates, and lipids. Membrane lipids are major targets of ROS, and lipid peroxidation may lead to membrane dysfunction and alterations in cell permeability.

Mitochondria are particularly vulnerable to oxidative damage because they are constantly exposed to high levels of ROS (Fig. 31.2). Mitochondrial DNA has been shown to undergo oxidative damage. In addition to lipid peroxidation, protein oxidation and nitration results in altered function of many metabolic enzymes in the mitochondrial matrix as well as those comprising the electron transport chain. A particularly relevant protein that loses function upon oxidation is SOD, which would further compromise antioxidant capacity and lead to further oxidative stress.

Increasing evidence suggests that ROS play a key role in promoting cytochrome c release from mitochondria.[2] Cytochrome c is normally bound to the inner mitochondrial membrane by association with cardiolipin.[3] Peroxidation of cardiolipin leads to dissociation of cytochrome c and its release through the outer mitochondrial membrane into the cytosol.[4] The mechanism by which cytochrome c is released through the outer membrane is not clear. One mechanism may involve

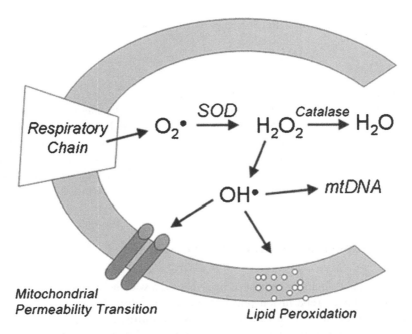

Fig. 31.2 Mitochondrial damage caused by reactive oxygen and nitrogen species. Free radicals generated by the electron transport chain can result in oxidative damage to mitochondrial DNA and proteins, lipid peroxidation, and opening of the mitochondrial permeability transition pore.

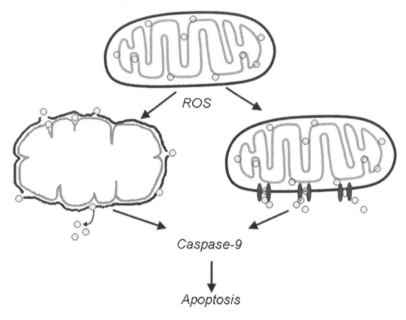

Fig. 31.3 Cytochrome c release from mitochondria. Cytochrome c (O) is normally associated with cardiolipin on the inner mitochondrial membrane. Cytochrome c is dissociated upon oxidation of cardiolipin and is believed to be released out of mitochondria either by mitochondrial permeability transition resulting in mitochondrial swelling and rupture of the outer membrane, or by channels formed by oligomerization of Bax. In the cytoplasm, cytochrome c activates caspase-9 and promotes apoptosis.

mitochondrial permeability transition (MPT), with swelling of the mitochondrial matrix and rupture of the outer membrane (Figure 3). ROS may promote MPT by causing oxidation of thiol groups on the adenine nucleotide translocator, which is believed to form part of the MPT pore.[5] Cytochrome c release may also occur via MPT-independent mechanisms and may involve an oligomeric form of Bax[6] (Fig. 31.3). Cytochrome c in the cytoplasm triggers the activation of caspase-9, which triggers the caspase cascade and ultimately leads to apoptosis.[7,8]

Diseases Associated With Oxidative Stress

Cellular oxidative injury is implicated in aging and a wide array of clinical disorders including ischemia-reperfusion injury, neurodegenerative diseases, diabetes, and inflammatory diseases such as atherosclerosis, arthritis, and hepatitis. Oxidative damage is also believed to play a role in drug-induced toxicity, including acetaminophen hepatotoxicity, methamphetamine neurotoxicity, cocaine hepatotoxicity, alcoholic fatty liver, and anthracycline toxicity.

Search for Effective Antioxidants

Large doses of antioxidants have been found to be effective in many animal models of diseases associated with oxidative damage. However, clinical trials with antioxidants such as vitamin E or recombinant human SOD have generally failed to demonstrate significant benefits, leading to the proposed antioxidant paradox.[9-11] One possible reason is that many of the antioxidants can also have prooxidant activity besides antioxidant activity, especially in the presence of transitional metals.[12] Another possibility is that some of the antioxidants do not reach the relevant sites of free radical generation. Large proteins such as SOD do not penetrate cell membranes and are therefore ineffective against intracellular ROS. Antioxidants such as vitamin E and coenzyme Q are very lipophilic and tend to be retained in cell membranes. The ideal antioxidant should be cell-permeable and be able to target mitochondria where they can protect mitochondria against oxidative damage. The conjugation of a triphenylalkylphosphonium cation to lipophilic antioxidants such as coenzyme Q (MitoQ) and vitamin E has been used to promote their delivery into mitochondria by taking advantage of the potential gradient across the inner mitochondrial membrane.[13] However, high concentrations of MitoQ have been shown to cause mitochondrial depolarization.[14,15]

Discovery of Cell-permeable, Mitochondria-targeted Peptide Antioxidants

A series of small, cell-permeable, mitochondria-targeted, antioxidant peptides that can protect mitochondria from oxidative damage was recently reported[16] (see Table 31.1).

Design for Free Radical Scavenging Properties

The structural motif of these SS (Szeto-Schiller) peptides centers on alternating aromatic residues and basic amino acids (aromatic-cationic peptides).[16] These SS peptides can scavenge H_2O_2 and $ONOO^-$ and inhibit lipid peroxidation in vitro as demonstrated by the inhibition of linoleic acid oxidation and low-density lipoprotein (LDL) oxidation (Fig. 31.4). Their antioxidant action can be attributed to the tyrosine, or dimethyltyrosine (Dmt), residue. Tyrosine can scavenge oxyradicals forming

Table 31.1 Cell-permeable, Mitochondria-targeted Peptides

SS-01	H-Tyr-D-Arg-Phe-Lys-NH₂
SS-02	H-Dmt-D-Arg-Phe-Lys-NH₂
SS-31	H-D-Arg-Dmt-Lys-Phe-NH₂
SS-20	H-Phe-D-Arg-Phe-Lys-NH₂

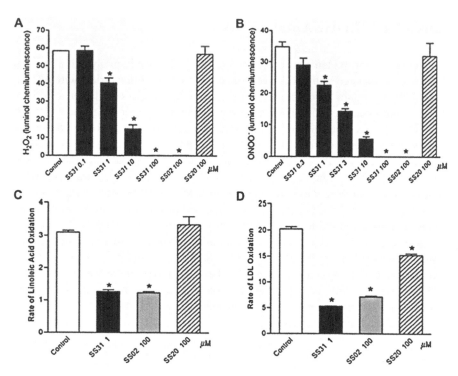

Fig. 31.4 Antioxidant properties of SS peptides. (A) Scavenging of H$_2$O$_2$ by SS-31 and SS-02 but not SS-20. H$_2$O$_2$ was measured by luminol chemiluminescence; (B) Scavenging of ONOO$^-$ by SS-31 and SS-02 but not SS-20. ONOO$^-$ was measured by luminol chemiluminescence; (C) Linoleic acid peroxidation was inhibited by SS-31 and SS-02 but not SS-20. Linoleic acid peroxidation was initiated by 2,2'-azobis(2-amidinopropane) and detected by formation of conjugated dienes measured by absorbance at 234 nm; and (D) LDL oxidation was inhibited by SS-31 and SS-02 but not SS-20. Human LDL was oxidized by CuSO$_4$, and the formation of conjugated dienes was measured by absorbance at 234 nm.

relatively unreactive tyrosyl radicals, which can be followed by radical-radical coupling to give dityrosine, or react with superoxide to form tyrosine hydroperoxide.[17] Dimethyltyrosine is more effective than tyrosine in scavenging of ROS. The specific location of the tyrosine or dimethyltyrosine residue is not important as SS-31 was found to be as effective as SS-02 in scavenging H$_2$O$_2$ and inhibiting LDL oxidation. However, replacement of Dmt with phenylalanine in SS-02 (SS-20) eliminated the scavenging ability (Fig. 31.4).

Method of Cell Uptake

These small peptides contain an amino acid sequence that allows them to freely penetrate cells despite carrying a 3+ net charge at physiologic pH.[18] These aromatic-cationic peptides are taken up into cells in an energy-independent nonsaturable manner. Uptake studies with [³H]SS-02 showed rapid uptake with steady-state achieved in less than 30 minutes.[16] This finding suggests that these peptides can freely pass through the plasma membrane in both directions. Unlike the larger cationic peptides such as *Tat* peptide,[19,20] there is no evidence of vesicular localization that would result from endocytosis.

Method of Mitochondria Targeting

These SS peptides have a sequence motif that targets them to mitochondria. Figure 5 shows the internalization and targeting of a fluorescent peptide analog (Dmt-D-Arg-Phe-atnDap-NH₂; atn = β-anthraniloyl-L-α,β-diaminopropionic acid) to mitochondria in living cells. The confocal images show that the pattern of localization of the fluorescent peptide analog is identical to that of Mitotracker TMRM, a fluorescent dye that is taken up into mitochondria in a potential-driven manner. Incubation of isolated mitochondria with [³H]SS-02 confirmed that it is taken up and concentrated >1000-fold in mitochondria.[16] Contrary to MitoQ, the uptake of these aromatic-cationic peptides into mitochondria is not dependent on mitochondrial potential, and they are localized to the inner mitochondrial membrane rather than in the matrix (see schematic in Fig. 31.5).

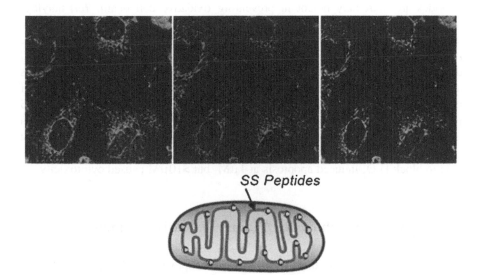

Fig. 31.5 Internalization and targeting of fluorescent SS peptide to mitochondria in living cells. Caco-2 cells were incubated with Dmt-D-Arg-Phe-atnDap-NH₂ (blue fluorescence) and TMRM (red fluorescence) at 37°C for 30 minutes and imaged by confocal laser scanning fluorescence microscopy.[16] Overlay of the 2 images shows colocalization of the fluorescent peptide and TMRM, suggesting mitochondrial targeting. (*See* also Color Insert).

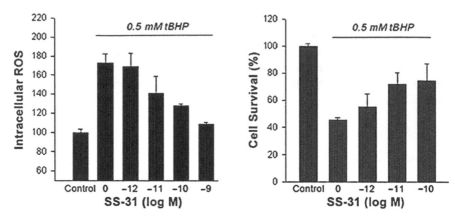

Fig. 31.6 Dose-dependent SS-31 reduced intracellular ROS and prevented cell death caused by *t*BHP. Neuroblastoma N₂A cells were treated with 0.5 mM *t*BHP for 40 minutes. Intracellular ROS was measured by 5-(and 6)-carboxy-2'7'-dichlorohydrofluorescein diacetate, and cell death was measured by the MTT assay.

Inhibition of Oxidative Cell Death

By targeting and partitioning in the inner mitochondrial membrane, these SS peptides are extremely potent in preventing oxidative cell death. *Tert*-butylhydroperoxide (*t*BHP) is a membrane-permeant oxidant compound that can induce cell death via apoptosis or necrosis.[21,22] *t*BHP is cell permeable and can generate *t*-butoxyl radicals via the Fenton reaction, resulting in lipid peroxidation and depletion of intracellular glutathione, followed by modification of protein thiols and loss of cell viability. Treatment of cells with *t*BHP causes rapid oxidation of pyridine nucleotides and increased ROS production in mitochondria.[23,24] The SS peptides are very potent in reducing intracellular ROS and preventing cell death after *t*BHP treatment, with EC$_{50}$ in the nM range (Fig. 31.6).[16] In contrast, most antioxidants require at least 100 μM to reduce oxidative cell death.[24-26] MitoQ was able to block H$_2$O$_2$-induced apoptosis at 1 μM, but >10 μM caused cytotoxicity.[15]

Protection of Mitochondria Against Oxidative Damage

Recent evidence suggest that *t*BHP-induced apoptosis is triggered by MPT.[22] Peroxidation of cardiolipin induces the dissociation of cytochrome *c* from the inner mitochondrial membrane and subsequent release into the cytoplasm as a result of the opening of the MPT pore. Calcium overload can also lead to increase in mitochondrial ROS and opening of the MPT pore. By reducing mitochondrial ROS, the scavenging SS peptides (SS-02 and SS-31) were able to inhibit MPT, prevent mitochondrial swelling, and reduce cytochrome *c* release in response to Ca^{2+} overload

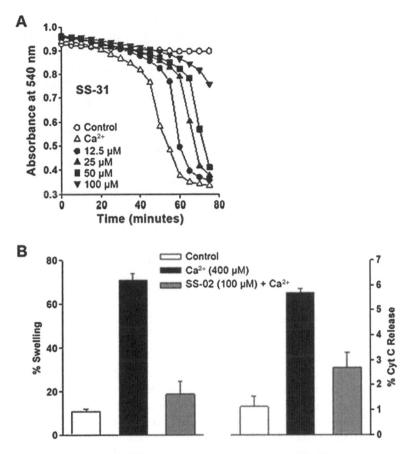

Fig. 31.7 SS peptides inhibited mitochondrial swelling (A) and prevented cytochrome c release (B) from isolated mitochondria subjected to calcium overload.[16] Isolated mouse liver mitochondria were exposed to 50 μM Ca^{2+} and swelling measured by absorbance at 540 nm. The amount of cytochrome c released was expressed as percentage of total cytochrome c in mitochondria.

(Fig. 31.7). On the other hand, the nonscavenging peptide, SS-20, did not prevent mitochondrial swelling at the same concentrations. These results support the proposal that ROS may potentiate MPT via oxidation of the adenine nucleotide translocator. The ability of SS peptides to prevent MPT will minimize MPT-induced ROS accumulation and further reduce oxidative damage on mitochondria.[27]

Protection Against Ischemia-Reperfusion Injury

ROS and mitochondrial permeability transition are thought to play a major role in ischemia-reperfusion injury.[28] In animal models, overexpression of SOD is associated with protection against reperfusion injury, while SOD knockout animals are more susceptible to reperfusion injury. However, although oxygen radical scavengers were found to be effective in several ex-vivo heart studies or animal studies, results from clinical trials have generally been disappointing. The efficacy of scavengers in preclinical studies may be attributed to their administration prior to ischemia in most studies rather than upon reperfusion as is usually done in patients with acute myocardial infarction or stroke. In addition, recombinant SOD is a large protein molecule that is unlikely to distribute across the endothelium and penetrate cells.

Small molecule SOD mimetics were found to be effective in canine studies but were associated with acute hypotension, and clinical trials of efficacy in humans have not been reported.

Both SS-02 and SS-31 were able to prevent myocardial stunning when administered upon reperfusion in the ex-vivo guinea pig heart.[16,29] In contrast, SS-20, which has no scavenging ability, was unable to prevent myocardial stunning when administered upon reperfusion. The ability of SS-02 to prevent myocardial stunning has been confirmed in rats in vivo.[30] These findings with the SS peptides support the proposal that ROS play a major role in reperfusion-induced myocardial stunning.

Pharmacokinetic Properties of SS Peptides

These antioxidant peptides are highly "druggable." They are small and easy to synthesize, readily soluble in water, and resistant to peptidase degradation. The presence of a D-amino acid in either the first or second position renders them resistant against aminopeptidase activity, and amidation of the C-terminus reduces hydrolysis from the C-terminus. Despite carrying 3+ net charge at physiological pH, these peptides have been shown to readily penetrate cell membranes of a variety of cell types.[18] Their cellular uptake appears to be concentration-dependent, nonsaturable, and not requiring energy.[18] In addition to cell uptake, SS-02 was shown to readily penetrate a monolayer of intestinal epithelial cells in both apical-basolateral and basolateral-apical directions. Furthermore, analgesia studies in mice suggest that SS-02 readily penetrates the blood-brain-barrier after subcutaneous administration.[31] This has also been confirmed by the detection of [^{3}H]SS-02 in mouse brain within 5 minutes after intravenous injection (Andrew Gifford, unpublished results, 2005). Finally, pharmacokinetic studies have revealed relatively long elimination half-life for SS-02 in sheep and rats.[32]

Conclusions

Oxidative damage is believed to be associated with aging and numerous degenerative diseases. However, available antioxidants have not proven to be particularly effective against many of these disorders. A possibility is that some of the antioxidants do not reach the relevant sites of free radical generation, especially if mitochondria are the primary source of ROS generation. The SS peptides represent a novel approach with targeted delivery of antioxidants to mitochondria. By protecting mitochondrial viability, these peptides can also minimize further ROS generation. By selectively concentrating in mitochondria, these peptides are extraordinarily potent in protecting against oxidative cell death. Preclinical studies support their potential use for ischemia-reperfusion injury and neurodegenerative disorders. Although peptides have often been considered to be poor drug candidates, these small peptides have excellent "druggable" properties, making them promising agents for many diseases with unmet needs.

Acknowledgments The SS peptides were developed in collaboration with Dr Peter W. Schiller of the Clinical Research Institute of Montreal, Montreal, Quebec, Canada. The majority of the work mentioned in this article was performed by Drs Kesheng Zhao, Guomin Zhao, Dunli Wu, and Yi Soong. The work was supported by the National Institute on Drug Abuse (NIDA, National Institutes of Health, Bethesda, MD, PO1 DA08924). Special thanks to Dr Dominic Desiderio (Charles B. Stout Mass Spectrometry Lab, University of Tennessee, Memphis, TN) and Dr Andrew Gifford (Brookhaven National Labs, Upton, NY) for their contributions to the pharmacokinetic studies. Dr Mun Hong (Department of Medicine, Weill Medical College of Cornell University) performed the in vivo studies with SS-02 in myocardial ischemia-reperfusion.

References

1. Turrens JF. Superoxide production by the mitochondrial respiratory chain. *Biosci Rep.* 1997;17:3-8.
2. Petrosillo G, Ruggiero FM, Pistolese M, Paradies G. Reactive oxygen species generated from the mitochondrial electron transport chain induce cytochrome c dissociation from beef-heart submitochondrial particles via cardiolipin peroxidation: possible role in the apoptosis. *FEBS Lett.* 2001;509:435-438.
3. Petrosillo G, Ruggiero FM, Paradies G. Role of reactive oxygen species and cardiolipin in the release of cytochrome c from mitochondria. *FASEB J.* 2003;17:2202-2208.
4. Shidoji Y, Hayashi K, Komura S, Ohishi N, Yagi K. Loss of molecular interaction between cytochrome c and cardiolipin due to lipid peroxidation. *Biochem Biophys Res Commun.* 1999;264:343-347.
5. Vieira HL, Belzacq AS, Haouzi D, et al. The adenine nucleotide translocator: a target of nitric oxide, peroxynitrite, and 4-hydroxynonenal. *Oncogene.* 2001;20:4305-4316.
6. Ott M, Robertson JD, Gogvadze V, Zhivotovsky B, Orrenius S. Cytochrome c release from mitochondria proceeds by a two-step process. *Proc Natl Acad Sci USA.* 2002;99:1259-1263.
7. Liu X, Kim CN, Yang J, Jemmerson R, Wang X. Induction of apoptotic program in cell-free extracts: requirement for dATP and cytochrome c. *Cell.* 1996;86:147-157.
8. Li P, Nijhawan D, Budihardjo I, et al. Cytochrome c and dATP-dependent formation of Apaf-1/caspase-9 complex initiates an apoptotic protease cascade. *Cell.* 1997;91:479-489.
9. Halliwell B. The antioxidant paradox. *Lancet.* 2000;355:1179-1180.
10. Patterson C, Madamanchi NR, Runge MS. The oxidative paradox: another piece in the puzzle. *Circ Res.* 2000;87:1074-1076.
11. Flaherty JT, Pitt B, Gruber JW, et al. Recombinant human superoxide dismutase (h-SOD) fails to improve recovery of ventricular function in patients undergoing coronary angioplasty for acute myocardial infarction. *Circulation.* 1994;89:1982-1991.
12. Maiorino M, Zamburlini A, Roveri A, Ursini F. Prooxidant role of vitamin E in copper induced lipid peroxidation. *FEBS Lett.* 1993;330:174-176.

13. Murphy MP, Smith RA. Drug delivery to mitochondria: the key to mitochondrial medicine. *Adv Drug Deliv Rev*. 2000;41:235-250.

14. Smith RA, Porteous CM, Coulter CV, Murphy MP. Selective targeting of an antioxidant to mitochondria. *Eur J Biochem*. 1999;263:709-716.

15. Kelso GF, Porteous CM, Coulter CV, et al. Selective targeting of a redox-active ubiquinone to mitochondria within cells: antioxidant and antiapoptotic properties. *J Biol Chem*. 2001;276:4588-4596.

16. Zhao K, Zhao GM, Wu D, et al. Cell-permeable peptide antioxidants targeted to inner mitochondrial membrane inhibit mitochondrial swelling, oxidative cell death, and reperfusion injury. *J Biol Chem*. 2004;279:34682-34690.

17. Winterbourn CC, Parsons-Mair HN, Gebicki S, Gebicki JM, Davies MJ. Requirements for superoxide-dependent tyrosine hydroperoxide formation in peptides. *Biochem J*. 2004;381: 241-248.

18. Zhao K, Luo G, Zhao GM, Schiller PW, Szeto HH. Transcellular transport of a highly polar 3+ net charge opioid tetrapeptide. *J Pharmacol Exp Ther*. 2003;304:425-432.

19. Drin G, Cottin S, Blanc E, Rees AR, Temsamani J. Studies on the internalization mechanism of cationic cell-penetrating peptides. *J Biol Chem*. 2003;278:31192-31201.

20. Derossi D, Calvet S, Trembleau A, Brunissen A, Chassaing G, Prochiantz A. Cell internalization of the third helix of the Antennapedia homeodomain is receptor-independent. *J Biol Chem*. 1996;271:18188-18193.

21. Haidara K, Morel I, Abalea V, Gascon BM, Denizeau F. Mechanism of tert-butylhydroperoxide-induced apoptosis in rat hepatocytes: involvement of mitochondria and endoplasmic reticulum. *Biochim Biophys Acta*. 2002;1542:173-185.

22. Piret JP, Arnould T, Fuks B, Chatelain P, Remacle J, Michiels C. Mitochondria permeability transition-dependent tert-butyl hydroperoxide-induced apoptosis in hepatoma HepG2 cells. *Biochem Pharmacol*. 2004;67:611-620.

23. Byrne AM, Lemasters JJ, Nieminen AL. Contribution of increased mitochondrial free Ca2+ to the mitochondrial permeability transition induced by tert-butylhydroperoxide in rat hepatocytes. *Hepatology*. 1999;29:1523-1531.

24. Nieminen AL, Byrne AM, Herman B, Lemasters JJ. Mitochondrial permeability transition in hepatocytes induced by t-BuOOH: NAD(P)H and reactive oxygen species. *Am J Physiol*. 1997;272:C1286-C1294.

25. Jauslin ML, Meier T, Smith RA, Murphy MP. Mitochondria-targeted antioxidants protect Friedreich Ataxia fibroblasts from endogenous oxidative stress more effectively than untargeted antioxidants. *FASEB J*. 2003;17:1972-1974.

26. Pias EK, Ekshyyan OY, Rhoads CA, Fuseler J, Harrison L, Aw TY. Differential effects of superoxide dismutase isoform expression on hydroperoxide-induced apoptosis in PC-12 cells. *J Biol Chem*. 2003;278:13294-13301.

27. Batandier C, Leverve X, Fontaine E. Opening of the mitochondrial permeability transition pore induces reactive oxygen species production at the level of the respiratory chain complex I. *J Biol Chem*. 2004;279:17197-17204.

28. Przyklenk K. Pharmacologic treatment of the stunned myocardium: the concepts and the challenges. *Coron Artery Dis*. 2001;12:363-369.

29. Wu D, Soong Y, Zhao GM, Szeto HH. A highly potent peptide analgesic that protects against ischemia- reperfusion-induced myocardial stunning. *Am J Physiol Heart Circ Physiol*. 2002;283:H783-H791.

30. Song W, Shin J, Lee J, et al. A potent opiate agonist protects against myocardial stunning during myocardial ischemia and reperfusion in rats. *Coron Artery Dis*. 2005;16:407-410.

31. Zhao GM, Wu D, Soong Y, et al. Profound spinal tolerance after repeated exposure to a highly selective mu-opioid peptide agonist: role of delta-opioid receptors. *J Pharmacol Exp Ther*. 2002;302:188-196.

32. Szeto HH, Lovelace JL, Fridland G, et al. In vivo pharmacokinetics of selective mu-opioid peptide agonists. *J Pharmacol Exp Ther*. 2001;298:57-61.

Chapter 32
Targeting Opioid Receptor Heterodimers: Strategies for Screening and Drug Development

Achla Gupta,[1] Fabien M. Décaillot,[1] and Lakshmi A. Devi[1]

Abstract G-protein-coupled receptors are a major target for the development of new marketable drugs. A growing number of studies have shown that these receptors could bind to their ligands, signal, and be internalized as dimers. Most of the evidence comes from in vitro studies, but recent studies using animal models support an important role for dimerization in vivo and in human pathologies. It is therefore becoming highly relevant to include dimerization in screening campaigns: the increased complexity reached by the ability to target 2 receptors should lead to the identification of more specific hits that could be developed into drugs with fewer side effects. In this review, we have summarized results from a series of studies characterizing the properties of G-protein-coupled receptor dimers using both in vitro and in vivo systems. Since opioid receptors exist as dimers and heterodimerization modulates their pharmacology, we have used them as a model system to develop strategies for the identification of compounds that will specifically bind and activate opioid receptor heterodimers: such compounds could represent the next generation of pain relievers with decreased side effects, including reduced drug abuse liability.

Keywords G-protein-coupled receptors, dimerization, allosteric interaction, high-throughput screening (HTS), secreted alkaline phosphatase (SEAP)

Introduction

The opioid system modulates several physiological processes, including analgesia, stress response, and neuroendocrine function. Three types of opioid receptors (μ, δ, and κ) have been pharmacologically characterized, and genes encoding

[1]Department of Pharmacology and Biological Chemistry, Mount Sinai School of Medicine, New York, NY 10029

Corresponding Author: Lakshmi A. Devi, Department of Pharmacology and Biological Chemistry, Mount Sinai School of Medicine, 19-84 Annenberg Building One Gustave L. Levy Place, New York, NY 10029. Tel: (212) 241-8345; Fax: (212) 996-7214; E-mail: lakshmi.devi@mssm.edu

R.S. Rapaka and W. Sadée (eds.), *Drug Addiction.*
© American Association of Pharmaceutical Scientists 2008

these receptors have been cloned.[1] Morphine, which predominantly binds to μ receptors, is currently administered to alleviate chronic pain in patients despite the fact that morphine elicits strong side effects, such as constipation, nausea, sedation, respiratory depression, and development of addiction. The analgesic effect is mainly due to the actions of morphine on μ opioid receptors in dorsal root ganglion and in the dorsal horn to inhibit nerve fibers that signal pain to the brain. These receptors are also expressed in different regions of the brain, in the gastrointestinal tract, and in the immune system, and when targeted by the agonist will lead to the development of side effects. This is a common problem encountered by researchers as well as pharmaceutical laboratories in the development of new drugs, since even the most specific molecule targeting a receptor has been found to cause severe side effects.

Opioid receptors belong to the G-protein-coupled receptor (GPCR) superfamily. GPCRs can form homo- (2 identical protomer partners) and hetero- (2 different protomer partners) dimers. An important discovery has been the observation that a pair of interacting GPCRs can have distinct pharmacological properties. Hence, dimerization could be seen as a way for an organism to increase the functional variety of GPCRs. It is likely that repertoires of heterodimers in different tissues are unique and that a specific dimer pair could represent a target potentially found in fewer tissues. A screen for molecules that interact and activate/inactivate specific heterodimers is becoming an attractive therapeutic target: only tissues expressing both GPCR protomers will be targeted by such molecules, with the potential for side effects greatly reduced.

This review contains a survey of literature suggesting the presence of and/or a role for GPCR dimers in vivo and describes strategies for screening assays targeting these dimers.

Dimers in Vitro

A large body of evidence for the existence of GPCRs as dimers and oligomers has rapidly accumulated in recent years. GPCR dimerization has been demonstrated to be a physiological process that modifies receptor pharmacology and regulates function.[2] Heterodimerization can generate receptors with novel characteristics, leading to altered pharmacological properties. The first demonstration of heterodimerization was using chimeric receptor molecules between α_{2c} adrenergic receptors and m_3 muscarinic receptors; this provided the first evidence to suggest that 2 nonfunctional chimeric receptors could physically associate to form a functional heterodimeric receptor with ligand binding and signaling capabilities.[3] The same strategy was followed by several other researchers demonstrating that heterodimerization occurs between many naturally occurring GPCRs. Indeed, this phenomenon has been shown to occur between both closely related GPCR types and distantly related receptors. In many cases, the resultant heterodimeric receptor complex has been found to have pharmacological properties different from those of both of the individual partner receptors.[4-7] Occasionally, heterodimerization of 2 receptors is necessary to form a functional receptor.[8] However, heterodimerization can also result in either an enhancement or a reduction in the activity of a fully functional receptor.[2,9,10]

In the opioid receptor family, δ opioid receptors have been shown to interact with both κ and μ opioid receptors to form heterodimers, and this leads to altered pharmacological properties.[11,12] In the case of interactions between κ and δ receptors, the resultant κ–δ heterodimers were found to have greatly reduced affinities for highly selective κ or δ receptor ligands.[11] In the presence of a δ-selective agonist, a κ-selective agonist bound to the receptors with high affinity, and reciprocally, a κ-selective agonist increased the binding of a δ-selective agonist. Cells coexpressing κ and δ receptors also exhibited synergistic effects on agonist-induced signaling (as measured by cAMP and phosphorylated mitogen-activated protein kinase levels). Finally, dimerization was found to affect the trafficking properties of these receptors because etorphine-induced trafficking of the δ receptor was significantly reduced in cells expressing κ–δ heterodimers, suggesting that δ receptors are retained at the cell surface as a result of dimerization with κ receptors.[11]

Studies with μ–δ heterodimers also demonstrated decreased binding affinity to selective synthetic agonists.[13] The rank order of agonist affinities for the heterodimeric receptors has been shown to be different from that of the individual receptors, suggesting allosteric modulation of the binding pocket.[12,13] In cells expressing μ–δ heterodimers, low doses of δ-selective ligands produce a significant increase in the binding of a μ-selective agonist. This treatment also enhances μ receptor-mediated signaling.[14] Thus physical interaction appears to modulate the binding pocket of opioid receptors. Ligands that selectively bind and activate μ–δ heterodimers will be useful in delineating the novel pharmacology of these receptors and will help address the physiological consequences of dimerization.

The opioid receptor has also been shown to heterodimerize with distantly related GPCRs such as somatostatin (SST_{2A}),[15] α_{2A}-adrenergic,[16,17] or substance P[18] receptors. These receptor heterodimers exhibit properties that are quite distinct from those of each individual receptor, again indicating that heterodimerization may increase the functional diversity of individual receptors. An interesting case is that of μ-α_{2A} heterodimers, in which coactivation of both receptors in heterologous cells leads to an increased detergent sensitivity and decreased signaling.[16] Decreased signaling by μ-α_{2A} heterodimers was also found to occur in primary spinal cord neurons, suggesting that these receptor interactions may play an important role in modulating pain transmission.[16] Taken together, these observations suggest that receptor homo- or heterodimerization leads to modulation of receptor pharmacology in a large variety of contexts. Therefore, the development of new drugs that selectively target receptor heterodimers seems to be an achievable goal. Such molecules would be important in the treatment of various pathologies involving GPCR dimers.

Dimers in Vivo

Although the identification of receptor dimers/heterodimers in vitro is well established, we are at only an early stage in the investigation of dimers in vivo and in the
understanding of their functional implications. Perhaps the most striking evidence
has been the observation of oligomeric arrays of rhodopsin dimers in isolated
mouse rod outer-segment membranes using atomic force microscopy.[19]

In an elegant set of experiments, Abdalla et al have shown a link between heterodimerization of bradykinin B_2 and angiotensin AT_1 receptors and hypertension
in preeclamptic women. They first observed an increased responsiveness of this
heterodimer to angiotensin as compared to AT_1 receptors alone in vitro.[20] They were
then able to isolate B_2-AT_1 heterodimers in higher quantity from platelets of preeclamptic women compared with controls.[21] This increase in B_2-AT_1 heterodimers
further correlates with increased G-protein activation, making this phenomenon a
good candidate to explain the increased sensitivity to angiotensin in these patients.
The same team also studied homodimerization of AT_1 receptors in monocytes of
hypertensive patients. They found an increased amount of cross-linked AT_1 receptors (formed through a covalent bond catalyzed by factor XIIIA) in patients with
higher risk of atherosclerosis: they observed that the AT_1 receptor dimer is more
sensitive to angiotensin and that this would lead to an enhanced adhesion of monocytes to endothelial cells.[22] These 2 examples are the only evidence of a functional
role (and even a pathological role) of dimerization in vivo. These observations were
made on more accessible nonneuronal cells. It is likely that similar pharmacological
changes can occur in other cells, including neurons. This would have implications
in central nervous system pathology.

We have shown that potentiation of a μ-opioid receptor agonist binding by a δ
antagonist observed in vitro leads to increased antinociceptive responses using a
classical analgesia test.[14] Similarly, such influence of a protomer over another could
exist between μ and NK1 receptors, which are known to interact and present a particular internalization pattern.[18] In vivo this interaction could be responsible for the
dramatic changes observed: the loss of morphine place preference in NK1 −/−
mice[23] and the alteration of NK1 internalization by substance P after chronic morphine treatment.[24] Hence, an emerging notion with GPCR dimerization in vivo is
that allosteric properties enabled by the interaction of 2 protomers could be used to
design new classes of compounds with more efficacious therapeutic properties.

Dimers Behave as Allosteric Complexes

GPCRs are natural allosteric proteins. Binding of an agonist to a GPCR causes
conformational changes within the core of the helical transmembrane domain that
are transmitted to the intracellular loops, resulting in G-protein activation.[25,26]
The presence of GPCRs in dimeric or oligomeric complexes makes allosteric

interactions between the protomer partners within the dimer possible. The most straightforward example of allosteric interactions between dimer partners is that of the $GABA_B$ receptors where several small-molecule allosteric modulators have been identified and characterized.[27] In these receptors, agonists bind to one of the protomers ($GABA_{B1}$), whereas G-protein activation occurs via the other ($GABA_{B2}$), implying that structural changes are transmitted across receptors.[28] Allosteric molecules that modulate this interaction have been shown to bind at the helical bundle of $GABA_{B2}$.[29] Importantly, one such allosteric ligand has been shown to induce anxiolytic effects in rats without the significant side effects (ie, sedation, hypolocomotion, and hypothermia) associated with baclofen administration.[30] Several allosteric modulators of family C[31-33] and family A GPCRs[34,35] have also been identified; the extent of regulation of receptor activity by binding to the heterodimer has yet to be determined.

As discussed earlier, we demonstrated the heterodimerization between δ and κ opioid receptors[11]; these heterodimers have pharmacological properties resembling those of the $κ_2$ receptor subtype characterized in vivo—that is, distinct from homodimers of either subunit. The δ–κ heterodimer not only exhibits decreased affinities for δ- or κ-selective agonists and antagonists but also synergistically binds certain partially selective agonists with high affinity. Synergy with respect to agonist binding is also reflected in the activation of signaling pathways, both inhibition of adenylyl cyclase and phosphorylation of mitogen activated protein kinase (MAPK).[11] Similarly, μ–δ heterodimers exhibit synergistic interactions in both binding and signaling.[12,13] Signaling via μ–δ heterodimers is insensitive to pertussis toxin, suggesting a shift in G-protein preference from Gi to pertussis-toxin-resistant subtypes.[13] Although all of these heterodimer effects on agonist binding and/or signaling can be interpreted as a result of domain swapping, they can also potentially reflect allosteric interactions between receptors within the homo- and heterodimers that are dependent on the location and/or specificity of the dimer interface.

Strategies for Screening and Drug Development

When carrying out a large-scale drug screen, one would choose a test with the fewest manipulations and the highest sensitivity. Changes occurring in ligand binding to a protomer by the coadministration of another ligand specific for the adjacent receptor have been described.[11,14] Binding assays are not suitable for drug screening because they require the use of radiolabeled ligands, which are expensive, may not be available for the receptors being studied, and generate radioactive waste that needs to be carefully discarded. Also, molecules that will allosterically change the binding of a chosen compound will not necessarily lead to an increase in the signaling potency. Functional tests more directly indicate whether a molecule has allosteric properties on the function of a GPCR dimer. We have shown that a δ antagonist is able to increase the efficacy of the μ agonist [D-Ala²,-N-Me-Phe⁴-Gly⁵-ol]enkephalin (DAMGO)[14] in the GTPγS binding assay. This assay is useful in that it provides a positive signal above the background for receptors that are coupled to Gi proteins. However, this assay is not highly sensitive and requires radiolabeled [^{35}S]GTPγS. Although fluorescent analogs of GTPγS have been developed, they display relatively low affinity for G proteins and exhibit nonspecific binding; these properties have made them unsuitable for high-throughput screening (HTS).[36] Assays that measure intracellular Ca^{2+} or cAMP have been increasingly used as screenings strategies and are discussed below.

Ca^{2+} Release Assay

Cell-based functional assays are now widely used for HTS since they provide a direct physiological measure for a candidate compound as opposed to traditional ligand-binding strategies. Among functional assays, monitoring Ca^{2+} release has proven to be very effective in screening for new GPCR ligands as well as identifying novel ligands for orphan receptors.[37,38] Furthermore, monitoring Ca^{++} release has also been successfully used in the identification of a positive modulator of mGluR1 receptors.[31] As an HTS test, this assay presents several advantages: (1) it is a sensitive nonradioactive fluorescence-based assay; (2) it can be miniaturized to a 384 well plate level; (3) it is easy to perform and can be automated; (4) it provides a positive signal over the background; and (5) it can be used to screen for ligands against receptors irrespective of the G-proteins they are coupled to (by the use of promiscuous G-proteins). Opioid receptors have been shown to elicit Ca^{2+} release in a variety of cells[39,40] through the action of βγ subunits. A previous study has shown that μ receptors are differentially coupled to a Ca^{2+} pathway in the presence of δ receptors in GH_3 cells.[41] This study suggests that the conventional Ca^{2+} assay could be sensitive enough to screen for allosteric modulation of the μ–δ heterodimer.

The screening for a compound that will specifically enhance the cellular response of a μ-δ heterodimer would require establishing cell lines that express each receptor individually and coexpress both receptors. Screening for a δ ligand that increases the Ca^{2+} response of a μ ligand (Fig. 32.1) should be done (1) on cells expressing only δ receptors to ascertain that the δ ligand does not increase Ca^{2+} by itself, and (2) on cells expressing μ receptors alone to show that this effect is solely due to the δ ligand's effect on δ receptors and it has no effect on μ receptors. Since opioid ligands represent a large and diverse family of molecules,[42] initial studies could be performed with known δ antagonists and inverse agonists. The data obtained using a combination of different μ-specific agonists with different δ ligands can be used to classify the latter as positive, negative, or neutral allosteric modulators. This in itself will provide important information on the existing ligands since the majority of selective δ ligands have been characterized mostly according to their selectivity or potency toward singly expressed receptors.[43,44] Some of these ligands may represent strong allosteric modulators of μ-δ heterodimers that could potentiate actions of μ agonists in vitro and in vivo. Previously, we have shown that the signaling by DAMGO or morphine can be potentiated by a variety of δ ligands as measured by the cAMP accumulation or GTPγS assays.[14] Since the Ca^{2+} release

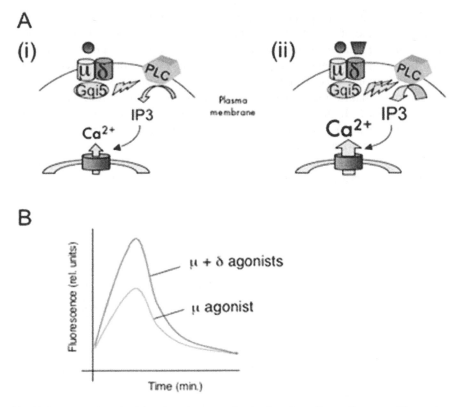

Fig. 32.1 Schematics of calcium-based strategy for the detection of heterodimer-specific agonists. (A) A chimeric Gαq protein (Gαqi5) couples opioid receptors to effectors, generating IP3 and leading to an increase in intracellular calcium that is monitored with cell-permeable calcium-sensitive fluorescent dyes. In the case of μ–δ heterodimers, presence of a μ agonist would produce a typical response (i) that would be further potentiated upon cotreatment with the δ ligand (ii). A graphic representation of the data is shown in B. IP3 indicates inositol triphosphate; Gqif, G-protein α_i subunit; PLC, phospholipase.

assay is based on the measurement of intracellular second messengers downstream in the transduction cascade, it tends to be more sensitive. Hence, the potentiation of DAMGO response observed using the less sensitive GTPγS binding should be even more pronounced using this Ca^{2+} release assay.

cAMP Accumulation Assay

Opioid receptors are known to be negatively coupled to adenylate cyclase through Gi/o proteins, and this leads to a decrease in the level of intracellular cAMP upon activation of the receptor. Hence, an alternative strategy to functionally screen new ligands for their allosteric potency would be to use the HTS version of cAMP detection assays. Some of the cAMP assay kits are now available in a 1536 well plate format, and the number of steps has been greatly reduced. A potential problem could be that these assays are typically less sensitive than other assays used for HTS. To overcome this, a highly sensitive gene reporter assay using secreted alkaline phosphatase (SEAP) has been used to measure intracellular cAMP (see Fig. 32.2A).[45] In this construct, 4 cAMP responsive element (CRE) elements are present upstream from the gene for alkaline phosphatase. An elevation of intracellular cAMP is known to activate protein kinase A, which translocates in the nucleus to phosphorylate CRE binding protein (CREB) transcription factors. The latter bind to CRE elements on the gene reporter to proportionally induce the translation of SEAP.

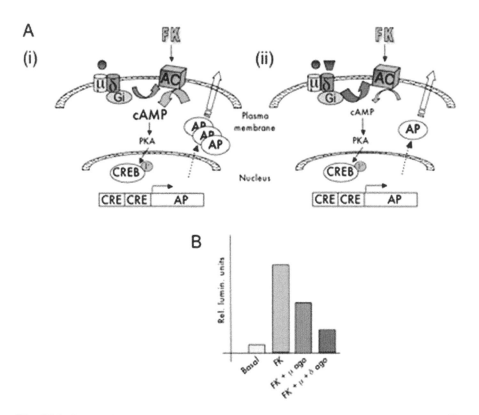

Fig. 32.2 Schematics of cAMP sensitive gene assay for detection of heterodimer-specific agonists. (A) FK activates AC, leading to increases in cAMP and activation of PKA followed by CREB phosphorylation and translation of the SEAP gene reporter to produce a secreted form of AP. FK alone will produce a signal that would be inhibited by the μ agonist (i), and this inhibition would be further potentiated by cotreatment with a δ ligand (ii). A graphical representation of the data is shown in B. FK indicates forskolin; AC, adenylyl cyclase; PKA, protein kinase A; CREB, CRE binding protein; AP, alkaline phosphatase; CRE, cAMP response element.

This enzyme has been designed to be able to diffuse directly into the supernatant. Hence, no cell lysis step is required: a sample of supernatant is transferred to another plate to determine SEAP enzyme activity using a colorimetric assay. The enzyme activity will therefore be proportional to the quantity of intracellular cAMP. In the case of opioid receptors, forskolin (FK) is added to enhance cAMP levels, and the extent of inhibition of this FK-stimulated cAMP by the μ agonist alone or with δ ligand is measured by the SEAP assay (Fig. 32.2B). Since this assay is performed on living cells, these cells can be used for additional tests after the ligands have been washed out.

Conclusion

With the discovery of GPCR dimerization, a new dimension in the pharmacology of GPCRs has been born. Binding, signaling, and internalization are due not only to the features presented by 1 receptor alone but also (and perhaps mainly) to a combination of receptors. We propose 2 known HTS and sensitive assays to screen for 1 or a combination of ligands that will be active at a particular pair of GPCRs. Among existing assays, a potentiation of a calcium response obtained using chimeric G proteins or the altered cAMP response monitored by the SEAP gene reporter is suitable for such screening. Studies performed thus far have focused on identification of a single ligand that is pharmacologically active at receptors in the heterodimer. For example, a compound that binds specifically to δ–κ heterodimers has recently been identified[46]; this compound shows a tissue-specific action since it has analgesic properties only when administered in spinal cord. Such compounds are likely to have fewer side effects. A comparison of binding of such ligands to heterodimers with binding to homodimers will provide insights into the molecular determinants required for selective activation of heterodimers.

Alternatively, the screening could be designed to identify a combination of ligands that target a specific set of receptor heterodimers. In addition to offering increased specificity, this strategy would allow the more direct identification of compounds that will potentiate a known cellular effect. Moreover, more candidates may be found using this approach since a large number of known δ antagonists are already able to potentiate the cellular response of DAMGO though μ receptors.[14] This could means that in a heterodimer, each receptor applies some structural constraints to the other and that the ligand binding releases some of these constraints, allowing the neighboring agonist-occupied receptor to signal better. The administration of 2 compounds will also increase the possibility for 1 of them to be active on its own, elsewhere in the body. To overcome this problem, allosteric modulators that by themselves have no activity but are able to enhance the action of endogenous ligands have been sought. These compounds bind to 1 protomer and enhance binding and signaling by the endogenous ligand to the other protomer.[28] Such allosteric modulators provide a very high specificity of action since the cellular effect is obtained only when the 2 receptors are activated[47] together.

The development of new sensitive and high-throughput functional assays is a very active area of investigation. Even though the identification of a ligand with a dimer-specific activity could be labor-intensive, the rate of screening and the size and complexity of libraries available make the isolation of such compounds feasible.[38] With the increased number of heterodimeric targets we should be able to successfully identify highly selective lead compounds that could be developed into drugs with better results when tested in clinical trials.

Acknowledgments We would like to thank Dr Ivone Gomes for her critical reading of the manuscript. This work is supported by the National Institutes of Health grants DA08863 and DA19521 (to L.A.D.).

References

1. Kieffer BL. Recent advances in molecular recognition and signal transduction of active peptides: receptors for opioid peptides. *Cell Mol Neurobiol.* 1995;15:615-635.
2. George SR, O'Dowd BF, Lee SP. G-protein-coupled receptor oligomerization and its potential for drug discovery. *Nat Rev Drug Discov.* 2002;1:808-820.
3. Maggio R, Vogel Z, Wess J. Coexpression studies with mutant muscarinic/adrenergic receptors provide evidence for intermolecular "cross-talk" between G-protein linked-receptors. *Proc Natl Acad Sci USA.* 1993;90:3103-3107.
4. Rios CD, Jordan BA, Gomes I, Devi LA. G-protein receptor dimerization: modulation of receptor function. *Pharmacol Ther.* 2001;92:71-87.
5. Angers S, Salahpour A, Bouvier M. Dimerization: an emerging concept for G-protein coupled receptor ontogeny and function. *Annu Rev Pharmacol Toxicol.* 2002;42:409-435.
6. Bai M. Dimerization of G-protein coupled receptors: roles in signal transduction. *Cell Signal.* 2004;16:175-186.
7. Kroeger KM, Pfleger KD, Eidne KA. G-protein coupled receptor oligomerization in neuroendocrine pathways. *Front Neuroendocrinol.* 2003;24:254-278.
8. Marshall FH, Jones KA, Kaupman K, Bettler B. GABA(B) receptors: the first 7TM heterodimers. *Trends Pharmacol Sci.* 1999;20:396-399.
9. Gomes I, Devi LA. Receptor-receptor interactions modulate opioid receptor function. In: Madras BH, Colvis CM, Pollock D, Rutter JL, Shurtleff D, Von Zastrow M, eds. *Cell Biology of Addiction.* New York, NY: Cold Spring Harbor Laboratory Press; 2005.
10. Bouvier M. Oligomerization of G-protein-coupled transmitter receptors. *Nat Rev Neurosci.* 2001;2:274-286.
11. Jordan BA, Devi LA. G-protein coupled receptor heterodimerization modulates receptor function. *Nature.* 1999;399:697-700.
12. Gomes I, Jordan BA, Gupta A, Trapaidze N, Nagy V, Devi LA. Heterodimerization of mu and delta opioid receptors: a role in opiate synergy. *J Neurosci.* 2000;20:RC110.
13. George SR, Fan T, Xie Z, et al. Oligomerization of mu and delta opioid receptors: generation of novel functional properties. *J Biol Chem.* 2000;275:26128-26135.
14. Gomes I, Gupta A, Filipovska J, Szeto HH, Pintar JE, Devi LA. A role for heterodimerization of μ and δ opiate receptors in enhancing morphine analgesia. *Proc Natl Acad Sci USA.* 2004;101:5135-5139.
15. Pfeiffer M, Koch T, Schroder H, Laugsch M, Hollt V, Schulz S. Heterodimerization of somatostatin and opioid receptors cross-modulates phosphorylation, internalization, and desensitization. *J Biol Chem.* 2002;277:19762-19772.
16. Jordan BA, Gomes I, Rios C, Filipovska J, Devi LA. Functional interactions between μ opioid and α_{2A}-adrenergic receptors. *Mol Pharmacol.* 2003;64:1317-1324.

17. Rios C, Gomes I, Devi LA. Interactions between delta opioid receptors and alpha-adrenoceptors. *Clin Exp Pharmacol Physiol.* 2004;31:833-836.
18. Pfeiffer M, Kirscht S, Stumm R, et al. Heterodimerization of substance P and mu-opioid receptors regulates receptor trafficking and resensitization. *J Biol Chem.* 2003;278:51630-51637.
19. Fotiadis D, Liang Y, Filipek S, Saperstein DA, Engel A, Palczewski K. Atomic-force microscopy: rhodopsin dimmers in native disc membranes. *Nature.* 2003;421:127-128.
20. AbdAlla S, Lother H, Quitterer U. AT1-receptor heterodimers show enhanced G-protein activation and altered receptor sequestration. *Nature.* 2000;407:94-98.
21. Abdalla S, Lother H, el Massiery A, Quitterer U. Increased AT(1) receptor heterodimers in preeclampsia mediate enhanced angiotensin II responsiveness. *Nat Med.* 2001;7:1003-1009.
22. Abdalla S, Lother H, Langer A, el Faramawy Y, Quitterer U. Factor XIIIA transglutaminase crosslinks AT1 receptor dimers of monocytes at the onset of atherosclerosis. *Cell.* 2004;119:343-354.
23. Murtra P, Sheasby AM, Hunt SP, De Felipe C. Rewarding effects of opiates are absent in mice lacking the receptor for substance P. *Nature.* 2000;405:180-183.
24. King T, Gardell LR, Wang R, et al. Role of NK-1 neurotransmission in opioid-induced hyperalgesia. *Pain.* 2005;116:276-288.
25. Hunyady L, Vauquelin G, Vanderheyden P. Agonist induction and conformational selection during activation of a G-protein-coupled receptor. *Trends Pharmacol Sci.* 2003;24:81-86.
26. Cherfils J, Chabre M. Activation of G-protein Galpha subunits by receptors through Galpha-Gbeta and Galpha-Ggamma interactions. *Trends Biochem Sci.* 2003;28:13-17.
27. Urwyler S, Pozza MF, Lingenhoehl K, et al. N,N'-Dicyclopentyl-2-methylsulfanyl-5-nitro-pyrimidine-4,6-diamine (GS39783) and structurally related compounds: novel allosteric enhancers of gamma-aminobutyric acidB receptor function. *J Pharmacol Exp Ther.* 2003;307:322-330.
28. Cryan JF, Kaupmann K. Don't worry 'B' happy!: a role for GABA(B) receptors in anxiety and depression. *Trends Pharmacol Sci.* 2005;26:36-43.
29. Binet V, Brajon C, Le Corre L, Acher F, Pin JP, Prezeau L. The heptahelical domain of GABA(B2) is activated directly by CGP7930, a positive allosteric modulator of the GABA(B) receptor. *J Biol Chem.* 2004;279:29085-29091.
30. Cryan JF, Kelly PH, Chaperon F, et al. Behavioral characterization of the novel GABAB receptor-positive modulator GS39783 (N,N'-dicyclopentyl-2-methylsulfanyl-5-nitro-pyrimidine-4,6-diamine): anxiolytic-like activity without side effects associated with baclofen or benzodiazepines. *J Pharmacol Exp Ther.* 2004;310:952-963.
31. Knoflach F, Mutel V, Jolidon S, et al. Positive allosteric modulators of metabotropic glutamate 1 receptor: characterization, mechanism of action, and binding site. *Proc Natl Acad Sci USA.* 2001;98:13402-13407.
32. Conigrave AD, Franks AH. Allosteric activation of plasma membrane receptors: physiological implications and structural origins. *Prog Biophys Mol Biol.* 2003;81:219-240.
33. Suzuki Y, Moriyoshi E, Tsuchiya D, Jingami H. Negative cooperativity of glutamate binding in the dimeric metabotropic glutamate receptor subtype 1. *J Biol Chem.* 2004;279:35526-35534.
34. Gao ZG, Kim SG, Soltysiak KA, Melman N, Ijzerman AP, Jacobson KA. Selective allosteric enhancement of agonist binding and function at human A3 adenosine receptors by a series of imidazoquinoline derivatives. *Mol Pharmacol.* 2002;62:81-89.
35. Trankle C, Weyand O, Voigtlander U, et al. Interactions of orthosteric and allosteric ligands with [3H]dimethyl-W84 at the common allosteric site of muscarinic M2 receptors. *Mol Pharmacol.* 2003;64:180-190.
36. Gille A, Seifert R. Low-affinity interactions of BODIPY-FL-GTPgammaS and BODIPY-FL-GppNHp with G(i)- and G(s)-proteins. *Naunyn Schmiedebergs Arch Pharmacol.* 2003;368:210-215.
37. Lembo PM, Grazzini E, Groblewski T, et al. Proenkephalin A gene products activate a new family of sensory neuron–specific GPCRs. *Nat Neurosci.* 2002;5:201-209.

38. Cacace A, Banks M, Spicer T, Civoli F, Watson J. An ultra-HTS process for the identification of small molecule modulators of orphan G-protein-coupled receptors. *Drug Discov Today.* 2003;8:785-792.
39. Chen L, Zou S, Lou X, Kang HG. Different stimulatory opioid effects on intracellular Ca(2+) in SH-SY5Y cells. *Brain Res.* 2000;882:256-265.
40. Yoon SH, Lo TM, Loh HH, Thayer SA. Delta-opioid-induced liberation of Gbetagamma mobilizes Ca2+ stores in NG108-15 cells. *Mol Pharmacol.* 1999;56:902-908.
41. Charles AC, Mostovskaya N, Asas K, Evans CJ, Dankovich ML, Hales TG. Coexpression of delta-opioid receptors with micro receptors in GH3 cells changes the functional response to micro agonists from inhibitory to excitatory. *Mol Pharmacol.* 2003;63:89-95.
42. Waldhoer M, Bartlett SE, Whistler JL. Opioid receptors. *Annu Rev Biochem.* 2004;73:953-990.
43. Schiller PW, Weltrowska G, Berezowska I, et al. The TIPP opioid peptide family: development of delta antagonists, delta agonists, and mixed mu agonist/delta antagonists. *Biopolymers.* 1999;51:411-425.
44. Bryant SD, Salvadori S, Cooper PS, Lazarus LH. New delta-opioid antagonists as pharmacological probes. *Trends Pharmacol Sci.* 1998;19:42-46.
45. Durocher Y, Perret S, Thibaudeau E, et al. A reporter gene assay for high-throughput screening of G-protein-coupled receptors stably or transiently expressed in HEK293 EBNA cells grown in suspension culture. *Anal Biochem.* 2000;284:316-326.
46. Waldhoer M, Fong J, Jones RM, et al. A heterodimer-selective agonist shows in vivo relevance of G protein-coupled receptor dimers. *Proc Natl Acad Sci USA.* 2005;102:9050-9055.
47. Mesnier D, Baneres JL. Cooperative conformational changes in a G-protein-coupled receptor dimer, the leukotriene B(4) receptor BLT1. *J Biol Chem.* 2004;279:49664-49670.

Chapter 33
Homology Modeling of Opioid Receptor-Ligand Complexes Using Experimental Constraints

Irina D. Pogozheva,[1] Magdalena J. Przydzial,[1] and Henry I. Mosberg[1]

Abstract Opioid receptors interact with a variety of ligands, including endogenous peptides, opiates, and thousands of synthetic compounds with different structural scaffolds. In the absence of experimental structures of opioid receptors, theoretical modeling remains an important tool for structure-function analysis. The combination of experimental studies and modeling approaches allows development of realistic models of ligand-receptor complexes helpful for elucidation of the molecular determinants of ligand affinity and selectivity and for understanding mechanisms of functional agonism or antagonism. In this review we provide a brief critical assessment of the status of such theoretical modeling and describe some common problems and their possible solutions. Currently, there are no reliable theoretical methods to generate the models in a completely automatic fashion. Models of higher accuracy can be produced if homology modeling, based on the rhodopsin X-ray template, is supplemented by experimental structural constraints appropriate for the active or inactive receptor conformations, together with receptor-specific and ligand-specific interactions. The experimental constraints can be derived from mutagenesis and cross-linking studies, correlative replacements of ligand and receptor groups, and incorporation of metal binding sites between residues of receptors or receptors and ligands. This review focuses on the analysis of similarity and differences of the refined homology models of μ, δ, and κ-opioid receptors in active and inactive states, emphasizing the molecular details of interaction of the receptors with some representative peptide and nonpeptide ligands, underlying the multiple modes of binding of small opiates, and the differences in binding modes of agonists and antagonists, and of peptides and alkaloids.

Keywords ligand docking, modeling, opioid receptors, opioid ligands, pharmacophore model

---

[1] Department of Medicinal Chemistry, College of Pharmacy, University of Michigan, Ann Arbor, MI 48109

Corresponding Author: Henry I. Mosberg, Department of Medicinal Chemistry, College of Pharmacy, University of Michigan, 428 Church St, Ann Arbor, MI 48109-1065. Tel: (734) 764-8117; Fax: (734) 763-5595.

R.S. Rapaka and W. Sadée (eds.), *Drug Addiction.*

559

Introduction

Clinical interest in opioid receptors (ORs) is related to the development of strong analgesics without potential for abuse or adverse side effects. This task, however, cannot be accomplished without understanding the differences in the OR subtypes as well as the modes of interactions of drugs/ligands with these receptors.

Research on ORs was significantly advanced by the cloning of δ-opioid (DOR), μ-opioid (MOR), and κ-opioid (KOR) receptors in the early 1990s.[1,2] Sequence comparison confirmed that ORs belong to the rhodopsin-like family of G-protein-coupled receptors (GPCRs).[1] ORs are composed of a core domain of 7 transmembrane (TM) α-helices and an adjacent, peripheral helix 8 (IL4), are connected by 3 extracellular (EL1, EL2, EL3) and 3 intracellular (IL1, IL2, IL3) loops, and contain glycosylated N-terminal and palmitoylated C-terminal domains of different sizes. ORs demonstrate high sequence identity in their TM domain (73%–76%) and in ILs (63%–66%) and large divergence in N- and C-terminal domains and ELs (34%–40% identity).

ORs are activated by either endogenous peptides or exogenous opiates. The endogenous opioid peptides such as β-endorphin, Leu- and Met-enkephalins, dynorphins, and many others are mainly derived from 3 precursors, pro-opiomelanocortin, proenkephalin, and prodynorphin. They are found mostly in central and peripheral neurons, and also in gut, lungs, spleen, heart, and blood cells.[3,4] In addition, several opioid peptides have been isolated from cow's milk and frog skin. The majority of opioid peptides contain the core tetrapeptide, Tyr-Gly-Gly-Phe, important for high affinity and bioactivity.[5] In frog-skin-derived peptides the "Gly-Gly" motif is substituted by D-stereoisomers of Ala, Met, or Ile. Pharmacological studies indicate that no family of endogenous peptides is exclusively associated with a particular receptor type.[6]

The need for highly selective and potent agonists and antagonists stimulated the design of numerous synthetic opioid peptides. Thousands of linear peptides have been synthesized, some of them demonstrating subtype selectivity. To improve ligand selectivity, conformational and topographical constraints have been incorporated into the peptide ligands, and several highly selective cyclic peptides have been generated.[5] The first highly δ-selective enkephalin analog, the cyclic peptapeptide Tyr-c[DPen-Gly-Phe-D-Pen]OH (DPDPE), was designed using cyclic bridging via a disulfide and the topographically constrained D-amino acid D-Pen (Pen, penicillamine, β'β-dimethylcysteine).[7] μ-Selective cyclic dodecapeptide antagonists lacking the characteristic "Tyr-Gly-Gly-Phe" motif were developed based on the somatostatin sequence.[8,9] Active cyclic analogs of dynorphin A(1–11) and (1–13) were also produced by incorporating disulfide cross-link between cysteines in positions 5–11, 5–10, 5–9, 4–9, 6–10, 8–12, 8–13, 5–13,[10] between L, D-Cys and L, D-Pen in positions 5–11,[11] or by introduction of a lactam bridge between residues in positions 2–5,[12] 2–6, 3–7, or 5–8.[13] Most of these cyclic dynorphin analogs demonstrated high κ- and μ-affinity, and some, such as c-[D-Asp3, Lys7]DynA(1–11)NH$_2$ were moderately κ-selective.[13] The properties of these cyclic opioid peptides have been reviewed in detail by Hruby and Agnes.[5]

Synthetic nonpeptide opioid ligands belong to several structural classes, such as morphine analogs, bimorphinans, benzomorphans, phenylpiperidines, phenylpiperazines, 4-anilinopiperidine, methadone analogs, and arylacetamides.[14] The correspondence of key structural elements between opioid peptides and nonpeptides is not always obvious.

Except for the recently crystallized rhodopsin,[15,16] structural data on individual GPCRs, including ORs, are limited; therefore theoretical modeling remains an important tool for structure-function analysis of these receptors.[17] Modeling of ligand-receptor complexes is usually performed to achieve several goals: to explain the experimental results of ligand-receptor interactions; to understand the molecular mechanism of ligand selectivity and ligand agonist or antagonist properties; or to propose a receptor-based pharmacophore model for agonists and antagonists that can provide a basis for virtual screening of future drug leads and for structure-based drug design.

Depending on the research goal, the modeling algorithm can include any of the following steps, which will be described in further detail: (1) identification of the bioactive conformation of the opioid ligands based on their structure activity relation (SAR) and theoretical and experimental conformational studies; (2) experimental studies of receptor-ligand interactions to uncover key ligand-receptor contacts; (3) homology modeling of the receptor using the rhodopsin template and additional experimental constraints appropriate for a specific receptor in its active or inactive states; (4) ligand docking using experimentally determined key interactions across a set of structurally similar and dissimilar ligands to develop, independently, pharmacophore models for agonist and antagonists.

Bioactive Conformation of Opioid Ligands

Small alkaloids, such as morphine analogs (eg, morphine, naltrindole (NTI), oxymorphinole (OMI), spiroindanyloxymorphone (SIOM), naloxone, naltrexone, etorphine) and benzomorphans (bremazocine), as well as the larger bimorphinans (norBNI) and phenylpiperazines (BW373U86) (Fig. 33.1), have relatively rigid structures that must represent their bioactive conformations.[18-21] Some rotational flexibility is allowed around a few rotatable bonds such as in the N-allyl or N-cyclopropylmethyl groups of morphinans, in C-7 substituents of oripavines, at fumatate moiety of β-FNA, and the diethylamide group of BW373U86. The possible uncertainties resulting from such limited flexibility can be analyzed during ligand docking.

Selective agonists based on the arylacetamide scaffold are more conformationally flexible. Rotation around 3 single bonds (ie, χ^1, χ^2, and χ^3 angles, see Fig. 33.1) dramatically changes the relative orientation of the key pharmacophore elements of U69,593: the ammonium moiety of its pyrrolidine ring, the amide carbonyl group, and the phenyl group. The bioactive conformation of arylacetamides can be deduced

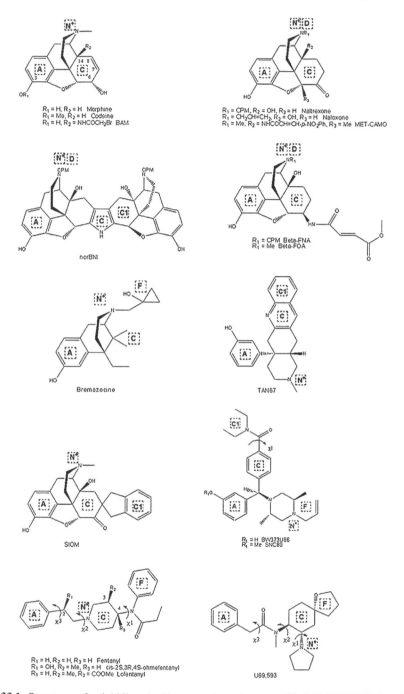

Fig. 33.1 Structures of opioid ligands. Pharmacophore elements, "N+," "A," "C," "C1," and "F" are indicated in the boxes.

from the superpositions of different analogs with structural restrictions introduced at the corresponding dihedral angles.[22] The reported X-ray structure of U69,593[23] overlaps well with all low-energy conformations of structurally restricted arylacetamides and therefore can be proposed as the bioactive conformation.

In the crystal structure of the μ-selective agonist cis(+)-3-methylfentanyl,[18] the central piperidine ring is in a chair conformation with 4-phenylpropanamide and N-phenethyl (in its extended conformation) in equatorial positions. Molecular dynamics simulations indicate high populations of different orientations of fentanyl analogs owing to torsional flexibility at 3 angles that define orientation of N-phenethyl (χ^1 and χ^2) and of N-phenylpropanamide (χ^3).[24] Docking of fentanyl analogs into a MOR model can be used to unequivocally identify the receptor-bound conformation of the ligand.

Linear opioid peptides are very flexible and can adopt a variety of different conformations in solution. To determine the bioactive conformations of opioid peptides, a great number of cyclic peptides have been synthesized.[5] Small cyclic peptides are particularly useful, as they adopt a restricted number of conformations that can be theoretically predicted or experimentally determined. Moreover, introduction of conformational constraints into small cyclic ligands allows exploration of the structural requirements for opioid peptides to effectively and selectively interact with ORs. During the past few years we have developed a large number of cyclic tetrapeptides with high affinity toward MOR, DOR, and KOR.[25-33] In particular, the cyclic tetrapeptides JOM13 (Tyr-c[D-Cys-Phe-D-Pen]OH, cyclized through a disulfide bond) and JOM6 (Tyr-c[D-Cys-Phe-D-Pen]NH2, cyclized via an ethylene dithioether), are highly potent and selective for DOR and MOR, respectively.[25] The design of κ-selective tetrapeptides based upon the same type scaffold as JOM13 and JOM6 has been more challenging. Although cyclic tetrapeptides with high κ-selectivity have not been obtained, the cyclic tetrapeptide, MP16 (Tyr-c[D-Cys-Phe-D-Cys]NH2, cyclized via a disulfide) demonstrates nanomolar affinity to KOR.[26]

Subsequent modifications of the parent tetrapeptides were directed toward elucidation of structural requirements for Tyr1 and Phe3 residues, which are key residues for recognition of cyclic tetrapeptides by ORs.[25-33] The following conclusions were derived from these studies (Table 33.1). First, the importance of aromatic residues in positions 1 and 3 was confirmed for all selective peptides. Second, cyclization via an ethylene dithioether bridge favors MOR binding, while the smaller disulfide-containing cycle is preferred for peptide recognition by DOR and KOR. Third, restriction of the Phe3 side chain in the *trans* ($\chi^1 \sim 180°$) rotamer is favorable for MOR and KOR high binding affinity, while restriction of the Phe3 side chain in the *gauche+* ($\chi^1 \sim -60°$) conformation provides improved DOR affinity. Fourth, the presence of a C-terminal amide is important for ligand binding to MOR and KOR, while a free C-terminal carboxylate enhances DOR affinity. Fifth, the presence of D-Cys4 in place of D-Pen4 in the tripeptide cycle dramatically increases binding affinity to KOR, while retaining high affinity to MOR and DOR. A combination of SAR, X-ray, and nuclear magnetic resonance (NMR) studies, and computational analysis of the cyclic tetrapeptides allowed us to deduce the bioactive conformations of JOM13,[25,31] JOM6,[32,34] and MP16,[26] which appeared to be complimentary to the binding pockets of modeled ORs.[26,34,35]

Table 33.1 Structural Requirements for Cyclic Tetrapeptides With High Affinity to μ-, δ-, and κ-receptors

Receptor (ligand)	$K_i \pm$ SEM (nM)	Residue 3	Residue 4	C-Terminus	Bridge	Side Chain Rotamer*		
						Residue 3	Residue 2	Residue 4
μ (JOM6)	0.17 ± 0.02	Phe³	D-Pen⁴	CONH₂	S-Et-S	trans	trans	trans
δ (JOM13)	1.3 ± 0.06	Phe³	D-Pen⁴	COO⁻	S-S	gauche+	trans	gauche+
κ (MP16)	38.7 ± 1.84	Phe³	D-Cys⁴	CONH₂	S-S	trans	gauche+	gauche−

*trans side chain rotamer corresponds to $\chi^1 \sim 180°$; gauche+ to $\chi^1 \sim -60°$; gauche− to $\chi^1 \sim +60°$.

Experimental Studies of Receptor-Ligand Interactions

Experimental studies useful for developing a crude topographical ligand-receptor interaction model include comparative affinity determination of ligands in receptor mutants, correlated replacements of ligand and receptor functional groups, covalent cross-linking of ligand to receptors, and the design of metal binding sites between ligand and receptors. Particularly important is the identification of specific interactions conferring ligand selectivity and agonist or antagonist properties.

Studies of OR chimeras and site-directed mutants revealed that the ligand binding pocket is located between TMs 2–7 and is covered by EL1, EL2, and EL3. Published mutagenesis data on ORs delineated a set of more than 20 residues in the TM α-bundle important for binding of opioid ligands.[36-38] It is assumed that conserved residues from TM 3–7 of ORs represent the common opioid pocket for the tyramine "message" part of opioid peptides and alkaloids, which triggers receptor transition to the active or inactive conformation, while subtype-specific residues from TMs 5–7, EL1, EL2, and EL3 contact the "address" part of the ligands, providing recognition of selective ligands by the corresponding receptors.[39,40]

The residues from the binding pocket, essential for ligand binding, are mostly conserved across the ORs and include Asp(3.32), Tyr(3.33), Lys(5.39), Phe(5.47), Trp(6.48), Ile(6.51), His(6.52), Ile(6.53), Ile(7.39), and Tyr(7.43).[41-50] Binding determinants for small alkaloids (morphine, codeine) reside in TMs 5–7.[51] Variable binding pocket residues confer selectivity. For example, Lys108 in EL1 of DOR prevents binding of the μ-selective DAMGO[52]; residues from EL2 and EL3 confer the selectivity of dynorphin to KOR[39,53-55]; and variable residues from EL3 and adjacent helices, particularly Lys303(6.58), Trp318(7.35), and His319(7.73) of MOR and the corresponding Trp284(6.58) and Leu300(7.35) and His301(7.36) of DOR are important for selective binding of morphine, DAMGO, and fentanyl analogs to MOR,[56-58] and of DPDPE, SNC80, and TAN67 to DOR.[37,59,60] Glu297(6.58) in KOR is involved in binding of norBNI.[61]

Several conserved residues in the binding pocket, such as Asp(3.32), Tyr(3.33), Lys(5.39), His(6.52), Trp(6.48), and Tyr(7.43), as well as divergent residues in positions 6.58 and 7.35, also participate in receptor activation.[42,44,47,56,62-65] Of interest, in the mutants D128K(3.32) of DOR and H297Q(6.52) of MOR, the antagonist naloxone demonstrates agonistic properties.[47,62] In addition, the H287Q(6.52) mutant of MOR is more resistant to β-FNA irreversible binding,[66] which acts at this mutant as a partial agonist.[66]

In many cases it is difficult to unequivocally distinguish between residues from the binding site, an allosteric regulation site, or those involved in receptor structural changes without detailed analysis of ligand-receptor interactions. To date, direct contacts between opioid ligands and corresponding receptor residues have been documented in only a few cases. Among these are interactions between the basic N$^+$ of the opioid ligand and Asp147(3.32) in MOR,[50] between the fumarate moiety of the irreversible μ-antagonist β-FNA and Lys233(5.39) in MOR,[67] and between the N-17' basic nitrogen of norBNI and the acidic Glu297(6.58) of KOR[61] or the corresponding K303E(6.58) of the MOR mutant.[68,69] Recently, MOR mutagenesis combined with comparison of affinity of different fentanyl analogs revealed interactions of the 2'-OH of cis(2'R,3R,4S)-ohmefentanyl and Tyr138(3.33), and the proximity of Trp318(7.35) and His319(7.36) to the pF-phenyl group of p-fluorofentanyl.[57,58]

Recent mutagenesis studies have allowed us to develop a topographical scheme of key ligand-receptor contacts between JOM6 and MOR,[34] which is presented in Fig. 33.2. These studies provided evidence for the formation of a metal binding site

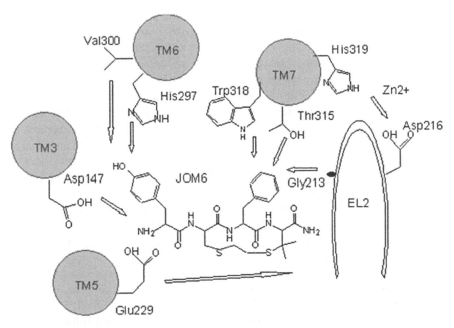

Fig. 33.2 Schematic drawing of the interactions of JOM6 with MOR.

by Asp216(EL2) and His319(7.36) near the peptide binding pocket of MOR and uncovered new interactions between MOR and its selective cyclic tetrapeptide, JOM6. In particular, Zn^{2+} binding sites were engineered between MOR mutants and His-substituted analogs of JOM6: [His1]JOM6-V300C-H297 and [His3]JOM6-G213C-T315C. Also, reciprocal substitution of receptor and ligand functional groups indicated the proximity between the C-terminal amide of JOM6 and Glu229 (5.35) and between Phe3 of JOM6 and Trp318 (7.35). Such unambiguous structural constraints between receptor and ligand atoms are essential for accurate modeling of the receptor ligand complexes. These constraints were recently employed for distance geometry calculations of complexes of MOR with the bimorphinan antagonist norBNI,[70] and with the cyclic tetrapeptide agonist JOM6.[34]

Homology Modeling of Opioid Receptors

During the mid to late 1990s several models of opioid receptors were proposed based on the nonhomologous bacteriorhodopsin or low resolution electron microscopy maps of rhodopsin.[22,24,57,71-77] We developed at that time a computational approach for modeling the transmembrane, 7 α-helical bundle of GPCRs that employed an iterative distance geometry refinement with an evolving system of interhelical hydrogen bonding constraints[78] and applied it to the modeling of MOR, DOR, and KOR[40] and other GPCRs.[79] The rhodopsin model calculated with this approach was close to the subsequently published crystal structure (root mean square deviation [rmsd] 2.88 Å for 186 Cα-atoms in the TM domain). Other methods for GPCR modeling that do not rely on a structural template include MembStruck[80] and PREDICT,[81] which also produced realistic models of rhodopsin (rmsd of 3.1 Å and 3.87 Å, respectively, vs the rhodopsin X-ray structure in the 7TM domain) and were used to model other GPCRs. Although such ab initio methods were able to achieve medium accuracy in the modeling of the α-helical TM domains of GPCRs, they failed to correctly predict the structure of the receptor loops.[80] This could seriously affect the analysis of ligand-receptor interactions, especially for peptide ligands since ELs are known to participate in contacts conferring ligand selectivity.[82,83] Nevertheless, these various methods yielded results that were consistent with available ligand SAR and confirmed the ligand-based pharmacophore models.[14,35]

It has been widely demonstrated that the most reliable computer-based technique for generating 3-dimensional models is via homology modeling.[84] The publication of the rhodopsin crystal structure[16,85] has made homology modeling of receptors from the rhodopsin-like family possible,[86-89] and several opioid receptor models based on the rhodopsin template have subsequently been produced.[37,65,88,90,91] Knowing the structural template, the homology models can be generated using MODELER,[92,93] or publicly available Web servers, such as SWISS-MODEL, EsyPred3D, Robetta, CPHmodels, or SDSC1,[94-98] or downloaded from databases, such as ModBase.[99]

The accuracy of comparative modeling is highly dependent on the sequence identity between the target sequence of interest and the template sequence. High accuracy comparative modeling (rmsd ~1 Å) can be achieved when the target and template proteins have sequence identity of more than 50%, while the accuracy drops when the identity of target and template sequences is less than 30%.[84] The opioid receptor sequences have only ~20% identity to rhodopsin for all residues and ~29% identity in TM segments. Therefore, automated homology modeling of ORs is likely to result in numerous errors. The major source of errors is from sequence misalignment,[81,100,101] which can be expected in areas of low sequence identity and in regions of helical distortions. Helical irregularities are indeed observed in the crystal structure of rhodopsin, which exhibits a fragment of 3_{10} helix in TM7 and α-aneurisms (one residue insertion) in TM2 and TM5, as well as proline-induced kinks in TMs 1, 2, 4, 5, 6, and 7.[102] These distortions in α-helices may not be present in other GPCRs. Other sources of errors are the divergent loops, which in many cases should be constructed ab initio.[103] Further, the α-helices of modeled proteins may have altered lengths, positions, and orientations relative to the template structure. Indeed, a sequence homology of ~20% between proteins suggests ~1.6 to 2.3 Å rmsd within the helical core, caused by helical shifts.[104]

Another problem is related to conformational rearrangement of the receptor during activation. The crystal structure of rhodopsin represents the inactive conformation in complex with the covalently bound inverse agonist, 11-cis-retinal. This structure can be used for homology modeling of the antagonist-bound inactive receptor state; however, the active states of rhodopsin and other GPCRs have been shown to differ from the inactive conformations.[15,105] The accumulated data from mutagenesis, cross-linking, electron paramagnetic resonance spectroscopy (EPR), and fluorescence studies suggest that different rhodopsin-like GPCRs share a common active conformation[106] in which TM6 undergoes a significant rigid-body motion in a counterclockwise direction, as viewed from the extracellular side.[107-109] This results in a significant shift of the intracellular end of TM6 outward from TM3[109,110] and TM7,[111,112] and toward TM5,[113] opening a cleft on the cytoplasmic surface of the α-bundle for binding of G-proteins.[105,114] A relatively smaller motion of TM3 and some conformational changes in the extracellular ends of TMs 1, 2, and 7 have also been observed.[109,115-120] Random mutagenesis of DOR provided evidence that the conformational transition originates at the ligand binding pocket near the extracellular ends of TM5, TM6, and EL3 and propagates through TMs 3, 6, and 7 down to a cytoplasmic switch between TMs 6 and 7.[65] Moreover, experimental studies of different GPCRs (eg, rhodopsin, β-adrenoreceptors, DOR) indicate that a conformational transition of the receptor may involve multiple intermediate states.[107,109,113,121-126] Therefore, agonists of different structural types may generate different activated states of receptors, which could be recognized by specific proteins involved in distinct transduction and regulation pathways.

Unfortunately, the existing methods for energy optimization, including molecular dynamics or distance geometry refinement, are unable to correct alignment errors or to reproduce helical shifts and distortions[127] and have been unsuccessful in modeling long irregular loops (>12 residues).[103] Some recent attempts demonstrated moderate improvement of homology models by combining several templates,[128] and some success in modeling helical shifts has resulted from using a new multiscale energy optimization algorithm.[129] Currently, model refinement requires human intervention and incorporation of additional information. For example, questionable target-template alignments in the area of helical distortions and in the loops of MOR have been clarified by mutagenesis data and construction of helix-loop metal binding sites.[34] In another example, initial homology models of tachykinin NK1 receptors were optimized in the area of the binding site by incorporation of distance constraints from the ligands in their bioactive conformation, using a new algorithm, MOBILE.[89,130] Accuracy of models of different functional states can also be improved by iterative distance geometry refinement with experimental interhelical restraints appropriate for only the active or inactive conformation derived from mutagenesis, cross-linking studies and design of metal binding sites together with ligand-receptor distance restraints.[70,88] For example, the important interhelical distance constraints for the positioning of TM6 in the activated receptor state can be deduced from recent data on the formation of disulfides between TM5 and TM6 in the m_3 muscarinic receptor upon agonist binding[131] and from the existence of an intrinsic allosteric Zn^{2+} binding site at the interface of TM5 and TM6 of the β_2-adrenergic receptor that facilitates agonist binding.[132] Additional constraints for adjusting helix packing in the activated state can be taken from the engineering of an activating metal-coordination center between TM3 and TM7 in β_2-adrenergic[133] and tachykinin receptors,[134] and also between TM2 and TM3 of the MC4 melanocortin receptor.[135]

Ligand Docking

Ligand docking should satisfy the surface complementarities between ligand and receptor and the key interactions deduced from mutagenesis studies of ligand-receptor interactions. In earlier modeling of receptor-ligand complexes, ligand docking was primarily done manually. In a recent review, Eguchi compared previously published models of receptor-ligand complexes for selective opioid agonists and antagonists that satisfied some experimental observations about receptor-ligand interactions and SAR of the ligands.[14] The comparison revealed that although the modeling was based on a common set of experimental data, the proposed models often contradicted each other in the manner of docking similar ligands, such as morphine and its analogs or κ-selective arylacetamides. It was unclear, however, whether such contradictions reflected the existence of multiple modes of ligand binding or appeared as a result of low accuracy of receptor modeling or inaccurate docking methods. Other important questions, such as differences between binding modes of peptides and alkaloids, and of agonists and antagonists were beyond the scope of the review by Eguchi. To answer these questions pharmacophore models should be developed separately for agonists and antagonists and docked to 3-D structures of the active and the inactive receptor conformations, respectively. Moreover, the models and docking algorithm should be relatively accurate.

Manual docking was recently used for homology- and knowledge-based models of inactive and activated GPCRs to find the position of ligands in the binding pockets that would agree with known ligand-receptor interactions.[88] The resulting models of antagonist-bound dopamine D_1, muscarinic m_1, and vasopressin V_{1a} and agonist-bound DOR, dopamine D_3, and β_2-adrenergic receptors appeared to be suitable for the virtual screening of drug leads from databases of drug-like compounds with hit rates from 2% to 37%, depending on docking algorithm and scoring function used.[88]

Numerous programs, based on different methods, have been developed to automatically dock small ligands into proteins. These programs include DOCK,[136] GOLD,[137] FlexX,[138] FDS,[139] Glide,[140] LigandFit,[141] ICM,[142] and others. To improve results, the best docking algorithms are combined with different scoring functions.[143] Program performance is largely dependent on the accuracy of the receptor structure (especially in the case of modeled structures), on the flexibility of the ligand (number of rotatable bonds), and on the nature of the binding site.[143-145]

Receptor flexibility presents the major complication for automated docking. Almost all currently used programs perform semiflexible ligand docking, where the ligand is considered as flexible and the protein, as rigid. Such an approach is known to cause errors in computational studies. A few algorithms perform flexible docking in which limited protein flexibility, such as side chain motions in the active site, is incorporated. Some recent algorithms use an ensemble of protein structures, pregenerated by molecular dynamic simulations, to account for backbone or side chain flexibility in structure-based drug design,[146] but they are very computationally intensive. In a recent approach incorporated in MOBILE,[130] an ensemble of homology models was generated much faster using MODELER,[92] and the ligands were docked into an averaged binding site representation using AutoDock. To improve the results obtained, the docking solution that better reproduced the experimentally determined key ligand-receptor interactions was selected and was further utilized for the iterative refinement of the ligand-bound homology models. The refined antagonist-bound homology model of tachykinin neurokinin 1 (NK1) receptor obtained in this manner was successfully employed for the virtual search of NK1 antagonists from a database of lead-like compounds.[89,147]

We have applied a similar method, employing structural constraints to produce a more reliable homology model of the agonist-bound receptor state of MOR in complex with the μ-selective cyclic peptide agonist, JOM6.[70] This approach complied with the SAR and key ligand-receptor interactions of relatively flexible peptide ligands, which is a more complicated task than the docking of more conformationally rigid alkaloids. To reproduce the agonist-bound state, the receptor was calculated together with the bioactive conformation of the cyclic tetrapeptide using experimental distance constraints between ligand and receptor functional groups (see Fig. 33.3). The active receptor conformation was calculated simultaneously using the interhelical distance constraints from the rhodopsin crystal structure to define the positions of TMs 1 to 5 and 7, receptor-specific H-bonds, and a set of experimental distance constraints between TMs 3 to 6 and TMs 5 to 6 to define the position of the largely flexible TM6. The latter constraints were derived from EPR,

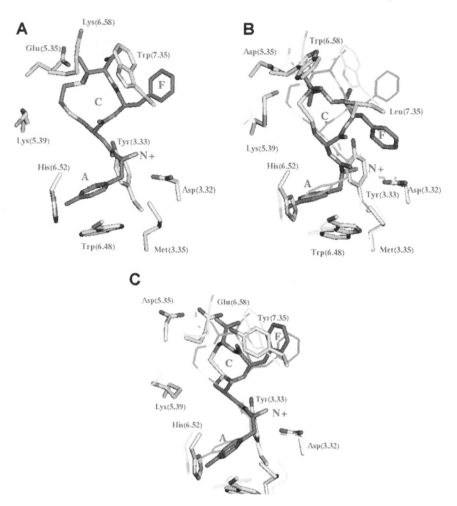

Fig. 33.3 JOM6 in the binding pocket of agonist-bound conformation of MOR (A) and its super-position with JOM13 in DOR binding pocket (B) or with MP16 in the KOR binding pocket (C). Ligands and several key residues, Asp(3.32), Tyr(3.33), Met(3.35), Glu/Asp/Asp(5.35), Lys(5.39), Trp(6.48), His(6.52), Lys/ Trp/Glu(6.58), and Trp/ Leu/ Tyr(7.35) from MOR/DOR/KOR, respectively, are shown. JOM6 and MOR residues on B and C are presented by thin lines. Pharmacophore elements are indicated by N+, A, C, and F.

cross-linking studies, and from engineered metal binding sites.[108,131,132] The agonist bound conformations of DOR with JOM13 and of KOR with MP16 have also been calculated based on the MOR-JOM6 complex.[25,26] The receptor-bound conformations of JOM13 appeared to be very similar to one of the crystal forms of JOM13,[31] while the receptor-bound conformation of MP16 requires a tripeptide cycle conformation that is ~2 kcal/mol higher in energy than the lowest energy state.[26]

The differences in binding cavity geometry among MOR, DOR, and KOR are related to the divergence in size, polarity, and charge of residues from the top of TMs 5 to 6, EL2, and EL3. The greatest difference is observed for KOR, whose 3-residue longer EL2 occupies more space between TM3 and TM7 and between TM3 and TM5. The binding pocket in KOR is consequently smaller in the regions between EL2 and TM7 and between EL2 and TM5. KOR also has several negatively charged side chains from EL2 (Asp204, Glu209, Asp216) and EL3 (Glu297) lining the binding cavity, which may have favorable ionic interactions with positively charged groups of κ-selective ligands.

In all 3 receptors, the positions of Tyr1 and of the central backbone cycle of tetrapeptide ligands are quite similar, but the orientations and interactions of the ligand Phe3 side chain are different (Fig. 33.3). The common Tyr1 of the tetrapeptides interacts with conserved charged, aromatic, and aliphatic side chains from the binding pockets; the positively charged amine group forms H-bond and ionic interactions with Asp(3.32) and participates in amine-aromatic interactions with Tyr(3.33); and the Tyr1 phenolic hydroxyl can either be an H-acceptor from His(6.52) or an H-donor to -C=O of Ala(5.46), which is excluded from the usual system of intrahelical H-bonds because of the presence of an α-aneurism in TM5. The Phe3 of JOM13 adopts a *gauche+* orientation that can be easily accommodated in the relatively hydrophobic environment of DOR between TM3, EL2, and TM7. In contrast, in MOR and KOR the corresponding area is partially filled by polar side chains from EL2. Therefore, the properties of the binding site in MOR and KOR favor the *trans* rotamer of Phe3, which is shifted closer to the extracellular surface. This is in agreement with the independently deduced pharmacophore model of cyclic tetrapeptides described above. In MOR, Trp318(7.35) forms an aromatic interaction with Phe3 of JOM6, supporting the important role of Trp318(7.35) in peptide binding to MOR.[56] Similarly, in KOR Tyr312(7.35) forms an aromatic interaction with Phe3 of MP16. The smaller size of the binding pocket in KOR relative to that in MOR, owing to extra residues inserted into EL2, prevents the binding of tetrapeptides with bulkier side chain substitutions in the Phe3 position. Indeed, the Trp3 analog of MP16, which cannot be accommodated between Phe214(EL2), Leu309(E3), and Tyr312(7.35) without some side chain and backbone shift, demonstrates decreased affinity.[26] On the other hand, the open space in MOR between the corresponding Phe221(EL2), Thr315(EL3), and Trp318(7.35) is large enough to accommodate the 1-Nal3-containing analog of JOM6, which shows high binding affinity.[148] The μ-, δ-, and κ-selectivity of opioid cyclic tetrapeptides is also largely affected by their C-terminal groups. The C-terminal -COO⁻ of JOM13 forms favorable ionic interaction with Nε⁺ of Lys214(5.39) inside the DOR binding pocket, thus explaining the preference of a C-terminal free carboxylate for δ-selectivity. In the receptor-bound conformations of JOM6 and MP16, their carboxamide groups are spatially shifted closer to Glu210(5.35) of MOR or to Glu297(6.58) of KOR. Therefore, in order to avoid electrostatic repulsion between negatively charged groups, a neutral C-terminus is required for high affinity of μ- and κ- peptides.

The calculated agonist-bound and inactive state models of MOR, DOR, and KOR[26,34,70] were used for subsequent docking of nonpeptide agonists and antagonists, respectively. The ligands were positioned to provide the best overlap of the message tyramine (or tyramine-like) moieties and to satisfy known SAR and key receptor-ligand interactions, starting with the largest rigid ligands. Ligands from each structural class were analyzed separately. To account for the intrinsic flexibility of the receptor an ensemble of 5 to 10 models, calculated with a distinct set of spatial constraints, was used for ligand docking.

All opioid ligands interact with the same binding pocket; however, smaller ligands only partially occupy the available space, leaving some empty areas, which could be filled by several flexible "rotating" side chains from TMs and loops. The key rotating residues in the binding pocket include Asp(3.32), Met(3.36), Trp(6.48), Lys/Trp/Glu(6.58), and Trp/Leu/Tyr(7.35), with most of these being implicated in receptor activation.[56,64,65]

Similar to the cyclic tetrapeptides, nonpeptide agonists form an H-bond and ionic interaction between their amine N+ and the *trans* rotamer of Asp(3.32), and a "stacking" interaction between aromatic tyramine ring and the indole ring of Trp(6.48), which can be slightly adjusted (χ^2~0 ± 20°) to better accommodate different ligands (Fig. 33.4). Unlike peptide ligands, the tyramine hydroxyl of nonpeptide agonists only interacts as an H-donor with backbone -C=O of Ala(5.46) but cannot interact with His(6.52). The functionally important α-hydroxyl or carbonyl at C-6 of opiates can form an H-bond with Lys(5.39) and Tyr(3.33), while a

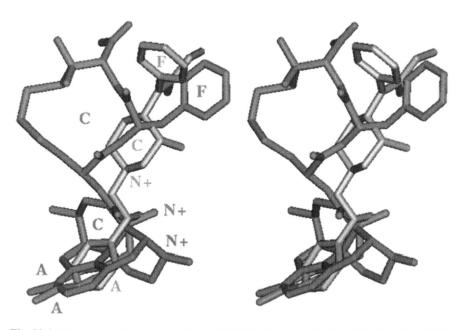

Fig. 33.4 Stereoview of the superposition of JOM6 (dark gray), morphine (black), and cis-2S,2R, 4S-ohmefentanyl (light gray) in the binding pocket of the agonist-bound conformation of MOR. Pharmacophore elements are indicated by N+, A, C, and F.

hydroxyl group at C-14 can form an H-bond with Tyr(3.33). The large aromatic moiety of δ-selective nonpeptide agonists (SIOM, TAN67) interacts with the indole ring of Trp284(6.58) of DOR, which is consistent with the important role of Trp284(6.58) in binding of these ligands, as suggested from DOR mutagenesis.[37,59,60] Morphine and its small analogs can be positioned similarly to the larger opiates. However, in the large MOR binding pocket they can also occupy certain alternative positions. In particular, these different positions can allow the irreversible morphine analogs, MET-CAMO,[149] BAM, or S-activated dihydromorphine derivatives[150] to form a covalent bond with Cys321(7.38). The fentanyl analog, cis-2S,3R,4S-ohmefentanyl, can be positioned in the MOR binding pocket in an extended conformation,[18] with its phenethyl group imitating the tyramine part of opiates and peptides, and its 4-phenylpropanamide, forming aromatic interactions with Trp318(7.35), similar to Phe3 of peptides. Positioned this way, the fentanyl analog's N+ can form an ionic interaction with Asp147(3.32) and an H-bond with Tyr148(3.33), while its 2~OH can form an H-bond with Tyr148(3.33). A similar arrangement of this fentanyl analog in MOR has been proposed[57] based on mutagenesis data.[57,58]

The comparison of the agonist-bound MOR[70] with our previously calculated inactive MOR[34] reveals that the major changes in the binding pocket are related to the side chain rotation of Trp293(6.48) from a rotamer with $\chi^1 \sim -60°$, $\chi^2 \sim 90°$ to a rotamer with $\chi^1 \sim -60°$ and $\chi^2 \sim 0°$ (Fig. 33.5). As a result, the indole ring of Trp293(6.48) relocates from the interface between TMs 6 to 7 to the interface between TMs 3 to 5–6, where it can form a "stacking" interaction with the aromatic ring of Tyr1 of JOM6.

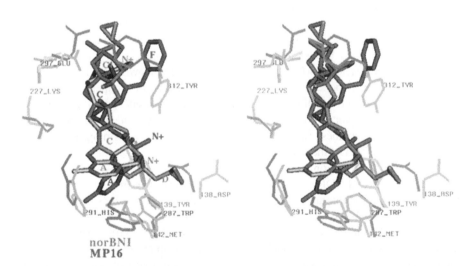

norBNI
MP16

Fig. 33.5 Stereoview of the superposition of MP16 in the binding pocket of the agonist-bound conformation of KOR (red) and norBNI in the binding pocket of the antagonist-bound conformation of KOR (blue). Only ligands and several important residues from MOR: Asp138(3.32), Tyr139(3.33), Met142(3.35), Lys227(5.39), Trp287(6.48), His291(6.52), Glu297(6.58), and Tyr312(7.35) are shown. Pharmacophore elements are indicated by N+, A, C, C1, and F. (*See* also Color Insert).

The agonist-induced Trp293(6.48) reorientation in MOR triggers a large TM6 rotation and shift, correlated reorientation of the Met151(3.35) side chain, ligand-dependent reorientations of the side chains of Asp147(3.32), Lys233(5.39), Lys303(6.35), and Trp318(7.35), and readjustment of some other helix positions. The important role of Trp(6.48) in the activation mechanism has been proposed previously based on muta-genesis data and on the experimentally documented movement of this side chain in photoactivated rhodopsin and in agonist-activated leukotriene receptors.[116,151-153] Of interest, the incorporation of different active state-specific experimental distance constraints between TMs 5 to 6[131,132] produced 5 different active conformations with deviation for the residues at the cytoplasmic ends of TM6 ranging from 7 to 11 Å, relative to the model of the inactive conformation.[34] Such flexibility of TM6 in the active conformation is consistent with the existence of ligand-dependent conforma-tional substates, which have been observed upon binding of different agonists, antagonists, and inverse agonists to DOR[123-126] and other GPCRs.[107,113,121,122]

Inactive and agonist-bound bound states of receptor also differ in the relative posi-tion of 2 key residues, Asp(3.32) and His(6.52), the suggested partners for the tyramine moiety of opioid ligands. In the inactive state Asp(3.32) assumes a *gauche+* rotamer ($\chi^1 \sim -60°$), which, instead of forming an H-bond/ionic interaction with the protonated amine of the ligand, participates in the formation of several H-bonds between residues of TMs 2, 3, 7: Thr(2.56), Gln(2.60), and Tyr(7.43). This H-bond network stabilizes the inactive receptor state. Indeed, D(3.32)N and D(3.32)K mutants that are incompat-ible with this H-bond network demonstrated increased constitutive activity.[44,62] In place of the agonist amine interaction with Asp(3.32), the positively charged amine of antagonists can instead form amine-aromatic interactions with the proximal Tyr(3.33), which is in agreement with the observed important role of this residue for ligand bind-ing.[43] In the inactive state of ORs, His(6.52) is located between TM6 and TM3, form-ing H-bond and van der Waals interactions with the tyramine moiety of antagonists. In the agonist-bound state, His(6.52) is shifted toward TM5 owing to TM6 rotation, which breaks the H-bond with the tyramine hydroxyl of nonpeptide agonists. Moreover, in the inactive or ligand-free receptor states Trp/Leu/Tyr(7.35) can be ori-ented inside the receptor ($\chi^1 \sim 180°$), filling the binding cavity, while in the presence of large peptide agonists these residues are reoriented ($\chi^1 \sim -60°$), forming hydrophobic interactions with Phe3 of the peptides (see above).

The comparison of agonist and antagonist positioning in the agonist-bound and the antagonist-bound KOR conformations is demonstrated in Fig. 33 5. Because of the differences in the interaction of the ligands with the key residues Asp138(3.32), Trp287(6.48), His291(6.52), and Tyr312(7.35), the antagonist norBNI is placed with its amine N+ shifted more deeply into the pocket relative to MP16. The antagonist activity of morphine analogs is usually associated with an N-allyl or N-cyclopropyl-methyl substituent on this amine N+, while an N-methyl substituent is associated with agonists.[154] Because of added steric bulk and the deeper positioning in the pocket, the N-cyclopropylmethyl group of norBNI locks Asp138(3.32) and indole ring of Trp287(6.48) in the "inactive" orientations. Moreover, the central part of the "address" moiety of norBNI, which overlaps with the cyclic ring of tetrapeptides, forms favorable hydrophobic interactions with the *trans* (ie, inactive) rotamer of

Tyr312(7.35), while its N-17 basic nitrogen forms an ionic interaction with Glu297(6.58), consistent with experimental observations.[61]

Such models of agonist and antagonist interactions with ORs can explain the observed larger effect of His(6.52) mutations and smaller effect of the D147A mutation on the binding of antagonists compared with agonists.[42,45] These models also provide a rationale for the recent observations that elimination of the N-terminal amino group converts several peptide agonists to antagonists.[155]

The analysis of modes of docking of peptide and nonpeptide agonists and antagonists into ORs using 3-D structures of ligands and receptors provides unique insights into pharmacophore features of agonists and antagonists. The key pharmacophore elements for agonist binding, found from superposition of peptide and nonpeptide agonists inside the receptor binding pocket (Figs. 33.3 and 33.4), include (1) positively charged amine ("N+") interacting with Asp(3.32) and, for peptides, with Tyr(3.33); (2) aromatic ring of tyramine ("A") forming "stacking" interactions with Trp(6.48); (3) the central hydrophobic core ("C") interacting with TM6 residues; and (4) the second aromatic ring ("F"). The aromatic ring "F" in μ-agonists forms essential aromatic interactions with Trp318(7.35). In κ-agonists, ring "F" can be smaller, because the corresponding space in KOR near Tyr312(7.35) is smaller and more polar. In δ-agonists, ring "F" may be shifted or may extend the central hydrophobic region (to "C1"), in order to form aromatic interactions with Trp284(6.58), which serves as the functional counterpart to Trp318(7.35) of MOR. The presence of polar groups (eg, hydroxyl of tyramine, hydroxyl or carbonyl at C-6, C-14 in opiates, 2'-OH of ohmefentanyl) can additionally contribute to the binding affinity of agonists. The key pharmacophore elements for antagonists (Figs. 33.1 and 33.5) include (1) positively charged ("N+") forming weaker ionic interactions with the more distant Asp(3.32) and amine-aromatic interactions with Tyr(3.33); (2) phenolic ring ("A") forming H-bond with His(6.52); (3) the central hydrophobic core ("C") contacting residues from TM3 and TM6; and (4) additional hydrophobic elements near N+ ("D"), which can lock Trp(6.48) in the "inactive" orientation. The presence of polar groups (hydroxyl at C-14, positively charged groups for κ-ligands) or an aromatic moiety ("C1") for δ-ligands can additionally contribute to antagonist binding affinity.

In contrast to previously developed ligand-based pharmacophore models of opioid ligands[156-159] these ligand and receptor-derived pharmacophore models not only clarify the available SAR of agonists and antagonists but suggest the role of specific ligand groups in the context of receptor structure and provide novel insights into aspects of the receptor environment that have not been previously explored.

Conclusions

The examples presented above demonstrate that accurate models of MOR, DOR, and KOR can be obtained using homology modeling based on the crystal structure of rhodopsin and distance geometry refinement with experimentally-derived constraints. Experimental information is required to verify the problematic areas, such as helix distortions and divergent extracellular loops included in the binding pocket. The incorporation of available constraints appropriate for distinct functional receptor states allows modeling of the inactive and agonist-activated receptor conformations separately. Accurate ligand docking guided by experimental ligand-receptor restraints helps explain the known SAR of opioid ligands and the differences between ligand-receptor interactions of peptide and nonpeptide agonists, as well as between agonists and antagonists. The resulting more complete and more contextual ligand and receptor-based pharmacophore models of agonists and antagonists should provide considerable advantages for rational design of compounds directed toward specific physiological responses.

Acknowledgments The authors are grateful to Dr Andrei Lomize for helpful discussions. These studies were supported by grant DA03910 from the National Institute on Drug Abuse (HIM) and University of Michigan College of Pharmacy Upjohn Research Award (IP).

References

1. Kieffer BL. Recent advances in molecular recognition and signal transduction of active peptides: receptors for opioid peptides. *Cell Mol Neurobiol*. 1995;15:615-635.
2. Waldhoer M, Bartlett SE, Whistler JL. Opioid receptors. *Annu Rev Biochem*. 2004;73:953-990.
3. Pasternak GW. Multiple opiate receptors: déjà vu all over again. *Neuropharmacology*. 2004;47:312-323.
4. Vaccarino AL, Kastin AJ. Endogenous opiates: 2000. *Peptides*. 2001;22:2257-2328.
5. Hruby VJ, Agnes RS. Conformation-activity relationships of opioid peptides with selective activities at opioid receptors. *Biopolymers*. 1999;51:391-410.
6. Mansour A, Hoversten MT, Taylor LP, Watson SJ, Akil H. The cloned mu, delta and kappa receptors and their endogenous ligands: evidence for two opioid peptide recognition cores. *Brain Res*. 1995;700:89-98.
7. Mosberg HI, Hurst R, Hruby VJ, et al. Conformationally constrained cyclic enkephalin analogs with pronounced delta opioid receptor agonist selectivity. *Life Sci*. 1983;32:2565-2569.
8. Pelton JT, Gulya K, Hruby VJ, Duckles S, Yamamura HI. Somatostatin analogs with affinity for opiate receptors in rat brain binding assay. *Peptides*. 1985;6:159-163.
9. Pelton JT, Kazmierski W, Gulya K, Yamamura HI, Hruby VJ. Design and synthesis of conformationally constrained somatostatin analogues with high potency and specificity for mu opioid receptors. *J Med Chem*. 1986;29:2370-2375.
10. Kawasaki AM, Knapp RJ, Walton A, et al. Syntheses, opioid binding affinities, and potencies of dynorphin A analogues substituted in positions 1, 6, 7, 8, and 10. *Int J Pept Protein Res*. 1993;42:411-419.
11. Meyer JP, Collins N, Lung FD, et al. Design, synthesis, and biological properties of highly potent cyclic dynorphin A analogues: analogues cyclized between positions 5 and 11. *J Med Chem*. 1994;37:3910-3917.
12. Arttamangkul S, Murray TF, DeLander GE, Aldrich JV. Synthesis and opioid activity of conformationally constrained dynorphin A analogues. 1. Conformational constraint in the "message" sequence. *J Med Chem*. 1995;38:2410-2417.
13. Lung FD, Collins N, Stropova D, et al. Design, synthesis, and biological activities of cyclic lactam peptide analogues of dynorphin A(1–11)-NH2. *J Med Chem*. 1996;39:1136-1141.

14. Eguchi M. Recent advances in selective opioid receptor agonists and antagonists. *Med Res Rev.* 2004;24:182-212.
15. Okada T, Ernst OP, Palczewski K, Hofmann KP. Activation of rhodopsin: new insights from structural and biochemical studies. *Trends Biochem Sci.* 2001;26:318-324.
16. Li J, Edwards PC, Burghammer M, Villa C, Schertler GF. Structure of bovine rhodopsin in a trigonal crystal form. *J Mol Biol.* 2004;343:1409-1438.
17. Flower DR. Modeling G-protein-coupled receptors for drug design. *Biochim Biophys Acta.* 1999;1422:207-234.
18. Flippen-Anderson JL, George C, Bertha CM, Rice KC. X-ray structure of potent opioid receptor ligands: etonitazene, cis-(+)-3-methylfentanyl, etorphine, diprenorphine, and buprenorphine. *Heterocycles.* 1994;39:751-766.
19. Urbanczyk-Lipkowska Z, Etter MC, Lipkowski AW, Portoghese PS. The crystal structure of a bimorphinan with highly selective kappa opioid receptor antagonist activity. *J Mol Struct.* 1987;159:287-295.
20. Griffin JF, Larson DL, Portoghese PS. Crystal structures of alpha- and beta-funaltrexamine: conformational requirement of the fumaramate moiety in the irreversible blockage of mu opioid receptors. *J Med Chem.* 1986;29:778-783.
21. Calderon SN, Rice KC, Rothman RB, et al. Probes for narcotic receptor mediated phenomena. 23. Synthesis, opioid receptor binding, and bioassay of the highly selective delta agonist (+)-4-[(alpha R)-alpha-((2S,5R)-4-Allyl-2,5-dimethyl-1-piperazinyl)-3-methoxybenzyl]-N,N-diethylbenzamide (SNC 80) and related novel nonpeptide delta opioid receptor ligands. *J Med Chem.* 1997;40:695-704.
22. Lavecchia A, Greco G, Novellino E, Vittorio F, Ronsisvalle G. Modeling of kappa-opioid receptor/agonists interactions using pharmacophore-based and docking simulations. *J Med Chem.* 2000;43:2124-2134.
23. Doi M, Ishida T, Inoue M. Conformational characteristics of opioid kappa-receptor agonist: crystal structure of (5S,7S,8S)-(-)-N-methyl-N-[7-(1-pyrrolidinyl)-1-oxaspiro[4.5]dec-8-yl]benzeneacetamide (U69,593), and conformational comparison with some kappa-agonists. *Chem Pharm Bull (Tokyo).* 1990;38:1815-1818.
24. Subramanian G, Patrelini MG, Portoghese PS, Ferguson DM. Molecular docking reveals a novel binding site model for fentanyl at the mu-opioid receptor. *J Med Chem.* 2000;43:381-391.
25. Mosberg HI, Fowler CB. Development and validation of opioid ligand-receptor interaction models: the structural basis of mu vs delta selectivity. *J Pept Res.* 2002;60:329-335.
26. Przydzial MJ, Pogozheva ID, Andrews SM, et al. Roles of residues 3 and 4 in cyclic tetrapeptide ligand recognition by the κ-opioid receptor. *J Pept Res.* 2005;65:333-342.
27. Mosberg HI, Omnaas JR, Medzihradsky F, Smith CB. Cyclic, disulfide- and dithioether-containing opioid tetrapeptides: development of a ligand with high delta opioid receptor selectivity and affinity. *Life Sci.* 1988;43:1013-1020.
28. Mosberg HI, Lomize AL, Wang C, et al. Development of a model for the δ-opioid receptor pharmacophore. 1. Conformationally restricted Tyr[1] replacements in the cyclic δ receptor selective tetrapeptide Tyr-c[D-Cys-Phe-D-Pen]OH (JOM-13). *J Med Chem.* 1994a ;37:4371-4383.
29. Mosberg HI, Omnaas JR, Lomize A, et al. Development of a model for the δ-opioid receptor pharmacophore. 2. Conformationally restricted Phe[3] replacements in the cyclic δ-receptor selective tetrapeptide Tyr-c[D-Cys-Phe-D-Pen]OH (JOM-13). *J Med Chem.* 1994b; 37:4384-4391.
30. Mosberg HI, Dua RK, Pogozheva ID, Lomize AL. Development of a model for the δ-opioid receptor pharmacophore. 4. Residue 3 dehydrophenyl-alanine analogs of Tyr-c[D-Cys-Phe-D-Pen]OH (JOM-13) confirm required gauche orientation of aromatic sidechain. *Biopolymers.* 1996;39:287-296.
31. Lomize AL, Flippen-Anderson JL, George C, Mosberg HI. Conformational analysis of the δ receptor-selective, cyclic opioid peptide,Tyr-c[D-Cys-Phe-D-Pen]OH(JOM-13): comparison of X-ray crystallographic structures, molecular mechanics simulations and ^{1}H NMR data. *J Am Chem Soc.* 1994;116:429-436.

32. Ho JC. *Development of a Model for the δ-opioid Receptor Pharmacophore [dissertation].* [thesis]. Ann Arbor, MI: University of Michigan; 1997.

33. McFadyen IJ, Ho JC, Mosberg HI, Traynor JR. Modifications of the cyclic mu receptor selective tetrapeptide Tyr-c[D-Cys-Phe-D-Pen]NH2 (Et): effects on opioid receptor binding and activation. *J Pept Res.* 2000;55:255-261.

34. Fowler CB, III, Pogozheva ID, III, Lomize AL, III, LeVine H, III, Mosberg HI. Complex of an active μ-opioid receptor with cyclic peptide agonist modeled from experimental constraints. *Biochemistry.* 2004a ;43:15796-15810.

35. Mosberg HI. Complementarity of delta opioid ligand pharmacophore and receptor models. *Biopolymers.* 1999;51:426-439.

36. Law PY, Loh HH. Regulation of opioid receptor activities. *J Pharmacol Exp Ther.* 1999;289:607-624.

37. Chaturvedi K, Christoffers KH, Singh K, Howells RD. Structure and regulation of opioid receptors. *Biopolymers.* 2000;55:334-346.

38. Chavkin C, McLaughlin JP, Celver JP. Regulation of opioid receptor function by chronic agonist exposure: constitutive activity and desensitization. *Mol Pharmacol.* 2001;60:20-25.

39. Coward P, Wada HG, Falk MS, et al. Controlling signaling with a specifically designed Gi-coupled receptor. *Proc Natl Acad Sci USA.* 1998;95:352-357.

40. Pogozheva ID, Lomize AL, Mosberg HI. Opioid receptor 3-dimensional structures from distance geometry calculations with hydrogen bonding constraints. *Biophys J.* 1998;75:612-634.

41. Surratt CK, Johnson PS, Moriwaki A, et al. Mu opiate receptor: charged transmembrane domain amino acids are critical for agonist recognition and intrinsic activity. *J Biol Chem.* 1994;269:20548-20553.

42. Befort K, Tabbara L, Bausch S, Chavkin C, Evans C, Kieffer BL. The conserved aspartate residue in the third putative transmembrane domain of the delta-opioid receptor is not the anionic counterpart for cationic opiate binding but is a constituent of the receptor binding site. *Mol Pharmacol.* 1996a;49:216-223.

43. Befort K, Tabbara L, Kling D, Maigret B, Kieffer BL. Role of aromatic transmembrane residues of the delta-opioid receptor in ligand recognition. *J Biol Chem.* 1996b;271:10161-10168.

44. Befort K, Zilliox C, Filliol D, Yue S, Kieffer BL. Constitutive activation of the delta opioid receptor by mutations in transmembrane domains III and VII. *J Biol Chem.* 1999;274:18574-18581.

45. Bot G, Blake AD, Li S, Reisine T. Mutagenesis of the mouse delta opioid receptor converts (-)-buprenorphine from a partial agonist to an antagonist. *J Pharmacol Exp Ther.* 1998a; 284:283-290.

46. Bot G, Blake AD, Li S, Reisine T. Mutagenesis of a single amino acid in the rat mu-opioid receptor discriminates ligand binding. *J Neurochem.* 1998b ;70:358-365.

47. Spivak CE, Beglan CL, Seidleck BK, et al. Naloxone activation of mu-opioid receptors mutated at a histidine residue lining the opioid binding cavity. *Mol Pharmacol.* 1997;52:983-992.

48. Mansour A, Taylor LP, Fine JL, et al. Key residues defining the mu-opioid receptor binding pocket: a site-directed mutagenesis study. *J Neurochem.* 1997;68:344–353.

49. Meng F, Ueda Y, Hoversten MT, et al. Creating a functional opioid alkaloid binding site in the orphanin FQ receptor through site-directed mutagenesis. *Mol Pharmacol.* 1998;53:772-777.

50. Li JG, Chen C, Yin J, et al. ASP147 in the third transmembrane helix of the rat mu opioid receptor forms ion-pairing with morphine and naltrexone. *Life Sci.* 1999;65:175-185.

51. Fukuda K, Terasako K, Kato S, Mori K. Identification of the amino acid residues involved in selective agonist binding in the first extracellular loop of the delta- and mu-opioid receptors. *FEBS Lett.* 1995;373:177-181.

52. Minami M, Onogi T, Nakagawa T, et al. DAMGO, a mu-opioid receptor selective ligand, distinguishes between mu-and kappa-opioid receptors at a different region from that for the distinction between mu- and delta-opioid receptors. *FEBS Lett.* 1995;364:23-27.

53. Wang JB, Johnson PS, Wu JM, Wang WF, Uhl GR. Human kappa opiate receptor second extracellular loop elevates dynorphin's affinity for human mu/kappa chimeras. *J Biol Chem.* 1994;269:25966-25969.
54. Xue JC, Chen C, Zhu J, et al. Differential binding domains of peptide and non-peptide ligands in the cloned rat kappa opioid receptor. *J Biol Chem.* 1994;269:30195-30199.
55. Ferguson DM, Kramer S, Metzger TG, Law PY, Portoghese PS. Isosteric replacement of acidic with neutral residues in extracellular loop-2 of the kappa-opioid receptor does not affect dynorphin A(1–13) affinity and function. *J Med Chem.* 2000;43:1251-1252.
56. Bonner G, Meng F, Akil H. Selectivity of mu-opioid receptor determined by interfacial residues near third extracellular loop. *Eur J Pharmacol.* 2000;403:37-44.
57. Xu H, Lu YF, Partilla JS, et al. Opioid peptide receptor studies. 11. Involvement of Tyr148, Trp318 and His319 of the rat mu-opioid receptor in binding of mu-selective ligands. *Synapse.* 1999;32:23-28.
58. Ulens C, Van Boven M, Daenens P, Tytgat J. Interaction of p-fluorofentanyl on cloned human opioid receptors and exploration of the role of Trp-318 and His-319 in mu-opioid receptor selectivity. *J Pharmacol Exp Ther.* 2000;294:1024-1033.
59. Pepin MC, Yue SY, Roberts E, Wahlestedt C, Walker P. Novel "restoration of function" mutagenesis strategy to identify amino acids of the delta-opioid receptor involved in ligand binding. *J Biol Chem.* 1997;272:9260-9267.
60. Valiquette M, Vu HK, Yue SY, Wahlestedt C, Walker P. Involvement of Trp-284, Val-296, and Val-297 of the human delta-opioid receptor in binding of delta-selective ligands. *J Biol Chem.* 1996;271:18789-18796.
61. Hjorth SA, Thirstrup K, Grandy DK, Schwartz TW. Analysis of selective binding epitopes for the kappa-opioid receptor antagonist nor-binaltorphimine. *Mol Pharmacol.* 1995;47:1089-1094.
62. Cavalli A, Babey AM, Loh HH. Altered adenylyl cyclase responsiveness subsequent to point mutations of Asp 128 in the third transmembrane domain of the delta-opioid receptor. *Neuroscience.* 1999;93:1025-1031.
63. Li J, Huang P, Chen C, de Riel JK, Weinstein H, Liu-Chen LY. Constitutive activation of the mu opioid receptor by mutation of D3.49(164), but not D3.32(147): D3.49(164) is critical for stabilization of the inactive form of the receptor and for its expression. *Biochemistry.* 2001;40:12039-12050.
64. Mouledous L, Topham CM, Moisand C, Mollereau C, Meunier JC. Functional inactivation of the nociceptin receptor by alanine substitution of glutamine 286 at the C terminus of transmembrane segment VI: evidence from a site-directed mutagenesis study of the ORL1 receptor transmembrane-binding domain. *Mol Pharmacol.* 2000;57:495-502.
65. DeCaillot FM, Befort K, Filliol D, Yue S, Walker P, Kieffer BL. Opioid receptor random mutagenesis reveals a mechanism for G protein-coupled receptor activation. *Nat Struct Biol.* 2003;10:629-636.
66. Spivak CE, Beglan CL, Zollner C, Surratt CK. Beta-Funaltrexamine, a gauge for the recognition site of wildtype and mutant H297Q mu-opioid receptors. *Synapse.* 2003;49:55-60.
67. Chen C, Yin J, Riel JK, et al. Determination of the amino acid residue involved in [3H]beta-funaltrexamine covalent binding in the cloned rat mu-opioid receptor. *J Biol Chem.* 1996;271:21422-21429.
68. Jones RM, Hjorth SA, Schwartz TW, Portoghese PS. Mutational evidence for a common kappa antagonist binding pocket in the wild-type kappa and mutant mu[K303E] opioid receptors. *J Med Chem.* 1998;41:4911-4914.
69. Larson DL, Jones RM, Hjorth SA, Schwartz TW, Portoghese PS. Binding of norbinaltorphimine (norBNI) congeners to wild-type and mutant mu and kappa opioid receptors: molecular recognition loci for the pharmacophore and address components of kappa antagonists. *J Med Chem.* 2000;43:1573-1576.
70. Fowler CB, III, Pogozheva ID, III, LeVine H, III, Mosberg HI. Refinement of a homology model of the μ-opioid receptor using distance constraints from intrinsic and engineered zinc-binding sites. *Biochemistry.* 2004b ;43:8700-8710.

71. Metzger TG, Paterlini MG, Portoghese PS, Ferguson DM. An analysis of the conserved residues between halobacterial retinal proteins and G-protein coupled receptors: implications for GPCR modeling. *J Chem Inf Comput Sci.* 1996;36:857-861.
72. Strahs D, Weinstein H. Comparative modeling and molecular dynamics studies of the delta, kappa and mu opioid receptors. *Protein Eng.* 1997;10:1019-1038.
73. Alkorta I, Loew GH. A 3D model of the delta opioid receptor and ligand-receptor complexes. *Protein Eng.* 1996;9:573-583.
74. Subramanian G, Paterlini MG, Larson DL, Portoghese PS, Ferguson DM. Conformational analysis and automated receptor docking of selective arylacetamide-based kappa-opioid agonists. *J Med Chem.* 1998;41:4777-4789.
75. Paterlini G, Portoghese PS, Ferguson DM. Molecular simulation of dynorphin A-(1–10) binding to extracellular loop 2 of the kappa-opioid receptor: a model for receptor activation. *J Med Chem.* 1997;40:3254-3262.
76. Filizola M, Laakkonen L, Loew GH. 3D modeling, ligand binding and activation studies of the cloned mouse delta, mu, and kappa opioid receptors. *Protein Eng.* 1999a ;12:927-942.
77. Filizola M, Carteni-Farina M, Perez JJ. Molecular modeling study of the differential ligand-receptor interaction at the mu, delta and kappa opioid receptors. *J Comput Aided Mol Des.* 1999b ;13:397-407.
78. Pogozheva ID, Lomize AL, Mosberg HI. The transmembrane 7 alpha-bundle of rhodopsin: distance geometry calculations with hydrogen bonding constraints. *Biophys J.* 1997;72:1963-1985.
79. Lomize AL, Pogozheva ID, Mosberg HI. Structural organization of G-protein-coupled receptors. *J Comput Aided Mol Des.* 1999;13:325-353.
80. Vaidehi N, Floriano WB, Trabanino R, et al. Prediction of structure and function of G protein-coupled receptors. *Proc Natl Acad Sci USA.* 2002;99:12622-12627.
81. Shacham S, Topf M, Avisar N, et al. Modeling the 3D structure of GPCRs from sequence. *Med Res Rev.* 2001;21:472-483.
82. Shi L, Javitch JA. The binding site of aminergic G protein-coupled receptors: the transmembrane segments and second extracellular loop. *Annu Rev Pharmacol Toxicol.* 2002;42:437-467.
83. Lawson Z, Wheatley M. The third extracellular loop of G-protein-coupled receptors: more than just a linker between 2 important transmembrane helices. *Biochem Soc Trans.* 2004;32:1048-1050.
84. Baker D, Sali A. Protein structure prediction and structural genomics. *Science.* 2001;294:93-96.
85. Palczewski K, Kumasaka T, Hori T, et al. Crystal structure of rhodopsin: a G protein-coupled receptor. *Science.* 2000;289:739-745.
86. Ballesteros JA, Shi L, Javitch JA. Structural mimicry in G protein-coupled receptors: implications of the high-resolution structure of rhodopsin for structure-function analysis of rhodopsin-like receptors. *Mol Pharmacol.* 2001;60:1-19.
87. Klabunde T, Hessler G. Drug design strategies for targeting G-protein-coupled receptors. *ChemBioChem.* 2002;3:928-944.
88. Bissantz C, Bernard P, Hibert M, Rognan D. Protein-based virtual screening of chemical databases. II. Are homology models of G-protein coupled receptors suitable targets? *Proteins.* 2003;50:5-25.
89. Evers A, Klebe G. Ligand-supported homology modeling of g-protein-coupled receptor sites: models sufficient for successful virtual screening. *Angew Chem Int Ed Engl.* 2004a ;43:248-251.
90. Horn F, Bettler E, Oliveira L, Campagne F, Cohen FE, Vriend G. GPCRDB information system for G protein-coupled receptors. *Nucleic Acids Res.* 2003;31:294-297.
91. Huang P, Li J, Chen C, Visiers I, Weinstein H, Liu-Chen LY. Functional role of a conserved motif in TM6 of the rat mu opioid receptor: constitutively active and inactive receptors result from substitutions of Thr6.34(279) with Lys and Asp. *Biochemistry.* 2001;40:13501-13509.
92. Sali A, Blundell TL. Comparative protein modeling by satisfaction of spatial restraints. *J Mol Biol.* 1993;234:779-815.

93. Fiser A, Sali A. Modeller: generation and refinement of homology-based protein structure models. *Methods Enzymol*. 2003;374:461-491.
94. Peitsch MC. ProMod and Swiss-Model: internet-based tools for automated comparative protein modelling. *Biochem Soc Trans*. 1996;24:274-279.
95. Lund O, Frimand K, Gorodkin J, et al. Protein distance constraints predicted by neural networks and probability density functions. *Protein Eng*. 1997;10:1241-1248.
96. 96. ShindyalovIN, BournePE. Improving alignments in HM protocol with intermediate sequences. In: Forth Meeting on the Critical Assessment of Techniques for Protein Structure Prediction; 2000: A-92.
97. Lambert C, Leonard N, De Bolle X, Depiereux E. ESyPred3D: prediction of proteins 3D structures. *Bioinformatics*. 2002;18:1250-1256.
98. Kim DE, Chivian D, Baker D. Protein structure prediction and analysis using the Robetta server. *Nucleic Acids Res*. 2004;32:W526-W531.
99. Pieper U, Eswar N, Braberg H, et al. MODBASE, a database of annotated comparative protein structure models, and associated resources. *Nucleic Acids Res*. 2004;32:D217-D222.
100. Eswar N, John B, Mirkovic N, et al. Tools for comparative protein structure modeling and analysis. *Nucleic Acids Res*. 2003;31:3375-3380.
101. John B, Sali A. Comparative protein structure modeling by iterative alignment, model building and model assessment. *Nucleic Acids Res*. 2003;31:3982-3992.
102. Riek RP, Rigoutsos I, Novotny J, Graham RM. Non-alpha-helical elements modulate polytopic membrane protein architecture. *J Mol Biol*. 2001;306:349-362.
103. Fiser A, Do RK, Sali A. Modeling of loops in protein structures. *Protein Sci*. 2000;9:1753-1773.
104. Chothia C, Lesk AM. Helix movements and the reconstruction of the haem pocket during the evolution of the cytochrome c family. *J Mol Biol*. 1985;182:151-158.
105 Meng EC, Bourne HR. Receptor activation: what does the rhodopsin structure tell us? *Trends Pharmacol Sci*. 2001;22:587-593.
106. Karnik SS, Gogonea C, Patil S, Saad Y, Takezako T. Activation of G-protein-coupled receptors: a common molecular mechanism. *Trends Endocrinol Metab*. 2003;14:431-437.
107. Ghanouni P, Steenhuis JJ, Farrens DL, Kobilka BK. Agonist-induced conformational changes in the G-protein-coupling domain of the beta 2 adrenergic receptor. *Proc Natl Acad Sci USA*. 2001a;98:5997-6002.
108. Farrens DL, Altenbach C, Yang K, Hubbell WL, Khorana HG. Requirement of rigid-body motion of transmembrane helices for light activation of rhodopsin. *Science*. 1996;274:768-770.
109. Gether U, Lin S, Ghanouni P, Ballesteros JA, Weinstein H, Kobilka BK. Agonists induce conformational changes in transmembrane domains III and VI of the beta2 adrenoceptor. *EMBO J*. 1997;16:6737-6747.
110. Dunham TD, Farrens DL. Conformational changes in rhodopsin: movement of helix F detected by site-specific chemical labeling and fluorescence spectroscopy. *J Biol Chem*. 1999;274:1683-1690.
111. Han M, Smith SO, Sakmar TP. Constitutive activation of opsin by mutation of methionine 257 on transmembrane helix 6. *Biochemistry*. 1998;37:8253-8261.
112. Cai K, Klein-Seetharaman J, Hwa J, Hubbell WL, Khorana HG. Structure and function in rhodopsin: effects of disulfide cross-links in the cytoplasmic face of rhodopsin on transducin activation and phosphorylation by rhodopsin kinase. *Biochemistry*. 1999;38:12893-12898.
113. Ghanouni P, Gryczynski Z, Steenhuis JJ, et al. Functionally different agonists induce distinct conformations in the G protein coupling domain of the beta 2 adrenergic receptor. *J Biol Chem*. 2001b;276:24433-24436.
114. Janz JM, Farrens DL. Rhodopsin activation exposes a key hydrophobic binding site for the transducin alpha-subunit C terminus. *J Biol Chem*. 2004;279:29767-29773.
115. Hubbell WL, Altenbach C, Hubbell CM, Khorana HG. Rhodopsin structure, dynamics, and activation: a perspective from crystallography, site-directed spin labeling, sulfhydryl reactivity, and disulfide cross-linking. *Adv Protein Chem*. 2003;63:243-290.

116. Lin SW, Sakmar TP. Specific tryptophan UV-absorbance changes are probes of the transition of rhodopsin to its active state. *Biochemistry*. 1996;35:11149-11159.

117. Altenbach C, Cai K, Khorana HG, Hubbell WL. Structural features and light-dependent changes in the sequence 306–322 extending from helix VII to the palmitoylation sites in rhodopsin: a site-directed spin-labeling study. *Biochemistry*. 1999a;38:7931-7937.

118. Altenbach C, Klein-Seetharaman J, Hwa J, Khorana HG, Hubbell WL. Structural features and light-dependent changes in the sequence 59–75 connecting helices I and II in rhodopsin: a site-directed spin-labeling study. *Biochemistry*. 1999b;38:7945-7949.

119. Altenbach C, Cai K, Klein-Seetharaman J, Khorana HG, Hubbell WL. Structure and function in rhodopsin: mapping light-dependent changes in distance between residue 65 in helix TM1 and residues in the sequence 306–319 at the cytoplasmic end of helix TM7 and in helix H8. *Biochemistry*. 2001a ;40:15483-15492.

120 Altenbach C, Klein-Seetharaman J, Cai K, Khorana HG, Hubbell WL. Structure and function in rhodopsin: mapping light-dependent changes in distance between residue 316 in helix 8 and residues in the sequence 60–75, covering the cytoplasmic end of helices TM1 and TM2 and their connection loop CL1. *Biochemistry*. 2001b ;40:15493-15500.

121. Gether U, Kobilka BK. G protein-coupled receptors. II. Mechanism of agonist activation. *J Biol Chem*. 1998;273:17979-17982.

122. Devanathan S, Yao Z, Salamon Z, Kobilka B, Tollin G. Plasmon-waveguide resonance studies of ligand binding to the human beta 2-adrenergic receptor. *Biochemistry*. 2004;43:3280-3288.

123. Salamon Z, Cowell S, Varga E, Yamamura HI, Hruby VJ, Tollin G. Plasmon resonance studies of agonist/antagonist binding to the human delta-opioid receptor: new structural insights into receptor-ligand interactions. *Biophys J*. 2000;79:2463-2474.

124. Salamon Z, Hruby VJ, Tollin G, Cowell S. Binding of agonists, antagonists and inverse agonists to the human delta-opioid receptor produces distinctly different conformational states distinguishable by plasmon-waveguide resonance spectroscopy. *J Pept Res*. 2002;60:322-328.

125. Alves ID, Ciano KA, Boguslavski V, et al. Selectivity, cooperativity, and reciprocity in the interactions between the delta-opioid receptor, its ligands, and G-proteins. *J Biol Chem*. 2004a;279:44673-44682.

126. Alves ID, Cowell SM, Salamon Z, Devanathan S, Tollin G, Hruby VJ. Different structural states of the proteolipid membrane are produced by ligand binding to the human delta-opioid receptor as shown by plasmon-waveguide resonance spectroscopy. *Mol Pharmacol*. 2004b; 65:1248-1257.

127. Tramontano A, Morea V. Exploiting evolutionary relationships for predicting protein structures. *Biotechnol Bioeng*. 2003;84:756-762.

128. Bates PA, Kelley LA, MacCallum RM, Sternberg MJ. Enhancement of protein modeling by human intervention in applying the automatic programs 3D-JIGSAW and 3D-PSSM. *Proteins*. 2001;39-46.

129. Li X, Jacobson MP, Friesner RA. High-resolution prediction of protein helix positions and orientations. *Proteins*. 2004;55:368-382.

130. Evers A, Gohlke H, Klebe G. Ligand-supported homology modelling of protein binding-sites using knowledge-based potentials. *J Mol Biol*. 2003;334:327-345.

131. Ward SD, Hamdan FF, Bloodworth LM, Wess J. Conformational changes that occur during M3 muscarinic acetylcholine receptor activation probed by the use of an in situ disulfide cross-linking strategy. *J Biol Chem*. 2002;277:2247-2257.

132. Swaminath G, Lee TW, Kobilka B. Identification of an allosteric binding site for Zn^{2+} on the beta2 adrenergic receptor. *J Biol Chem*. 2003;278:352-356.

133. Elling CE, Thirstrup K, Holst B, Schwartz TW. Conversion of agonist site to metal-ion chelator site in the beta(2)-adrenergic receptor. *Proc Natl Acad Sci USA*. 1999;96:12322-12327.

134. Holst B, Elling CE, Schwartz TW. Partial agonism through a zinc-ion switch constructed between transmembrane domains III and VII in the tachykinin NK(1) receptor. *Mol Pharmacol*. 2000;58:263-270.

135. Lagerstrom MC, Klovins J, Fredriksson R, et al. High affinity agonistic metal ion binding sites within the melanocortin 4 receptor illustrate conformational change of transmembrane region 3. *J Biol Chem.* 2003;278:51521-51526.
136. Ewing TJ, Makino S, Skillman AG, Kuntz ID. DOCK 4.0: search strategies for automated molecular docking of flexible molecule databases. *J Comput Aided Mol Des.* 2001;15:411-428.
137. Jones G, Willett P, Glen RC, Leach AR, Taylor R. Development and validation of a genetic algorithm for flexible docking. *J Mol Biol.* 1997;267:727-748.
138. Rarey M, Wefing S, Lengauer T. Placement of medium-sized molecular fragments into active sites of proteins. *J Comput Aided Mol Des.* 1996;10:41-54.
139. Taylor RD, Jewsbury PJ, Essex JW. FDS: flexible ligand and receptor docking with a continuum solvent model and soft-core energy function. *J Comput Chem.* 2003;24:1637-1656.
140. Halgren TA, Murphy RB, Friesner RA, et al. Glide: a new approach for rapid, accurate docking and scoring. 2. Enrichment factors in database screening. *J Med Chem.* 2004;47:1750-1759.
141. Venkatachalam CM, Jiang X, Oldfield T, Waldman M. LigandFit: a novel method for the shape-directed rapid docking of ligands to protein active sites. *J Mol Graph Model.* 2003;21:289-307.
142. Cavasotto CN, Abagyan RA. Protein flexibility in ligand docking and virtual screening to protein kinases. *J Mol Biol.* 2004;337:209-225.
143. Perola E, Walters WP, Charifson PS. A detailed comparison of current docking and scoring methods on systems of pharmaceutical relevance. *Proteins.* 2004;56:235-249.
144. Halperin I, Ma B, Wolfson H, Nussinov R. Principles of docking: an overview of search algorithms and a guide to scoring functions. *Proteins.* 2002;47:409-443.
145. Kontoyianni M, McClellan LM, Sokol GS. Evaluation of docking performance: comparative data on docking algorithms. *J Med Chem.* 2004;47:558-565.
146. Carlson HA, McCammon JA. Accommodating protein flexibility in computational drug design. *Mol Pharmacol.* 2000;57:213-218.
147. Evers A, Klebe G. Successful virtual screening for a submicromolar antagonist of the neurokinin-1 receptor based on a ligand-supported homology model. *J Med Chem.* 2004b ;47:5381-5392.
148. Heyl DL, Mosberg HI. Modification of the Phe3 aromatic moiety in delta receptor-selective dermorphin/deltorphin-related tetrapeptides: effects on opioid receptor binding. *Int J Pept Protein Res.* 1992;39:450-457.
149. Sebastian A, Bidlack JM, Jiang Q, et al. 14 beta-[(p-nitrocinnamoyl)amino]morphinones, 14 beta-[(p-nitrocinnamoyl)amino]-7,8-dihydromorphinones, and their codeinone analogues: synthesis and receptor activity. *J Med Chem.* 1993;36:3154-3160.
150. Sagara T, Egashira H, Okamura M, Fujii I, Shimohigashi Y, Kanematsu K. Ligand recognition in mu opioid receptor: experimentally based modeling of mu opioid receptor binding sites and their testing by ligand docking. *Bioorg Med Chem.* 1996;4:2151-2166.
151. Chabre M, Breton J. Orientation of aromatic residues in rhodopsin: rotation of one tryptophan upon the meta I to meta II transition after illumination. *Photochem Photobiol.* 1979;30:295-299.
152. Baneres JL, Martin A, Hullot P, Girard JP, Rossi JC, Parello J. Structure-based analysis of GPCR function: conformational adaptation of both agonist and receptor upon leukotriene B4 binding to recombinant BLT1. *J Mol Biol.* 2003;329:801-814.
153. Ruprecht JJ, Mielke T, Vogel R, Villa C, Schertler GF. Electron crystallography reveals the structure of metarhodopsin I. *EMBO J.* 2004;23:3609-3620.
154. Sammes PG, Taylor JB. Opioid receptors. In: Hansch C, ed. *Comprehensive Medicinal Chemistry* Oxford, UK: Pergamon Press; 1990:805-844.
155. Schiller PW, Weltrowska G, Nguyen TM-D, Lemieux C, Chung NN, Lu Y. Conversion of μ-, δ- and κ-receptor selective opioid peptide agonists into μ-, δ-, and κ-receptor selective antagonists. *Life Sci.* 2003;73:691-698.

156. Huang P, Kim S, Loew G. Development of a common 3D pharmacophore for delta-opioid recognition from peptides and non-peptides using a novel computer program. *J Comput Aided Mol Des*. 1997;11:21-28.
157. Filizola M, Villar HO, Loew GH. Molecular determinants of non-specific recognition of delta, mu, and kappa opioid receptors. *Bioorg Med Chem*. 2001a ;9:69-76.
158. Filizola M, Villar HO, Loew GH. Differentiation of delta, mu, and kappa opioid receptor agonists based on pharmacophore development and computed physicochemical properties. *J Comput Aided Mol Des*. 2001b ;15:297-307.
159. Bernard D, Jr, Coop A, Jr, MacKerell AD, Jr. 2D conformationally sampled pharmacophore: a ligand-based pharmacophore to differentiate delta opioid agonists from antagonists. *J Am Chem Soc*. 2003;125:3101-3107.

Chapter 34
Molecular Recognition of Opioid Receptor Ligands

Brian E. Kane,[1] Bengt Svensson,[1] and David M. Ferguson[1]

Abstract The cloning of the opioid receptors and subsequent use of recombinant DNA technology have led to many new insights into ligand binding. Instead of focusing on the structural features that lead to increased affinity and selectivity, researchers are now able to focus on why these features are important. Site-directed mutagenesis and chimeric data have often been at the forefront in answering these questions. Herein, we survey pharmacophores of several opioid ligands in an effort to understand the structural requirements for ligand binding and selectivity. Models are presented and compared to illustrate key sites of recognition for both opiate and nonopiate ligands. The results indicate that different ligand classes may recognize different sites within the receptor, suggesting that multiple epitopes may exist for ligand binding and selectivity.

Keywords Opioid, structure-function, pharmacophore, mutagenesis, chimeric

Introduction

Over the years, a great amount of effort has been devoted to the development of structural models that predict ligand binding and selectivity for the μ, δ, and κ opioid receptors. In the absence of crystallographic data, indirect methods, which include site-directed mutagenesis, chimeric studies, the substituted cysteine accessibility method, and affinity labeling studies, have been instrumental in locating key contacts for molecular recognition. One of the most informative methods has been the engineering of chimeric receptors. By interchanging sequences of the μ, δ, and κ receptors, researchers have identified regions of the receptor responsible for

[1]University of Minnesota, College of Pharmacy, Department of Medicinal Chemistry, Minneapolis, MN 55455

Corresponding Author: David M. Ferguson, Department of Medicinal Chemistry, University of Minnesota, 308 Harvard St SE, 8-101 Weaver-Densford Hall, Minneapolis, MN 55455. Tel: (612) 626-2601; Fax: (612) 624-0139; E-mail: ferguson@umn.edu

R.S. Rapaka and W. Sadée (eds.), *Drug Addiction*.
© American Association of Pharmaceutical Scientists 2008

discriminating differences between peptide and nonpeptide recognition, as well as regions necessary for selectivity.[1-4] For example, chimeric studies have shown that the second extracellular loop (EL-2) of the κ receptor is essential for the activity of the selective peptide agonist dynorphin A (Dyn A).[5,6] When EL-2 from μ or δ was inserted into the κ sequence, Dyn A lost activity. Conversely, when EL-2 from κ was inserted into μ or δ sequences, Dyn A gained activity.

Whereas chimeric studies generally paint a broad picture of what regions of the receptor may be important for binding, site-directed mutagenesis studies implicate individual residues. Thus, results often indicate how ligand recognition may be occurring at the molecular level. By the time opioid receptors were cloned, such studies were commonly used in the study of other receptor systems.[7,8] Important for the opioid receptor family were those on the β-adrenergic receptor, another G-protein coupled receptor (GPCR).[9] This GPCR binds epinephrine and numerous catecholamine analogs. Since opiates and opioid peptides share common structural features with epinephrine (Fig. 34.1), it was suggested that they share similar interactions for their respective receptors.

One such interaction involves an aspartate residue in transmembrane helix III. This aspartate (Asp III:08, see Fig. 34.2 for an explanation of the nomenclature) is conserved among all biogenic amine receptor families, including the β-adrenergic and opioid receptors.[10] When this residue in the β-adrenergic receptor was mutated to its neutral isostere asparagine (Asn), a large decrease in epinephrine binding was seen.[11] This suggested that a salt bridge between the amine of epinephrine and the carboxylate of the Asp had been disrupted. Since opioid ligands also possess an amine, a homologous interaction was proposed. When Asp III:08 in the μ receptor was mutated to Asn, several opioid receptor ligands did not bind, indicating a salt bridge.[1]

Further insight on opioid ligand recognition was realized by analyzing similar results from the β-adrenergic receptor system. For example, site-directed mutagenesis results suggested that conserved serine residues (V:09 and V:12) were hydrogen bonding to epinephrine's catechol moiety.[12] Since the structurally similar phenolic group is often essential for opiate and opioid activity,[13] it was believed that the formation of a hydrogen bond might be important in the opioid receptor family as well.

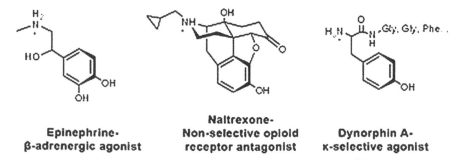

Epinephrine-
β-adrenergic agonist

Naltrexone-
Non-selective opioid
receptor antagonist

Dynorphin A-
κ-selective agonist

Fig. 34.1   Epinephrine contains a *p*-hydroxyphenethylamine (tyramine) moiety, as do many opiates and opioid peptide ligands. Gly indicates glycine; Phe, phenylalanine.

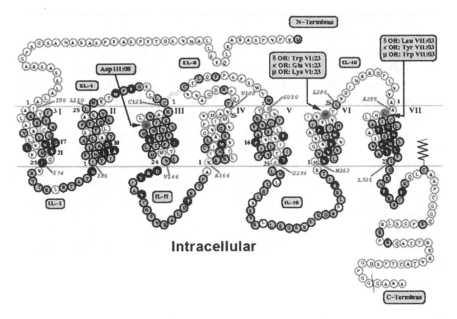

Fig. 34.2 Serpentine model of the δ receptor. Circles contain the 1-letter code for the given amino acid. Horizontal lines indicate the beginning and ends of the helices. The gray circles indicate the residues that are conserved among all 3 receptor types (μ, δ, and κ), while the black circles indicate the residues that are highly conserved among the rhodopsin subclass of G-protein coupled receptors. Each transmembrane (TM) region is indicated by a roman numeral. At the beginning and end of each helix there are Arabic numbers starting with 1 and ending at 25 (variable, depending on helix length). These numbers correspond to the position of the residue within the helix. For example, the Asp in TM III is denoted as III:08. Asp indicates aspartate; EL, extracellular loop; Glu, glutamine; IL, intracellular loop; Leu, leucine; Lys, lysine; OR, opioid receptor; Trp, tryptophan; Tyr, tyrosine.

However, since opioid receptors lack residues capable of forming hydrogen bonds at positions V:09 and V:12, an alternative site had to be considered. Presumably, this residue needed to be conserved, needed to be able to hydrogen-bond, and needed to be positioned at an appropriate distance from Asp III:08. A histidine located in TM VI (His VI:17) satisfied all these criteria. When this residue (in the μ receptor) was replaced with a residue incapable of forming hydrogen bonds (eg, alanine) decreases in binding occurred.[14] On the other hand, conservative mutations (ie, those that do not disrupt hydrogen bonding interactions, eg, histamine or glutamine to asparagine), had only minor effects on ligand binding.[15] From these results, it was suggested that His VI:17 hydrogen-bonds to the opioids' phenol.

Just as common structural moieties interact with conserved residues, uncommon moieties interact with variable residues within the receptor. This is best explained by the "message-address" concept.[16] In short, the message-address concept states that ligands contain different recognition elements that are responsible for their differential binding activities. Their shared, or universal, portion represents the "message," while their unique, or variable, portion represents the "address." For the opiates, the tyramine moiety (the amine and phenol) represents the message, while large substituents on the C ring represent the address (Fig. 34.3).[17] The nonselective ligand naltrexone (NTX)[18] does not contain an address and thus is not selective. Meanwhile, the δ-selective ligand naltrindole[19] (NTI) contains indole moiety, and the κ-selective ligand 5-guanidinylnaltrindole[20] (gNTI) contains a guanidinyl moiety that acts as the address to confer selectivity.

It should be noted that the opiates are exceptional examples of the message-address theory, because both the message and address moieties are well defined. In contrast, nonopiates such as fentanyl[21] (μ-selective agonist), U50,488,[22] and U69,593[23] (κ-selective agonists) do not contain a traditional message and address. For these 2 ligand classes (the fentanyls and arylacetamides), docking studies predict a unique epitope that has minimal overlap with the opiate pharmacophore.[24-30] Thus, this review is broken up into sections based on ligand class. For each class, molecular recognition will be discussed in terms of how specific interactions assist ligand binding.

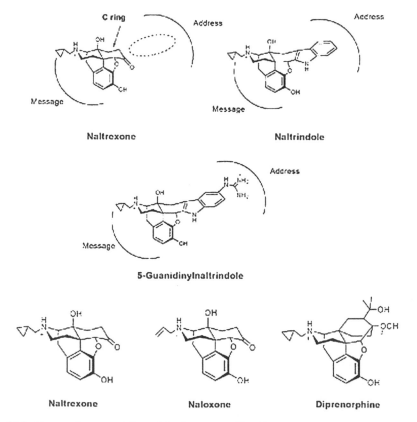

Fig. 34.3 Structural representation of the "message-address" concept.

Opioid Receptors: Model Development

Before the molecular recognition of opioids is presented, a general discussion of opioid receptors must be undertaken. Because opioid receptors do not have a crystal structure, sequence analysis methods have been important in revealing many of the receptors' general characteristics. These methods, which include hydropathy plots and multiple sequence alignments, have classified the opioid receptors (μ, δ, and κ) into the class A GPCRs resembling rhodopsin.[31] These membrane-bound proteins contain an extracellular N-terminus, 7 transmembrane helices, and an intracellular C-terminus (Fig. 34.2). The helices are bundled in a counterclockwise fashion and connected intra- and extracellularly by loops that vary in size and composition.

Also evident from Fig. 34.2 is the high sequence homology between the 3 opioid receptor types (indicated by gray and black circles). The transmembrane helices show ~70% identity, and the loops show ~60% identity.[31] In both cases, however, sequence identity is dependent on the region of the receptor being analyzed. For example, while the intracellular loops share ~90% homology, the N-terminus, EL-2, EL-3, and the C-terminus share little to no homology. Likewise, TM helices II, III, and VII have ~75% identity, while helices IV, V, and VI share considerably less sequence identity.

Each receptor type has also been further characterized into subtypes. Pharmacological and radioligand studies point toward at least 2 variants for each receptor type, namely μ_1/μ_2, δ_1/δ_2, and κ_1/κ_2.[31] The δ_1 receptor, for example, has been characterized based on the ability of 7-benzylidenenaltrexone and the enkephalin analog DALCE to selectively antagonize the antinociceptive activity of DPDPE and DADLE.[32] Meanwhile, δ_2 is characterized based on the ability of naltriben and 5'-NTII (naltrindole isothiocyanate) to selectively antagonize deltorphin II and DSLET.[33] Since both receptor subtypes share the same amino acid sequence, the unique binding profiles have been speculated to be the result of different posttranslational modifications, distinct cellular localizations, and varying interactions with other associated proteins.[34] It remains largely unknown how these interactions contribute to the receptor's overall conformation. Thus, even as newer models (derived from the more recently acquired high-resolution crystal structure rhodopsin)[35,36] replace older bacteriorhodopsin-derived models, the connection between receptor conformation and resultant biological activity has not been resolved.[30,31,37-39]

Despite this fact, the development of pharmacophores for opioid receptor ligands has flourished. One approach to identifying these pharmacophores uses automated docking simulations (eg, the DOCK[40] suite of programs) to predict binding modes. Flexible ligands often produce a larger number of different but plausible binding site models. Thus, narrowing down the binding modes is often more difficult. In some instances, biophysical data are available to support one of the proposed pharmacophores or to reject the existence of another. Much of the time, such data do not exist and the selection of a binding mode is based on the researcher's interpretation. This can lead to pharmacophores that vary tremendously. Conversely, the models developed for the more rigid opiates are very similar to one another. These models are also supported by more extensive biophysical data. Since it is thought that nonopiates bind in a similar pocket, the more refined opiate models have often been the starting structure for docking studies for nonopiates. Thus, they will be discussed first to provide a basis for the other opioid receptor models.

Pharmacophoric Models

Nonselective Opiates

Naltrexone is a known as a universal opiate antagonist. It and the closely related nonselective opiates naloxone[41] and diprenorphine[42] all bind to the μ, δ, and κ receptors with very high affinity. Furthermore, these ligands share structural similarities that are thought to be the source of their activities. First, they contain an amine that is thought to be protonated at physiological pH; second, they contain a phenolic ring. Together, these components form a tyramine or "message" moiety. Lastly, these opiates contain a hydrophobic portion. Approximately 50 years ago, Beckett and Casy proposed a crude receptor model that encompassed these 3 characteristics (Fig. 34.4).[43]

Beckett and Casy's 3-point model was invaluable for explaining generic receptor-ligand interactions; however, it did not take into account the specific interactions responsible for ligand recognition. Since the success of drug discovery often lies in determining such details, transforming this model into a contemporary pharmacophore that could implicate individual residues was essential. As mentioned in the introduction, comparisons of opiates to the catecholamines suggested that binding occurs within conserved regions of the transmembrane helices, specifically using interactions between an amine and Asp III:08, and a phenol and His VI:17.[1,14] These interactions accounted for two thirds of the 3-point model, but the determination of the residues suggested to interact with the hydrophobic region still remained.

Given the relatively small nature of the nonselective opiates, it was presumed that a hydrophobic pocket might be found in close proximity to Asp III:08 and His VI:17. Sequence analysis revealed that a cluster of conserved hydrophobic residues existed approximately halfway down TM helices III to VI (Trp IV:10, Phe V:13, Phe VI:09, and Trp VI:13).[44] These residues were mutated in order to determine the role of aromatic transmembrane residues of the δ receptor in ligand binding.[45] Results suggested that the residues Trp V:10, Phe V:13, and Trp VI:13 might help form the putative hydrophobic pocket. Since these residues are conserved, it was suggested that these residues play a similar role in the μ and κ receptors as well. A summary of these interactions, using naltrexone as a representative ligand, is shown in Fig. 34.5.

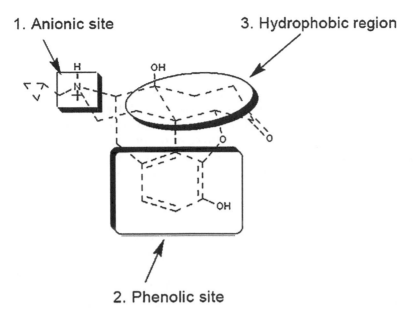

1. Anionic site

3. Hydrophobic region

2. Phenolic site

Fig. 34.4 Above: Nonselective antagonists naltrexone, naloxone, and diprenorphine. Below: Beckett and Casy's 3-point receptor model shown with naltrexone as a representative ligand. It is suggested that the first 2 points of the model, the anionic and phenolic site, interact with the tyramine "message" moiety. The third point of the receptor model suggests that a hydrophobic region within the receptor stabilizes the remaining alkaloid scaffold, specifically rings C to E.

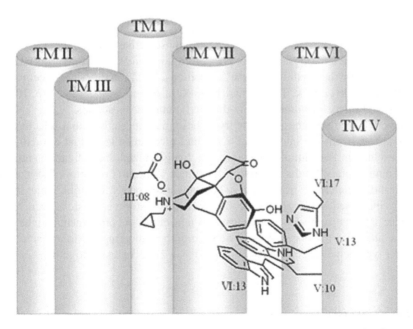

Fig. 34.5 The pharmacophore of the nonselective opiate naltrexone. The tyramine "message" moiety forms a salt bridge with Asp III:08 and a hydrogen bond with His VI:17. Aromatic residues that stabilize the hydrophobic core include Trp V:10, Phe V:13, and Trp VI:13. Asp indicates aspartate; His, histidine; Phe, phenylalanine; TM, transmembrane; Trp, tryptophan.

Selective Opiates

The 3-point model is well suited to describe the interactions of nonselective opiates. However, it does not account for interactions of the "address" moieties found in selective opiates like NTI and gNTI (Fig. 34.3). For these ligands, an address locus containing variable residues is believed to be responsible for conferring selectivity. Experimental data support this hypothesis. Specifically, chimeric studies have revealed that the highly variable region from the top of TM VI to the C-terminus is required for high affinity binding of the κ-selective antagonist norbinaltorphimine (norBNI).[46] Additionally, chimeric studies have determined that the same region is implicated for δ-selective opiates.[4]

Once this region had been implicated as an "address" locus, it was hypothesized that individual residues within this region were responsible for conferring selectivity. In general, 2 techniques, alanine scanning and directed mutation, were applied to determine what residues, if any, were involved. The former method is a technique in which a side chain is individually and randomly mutated to alanine. It is hypothesized that if a large change in binding is observed, then the residue may be involved in ligand binding, thus warranting further investigation. Results from this method revealed that 3 residues near the top of TM VI and VII were implicated in binding to a wide variety of δ-selective ligands (these individual sites and their importance to ligand binding will be discussed in detail in the section concerning δ-selectivity).[47] The other method, directed mutation, uses molecular models to determine which residues to mutate. Under the assumption that the shared alkaloid scaffold of selective opiates binds in a similar manner as the nonselective opiates, the models suggested that there are 2 positions that are both unique and oriented appropriately for interaction with the ligands.[45] These 2 positions, VI:23 and VII:03, occupied by Glu297 and Tyr312 in κ, Trp284 and Leu300 in δ, and Lys303 and Trp318 in μ, became the targets for numerous site-directed mutagenesis studies.

Site-directed mutagenesis results from these mutants suggest that selectivity for opiates arises from the interplay of 2 distinct mechanisms, mutual attraction and steric exclusion. For mutual attraction, it is hypothesized that a ligand is attracted to a complimentary residue or group of residues within the receptor. The incurring stabilization, generally from charge neutralization or hydrophobic interactions, leads to increased binding. The second mechanism, steric exclusion, occurs when a residue or a group of residues does not allow a favorable or complimentary interaction (mutual attraction) to occur. As will be seen in the following sections, each opioid receptor type achieves selectivity by using these 2 mechanisms together.

Kappa-Selective Opiates

Ligand recognition of gNTI and norBNI[48] (Fig. 34.6) has been studied extensively. One obvious difference between these κ-selective opiates and the nonselective opiates is the presence of a second basic moiety found in the "address." This basic moiety has been implicated in forming a salt bridge with a unique glutamate within the κ receptor, Glu VI:23.[20,49] Specifically, when Glu was mutated to a lysine (the homologous residue found in μ), a significant decrease in binding for norBNI and gNTI was observed. Meanwhile, no significant changes were observed for the nonspecific ligands naloxone (NLX) and naltrexone (NTX). Furthermore, when the homologous position in μ (K303) was mutated to glutamate (as to mimic the κ receptor), norBNI and gNTI's activity was comparable to that of wild-type κ.[20] Studies conducted in mutant δ receptors also exhibited similar trends. For example, when Trp VI:23 was mutated to glutamate, activity for norBNI and gNTI was significantly enhanced.[20]

Although mutation of Glu VI:23 had profound effects on norBNI and gNTI activity, it was postulated that other variant residues may help to confer selectivity through mechanisms of steric exclusion. One method of testing this hypothesis was by generating mutations that would give selective ligands enhanced affinity for their nonpreferred wild-type receptors. As a general example, if a bulky residue is blocking the access of a binding pocket, then replacement of this large residue with a smaller residue would significantly alter the binding affinity. On the other hand, small residues that allow numerous ligands access could be mutated to bulky residues so as to limit the number of ligands. One position that was hypothesized to play such a role was that of VII:03. When this position in κ was mutated, Tyr VII:03 to alanine (Ala), small changes in norBNI and gNTI binding were observed.[49] This suggested that the tyrosine was not directly involved in ligand binding. However, when the homologous residue in μ was mutated, Trp VII:03 to Ala, a significant increase in binding was observed.[49] Thus, it was suggested that the tryptophan in μ sterically excludes opiates with large address moieties from binding. The proposed pharmacophore for gNTI is presented in Fig. 34.7 (the conserved aromatic residues from Fig. 34.5 have been excluded for clarity).

Delta-Selective Opiates

The molecular recognition of the prototypical δ-selective opiates NTI and 7-spiro-indanyloxymorphone[50] (SIOM) (Fig. 34.8) has also been well studied. Like their κ counterparts, δ-selective opiates have a distinctive "address" moiety. For these

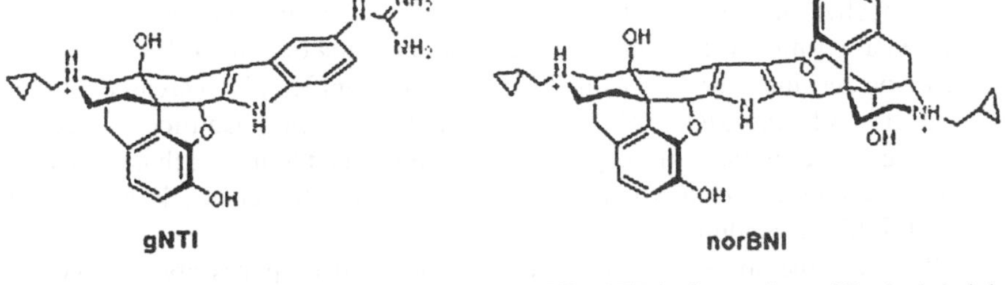

Fig. 34.6 Kappa-selective opiates gNTI and norBNI. gNTI indicates 5-guanidinylnaltrindole; norBNI, norbinaltorphimine.

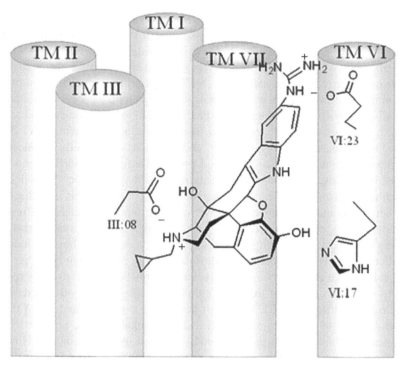

Fig. 34.7 The pharmacophore of gNTI in the κ receptor. The "message" moiety forms a salt bridge with Asp III:08 and a hydrogen bond with His VI:17. The positively charged guanidinyl group is thought to form a salt bridge with Glu VI:23. This interaction is the basis for selectivity. Asp indicates aspartate; His, histidine; Glu, glutamine; TM, transmembrane.

δ-selective ligands, however, a hydrophobic group such as an indole or spiroindane forms the address (NTI and SIOM, respectively). As mentioned previously, an alanine scan was conducted to determine whether residues within the address locus could be implicated in ligand binding. For naltrindole, the mutations that had the most pronounced effects were Trp VI:23, Leu VII:-04, and Ala VII:-01 (to glycene [Gly]).[47] Although no specific interaction with NTI was proposed, it is generally believed that these residues form a hydrophobic pocket that helps to stabilize the indolic moiety of NTI.

Similar to κ-selective opiates, δ-selective opiates appear to obtain their selectivity through mechanisms of exclusion. Again, site-directed mutagenesis studies were conducted at position VII:03. In the μ receptor, mutation of Trp VII:03 to Ala, Lys, or Leu (the residue found in wildtype δ) led to significantly increased binding affinities for NTI and SIOM.[49,51] This suggested that tryptophan blocks access of δ-selective opiates to the μ binding cavity. Also important to note is that the activity of NTI was similar for all 3 mutants, suggesting that the leucine is not directly involved in ligand binding.

Collectively, the above studies suggest that δ-selective opiates obtain selectivity through 2 main mechanisms. The first involves hydrophobic stabilization by residues

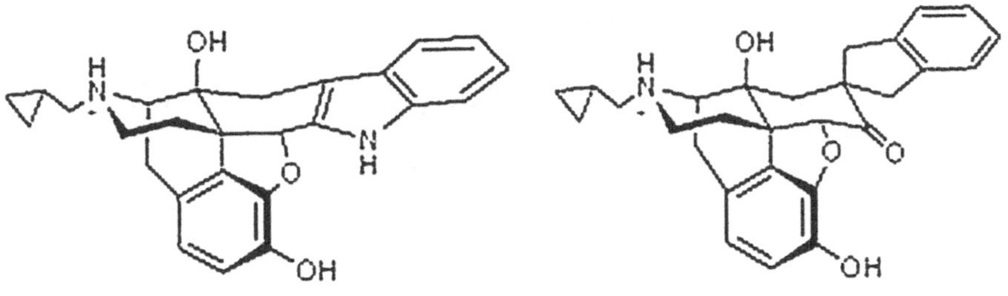

Fig. 34.8 Delta-selective opiates NTI and SIOM. NTI indicates naltrindole; SIOM, 7-spiroindanyloxymorphone.

unique to the δ receptor found at the top of TM VI and VII (Trp VI:23, Leu VII:-04, Ala VII:-01). The second mechanism implicates a tryptophan residue in μ that creates too much steric bulk. A depiction of these interactions appears in Fig. 34.9.

Mu-Selective Opiates

In the previous sections on κ and δ selectivity, it was apparent that one particular chemical moiety, the address, conferred selectivity. The μ-selective opiates morphine and β-funaltrexamine (β-FNA) (Fig. 34.10) lack a common chemical moiety; thus, it is unlikely that common mechanisms exist for their molecular recognition. For this reason, they will be examined independently so that their unique structural features and their role in conferring selectivity can be discussed.

Morphine, the prototypical μ opiate, has been studied extensively. X-ray studies have determined that the C ring adopts a boat conformation, placing the 6α-hydroxyl group in an equatorial position.[13] It is often suggested that this hydroxyl group plays a role in selectivity. However, inversion of the hydroxyl group to the 6β diastereomer leads to only minor changes in selectivity.[13] Thus, it remains unclear how the hydroxyl group confers selectivity. One docking study suggests that it hydrogen-bonds to Asn V:02, a unique residue of the μ receptor.[30] Mutation of this residue to a leucine or a threonine moderately increases morphine's activity, thus casting serious doubts about this asparagine's putative role.[52] Another study used S-activated dihydromorphine derivatives, in combination with molecular mechanics, to create a pharmacophore. This model suggests that the 6α-hydroxyl group interacts with residues at the top of TM VII (near cysteine [Cys] VII:06), while the phenolic ring interacts with Tyr VI:19.[53] Although this model is plausible, it also lacks compelling site-directed mutagenesis data to support its claims, thereby diminishing its reliability.

The affinity label β-FNA is an irreversible μ antagonist. Although K_i values in the guinea pig brain show only slight selectivity for μ over κ, it has been shown that

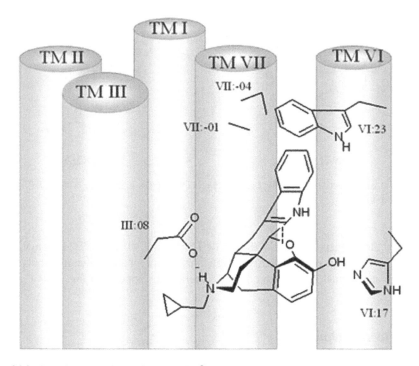

Fig. 34.9 The pharmacophore of NTI in the δ receptor. Again, Asp III:08 and VI:17 anchor the tyramine moiety. Residues unique to the δ receptor at the top of TM VI and VII (Trp VI:23, Leu VII:-04, Ala VII:-01) confer selectivity. Presumably these residues form a hydrophobic pocket around the indolic moiety of NTI. Ala indicates alanine; Asp, aspartate; Leu, leucine; NTI, naltrindole; TM, transmembrane; Trp, tryptophan.

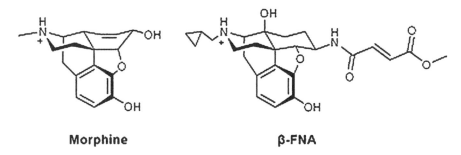

Morphine   **β-FNA**

Fig. 34.10 Mu-selective opiates morphine and β-FNA. β-FNA indicates β-funaltrexamine.

at low concentrations [³H] β-FNA covalently labels the μ receptor with high specificity.[54]Kinetic studies have suggested that the molecular recognition of this irreversible antagonist involves 2 steps.[54] First, reversible binding occurs within the binding pocket. This positions the reactive affinity label in the proper orientation to irreversibly react with a nucleophilic site within the receptor. Site-directed mutagenesis

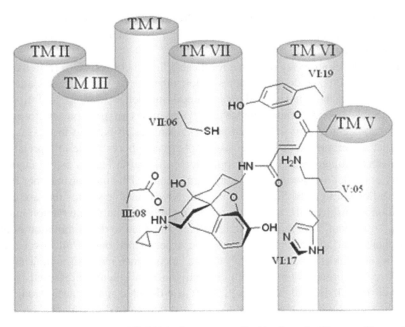

Fig. 34.11 The pharmacophore of β-FNA in the μ receptor. Besides the typical "message" interactions, little is known about the residues that confer selectivity to this ligand. It has been suggested that Lys V:05 attacks the affinity label. Other residues in this putative pocket include those that were deemed important for morphine's recognition (Tyr VI:19 and Cys VII:06). β-FNA indicates β-funaltrexamine; Cys, cysteine; Lys, lysine; TM, transmembrane; Tyr, tyrosine.

results have indicated that Lys V:05 is responsible for this attack.[55] Surprisingly, a lysine present at the homologous position of the κ receptor does not form a covalent bond with β-FNA. The molecular basis behind this puzzling result remains undetermined but presumably involves residues near Lys V:05 that alter the local environment of the κ binding pocket. β-FNA's interactions are highlighted in the pharmacophore in Fig. 34.11.

Selective Nonopiate Ligands

In contrast to the opiates, there have not been any small-molecule ligands that show a high affinity for all 3 receptor types. Therefore, the remainder of this review will focus on the molecular recognition of the prototypical small-ligand agonists for each receptor type: the δ-selective diarylpiperazines (SNC 80[56] and analogs), the μ-selective fentanyls, and the κ-selective arylacetamides. Although exhaustive structure-activity relationships (SAR) data has determined which structural features are necessary for activity, the interactions that confer their selectivity are not well understood. In fact, conflicting pharmacophores have been proposed for each ligand class.[24-30] For the δ-selective SNC 80 derivatives, controversy exists over whether the pharmacophoric determinants of SNC 80 (and analogs) are the same as those for the δ-selective opiates NTI and SIOM.[57-59] For the fentanyls and arylacetamides, different yet important discrepancies exist.

Much of the controversy observed for these 3 ligand classes stems from the interpretation of automated docking studies. Their inherent flexibility creates numerous issues. Whereas the opiates produce a limited number of binding conformations, these flexible ligands often produce large ensembles of possible conformations within the receptor. This often leads to discrepancies in binding modes. Another issue that sometimes leads to inconsistent pharmacophores is the interpretation of site-directed mutagenesis. It is generally accepted that at least a 5-fold change in activity is needed before one can imply significance. This may or may not be true for such flexible ligands. Since these ligands have rotatable groups that are able to reposition themselves, the elimination of a single hydrophobic interaction may not give a "significant" difference in binding. This may lead to the elimination of pharmacophores that are presumed to not fit the experimental data. Collectively, all of these factors make the search for an "address" locus much more difficult. The scope of this review prevents an in-depth comparison of all details presented by each proposed model. Instead, key results from site-directed mutagenesis studies and chimeric studies will be highlighted to present a generalized pharmacophore.

SNC 80 and Analogs

The δ-selective agonist SNC 80 and its analogs (eg, compounds **1**[60] and **2**[61]) share several common structural features (Fig. 34.12). One common feature is the presence of a piperidine or piperazine ring (ring A). Although substitution of this ring is not necessary, the addition of small hydrophobic groups sometimes leads to slightly enhanced binding affinity or selectivity.[62] Also common to these ligands are 2 aromatic rings (B and C). Ring B is generally substituted with a diethyl amide and ring C with a hydroxyl or methoxyether group. For a complete overview on SAR, the reader is referred to reviews by Calderon[63] and Knapp.[62]

Inspection of these ligands has suggested that they have structural similarities to δ-selective opiates NTI and SIOM.[64] A side-by-side comparison between **1** and SIOM reveals that rings A and C may mimic the classical opiate "message." Similarly, ring B and the diethyl amide mimic the spirocyclic address group of SIOM (Fig. 34.13). Accordingly, it was suggested that the ligands may be binding in a similar orientation, using the same residues that were found to impart δ-selectivity for the opiates. Based on this hypothesis, Dondio et al designed the SNC 80-indolomorphan mimic SB-220718.[65]

Despite Dondio's successful application of the proposed hypothesis, several studies have questioned the validity of such a simplistic model.[65-67] One area of disagreement lies in the analysis of SAR data. It is argued that since the diethyl amide in SB-220718 can be modified to an ester or a thioamide without a significant decrease in activity,[66] similar results should be seen for SNC 80 analogs with the

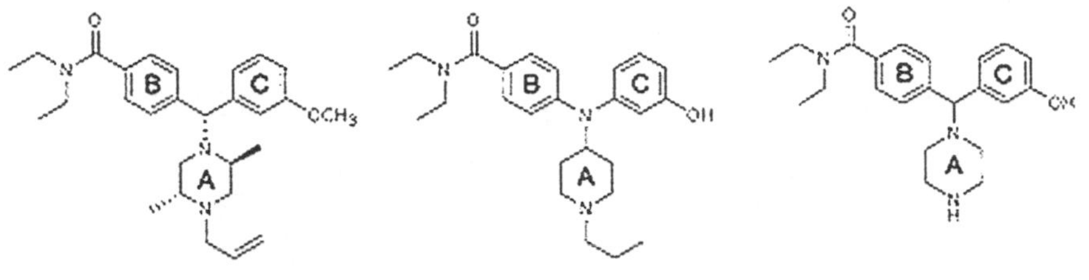

Fig. 34.12 SNC 80 and its δ-selective analogs.

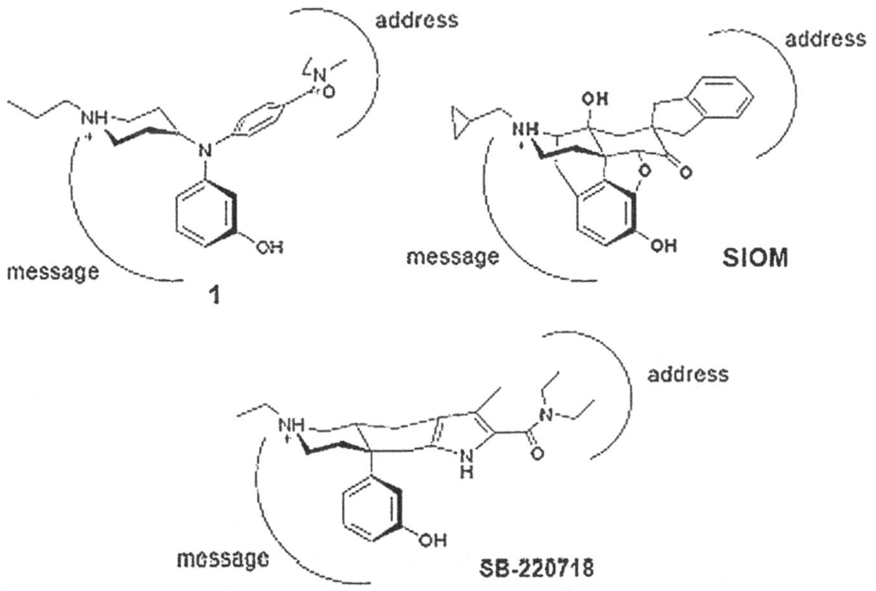

Fig. 34.13 Message-address concept applied to δ-selective ligands lacking the traditional opiate core. SIOM indicates 7-spiroindanyloxymorphone.

same substitutions. However, this is not the case.[61] Other SAR inconsistencies are believed to occur at the 3' position. In the opiates, the presence of a hydroxyl group is essential for activity,[13] but for SNC 80 it is not. Important to note is that this discrepancy is not consistent for all SNC 80 analogs. For example, the methoxy analog of **1** is nearly 100-fold less active than the hydroxyl analog.[62] Other analogs also show selectivity profiles in which the presence of a hydroxyl group is much greater.[65] This suggests that variations between structurally similar molecules (SNC 80 and **1**) can result in quite different SAR data.

Site-directed mutagenesis results also give clues that suggest whether these SNC 80 analogs share pharmacophoric overlap with the opiates.[55] As mentioned previously, a collection of residues near the putative δ address locus were randomly

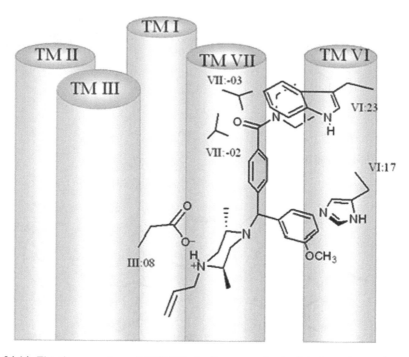

Fig. 34.14 The pharmacophore of SNC 80 in the δ receptor. A selectivity locus is near the top of TM VI and VII. Presumably Trp VI:23, Val VII:-02, and Val VII:-03 form a hydrophobic pocket that stabilizes the diethylamide moiety. His VI:17 may participate in hydrophobic stacking or may hydrogen-bond when applicable. Additional selectivity may be observed depending on which interaction occurs.

mutated to alanines. Binding results from this study revealed that Trp VI:23, Leu VII:-04, and Ala VII:-01 were important for NTI binding. The same study also reported that Trp VI:23, valine (Val) VII:-02, and Val VII:-03 were important for SNC 80 binding. Although Val VII:-02 and Val VII:-03 are not part of the 3 residues that were deemed to be important for NTI binding, they are located next to the ones that have been implicated. Therefore, it is reasonable to suggest that SNC 80 and its analogs share the same binding pocket as NTI but are oriented slightly differently (Fig. 34.14).

Fentanyl and Analogs

Fentanyl and its congeners (the fentanyls) (Fig. 34.15) are well known for their tremendous analgesic properties. Key to their pharmacological activity (μ-selective agonism) is the N-phenyl-N-piperidinyl propionamide moiety. Another group that is required for activity is a phenethyl group (although the phenyl ring can be substituted with a thiophene or methyl ester, as in the case of sufentanil and remifentanil).

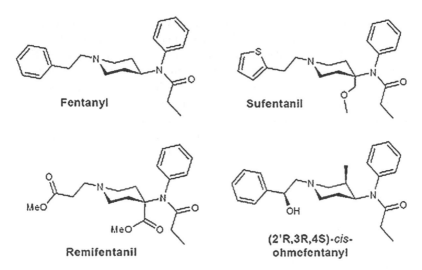

Fig. 34.15 Fentanyl and its μ-selective analogs.

Other modifications that modulate activity include small moieties at the 3 or 4 position of the piperidine ring and a β-hydroxyl substitution. For an extensive overview on the SAR associated with these ligands, the reader is referred to a review by Casy et al.[67]

Despite exhaustive SAR data, the molecular recognition of the fentanyls remains largely unknown. Although it is accepted that the aminergic nitrogen interacts with Asp III:08, the nature of the interactions that confer fentanyl's selectivity is highly disputed. Mutational data from Lys VI:23 and Trp VII:03 (positions that were important for selective opiate recognition) suggest that these 2 residues are not involved in fentanyl's binding.

Docking methods have been used to suggest an alternative binding pocket. Unfortunately, fentanyl's flexibility makes such methods very difficult to interpret.[24-26] Potential bioactive conformations have been analyzed, yet the findings have not been conclusive.[30,68-70] In particular, the conformation of the phenethyl group has been the topic of numerous discussions. Although it has been predicted that the fentanyls prefer extended conformation, it is unclear whether the extended conformation is the bioactive form. One docking study suggests that the β-hydroxy group of the fentanyl interacts with Tyr III:09.[71] However, when this residue was mutated to phenylalanine, only a minor difference in binding was observed.[72] Another study suggests that the phenethyl group points up toward Lys III:02.[30] A third study suggests that the phenethyl moiety is projected deep within the cavity of TM II, III, and VII.[24] This final pharmacophoric model is the only one that maintains the phenethyl moiety in an extended conformation. Therefore, it will be the focus of the highlighted pharmacophore.

A notable feature of this pharmacophore (Fig. 34.16) is the addition of an alternative address locus located deep within the cavity between TM II, III, and VII. This locus is supported by the increased μ activity of several compounds containing large aromatic moieties (generally phenethyl) positioned on the piperidine ring.[24,72] For example, the δ-selective ligand **1** shows enhanced activity for the μ receptor when a phenethyl moiety replaces the propyl-containing lead.[72] Additionally, it has been shown that N-phenethylmorphine shows greater potency than its parent compound morphine.[73] Also important to note is that this pocket contains several residues that can hydrogen-bond with the hydroxyl group of ohmefentanyl, specifically a threonine in TM II. However, since this residue is conserved, it is not apparent how it might contribute to ohmefentanyl's increased selectivity. Undoubtedly, more site-directed mutagenesis studies need to be conducted to help validate this pharmacophore.

Arylacetamides

The arylacetamides U50,488, U69,593, and CI-977[74] are potent κ-selective agonists (Fig. 34.17). Structure-activity relationships have elucidated the chemical features necessary for binding.[75] In summary, SAR reveals that the transconfiguration of the amine and the amide moiety is essential. Compounds with altered stereochemistry at this position do not retain activity. The location of the amide moiety with respect to the aromatic moiety is also key. Reversing the amide or shortening the phenacetyl derivative to a benzamide derivative changes the binding activity significantly. SAR data also indicate that the pyrrolidine ring is optimal for both high affinity and selectivity.

Comparison of the arylacetamides to the κ-selective opiates does not lead to obvious similarities. Despite this fact, numerous attempts have been made to compare the 2.[76,77] Presumably, if a link between these 2 ligand classes could be established, it would be easier to model and design new κ-selective ligands. A study by Rajagopalan et al prepared numerous tetrahydronaphthalenes-U50,488 mimics.[78] This study observed that hydroxyl substitution on the 6′ position led to compounds that achieved high affinity to both κ and μ receptors. When the 6′ position was substituted with a methoxy ether (DuP-747), selectivity for the κ receptor was obtained, with little effect on the activity.[78]These tetrahydronapthalene-U50,488 mimics have since been used in molecular modeling studies[28] and compared with ethylketocyclazocine, a benzomorphan with slight κ-selectivity (Fig. 34.18). Although it has been suggested that the molecular basis behind the increased κ activity is attributable to the interaction of the phenolic moiety with His VI:17, no attempts were made at determining the interactions responsible for cross-selectivity.[28]

Also important to note about the arylacetamides is the lack of a second cationic moiety. Thus, it was not unexpected when a mutation introduced at the traditional κ address site, Glu VI:23, led to only minimal effects on arylacetamide binding, suggesting no interaction.[79] However, other mutations in the traditional address locus did reveal significant changes in binding. For example, mutation of Tyr VII:03 to Ala led to significantly lower binding affinities.[79] Another mutation in this region that has shown importance is Ile VI:20. Mutation of this residue to lysine

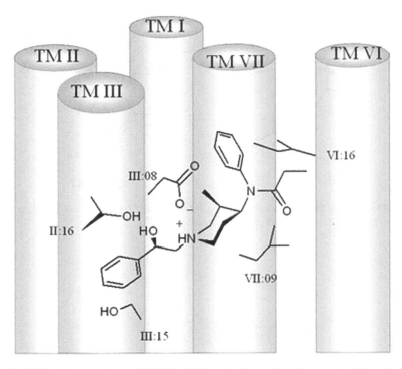

Fig. 34.16 The pharmacophore of (2′R,3R,4S)-cis-ohmefentanyl in the μ receptor. The piperidine forms a salt bridge with Asp II:08. A putative hydrogen bonding interaction is thought to occur for Thr II:16. Other important interactions include Ile VI:16, Leu VII:09, and Ser III:15. Asp indicates aspartate; Ile, isoleucine; Leu, leucine; Ser, serine; Thr, threonine; TM, transmembrane.

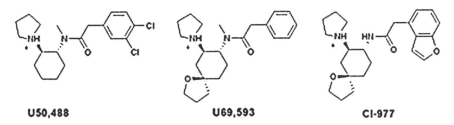

U50,488   **U69,593**   **CI-977**

Fig. 34.17 The κ-selective arylacetamides U50,488, U69,593, and CI-977.

resulted in a decrease of CI-977's affinity by over 100-fold. Collectively, these results point toward a novel arylacetamide binding epitope that has the amine interacting with Asp III:08 and has residues Ile VI:20 and Tyr VII:03 playing distinct, albeit unknown roles (Fig. 34.19). Binding models also suggest that Leu VI:21 and Ala VI 24 also help to stabilize the arylacetamides.[28] With the exception of Asp III:08, all of these residues are unique to the κ receptor.

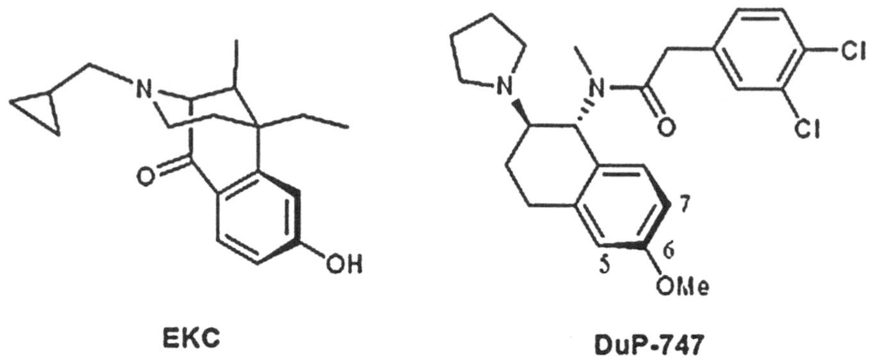

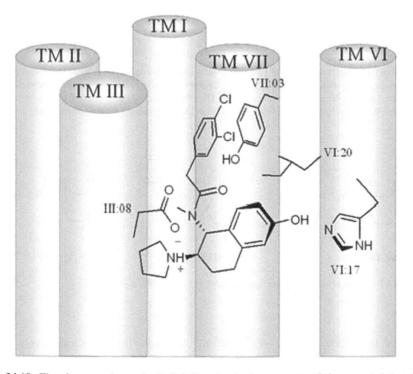

Fig. 34.18 EKC and DuP 747, a κ-selective ligand structurally similar to the arylacetamides and benzomorphans. EKC indicates ethylketocyclazocine.

Fig. 34.19 The pharmacophore of a DuP 747 analog in the κ receptor. It is suggested that Asp III:08 forms a salt bridge with the pyrrolidine ring. The phenolic ring is thought to interact with His VI:17. Other residues that have been implicated in binding (via site-directed mutagenesis) include Ile VI:20 and Tyr VII:03.

Conclusions

Pharmacophores have been presented for the prototypical opiate and nonopiate ligands (excluding peptides). For each ligands class, an attempt was made to present the model that, as far as we know, most accurately reflects the most current experimental data. However, since the interpretation of docking studies and site-directed mutation results often is subjective, there can be some debate as to whether the proposed model accurately depicts the true interactions. In some cases, such as that of gNTI, the experiments paint a clear picture of structure and function. However, for the majority of ligands, it is fairly clear that multiple sites of recognition exist. Comparisons between arylacetamides and SNC80 analogs, for example, indicate that these compounds most likely recognize different sites of selectivity within the opioid receptors. It is hoped that in the future, these ligand-specific sites will be identified and applied to design the next generation of opioid ligands.

References

1. Haeyoung K, Raynor K, Reisine T. Amino acids in the cloned mouse kappa receptor that are necessary for high affinity agonist binding but not antagonist binding. *Regul Pept.* 1994;54:155-156.
2. Meng F, Hoversten MT, Thompson RC, Taylor L, Watson SJ, Akil H. A chimeric study of the molecular basis of affinity and selectivity of the κ and the δ opioid receptors: potential role of extracellular domains. *J Biol Chem.* 1995;270:12730-12736.
3. Xue JC, Chen C, Zhu J, et al. The third extracellular loop of the μ opioid receptor is important for agonist selectivity. *J Biol Chem.* 1995;270:12977-12979.
4. Meng F, Ueda Y, Hoversten MT, et al. Mapping the receptor domains critical for the binding selectivity of delta-opioid receptor ligands. *Eur J Pharmacol.* 1996;311:285-292.
5. Wang JB, Johnson PS, Wu JM, Wang WF, Uhl GR. Human κ opiate receptor second extracellular loop elevates dynorphin's affinity for human μ/κ chimeras. *J Biol Chem.* 1994;269:25966-25969.
6. Teschemacher H, Opheim KE, Cox BM, Goldstein A. Peptidelike substance from pituitary that acts like morphine, I: isolation. *Life Sci.* 1975;16:1771-1775.
7. Strader CD, Sigal IS, Dixon RA. Structural basis of β-adrenergic receptor function. *FASEB J.* 1989;3:1825-1832.
8. Hibert MF, Trumpp-Kallmeyer S, Bruinvels A, Hoflack J. Three-dimensional models of neurotransmitter G-binding protein-coupled receptors. *Mol Pharmacol.* 1991;40:8-15.
9. Trumpp-Kallmeyer S, Hoflack J, Bruinvels A, Hibert M. Modeling of G-protein-coupled receptors: application to dopamine, adrenaline, serotonin, acetylcholine, and mammalian opsin receptors. *J Med Chem.* 1992;35:3448-3462.
10. Baldwin JM. The probable arrangement of the helices in G protein-coupled receptors. *EMBO J.* 1993;12:1693-1703.
11. Strader CD, Sigal IS, Candelore MR, Rands E, Hill WS, Dixon RAF. Conserved aspartic acid residues 79 and 113 of the β-adrenergic receptor have different roles in receptor function. *J Biol Chem.* 1988;263:10267-10271.
12. Strader CD, Candelore MR, Hill WS, Sigal IS, Dixon RA. Identification of two serine residues involved in agonist activation of the β-adrenergic receptor. *J Biol Chem.* 1989;264:13572-13578.
13. Lenz GR, Evans SM, Walters DE, Hopfinger AJ. *Opiates.* Orlando, FL: Academic Press; 1986.

14. Surratt CK, Johnson PS, Moriwaki A, et al. Mu opiate receptor. Charged transmembrane domain amino acids are critical for agonist recognition and intrinsic activity. *J Biol Chem.* 1994;269:20548-20553.

15. Spivak CE, Beglan CL, Seidleck BK, et al. Naloxone activation of μ-opioid receptors mutated at a histidine residue lining the opioid binding cavity. *Mol Pharmacol.* 1997;52:983-992.

16. Schwyzer R, Eberle A. On the molecular mechanism of α-MSH receptor interactions. *Front Horm Res.* 1977;4:18-25.

17. Portoghese PS, Sultana M, Takemori AE. Design of peptidomimetic δ opioid receptor antagonists using the message-address concept. *J Med Chem.* 1990;33:1714-1720.

18. Resnick RB, Volavka J, Freedman AM, Thomas M. Studies of EN-1639A (naltrexone): a new narcotic antagonist. *Am J Psychiatry.* 1974;131:646-650.

19. Portoghese PS, Sultana M, Takemori AE. Naltrindole: a highly selective and potent non-peptide delta opioid receptor antagonist. *Eur J Pharmacol.* 1988;146:185-186.

20. Jones RM, Hjorth SA, Schwartz TW, Portoghese PS. Mutational evidence for a common κ antagonist binding pocket in the wild-type κ and mutant μ[K303E] opioid receptors. *J Med Chem.* 1998;41:4911-4914.

21. Magnan J, Paterson SJ, Tavani A, Kosterlitz HW. The binding spectrum of narcotic analgesic drugs with different agonist and antagonist properties. *Naunyn Schmiedebergs Arch Pharmacol.* 1982;319:197-205.

22. Szmuszkovicz J, Von Voightlander PF. Benzeneacetamide amines: structurally novel non-μ-opioids. *J Med Chem.* 1982;25:1125-1126.

23. Lahti RA, Mickelson MM, McCall JM, Von Voigtlander PF. [³H]U-69593 a highly selective ligand for the opioid kappa receptor. *Eur J Pharmacol.* 1985;109:281-284.

24. Subramanian G, Paterlini MG, Portoghese PS, Ferguson DM. Molecular docking reveals a novel binding site model for fentanyl at the μ-opioid receptor. *J Med Chem.* 2000;43:381-391.

25. Xu H, Lu YF, Partilla JS, et al. Opioid peptide receptor studies, 11: involvement of Tyr149, Trp318 and His319 of the rat μ-opioid receptor in binding of μ-selective ligands. *Synapse.* 1999;32:23-28.

26. Jiang HL, Huang XQ, Rong SB, et al. Theoretical studies on opioid receptors and ligands, I: molecular modeling and QSAR studies on the interaction mechanism of fentanyl analogs binding to μ-opioid receptor. *Int J Quantum Chem.* 2000;78:285-293.

27. Subramanian G, Paterlini MG, Larson DL, Portoghese PS, Ferguson DM. Conformational analysis and automated receptor docking of selective arylacetamide-based κ-opioid agonists. *J Med Chem.* 1998;41:4777-4789.

28. Lavecchia A, Greco G, Novellino E, Vittorio F, Ronsisvalle G. Modeling of κ-opioid receptor/agonists interactions using pharmacophore-based and docking simulations. *J Med Chem.* 2000;43:2124-2134.

29. Cappelli A, Anzini M, Vomero S, et al. Synthesis, biological evaluation, and quantitative receptor docking simulations of 2-[(acylamino)ethyl]-1,4-benzodiazepines as novel tifluadom-like ligands with high affinity and selectivity for κ-opioid receptors. *J Med Chem.* 1996;39:860-872.

30. Pogozheva ID, Lomize AL, Mosberg HI. Opioid receptor three-dimensional structures from distance geometry calculations with hydrogen bonding constraints. *Biophys J.* 1998;75:612-634.

31. Knapp RJ, Malatynska E, Collins N, et al. Molecular biology and pharmacology of cloned opioid receptors. *FASEB J.* 1995;9:516-525.

32. Jiang Q, Takemori AE, Sultana M, et al. Differential antagonism of opioid delta antinociception by [D-Ala2,Leu5,Cys6]enkephalin and naltrindole 5'-isothiocyanate: evidence for delta receptor subtypes. *J Pharmacol Exp Ther.* 1991;257:1069-1075.

33. Sofuoglu M, Portoghese PS, Takemori AE. 7-Benzylidenenaltrexone (BTNX): a selective Δ_1 opioid receptor antagonist in the mouse spinal cord. *Life Sci.* 1993;52:769-775.

34. Zaki PA, Bilsky EJ, Vanderah TW, Lai J, Evans CJ, Porreca F. Opioid receptor types and subtypes: the δ receptor as a model. *Annu Rev Pharmacol Toxicol.* 1996;36:379-401.

35. Stenkamp RE, Filipek S, Driessen CA, Teller DC, Palczewski K. Crystal structure of rhodopsin: a template for cone visual pigments and other G protein-coupled receptors. *Biochim Biophys Acta.* 2002;1565:168-182.

36. Filipek S, Teller DC, Palczewski K, Stenkamp R. The crystallographic model of rhodopsin and its use in studies of other G protein-coupled receptors. *Annu Rev Biophys Biomol Struct.* 2003;32:375-397.
37. Metzger TG, Paterlini MG, Portoghese PS, Ferguson DM. Application of the message-address concept of the docking of naltrexone and selective naltrexone-derived opioid antagonists into opioid receptor models. *Neurochem Res.* 1996;21:1287-1294.
38. Alkorta I, Loew GH. A 3D model of the δ opioid receptor and ligand-receptor complexes. *Protein Eng.* 1996;9:573-583.
39. Strahs D, Weinstein H. Comparative modeling and molecular dynamics studies of the δ, κ and μ opioid receptors. *Protein Eng.* 1997;10:1019-1038.
40. Meng EC, Shoichet BK, Kuntz ID. Automated docking with grid-based energy evaluation. *J Comput Chem.* 1992;13:505-524.
41. Blumberg H, Dayton HB, Wolf PS. Counteraction of narcotic antagonist analgesics by the narcotic antagonist naloxone. *Proc Soc Exp Biol Med.* 1966;123:755-758.
42. Pasternak GW, Snyder SH. Opiate receptor binding: enzymic treatments that discriminate between agonist and antagonist interactions. *Mol Pharmacol.* 1975;11:478-484.
43. Beckett AH, Casy AF. Synthetic analgesics: stereochemical considerations. *J Pharm Pharmacol.* 1954;6:986-1001.
44. Attwood TK, Findlay JBC. Fingerprinting G-protein-coupled receptors. *Protein Eng.* 1994;7:195-203.
45. Befort K, Tabbara L, Kling D, Maigret B, Kieffer BL. Role of aromatic transmembrane residues on the δ-opioid receptor in ligand recognition. *J Biol Chem.* 1996;271:10161-10168.
46. Hjorth SA, Thirstrup K, Grandy DK, Schwartz TW. Analysis of selective binding epitopes for the κ-opioid receptor antagonist nor-binaltorphimine. *Mol Pharmacol.* 1995;47:1089-1094.
47. Valiquette M, Vu HK, Yue SY, Wahlestedt C, Walker P. Involvement of Trp-284, Val-296, and Val-297 of the human δ-opioid receptor in binding of δ-selective ligands. *J Biol Chem.* 1996;271:18789-18796.
48. Portoghese AS, Lipkowski AW, Takemori AE. Bimorphinans as highly selective, potent κ opioid receptor antagonists. *J Med Chem.* 1987;30:238-239.
49. Metzger TG, Paterlini MG, Ferguson DM, Portoghese PS. Investigation of the selectivity of oxymorphone- and naltrexone-derived ligands via site-directed mutagenesis of opioid receptors: exploring the 'address' recognition locus. *J Med Chem.* 2001;44:857-862.
50. Portoghese PS, Moe ST, Takemori AE. A selective δ₁ opioid receptor agonist derived from oxymorphone. Evidence for separate recognition sites for δ₁ opioid receptor agonists and antagonists. *J Med Chem.* 1993;36:2572-2574.
51. Bonner G, Meng F, Akil H. Selectivity of μ-opioid receptor determined by interfacial residues near third extracellular loop. *Eur J Pharmacol.* 2000;403:37-44.
52. Pil J, Tytgat J. The role of the hydrophilic Asn230 residue of the μ-opioid receptor in the potency of various opioid agonists. *Br J Pharmacol.* 2001;134:496-506.
53. Kanematsu K, Sagara T. An approach to the rational design of opioid receptor ligands: non-narcotic κ-opioid receptor ligand KT-95 free from euphoria and/or dysphoria. *Curr Med Chem CNS Agents.* 2001;1:1-25.
54. Liu-Chen LY, Li SX, Tallarida RJ. Studies on kinetics of [³H]β-funaltrexamine binding to μ opioid receptor. *Mol Pharmacol.* 1990;37:243-250.
55. Chen C, Yin J, Riel JK, et al. Determination of the amino acid residue involved in [³H]β-funaltrexamine covalent binding in the cloned rat μ-opioid receptor. *J Biol Chem.* 1996;271:21422-21429.
56. Calderon SN, Rothman RB, Porreca F, et al. Probes for narcotic receptor mediated phenomena, 19: synthesis of (+)-4-[(αR)-α-((2S,5R)-4-allyl-2,5-dimethyl-1-piperazinyl)-3-methoxybenzyl]-N,N-diethylbenzamide (SNC 80): a highly selective, nonpeptide δ opioid receptor agonist. *J Med Chem.* 1994;37:2125-2128.
57. Liao S, Alfaro-Lopez J, Shenderovich MD, et al. De novo design, synthesis, and biological activities of high-affinity and selective non-peptide agonists of the delta-opioid receptor. *J Med Chem.* 1998;41:4767-4776.

58. Coop A, Jacobson AE. The LMC delta opioid recognition pharmacophore: comparison of SNC80 and oxymorphindole. *Bioorg Med Chem Lett*. 1999;9:357-362.
59. Bernard D, Coop A, MacKerell AD. 2D conformationally sampled pharmacophore: a ligand-based pharmacophore to differentiate delta opioid agonists from antagonists. *J Am Chem Soc*. 2003;125:3101-3107.
60. Carson J, Carmosin F, Fitzpatrick L, Reitz A, Jetter M, inventors. 4-[aryl(piperidin-4-yl)]aminobenzamides. US patent 6 436 959. December 23, 1998.
61. Wei ZY, Brown W, Takasaki B, et al. N,N-Diethyl-4-(phenylpiperidin-4-ylidenemethyl) benzamide: a novel, exceptionally selective, potent δ opioid receptor agonist with oral bioavailability and its analogues. *J Med Chem*. 2000;43:3895-3905.
62. Knapp RJ, Santoro G, De Leon IA, et al. Structure-activity relationships for SNC80 and related compounds at cloned human delta and mu opioid receptors. *J Pharmacol Exp Ther*. 1996;277:1284-1291.
63. Calderon SN, Coop A. SNC 80 and related δ opioid agonists. *Curr Pharm Des*. 2004;10:733-742.
64. Podlogar BL, Poda GI, Demeter DA, et al. Synthesis and evaluation of 4-(N,N-diarylamino)piperidines with high selectivity to the δ-opioid receptor: a combined 3D-QSAR and ligand docking study. *Drug Des Discov*. 2000;17:34-50.
65. Dondio G, Ronzoni S, Eggleston DS, et al. Discovery of a novel class of substituted pyrrolooctahydroisoquinolines as potent and selective δ opioid agonists, based on an extension of the message-address concept. *J Med Chem*. 1997;40:3192-3198.
66. Dondio G, Ronzoni S, Petrillo P, Desjarlais RL, Raveglia LF. Pyrrolooctahydroisoquinolines as potent and selective δ opioid receptor ligands: SAR analysis and docking studies. *Bioorg Med Chem Lett*. 1997;7:2967-2972.
67. Casy AF, Parfitt RT. *Opioid Analgesics: Chemistry and Receptors*. New York, NY: Plenum Press; 1986.
68. Subramanian G, Ferguson DM. Conformational landscape of selective μ-opioid agonists in gas phase and in aqueous solution: the fentanyl series. *Drug Des Discov*. 2000;17:55-67.
69. Cometta-Morini C, Loew GH. Development of a conformational search strategy for flexible ligands: a study of the potent mu-selective opioid analgesic fentanyl. *J Comput Aided Mol Des*. 1991;5:335-356.
70. Brandt W, Barth A, Holtje HD. A new consistent model explaining structure (conformation)-activity relationships of opiates with μ-selectivity. *Drug Des Discov*. 1993;10:257-283.
71. Tang Y, Chen KX, Jiang HL, Wang ZX, Ji RY, Chi ZQ. Molecular modeling of μ opioid receptor and its interaction with ohmefentanyl. *Zhongguo Yao Li Xue Bao*. 1996;17:156-160.
72. Xu H, Lu YF, Partilla JS, et al. Opioid peptide receptor studies, 11: involvement of Tyr149, Trp318 and His319 of the rat μ-opioid receptor in binding of μ-selective ligands. *Synapse*. 1999;32:23-28.
73. Winter CA, Orahovats PD, Lehman EG. Analgesic activity and morphine antagonism of compounds related to nalorphine. *Arch Int Pharmacodyn Ther*. 1957;110:186-202.
74. Hunter JC, Leighton GE, Meecham KG, et al. CI-977, a novel and selective agonist for the κ-opioid receptor. *Br J Pharmacol*. 1990;101:183-189.
75. Rees DC. Chemical structures and biological activities of non-peptide selective kappa opioid ligands. *Prog Med Chem*. 1992;29:109-139.
76. Froimowitz M, DiMeglio CM, Makriyannis A. Conformational preferences of the κ-selective opioid agonist U50488. A combined molecular mechanics and nuclear magnetic resonance study. *J Med Chem*. 1992;35:3085-3094.
77. Higginbottom M, Nolan W, O'Toole J, Ratcliffe GS, Rees DC, Roberts E. The design and synthesis of κ opioid ligands based on a binding model for κ agonists. *Bioorg Med Chem Lett*. 1993;3:841-846.
78. Rajagopalan P, Scribner RM, Pennev P, et al. Dup 747: sar study. *Bioorg Med Chem Lett*. 1992;2:721-726.
79. Thirstrup K, Hjorth SA, Schwartz TW. Investigation of the binding pocket in the kappa opioid receptor by a combination of alanine substitutions and steric hindrance mutagenesis. Poster M30. 27th Meeting of the International Narcotics Research Conference; July 21–26, 1996; Long Beach, CA.

Chapter 35
Role of Morphine's Metabolites in Analgesia: Concepts and Controversies

Erica Wittwer[1] and Steven E. Kern[1,2]

Abstract The metabolites of morphine, morphine-6-glucuronide (M6G) and morphine-3-glucuronide (M3G), have been extensively studied for their contribution to clinical effects following administration of morphine. Those contributions to both the desired effect (ie, analgesia) and the undesired effects (eg, nausea, respiratory depression) are the subject of clinical controversy. Much attention and effort have been directed at investigating the properties of M6G because of interest in this substance as a possible substitute for morphine. It exhibits increased potency and the possibility of a better side effect profile compared with morphine, although the reported relative benefits vary widely. M3G is not analgesic, but its role in producing side effects, including the development of clinical tolerance, has been proposed. This review is focused on M6G and the factors that contribute to its clinical utility. The formation and distribution of M6G are presented, as are the analgesic effect and the onset of this effect. The impact of genetics, age, and gender on M6G and its effects is also reviewed.

Keywords Morphine, morphine-6-glucuronide, clinical pharmacology, clinical covariates

Introduction

Morphine, the prototypical opioid analgesic, is metabolized in vivo primarily to morphine-3-glucuronide (M3G) and morphine-6-glucuronide (M6G). These metabolic products account for ~65% of a dose of morphine, with the remaining drug biotransformed to

[1]Department of Pharmaceutics and Pharmaceutical Chemistry, College of Pharmacy, University of Utah, Salt Lake City, UT

[2]Department of Anesthesiology, School of Medicine, University of Utah, Salt Lake City, UT

Corresponding Author: Steven E. Kern, Assistant Professor and Interim Chair, Department of Pharmaceutics and Pharmaceutical Chemistry, University of Utah, 421 Wakara Way, Suite 318, Salt Lake City, UT 84108. Tel: (801) 585-5958; Fax: (801) 585-3614; E-mail: Steven.Kern@hsc.utah.edu

R.S. Rapaka and W. Sadée (eds.), *Drug Addiction*.
© American Association of Pharmaceutical Scientists 2008

multiple minor species or excreted unchanged.[1] These primary metabolites have been the focus of extensive basic and clinical evaluation for more than 25 years as investigators seek to better understand factors that contribute to opioids' analgesic effect and side effects. We have also been addressing issues related to the impact these metabolites may play on differences between patients who receive a standard dose of morphine.[2] While much is still unknown about the clinical pharmacology of morphine metabolites, what emerges from this body of literature is an understanding of the physicochemical and pharmacologic differences between the metabolites and the parent drug that explain their unique pharmacology and provide insight into both genetic and demographic differences (eg, gender, age) that exist for these therapeutic compounds.

Endogenous Metabolite Formation

Morphine is primarily metabolized in the liver by urldine-5′-diphosphate (UDP) glucuronosyltransferase, with specific affinity for the UGT2B7 isozyme. This isozyme is responsible for the formation of both glucuronide species. The differential amounts of metabolite formation (5 times more M3G is formed than M6G) have lead researchers to postulate that there is another metabolic isozyme that primarily forms M3G. Although in vitro results have indicated a possible role of UGT1A1 in the formation of M3G, in vivo the 2B7 isozyme is the primary morphine metabolite location.[3] The difference in formation of these 2 metabolites is more likely due to physicochemical and steric issues that affect the binding of morphine to the phase II enzyme.[1]

UGT2B7 is the primary enzyme for morphine metabolism, but it is also responsible for the metabolism of several endogenous and exogenous compounds. Chief among them are the steroid hormones, and also bilirubin in newborn infants. While these compounds are substrates for UGT2B7, they are also metabolized by other liver enzymes. Thus, these compounds could interfere with the production of morphine metabolites in vivo. Several substances can also serve in this capacity, including ranitidine, naltrexone, naloxone, and ethanol.[1,4,5]

Repeated injections of heroin in rats were shown to increase plasma levels of M6G (which were undetectable in the rats that received morphine instead of heroin) and to decrease the plasma levels of M3G. After the heroin injections were discontinued, the metabolism of morphine returned to normal.[6] This phenomenon was also seen in humans. Long-term intravenous heroin abusers given morphine or street heroin made more M6G and less M3G than nonheroin users given morphine.[7] Although heroine is a prodrug for morphine, the rationale for the influence of heroin on M6G formation is not known.

Analgesic Onset of Effect

In terms of pharmacological activity, M6G is an opioid agonist with a potency that is 2 to 4 times greater than morphine's, although these values vary widely depending on the study design used to assess drug effect. While relative potency in animals has been reported to range from 1:1 to 678:1, the range in humans is consistently reported to be in this lower range of 2 to 4:1.[8] In contrast, M3G is inactive and is reported to have little pharmacologic activity, although its role in contributing to analgesic effect and side effects is disputed.[9-14]

This increased potency of the M6G metabolite relative to morphine has been postulated to be related to the ability of M6G to exist at higher concentrations at the receptor sites in the central nervous system (CNS), rather than reflecting a significant difference in pharmacologic potency.[15] M6G is significantly less lipophilic than morphine, which substantially reduces its relative blood-brain barrier permeability. Yet its CNS uptake rate is greater than would be predicted based on the reduced level of lipophilicity and permeability. This suggests that M6G may be taken up into the CNS by an active transport mechanism.[16]

M6G crosses the blood-brain barrier slowly, showing a maximum concentration in the range of 6 hours for human volunteers after an intravenous dose.[17] The analgesic effect from M6G persists for a longer period of time than suggested by its elimination from the plasma. This is due to a significantly prolonged CNS clearance compared with systemic levels.[18] The effect may be prolonged in patients with renal failure because of metabolite buildup even though the metabolite is cleared from the blood during hemodialysis.

Experimental evidence from rats regarding factors that influence the effect of M6G on analgesia found that the delay in CNS effect was due to transport across the blood-brain barrier and also to distribution in the brain tissue or rate-limiting mechanisms at the receptor level.[19] In situ experiments using mouse brain found that M6G is not transported by P-glycoprotein or multidrug resistance protein 1 but is transported by GLUT-1 and a digoxin-sensitive transporter. These transporters are found on the luminal and abluminal sides of the brain endothelial cells, which may allow for bidirectional transport of M6G.[20] Although the previous study did not show that M6G was transported by P-glycoprotein, it has been shown that when the P-glycoprotein inhibitor PSC833 was given to rats receiving M6G, spinal cord tissue concentrations of M6G and antinociceptive effects were increased,[21] which was probably (as with probenecid) a secondary consequence of reduced systemic clearance rather than altered transport across the blood-brain barrier.[18]

Analgesic Activity

Experimental evidence from volunteer studies has shown that when M6G is administered intravenously, it has significant analgesic activity.[22] This result is in contrast to results from a study comparing morphine sulfate to M6G in patients undergoing major joint replacement surgery; it was found that patients receiving M6G had higher pain scores at 30 minutes and 1 hour postsurgery.[23] Furthermore, in a study comparing a single dose of morphine to a single dose of M6G at the end of open knee surgery, it was found that the placebo group and the M6G group required greater amounts of morphine from a patient-controlled analgesia pump than did the group that received the dose of morphine.[24] These conflicting reports exist for both clinical trials and volunteer experiments. While these differences are not fully understood, it appears that when M6G is directly administered intravenously in patients, the concentrations that produce acute analgesia are an order of magnitude higher than the concentrations that result from its metabolism from morphine.[8] Given M6G's relatively long time to peak effect, large doses of M6G may be needed to produce adequate concentrations in the CNS for acute analgesia. The conflicting reports on its efficacy after intravenous administration may indicate that too small a dose was administered or too short a time was allowed for assessment of its effect.[8] When M6G is given intrathecally, it produces profound analgesia in both animal and human clinical studies.[25,26] This further supports the idea that factors that affect the ability of M6G to cross the blood-brain barrier after direct intravenous administration may contribute to reported differences in its analgesic effect.

In addition to the liver, human brain homogenates have been shown to metabolize morphine at nanomolar concentrations to M3G and M6G, supporting the idea that M6G in the CNS may be formed there directly from morphine, which penetrates the blood-brain barrier at a greater rate than M6G.[27] Interestingly, this study also found a concentration dependency in the M3G/M6G ratio formed by the brain homogenate. At lower concentrations of morphine, the M3G/M6G ratio was lower, perhaps indicating a preference for forming M6G when less morphine is present.[27] These factors add to the complexity of understanding the relative contribution of M6G to analgesia when it is formed from morphine and comparing it with M6G's direct administration as an analgesic agent. It is clear that M6G has a very different absorption, distribution, metabolism, and excretion profile from morphine both systemically and at the site of drug effect; these differences contribute to the complexity of understanding the clinical pharmacology of this analgesic.

Further work is required to examine the clinical pharmacology profile of M6G. There is evidence that M6G reduces the severity of respiratory depression and nausea compared with morphine.[26,28,29] Whether M6G penetrates differentially to areas of the brain involved in pain, nausea, vomiting, and respiratory control or whether various opioid receptors in these brain areas differ in their pharmacology remains to be determined.[15,30] For instance, it has been shown that M6G has greater affinity for the μ_1 receptor subtype than for μ_2, the latter of which is thought to contribute to the negative side effects caused by opioids.[8] Furthermore, the opioid receptor is coded by a single gene that has at least several exons.[31] Knockout studies have shown that M6G and morphine have different sensitivities when alterations at exons 1 through 3 are evaluated.[32,33] These authors postulate the presence of a distinct receptor for M6G that may be important in the regulation of endogenous opioids, a premise supported by other groups as well.[16]

Genetics

Studies that relate differences in the genes that code for the enzyme for metabolizing morphine to M6G and for the mu opioid receptor have been conducted to determine whether these factors may contribute to the differential pharmacology of morphine and M6G. An extensive review of this literature was recently published by Lotsch et al.[21] With regard to morphine metabolism and M6G formation, the primary results have shown that morphine glucuronidation is unaffected by numerous UGT2B7 mutations, including the UGT2B7 H268Y polymorphism.[21] Interethnic differences have been seen between Caucasians and Native Americans, with the latter forming less M6G for an equivalent dose.[21] Multidrug resistance protein 3 (MRP3) polymorphisms may account for differences between individuals in M3G and M6G levels. MRP3 is the only transporter of M3G out of liver cells into plasma. In its absence, M3G is excreted in the bile in rats.[34]

Variants in the gene that codes for the mu opioid receptor have been linked to clinically measurable differences in the opioid effect of M6G. In particular, M6G was shown to have decreased efficacy with the A118G allele of the OPRM1 gene in homozygous carriers of the mutation when compared with the wild-type allele.[35] The same group found a decreased potency of M6G in both heterozygous and homozygous A118G carriers, with a larger decrease seen in the homozygous carrier.[36] Another group found that while the analgesic efficacy of M6G is reduced in those carriers of this mutation, it does not protect against respiratory effects.[37] A fascinating observation shown to occur in both mice and red-haired humans was that a mutation resulting in loss of function at the melanocortin 1 receptor gene was associated with greater analgesia from M6G.[38] This finding was gender independent, which contrasts with previous findings related to this mutation that showed a greater impact in women compared with men for predominantly the κ–opioid agonist pentazocine. These results indicate that differences in effect for a given dose of morphine may be related to both pharmacokinetic and pharmacodynamic phenotypes; these factors need to be independently assessed to better understand the role of M6G in the level of analgesia produced by morphine.

Impact of Gender and Age

Both gender and age contribute to differences in the pharmacokinetics of M6G and morphine that will ultimately affect pharmacologic effect. Results from our group showed that elderly women had higher levels of morphine metabolites compared with elderly men and that their clearance of the metabolites was reduced.[2] Further analysis revealed that progesterone levels may affect the clearance rates for the M3G metabolite in particular, which could contribute to its accumulation in elderly women who are on chronic opioid therapy.[39] Since the metabolites of morphine are cleared renally, it is anticipated that decreased renal function with age would also result in lower systemic clearance of both metabolite species, leading to longer accumulation of M6G and potentially extended effect.

Murthy et al constructed a model to investigate the contribution of M6G to morphine analgesia in humans.[40] Their study included 8 volunteers, 3 males and 5 females, and found that M6G contribution was extremely variable, ranging from <0.1% to 66%. They also found a gender difference in the contribution of M6G to analgesia, with the average contribution in males being 32% and in females 13%. The M6G contribution was inversely related to the overall effect elicited by the morphine dose.[40]

Conclusions

M6G is formed endogenously from the metabolism of morphine by the UGT2B7 isozyme. While M6G has a greater analgesic effect than morphine when administered intrathecally, the effects of exogenous M6G when administered intravenously are complex. The passage of M6G across the blood-brain barrier is slow and appears to be one of the primary factors in the difference in analgesic effect between systemic morphine and M6G. Additionally, evidence suggests that morphine is metabolized to M6G in the brain, which further complicates the evaluation of M6G as an analgesic compared with morphine.

The differences between the side effect profiles of M6G and morphine are encouraging for the potential therapeutic use of M6G, but they need further confirmation. These differences may be due to different effects at the same receptor or actions of M6G at a distinct receptor. M6G's effect has been shown to be influenced by variants in the gene that codes for the mu opioid receptor, particularly in the A118G allele of the OPRM1 gene. The presence of this allele is associated with decreased efficacy. Gender and age are both important factors in the analgesic effect of morphine and M6G. Continued investigation is necessary to resolve the controversies surrounding M6G and to further our understanding of its actions and interactions in the body.

References

1. Coffman B, King C, Rios G, Tephly T. The glucuronidation of opioids, other xenobiotics, and androgens by human UGT2B7Y(268) and UGT2B7H(268). *Drug Metab Dispos.* 1998;26:73-77.
2. Ratka A, Wittwer E, Baker L, Kern S. Pharmacokinetics of morphine, morphine-3-glucuronide, and morphine-6-glucuronide in healthy older men and women. *Am J Pain Manage.* 2004;14:45-55.
3. Stone A, Mackenzie P, Galetin A, Houston J, Miners J. Isoform selectivity and kinetics of morphine 3- and 6-glucuronidation by human UDP-glucuronosyltransferases: evidence for atypical glucuronidation kinetics by UGT2B7. *Drug Metab Dispos.* 2003;31:1086-1089.
4. Aasmundstad T, Storset P. Influence of ranitidine on the morphine-3-glucuronide to morphine-6-glucuronide ratio after oral administration of morphine in humans. *Hum Exp Toxicol.* 1998;17:347-352.
5. Faura C, Collins S, Moore R, McQuay H. Systematic review of factors affecting the ratio of morphine and its major metabolites. *Pain.* 1998;74:43-53.
6. Antonilli L, Suriano C, Paolone G, Badiani A, Nencini P. Repeated exposures to heroin and/or cadmium alter the rate of formation of morphine glucuronides in the rat. *J Pharmacol Exp Ther.* 2003;307:651-660.

7. Antonilli L, Semeraro F, Suriano C, Signore L, Nencini P. High levels of morphine-6-glucuronide in street heroin addicts. *Psychopharmacology (Berl)*. 2003;170:200-204.
8. Lotsch J, Geisslinger G. Morphine-6-glucuronide: an analgesic of the future? *Clin Pharmacokinet*. 2001;40:485-499.
9. Smith G, Smith M. Morphine-3-glucuronide: evidence to support its putative role in the development of tolerance to the antinociceptive effects of morphine in the rat. *Pain*. 1995;62:51-60.
10. Vaughan CW, Connor M. In search of a role for the morphine metabolite morphine-3-glucuronide. *Anesth Analg*. 2003;97:311-312.
11. Andersen G, Christrup L, Sjogren P. Relationships among morphine metabolism, pain and side effects during long-term treatment: an update. *J Pain Symptom Manage*. 2003;25:74-91.
12. Ashby M, Fleming B, Wood M, Somogyi A. Plasma morphine and glucuronide (M3G and M6G) concentrations in hospice inpatients. *J Pain Symptom Manage*. 1997;14:157-167.
13. Baker L, Hyrien O, Ratka A. Contributions of morphine-3-glucuronide and morphine-6-glucuronide to differences in morphine analgesia in humans. *Am J Pain Manage*. 2003;13:16-28.
14. Hemstapat K, Monteith G, Smith D, Smith M. Morphine-3-glucuronide's neuro-excitatory effects are mediated by indirect activation of NMDA receptors: mechanistic studies in embryonic cultured hippocampal neurones. *Anesth Analg*. 2003;97:494-505.
15. Okura T, Saito M, Nakanishi M, et al. Different distribution of morphine and morphine-6β-glucuronide after intracerebroventricular injection in rats. *Br J Pharmacol*. 2003;140: 211-217.
16. Mantione KJ, Goumon Y, Esch T, Stefano GB. Morphine 6B glucuronide: fortuitous morphine metabolite or preferred peripheral regulatory opiate? *Med Sci Monit*. 2005;11:MS43-MS46.
17. Lotsch J, Skarke C, Darimont J, Schmidt H, Geisslinger G. The transfer half-life of morphine-6-glucuronide from plasma to effect site assessed by pupil size measurement in healthy volunteers. *Anesthesiology*. 2001;95:1329-1338.
18. Tunblad K, Hammarlund-Udenaes M, Jonsson EN. Influence of probenecid on the delivery of morphine-6-glucuronide to the brain. *Eur J Pharm Sci*. 2005;24:49-57.
19. Bouw MRXR, Tunblad K, Hammarlund-Udenaes M. Blood-brain barrier transport and brain distribution of morphine-6-glucuronide in relation to the antinociceptive effect in rats—pharmacokinetic/pharmacodynamic modelling. *Br J Pharmacol*. 2001;134:1796-1804.
20. Bourasset F, Cisternino S, Temsamani J, Scherrmann JM. Evidence for an active transport of morphine-6-β-D-glucuronide but not P-glycoprotein-mediated at the blood-brain barrier. *J Neurochem*. 2003;86:1564-1567.
21. Lotsch J, Skarke C, Liefhold J, Geisslinger G. Genetic predictors of the clinical response to opioid analgesics. *Clin Pharmacokinet*. 2004;43:983-1013.
22. Buetler TMW, Wilder-Smith OH, Wilder-Smith CH, Aebi S, Cerny T, Brenneisen R. Analgesic action of i.v. morphine-6-glucuronide in healthy volunteers. *Br J Anaesth*. 2000;84:97-99.
23. Hanna MHEK, Fung M. Randomized, double-blind study of the analgesic efficacy of morphine-6-glucuronide versus morphine sulfate for postoperative pain in major surgery. *Anesthesiology*. 2005;102:815-821.
24. Motamed C, Mazoit X, Ghanouchi K, et al. Preemptive intravenous morphine-6-glucuronide is ineffective for postoperative pain relief. *Anesthesiology*. 2000;92:355-360.
25. Langlade A, Carr DB, Serrie A, Silbert BS, Szyfelbein SK, Lipkowski AW. Enhanced potency of intravenous, but not intrathecal, morphine and morphine-6-glucuronide after burn trauma. *Life Sci*. 1994;54:1699-1709.
26. Grace D, Fee J. A comparison of intrathecal morphine-6-glucuronide and intrathecal morphine sulfate as analgesics for total hip replacement. *Anesth Analg*. 1996;83:1055-1059.
27. Yamada H, Ishii K, Ishii Y, et al. Formation of highly analgesic morphine-6-glucuronide following physiologic concentration of morphine in human brain. *J Toxicol Sci*. 2003;28:395-401.
28. Cann C, Curran J, Milner T, Ho B. Unwanted effects of morphine-6-glucuronide and morphine. *Anaesthesia*. 2002;57:1200-1203.
29. Romberg R, Olofsen E, Sarton E, Teppema L, Dahan A. Pharmacodynamic effect of morphine-6-glucuronide versus morphine on hypoxic and hypercapnic breathing in healthy volunteers. *Anesthesiology*. 2003;99:788-798.

30. Kilpatrick G, Smith T. Morphine-6-glucuronide: actions and mechanisms. *Med Res Rev.* 2005;25:521-544.
31. Pasternak G. Incomplete cross tolerance and multiple mu opioid peptide receptors. *Trends Pharmacol Sci.* 2001;22:67-70.
32. Rossi GC, Pan YX, Brown GP, Pasternak GW. Antisense mapping the MOR-1 opioid receptor: evidence for alternative splicing and a novel morphine-6 beta-glucuronide receptor. *FEBS Lett.* 1995;369:192-196.
33. Rossi GC, Leventhal L, Pan YX, et al. Antisense mapping of MOR-1 in rats: distinguishing between morphine and morphine-6beta-glucuronide antinociception. *J Pharmacol Exp Ther.* 1997;281:109-114.
34. Zelcer N, Wetering K, Hillebrand M, et al. Mice lacking multidrug resistance protein 3 show altered morphine pharmacokinetics and morphine-6-glucuronide antinociception. *Proc Natl Acad Sci USA.* 2005;102:7274-7279.
35. Lotsch J, Zimmermann M, Darimont J, et al. Does the A118G polymorphism at the μ-opioid receptor gene protect against morphine-6-glucuronide toxicity? *Anesthesiology.* 2002;97:814-819.
36. Lotsch J, Skarke C, Grosch S, Darimont J, Schmidt H, Geisslinger G. The polymorphism A118G of the human mu-opioid receptor gene decreased the pupil constrictory effect of morphine-6-glucuronide but not that of morphine. *Pharmacogenetics.* 2002;12:3-9.
37. Romberg R, Olofsen E, Bijl H, et al. Polymorphism of mu-opioid receptor gene (OPRM1: c.118A>G) does not protect against opioid-induced respiratory depression despite reduced analgesic response. *Anesthesiology.* 2005;102:522-530.
38. Mogil JSSS, Strasburg K, Kaplan L, et al. Melanocortin-1 receptor gene variants affect pain and μ-opioid analgesia in mice and humans. *J Med Genet.* 2005;42:583-587.
39. Wittwer E, Ratka A, Kern S. The impact of endogenous steroidal hormones on the pharmacokinetics of oral morphine: a population analysis. Proceedings of the 79th IARS Clinical and Scientific Conference. 79th IARS Clinical and Scientific Conference; March 20-22, 2005; Honolulu, HI. Philadelphia, PA: LWW Publishers; 2004: PR04-R58.
40. Murthy BR, Pollack GM, Brouwer KL. Contribution of morphine-6-glucuronide to antinociception following intravenous administration of morphine to healthy volunteers. *J Clin Pharmacol.* 2002;42:569-576.

Chapter 36
Mu Opioid Receptor Regulation and Opiate Responsiveness

Kirsten M. Raehal[1] and Laura M. Bohn[1]

Abstract Opiate drugs such as morphine are well known for their ability to produce potent analgesia as well as such unwanted side effects as tolerance, physical dependence, respiratory suppression and constipation. Opiates act at opioid receptors, which belong to the family of G protein-coupled receptors. The mechanisms governing mu opioid receptor (μOR) regulation are of particular interest since morphine and other clinically important analgesics produce their pharmacological effects through this receptor. Here we review recent advances in understanding how opioid receptor regulation can impart differential agonist efficacy produced in vivo.

Introduction

Of the three major classes of opioid receptors, mu (μ), delta (δ), and kappa (κ), the μOR has proven to be the major target of opiate analgesics (for reviews see[1-3]). The opioid receptors belong to the family of G protein-coupled receptors (GPCRs), and like most GPCRs, they can be regulated by multiple mechanisms including receptor desensitization, internalization, resensitization and downregulation. G protein-coupled receptor regulatory elements such as GPCR kinases (GRKs) and βarrestins are important mediators of these processes. Agonist stimulation of GPCRs promotes receptor phosphorylation by GRKs and leads to recruitment of βarrestins which effectively uncouple the receptor and G proteins, thus preventing further signaling.[4-6] In addition to mediating

[1] Departments of Pharmacology & Psychiatry, The Ohio State University College of Medicine and Public Health, Columbus, OH 43210

Corresponding Author: Laura M. Bohn, Assistant Professor, Departments of Pharmacology & Psychiatry, The Ohio State University, College of Medicine & Health Science, 5184A Graves Hall, 333 W 10th Ave, Columbus, OH 43210-1239. Tel: 614-292-1303; Fax: 614-292-7232; E-mail: Bohn.24@osu.edu

R.S. Rapaka and W. Sadée (eds.), *Drug Addiction*.
© American Association of Pharmaceutical Scientists 2008

receptor desensitization, βarrestins also facilitate the internalization of inactivated receptors which can promote receptor recycling to the plasma membrane or lead to downregulation by receptor degradation.[4-6] βarrestins were first described for their ability to negatively regulate GPCR signaling (i.e, desensitization).[7,8] However, βarrestins can also play a more complex role in mediating receptor signaling and increasing evidence suggests that the complement of certain scaffolding proteins within the cellular environment may play a major role in determining overall receptor responsiveness to different agonists in particular cell types.[5,6]

The role of βarrestins in regulating the μOR has been studied at both the molecular level in vitro and at the pharmacological level in vivo (for reviews see[9-12]). Early in vitro studies in transfected HEK-293 cells revealed that the μOR, upon activation with morphine, does not robustly recruit βarrestins to the membrane while other opioid agonists, such as etorphine, do.[13] Since agonist activation of GPCRs typically induces βarrestin recruitment, morphine's actions at the μOR are unusual. These early observations suggested that the morphine-bound μOR may not be regulated by βarrestins. However, the physiological importance of μOR-βarrestin interactions was soon revealed when morphine-induced behaviors were evaluated in mice lacking βarrestin2.

Mice lacking βarrestin2 appear normal, although this molecule has been implicated in regulating numerous GPCRs that are expressed throughout the body. When morphine is administered to these animals, striking differences become immediately apparent when they are compared with normal, wild-type (WT) mice. βarrestin2-knockout (βarr2-KO) mice display enhanced and prolonged morphine-induced analgesia in both hot-plate and tail-flick antinociceptive tests.[14,15] Moreover, morphine-induced striatal extracellular dopamine levels as well as drug reinforcement are enhanced in the βarr2-KO mice compared with their WT counterparts.[16] Further investigation into behaviors in the absence of drug, revealed that basal tail-flick nociceptive response latencies are prolonged and this effect can be blocked by the opiate antagonist, naltrexone.[15] This suggests that the μOR-βarrestin2 interaction may not only be important for regulating the morphine-activated receptor, but may also help to establish the basal tone of receptor signaling. This finding also correlates with the observation that μOR agonist stimulated G protein-coupling is elevated in βarr2-KO mouse brain regions (periaqueductal gray, brainstem) as well as spinal cord.[14,15,17] In the absence of agonist stimulation, the basal degree of μOR-G protein-coupling is also significantly higher in brain regions in βarr2-KO compared with WT mice (LM Bohn, D Wang, W Sadée, unpublished observations). Therefore, the role of βarrestin2 in regulating the μOR is important for setting the basal tone as well as determining the potential for agonist-activated receptor signaling.

In the presence of persistent agonist treatment, GPCRs are subject to desensitization. Chronic morphine treatment, in vivo, leads to the development of opiate antinociceptive tolerance and physical dependence. Antinociceptive tolerance has previously been correlated with μOR desensitization[18,19] yet this has been difficult to test experimentally since there are no pharmacological tools which directly block desensitization. The βarr2-KO mice, after several different regimens of chronic morphine treatment, do not develop morphine-induced tolerance in the hot plate test, and display greatly attenuated tolerance in the tail-flick test.[15,17] Moreover, G protein-coupling in periaqueductal gray and brainstem of mice chronically treated with morphine reveal that while the μOR is significantly uncoupled from G proteins in WT mice, coupling is preserved in the βarr2-KO mice.[17] In another set of studies, Przewlocka et al.[20] showed that intrathecal administration of βarrestin2-specific antisense oligonucleotides could delay the onset of morphine antinociceptive tolerance in mice. Taken together, the biochemical and behavioral data suggest that βarrestin2 acts as a negative regulator, or desensitizing component, of μOR signaling in vivo.

While many of the morphine-induced responses in the βarr2-KO mice support the classically defined role of βarrestins as negative regulators of GPCR signaling, other physiological and behavioral responses to morphine do not. Morphine is known to activate locomotor activity in mice; however, the βarr2-KO mice display *less* activation of locomotion compared with their WT counterparts despite increased extracellular dopamine levels in striatum.[16] Moreover, while the βarr2-KO mice are resistant to morphine-induced antinociceptive tolerance, both genotypes develop a similar extent of physical dependence.[17] Current studies of respiratory suppression and gastrointestinal transit suggest that morphine-induced side effects are also not enhanced and may be less severe in mice lacking βarrestin2[21].

The question arises as to whether βarrestin2 may also be playing a role as a positive mediator of μOR signaling in vivo. Although βarrestins are traditionally viewed as negative regulators of GPCR signaling, βarrestins also function as scaffolding molecules that mediate GPCR signaling by facilitating interactions between signaling proteins and the receptor. In this scenario, μOR signaling may differ in certain cell types wherein the receptor's fate may be determined by the cellular complement of proteins within the receptor's immediate environment. Several in vitro studies have demonstrated that βarrestins act as adaptors between GPCRs and intracellular signaling proteins including the non-receptor tyrosine kinase, c-Src,[22-28] extracellular signal-regulated kinases (ERK)[22,25,29-32] and c-Jun N-terminal kinase (JNK).[33] The role of βarrestin2 in modulating receptor signaling in vivo has been demonstrated by a recent study by Wang et al.[34] wherein βarr2-KO mice developed *less* sedation with the alpha adrenergic 2A receptor agonist UK 14,304 in the rotorod test, suggesting that βarrestin2 may be directly involved in promoting this response rather then attenuating it.

The unbiquitination of βarrestins is yet another mechanism that plays a role in regulating βarrestin-mediated internalization and/or signaling via GPCRs. Agonist-stimulated ubiquitination of βarrestin2 has been implicated in co-trafficking and subsequent endocytosis of several GPCRs.[35-37] The ubiquitinated receptor-βarrestin complex may also be important for initiating βarrestin-mediated signal transduction wherein endosomes containing receptor-βarrestin complexes may act as 'signalsomes' by promoting receptor endocytosis as well as G-protein independent signaling.[37] However, such a role for βarrestins has yet to be demonstrated in μOR signaling.

It is apparent that the current understanding of GPCR signaling is rapidly expanding past the classical models of G-protein coupling and βarrestin-mediated desensitization. The complexity of determining receptor conformation, signaling and regulation is compounded by the organization of GPCRs into dimers and multimers. Interactions between receptors, as homo-, hetero- or oligo-mers, could change receptor expression profiles, ligand binding, and receptor signaling as well as trafficking and regulation. Cvejic and Devi[38] reported that δ opioid receptors (δORs) can exist as dimers in vitro and that the dimer complex can be desensitized in an agonist-dependent manner. Heterodimerization between δ- and κORs confers different receptor properties with distinct binding and signal transduction profiles compared with either the κ- or δOR alone.[39] The μ- and δORs can heterodimerize and, in the presence of δ-antagonists, μOR agonist binding and signaling is enhanced.[40] This finding was extended to animals wherein δ-antagonists significantly augmented morphine-induced analgesia in mice.[40] Recently, Wang et al.[41] demonstrated that all three opioid receptors (μ, δ, κ) have an equal potential to form homo- or heterodimers with each other. Interactions between opioid receptors and other receptor types including the β$_2$-adrenergic,[42] nociceptin/orphanin FQ,[43] somatostatin receptors[44,45] and substance P receptors[46] have been reported in vitro and may further increase the level of complexity in conferring opioid receptor responsiveness.

Signaling via the μOR, therefore, has the potential to be regulated by multiple means. Even if the μOR is regulated by the classical desensitization paradigm by βarrestin2 in some neurons this may not hold true for other cell types. For example, the μOR is widely distributed throughout the CNS and periphery and therefore, μORs expressed in one particular cell type (i.e medium spiny neurons) may not be subject to the same regulatory mechanisms as μORs expressed in other cell types (i.e, enteric neurons). Studies have shown decreased μOR-G protein coupling following morphine treatment in several brainstem regions of rat including the dorsal raphe nucleus, locus coeruleus, parabrachial nuclei, and the commissural nucleus tractus solitatius while no changes in μOR-G protein-coupling were observed in other regions such as the nucleus accumbens, amygdala, thalamus, and substania nigra.[19] Decreases in μOR activated G protein-coupling in the same regions affected by morphine (periaqueductal gray, locus coeruleus, and lateral parabrachial nucleus) were also seen in rats self-administering heroin.[47] Further, chronic morphine has been shown to induce desensitization of the μOR as measured by adenylyl cyclase inhibition in thalamus and periaqueductal gray brain regions but not in caudate putamen or nucleus accumbens.[18] These observations suggest that while the μOR is expressed in these brain regions, it is not desensitized to the same extent following chronic morphine treatment and demonstrates that the μOR can be differentially regulated in different cellular environments.

The relative responsiveness of the μOR is not only dependent on agonist occupancy but can vary with distinct opiate agonists. Several groups have demonstrated in vitro that while agonists such as morphine, DAMGO, etorphine, methadone and fentanyl can activate μOR signaling with similar efficacy they differ in their ability to promote receptor desensitization and internalization.[48-50] For example, morphine and heroin do not promote robust βarrestin2 translocation or receptor endocytosis in HEK-293 cells while other opiate agonists including DAMGO, etorphine, methadone and fentanyl do.[13,50-55] The inability of morphine and heroin to induce βarrestin2 translocation could however be overcome by the overexpression of

GRK2.[13,54] Studies in mouse embryonic fibroblasts lacking endogenous βarrestin1 and βarrestin2 suggest that the morphine-bound μOR preferentially interacts with βarrestin2.[54] This concept is further strengthened by the finding that the enhanced morphine analgesia in βarr2-KO mice could not be recapitulated in mice lacking βarrestin1, indicating that βarrestin2, rather than βarrestin1, may preferentially regulate the μOR in vivo.[54] Cheng et al.[56] showed that βarrestin1 interferes with δ- and κOR stimulated G protein-coupling but had no effect on μOR activation of G proteins further supporting a selective interaction between the μOR and βarrestin2 rather than βarrestin1.

Studies in cell culture reveal that the morphine-bound μOR is weakly phosphorylated, a poor substrate for βarrestins, and does not internalize. However, the overexpression of βarrestins or GRKs can overcome these apparent limitations.[13,53,54] Therefore, it is reasonable that if a certain neuron expresses higher levels of βarrestins or GRKs, the μOR may be able to internalize with morphine binding. While studies have nicely shown different levels of GRK and βarrestin mRNA expression in certain brain regions,[57] a lack of selective antibody tools have made it difficult to quantify protein expression patterns of each GRK and βarrestin type. Furthermore, GRK and βarrestin levels are dynamic and opiate agonists have been shown to alter their expression patterns throughout the CNS. Terwilliger et al.[58] reported that βarrestin1 and βarrestin2 levels increase in locus coeruleus neurons in response to chronic morphine treatment. In addition, acute and chronic morphine treatment also differentially alters βarrestin1 and βarrestin2 mRNA expression patterns in hippocampal, cerebral cortex, periaqueductal gray and locus coeruleus.[59] Mice acutely or chronically treated with the opiate agonist sufentanil have upregulated GRK2, GRK6 and βarrestin2 levels in brain while GRK3 levels are only elevated after acute treatment.[60] Increased levels of GRK2, GRK3, GRK6 and βarrestin2 in the cortex and striatum have also been observed following chronic opioid antagonist treatment with naloxone and naltrexone.[61] Finally, decreases in μOR density as well as GRK2, GRK6 and βarrestin2 levels in the prefrontal cortex have been observed in post-mortem brains of opiate addicts.[62]

Overall, there is a great deal of evidence supporting the dynamic expression of GRKs and βarrestins in the central nervous system. Therefore, μOR regulation profiles may also be dynamic, dependent not only on the site of expression but also upon drug exposure. Recently, Haberstock-Debic et al.[63] reported that while morphine-bound μORs do not internalize in the cell body of neurons, receptor internalization does occur in the dendrites of the same hippocampal neuron. This observation further emphasizes and points to the importance of the immediate cellular environment to the overall receptor regulation. Upon considering both the cell culture and animal studies in parallel, it is apparent that opioid receptor regulation can have profound impacts on overall agonist responsiveness. The complexity governing such diverse potential regulatory mechanisms emphasizes the need to study receptor signaling in the endogenous environment as this may ultimately determine the physiological response to the drug. As these complexities are revealed, novel therapeutic targets may become available to enhance and fine-tune opioid receptor pharmacology for the treatment of pain and addiction.

References

1. Mansour A, Watson SJ, Akil H. Opioid receptors: Past, present and future. *Trends Neurosci.* 1995;18:69-70.
2. Kieffer BL. Opioids: First lessons from knockout mice. *Trends Pharmacol Sci.* 1999; 20:19-26.
3. Kieffer BL, Gaveriaux-Ruff C. Exploring the opioid system by gene knockout. *Prog Neurobiol.* 2002;66:285-306.
4. Ferguson SS, Zhang J, Barak LS, Caron MG. Role of beta-arrestins in the intracellular trafficking of G-protein-coupled receptors. *Adv Pharmacol.* 1998;42:420-424.
5. Luttrell LM, Lefkowitz RJ. The role of beta-arrestins in the termination and transduction of G-protein-coupled receptor signals. *J Cell Sci.* 2002;115:455-465.
6. Perry SJ, Lefkowitz RJ. Arresting developments in heptahelical receptor signaling and regulation. *Trends Cell Biol.* 2002;12:130-138.
7. Benovic JL, Kuhn H, Weyand I, Codina J, Caron MG, Lefkowitz RJ. Functional desensitization of the isolated beta-adrenergic receptor by the beta-adrenergic receptor kinase: Potential role of an analog of the retinal protein arrestin (48-kDa protein). *Proc Natl Acad Sci USA.* 1987;84:8879-8882.
8. Lohse MJ, Benovic JL, Codina J, Caron MG, Lefkowitz RJ. Beta-Arrestin: A protein that regulates beta-adrenergic receptor function. *Science.* 1990;248:1547-1550.
9. Chavkin C, McLaughlin JP, Celver JP. Regulation of opioid receptor function by chronic agonist exposure: constitutive activity and desensitization. *Mol Pharmacol.* 2001;60:20-25.
10. Connor M, Osborne PB, Christie MJ. Mu-opioid receptor desensitization: Is morphine different? *Br J Pharmacol.* 2004;143:685-696.
11. Bohn LM, Gainetdinov RR, Caron MG. G protein-coupled receptor kinase/beta-arrestin systems and drugs of abuse: Psychostimulant and opiate studies in knockout mice. *Neuromolecular Med.* 2004;5:41-50.
12. Gainetdinov RR, Premont RT, Bohn LM, Lefkowitz RJ, Caron MG. Desensitization of G protein-coupled receptors and neuronal functions. *Annu Rev Neurosci.* 2004;27:107-144.
13. Zhang J, Ferguson SS, Barak LS, et al. Role for G protein-coupled receptor kinase in agonist-specific regulation of mu-opioid receptor responsiveness. *Proc Natl Acad Sci USA.* 1998;95:7157-7162.
14. Bohn LM, Lefkowitz RJ, Gainetdinov RR, Peppel K, Caron MG, Lin FT. Enhanced morphine analgesia in mice lacking beta-arrestin 2. *Science.* 1999;286:2495-2498.
15. Bohn LM, Lefkowitz RJ, Caron MG. Differential mechanisms of morphine antinociceptive tolerance revealed in beta-arrestin2 knock-out mice. *J Neurosci.* 2002;22:10494-10500.
16. Bohn LM, Gainetdinov RR, Sotnikova TD, et al. Enhanced rewarding properties of morphine, but not cocaine, in beta-arrestin2 knock-out mice. *J Neurosci.* 2003;23:10265-10273.
17. Bohn LM, Gainetdinov RR, Lin FT, Lefkowitz RJ, Caron MG. Mu-opioid receptor desensitization by beta-arrestin2 determines morphine tolerance but not dependence. *Nature.* 2000;408:720-723.
18. Noble F, Cox BM. Differential desensitization of mu- and delta- opioid receptors in selected neural pathways following chronic morphine treatment. *Br J Pharmacol.* 1996;117: 161-169.
19. Sim LJ, Selley DE, Dworkin SI, Childers SR. Effects of chronic morphine administration on mu opioid receptor-stimulated [35S]GTPgammaS autoradiography in rat brain. *J Neurosci.* 1996;16:2684-2692.
20. Przewlocka B, Sieja A, Starowicz K, Maj M, Bilecki W, Przewlocki R. Knockdown of spinal opioid receptors by antisense targeting beta-arrestin reduces morphine tolerance and allodynia in rat. *Neurosci Lett.* 2002;325:107-110.
21. Raehal KM, Walker JKL, Bohn LM. Morphine side-effects in b-arrestin-2 knockout mice. *J Pharmacol Exp Ther.* 2005;314:1195-1201.

22. Luttrell LM, Ferguson SS, Daaka Y, et al. Beta-arrestin-dependent formation of beta2 adrenergic receptor-Src protein kinase complexes. *Science*. 1999;283:655-661.
23. Luttrell LM, Daaka Y, Lefkowitz RJ. Regulation of tyrosine kinase cascades by G-protein-coupled receptors. *Curr Opin Cell Biol*. 1999;11:177-183.
24. Ahn S, Maudsley S, Luttrell LM, Lefkowitz RJ, Daaka Y. Src-mediated tyrosine phosphorylation of dynamin is required for beta2-adrenergic receptor internalization and mitogen-activated protein kinase signaling. *J Biol Chem*. 1999;274:1185-1188.
25. DeFea KA, Vaughn ZD, O'Bryan EM, Nishijima D, Dery O, Bunnett NW. The proliferative and antiapoptotic effects of substance P are facilitated by formation of a beta -arrestin-dependent scaffolding complex. *Proc Natl Acad Sci USA*. 2000;97:11086-11091.
26. Miller WE, Maudsley S, Ahn S, Khan KD, Luttrell LM, Lefkowitz RJ. beta-arrestin1 interacts with the catalytic domain of the tyrosine kinase c-SRC. Role of beta-arrestin1-dependent targeting of c-SRC in receptor endocytosis. *J Biol Chem*. 2000;275:11312-11319.
27. Barlic J, Andrews JD, Kelvin AA, et al. Regulation of tyrosine kinase activation and granule release through beta-arrestin by CXCR1. *Nat Immunol*. 2000;1:227-233.
28. Imamura T, Huang J, Dalle S, et al. beta -Arrestin-mediated recruitment of the Src family kinase Yes mediates endothelin-1-stimulated glucose transport. *J Biol Chem*. 2001;276:43663-43667.
29. DeFea KA, Zalevsky J, Thoma MS, Dery O, Mullins RD, Bunnett NW. beta-arrestin-dependent endocytosis of proteinase-activated receptor 2 is required for intracellular targeting of activated ERK1/2. *J Cell Biol*. 2000;148:1267-1281.
30. Luttrell LM, Roudabush FL, Choy EW, et al. Activation and targeting of extracellular signal-regulated kinases by beta-arrestin scaffolds. *Proc Natl Acad Sci USA*. 2001;98:2449-2454.
31. Tohgo A, Pierce KL, Choy EW, Lefkowitz RJ, Luttrell LM. Beta-Arrestin scaffolding of the ERK cascade enhances cytosolic ERK activity but inhibits ERK-mediated transcription following angiotensin AT1a receptor stimulation. *J Biol Chem*. 2002;277:9429-9436.
32. Tohgo A, Choy EW, Gesty-Palmer D, et al. The stability of the G protein-coupled receptor-beta-arrestin interaction determines the mechanism and functional consequence of ERK activation. *J Biol Chem*. 2003;278:6258-6267.
33. McDonald PH, Chow CW, Miller WE, et al. Beta-arrestin2: A receptor-regulated MAPK scaffold for the activation of JNK3. *Science*. 2000;290:1574-1577.
34. Wang Q, Zhao J, Brady AE, et al. Spinophilin blocks arrestin actions in vitro and in vivo at G protein-coupled receptors. *Science*. 2004;304:1940-1944.
35. Shenoy SK, McDonald PH, Kohout TA, Lefkowitz RJ. Regulation of receptor fate by ubiquitination of activated beta 2-adrenergic receptor and beta-arrestin. *Science*. 2001;294:1307-1313.
36. Shenoy SK, Lefkowitz RJ. Trafficking patterns of beta-arrestin and G protein-coupled receptors determined by the kinetics of beta-arrestin deubiquitination. *J Biol Chem*. 2003;278:14498-14506.
37. Shenoy SK, Lefkowitz RJ. Receptor-specific ubiquitination of beta-arrestin directs assembly and targeting of 7TM receptor-signalosomes. *J Biol Chem*. 2005;280:15315-15324.
38. Cvejic S, Devi LA. Dimerization of the delta opioid receptor: Implication for a role in receptor internalization. *J Biol Chem*. 1997;272:26959-26964.
39. Jordan BA, Devi LA. G-protein-coupled receptor heterodimerization modulates receptor function. *Nature*. 1999;399:697-700.
40. Gomes I, Gupta A, Filipovska J, Szeto HH, Pintar JE, Devi LA. A role for heterodimerization of mu and delta opiate receptors in enhancing morphine analgesia. *Proc Natl Acad Sci USA*. 2004;101:5135-5139.
41. Wang D, Sun X, Bohn LM, Sadee W. Opioid receptor homo- and hetero-dimerization in living cells by quantitative bioluminescence resonance energy transfer. *Mol Pharmacol*. 2005;67:2173-2184.
42. Jordan BA, Trapaidze N, Gomes I, Nivarthi R, Devi LA. Oligomerization of opioid receptors with beta 2-adrenergic receptors: a role in trafficking and mitogen-activated protein kinase activation. *Proc Natl Acad Sci USA*. 2001;98:343-348.

43. Pan YX, Bolan E, Pasternak GW. Dimerization of morphine and orphanin FQ/nociceptin receptors: Generation of a novel opioid receptor subtype. *Biochem Biophys Res Commun.* 2002;297:659-663.

44. Pfeiffer M, Koch T, Schroder H, et al. Homo- and heterodimerization of somatostatin receptor subtypes. Inactivation of sst(3) receptor function by heterodimerization with sst(2A). *J Biol Chem.* 2001;276:14027-14036.

45. Pfeiffer M, Koch T, Schroder H, Laugsch M, Hollt V, Schulz S. Heterodimerization of somatostatin and opioid receptors cross-modulates phosphorylation, internalization, and desensitization. *J Biol Chem.* 2002;277:19762-19772.

46. Pfeiffer M, Kirscht S, Stumm R, et al. Heterodimerization of substance P and mu-opioid receptors regulates receptor trafficking and resensitization. *J Biol Chem.* 2003;278:51630-51637.

47. Yu Y, Zhang L, Yin X, Sun H, Uhl GR, Wang JB. Mu opioid receptor phosphorylation, desensitization, and ligand efficacy. *J Biol Chem.* 1997;272:28869-28874.

48. Sim-Selley LJ, Selley DE, Vogt LJ, Childers SR, Martin TJ. Chronic heroin self-administration desensitizes mu opioid receptor-activated G-proteins in specific regions of rat brain. *J Neurosci.* 2000;20:4555-4562.

49. Yabaluri N, Medzihradsky F. Down-regulation of mu-opioid receptor by full but not partial agonists is independent of G protein coupling. *Mol Pharmacol.* 1997;52:896-902.

50. Arden JR, Segredo V, Wang Z, Lameh J, Sadee W. Phosphorylation and agonist-specific intracellular trafficking of an epitope-tagged mu-opioid receptor expressed in HEK 293 cells. *J Neurochem.* 1995;65:1636-1645.

51. Keith DE, Murray SR, Zaki PA, et al. Morphine activates opioid receptors without causing their rapid internalization. *J Biol Chem.* 1996;271:19021-19024.

52. Sternini C, Spann M, Anton B, et al. Agonist-selective endocytosis of mu opioid receptor by neurons in vivo. *Proc Natl Acad Sci USA.* 1996;93:9241-9246.

53. Whistler JL, von Zastrow M. Morphine-activated opioid receptors elude desensitization by beta-arrestin. *Proc Natl Acad Sci USA.* 1998;95:9914-9919.

54. Bohn LM, Dykstra LA, Lefkowitz RJ, Caron MG, Barak LS. Relative opioid efficacy is determined by the complements of the G protein-coupled receptor desensitization machinery. *Mol Pharmacol.* 2004;66:106-112.

55. Koch T, Widera A, Bartzsch K, et al. Receptor endocytosis counteracts the development of opioid tolerance. *Mol Pharmacol.* 2005;67:280-287.

56. Cheng ZJ, Yu QM, Wu YL, Ma L, Pei G. Selective interference of beta-arrestin 1 with kappa and delta but not mu opioid receptor/G protein coupling. *J Biol Chem.* 1998;273:24328-24333.

57. Gurevich EV, Benovic JL, Gurevich VV. Arrestin2 expression selectively increases during neural differentiation. *J Neurochem.* 2004;91:1404-1416.

58. Terwilliger RZ, Ortiz J, Guitart X, Nestler EJ. Chronic morphine administration increases beta-adrenergic receptor kinase (beta ARK) levels in the rat locus coeruleus. *J Neurochem.* 1994;63:1983-1986.

59. Fan XL, Zhang JS, Zhang XQ, Yue W, Ma L. Differential regulation of beta-arrestin 1 and beta-arrestin 2 gene expression in rat brain by morphine. *Neuroscience.* 2003;117:383-389.

60. Hurle MA. Changes in the expression of G protein-coupled receptor kinases and beta-arrestin 2 in rat brain during opioid tolerance and supersensitivity. *J Neurochem.* 2001;77:486-492.

61. Diaz A, Pazos A, Florez J, Ayesta FJ, Santana V, Hurle MA. Regulation of mu-opioid receptors, G-protein-coupled receptor kinases and beta-arrestin 2 in the rat brain after chronic opioid receptor antagonism. *Neuroscience.* 2002;112:345-353.

62. Ferrer-Alcon M, La Harpe R, Garcia-Sevilla JA. Decreased immunodensities of micro-opioid receptors, receptor kinases GRK 2/6 and beta-arrestin-2 in postmortem brains of opiate addicts. *Brain Res Mol Brain Res.* 2004;121:114-122.

63. Haberstock-Debic H, Wein M, Barrot M, et al. Morphine acutely regulates opioid receptor trafficking selectively in dendrites of nucleus accumbens neurons. *J Neurosci.* 2003;23:4324-4332.

Chapter 37
Agmatine: Biological Role and Therapeutic Potentials in Morphine Analgesia and Dependence

Soundar Regunathan[1]

Abstract Agmatine is an amine that is formed by decarboxylation of L-arginine by the enzyme arginine decarboxylase (ADC) and hydrolyzed by the enzyme agmatinase to putrescine. Agmatine binds to several target receptors in the brain and has been proposed as a novel neuromodulator. In animal studies, agmatine potentiated morphine analgesia and reduced dependence/withdrawal. While the exact mechanism is not clear, the interactions with N-methyl-D-aspartate (NMDA) receptors, α2-adrenergic receptors, and intracellular cyclic adenosine monophosphate (cAMP) signaling have been proposed as possible targets. Like other monoamine transmitter molecules, agmatine is rapidly metabolized in the periphery and has poor penetration into the brain, which limits the use of agmatine itself as a therapeutic agent. However, the development of agmatinase inhibitors will offer a useful method to increase endogenous agmatine in the brain as a possible therapeutic approach to potentiate morphine analgesia and reduce dependence/withdrawal. This review provides a succinct discussion of the biological role/therapeutic potential of agmatine during morphine exposure/pain modulation, with an extensive amount of literature cited for further details.

Keywords agmatine, morphine, opioids, analgesia, withdrawal

Introduction

Agmatine is an amine that is formed by decarboxylation of L-arginine by the enzyme arginine decarboxylase (ADC) and hydrolyzed by the enzyme agmatinase (agmatine uryl hydrolase) to putrescine. After an initial report in 1994,[1] several

---

[1]Division of Neurobiology and Behavior Research, Department of Psychiatry and Human Behavior, University of Mississippi Medical Center, Jackson, MS

Corresponding Author: Soundar Regunathan, Division of Neurobiology and Behavior Research, Department of Psychiatry and Human Behavior, University of Mississippi Medical Center, 2500 N State Street, Jackson, MS 39216. Tel: (601) 984-5471; Fax: (601) 984-5899; E-mail: sregunathan@psychiatry.umsmed.edu

R.S. Rapaka and W. Sadée (eds.), *Drug Addiction.*
© American Association of Pharmaceutical Scientists 2008

laboratories confirmed the presence of agmatine in the brain and its interaction with several target receptors such as α2-adrenergic, imidazoline, and NMDA receptors.[1-4] These observations suggested that agmatine may have functions of a novel neurotransmitter/neuromodulator.[5] Using specific antibodies to agmatine,[6] we have shown by immunocytochemical studies that in the brain agmatine (1) is stored in the perikarya of a specific population of central neurons,[7] and (2) is found in small vesicles of axon terminals[8,9] that form synaptic contacts and is presumably costored and released with traditional transmitters/modulators, including l-glutamate and arginine vasopressin.[9] Agmatine is synthesized by a mammalian form of ADC[10,11] whose complementary DNA (cDNA) sequence has been recently identified.[12] Agmatine can be degraded by agmatinase in the brain[13] and by diamine oxidase in peripheral tissues.[14] The physiological role of agmatine in normal brain function is still unknown, in part because of the absence of adequate pharmacological tools to manipulate its synthesis and degradation. Moreover, since agmatine has several molecular targets and acts as an antagonist in most targets, it has been difficult to evaluate the function of endogenous agmatine in the whole organism. However, as discussed below, studies of the actions of exogenous agmatine have identified several intriguing neurally relevant functions of the amine that are of potential therapeutic importance. Agmatine administered intrathecally, locally or systemically, reduces the neuronal injury produced by excitotoxins,[15,16] global/focal ischemia,[17-19] spinal cord injury,[17,20] and hypoxic ischemic injury.[21] Another notable effect of agmatine is its ability to reduce chemically and electrically induced convulsive seizures.[22-24] Agmatine has also been proposed as an adjunct in the treatment of several chronic pain syndromes, and as effective in facilitating the action of morphine while profoundly reducing the development of tolerance.[25] Agmatine administered intrathecally or intraperitoneally (IP) blocks the development of morphine tolerance[20,25] and inhibits naloxone-precipitated signs of morphine withdrawal in rats.[26-29] Agmatine also has notable effects on learning behavior in fear-conditioning models[30,31] and antidepressant-like effects in depression models.[32-34]

Exogenous Agmatine, Morphine, and Analgesia

Several studies have reported the in vivo effects of agmatine on morphine analgesia/dependence, nociceptive responses, neuronal injury, and other behavioral effects in several animal models, as recently reviewed by Nguyen et al.[29] The first study, from the Pasternak laboratory, showed that agmatine at the dose of 10 mg/kg (subcutaneous) potentiated morphine analgesia and prevented the development of tolerance to chronic morphine.[25] Subsequently, several studies have confirmed the effects of agmatine on morphine pain tolerance and withdrawal symptoms with doses ranging from 1 to 25 mg/kg.[26,35,36] Most intriguing is agmatine's ability to potentiate the analgesic effect of morphine while also reducing the withdrawal symptoms after chronic exposure.[35,37] Thus, acute injection of agmatine by the peripheral route increases the analgesic effects of morphine and reduces tolerance to repeated morphine injection. Agmatine has been shown to reduce symptoms of withdrawal from morphine as measured by physical dependence in animal models. The reduction of central symptoms required the expression of functional neuronal nitric oxide synthase activity.[38] In related studies, intravenous agmatine was shown to evoke the escalation of fentanyl, but not cocaine, self-administration.[39] Besides potentiating morphine analgesia, agmatine, by itself, also has noted effects on nociceptive responses.[20,27,40-43] For example, agmatine can act like an antihyperalgesic agent in reducing the mechanical and inflammation-induced hypersensitivity to pain stimulation.[20] It is also important to point out that in all animal studies reported, agmatine had no effect on normal behavior, motor activity, or cardiovascular parameters and had no other toxic effects in normal animals in doses up to 100 mg/kg.

Molecular Targets of Agmatine Action

As agmatine does not bind to opiate receptors, the analgesic effects and the reduction of withdrawal to morphine are not likely to be mediated by a direct effect on opiate receptors.[44] However, agmatine interacts with several other target proteins that could mediate its effects. Agmatine binds to NMDA receptors and acts as an antagonist at NMDA receptor channels,[8,16,45-47] and NMDA antagonists are known to block opioid withdrawal symptoms.[48] Agmatine also binds to $\alpha2$-adrenergic receptors, and agonists of $\alpha2$-adrenergic receptors have been known to inhibit opioid withdrawal. The activation of $\alpha2$-adrenergic receptors by agonists like clonidine inhibits dependence and withdrawal. While agmatine was discovered because of its ability to bind to $\alpha2$-adrenergic receptors,[1] several subsequent functional studies reported that agmatine is not an agonist at this site.[4,49] Moreover, administration of $\alpha2$-adrenergic agonists like clonidine, while blocking opiate withdrawal, causes sympathetic inhibition and reduction in arterial pressure.[50-52] In several animal models, agmatine, administered intracerebroventricular (i.c.v.) or IP, has not been shown to lower arterial pressure,[53-55] thus ruling out the possibility of $\alpha2$-adrenergic receptor activation in this action of agmatine. Thus, the actions of agmatine on morphine pain response and withdrawal are most likely mediated by its ability to block NMDA receptor channels.[56] Meanwhile, other studies have suggested that the blockade of NMDA receptors may not be the only mechanism by which agmatine regulates glutamatergic neurotransmission during acute or chronic morphine exposure. Agmatine has been shown to modulate presynaptic calcium channels,[57,58] and such an effect could lead to lower glutamate release after acute agmatine injection. Our recent results indicate that acute agmatine administration reduces extracellular glutamate during pentylenetetrazole (PTZ)-induced convulsive seizures as measured by in vivo microdialysis.[59] Thus, agmatine may also regulate the release of glutamate during morphine withdrawal.

In initial behavior studies in rats and mice, symptoms of withdrawal from morphine, induced by naloxone, were reduced by agmatine when it was injected with naloxone,[25,35] probably because the agmatine directly inhibited NMDA receptors. More recently, we showed that chronic injection of agmatine during morphine exposure (lasting 7 days), but not at the time of inducing withdrawal by naloxone, substantially reduced the withdrawal symptoms.[37] Since agmatine was not present during the induction of withdrawal, direct inhibition of NMDA receptors could not be involved in this mode of agmatine action. Therefore, it appears that agmatine, administered during the development of morphine dependence, blocks the events leading to a hyperexcitable state of the neurons during chronic morphine exposure, thereby reducing withdrawal. This idea was conceived based on several reports indicating intracellular effects of agmatine. These effects include inhibition of cellular proliferation in kidney and vascular smooth muscle cells,[60,61] inflammatory signaling in macrophages and glial cells,[62-64] and morphine-induced cAMP super-activation in NG108-15 cells[65] and the rat brain.[37]

The cellular and molecular mechanisms for opiate tolerance/dependence and withdrawal have been fairly well documented. Electrophysiological and neuro-chemical studies have indicated that a hyperexcitable state of neurons in the locus coeruleus (LC), the ventral tegmental area (VTA), and the nucleus accumbens after chronic morphine exposure contributes to dependence and withdrawal. These changes occur because of a cycle of molecular events of higher phosphorylation and gene expression, resulting in adaptive upregulation of the cAMP system after chronic morphine abuse.[66] This upregulation has been shown in in vitro model systems including NG108-15 cells and cells transfected with μ-opioid receptors, as well as in in vivo animal models.[67-70] The resulting higher cAMP causes increased protein kinase A (PKA) activity, which phosphorylates several target proteins, including tyrosine hydroxylase (TH) and cAMP response element binding protein (CREB). The phosphorylated CREB subsequently acts as a transcription factor increasing the expression of several proteins, including adenylate cyclase and TH.[71] There is also evidence that initial suppression of cAMP production by morphine could increase the expression of specific subunits of PKA.[71] All these molecular changes initiate the cycle of events resulting in higher TH, adenylate cyclase, PKA, and several phosphorylated proteins, including membrane sodium channels, causing the hyperexcitable state of the neurons. We hypothesized that chronic administration of agmatine along with morphine interferes with some step in these intracellular signal transduction pathways, thereby reducing dependence/withdrawal. In fact, one previous study reported that agmatine inhibited the increase in cAMP in morphine-exposed NG108-15 cells when the cells were challenged with naloxone.[65] Our recent report confirmed this finding in brain cortical slices of rats chronically exposed to morphine and agmatine.[37] We have also observed that agmatine inhibits the higher expression of TH during chronic morphine exposure in rat LC and striatum (S. Regunathan and F. Aricoglu, unpublished data, December 2004). These initial findings support our hypothesis, but further studies are required to investigate how agmatine regulate the downstream events of cAMP signaling.

Morphine Exposure and Endogenous Agmatine

While exogenous agmatine is clearly effective in modulating opiate analgesia/dependence, whether endogenous agmatine has a similar function is not known. It is important to note that all the brain structures that are involved in drugs of abuse—the VTA, the nucleus accumbens, the amygdala, and the LC—contain substantial agmatine immunoreactive neurons.[7] Agmatine and ADC activity are known to be regulated in certain other conditions, such as inflammatory neuropathic pain, ischemic stroke, and depression.[18,20,72,73] Our initial studies have indicated that agmatine levels and ADC activity are lower in the rat brain and other tissues after 3 days of exposure to morphine.[74] Studies on the in vivo release of agmatine during morphine exposure and withdrawal should provide some evidence for the role of endogenous agmatine in opiate drug abuse. However, the ultimate proof will be to show that increasing endogenous agmatine levels reduces symptoms of morphine withdrawal and decreasing these levels exacerbates symptoms of morphine withdrawal. Blocking the biosynthetic enzyme, ADC, could be the direct approach to reducing endogenous agmatine levels. Although no selective inhibitor of mammalian ADC is presently available, other means of decreasing ADC activity are feasible. For example, the cDNA sequence of mammalian ADC can be used to design RNA interference (small double-stranded RNA) to degrade ADC messenger RNA (mRNA), thereby lowering the expression of ADC activity and levels of agmatine. We have recently produced small interfering ribonucleic aid (siRNA) capable of reducing ADC mRNA levels and agmatine production in cultured neurons and glial cells.[75]

Another approach that is currently being used successfully is blocking the action of endogenous agmatine by selective agmatine antibodies. In a recent study, Fairbanks et al showed that antiagmatine immunoglobulin G (IgG), but not normal IgG, reversed exogenous agmatine-mediated, but not MK801-mediated, inhibition of NMDA-evoked behavior in mice and induced tolerance to opioid agonists at lower doses.[76] These findings were interpreted to mean that sequestration of endogenous agmatine by agmatine-selective IgG increases the susceptibility to tolerance induced by opioid agonists. This strategy has been used previously[77] to show that an antiserum raised against [Leu5]enkephalin prevents the increase in morphine potency induced by exogenous i.c.v. administration of [Leu5]enkephalin. These results validate the approach of determining the physiological effects of inactivating endogenous agmatine by administering exogenous antisera.

Obviously, further studies using the approach of increasing or decreasing endogenous agmatine are required to establish the proof-of-concept that agmatine is an endogenous protective molecule against morphine/opiate dependence/withdrawal and that increasing its levels in the brain benefits the system. Such observations will also provide a basis for the use of drugs to increase endogenous agmatine levels as a way to potentiate morphine analgesia and reduce morphine dependence/tolerance. Although agmatine is effective in animal models, it is unlikely to be a useful drug candidate because of its rapid metabolism, high turnover, and poor penetration into the brain. Frequent administration of high doses of exogenous agmatine is required to observe the effect in animal models. Thus, increasing endogenous agmatine by other means will be a valuable way to sustain higher levels of agmatine in the brain. One approach would be the use of inhibitors of agmatinase, the major degradative enzyme for agmatine in the brain.[78] The inhibitors of mammalian agmatinase are currently being evaluated,[34] and these initial efforts have identified a certain class of compounds as potential targets. It is important to identify selective agmatinase inhibitors since many structural analogs of agmatine are also potent inhibitors of NMDA receptors. For example, arcaine (diguanido butane), a potent inhibitor of agmatinase,[34] is a well-known NMDA antagonist.[45] From our initial screening of selective compounds, we have identified 3-aminoprpopyl guanidine as a potent inhibitor of agmatinase in vitro with no binding to NMDA receptors.[34] Further studies are under way to determine whether agmatinase inhibitors can actually increase endogenous agmatine levels in the brain in vivo. The use of agmatinase inhibitors along with exogenous agmatine will be a very useful approach to sustaining higher levels of agmatine in the brain.

Conclusions

One of the most fascinating aspects of agmatine, an endogenous molecule, is its ability to potentiate the analgesic effect of morphine while also reducing morphine dependence and withdrawal symptoms. At the same time, agmatine has absolutely no effect in naive animals on behavior, locomotion, or cardiovascular functions. Here, therefore, we have the opportunity to manipulate a system that is activated only when the normal homeostasis of the brain/cells/neurons is altered, for example, in the hyperexcitable state after chronic morphine exposure. Moreover, as agmatine has multiple molecular targets with low affinity and, thus, is easily reversible in functional actions with no toxic effects, it has tremendous therapeutic potential. The use of agmatine by itself or along with selective agmatinase inhibitors will be a valuable therapeutic approach for several targets, including ischemic injury, convulsive seizures, and opiate analgesia with reduced risk of dependence.

References

1. Li G, Regunathan S, Barrow CJ, Eshraghi J, Cooper R, Reis DJ. Agmatine: an endogenous clonidine-displacing substance in the brain. *Science.* 1994;263:966-969.
2. Piletz JE, Chikkala DN, Ernsberger P. Comparison of the properties of agmatine and endogenous clonidine-displacing substance at imidazoline and alpha-2 adrenergic receptors. *J Pharmacol Exp Ther.* 1995;272:581-587.
3. Pinthong D, Hussain JF, Kendall DA, Wilson VG. Comparison of the interaction of agmatine and crude methanolic extracts of bovine lung and brain with alpha 2-adrenoceptor binding sites. *Br J Pharmacol.* 1995;115:689-695.
4. Pinthong D, Wright IK, Hanmer C, et al. Agmatine recognizes alpha 2-adrenoceptor binding sites but neither activates nor inhibits alpha 2-adrenoceptors. *Naunyn Schmiedebergs Arch Pharmacol.* 1995;351:10-16.

5. Reis DJ, Regunathan S. Is agmatine a novel neurotransmitter in brain? *Trends Pharmacol Sci.* 2000;21:187-193.
6. Wang H, Regunathan S, Youngson C, Bramwell S, Reis DJ. An antibody to agmatine localizes the amine in bovine adrenal chromaffin cells. *Neurosci Lett.* 1995;183:17-21.
7. Otake K, Ruggiero DA, Regunathan S, Wang H, Milner TA, Reis DJ. Regional localization of agmatine in the rat brain: an immunocytochemical study. *Brain Res.* 1998;787:1-14.
8. Yang X-C, Reis DJ. Agmatine selectively blocks the NMDA subclass of glutamate receptor channels in cultured mouse hippocampal neurons. *J Pharmacol Exp Ther.* 1999;288:544-549.
9. Gorbatyuk OS, Milner TA, Wang G, Regunathan S, Reis DJ. Localization of agmatine in vasopressin and oxytocin neurons of the rat hypothalamic paraventricular and supraoptic nuclei. *Exp Neurol.* 2001;171:235-245.
10. Li G, Regunathan S, Reis DJ. Agmatine is synthesized by a mitochondrial arginine decarboxylase in rat brain. *Ann N Y Acad Sci.* 1995;763:325-329.
11. Lortie MJ, Novotny WF, Peterson OW, et al. Agmatine, a bioactive metabolite of arginine. *J Clin Invest.* 1996;97:413-420.
12. Zhu MY, Iyo A, Piletz JE, Regunathan S. Expression of human arginine decarboxylase, the biosynthetic enzyme for agmatine. *Biochim Biophys Acta.* 2004;1670:156-164.
13. Sastre M, Regunathan S, Reis DJ. Agmatinase activity in rat brain: a metabolic pathway for the degradation of agmatine. *J Neurochem.* 1996;67:1761-1765.
14. Holt A, Baker GB. Metabolism of agmatine (clonidine-displacing substance) by diamine oxidase and the possible implications for studies of imidazoline receptors. *Prog Brain Res.* 1995;106:187-197.
15. Olmos G, DeGregorio-Rocasolano N, Regalado MP, et al. Protection by imidazol(ine) drugs and agmatine of glutamate-induced neurotoxicity in cultured cerebellar granule cells through blockade of NMDA receptor. *Br J Pharmacol.* 1999;127:1317-1326.
16. Zhu MY, Piletz JE, Halaris A, Regunathan S. Effect of agmatine against cell death induced by NMDA and glutamate in neurons and PC12 cells. *Cell Mol Neurobiol.* 2003;23:865-872.
17. Gilad GM, Gilad VH. Accelerated functional recovery and neuroprotection by agmatine after spinal cord ischemia in rats. *Neurosci Lett.* 2000;296:97-100.
18. Gilad GM, Gilad VH, Rabey JM. Arginine and ornithine decarboxylation in rodent brain—coincidental changes during development and after ischemia. *Neurosci Lett.* 1996;216:33-36.
19. Kim JH, Yenari MA, Giffard RG, Cho SW, Park KA, Lee JE. Agmatine reduces infarct area in a mouse model of transient focal cerebral ischemia and protects cultured neurons from ischemia-like injury. *Exp Neurol.* 2004;189:122-130.
20. Fairbanks CA, Schreiber KL, Brewer KL, et al. Agmatine reverses pain induced by inflammation, neuropathy, and spinal cord injury. *Proc Natl Acad Sci USA.* 2000;97:10584-10589.
21. Feng Y, Piletz JE, Leblanc MH. Agmatine suppresses nitric oxide production and attenuates hypoxic-ischemic brain injury in neonatal rats. *Pediatr Res.* 2002;52:606-611.
22. Bence AK, Worthen DR, Stables JP, Crooks PA. An in vivo evaluation of the antiseizure activity and acute neurotoxicity of agmatine. *Pharmacol Biochem Behav.* 2003;74:771-775.
23. Su RB, Wei XL, Zheng JQ, Liu Y, Lu XQ, Li J. Anticonvulsive effect of agmatine in mice. *Pharmacol Biochem Behav.* 2004;77:345-349.
24. Aricioglu F, Kan B, Yillar O, Korcegez E, Berkman K. Effect of agmatine on electrically and chemically induced seizures in mice. *Ann N Y Acad Sci.* 2003;1009:141-146.
25. Kolesnikov Y, Jain S, Pasternak GW. Modulation of opioid analgesia by agmatine. *Eur J Pharmacol.* 1996;296:17-22.
26. Aricioglu-Kartal F, Uzbay IT. Inhibitory effect of agmatine on naloxane-precipitated abstinence syndrome. *Life Sci.* 1997;61:1775-1781.
27. Fairbanks CA, Brewer KL, Stone LS, et al. The behavioral and neuroprotective effects of agmatine in different models of pain and neuronal injury in rodents. *Soc Neurosci Abstr.* 1998;24:1253.
28. Li J, Li X, Pei G, Qin BY. Agmatine inhibited tolerance to and dependence on morphine in guinea pig ileum in vitro. *Zhongguo Yao Li Xue Bao.* 1998;19:564-568.

29. Nguyen HO, Goracke-Postle CJ, Kaminski LL, Overland AC, Morgan AD, Fairbanks CA. Neuropharmacokinetic and dynamic studies of agmatine (decarboxylated arginine). *Ann N Y Acad Sci.* 2003;1009:82-105.

30. Arteni NS, Lavinsky D, Rodrigues AL, Frison VB, Netto CA. Agmatine facilitates memory of an inhibitory avoidance task in adult rats. *Neurobiol Learn Mem.* 2002;78:465-469.

31. Lavinsky D, Arteni NS, Netto CA. Agmatine induces anxiolysis in the elevated plus maze task in adult rats. *Behav Brain Res.* 2003;141:19-24.

32. Zomkowski AD, Hammes L, Calixto JB, Lin J, Santos AR, Rodrigues AL. Agmatine produces antidepressant-like effects in two models of depression in mice. *Neuroreport.* 2002;13:387-391.

33. Sauve Y, Reader TA. Effects of alpha-methyl-p-tyrosine on monoamines and catecholamine receptors in rat cerebral cortex and neostriatum. *Neurochem Res.* 1988;13:807-815.

34. Dias Elpo Zomkowski A, Oscar Rosa A, Lin J, Santos AR, Calixto JB, Lucia Severo Rodrigues A. Evidence for serotonin receptor subtypes involvement in agmatine antidepressant like-effect in the mouse forced swimming test. *Brain Res.* 2004;1023:253-263.

35. Li J, Li X, Pei G, Qin BY. Effects of agmatine on tolerance to and substance dependence on morphine in mice. *Zhongguo Yao Li Xue Bao.* 1999;20:232-238.

36. Uzbay IT, Yesilyurt O, Celik T, Ergun H, Isimer A. Effects of agmatine on ethanol withdrawal syndrome in rats. *Behav Brain Res.* 2000;107:153-159.

37. Aricioglu F, Means A, Regunathan S. Effect of agmatine on the development of morphine dependence in rats: potential role of cAMP system. *Eur J Pharmacol.* 2004;504:191-197.

38. Aricioglu F, Paul IA, Regunathan S. Agmatine reduces only peripheral-related behavioral signs, not the central signs, of morphine withdrawal in nNOS deficient transgenic mice. *Neurosci Lett.* 2004;354:153-157.

39. Morgan AD, Campbell UC, Fons RD, Carroll ME. Effects of agmatine on the escalation of intravenous cocaine and fentanyl self-administration in rats. *Pharmacol Biochem Behav.* 2002;72:873-880.

40. Aricioglu F, Korcegez E, Bozkurt A, Ozyalcin S. Effect of agmatine on acute and mononeuropathic pain. *Ann N Y Acad Sci.* 2003;1009:106-115.

41. Onal A, Delen Y, Ulker S, Soykan N. Agmatine attenuates neuropathic pain in rats: possible mediation of nitric oxide and noradrenergic activity in the brainstem and cerebellum. *Life Sci.* 2003;73:413-428.

42. Yu CG, Fairbanks CA, Wilcox GL, Yezierski RP. Effects of agmatine, interleukin-10, and cyclosporin on spontaneous pain behavior after excitotoxic spinal cord injury in rats. *J Pain.* 2003;4:129-140.

43. Santos AR, Gadotti VM, Oliveira GL, et al. Mechanisms involved in the antinociception caused by agmatine in mice. *Neuropharmacology.* 2005;48:1021-1034.

44. Bradley KJ, Headley PM. Effect of agmatine on spinal nociceptive reflexes: lack of interaction with alpha2-adrenoceptor or mu-opioid receptor mechanisms. *Eur J Pharmacol.* 1997;331:133-138.

45. Reynolds IJ. Arcaine uncovers dual interactions of polyamines with the n-methyl-d-aspartate receptor. *J Pharmacol Exp Ther.* 1990;255:1001-1007.

46. Gibson DA, Harris BR, Rogers DT, Littleton JM. Radioligand binding studies reveal agmatine is a more selective antagonist for a polyamine-site on the NMDA receptor than arcaine or ifenprodil. *Brain Res.* 2002;952:71-77.

47. Askalany AR, Yamakura T, Petrenko AB, Kohno T, Sakimura K, Baba H. Effect of agmatine on heteromeric N-methyl-d-aspartate receptor channels. *Neurosci Res.* 2005;52:387-392.

48. Trujillo KA, Akil H. Inhibition of opiate tolerance by non-competitive N-methyl-D-aspartate receptor antagonists. *Brain Res.* 1994;633:178-188.

49. Jurkiewicz NH, do Carmo LG, Hirata H, da Costa Santos W, Jurkiewicz A. Functional properties of agmatine in rat vas deferens. *Eur J Pharmacol.* 1996;307:299-304.

50. Gatti PJ, Hill KJ, Da Silva AM, Norman WP, Gillis RA. Central nervous system site of action for the hypotensive effect of clonidine in the cat. *J Pharmacol Exp Ther.* 1988;245:373-380.

51. Hansson BG, Hokfelt B. Changes in blood pressure, plasma catecholamines and plasma renin activity during and after treatment with tiamenidine and clonidine. *Br J Clin Pharmacol.* 1981;11:73-77.
52. Hieble JP, Kolpak DC. Mediation of the hypotensive action of systemic clonidine in the rat by alpha 2-adrenoceptors. *Br J Pharmacol.* 1993;110:1635-1639.
53. Sun MK, Regunathan S, Reis DJ. Cardiovascular responses to agmatine, a clonidine-displacing substance, in anesthetized rat. *Clin Exp Hypertens.* 1995;17:115-128.
54. Szabo B, Urban R, Limberger N, Starke K. Cardiovascular effects of agmatine, a "clonidine-displacing substance", in conscious rabbits. *Naunyn Schmiedebergs Arch Pharmacol.* 1995;351:268-273.
55. Raasch W, Schafer U, Qadri F, Dominiak P. Agmatine, an endogenous ligand at imidazoline binding sites, does not antagonize the clonidine-mediated blood pressure reaction. *Br J Pharmacol.* 2002;135:663-672.
56. Tokuyama S, Zhu H, Oh S, Ho IK, Yamamoto T. Further evidence for a role of NMDA receptors in the locus coeruleus in the expression of withdrawal syndrome from opioids. *Neurochem Int.* 2001;39:103-109.
57. Wang G, Gorbatyuk O, Dayanithi G, et al. Evidence for endogenous agmatine in hypothalamo-neurohypophysial tract and its modulation on vasopressin release and Ca2+ channels. *Brain Res.* 2002;932:25-36.
58. Zheng JQ, Weng XC, Gai XD, Li J, Xiao WB. Mechanism underlying blockade of voltage-gated calcium channels by agmatine in cultured rat hippocampal neurons. *Acta Pharmacol Sin.* 2004;25:281-285.
59. Feng Y, Leblanc MH, Regunathan S. Agmatine reduces extracellular glutamate during pentylenetetrazole-induced seizures in rat brain: a potential mechanism for the anticonvulsive effects. *Neurosci Lett.* 2005;390:129-133.
60. Regunathan S, Youngson C, Raasch W, Wang H, Reis DJ. Imidazoline receptors and agmatine in blood vessels: a novel system inhibiting vascular smooth muscle proliferation. *J Pharmacol Exp Ther.* 1996;276:1272-1282.
61. Satriano J, Matsufuji S, Murakami Y, et al. Agmatine suppresses proliferation by frameshift induction of antienzyme and attenuation of cellular polyamine levels. *J Biol Chem.* 1998;273:15313-15316.
62. Abe K, Abe Y, Saito H. Agmatine suppresses nitric oxide production in microglia. *Brain Res.* 2000;872:141-148.
63. Satriano J, Schwartz D, Ishizuka S, et al. Suppression of inducible nitric oxide generation by agmatine aldehyde: beneficial effects in sepsis. *J Cell Physiol.* 2001;188:313-320.
64. Regunathan S, Piletz JE. Regulation of inducible nitric oxide synthase and agmatine synthesis in macrophages and astrocytes. *Ann N Y Acad Sci.* 2003;1009:20-29.
65. Li J, Li X, Pei G, Qin BY. Influence of agmatine in adaptation of cAMP signal transduction system of opiate receptors. *Zhongguo Yao Li Xue Bao.* 1999;20:592-596.
66. Nestler EJ. Molecular neurobiology of addiction. *Am J Addict.* 2001;10:201-217.
67. Copeland RL, Pradhan SN, Dillon-Carter O, Chuang DM. Rebound increase of basal cAMP level in NG108-15 cells during chronic morphine treatment: effects of naloxane and chloramphenicol. *Life Sci.* 1989;44:1107-1116.
68. Mehta CS, Strada SJ. Effects of acute and continuous administration of morphine on the cAMP response induced by norepinephrine in rat brain slices. *Life Sci.* 1994;55:35-42.
69. Avidor-Reiss T, Bayewitch M, Levy R, Matus-Leibovitch N, Nevo I, Vogel Z. Adenylylcyclase supersensitization in mu-opioid receptor-transfected Chinese hamster ovary cells following chronic opioid treatment. *J Biol Chem.* 1995;270:29732-29738.
70. Guitart X, Nestler EJ. Second messenger and protein phosphorylation mechanisms underlying opiate addiction: studies in the rat locus coeruleus. *Neurochem Res.* 1993;18:5-13.
71. Lane-Ladd SB, Pineda J, Boundy VA, et al. CREB (cAMP response element-binding protein) in the locus coeruleus: biochemical, physiological, and behavioral evidence for a role in opiate dependence. *J Neurosci.* 1997;17:7890-7901.

72. Feng Y, Leblanc MH. Effect of agmatine on the time course of brain inflammatory cytokines after injury in rat pups. *Ann N Y Acad Sci.* 2003;1009:152-156.
73. Halaris A, Zhu H, Feng Y, Piletz JE. Plasma agmatine and platelet imidazoline receptors in depression. *Ann N Y Acad Sci.* 1999;881:445-451.
74. Aricioglu-Kartal F, Regunathan S. Effect of chronic morphine treatment on the biosynthesis of agmatine in rat brain and other tissues. *Life Sci.* 2002;71:1695-1701.
75. Iyo AH, Zhu MY, Ordway GA, Regunathan S. Expression of arginine decarboxylase in brain regions and neuronal cells. *J Neurochem.* 2006;96:1042-1050.
76. Fairbanks CA, Kaminski LL, Nguyen HO, et al. Pretreatment with antisera raised against agmatine sensitizes mice to plasticity-mediated events [abstract]. *Soc Neurosci Abstr [serial online].* 2001;27:.
77. Vanderah TW, Wild KD, Takemori AE, et al. Modulation of morphine antinociception by swim-stress in the mouse: involvement of supraspinal opioid delta-2 receptors. *J Pharmacol Exp Ther.* 1993;267:449-455.
78. Huang M-J, Regunathan S, Botta M, et al. Structure-activity analysis of guanidine group in agmatine for brain agmatinase. *Ann N Y Acad Sci.* 2003;1009:52-63.

Part V
Cannabinoid

Chapter 38
The Therapeutic Potential of Drugs that Target Cannabinoid Receptors or Modulate the Tissue Levels or Actions of Endocannabinoids

Roger G. Pertwee[1]

Abstract There are at least 2 types of cannabinoid receptor, CB_1 and CB_2, both G protein coupled. CB_1 receptors are expressed predominantly at nerve terminals and mediate inhibition of transmitter release, whereas CB_2 receptors are found mainly on immune cells, their roles including the modulation of cytokine release and of immune cell migration. Endogenous agonists for cannabinoid receptors also exist. These "endocannabinoids" are synthesized on demand and removed from their sites of action by cellular uptake and intracellular enzymic hydrolysis. Endocannabinoids and their receptors together constitute the endocannabinoid system. This review summarizes evidence that there are certain central and peripheral disorders in which increases take place in the release of endocannabinoids onto their receptors and/or in the density or coupling efficiency of these receptors and that this upregulation is protective in some disorders but can have undesirable consequences in others. It also considers therapeutic strategies by which this upregulation might be modulated to clinical advantage. These strategies include the administration of (1) a CB_1 and/or CB_2 receptor agonist or antagonist that does or does not readily cross the blood brain barrier; (2) a CB_1 and/or CB_2 receptor agonist intrathecally or directly to some other site outside the brain; (3) a partial CB_1 and/or CB_2 receptor agonist rather than a full agonist; (4) a CB_1 and/or CB_2 receptor agonist together with a noncannabinoid, for example, morphine or codeine; (5) an inhibitor or activator of endocannabinoid biosynthesis, cellular uptake, or metabolism; (6) an allosteric modulator of the CB_1 receptor; and (7) a CB_2 receptor inverse agonist.

Keywords cannabinoid receptors, endocannabinoids, fatty acid amide hydrolase inhibitors, autoprotection, therapeutic strategies

[1] School of Medical Sciences, Institute of Medical Sciences, University of Aberdeen, Foresterhill, Aberdeen AB25 2ZD, Scotland, UK

Corresponding Author: Roger G. Pertwee, School of Medical Sciences, Institute of Medical Sciences, University of Aberdeen, Foresterhill, Aberdeen AB25 2ZD, Scotland.
Tel: + 44-1224-555740; Fax: + 44-1224-555844; E-mail: rgp@abdn.ac.uk

R.S. Rapaka and W. Sadée (eds.), *Drug Addiction.*
© American Association of Pharmaceutical Scientists 2008

Introduction

Mammalian tissues are now known to express at least 2 types of cannabinoid receptor, both of which are G-protein coupled.[1,2] These are CB_1 receptors, cloned in Tom Bonner's laboratory in 1990 (Matsuda et al[3]), and CB_2 receptors, cloned by Sean Munro in 1993.[4] Although CB_1 receptors are expressed by certain nonneuronal cells and tissues, for example, the pituitary gland, immune cells, and reproductive tissues, they are found predominantly at central and peripheral nerve terminals where they mediate inhibition of transmitter release. CB_2 receptors occur mainly on immune cells, their functions including the modulation, both within and outside the central nervous system, of cytokine release and immune cell migration. Thus, one common role of CB_1 and CB_2 receptors appears to be the regulation of ongoing release of chemical messengers, CB_1 receptors mainly from neurones and CB_2 receptors from immune cells. The finding that mammalian tissues express cannabinoid receptors was followed by the discovery of endogenous ligands for these receptors (*Endocannabinoids* section). These endogenous cannabinoids or endocannabinoids are all eicosanoids, 2 notable examples being *N*-arachidonoylethanolamine (anandamide) and 2-arachidonoyl glycerol. Endocannabinoids together with cannabinoid CB_1 and CB_2 receptors constitute the endocannabinoid system.

The discovery of the endocannabinoid system has prompted research directed at establishing its physiological and pathophysiological roles. This research has provided evidence first, that there are certain disorders in which endocannabinoid levels, cannabinoid receptor density, and/or cannabinoid receptor coupling efficiency increase in particular tissues, and second, that this upregulation of the endocannabinoid system often leads to a suppression of unwanted signs and symptoms, and so is autoprotective. The main objectives of this review are to summarize the evidence that the endocannabinoid system can be protective, and then to go on to consider possible therapeutic strategies by which such protection might best be exploited in the clinic. These are strategies in which endocannabinoid-induced protection is mimicked with directly acting CB_1 and/or CB_2 receptor agonists or in which it is augmented with drugs expected to delay the disappearance of endocannabinoids following their endogenous release or to induce an allosteric enhancement of cannabinoid receptor activation by released endocannabinoids. Evidence that the endocannabinoid system may sometimes be responsible for the production of undesirable effects is also briefly discussed. The review begins with short overviews of first, the pharmacological actions of important cannabinoid receptor ligands; second, the processes by which endocannabinoids are produced and then removed from their sites of action; and third, the progress that has been made to date in the development of drugs that can selectively inhibit one or other of these removal processes.

Cannabinoid Receptor Ligands

Several ligands that bind selectively to cannabinoid receptors are now available.[1,2] These fall essentially into 2 categories: the exogenous cannabinoids that are found in cannabis or have been designed and synthesized by chemists and the endogenous cannabinoids that occur naturally in mammalian tissues.

Exogenous Ligands

As detailed elsewhere,[1,2] a large number of CB_1 and CB_2 receptor agonists and antagonists have now been developed. Among the agonists are several compounds that bind more or less equally well to CB_1 and CB_2 receptors, examples being the "classical" cannabinoids, Δ^9-THC and (−)-11-hydroxy-Δ^8-THC-dimethylheptyl (HU-210), the "nonclassical" cannabinoid, CP55940, and the aminoalkylindole cannabinoid, R-(+)-WIN55212, which has marginally greater CB_2 than CB_1 affinity. Of these nonselective agonists, HU-210, CP55940, and R-(+)-WIN55212 have the highest CB_1 and CB_2 relative intrinsic activities, and HU-210 has the highest affinity for both CB_1 and CB_2 receptors. Δ^9-THC, which is the main psychotropic constituent of cannabis, has lower CB_1 and CB_2 affinities and relative intrinsic activities than these other cannabinoids. Indeed, at both receptor types, Δ^9-THC exhibits the mixed agonist-antagonist properties that are typical of a partial agonist. Another cannabis constituent, the classical cannabinoid cannabinol, also behaves as a partial agonist, at least at CB_1 receptors.[5] Agonists with significant selectivity for CB_1 or CB_2 receptors have also been developed. Notable CB_1-selective agonists include the eicosanoids R-(+)-methanandamide, arachidonyl-2′-chloroethylamide (ACEA), arachidonylcyclopropylamide (ACPA), and O-1812, which are all analogs of the endocannabinoid, anandamide (*Endocannabinoids* section). CB_2-selective agonists include L-759633, L-759656, and JWH-133, all structural analogs of Δ^9-THC; other notable examples are the nonclassical cannabinoid, HU-308, and the aminoalkylindoles, JWH-015 and AM1241.

Turning now to cannabinoid receptor antagonists, the compounds most commonly used in research are the CB_1-selective SR141716A, AM251, and AM281 and the CB_2-selective SR144528 and AM630. These are usually all classified as inverse agonists since they can, in at least some cannabinoid receptor-containing systems, produce effects by themselves that are opposite in direction from those produced by agonists for these receptors.[6] It is thought that they may produce these inverse cannabimimetic effects by shifting cannabinoid receptors from a constitutively active "on" state to one or more constitutively inactive "off" states. This putative mechanism relies on the assumption that cannabinoid receptors can exist in a constitutively active state in which they undergo some degree of spontaneous coupling to their effector mechanisms even in the absence of an endogenously released or exogenously added agonist. "Neutral" antagonists have also been developed.[6] These share the ability of the inverse agonists to block responses to cannabinoid receptor agonists but lack the apparent ability of inverse agonists to produce inverse cannabimimetic effects in cannabinoid receptor-containing systems in the absence of any endogenously released or exogenously added cannabinoid receptor agonist. Neutral antagonists are, however, expected to share the ability of CB_1 and CB_2 receptor inverse agonists to produce inverse cannabimimetic effects in tonically active biological systems when this tonic activity arises from ongoing endocannabinoid release onto cannabinoid receptors.

There is evidence that some established exogenous cannabinoid receptor agonists and antagonists have non-CB_1, non-CB_2 pharmacological targets.[2,6,7] These include TRPV1 (vanilloid VR1) receptors for some eicosanoid agonists (see also *Endocannabinoids* section), adenosine A_1 receptors for SR141716A and AM251, and possibly also the following:

- central putative TRPV1-like receptors for CP55940, *R*-(+)-WIN55212 and SR141716A but not AM251;
- central putative non-CB_1, non-CB_2, non-TRPV1 G protein-coupled receptors for *R*-(+)-WIN55212 but not Δ^9-THC, HU-210, or CP55940;
- putative non-CB_1, non-CB_2, non-TRPV1 receptors on perivascular sensory neurons for Δ^9-THC and cannabinol but not HU-210 or CP55940;
- putative non-I_1, non-I_2 imidazoline receptors for CP55940, *R*-(+)-WIN55212, and SR141716A;
- putative abnormal-cannabidiol receptors on mesenteric arteries for *R*-(+)-methanandamide and SR141716A but not for Δ^9-THC or *R*-(+)-WIN55212;
- gap junctions and L-type Ca^{2+} channels for SR141716A;
- Ca^{2+}-activated (BK_{Ca}) and ATP-sensitive potassium channels for SR141716A; and
- putative allosteric sites for certain exogenous cannabinoid receptor ligands on muscarinic M_1 and M_4, 5-HT_2 and 5-HT_3 receptors.

Evidence has also recently emerged for the presence of an allosteric site on the CB_1 receptor. Thus, we have found a series of novel compounds to behave as allosteric CB_1 receptor modulators. These compounds do not displace [^{3}H]CP55940 from CB_1 binding sites but do modulate the rate at which [^{3}H]CP55940 dissociates from these sites.[8] Whether there are also allosteric sites on CB_2 receptors remains to be established.

Endocannabinoids

The most investigated of the endocannabinoids have been the polyunsaturated fatty acid amide, *N*-arachidonoylethanolamine (anandamide), and the polyunsaturated monoacylglycerol, 2-arachidonoyl glycerol.[1,2,9] Of these, anandamide has marginally greater CB_1 than CB_2 affinity and, like the exogenous cannabinoid Δ^9-THC, exhibits relatively low efficacy at CB_1 and CB_2 receptors, behaving as a partial agonist at both receptor types. As to 2-arachidonoyl glycerol, this has been found in several investigations to have affinities for CB_1 and CB_2 receptors similar to those of anandamide but to exhibit higher CB_1 and CB_2 efficacy than anandamide. There has, however, been one recent investigation with human CB_1 receptor-containing tissue in which 2-arachidonoyl glycerol was found both to exhibit lower CB_1 receptor affinity than anandamide and to lack detectable CB_1 receptor efficacy at concentrations of up to $10\,\mu M$.[10]

It is likely that anandamide and/or 2-arachidonoyl glycerol have neuromodulatory roles (eg, by serving as retrograde synaptic messengers) and immunomodulatory roles (eg, through the regulation of cytokine release and immune cell migration).[1,2,11-13] It is also likely that both these endocannabinoids play a part in certain pathological processes both within and without the central nervous system.

Cannabinoid CB_1 and CB_2 receptors are not the only pharmacological targets for anandamide.[2,7,14-16] Thus, it is generally accepted that the TRPV1 receptor is activated by anandamide and by synthetic analogs of this endocannabinoid such as methanandamide, arachidonyl-2′-chloroethylamide, and N-(4-hydroxybenzyl)arachidonoylamine (AM404), although not by 2-arachidonoyl glycerol or by noneicosanoid cannabinoid receptor agonists such as R-(+)-WIN55212, CP55940, or HU-210. As detailed elsewhere,[2,7] additional targets that have been proposed for anandamide include

- central putative non-CB_1, non-CB_2, non-TRPV1 G protein-coupled receptors that are also activated by R-(+)-WIN55212;
- putative non-CB_1, non-TRPV1 receptors on neurons of the small intestine;
- putative non-I_1, non-I_2 imidazoline receptors that are also activated by CP55940 and R-(+)-WIN55212;
- putative abnormal-cannabidiol receptors on mesenteric arteries that are also activated by R-(+)-methanandamide but not by 2-arachidonoyl glycerol;
- putative non-CB_1, non-CB_2, non-TRPV1 receptors on coronary arteries;
- allosteric sites on muscarinic M_1 and M_4 receptors and on 5-HT_3 receptors that are also activated by certain exogenous cannabinoids; and
- allosteric sites on glutamate GLU_{A1} and GLU_{A3} receptors.

Other endocannabinoids are the anandamide analogs, dihomo-γ-linolenoylethanolamide, docosatetraenoylethanolamide, and possibly the CB_1-selective agonist 2-arachidonylglyceryl ether (noladin ether).[9] N-arachidonoyl dopamine, N-oleoyl dopamine, and oleamide may also be endocannabinoids as there are reports that these endogenous compounds can bind to CB_1 receptors with K_i values that are in the midnanomolar (N-arachidonoyl dopamine) or low micromolar range.[9,17,18] N-arachidonoyl dopamine can induce both antinociception in the mouse hot-plate test and thermal hyperalgesia, is distributed differently from anandamide in the brain, and shares the ability of anandamide to activate TRPV1 receptors.[9,17] N-oleoyl dopamine is also a TRPV1 receptor agonist. Indeed, it activates these receptors with particularly high potency and has also been found to induce both thermal hyperalgesia and allodynia.[9] The mono-unsaturated fatty acid amide, oleamide, has been shown to activate CB_1 receptors at concentrations above 10 or 100 nM, to block gap junction-mediated cell-cell communication, and to increase food intake, and has been postulated to be involved in sleep regulation.[9,18] One other endogenous fatty acid amide that interacts with cannabinoid receptors at concentrations in the low micromolar range is O-arachidonoylethanolamine (virodhamine).[9] In one investigation this ligand was found to activate CB_2 receptors but to exhibit either partial agonist or antagonist activity at CB_1 receptors,[19] whereas in another it behaved as a CB_1 receptor antagonist/inverse agonist.[10]

The Fate of Endocannabinoids and Its Modulation by Drugs

The Biosynthesis and Fate of Endocannabinoids

The biosynthesis of anandamide takes place on demand in response to elevations of intracellular calcium. The immediate precursor to anandamide is N-arachidonoyl phosphatidylethanolamine, which is formed from phosphatidylcholine and phosphatidylethanolamine and is converted to anandamide by the action of N-arachidonoyl phosphatidylethanolamine-phospholipase D.[16,20] Anandamide is removed from its sites of action by cellular uptake processes that may involve a transmembrane carrier protein, membrane-associated binding proteins, and/or simple diffusion.[21] It is then metabolized intracellularly. In most tissues, this metabolism is catalyzed by fatty acid amide hydrolase (FAAH),[16,22,23] an enzyme that in central neurons is located mainly on the cytosolic surfaces of smooth endoplasmic reticulum cisternae and mitochondria.[24] Anandamide is also sometimes metabolized by another intracellular enzyme, palmitoylethanolamide-preferring acid amidase (PAA),[22,25,26] and indeed, there is evidence that it is PAA rather than FAAH that is primarily responsible for deactivating anandamide in the mouse duodenum.[27] Other enzymes that can metabolize anandamide are cyclooxygenase-2, lipoxygenases, and cytochrome P450.[28]

Like anandamide, 2-arachidonoyl glycerol is not stored but rather synthesized on demand in a manner that can be triggered by elevations of intracellular calcium.[16,20] Its synthesis depends on the conversion of 2-arachidonate-containing phosphoinositides to diacylglycerols (DAGs), which are then converted to 2-arachidonoyl glycerol by the action of DAG lipase. Also, like anandamide, 2-arachidonoyl glycerol is thought to be removed from its sites of action by cellular uptake and then to be metabolized intracellularly.[16,20,28] Although 2-arachidonoyl glycerol can readily be metabolized by FAAH as well as by cyclooxygenase-2 and lipoxygenases, there is evidence that the enzyme mainly responsible for its metabolism in vivo may be monoacyl glycerol (MAG) lipase.[20,22,29,30] FAAH, MAG lipase, and cannabinoid CB_1 receptors have broadly similar distribution patterns, at least within some brain areas.[24] It is noteworthy, however, that while MAG lipase and cannabinoid CB_1 receptors are located mainly presynaptically in these brain areas, FAAH is found mainly postsynaptically in somata and dendrites of principal neurons. Unlike polyunsaturated fatty acid amides, mono-unsaturated and saturated fatty acid amides are thought to be poor substrates for the putative anandamide transporter.[27] In contrast, cellular uptake may be the main means by which noladin ether is removed from its site of action as this putative endocannabinoid is considered not to be a likely substrate for enzymic hydrolysis.[31] N-oleoyl dopamine is also thought to be recognized by the putative anandamide transporter and to be only a poor FAAH substrate.[9] However, 3 other putative endocannabinoids, oleamide, N-arachidonoyl dopamine, and virodhamine, all appear to be reasonable FAAH substrates.[23]

Several endogenous fatty acid amides, in addition to anandamide, are metabolized by FAAH.[22,23,26,27] These include not only polyunsaturated fatty acid amides such as N-arachidonoyl dopamine but also a range of mono-unsaturated and saturated compounds. One endogenous saturated fatty acid amide that serves as a substrate for FAAH, and also for PAA, is palmitoylethanolamide.[22,25] This has antiinflammatory and antinociceptive properties, can potentiate anandamide-induced antinociception and TRPV1 receptor activation, lacks significant affinity for CB_1 or CB_2 receptors, and is thought to be an agonist for the PPAR-α receptor and possibly also for a putative "CB_2-like" receptor.[7,26,32] A second pharmacologically active endogenous substrate of FAAH and PAA is the mono-unsaturated fatty acid amide, oleoylethanolamide, which can inhibit both anandamide cellular uptake and metabolism. Like palmitoylethanolamide, oleoylethanolamide can activate PPAR-α receptors and has negligible affinity for CB_1 or CB_2 receptors.[9] There is evidence that oleoylethanolamide serves as a satiety hormone, that it is released in the upper small intestine in response to food intake, and that it induces hypophagia by acting through intestinal PPAR-α receptors to activate vagal sensory afferent neurons that innervate higher brain structures involved in the control of energy balance.[26,27] Oleoylethanolamide is also a TRPV1 receptor agonist.[9]

Other pharmacologically active endogenous fatty acid amides include linoleamide, which is a FAAH substrate, may be involved in sleep regulation, and does not interact appreciably with cannabinoid receptors; N-arachidonoyl serine, which activates the putative abnormal-cannabidiol receptor; and N-palmitoyl dopamine and N-stearoyl dopamine, which potentiate anandamide at TRPV1 receptors but do not inhibit its cellular uptake or its metabolism by FAAH.[9] Two other endogenous ligands of interest are N-arachidonoyl glycine and the unsaturated fatty acid amide, linoleoylethanolamide, as both have been reported to inhibit FAAH. It has also been found that N-arachidonoyl glycine has antinociceptive and anti-edema activity, that it lacks significant affinity for cannabinoid CB_1 receptors, and that it is a FAAH substrate.[9,23,33]

Finally, it is noteworthy that some effects of endogenously released anandamide and 2-arachidonoyl glycerol may be enhanced through an "entourage effect" that relies on the corelease of other endogenous fatty acid derivatives. These derivatives include palmitoylethanolamide and oleamide, which can potentiate anandamide, and 2-linoleyl glycerol and 2-palmitoyl glycerol, which can potentiate 2-arachidonoyl glycerol.[2]

Inhibitors of Endocannabinoid Cellular Uptake and Intracellular Metabolism

The finding that the actions of anandamide and 2-arachidonoyl glycerol are terminated by cellular uptake and intracellular enzymic hydrolysis has been followed by the discovery of several drugs that will inhibit one or other of these processes.[16,23] Several of these inhibitors have been used as pharmacological tools in animal experiments directed at elucidating the physiological and pathological roles of anandamide or 2-arachidonoyl glycerol when these are released endogenously. These compounds are

- palmitylsulphonyl fluoride (AM374), an irreversible FAAH inhibitor (IC_{50} = 13 or 50 nM) that inhibits this enzyme at concentrations below those at which it binds to CB_1 receptors (K_i = 520 nM)[23];
- methyl arachidonoyl fluorophosphonate (MAFP), an irreversible FAAH inhibitor (IC_{50} = 1 to 3 nM) that has been reported also to inhibit MAG lipase (IC_{50} = 2 to 800 nM) in brain tissue, to bind irreversibly to CB_1 receptors at concentrations in the low nanomolar range,[23] and to behave as an irreversible CB_1 receptor antagonist in one investigation[34] but not in another[35];
- diazomethylarachidonoylketone (DAK), an irreversible FAAH inhibitor (IC_{50} = 500 nM), that has been reported also to inhibit MAG lipase in vitro at 1 μM and to bind to CB_1 receptors (IC_{50} = 1.3 μM)[23,36];
- the alkylcarbamic acid aryl esters, URB532 and URB597, that are irreversible FAAH inhibitors (IC_{50} = 63 and 4.6 nM, respectively) that do not inhibit MAG lipase, acetylcholinesterase, butyrylcholinesterase, or the putative anandamide membrane transporter at concentrations of up to 30 or 300 μM and lack significant affinity both for CB_1 and CB_2 receptors and for several other established receptors[37];
- the α-ketoheterocycle, 1-oxo-1[5-(2-pyridyl)-2-yl]-7-phenylheptane (OL-135), that is a potent reversible FAAH inhibitor (IC_{50} = 2.1 nM), has less potency as an inhibitor of triacylglycerol hydrolase (IC_{50} = 620 nM), and does not inhibit MAG lipase or a selection of other serine hydrolases at concentrations of up to 10 μM or exhibit significant affinity for CB_1 or CB_2 receptors (K_i > 10 μM)[38];
- N-arachidonoyl glycine, a FAAH substrate that is found endogenously, inhibits anandamide metabolism (IC_{50} = 4.1 or 7 μM), and lacks significant affinity for CB_1 receptors (K_i > 10 μM)[33,39];
- N-arachidonoyl serotonin that inhibits anandamide metabolism (IC_{50} = 5.6, 9, or 12 μM), does not significantly inhibit anandamide cellular uptake at 25 μM, and lacks significant affinity for CB_1 receptors (K_i > 50 μM)[40,41];
- palmitoylisopropylamide that inhibits FAAH (IC_{50} = 12.9 μM) and probably also anandamide cellular uptake and does not readily displace [³H]CP55940 or [³H]R-(+)-WIN55212 from CB_1 or CB_2 receptors (IC_{50} > 100 μM)[42];
- N-(4-hydroxybenzyl)arachidonoylamine (AM404), an inhibitor of anandamide cellular uptake (IC_{50} = 1 to 11 μM) that, however, also inhibits FAAH (IC_{50} = 0.5–5.9 μM or 22 μM or >30 μM), binds to CB_1 receptors (K_i = 1.76 μM), and potently activates TRPV1 receptors (EC_{50} = 26 to 50 nM)[43-48];

- Two structural analogs of AM404, VDM11 and VDM13, that inhibit anandamide cellular uptake (IC_{50} = 6.1 to 11 μM, and 12 μM, respectively), have less potency as TRPV1 receptor agonists (EC_{50} >> 10 μM) and also as FAAH inhibitors in some experiments (IC_{50} > 50 μM and = 27 μM, respectively) but not others (VDM11 IC_{50} = 1.2 to 3.7 μM, and bind to CB_1 and CB_2 receptors with K_i values that exceed 5 or 10 μM[47,48];
- the (S)- and (R)-1'-(4-hydroxybenzyl) derivatives of N-oleoylethanolamine (OMDM-1 and OMDM-2 respectively) that inhibit anandamide cellular uptake (K_i = 2.4 and 3 μM, respectively; IC_{50} = 2.6 or >20 μM, and 3.2 or 17 μM, respectively), have less potency as FAAH inhibitors (K_i or IC_{50} >50 or >100 μM) or as TRPV1 receptor agonists (EC_{50} ≥ 10 μM) and bind to CB_1 receptors (K_i = 12 μM and 5 μM, respectively)[48,49];
- N-(3-furylmethyl)arachidonoylamine (UCM707) that inhibits anandamide cellular uptake (K_i = 0.8, 25, 41, or >100 μM), is a FAAH substrate and inhibitor (IC_{50} = 30 μM or >100 μM), binds to CB_1 (K_i = 4.7 μM) and CB_2 receptors (K_i = 67 nM), and lacks appreciable affinity for TRPV1 receptors (K_i > 5 μM).[48,50,51]

AM374 is an analog of the irreversible serine protease inhibitor, phenylmethyl-sulphonyl fluoride (PMSF), which itself inhibits both FAAH (IC_{50} = 290 nM to 15 μM) and MAG lipase (IC_{50} = 155 μM or >500 μM).[23] MAG lipase inhibitors with sufficient potency and selectivity for use as pharmacological tools have yet to be developed.[23]

Results obtained with the FAAH and cellular uptake inhibitors listed above should be interpreted with particular caution as the pharmacological characterization of these compounds is far from complete. An added complication for some of these inhibitors is that they can activate TRPV1 receptors, an action that is known to stimulate anandamide biosynthesis, presumably by increasing the intracellular concentration of calcium,[16] and that will most likely also stimulate the biosynthesis of other endocannabinoids including 2-arachidonoyl glycerol. Based on the available data, compounds that currently show greatest promise as pharmacological tools are AM374, URB532, URB597, and OL-135 for FAAH inhibition, and OMDM-1 for inhibition of the cellular uptake of anandamide.

Evidence for an Upregulation of the Endocannabinoid System in Some Disorders

Since the discovery of anandamide in 1992, there have been several reports that tissue concentrations of this endogenous fatty acid amide increase in some human disorders and in animal models of certain diseases or disorders. More specifically, such increases have been detected in

- brain, blood, or circulating monocytes of patients with disorders that include schizophrenia, stroke, endotoxic (septic) shock, embryo implantation failure, and cancer (Table 38.1);

Table 38.1 Effects of Certain Diseases and Syndromes on the Human Endocannabinoid System*

Disease or Syndrome	Effect of Disease or Syndrome					
	EC Concentration		Protein Expression or Binding Site Density		Activity or Protein Expression	Reference
	AEA	2-AG	CB$_1$	CB$_2$	FAAH	
Alzheimer's disease (postmortem entorhinal and parahippocampal cortices)	ND	ND	0†(expression)	+†(expression)	+†(activity and expression)	52
Alzheimer's disease (postmortem frontal cortex)	ND	ND	−‡(expression)	+‡(expression)	ND	53
Paranoid-type schizophrenia (csf)	+	ND	ND	ND	ND	54
Schizophrenia with psychotic symptoms (csf)	+	0	ND	ND	ND	55
Schizophrenia (postmortem dorsolateral prefrontal cortex)	ND	ND	+ (binding)	§	ND	56
Schizophrenia (postmortem anterior cingulate cortex)	ND	ND	+ (binding)	ND	ND	57
Acute schizophrenia (human blood)	+	ND	ND||	ND||	ND||	58
Depressed suicide (postmortem dorsolateral prefrontal cortex)	ND	ND	+¶ § (expression and binding)	§	ND	59
Alcoholism + suicide (postmortem dorsolateral prefrontal cortex)	+	+	+¶ § (expression and binding)	§	ND	60
Parkinson's disease (postmortem caudate nucleus and putamen)	ND	ND	+¶ § (binding)	§	ND	61
Huntington's disease (postmortem substantia nigra, globus pallidus, putamen, and caudate nucleus)	ND	ND	− § (binding)	§	ND	62,63
Hemispheric stroke (stroke penumbra; microdialysis)	+#	ND	ND	ND	ND	64
Miscarriage (peripheral lymphocytes)	ND	ND	ND	ND	−	65
Implantation failure after in vitro fertilization and embryo transfer (AEA and 2-AG in blood; cannabinoid receptor binding and FAAH in peripheral lymphocytes)	+	0	0§ (binding)	0§ (binding)	− (activity and expression)	66
Endotoxic shock (serum)	+	+	ND	ND	ND	67
Advanced liver cirrhosis: (a) monocytes and (b) hepatic arterial endothelial cells	(a) +	ND	(b) + (mRNA and binding)	ND	ND	68
Liver cirrhosis (plasma)	+	ND	ND	ND	ND	69

Liver cirrhosis (fibrogenic cells in human liver biopsy specimens)	ND	ND	ND	+ (expression)	ND	70
Atherosclerosis (human and mouse atherosclerotic plaques)	ND	ND	0 (expression)	+ (expression)	ND	71
Cancer (human adenomas and/or carcinomas; colorectal biopsies)	+	+	0 (mRNA and expression)	0 (mRNA and expression)	0 (mRNA)	41
Cancer (meningiomas; resected human brain tissue)	−	0	ND	ND	ND	72
Cancer: (a) glioblastomas and (b) meningiomas; resected human brain tissue	(a) + (b) 0	(a) 0 (b) +	ND	ND	(a) - (activity) (b) - (activity)	73
Cancer (human pituitary adenomas; postmortem)	+	+	**(mRNA and expression)	ND	ND	74
Prostate cancer (human cell lines)	ND	ND	+ (expression)	+ (expression)	ND	75
Bone cement implantation syndrome (blood)	+	+	ND	ND	ND	76

*2-AG indicates 2-arachidonoyl glycerol; AEA, anandamide; EC, endocannabinoid; FAAH, fatty acid amide hydrolase; csf, cerebral spinal fluid; ND, not determined.

†FAAH protein and enzyme activity were overexpressed in neuritic plaque-associated astrocytes; CB_2 receptor protein was overexpressed in neuritic plaque-associated microglia; no change in CB_1 receptor protein density or location in the vicinity of neuritic plaques.

‡Signs of microglial activation; CB_2 receptor protein expressed in tangle-like neurons and dystrophic neurites and CB_1 and CB_2 receptor protein in senile plaques; CB_1-positive neuron density was greatly reduced in areas of microglial activation; cannabinoid receptor coupling efficiency was decreased.

§Binding experiments were perfomed with $[^3H]CP55940$, which binds equally well to CB_1 and CB_2 receptors.

‖Pharmacologically-induced clinical improvement was accompanied by decreases in blood levels of anandamide and in FAAH mRNA and CB_2 receptor mRNA but not CB_1 receptor mRNA in mononuclear cells.

¶Increased CB_1 receptor immunoreactivity (not reference 61) and cannabinoid receptor binding site density and coupling efficiency.

#Increased levels of palmitoylethanolamide and oleoylethanolamide were also detected.

**CB_1 receptors were detected in most but not all types of adenoma.

- blood in bone cement implantation syndrome (Table 38.1);
- brain and spinal cord in a mouse model of multiple sclerosis (Table 38.2);
- lumbar spinal cord in a mouse model of amyotrophic lateral sclerosis (Table 38.2);
- basal ganglia in a rat model of Parkinson's disease (Table 38.2);
- ventral mesencephalon in a rat model of Huntington's disease (Table 38.2);
- periaqueductal gray in a rat model of inflammatory pain (Table 38.2);
- urinary bladder in a rat model of painful hemorrhagic cystitis (Table 38.2);
- hypothalamus and uterus in mouse models of obesity (Table 38.2);
- cardiovascular tissue in experimental models of septic shock, cardiogenic shock, and biliary cirrhosis (Table 38.3);
- small intestine in rodent models of paralytic ileus, ileitis, and secretory diarrhea (Table 38.3); and
- lesioned brain areas in rat models of cerebral ischemia and excitotoxicity (Table 38.4).

In some of these investigations, tissue levels of 2-arachidonoyl glycerol were also monitored. These were found to increase in human colorectal and pituitary adenomas or carcinomas (Table 38.1); in bone cement implantation syndrome (Table 38.1); in mouse models of multiple sclerosis, amyotrophic lateral sclerosis, aversive memory extinction, and obesity (Tables 38.2 and 38.3); in rat models of hepatic ischemia-reperfusion injury, myocardial infarction, and ileitis (Table 38.4); and in a model of cardiogenic shock (Table 38.3). Usually these increases were detected in the same tissues as those in which increases in anandamide levels occurred. However, there have been at least 2 instances in which increases in anandamide and 2-arachidonoyl glycerol were found to have taken place in different cell-types: in a mouse model of septic shock[113] and in experiments with human cancer cells[73] (Tables 38.1 and 38.3). There have also been a few instances in which increases in anandamide levels were found not to have been paralleled by any detectable increases in 2-arachidonoyl glycerol (Tables 38.1, 38.2, 38.3, and 38.4) or in which an increase in 2-arachidonoyl glycerol was not accompanied by any increase in anandamide (Tables 38.2, 38.3, and 38.4). Increased levels of 2-arachidonoyl glycerol in brain tissue have sometimes been observed in experiments in which anandamide levels were not also monitored, for example, in experiments with a mouse model of closed head injury and with a rat model of excitotoxicity (Table 38.4).

Increases in tissue levels of anandamide and 2-arachidonoyl glycerol are most likely usually triggered by increases in intracellular calcium. However, there is evidence that these increases are sometimes further modulated by changes in the ability of tissues to synthesize these compounds and/or to dispose of them by cellular uptake or subsequent enzymic degradation. Thus, for example, in a mouse model of obesity in which increases in uterine levels of both anandamide and 2-arachidonoyl glycerol were detected, these increases were found to be accompanied by a decrease in uterine tissue both of FAAH and MAG lipase activity and of anandamide transport across membranes[104] (Table 38.2). An increase in uterine DAG lipase activity was noted as well, suggesting that the increased uterine levels of 2-arachidonoyl glycerol observed in these experiments were partly attributable to an increase in the capacity of the uterus to synthesize this endocannabinoid.

Table 38.2 Signs of Upregulation or Downregulation of the Endocannabinoid System in Animal In Vivo Models of Multiple Sclerosis. Amyotrophic Lateral Sclerosis, Encephalitis, Alzheimer's Disease, Parkinson's Disease, Huntington's Disease, Pain, Obesity, Feeding, and Fasting*

Experimental Model	Effect Observed in Experimental Model					Reference
	EC Concentration		Protein Expression, mRNA or Binding Site Density	Activity or Protein Expression		
	AEA	2-AG	CB_1	FAAH	AMT	
CREAE model of multiple sclerosis (mouse brain and spinal cord)	+†	+†	ND	ND	ND	77
EAE model of multiple sclerosis (rat caudate putamen and/or cerebral cortex)	ND	ND	−§ ‖ (mRNA and binding)	ND	ND	78
EAU model of uveoretinitis (mouse retina)	ND	ND	‡ND	ND	ND	79
Model of amyotrophic lateral sclerosis (lumbar spinal cords of transgenic mice)	+	+	ND	ND	ND	80
Human immunodeficiency virus-induced encephalitis (macaque cerebral cortex)	ND	ND	0 ¶ (expression)	+¶ (expression)	ND	81
β-Amyloid peptide model of Alzheimer's disease (rat cerebral cortex)	ND	ND	- (expression)	ND	ND	53
Attention-deficit hyperactivity disorder ("Impulsive" spontaneously hypertensive adolescent rats; prefrontal cortex)	ND	ND	- (expression)	ND	ND	82
Reserpine model of Parkinson's disease (rat globus pallidus)	0	+	ND	ND	ND	83
6-Hydroxydopamine model of Parkinson's disease (rat striatum)	+	0	0‖ (binding)	- (activity)	- (activity)	84,85
6-Hydroxydopamine model of Parkinson's disease (rat striatum)	ND	ND	ND	- (activity)	ND	86
6-Hydroxydopamine model of Parkinson's disease (rat striatum)	ND	ND	+ or 0# (mRNA)	ND	ND	89-91
MPTP model of Parkinson's disease (marmoset striatum)	ND	ND	+‖ # (binding)	ND	ND	61

(continued)

Table 38.2 (continued)

Experimental Model	EC Concentration		Protein Expression, mRNA or Binding Site Density	Activity or Protein Expression		Reference
	AEA	2-AG	CB₁	FAAH	AMT	
Huntington's disease (lateral striata of transgenic mice)	ND	ND	- (mRNA)	ND	ND	92
3-NP model of Huntington's disease (rat basal ganglia)	ND	ND	−∥ (binding)	ND	ND	93
3-NP model of Huntington's disease (rat striatum)	−	−	0∥ ** (binding)	ND	ND	94
3-NP model of Huntington's disease (rat ventral mesencephalon)	+	0	0∥ ** (binding)	ND	ND	94
3-NP model of Huntington's disease (rat striatum)	ND	ND	−∥ ** (mRNA and binding)	ND	ND	95
3-NP model of Huntington's disease (rat striatum and/or globus pallidus)	ND	ND	−∥ (mRNA and binding)	ND	ND	96
Transgenic model of Huntington's disease (mouse basal ganglia)	ND	ND	−∥ **(mRNA and binding)	ND	ND	97
Formalin paw model of inflammatory pain (rat periaqueductal gray)	+	ND	ND	ND	ND	98
Neuropathic pain model (rat spinal cord dorsal horn)	ND	ND	+ (expression)	ND	ND	99
Neuropathic pain model (rat lumbar spinal cord)	ND	ND	††ND	ND	ND	100
Cyclophosphamide model of painful hemorrhagic cystitis (rat bladder)	+	ND	ND	ND	ND	101
Obesity model (Zucker *fa/fa* rat hypothalamus)	0	+†	ND	ND	ND	102
Obesity model (*db/db* mouse hypothalamus)	+	+†	ND	ND	ND	
Obesity model (*ob/ob* mouse hypothalamus)	0	+	ND	ND	ND	
Obesity model (obese *fa/fa* rat adipose tissue and mouse cultured differentiated 3T3 F442A adipocyte cells)	ND	ND	+ (mRNA or expression)	ND	ND	103
Obesity model (*ob/ob* mouse uterus)	+	+†	0∥	- (activity; also MAG lipase)	–	104

Feeding (a) and fasting (b) (rat limbic forebrain and/or hypothalamus)	(a) 0 (b) +	(a) – (b) +	ND	ND	ND	ND [105]

* AMT indicates anandamide membrane tranport; CREAE, chronic relapsing experimental allergic encephalomyelitis; EAE, experimental allergic encephalomyelitis; EAU, experimental autoimmune uveoretinitis; MAG lipase, monoacyl glycerol lipase; MPTP, 1-methyl-4-phenyl-1,2,3,6-tetrahydropyridine; 3-NP,3-nitropropionic acid; TMEV -IDD, Theiler murine encephalomyelitis virus-induced demyelinating disease. (See first footnote to Table 1 for additional definitions.)

†Increased levels of palmitoylethanolamide were also detected in CREAE mouse spinal cord but not in CREAE mouse brain or in *fa/fa* rat or *db/db* mouse hypothalamus or *ob/ob* mouse uterus.

‡Retinal infiltrated cells, predominantly T cells and macrophages, were positive for the CB_2 receptor.

§ Increased cannabinoid receptor coupling efficiency in caudate putamen and cerebral cortex.

‖These binding experiments were perfomed with [³H]CP55940, [³H]R-(+)-WIN55212 or [³H]anandamide which have significant affinities for both CB_1 and CB_2 receptors.

¶ FAAH overexpressed in perivascular astrocytes and astrocytic processes and CB_2 receptor immunoreactivity detected in cerebrocortical perivascular macrophages, microglial nodules and T-lymphocytes.

Increase[61] or no change[89] in cannabinoid receptor coupling efficiency.

** Decrease in cannabinoid receptor coupling efficiency in the globus pallidus[97] or in the area(s) indicated in the left hand column.

†† CB_2 expression detected in the lumbar spinal cord undergoing neuronal damage (CB_2 mRNA and immunoreactivity, probably on activated microglia); CB_2 mRNA was not detected in the spinal cords of rats with inflamed paws.

Table 38.3 Signs of Upregulation or Downregulation of the Endocannabinoid System in Animal Models of Stress, Memory, Aging, Hypertension, Cirrhosis, Septic Shock, Cardiogenic Shock, and Various Intestinal Disorders*

Experimental Model	EC Concentration		Protein Expression, mRNA, cDNA, Enzymic Activity or Binding Site Density		Reference
	AEA	2-AG	CB_1	FAAH	
Chronic unpredictable stress (rat hippocampus)	0	–	-† (expression and binding)	ND	106
Mouse forebrain after (a) acute or (b) repeated restraint stress or mouse amygdala after (c) acute or (d) repeated restraint stress	(a) 0 (b) 0 (c) – (d) –	(a) 0 (b) + (c) 0 (d) +	ND	ND	107
Extinction of aversive memories (mouse amygdala)	+	+	ND	ND	108
Age: (a) rat entorhinal and temporal cortices and (b) rat postrhinal cortex	ND	ND	(a) + (b) – (expression)	ND	109
Exercise (human plasma)	+	0	ND	ND	110
Spontaneously hypertensive rats (myocardial or aortic tissue)	–	0	+ (expression)	+ (expression)	111
Biliary cirrhosis and hypotension (rat monocytes)	+	ND	ND	ND	68
Cirrhosis (rat mesenteric arteries)	ND	ND	+ (expression)	ND	112
LPS model of septic shock/hypotension: (a) mouse platelets or (b) mouse macrophages	(a) 0 (b) +	(a) +	ND	ND	113
LPS model of septic shock/hypotension (mouse macrophages)	+	0	ND	+ (mRNA and activity)	114
LPS model of septic shock/hypotension (human lymphocytes)	+	ND	0† ‡ (cDNA and binding)	- (expression, cDNA and activity)	115
Cardiogenic shock/hypotension (human monocytes and platelets)	+	+	ND	ND	116
Intestinal inflammation and hypermotility (mouse small intestine)	0§	0§	+ (expression)	+ (activity)	117
Colitis (mouse colon)	ND	ND	+ (mRNA)	ND	118

Cholera toxin-induced secretory diarrhea (mouse small intestine)	+	0§||	+ (mRNA and expression)	0 (activity)	119
Clostridium difficile toxin A model of ileitis (rat ileum)	+	+	ND	ND	120
Paralytic ileus (mouse small intestine)	+	0§||	+ (expression)	0 (activity)	121

* LPS indicates lipopolysaccharide. (See first footnote to Table 38.1 for additional definitions.)

† These binding experiments were performed with [^{3}H]CP55940 which has significant affinity for both CB$_1$ and CB$_2$ receptors.

‡ Similar CB$_2$ receptor data were obtained.

§ No higher than in controls in which significant levels were detected.

\|\| No increased levels of palmitoylethanolamide.

Table 38.4 Signs of Upregulation or Downregulation of the Endocannabinoid System in Animal Models of Cerebral Ischemia, Myocardial Infarction, Neurotoxicity, and Febrile Seizures*

Experimental Model	EC Concentration		Protein Expression, mRNA, Enzymic Activity or Binding Site Density		Reference
	AEA	2-AG	CB$_1$	FAAH	
Focal cerebral ischemia induced by transient left middle cerebral artery occlusion (rat cortical neurons)	ND	ND	+† (expression)	ND	122
Focal cerebral ischemia induced by transient left middle cerebral artery occlusion (rat brain)	+	0	ND	ND	123
Hepatic ischemia-reperfusion injury (rat plasma): (a) short ischemia (b) long ischemia	(a) + (b) 0	(a) + (b) +	ND	ND	124
Acute myocardial infarction (rat monocytes and platelets)	+	+	ND	ND	116
(a) Excitotoxicity (intracerebral NMDA) or (b) traumatic head injury (rat pup brain areas)	(a) +‡ (b) +	(a) 0 (b) 0	(a) −§ (b) +§ (mRNA or binding)	ND	125
Traumatic brain injury (closed head injury; mouse brain)	ND	+	ND	ND	126
Picrotoxinin-induced excitotoxicity (rat brain)	ND	+‖	ND	ND	127
Kainic acid-induced excitotoxicity (rat hippocampus)	+	0	ND	ND	128v
Febrile seizures (rat hippocampus)	0	0	+ (expression)	0¶ (activity)	129
Human immunodeficiency virus type-1 coat glycoprotein gp120-induced neurotoxicity (rat cerebral cortex)	−	ND	0§ (binding)	+# (expression and activity)	130

*NMDA indicates N-methyl-D-aspartate. (See footnote to Table 1 for additional definitions.)

†In the ischemic boundary zone of the cortical mantle but not in the cortical or striatal sectors of the ischemic core.

‡Increased levels of 16:0, 18:0, 18:1, and 18:2 acyl ethanolamides were also detected.

§These binding experiments were perfomed with [³H]CP55940 or [³H]anandamide which have significant affinity for both CB$_1$ and CB$_2$ receptors.

‖Increased levels of 1(3)-arachidonoyl glycerol but not of other acyl glycerols such as 2-palmitoyl or 2-oleoyl glycerol were also detected.

¶The activity of MAG lipase was also not affected.

#There was also an increase in anandamide membrane transport.

A decrease in FAAH activity has also been observed to accompany increases in anandamide levels in the peripheral lymphocytes of women with implantation failure (Table 38.1) and in rat striatal tissue in a model of Parkinson's disease (Table 38.2). Also observed in these rat experiments was a decrease in anandamide cellular uptake. However, in experiments using a lipopolysaccharide (LPS) model of endotoxic shock, in one study LPS-induced increases in anandamide levels were reported to be paralleled by a decrease in the gene expression and activity of FAAH (in human peripheral lymphocytes),[115] while in another study, in which a much lower concentration of LPS was used, increases in anandamide levels were found to be paralleled by an *increase* in the expression and activity of this enzyme (in mouse macrophages)[114] (Table 38.3). In the second of these investigations, increases were also detected in the activities of 2 enzymes that can catalyze anandamide biosynthesis (N-acyltranferase and N-arachidonoyl phosphatidyleth-anolamine-phospholipase D). An increase in FAAH activity has also been detected in the small intestine of mice in which intestinal inflammation and increased motility had been induced by orally administered croton oil[117] (Table 38.3). In these experiments, high levels of anandamide (and 2-arachidonoyl glycerol) were detected in the small intestine of both croton oil-treated and control mice. Some increases in anandamide tissue levels take place in the absence of changes in FAAH expression or activity. Thus, for example, in experiments with human colorectal cancer biopsies (Table 38.1) and with mouse models of diarrhea and paralytic ileus (Table 38.3), elevations in anandamide levels observed in the cancerous tissue and in mouse small intestine were not associated with any detectable changes in FAAH expression or activity.

In some disorders or animal models in which endocannabinoid tissue concentrations have been reported to be high, elevated expression levels and/or densities of cannabinoid CB_1 receptors have also been detected. Such upregulation of the CB_1 receptor has been observed in the following:

- postmortem cerebral cortical tissue of suicide victims (Table 38.1),
- tissue from humans with advanced liver cirrhosis (Table 38.1),
- brain tissue in a rat model of traumatic head injury (Table 38.4), and
- small intestine in mouse models of intestinal inflammation, secretory diarrhea, and paralytic ileus (Table 38.3).

Increases in CB_1 receptor density have also sometimes been detected in experiments in which no increases in endocannabinoid levels were observed or no measurements of endocannabinoid tissue concentrations made. These increases in receptor density were detected in the following:

- brain tissue taken postmortem from patients with schizophrenia or Parkinson's disease (Table 38.1),
- the striatum in marmoset and rat models of Parkinson's disease (Table 38.2),
- the spinal cord in a rat model of neuropathic pain (Table 38.2),
- cortical neurons in a rat model of focal cerebral ischemia (Table 38.4),
- the hippocampus in a rat febrile seizure model (Table 38.4),

- the colon in a mouse model of colitis (Table 38.3),
- mesenteric arteries in a rat model of cirrhosis (Table 38.3), and
- human prostate cancer cells (Table 38.1).

It is noteworthy that spontaneously hypertensive rats have been reported to exhibit increased CB_1 receptor density in myocardium and aorta but a decrease in myocardial anandamide levels[111] (Table 38.3). Conversely, excitotoxicity induced by N-methyl-D-aspartate (NMDA) in rats has been found to provoke not only a rise in anandamide concentrations but a fall in CB_1 receptor density and expression level in some brain areas (Table 38.4). A fall in CB_1 receptor density has also been detected in cerebral cortex and caudate putamen in a rat model of multiple sclerosis (Table 38.2). However, in this investigation, the reduced population of cannabinoid receptors was found to signal with increased efficiency. Increases in the efficiency of CB_1 receptor signaling have also been observed in postmortem brain tissue of patients who had suffered from Parkinson's disease or were suicide victims (Table 38.1) and in the striatum in a marmoset model of Parkinson's disease (Table 38.2). Additional examples of human disorders or of animal models of disorders in which signs of *downregulation* rather than upregulation of the endocannabinoid system have been observed are to be found in Tables 38.1 to 38.4.

It is likely that expression levels of CB_2 receptors also change in certain disorders. Indeed, Zhang et al[100] have found that when signs of neuropathic pain were produced in rats by sciatic nerve ligation, nonneuronal CB_2-expressing cells became detectable in the lumbar spinal cord. These cells were probably activated microglia that had migrated into this region of the cord. CB_2 expression was detectable only in certain regions of the dorsal and ventral horns, the precise distribution pattern of these receptors within the spinal cord varying with the model of experimental neuropathic pain used. No change in CB_2 expression was observed in the spinal cords of rats with inflamed paws. There have also been reports that

- in Alzheimer's disease brain tissue, CB_2 receptors are selectively overexpressed in neuritic plaque-associated microglia and are also expressed in tangle-like neurons and dystrophic neurites but not in normal brain tissue[52,53] (see also Table 38.1),
- CB_2-expressing immune cells are present in brain tissue samples from macaques with simian immunodeficiency virus-induced encephalitis but not in samples from control animals[81] (see also Table 38.2),
- CB_2 receptors are expressed in atherosclerotic plaques of human and mouse diseased arteries but not in nondiseased arteries (Table 38.1),
- CB_2 receptors are highly upregulated in human cirrhotic liver (Table 38.1),
- CB_2 (and CB_1) receptor expression is higher in human prostate cancer cells than in normal cells[75] (see also Table 38.1), and
- CB_2 but not CB_1 receptor expression is higher in biopsies from human astrocytomas exhibiting high-grade malignancy than in biopsy tissue exhibiting lower grade malignancy.[131]

Finally, it is important to bear in mind that changes in endocannabinoid tissue levels or in the expression level or density of cannabinoid receptors seems to take place in response not only to certain pathological insults but also to some nonpathological processes or stimuli such as fasting, feeding, stress, aging, and exercise (Tables 38.2 and 38. 3).

Evidence That the Endocannabinoid System Is Autoprotective

There is evidence not only that tissue concentrations of endocannabinoids, cannabinoid receptor density and/or cannabinoid receptor coupling efficiency increase in a range of different disorders but also that these increases serve to reduce the severity of signs and symptoms of some of these disorders or even to oppose disease progression. Support for the hypothesis that the endocannabinoid system has such an "autoprotective" role has so far come mainly from experiments concerned with pain, multiple sclerosis, cancer, intestinal, mental and cardiovascular disorders, excitotoxicity, traumatic head injury, and Parkinson's disease.

Pain

Reports are emerging that FAAH inhibitors such as OL-135, URB532, URB597, and N-arachidonoylglycine are antinociceptive in various rodent models of pain. These models are the formalin paw test of persistent inflammatory pain[38,39] in which it is already known that central nervous system (CNS) levels of anandamide rise above control values in response to the formalin (Table 38.2), and the tail-immersion and hot-plate tests of acute thermal pain.[37,38,132] There are reports too that the endocannabinoid cellular uptake inhibitors, OMDM-2 and VDM11, produce antinociception in the rat hot-plate test.[133]

That the antinociception induced by inhibitors of FAAH or endocannabinoid cellular uptake is mediated by endogenous fatty acid ethanolamides is supported by several findings. These include the observations that OL-135, URB597, and N-arachidonoylglycine elevate endogenous levels of these amides in rodents[37,38,134] and that exogenously administered anandamide can be potentiated by OL-135 in the mouse tail-immersion test[38] and by AM404 in the mouse hot-plate test.[44] Also consistent with this hypothesis are the findings first, that mice from which FAAH has been genetically deleted (FAAH$^{-/-}$ mice) exhibit reduced sensitivity to noxious stimuli when these are applied in the tail-immersion, hot-plate, or formalin paw test or in the carrageenan model of inflammatory pain[135,136]; and second, that FAAH$^{-/-}$ mice have elevated tissue levels of anandamide and other fatty acid ethanolamides and exhibit greater sensitivity than wild-type mice to the antinociceptive effect of exogenously administered anandamide.[135]

Some experiments have been performed with transgenic (FAAH-NS) mice that express FAAH only within the nervous system. These differ from FAAH$^{-/-}$ mice in not exhibiting enhanced levels of anandamide and other fatty acid ethanolamides in the CNS or reduced nociception in the tail-immersion or hot-plate plate test.[137] Consequently, it is likely that signs of hypoalgesia in these tests that are observed in FAAH$^{-/-}$ mice or are induced by FAAH or endocannabinoid cellular uptake inhibitors in wild-type mice depend on the activation of targets located in the nervous system. It is also likely that these targets are mainly or wholly cannabinoid CB$_1$ receptors. Thus, Kathuria et al[37] found that the antinociceptive effects of URB532 and URB597 in the mouse hot-plate test were attenuated by SR141716A at a dose that by itself had no effect on nociception. Similarly, it was found by Lichtman et al[38] that SR141716A attenuated OL-135 induced-antinociception in mice in the tail-immersion, hot-plate, and formalin paw tests. None of the FAAH inhibitors used in these 2 investigations exhibited significant affinity for CB$_1$ (or CB$_2$) receptors, suggesting that these inhibitors did not produce antinociception by activating cannabinoid receptors directly. It has also been found that after they have been injected with SR141716A, FAAH$^{-/-}$ mice no longer exhibit hypoalgesic responses to noxious stimuli in the tail-immersion test, the hot-plate test, or the formalin paw test (both phases).[135,136] There is good evidence that CB$_2$ receptor activation can induce antinociception in the second phase of the formalin paw test (see below). Even so, it is unlikely that the signs of hypoalgesia that are exhibited by FAAH$^{-/-}$ mice in this pain model are mediated by CB$_2$ receptors as the ability of SR141716A to eliminate these signs in such animals is not shared by SR144528.[136]

The concept that cannabinoid CB$_1$ receptors can mediate antinociception produced by inhibitors of FAAH or endocannabinoid cellular uptake or by genetic deletion of FAAH is consistent with several findings that have been extensively reviewed elsewhere.[20,138-140] Briefly, these findings are first, that CB$_1$ receptors are located on pain pathways in the brain and spinal cord and on the central and peripheral terminals of primary afferent neurons that mediate both neuropathic and nonneuropathic pain, and second, that cannabinoid receptor agonists can induce signs of antinociception when injected either systemically or directly onto a CB$_1$ receptor-expressing region of a pain pathway. CB$_1$ receptor agonists exhibit antinociceptive activity in a wide range of experimental pain models and this antinociception has often been found to be antagonized by SR141716A, albeit sometimes in models in which this antagonist produces signs of hyperalgesia when administered by itself. This hyperalgesia could reflect either antagonism of endocannabinoids released onto CB$_1$ receptors or an ability of SR141716A to reduce the extent to which CB$_1$ receptors couple spontaneously to their effector mechanisms (*Exogenous Ligands* section) or both of these actions. Since SR141716A-induced inverse agonism is expected to occur particularly in tissues in which there is a relatively high expression of CB$_1$ receptors, it is noteworthy that CB$_1$ receptor expression levels in the spinal cord increase in a rat model of neuropathic pain in which SR141716A has been found to be hyperalgesic[99,141] (see also Table 38.2).

That CB$_1$ receptors have a role in pain perception is also supported by the results from experiments in which antisense methods have been used to achieve a "knockdown" of CB$_1$ receptors in the brain or spinal cord.[142-144] Additional support comes from findings that mice from which the CB$_1$ receptor has been genetically deleted (CB$_1$$^{-/-}$ mice) exhibit reduced antinociception following a forced swim in water at

$34°C$[145] and increased tactile sensitivity.[146] Unexpectedly though, there are also reports that compared with wild-type animals, $CB_1^{-/-}$ mice exhibit either no differences in nociceptive behavior in hot-plate, tail-immersion, tail-flick, tail-pressure, or abdominal-stretch tests[146-148] or even signs of hypoalgesia in the hot-plate test and the first phase of the formalin paw test.[148]

There is evidence that CB_2 receptors can also mediate analgesia. Thus, for example, when administered systemically to rats or mice the CB_2-selective agonists HU308, GW405833, and AM1241 have all been found to exhibit antinociceptive activity in various pain models in a manner that is opposed by a CB_2-selective antagonist. Such apparent CB_2-mediated antinociception has been observed for HU308 in the second phase of the mouse formalin paw test,[149] for GW405833 in rat carrageenan and rat and mouse Freund's complete adjuvant models of inflammatory pain and in rat models of neuropathic and incisional pain,[150,151] and for AM1241 in rat models of allodynia and of thermal and inflammatory pain and in mouse and rat models of neuropathic pain.[146,152-155] It is unlikely that these CB_2-selective agonists were also activating CB_1 receptors, as AM1241 was no less effective in reducing signs of neuropathic pain in $CB_1^{-/-}$ mice than in wild-type animals[146] and as HU-308 and AM1241 were not antagonized by CB_1-selective antagonists. It is possible that CB_2 receptors that mediate antinociception are located on nonneuronal cells in the skin and that, when activated, these receptors modulate the endogenous release of molecules that target peripheral nociceptors.[152] Indeed, evidence has recently emerged that suggests that one mechanism by which CB_2 selective agonists such as AM1241 produce antinociception, at least in a rat model of thermal pain, may be by stimulating the release of β-endorphin from CB_2-expressing cells in the skin such as keratinocytes onto μ-opioid receptors located on the terminals of primary afferent neurons.[156] However, it would be premature to exclude other possibilities, for example, that CB_2 receptors can also be expressed by sensory neurons[157] and that such CB_2 receptors, or indeed microglial CB_2 receptors that appear in the spinal cord after nerve injury[100] (see also Table 38.2), can mediate antinociceptive effects. It also remains possible that CB_2-selective agonists can produce antinociception in at least some pain models by activating "CB_2-like" receptors, putative receptors at which the endogenous fatty acid amide palmitoylethanolamide may induce hypoalgesia (reviewed elsewhere[7,139]).

In some pain models, signs of hypoalgesia that seem to be produced by endogenously released endocannabinoids appear to be entirely CB_1 receptor mediated. However, there is also some evidence that antinociception may sometimes be induced instead by endogenous activation of CB_2 or (CB_2-like) receptors. Thus, in $FAAH^{-/-}$ mice, there is an elevation in the tissue levels of palmitoylethanolamide,[135] which may produce antinociception by acting on a CB_2-like receptor, and in the carrageenan model of inflammatory pain, although not in the formalin paw test (see preceding paragraph), these knockout mice exhibit signs of hypoalgesia that are not reduced by SR141716A but are lessened, albeit only partially, by SR144528.[136] It has also been reported that URB597 decreases carrageenan-induced mouse paw edema in an SR144528-sensitive manner.[158] Moreover, when administered by itself, this CB_2-selective antagonist has been found to produce signs of hyperalgesia in rats both in the carrageenan model[150] and in the first phase of the formalin paw test.[159] However, there are also several reports that CB_2 receptor antagonists are not hyperalgesic in these rat models of inflammatory pain or in models of allodynia or thermal pain.[152-155,160] A CB_1- or CB_2 receptor antagonist may of course sometimes fail to enhance signs of pain in an experimental model because the pain score is already maximal. Conversely, it remains possible that in experiments in which SR144528 was hyperalgesic, it was acting as an inverse agonist rather than as an antagonist of endogenously released endocannabinoids.

There is evidence that cannabinoid receptor agonists can also relieve pain in humans, for example, in patients with neuropathic pain[161] and in some patients with cancer, multiple sclerosis, spinal cord injury, blepharospasm, brachial plexus damage, or pain from limb amputation.[161-169] Whether inhibitors of endocannabinoid metabolism or cellular uptake will also be able to induce analgesia in the clinic has still to be established.

Finally, there is evidence that CB_2 receptor *inverse* agonists have therapeutic potential as antiinflammatory agents. Thus, although there is little doubt that CB_2 receptor agonists can produce antinociception in experimental models of various kinds of pain that include inflammatory pain, it has also been found that the CB_2 receptor inverse agonists, SR144528 and JTE-907, can inhibit carrageenan-induced mouse paw edema,[170] indicating them to be antiinflammatory agents, and that a third CB_2 receptor inverse agonist, Schering-Plough's compound 4j, inhibits immune cell migration both in vitro and in vivo.[171,172] There is also some evidence that although FAAH inhibitors may be effective against thermal and inflammatory pain, they lack potential for the management of neuropathic pain. Thus, in experiments with sciatic nerve ligation models, it has been observed that FAAH$^{-/-}$ mice do not show signs of hypoalgesia[136] and that rats exhibit an antinociceptive response to URB597 only when this is administered at a dose well above its threshold dose for FAAH inhibition.[173]

Multiple Sclerosis

There are 2 reports that in a mouse model of multiple sclerosis, spasticity can be ameliorated both by the FAAH inhibitor, AM374, and by the inhibitors of endocannabinoid cellular uptake, AM404, VDM11, OMDM-1, and OMDM-2.[77,133] The model used, the chronic relapsing experimental allergic encephalomyelitis (CREAE) model, is one in which levels of anandamide and 2-arachidonoyl glycerol in both brain and spinal cord are higher than in unlesioned animals (Table 38.2). In another model of multiple sclerosis in which mice are inoculated intracerebrally with Theiler's murine encephalomyelitis virus (TMEV), OMDM-1 has been found to oppose the impaired rotarod performance and reductions in spontaneous motor activity exhibited by the lesioned animals and to enhance levels of anandamide although not 2-arachidonoyl glycerol in the spinal cords of these animals.[174]

There are several reasons for believing that the amelioration of spasticity induced in CREAE mice by inhibitors of FAAH or endocannabinoid cellular uptake is mediated at least in part by CB_1 and possibly also by CB_2 receptors. First, the antispastic effect of the FAAH inhibitor, AM374, has been found to be blocked by SR141716A and SR144528.[77] As AM374 is not itself expected to bind to cannabinoid receptors at the dose used, this finding suggests that it produced its inhibitory effect on spasticity indirectly by enhancing endocannabinoid concentrations at these receptors. Second, Pryce et al[175] have found that compared with wild-type CREAE mice, $CB_1^{-/-}$ CREAE mice exhibit an earlier onset of spasticity, more immobility, residual paresis, spinal cord axonal loss and spinal neurodegeneration, and greater mortality. Third, there have been several reports that the exogenous administration to lesioned rodents of cannabinoid receptor agonists, including anandamide and 2-arachidonoyl glycerol, R-(+)-WIN55212 and Δ^9-THC, the CB_1-selective agonists, R-(+)-methanandamide and ACEA, and the CB_2-selective agonists, JWH-133 and JWH-015, can reduce spasticity or other signs of neurological damage such as tremor and spasm[77,176-178] or ameliorate atonia, ataxia, gait abnormalities, paralysis, moribundity, and mortality[179-181] or improve rotarod performance.[182] These experiments were performed with rodent models of multiple sclerosis in which demyelination was induced by inoculation either with TMEV[181,182] or with mixtures containing CNS tissue or myelin basic protein (CREAE/EAE models). Finally, the CB_1/CB_2 receptor agonist R-(+)-WIN55212 has been found to ameliorate clinical signs of demyelination in mice in a manner that is both stereoselective (CREAE and TMEV mice) and susceptible to antagonism by SR141716A and SR144528 (CREAE mice).[176,177,181]

Evidence that cannabinoids can reduce the spasms, spasticity, or tremor of multiple sclerosis has also been obtained in clinical trials with multiple sclerosis patients[165,166,183,184] (also reviewed elsewhere[164]). The degree of spasm or spasticity was either scored by the investigators using an objective measure or assessed subjectively by the patients themselves. The negative results sometimes obtained in such experiments when spasticity has been scored objectively[166,184,185] may well be a reflection of the low sensitivity of the available methods.

Further support for the hypothesis that CREAE mice release endocannabinoids onto cannabinoid receptors and that the resultant activation of these receptors reduces spasticity comes from the finding that CREAE mice with mild spasticity became significantly more spastic when injected with SR141716A alone or in combination with SR144528.[176] However, since these agents are both inverse agonists, it is also possible that they acted in an endocannabinoid-independent manner by reducing the extent to which cannabinoid receptors were coupling spontaneously to their effector mechanisms. Because SR141716A and SR144528 increase spasticity in CREAE mice, the finding that these cannabinoid receptor antagonists oppose R-(+)-WIN55212-induced reductions in the spasticity of CREAE mice should be interpreted with caution.

Results obtained with CREAE/EAE or TMEV models of multiple sclerosis also suggest that cannabinoid CB_1 or CB_2 receptor activation by exogenously administered or endogenously released agonists may oppose the progression of multiple sclerosis by slowing the neurodegenerative process,[175] reducing inflammation,[174,179,181,182] and promoting remyelination.[182]

Cancer

Evidence is emerging that certain types of cancer cells overproduce anandamide and/or 2-arachidonoyl glycerol (Table 38.1), that these endocannabinoids act through cannabinoid receptors to inhibit cancer cell proliferation or invasion, and that this inhibitory effect can be enhanced by inhibitors of endocannabinoid metabolism or cellular uptake.

Ligresti et al[41] have detected both these endocannabinoids in biopsy specimens from human CB_1-, CB_2-, and FAAH-expressing colorectal tissue and found that the levels of anandamide and 2-arachidonoyl glycerol were highest in precancerous adenomatous polyps, lower in carcinomas, and lowest in normal tissue. Experiments were also performed with cultured colorectal cancer cells (CaCo-2 cells) that express CB_1 receptors and FAAH but not CB_2 receptors and contain anandamide and 2-arachidonoyl glycerol. The proliferation of these cells was inhibited by anandamide, by 2-arachidonoyl glycerol, by certain synthetic CB_1 receptor agonists, by the FAAH inhibitor *N*-arachidonoyl serotonin, and by the endocannabinoid cellular uptake inhibitors, VDM11 and VDM13, in a manner that was sensitive to antagonism by SR141716A. Of interest, anandamide did not inhibit the proliferation of CaCo-2 cells that had differentiated into enterocytes. These differentiated cells exhibit much lower malignancy and invasiveness, have a lower endocannabinoid content, and express more FAAH than undifferentiated CaCo-2 cells.

More recently, Bifulco et al[186] showed that in vivo growth of rat thyroid tumors in athymic mice could be inhibited by intratumoral injections of VDM11 or *N*-arachidonoyl serotonin. The tumor content of 2-arachidonoyl glycerol was increased by both these drugs, whereas the tumor content of anandamide (and palmitoylethanolamide) was increased only by *N*-arachidonoyl serotonin. It was also found that in vitro proliferation of these tumor cells was inhibited both by VDM11 and by the cannabinoid receptor agonist, 2-methyl-arachidonyl-2'-fluoro-ethylamide, and that this inhibition was blocked by SR141716A but not by SR144528. 2-Arachidonoyl glycerol and *N*-arachidonoyl serotonin, which also inhibited the in vitro proliferation of these cells, were less susceptible to antagonism by SR141716A. These findings are in line with evidence from previous investigations that both cancer cell proliferation in vitro and angiogenesis, tumor growth, and metastatic spreading of cancer cells in vivo can be decreased by CB_1 receptor activation.[187-191] Evidence that CB_2 receptors mediate antitumor effects also exists.[188,190,191] Intriguingly, it is likely that as well as acting through CB_1 receptors to inhibit the growth of tumors in vivo and cancer cell proliferation in vitro, the anandamide analog, 2-methyl-arachidonyl-2'-fluoro-ethylamide, increases expression of CB_1 receptors in these tumors and cancer cells but decreases the levels of these receptors in healthy, noncancerous cells.[187,189] Such an action would presumably be shared by other cannabinoid receptor agonists when these are exogenously administered or endogenously released.

In another recent investigation, Nithipatikom et al[36] found first, that certain CB_1 and CB_2-expressing human cultured androgen-independent prostate cancer cells produce 2-arachidonoyl glycerol at high concentrations, and second, that in vitro invasion of these cells could be inhibited by 2-arachidonoyl glycerol, noladin ether, R-(+)-WIN55212 and R-(+)-methanandamide, and also by 2 inhibitors of 2-arachidonoyl glycerol metabolism, MAFP and DAK. SR141716A but not SR144528 increased invasion of the prostate cancer cells and reversed the inhibitory effect of MAFP. It was also found that MAFP-induced inhibition of invasion of these cells could be enhanced by 2-arachidonoyl glycerol. Evidence has also recently been obtained from experiments with human cultured androgen-sensitive prostate cancer cells for a CB_1 and CB_2 receptor-mediated induction of apoptosis and inhibition of cell growth by R-(+)-WIN55212 and for the reduction by this cannabinoid receptor agonist of angiogenesis.[75]

Intestinal Disorders

There is evidence first, that certain disorders characterized by inflammation of the gastrointestinal tract or by diarrhea may be associated with an increase in intestinal endocannabinoid levels and/or in the expression of CB_1 receptors by myenteric neurons (Table 38.3), second, that the resultant hyperactivity of the endocannabinoid system ameliorates at least some of the symptoms of these diseases and, third, that this amelioration can be mimicked by CB_1 receptor agonists or enhanced by inhibitors of endocannabinoid metabolism.[192]

Izzo et al[119] have obtained evidence that the endocannabinoid system acts through overexpressed CB_1 receptors to oppose cholera toxin-induced accumulation of intestinal fluid in mice. Thus, levels of anandamide, although not of 2-arachidonoyl glycerol or palmitoylethanolamide, increased in the small intestine in response to cholera toxin as did the expression of CB_1 receptors. The intestinal fluid accumulation induced by cholera toxin was increased by SR141716A but not by SR144528 and was reduced by CP55940 and ACEA pretreatment in a manner that was sensitive to antagonism by SR141716A but not SR144528. Intestinal fluid accumulation was also prevented by VDM11 in an SR141716A-sensitive manner but was unaffected by the CB_2-selective agonist JWH-015 or by the TRPV1 antagonist capsazepine.

Results obtained by Massa et al[118] from experiments with $CB_1^{-/-}$, FAAH$^{-/-}$, and wild-type mice suggest that the CB_1 component of the endogenous cannabinoid system decreases colonic inflammation induced by intrarectal administration of 2,4-dinitrobenzene sulphonic acid (DNBS). DNBS-induced colitis was more marked in $CB_1^{-/-}$ mice and less marked in FAAH$^{-/-}$ mice than in wild-type mice. Moreover, in wild-type mice, DNBS-induced colitis was reduced by HU-210 and enhanced by SR141716A and provoked an increase in the number of CB_1-expressing cells in mouse colonic myenteric plexus. There is also a report that intestinal inflammation and hypermotility induced by oral croton oil is associated with an increase in CB_1 expression level in mouse jejunum.[117] The sensitivity of croton oil-treated mice to CP55940 and cannabinol-induced inhibition of gastrointestinal transit of an orally administered charcoal suspension increased as well. High levels of anandamide and 2-arachidonoyl glycerol were detected in the small intestines of both croton oil-treated and control mice, even though FAAH activity was 2-fold *higher* in inflamed small intestine than in control tissue.

Mental Disorders

Giuffrida et al[54] have found that levels of anandamide but not of palmitoylethanolamide or oleoylethanolamide are markedly higher in the cerebrospinal fluid of antipsychotic-naïve first-episode paranoid schizophrenics and of schizophrenics taking "atypical" antipsychotics than in the cerebrospinal fluid of healthy controls. In contrast, anandamide levels were not elevated in schizophrenics taking "typical" antipsychotics or in patients with dementia or affective disorders. In the antipsychotic-naïve schizophrenics there was a negative correlation between anandamide levels and severity of symptoms, a finding that is at least consistent with the hypothesis that anandamide has a *protective* role in schizophrenia. These findings raise the possibility that in schizophrenia, exaggerated dopamine release onto postsynaptic D_2-like receptors triggers release of anandamide, which then acts as a retrograde messenger to induce a CB_1 receptor-mediated attenuation of dopamine release. This chain of events would most likely be prevented by typical antipsychotics as these block D_2-like receptors but be unaffected by atypical antipsychotics as these act mainly on $5-HT_{2A}$ receptors. Giuffrida et al[54] have also suggested that heavy cannabis use may promote psychotic episodes in vulnerable individuals by desensitizing CB_1 receptors such that the ability of endogenously released anandamide to ameliorate signs and symptoms of schizophrenia is compromised.

Marsicano et al[108] performed experiments with an aversive memory model in which mice are trained to associate a tone with a foot-shock such that once they are conditioned, they freeze when re-exposed just to the tone. Their main findings were that this tone provoked an increase in anandamide and 2-arachidonoyl glycerol levels in the basolateral amygdala complex but not the medial prefrontal cortex of conditioned mice, that extinction of tone-induced freezing behavior was more pronounced in wild-type than $CB_1^{-/-}$ mice, and that extinction was also impaired by SR141716A in wild-type mice. These results prompted the suggestion that the endocannabinoid system could represent a therapeutic target for the treatment of diseases associated with inappropriate retention of aversive memories or with inadequate responses to aversive situations such as post-traumatic stress disorders or phobias.

Excitotoxicity and Traumatic Brain Injury

There is some evidence from experiments with mice that anandamide is released onto CB_1 receptors during excitotoxicity (Table 38.4) and that this release has a protective role.[128] More specifically, it has been found that kainic acid elevates anandamide but not 2-arachidonoyl glycerol or palmitoylethanolamide in the hippocampus, that this excitotoxin induces more severe seizures when the CB_1 receptor is genetically deleted or blocked with SR141716A, and that CB_1 receptor-expressing mice can be protected from kainic acid-induced seizures by the endo-cannabinoid cellular uptake inhibitor, UCM707. In addition, the data obtained suggest that the CB_1 receptors mediating this protective effect are located on prin-cipal forebrain neurons rather than on GABAergic interneurons, the likely end result of anandamide-induced activation of these receptors being inhibition of glutamate release.

There is also evidence that the endocannabinoid system may protect against the consequences of traumatic brain injury, although in this case through the release of 2-arachidonoyl glycerol. Thus, results obtained using a mouse model of closed head injury suggest that brain levels of 2-arachidonoyl glycerol increase in response to traumatic brain injury (Table 38.4) and that when administered exogenously, this endocannabinoid can act through CB_1 receptors to reduce brain edema and improve neurobehavioral function and clinical recovery.[126,193]

Parkinson's Disease

It has been postulated that it may prove possible to alleviate symptoms of Parkinson's disease by using inhibitors of the metabolism or cellular uptake of anandamide to raise endogenous levels of this fatty acid amide so that its inhibitory effect on glutamate release from corticostriatal neurons is enhanced.[84,85] This hypothesis was prompted by results obtained in experiments using a rat model of Parkinson's disease in which nigrostriatal dopaminergic neurons are destroyed unilaterally by injecting 6-hydrox-ydopamine close to the substantia nigra on one side of the brain. These experiments showed that the frequency of glutamatergic spontaneous excitatory postsynaptic potentials (sEPSPs) was greater in corticostriatal slices of lesioned than of control (sham-operated) animals and that this in creased rate of firing could be reduced by the fatty acid amide hydrolase inhibitors, PMSF and MAFP, and by the anandamide cellular uptake inhibitors, AM404 and VDM11. The direct CB_1 receptor agonist, HU-210, was found to mimic this effect of these inhibitors, while the CB_1-selective antagonist, SR141716A prevented the effects of AM404 and PMSF. It was also found that 6-hydroxydopamine elevates levels of anandamide in the striatum but not in the cerebellum. Striatal and cerebellar levels of 2-arachidonoyl glycerol were unaffected. That inhibitors of anandamide metabolism or cellular uptake may alleviate symptoms of Parkinson's disease is also supported by a report that intraperitoneally administered AM404 ameliorates akinesia and sensorimotor orientation and reduces amphetamine-induced turning behavior in 6-hydroxydopamine-lesioned rats.[86] The effect of AM404 on amphetamine-induced turning behavior was abolished by the CB_1-selective antagonist, AM251. There is also evidence from experiments with 6-hydroxydopamine-lesioned rats that drugs that enhance the activity of the endo-cannabinoid system may have the capacity to suppress or prevent unwanted dyskinesias that are often induced in parkinsonian patients by the therapeutic agent, L-dihydroxy-phenylalanine (L DOPA).[87]

Results from other investigations have raised the possibility that symptoms of Parkinson's disease could be alleviated by CB_1 receptor antagonists. Thus there are 2 reports from the same laboratory that the akinesia, sensorimotor orientation, and asymmetric motor behavior exhibited by rats with 6-hydroxydopamine-induced unilateral nigral lesions can be significantly attenuated by SR141716A or AM251 when these are given either systemically or unilaterally into the striatum or globus pallidus on the lesioned side of the brain.[194,195] An additional finding, that inhibitory effects of systemic SR141716A or AM251 on amphetamine-induced asymmetric motor behavior could be prevented by AM404, was taken as evidence for the presence of a CB_1 receptor-mediated modulation of nigrostriatal dopaminergic tone in the lesioned animals and also suggests that these antagonists were acting to reduce this tone. SR141716A and AM251 were most effective when given to rats exhibiting particularly severe behavioral signs of nigral degeneration, suggesting that cannabinoid CB_1 receptor antagonists might be useful for treating advanced stages of Parkinson's disease in humans.[195] That CB_1 receptor antagonists could be used for the management of Parkinson's disease has also been proposed by Lastres-Becker et al.[61] This suggestion was prompted by results they obtained in experiments with tissue both from parkinsonian patients and from marmosets lesioned with 1-methyl-4-phenyl-1,2,3,6-tetrahydropyridine (MPTP). More specifically, they found that CB_1 receptors in parkinsonian and MPTP-lesioned basal ganglia bind more [^{3}H]CP55940 and exhibit greater coupling efficiency than control tissue and that these changes were less marked in the basal ganglia of MPTP-treated animals that had been exposed to L-DOPA. It is noteworthy, however, that Meschler et al[196] have reported that SR141716A does not alleviate motor deficits induced by MPTP in cynomolgus monkeys.

Clearly no firm conclusions can yet be drawn about the role of the endocannabinoid system in Parkinson's disease or about the extent to which modulation of this system with drugs could alleviate undesirable symptoms associated either with the disease itself or with the established anti-parkinsonian drug, L-DOPA.

Cardiovascular Disorders

There is evidence that anandamide and 2-arachidonoyl glycerol are major contributors to hypotension associated with hemorrhagic, septic, or cardiogenic shock. Thus first, it has been found that hypotension induced in anaesthetized rats by bleeding, by acute myocardial infarction, or by intravenous administration of bacterial lipopolysaccharide (LPS), a major pathogenic factor in septic shock, can be opposed by SR141716A or AM281, whereas exogenous 2-arachidonoyl glycerol administration induces hypotension in anaesthetized normotensive animals.[113,116,197,198]

Second, there are reports that macrophages obtained from the blood of rats that are normotensive or in hemorrhagic shock can synthesize anandamide[197] and that in vitro administration of LPS elevates levels of 2-arachidonoyl glycerol in rat platelets and of anandamide in rat and mouse macrophages and human lymphocytes[113-115] (Table 38.3). There is also a report that anandamide and 2-arachidonoyl glycerol are detectable in monocytes and platelets isolated from rats after acute myocardial infarction but not in cells obtained from control animals[116] (Table 38.3). Third, blood from hemorrhaged rats and cells isolated from rat blood after acute myocardial infarction or onset of LPS-induced hypotension can cause prolonged hypotension in anaesthetized normotensive rats.[113,116,197] This hypotension was found to be considerably attenuated or completely abolished by SR141716A, pointing to an involvement of CB_1 receptors. Moreover the ability of LPS to increase anandamide levels in mouse macrophages in vitro can be enhanced by the nonselective FAAH inhibitor, PMSF, and a much greater decrease in blood pressure can be elicited by LPS-treated peritoneal macrophages when these cells are obtained from FAAH$^{-/-}$ rather than from FAAH$^{+/+}$ mice.[114]

It is possible that CB_1-mediated hypotension may aid survival in hemorrhagic and cardiogenic shock. Thus, as well as attenuating hypotension induced in urethane-anaesthetized rats by bleeding or acute myocardial infarction, SR141716A has been found to reduce the survival time of these animals.[116,197] Conversely, survival of hemorrhaged rats is significantly increased by the cannabinoid receptor agonists, Δ^9-THC and HU-210.[197] In LPS-treated rats, however, survival can be improved both by Δ^9-THC and by SR141716A or AM281.[113,198]

There is also evidence that CB_1 receptors may mediate a protective hypotensive effect in spontaneously hypertensive rats.[111] These are animals in which it has been found that blood pressure is elevated by SR141716A and reduced by the FAAH inhibitor, URB597, and by 2 inhibitors of endocannabinoid cellular uptake, AM404 and OMDM-2. The blood pressure of normotensive rats was not affected by any of these drugs. Compared with normotensive rats, spontaneously hypertensive rats also express more CB_1 receptors in the myocardium and aorta (Table 38.3) and show greater sensitivity to anandamide- and HU-210-induced hypotension.[111] However, FAAH expression is higher and myocardial levels of anandamide (but not of 2-arachidonoyl glycerol) are lower in spontaneously hypertensive rats than in normotensive animals (Table 38.3), raising the possibility that the endocannabinoid system may protect against hypertension in this animal model by increasing "target organ sensitivity" rather than by increasing endocannabinoid levels.[111]

Finally, it is possible that the endocannabinoid system may protect against atherosclerosis as first, CB_2 receptors are expressed by macrophages and T-lymphocytes within atherosclerotic plaques of human and mouse diseased arteries (Table 38.1), and second, there is evidence that when administered orally at 1 mg/kg per day, Δ^9-THC can act through CB_2 receptors to produce a significant inhibition of atherosclerosis progression in mice.[71]

Therapeutic Strategies

It is clear from the preceding 2 sections of this review that the endocannabinoid system is thought to upregulate in some disorders and that one consequence of this upregulation may be the alleviation of symptoms or even the removal of the underlying causes of some of these symptoms. This section begins by considering how direct agonists might best be used in the clinic to mimic protective effects of the endocannabinoid system. It then goes on to discuss some alternative potential strategies that would augment these protective effects indirectly by potentiating endogenously released endocannabinoids through effects on their metabolism, cellular uptake, or receptors.

Direct Cannabinoid Receptor Agonists

Two CB_1/CB_2 cannabinoid receptor agonists have been licensed for clinical use in some countries for several years. These are dronabinol (Marinol; Δ^9-THC) and the synthetic Δ^9-THC analog, nabilone, which can be prescribed as antiemetics (both drugs) and to stimulate appetite (dronabinol).[199] Both these drugs are administered orally. In addition, Sativex, a medicine that contains Δ^9-THC and cannabidiol, was recently licensed for the management of neuropathic pain associated with multiple sclerosis. [199,200] A significant number of patients also claim to obtain relief from symptoms of multiple sclerosis and, indeed, from various kinds of chronic pain, from arthritis and/or from neuropathy by self-medicating with cannabis.[201,202] As to novel synthetic CB_1/CB_2 or CB_2 cannabinoid receptor agonists that exhibit antinociceptive activity in animal models of pain, there are as yet no clinical data, although several of these have been synthesized and investigated preclinically by drug companies (eg, by GlaxoSmithKlein[150,151] and by Bayer[203]).

A strong case can be made for using cannabinoid receptor direct agonists in the clinic now, particularly to relieve neuropathic pain and to ameliorate the spasms and spasticity of multiple sclerosis. However, a strong argument can also be made for conducting research directed at establishing how in the longer term the benefit-to-risk ratio of drugs that rely on the activation of cannabinoid receptors for their sought-after clinical effects can be improved. Some potential strategies for meeting this objective are listed below.

- Exploit the ability of cannabinoid CB_1 receptors expressed outside the central nervous system to mediate sought-after effects such as pain relief (reviewed elsewhere[139,140]), the inhibition of cancer cell proliferation and spread (*Cancer* section) and the amelioration of certain intestinal and cardiovascular disorders (*Intestinal Disorders* and *Cardiovascular Disorders* sections). One possibility would be to administer CB_1 receptor agonists transdermally and, indeed, there is already evidence that this strategy is effective in human subjects for reducing experimental pain.[204,205] A second possibility would be to develop CB_1 receptor agonists that do not readily cross the blood-brain barrier.

- Exploit the ability of cannabinoid CB_1 receptors expressed in the spinal cord to mediate pain relief by administering CB_1 receptor agonists intrathecally (reviewed elsewhere[139,140]). This is already an accepted procedure that is, for example, used for the self-administration of baclofen by some multiple sclerosis patients.
- Exploit the ability of cannabinoid CB_2 receptors to mediate pain relief by administering a CB_2-selective agonist (*Pain* section). This would of course avoid all unwanted consequences of CB_1 receptor activation, provided the dose of agonist used was not excessive.
- Exploit the ability of a low dose of a cannabinoid receptor agonist such as Δ^9-THC both to interact synergistically with a low dose of an opioid such as morphine or codeine for the production of analgesia and to oppose onset of opioid tolerance (reviewed elsewhere[139,206]). The success of this approach will depend on the extent to which these drugs interact synergistically in the clinic to produce undesirable effects. It is worth noting that there is already a report that orally-administered Δ^9-THC had a "morphine-sparing effect" for a patient with severe abdominal pain.[207]
- Exploit the apparent ability of drugs such as the nonpsychotropic cannabinoid, cannabidiol, to reduce some of the undesirable effects of CB_1 receptor activation and perhaps also provide additional beneficial effects.[208] Indeed, the licensed medicine, Sativex, contains both cannabidiol and Δ^9-THC.[199,200]

For some clinical applications it may be advantageous to combine 2 or more of these potential strategies. For example, neuropathic pain might sometimes best be relieved by targeting both CB_1 and CB_2 receptors, perhaps by administering a CB_2 receptor agonist together with a CB_1 agonist that does not readily cross the blood-brain barrier.

Any agonist that possesses CB_1 or CB_2 selectivity is expected to target CB_1 or CB_2 receptors selectively only within a finite dose range and to activate both receptor types when administered at a dose that lies above this range. Such a finding has, for example, been made with the CB_2-selective agonist GW405833.[151] For any particular agonist, the width of its CB_1 or CB_2 selectivity window will of course be affected by the CB_1 to CB_2 receptor ratios of the tissues in which sought-after (or unwanted) effects are induced by CB_1 or CB_2 receptor activation. It is noteworthy, therefore, that not all tissues express CB_1 and CB_2 receptors in equal numbers in health and that there is also evidence that disparate changes in CB_1 and CB_2 expression levels may be induced in some cells or tissues either pathologically or pharmacologically. Consequently, when an agonist that binds more readily either to CB_1 or to CB_2 receptors is administered to patients, it is likely that the CB_1 or CB_2 selectivity of this ligand will not be the same in all tissues that express both receptor types and also that any selectivity will be lost when a certain dose level is exceeded. It is also important to bear in mind that there is evidence that some cannabinoid receptor agonists can activate non-CB_1, non-CB_2 pharmacological targets. Since cannabinoid receptor agonists differ in the extent to which they appear to interact with each of these proposed additional targets, it follows that some ligands with apparently similar abilities to activate CB_1 and/or CB_2 receptors are likely to possess different pharmacological profiles.

Indirect Cannabinoid Receptor Agonists

Existing indirect cannabinoid receptor agonists are all drugs that delay the removal of endocannabinoid molecules from their sites of action. They can be subdivided into FAAH inhibitors that inhibit the metabolism of anandamide and certain other fatty acid amides, MAG-lipase inhibitors that inhibit the metabolism of 2-arachidonoyl glycerol and related compounds, and drugs that inhibit endocannabinoid cellular uptake (*Inhibitors of Endocannabinoid Cellular Uptake and Intracellular Metabolism* section). Following the discovery of allosteric sites on CB_1 receptors, it may also prove possible to develop a second category of indirect cannabinoid receptor agonists that act by allosterically enhancing the ability of endogenously released (and exogenously administered) ligands to activate cannabinoid CB_1 receptors. The argument for using indirect agonists as therapeutic agents is that there are disorders in which endocannabinoids appear to be released selectively onto just certain populations of cannabinoid receptors, some or all of which mediate symptom relief. Consequently, drugs that potentiate endocannabinoids are expected to augment the relief of symptoms produced by such disorders without eliciting as many unwanted cannabinoid receptor-mediated responses as direct agonists that of course will activate all accessible CB_1 and/or CB_2 receptors.

Currently, much attention is being directed at the possibility of developing FAAH inhibitors as medicines. As a result FAAH inhibitors with some degree of selectivity have been developed, and the ability of these compounds to ameliorate symptoms in animal models of pain, multiple sclerosis, excitotoxicity, Parkinson's disease, and hypertension and to reduce cancer cell proliferation has been demonstrated. There is also evidence from animal experiments that FAAH inhibitors are more selective than direct CB_1 receptor agonists, at least after single administration. Thus, for example, in contrast to direct CB_1 agonists, FAAH inhibitors can produce antinociception in mice at doses that do not also induce hypomotility, hypothermia, or catalepsy.[20,37,38] It is noteworthy, however, that there are as yet no published clinical data for this group of compounds. Also, although FAAH inhibitors can induce signs of analgesia in animal models of acute and inflammatory pain, there is some doubt as to whether they would be effective against neuropathic pain. Some important pharmacological considerations that relate to FAAH inhibitors are listed below.

- Inhibition of FAAH is likely to augment anandamide levels not only at cannabinoid receptors but also at its other targets, for example the vanilloid TRPV1 receptor and the putative abnormal cannabidiol receptor, if this endocannabinoid is being released onto these other targets.
- Inhibition of FAAH is also likely to augment levels of certain other endogenous fatty acid amides when these are undergoing release. These amides include 2 cannabinoid receptor ligands, oleamide which might well increase drowsiness if its levels in the brain are elevated,[209] and *N*-arachidonoyl dopamine. They also include ligands that do not readily bind to cannabinoid receptors such as palmitoyl-ethanolamide, which produces antinociception possibly by acting on peripheral "CB_2-like" receptors (*Pain* section), oleoylethanolamide, which is thought

to stimulate fat utilization through activation of PPAR-α receptors, and *N*-arachidonoyl glycine, which is itself a FAAH inhibitor that can induce antinociception in animals when administered exogenously.

- A FAAH inhibitor is not expected to enhance the ability all endocannabinoids to induce symptom relief. Thus, some putative endocannabinoids are metabolically stable (eg, noladin ether) or are metabolized mainly by enzymes other than FAAH (eg, 2-arachidonoyl glycerol).
- Inhibition of FAAH may increase the extent to which the fatty acid amide substrates of this enzyme are degraded by other enzymes. For example, anandamide is known also to be metabolized by PAA, by cyclo-oxygenase-2, by lipoxygenases, and by cytochrome P450. Moreover, as there is evidence that the lipoxygenase metabolites of anandamide are more potent than their parent compound as TRPV1 agonists,[210] it is possible that some patients receiving a FAAH inhibitor would experience either hyperalgesia due to TRPV1 activation or analgesia resulting from TRPV1 desensitization.

Turning now to inhibitors of endocannabinoid cellular uptake, there is evidence that these too have therapeutic potential. This comes from experiments in which such inhibitors have been found to decrease cancer cell proliferation and tumor growth and to ameliorate symptoms in animal models of pain, multiple sclerosis, excitotoxicity, Parkinson's disease, cholera toxin-induced diarrhea, and hypertension. As to MAG lipase inhibitors, any assessment of their therapeutic potential must await the development of suitable compounds, there being a need for compounds that inhibit MAG lipase at doses that do not also inhibit FAAH or interact directly with cannabinoid receptors or with other pharmacological targets that might compromise their selectivity. There is also an urgent need for an allosteric enhancer of the CB_1 receptor that exhibits appropriate efficacy and selectivity. Such an enhancer will most likely differ from a FAAH inhibitor in the following ways:

- by possessing the ability to produce greater symptom alleviation in at least some disorders through the augmentation of CB_1 receptor-mediated responses to all endocannabinoids no matter how their actions are terminated and
- by lacking the ability to augment the activation by anandamide or other fatty acid amides of targets other than CB_1 receptors.

Cannabinoid Receptor Expression Levels and Signaling

There is evidence that upregulation of the endocannabinoid system leading to an alleviation of symptoms can take the form not only of enhanced endocannabinoid release but also of an increase in cannabinoid receptor density or coupling efficiency in tissues in which these receptors mediate symptom relief or inhibition of disease progression when activated by endogenously released endocannabinoids or by exogenously administered cannabinoid receptor agonists. Indeed, results from rat experiments suggest that the endocannabinoid system may protect against hypertension through an increase in CB_1 receptor density/sensitivity rather than through an increase in endocannabinoid release (*Cardiovascular Disorders* section). Other seemingly protective increases in CB_1 and/or CB_2 receptor density or coupling efficiency have been detected in human and mouse atherosclerotic plaques, in human prostate cancer cells, and in animal models of Parkinson's disease, neuropathic pain, diarrhea, intestinal inflammation, and colitis.

It has been reported that cannabinoid receptor expression is higher in some cancer cells than in normal cells[75,187,189] and also that it sometimes correlates with the degree of cancer cell malignancy.[131] It will be important to identify other disorders in which cannabinoid receptor upregulation is confined entirely or mainly to tissues in which activation of cannabinoid receptors is expected to alleviate symptoms or to inhibit disease progression. This is because such a pattern of receptor upregulation may well improve the selectivity of cannabinoid receptor agonists by enhancing their potency for the production of sought-after effects more than their potency for the production of unwanted effects. Selectivity improvements resulting from an uneven cannabinoid receptor upregulation of this kind are expected to be most evident for partial agonists such as Δ^9-THC and cannabinol. Thus although an increase in receptor density will augment the potencies of both full and partial agonists, it will often also increase the size of the maximal response to a partial agonist without affecting the maximal response to a full agonist. This difference between the pharmacology of full and partial agonists can be seen in results from experiments with cannabinol and CP55940 in which an increase in the intestinal expression of CB_1 receptors (and intestinal inflammation) had been induced in mice by oral croton oil and in which the measured response was cannabinoid-induced CB_1 receptor-mediated inhibition of upper gastrointestinal transit of a charcoal suspension.[117] Thus, it was found that this increase in CB_1 expression level was accompanied not only by a leftward shift in the log dose-response curve of cannabinol but also by an increase in the size of the maximal effect of this partial agonist. In contrast, the higher efficacy agonist, CP55940, exhibited an increase in its potency but no change in its maximal effect.

The upregulation of a subpopulation of cannabinoid receptors that alleviates symptoms or inhibits disease progression when activated should of course also augment protective effects of endogenously released endocannabinoids and hence of FAAH inhibitors and other types of indirect agonist. For anandamide, cannabinoid receptor upregulation is likely to produce an increase in maximal effect as well as potency as this endocannabinoid is a CB_1 and CB_2 receptor partial agonist. On the other hand, 2-arachidonoyl glycerol would be expected to exhibit only an increase in potency as it has been found in several investigations to exhibit much higher CB_1 and CB_2 receptor efficacy than anandamide (*Endocannabinoids* section).

Tolerance can develop to CB_1 receptor agonists and there is evidence that this is often caused by a reduction in CB_1 receptor density or signaling.[211] Consequently, it is tempting to speculate that if a particular disease causes an increase in cannabinoid receptor density or signaling this receptor upregulation may oppose the ability of endogenously released or exogenously administered cannabinoid receptor agonists to induce tolerance. If such receptor upregulation is restricted largely to receptors that mediate an alleviation of symptoms or an inhibition of disease progression, then patients would be protected from the development of tolerance to sought-after but not to unwanted effects of a cannabinoid receptor agonist in a manner that would lead to a broadening of the agonist's therapeutic window in response to its repeated administration. There is already good evidence that tolerance develops less readily to some effects of cannabinoid receptor agonists than to others (reviewed elsewhere[212]) and, indeed, that some sought-after therapeutic effects of a CB_1 receptor agonist may be more resistant to tolerance development than some of its unwanted effects.[213] CB_1 receptor agonists may also sometimes widen their own therapeutic windows by inducing a selective increase in the density of CB_1 receptors that are mediating a sought-after effect such as inhibition of the growth and proliferation of cancer cells.

Damaging Upregulation of the Endocannabinoid System?

There are some disorders in which the endocannabinoid system appears to upregulate to induce *undesirable* symptoms, an indication that this system may sometimes malfunction. For example, it has been postulated that upregulation of the endocannabinoid system can

- impair fertility in some women as there are reports (1) that FAAH activity and expression fall in the lymphocytes of some women who miscarry or who fail to become pregnant after in vitro fertilization (IVF) and embryo transfer, (2) that this fall is accompanied in the IVF-embryo transfer group of women by a corresponding rise in blood anandamide[65,66] (see also Table 38.1), and (3) that anandamide can impair embryo implantation and development in mice[214];
- contribute toward obesity in some individuals as, for example, it has been found that hypothalamic levels of anandamide and/or 2-arachidonoyl glycerol are raised in obese *db/db* and *ob/ob* mice and *fa/fa* rats (Table 38.2), that CB_1 receptor expression levels are elevated in the adipose tissue of obese *fa/fa* rats (Table 38.2), and that SR141716A reduces the food intake of *db/db* and *ob/ob* mice, reduces the body weight of *db/db* mice, and decreases the food intake, body weight, and waist circumference of obese humans[102,215];
- contribute toward osteoporosis and other diseases in which there is bone loss, as bone mineral density is greater in $CB_1^{-/-}$ mice than in wild type animals, as ovariectomy does not induce bone loss in $CB_1^{-/-}$ mice, as AM251 and SR144528 protect against ovariectomy-induced bone resorption, as CB_1 and CB_2 receptor antagonists/inverse agonists significantly inhibit evoked osteoclast formation in CB_1 and CB_2 receptor-expressing mouse bone marrow cultures, and as anandamide and CP55940 can stimulate osteoclast formation in these cultures[216];
- contribute toward the production of cerebral injury in stroke as unilateral ischemia/reperfusion injury induced in rats by transient middle cerebral artery occlusion has been reported to be associated with an elevation of whole brain

anandamide and as infarct volume and neurological impairment in lesioned rats were both found to be less after pretreatment with selective CB_1 receptor antagonists[123] (see also Table 38.4);

- contribute toward the life-threatening excessive hypotension of endotoxaemic shock triggered by advanced liver cirrhosis[68,112] (Table 38.3) or by the cemented hip arthroplasty procedure[76] (Table 38.1) (but may aid survival in hemorrhagic, septic, and cardiogenic shock);

- contribute toward the development of hyperreflexia and hyperalgesia during cystitis as it has been found that urinary bladder levels of anandamide increase in a rat model of this disorder (Table 38.2) and that reflex activity increased both when anandamide was applied to healthy bladders and when the FAAH/anandamide cellular uptake inhibitor, palmitoylisopropylamide, was applied to healthy or inflamed bladders[101];

- contribute toward intestinal inflammation in ileitis as there is a report that ileal levels of anandamide (and 2-arachidonoyl glycerol) increase in a rat model of this disorder (Table 38.3), as inflammation and fluid accumulation in the rat ileum increase in response to intraluminal injection of either of these endocannabinoids, and as intraluminal injections of the FAAH/MAG lipase inhibitors, PMSF or MAFP, augment intra-ileal fluid accumulation induced by *Clostridium difficile* toxin A[120];

- contribute toward intestinal hypomotility in paralytic ileus as reductions in mouse intestinal motility induced by peritoneal irritation with acetic acid has been shown to be counteracted by SR141716A (although not by SR144528), to be exacerbated by the anandamide cellular uptake inhibitor, VDM11, in an SR141716A-sensitive manner, and to be accompanied in the small intestine by increases in anandamide levels and in the neural density of CB_1 receptor immunoreactivity[121] (see also Table 38.3).

Endocannabinoids appear to produce many of their unwanted effects by interacting with cannabinoid CB_1 receptors. Thus, results from animal experiments suggest that endocannabinoids act on these receptors to induce (1) impairment of embryo implantation and development (reviewed elsewhere[214]), (2) increases in food intake and body weight associated with obesity,[102] (3) cerebral injury in stroke,[123] (4) hypotension in liver cirrhosis,[68] and (5) intestinal hypomotility in paralytic ileus.[121] As to the CB_2 component of the endocannabinoid system, evidence is emerging that this too may sometimes induce unwanted effects by promoting inflammation in a manner that can be counteracted by CB_2 receptor inverse agonism. There are also unwanted effects of the endocannabinoids that appear to be mediated by TRPV1 rather than CB_1 or CB_2 receptors. These are urinary bladder hyperreflexia in cystitis, and intestinal inflammation and fluid accumulation in ileitis.[101,120] In these instances the undesirable effects can be attenuated by TRPV1 receptor antagonism but not CB_1 receptor antagonism which, indeed, was found to exacerbate anandamide-induced bladder hyperreflexia. Clearly then, there may be a place in the clinic for CB_1 and TRPV1 receptor antagonists and possibly also for CB_2 receptor inverse antagonists. Indeed, the CB_1 receptor antagonist, SR14171A (rimonabant; Acomplia), is already in the final stages of development as an anti-obesity agent.[215] Selective inhibitors of endocannabinoid biosynthesis, activators of endocannabinoid-metabolizing enzymes, and allosteric antagonists of the CB_1 receptor also have therapeutic potential for the management of some disorders with symptoms that are induced by endogenously released cannabinoids. However, such drugs have yet to be developed.

Future Directions

There is no doubt that the endocannabinoid system upregulates both in response to certain pathological changes or to stress and during normal physiological events such as aging, feeding, fasting, and exercise. There is also good evidence that this upregulation can take the form of an increase both in the release of endocannabinoid molecules onto their receptors and in the density or coupling efficiency of some of these receptors. Often, this upregulation appears to protect the organism from unwanted symptoms or even to slow the progression of a disease. However, there is also evidence that upregulation of the endocannabinoid system can sometimes trigger unwanted symptoms, an indication that this system has its own pathology and possibly also that it is sometimes influenced detrimentally by pathological events taking place in some other system from which it receives input.

As to the future, it will be important to obtain a more complete list of pathological processes that are modulated by the endocannabinoid system and to determine for each of these processes whether this modulation has desirable or undesirable consequences. It will also be important to establish both the nature of this modulation and the extent to which it is confined to tissues in which cannabinoid receptor activation affects symptoms or disease progression. This in turn will help identify the best pharmacological strategy for the management of any particular disorder in which the endocannabinoid system has upregulated, be this to administer a CB_1 and/or CB_2 receptor agonist or antagonist that does or does not readily cross the blood-brain barrier, a CB_1 and/or CB_2 receptor agonist intrathecally or directly to some other site outside the brain, a partial CB_1 and/or CB_2 receptor agonist rather than a full agonist, a CB_1 and/or CB_2 receptor agonist together with a noncannabinoid, an inhibitor or activator of endocannabinoid biosynthesis, cellular uptake or metabolism, an allosteric modulator of the CB_1 receptor, or a CB_2 receptor inverse agonist. Other important objectives for future research are

- to obtain a more complete understanding of the processes that determine the biosynthesis, release, and fate of endocannabinoids,
- to identify those drugs that are best at modulating these processes selectively or at producing selective allosteric enhancement or antagonism of cannabinoid receptors,
- to characterize the pharmacology of these drugs and to test them in the clinic,
- to investigate the extent to which tolerance develops over time to protective effects of endocannabinoids when these are released by themselves or in the presence of drugs that augment the tissue levels of released endocannabinoids,

- to establish in greater detail the part played by non-CB_1, non-CB_2 targets in both the protective and the undesirable consequences of endogenous cannabinoid release, and
- to gain a better understanding of the part played by spinal or peripheral CB_1 and CB_2 receptors in modulating the symptoms and progression of particular diseases.

Finally, since the completion of this review, evidence has emerged that the orphan G protein-coupled receptor, GPR55, is a cannabinoid receptor,[217,218] prompting a need for research that will identify the physiological and/or pathological roles of this receptor and characterize its pharmacology. The discovery of a selective MAG lipase inhibitor, URB602, has also just been announced.[219]

Acknowledgments The writing of this review was supported by grants from NIDA (DA09789) and from GW Pharmaceuticals (Salisbury, Wiltshire, UK).

References

1. Howlett AC, Barth F, Bonner TI, et al. International Union of Pharmacology. XXVII. Classification of cannabinoid receptors. *Pharmacol Rev.* 2002;54:161-202.
2. Pertwee RG. Pharmacological actions of cannabinoids. In: Pertwee RG, ed. *Cannabinoids, Handbook of Experimental Pharmacolology.* Heidelberg, Germany: Springer-Verlag; 2005;168:1-51.
3. Matsuda LA, Lolait SJ, Brownstein MJ, Young AC, Bonner TI. Structure of a cannabinoid receptor and functional expression of the cloned cDNA. *Nature.* 1990;346:561-564.
4. Munro S, Thomas KL, Abu-Shaar M. Molecular characterization of a peripheral receptor for cannabinoids. *Nature.* 1993;365:61-65.
5. Pertwee RG. Pharmacology of cannabinoid receptor ligands. *Curr Med Chem.* 1999;6:635-664.
6. Pertwee RG. Inverse agonism and neutral antagonism at cannabinoid CB_1 receptors. *Life Sci.* 2005;76:1307-1324.
7. Pertwee RG. Novel pharmacological targets for cannabinoids. *Curr Neuropharmacol.* 2004;2:9-29.
8. Price MR, Baillie G, Thomas A, et al. Allosteric modulation of the cannabinoid CB_1 receptor. *Mol Pharmacol.* In press.
9. Bradshaw HB, Walker JM. The expanding field of cannabimimetic and related lipid mediators. *Br J Pharmacol.* 2005;144:459-465.
10. Steffens M, Zentner J, Honegger J, Feuerstein TJ. Binding affinity and agonist activity of putative endogenous cannabinoids at the human neocortical CB_1 receptor. *Biochem Pharmacol.* 2005;69:169-178.
11. Cabral GA, Staab A. Effects on the immune system. In: Pertwee RG, ed. *Cannabinoids, Handbook of Experimental Pharmacolology.* Heidelberg, Germany: Springer-Verlag; 2005;168:385-423.
12. Szabo B, Schlicker E. Effects of cannabinoids on neurotransmission. In: Pertwee RG, ed. *Cannabinoids, Handbook of Experimental Pharmacolology.* Heidelberg, Germany: Springer-Verlag; 2005;168:327-365.
13. Vaughan CW, Christie MJ. Retrograde signalling by endocannabinoids. In: Pertwee RG, ed. *Cannabinoids, Handbook of Experimental Pharmacolology.* Heidelberg, Germany: Springer-Verlag; 2005;168:367-383.
14. Price TJ, Patwardhan A, Akopian AN, Hargreaves KM, Flores CM. Modulation of trigeminal sensory neuron activity by the dual cannabinoid-vanilloid agonists anandamide, *N*-arachidonoyl-dopamine and arachidonyl-2-chloroethylamide. *Br J Pharmacol.* 2004;141:1118-1130.

15. Baker CL, McDougall JJ. The cannabinomimetic arachidonyl-2-chloroethylamide (ACEA) acts on capsaicin-sensitive TRPV1 receptors but not cannabinoid receptors in rat joints. *Br J Pharmacol.* 2004;142:1361-1367.
16. Di Marzo V, De Petrocellis L, Bisogno T. The biosynthesis, fate and pharmacological properties of endocannabinoids. In: Pertwee RG, ed. *Cannabinoids, Handbook of Experimental Pharmacolology.* Heidelberg, Germany: Springer-Verlag; 2005;168:147-185.
17. Bisogno T, Melck D, Bobrov MY, et al. *N*-acyl-dopamines: novel synthetic CB_1 cannabinoid-receptor ligands and inhibitors of anandamide inactivation with cannabimimetic activity *in vitro* and *in vivo*. *Biochem J.* 2000;351:817-824.
18. Leggett JD, Aspley S, Beckett SRG, D'Antona AM, Kendall DA, Kendall DA. Oleamide is a selective endogenous agonist of rat and human CB_1 cannabinoid receptors. *Br J Pharmacol.* 2004;141:253-262.
19. Porter AC, Sauer J-M, Knierman MD, et al. Characterization of a novel endocannabinoid, virodhamine, with antagonist activity at the CB_1 receptor. *J Pharmacol Exp Ther.* 2002;301:1020-1024.
20. Cravatt BF, Lichtman AH. The endogenous cannabinoid system and its role in nociceptive behavior. *J Neurobiol.* 2004;61:149-160.
21. Hillard CJ, Jarrahian A. Cellular accumulation of anandamide: consensus and controversy. *Br J Pharmacol.* 2003;140:802-808.
22. Ueda N. Endocannabinoid hydrolases. *Prostaglandins Other Lipid Mediat.* 2002;68-9: 521-534.
23. Ho W-SV, Hillard CJ. Modulators of endocannabinoid enzymic hydrolysis and membrane transport. In: Pertwee RG, ed. *Cannabinoids, Handbook of Experimental Pharmacolology.* Heidelberg, Germany: Springer-Verlag; 2005;168:187-207.
24. Gulyas AI, Cravatt BF, Bracey MH, et al. Segregation of 2 endocannabinoid-hydrolyzing enzymes into pre- and postsynaptic compartments in the rat hippocampus, cerebellum and amygdala. *Eur J Neurosci.* 2004;20:441-458.
25. Ueda N, Yamanaka K, Yamamoto S. Purification and characterization of an acid amidase selective for *N*-palmitoylethanolamine, a putative endogenous anti-inflammatory substance. *J Biol Chem.* 2001;276:35552-35557.
26. Lo Verme J, Gaetani S, Fu J, Oveisi F, Burton K, Piomelli D. Regulation of food intake by oleoylethanolamide. *Cell Mol Life Sci.* 2005;62:708-716.
27. Fegley D, Gaetani S, Duranti A, et al. Characterization of the fatty acid amide hydrolase inhibitor cyclohexyl carbamic acid 3′-carbamoyl-biphenyl-3-yl ester (URB597): effects on anandamide and oleoylethanolamide deactivation. *J Pharmacol Exp Ther.* 2005;313:352-358.
28. Kozak KR, Marnett LJ. Oxidative metabolism of endocannabinoids. *Prostaglandins Leukot Essent Fatty Acids.* 2002;66:211-220.
29. Saario SM, Savinainen JR, Laitinen JT, Järvinen T, Niemi R. Monoglyceride lipase-like enzymatic activity is responsible for hydrolysis of 2-arachidonoylglycerol in rat cerebellar membranes. *Biochem Pharmacol.* 2004;67:1381-1387.
30. Dinh TP, Kathuria S, Piomelli D. RNA interference suggests a primary role for monoacylglycerol lipase in the degradation of the endocannabinoid 2-arachidonoylglycerol. *Mol Pharmacol.* 2004;66:1260-1264.
31. Fezza F, Bisogno T, Minassi A, Appendino G, Mechoulam R, Di Marzo V. Noladin ether, a putative novel endocannabinoid: inactivation mechanisms and a sensitive method for its quantification in rat tissues. *FEBS Lett.* 2002;513:294-298.
32. De Petrocellis L, Davis JB, Di Marzo V. Palmitoylethanolamide enhances anandamide stimulation of human vanilloid VR1 receptors. *FEBS Lett.* 2001;506:253-256.
33. Sheskin T, Hanus L, Slager J, Vogel Z, Mechoulam R. Structural requirements for binding of anandamide-type compounds to the brain cannabinoid receptor. *J Med Chem.* 1997;40:659-667.
34. Fernando SR, Pertwee RG. Evidence that methyl arachidonyl fluorophosphonate is an irreversible cannabinoid receptor antagonist. *Br J Pharmacol.* 1997;121:1716-1720.
35. Savinainen JR, Saario SM, Niemi R, Järvinen T, Laitinen JT. An optimized approach to study endocannabinoid signaling: evidence against constitutive activity of rat brain adenosine A_1 and cannabinoid CB_1 receptors. *Br J Pharmacol.* 2003;140:1451-1459.

36. Nithipatikom K, Endsley MP, Isbell MA, et al. 2-Arachidonoylglycerol: a novel inhibitor of androgen-independent prostate cancer cell invasion. *Cancer Res.* 2004;64:8826-8830.
37. Kathuria S, Gaetani S, Fegley D, et al. Modulation of anxiety through blockade of anandamide hydrolysis. *Nat Med.* 2003;9:76-81.
38. Lichtman AH, Leung D, Shelton CC, et al. Reversible inhibitors of fatty acid amide hydrolase that promote analgesia: evidence for an unprecedented combination of potency and selectivity. *J Pharmacol Exp Ther.* 2004;311:441-448.
39. Huang SM, Bisogno T, Petros TJ, et al. Identification of a new class of molecules, the arachidonyl amino acids, and characterization of one member that inhibits pain. *J Biol Chem.* 2001;276:42639-42644.
40. Bisogno T, Melck D, De Petrocellis L, et al. Arachidonoylserotonin and other novel inhibitors of fatty acid amide hydrolase. *Biochem Biophys Res Commun.* 1998;248:515-522.
41. Ligresti A, Bisogno T, Matias I, et al. Possible endocannabinoid control of colorectal cancer growth. *Gastroenterology.* 2003;125:677-687.
42. Jonsson K-O, Vandevoorde S, Lambert DM, Tiger G, Fowler CJ. Effects of homologues and analogues of palmitoylethanolamide upon the inactivation of the endocannabinoid anandamide. *Br J Pharmacol.* 2001;133:1263-1275.
43. Khanolkar AD, Abadji V, Lin S, et al. Head group analogs of arachidonylethanolamide, the endogenous cannabinoid ligand. *J Med Chem.* 1996;39:4515-4519.
44. Beltramo M, Stella N, Calignano A, Lin SY, Makriyannis A, Piomelli D. Functional role of high-affinity anandamide transport, as revealed by selective inhibition. *Science.* 1997;277:1094-1097.
45. Jarrahian A, Manna S, Edgemond WS, Campbell WB, Hillard CJ. Structure-activity relationships among *N*-arachidonylethanolamine (anandamide) head group analogues for the anandamide transporter. *J Neurochem.* 2000;74:2597-2606.
46. Zygmunt PM, Chuang H, Movahed P, Julius D, Högestätt ED. The anandamide transport inhibitor AM404 activates vanilloid receptors. *Eur J Pharmacol.* 2000;396:39-42.
47. De Petrocellis L, Bisogno T, Davis JB, Pertwee RG, Di Marzo V. Overlap between the ligand recognition properties of the anandamide transporter and the VR1 vanilloid receptor: inhibitors of anandamide uptake with negligible capsaicin-like activity. *FEBS Lett.* 2000;483:52-56.
48. Fowler CJ, Tiger G, Ligresti A, López-Rodríguez ML, Di Marzo V. Selective inhibition of anandamide cellular uptake versus enzymatic hydrolysis—a difficult issue to handle. *Eur J Pharmacol.* 2004;492:1-11.
49. Ortar G, Ligresti A, De Petrocellis L, Morera E, Di Marzo V. Novel selective and metabolically stable inhibitors of anandamide cellular uptake. *Biochem Pharmacol.* 2003;65:1473-1481.
50. López-Rodríguez ML, Viso A, Ortega-Gutiérrez S, et al. Design, synthesis and biological evaluation of new endocannabinoid transporter inhibitors. *Eur J Med Chem.* 2003;38:403-412.
51. Ruiz-Llorente L, Ortega-Gutiérrez S, Viso A, et al. Characterization of an anandamide degradation system in prostate epithelial PC-3 cells: synthesis of new transporter inhibitors as tools for this study. *Br J Pharmacol.* 2004;141:457-467.
52. Benito C, Núñez E, Tolón RM, et al. Cannabinoid CB_2 receptors and fatty acid amide hydrolase are selectively overexpressed in neuritic plaque-associated glia in Alzheimer's disease brains. *J Neurosci.* 2003;23:11136-11141.
53. Ramírez BG, Blázquez C, Gómez del Pulgar T, Guzmán N, de Ceballos ML. Prevention of Alzheimer's disease pathology by cannabinoids: neuroprotection mediated by blockade of microglial activation. *J Neurosci.* 2005;25:1904-1913.
54. Giuffrida A, Leweke FM, Gerth CW, et al. Cerebrospinal anandamide levels are elevated in acute schizophrenia and are inversely correlated with psychotic symptoms. *Neuropsychopharmacology.* 2004;29:2108-2114.
55. Leweke FM, Giuffrida A, Wurster U, Emrich HM, Piomelli D. Elevated endogenous cannabinoids in schizophrenia. *Neuroreport.* 1999;10:1665-1669.
56. Dean B, Sundram S, Bradbury R, Scarr E, Copolov D. Studies on [^{3}H]CP-55940 binding in the human central nervous system: regional specific changes in density of cannabinoid-1 receptors associated with schizophrenia and cannabis use. *Neuroscience.* 2001;103:9-15.

57. Zavitsanou K, Garrick T, Huang XF. Selective antagonist [^{3}H]SR141716A binding to cannabinoid CB$_1$ receptors is increased in the anterior cingulate cortex in schizophrenia. *Prog Neuropsychopharmacol Biol Psychiatry.* 2004;28:355-360.

58. De Marchi N, De Petrocellis L, Orlando P, Daniele F, Fezza F, Di Marzo V. Endocannabinoid signalling in the blood of patients with schizophrenia. *Lipids Health Dis.* 2003;2:1-9.

59. Hungund BL, Vinod KY, Kassir SA, et al. Upregulation of CB$_1$ receptors and agonist-stimulated [^{35}S]GTPγS binding in the prefrontal cortex of depressed suicide victims. *Mol Psychiatry.* 2004;9:184-190.

60. Vinod KY, Arango V, Xie S, et al. Elevated levels of endocannabinoids and CB$_1$ receptor-mediated G-protein signaling in the prefrontal cortex of alcoholic suicide victims. *Biol Psychiatry.* 2005;57:480-486.

61. Lastres-Becker I, Cebeira M, de Ceballos ML, et al. Increased cannabinoid CB$_1$ receptor binding and activation of GTP-binding proteins in the basal ganglia of patients with Parkinson's syndrome and of MPTP-treated marmosets. *Eur J Neurosci.* 2001;14:1827-1832.

62. Glass M, Faull R, Dragunow M. Loss of cannabinoid receptors in the substantia-nigra in Huntington's disease. *Neurosci.* 1993;56:523-527.

63. Richfield EK, Herkenham M. Selective vulnerability in Huntington's disease: preferential loss of cannabinoid receptors in lateral globus pallidus. *Ann Neurol.* 1994;36:577-584.

64. Schäbitz W-R, Giuffrida A, Berger C, et al. Release of fatty acid amides in a patient with hemispheric stroke: a microdialysis study. *Stroke.* 2002;33:2112-2114.

65. Maccarone M, Valensise H, Bari M, Lazzarin N, Romanini C, Finazzi-Agricò A. Relation between decreased anandamide hydrolase concentrations in human lymphocytes and miscarriage. *Lancet.* 2000;355:1326-1329.

66. Maccarone M, Bisogno T, Valensise H, et al. Low fatty acid amide hydrolase and high anandamide levels are associated with failure to achieve an ongoing pregnancy after IVF and embryo transfer. *Mol Hum Reprod.* 2002;8:188-195.

67. Wang Y, Liu Y, Ito Y, et al. Simultaneous measurement of anandamide and 2- arachidonoylglycerol by polymyxin B-selective adsorption and subsequent high-performance liquid chromatography analysis: increase in endogenous cannabinoids in the sera of patients with endotoxic shock. *Anal Biochem.* 2001;294:73-82.

68. Bátkai S, Járai Z, Wagner JA, et al. Endocannabinoids acting at vascular CB$_1$ receptors mediate the vasodilated state in advanced liver cirrhosis. *Nat Med.* 2001;7:827-832.

69. Fernández-Rodriguez CM, Romero J, Petros TJ, et al. Circulating endogenous cannabinoid anandamide and portal, systemic and renal hemodynamics in cirrhosis. *Liver Int.* 2004;24:477-483.

70. Julien B, Grenard P, Teixeira-Clerc F, et al. Antifibrogenic role of the cannabinoid receptor CB$_2$ in the liver. *Gastroenterology.* 2005;128:742-755.

71. Steffens S, Veillard NR, Arnaud C, et al. Low dose oral cannabinoid therapy reduces progression of atherosclerosis in mice. *Nature.* 2005;434:782-786.

72. Maccarone M, Attinà M, Cartoni A, Bari M, Finazzi-Agricò A. Gas chromatography-mass spectrometry analysis of endogenous cannabinoids in healthy and tumoral human brain and human cells in culture. *J Neurochem.* 2001;76:594-601.

73. Petersen G, Moesgaard B, Schmid PC, et al. Endocannabinoid metabolism in human glioblastomas and meningiomas compared to human non-tumour brain tissue. *J Neurochem.* 2005;93:299-309.

74. Pagotto U, Marsicano G, Fezza F, et al. Normal human pituitary gland and pituitary adenomas express cannabinoid receptor type 1 and synthesize endogenous cannabinoids: first evidence for a direct role of cannabinoids on hormone modulation at the human pituitary level. *J Clin Endocrinol Metab.* 2001;86:2687-2696.

75. Sarfaraz S, Afaq F, Adhami VM, Mukhtar H. Cannabinoid receptor as a novel target for the treatment of prostate cancer. *Cancer Res.* 2005;65:1635-1641.

76. Motobe T, Hashiguchi T, Uchimura T, et al. Endogenous cannabinoids are candidates for lipid mediators of bone cement implantation syndrome. *Shock.* 2004;21:8-12.

77. Baker D, Pryce G, Croxford JL, et al. Endocannabinoids control spasticity in a multiple sclerosis model. *FASEB J.* 2001;15:300-302.

78. Berrendero F, Sánchez A, Cabranes A, et al. Changes in cannabinoid CB_1 receptors in striatal and cortical regions of rats with experimental allergic encephalomyelitis, an animal model of multiple sclerosis. *Synapse*. 2001;41:195-202.

79. Cheng BC, Xu H, Calbay L, Pertwee RG, Coutts A, Forrester JV. Specific CB_2 receptor agonist suppresses the murine model of experimental autoimmune uveitis. *Invest Ophthalmol Vis Sci*. 2004;45:552.

80. Witting A, Weydt P, Hong S, Kliot M, Möller T, Stella N. Endocannabinoids accumulate in spinal cord of SOD1^{G93A} transgenic mice. *J Neurochem*. 2004;89:1555-1557.

81. Benito C, Kim W-K, Chavarria I, et al. A glial endogenous cannabinoid system is upregulated in the brains of macaques with simian immunodeficiency virus-induced encephalitis. *J Neurosci*. 2005;25:2530-2536.

82. Adriani W, Caprioli A, Granstrem O, Carli M, Laviola G. The spontaneously hypertensive-rat as an animal model of ADHD: evidence for impulsive and non-impulsive subpopulations. *Neurosci Biobehav Rev*. 2003;27:639-651.

83. Di Marzo V, Hill MP, Bisogno T, Crossman AR, Brotchie JM. Enhanced levels of endogenous cannabinoids in the globus pallidus are associated with a reduction in movement in an animal model of Parkinson's disease. *FASEB J*. 2000;14:1432-1438.

84. Gubellini P, Picconi B, Bari M, et al. Experimental parkinsonism alters endocannabinoid degradation: implications for striatal glutamatergic transmission. *J Neurosci*. 2002;22: 6900-6907.

85. Maccarone M, Gubellini P, Bari M, et al. Levodopa treatment reverses endocannabinoid system abnormalities in experimental parkinsonism. *J Neurochem*. 2003;85:1018-1025.

86. Fernandez-Espejo E, Caraballo I, Rodriguez de Fonseca F, et al. Experimental parkinsonism alters anandamide precursor synthesis, and functional deficits are improved by AM404: a modulator of endocannabinoid function. *Neuropsychopharmacology*. 2004;29:1134-1142.

87. Ferrer B, Asbrock N, Kathuria S, Piomelli D, Giuffrida A. Effects of levodopa on endocannabinoid levels in rat basal ganglia: implications for the treatment of levodopa-induced dyskinesias. *Eur J Neurosci*. 2003;18:1607-1614.

88. Herkenham M, Lynn AB, de Costa BR, Richfield EK. Neuronal localization of cannabinoid receptors in the basal ganglia of the rat. *Brain Res*. 1991;547:267-274.

89. Romero J, Berrendero F, Pérez-Rosado A, et al. Unilateral 6-hydroxydopamine lesions of nigrostriatal dopaminergic neurons increased CB_1 receptor mRNA levels in the caudate-putamen. *Life Sci*. 2000;66:485-494.

90. Mailleux P, Vanderhaeghen J-J. Dopaminergic regulation of cannabinoid receptor mRNA levels in the rat caudate-putamen: an in situ hybridization study. *J Neurochem*. 1993;61:1705-1712.

91. Zeng B-Y, Dass B, Owen A, et al. Chronic L-DOPA treatment increases striatal cannabinoid CB_1 receptor mRNA expression in 6-hydroxydopamine-lesioned rats. *Neurosci Lett*. 1999;276:71-74.

92. McCaw EA, Hu H, Gomez GT, Hebb ALO, Kelly MEM, Denovan-Wright EM. Structure, expression and regulation of the cannabinoid receptor gene (*CB1*) in Huntington's disease transgenic mice. *Eur J Biochem*. 2004;271:4909-4920.

93. Page KJ, Besret L, Jain M, Monaghan EM, Dunnett SB, Everitt BJ. Effects of systemic 3-nitropropionic acid-induced lesions of the dorsal striatum on cannabinoid and μ-opioid receptor binding in the basal ganglia. *Exp Brain Res*. 2000;130:142-150.

94. Lastres-Becker I, Fezza F, Cebeira M, et al. Changes in endocannabinoid transmission in the basal ganglia in a rat model of Huntington's disease. *Neuroreport*. 2001;12:2125-2129.

95. Lastres-Becker I, Bizat N, Boyer F, Hantraye P, Fernández-Ruiz J, Brouillet E. Potential involvement of cannabinoid receptors in 3-nitropropionic acid toxicity *in vivo*. *Neuroreport*. 2004;15:2375-2379.

96. Lastres-Becker I, Hansen HH, Berrendero F, et al. Alleviation of motor hyperactivity and neurochemical deficits by endocannabinoid uptake inhibition in a rat model of Huntington's disease. *Synapse*. 2002;44:23-35.

97. Lastres-Becker I, Berrendero F, Lucas JJ, et al. Loss of mRNA levels, binding and activation of GTP-binding proteins for cannabinoid CB_1 receptors in the basal ganglia of a transgenic model of Huntington's disease. *Brain Res*. 2002;929:236-242.

98. Walker JM, Huang SM, Strangman NM, Tsou K, Sañudo-Peña MC. Pain modulation by release of the endogenous cannabinoid anandamide. *Proc Natl Acad Sci USA*. 1999;96:12198-12203.
99. Lim G, Sung B, Ji R-R, Mao J. Upregulation of spinal cannabinoid-1-receptors following nerve injury enhances the effects of Win 55,212-2 on neuropathic pain behaviors in rats. *Pain*. 2003;105:275-283.
100. Zhang J, Hoffert C, Vu HK, Groblewski T, Ahmad S, O'Donnell D. Induction of CB_2 receptor expression in the rat spinal cord of neuropathic but not inflammatory chronic pain models. *Eur J Neurosci*. 2003;17:2750-2754.
101. Dinis P, Charrua A, Avelino A, et al. Anandamide-evoked activation of vanilloid receptor 1 contributes to the development of bladder hyperreflexia and nociceptive transmission to spinal dorsal horn neurons in cystitis. *J Neurosci*. 2004;24:11253-11263.
102. Di Marzo V, Goparaju SK, Wang L, et al. Leptin-regulated endocannabinoids are involved in maintaining food intake. *Nature*. 2001;410:822-825.
103. Bensaid M, Gary-Bobo M, Esclangon A, et al. The cannabinoid CB_1 receptor antagonist SR141716 increases Acrp30 mRNA expression in adipose tissue of obese fa/fa rats and in cultured adipocyte cells. *Mol Pharmacol*. 2003;63:908-914.
104. Maccarrone M, Fride E, Bisogno T, et al. Up-regulation of the endocannabinoid system in the uterus of leptin knockout (*ob/ob*) mice and implications for fertility. *Mol Hum Reprod*. 2005;11:21-28.
105. Kirkham TC, Williams CM, Fezza F, Di Marzo V. Endocannabinoid levels in rat limbic forebrain and hypothalamus in relation to fasting, feeding and satiation: stimulation of eating by 2-arachidonoyl glycerol. *Br J Pharmacol*. 2002;136:550-557.
106. Hill MN, Patel S, Carrier EJ, et al. Downregulation of endocannabinoid signaling in the hippocampus following chronic unpredictable stress. *Neuropsychopharmacology*. 2005;30: 508-515.
107. Patel S, Roelke CT, Rademacher DJ, Hillard CJ. Inhibition of restraint stress-induced neural and behavioural activation by endogenous cannabinoid signalling. *Eur J Neurosci*. 2005;21: 1057-1069.
108. Marsicano G, Wotjak CT, Azad SC, et al. The endogenous cannabinoid system controls extinction of aversive memories. *Nature*. 2002;418:530-534.
109. Liu P, Bilkey DK, Darlington CL, Smith PF. Cannabinoid CB_1 receptor protein expression in the rat hippocampus and entorhinal, perirhinal, postrhinal and temporal cortices: regional variations and age-related changes. *Brain Res*. 2003;979:235-239.
110. Sparling PB, Giuffrida A, Piomelli D, Rosskopf L, Dietrich A. Exercise activates the endocannabinoid system. *Neuroreport*. 2003;14:2209-2211.
111. Bátkai S, Pacher P, Osei-Hyiaman D, et al. Endocannabinoids acting at cannabinoid-1 receptors regulate cardiovascular function in hypertension. *Circulation*. 2004;110:1996-2002.
112. Domenicali M, Ros J, Fernández-Varo G, et al. Increased anandamide induced relaxation in mesenteric arteries of cirrhotic rats: role of cannabinoid and vanilloid receptors. *Gut*. 2005;54:522-527.
113. Varga K, Wagner JA, Bridgen DT, Kunos G. Platelet- and macrophage-derived endogenous cannabinoids are involved in endotoxin-induced hypotension. *FASEB J*. 1998;12:1035-1044.
114. Liu J, Bátkai S, Pacher P, et al. Lipopolysaccharide induces anandamide synthesis in macrophages via CD14/MAPK/phosphoinositide 3-kinase/NF-κB independently of platelet-activating factor. *J Biol Chem*. 2003;278:45034-45039.
115. Maccarrone M, De Petrocellis L, Bari M, et al. Lipopolysaccharide downregulates fatty acid amide hydrolase expression and increases anandamide levels in human peripheral lymphocytes. *Arch Biochem Biophys*. 2001;393:321-328.
116. Wagner JA, Hu K, Bauersachs J, et al. Endogenous cannabinoids mediate hypotension after experimental myocardial infarction. *J Am Coll Cardiol*. 2001;38:2048-2054.
117. Izzo AA, Fezza F, Capasso R, et al. Cannabinoid CB_1-receptor mediated regulation of gastrointestinal motility in mice in a model of intestinal inflammation. *Br J Pharmacol*. 2001; 134:563-570.
118. Massa F, Marsicano G, Hermann H, et al. The endogenous cannabinoid system protects against colonic inflammation. *J Clin Invest*. 2004;113:1202-1209.

119. Izzo AA, Capasso F, Costagliola A, et al. An endogenous cannabinoid tone attenuates cholera toxin-induced fluid accumulation in mice. *Gastroenterology*. 2003;125:765-774.
120. McVey DC, Schmid PC, Schmid HHO, Vigna SR. Endocannabinoids induce ileitis in rats via the capsaicin receptor (VR1). *J Pharmacol Exp Ther*. 2003;304:713-722.
121. Mascolo N, Izzo AA, Ligresti A, et al. The endocannabinoid system and the molecular basis of paralytic ileus in mice. *FASEB J*. 2002;16:U131-U51.
122. Jin KL, Mao XO, Goldsmith PC, Greenberg DA. CB$_1$ cannabinoid receptor induction in experimental stroke. *Ann Neurol*. 2000;48:257-261.
123. Muthian S, Rademacher DJ, Roelke CT, Gross GJ, Hillard CJ. Anandamide content is increased and CB$_1$ cannabinoid receptor blockade is protective during transient, focal cerebral ischemia. *Neuroscience*. 2004;129:743-750.
124. Kurabayashi M, Takeyoshi I, Yoshinari D, Matsumoto K, Maruyama I, Morishita Y. 2-Arachidonoylglycerol increases in ischemia-reperfusion injury of the rat liver. *J Invest Surg*. 2005;18:25-31.
125. Hansen HH, Schmid PC, Bittigau P, et al. Anandamide, but not 2-arachidonoylglycerol, accumulates during *in vivo* neurodegeneration. *J Neurochem*. 2001;78:1415-1427.
126. Panikashvili D, Simeonidou C, Ben-Shabat S, et al. An endogenous cannabinoid (2-AG) is neuroprotective after brain injury. *Nature*. 2001;413:527-531.
127. Sugiura T, Yoshinaga N, Kondo S, Waku K, Ishima Y. Generation of 2-arachidonoylglycerol, an endogenous cannabinoid receptor ligand, in picrotoxinin-administered rat brain. *Biochem Biophys Res Commun*. 2000;271:654-658.
128. Marsicano G, Goodenough S, Monory K, et al. CB$_1$ cannabinoid receptors and on-demand defense against excitotoxicity. *Science*. 2003;302:84-88.
129. Chen K, Ratzliff A, Hilgenberg L, et al. Long-term plasticity of endocannabinoid signaling induced by developmental febrile seizures. *Neuron*. 2003;39:599-611.
130. Maccarone M, Piccirilli S, Battista N, et al. Enhanced anandamide degradation is associated with neuronal apoptosis induced by the HIV-1 coat glycoprotein gp120 in the rat neocortex. *J Neurochem*. 2004;89:1293-1300.
131. Sánchez C, de Ceballos ML, Gómez del Pulgar T, et al. Inhibition of glioma growth in vivo by selective activation of the CB$_2$ cannabinoid receptor. *Cancer Res*. 2001;61:5784-5789.
132. Burstein SH, Rossetti RG, Yagen B, Zurier RB. Oxidative metabolism of anandamide. *Prostaglandins Other Lipid Mediat*. 2000;61:29-41.
133. de Lago E, Ligresti A, Ortar G, et al. In vivo pharmacological actions of 2 novel inhibitors of anandamide cellular uptake. *Eur J Pharmacol*. 2004;484:249-257.
134. Burstein SH, Huang SM, Petros TJ, Rossetti RG, Walker JM, Zurier RB. Regulation of anandamide tissue levels by *N*-arachidonylglycine. *Biochem Pharmacol*. 2002;64:1147-1150.
135. Cravatt BF, Demarest K, Patricelli MP, et al. Supersensitivity to anandamide and enhanced endocannabinoid signaling in mice lacking fatty acid amide hydrolase. *Proc Natl Acad Sci USA*. 2001;98:9371-9376.
136. Lichtman AH, Shelton CC, Advani T, Cravatt BF. Mice lacking fatty acid amide hydrolase exhibit a cannabinoid receptor-mediated phenotypic hypoalgesia. *Pain*. 2004;109:319-327.
137. Cravatt BF, Saghatelian A, Hawkins EG, Clement AB, Bracey MH, Lichtman AH. Functional disassociation of the central and peripheral fatty acid amide signaling systems. *Proc Natl Acad Sci USA*. 2004;101:10821-10826.
138. Martin BR, Lichtman AH. Cannabinoid transmission and pain perception. *Neurobiol Dis*. 1998;5:447-461.
139. Pertwee RG. Cannabinoid receptors and pain. *Prog Neurobiol*. 2001;63:569-611.
140. Walker JM, Hohman AG. Cannabinoid mechanisms of pain suppression. In: Pertwee RG, ed. *Cannabinoids, Handbook of Experimental Pharmacolology*. Heidelberg, Germany: Springer-Verlag; 2005;168:509-54.
141. Herzberg U, Eliav E, Bennett GJ, Kopin IJ. The analgesic effects of R(+)-WIN 55,212-2 mesylate, a high affinity cannabinoid agonist, in a rat model of neuropathic pain. *Neurosci Lett*. 1997;221:157-160.

142. Edsall SA, Knapp RJ, Vanderah TW, Roeske WR, Consroe P, Yamamura HI. Antisense oligodeoxynucleotide treatment to the brain cannabinoid receptor inhibits antinociception. *Neuroreport.* 1996;7:593-596.
143. Richardson JD, Aanonsen L, Hargreaves KM. Hypoactivity of the spinal cannabinoid system results in NMDA-dependent hyperalgesia. *J Neurosci.* 1998;18:451-457.
144. Dogrul A, Gardell LR, Ma S, Ossipov MH, Porreca F, Lai J. 'Knock-down' of spinal CB$_1$ receptors produces abnormal pain and elevates spinal dynorphin content in mice. *Pain.* 2002;100:203-209.
145. Valverde O, Ledent C, Beslot F, Parmentier M, Roques BP. Reduction of stress-induced analgesia but not of exogenous opioid effects in mice lacking CB$_1$ receptors. *Eur J Neurosci.* 2000;12:533-539.
146. Ibrahim MM, Deng H, Zvonok A, et al. Activation of CB$_2$ cannabinoid receptors by AM1241 inhibits experimental neuropathic pain: pain inhibition by receptors not present in the CNS. *Proc Natl Acad Sci USA.* 2003;100:10529-10533.
147. Ledent C, Valverde O, Cossu G, et al. Unresponsiveness to cannabinoids and reduced addictive effects of opiates in CB$_1$ receptor knockout mice. *Science.* 1999;283:401-404.
148. Zimmer A, Zimmer AM, Hohmann AG, Herkenham M, Bonner TI. Increased mortality, hypoactivity, and hypoalgesia in cannabinoid CB$_1$ receptor knockout mice. *Proc Natl Acad Sci USA.* 1999;96:5780-5785.
149. Hanus L, Breuer A, Tchilibon S, et al. HU-308: a specific agonist for CB$_2$, a peripheral cannabinoid receptor. *Proc Natl Acad Sci USA.* 1999;96:14228-14233.
150. Clayton N, Marshall FH, Bountra C, O'Shaughnessy CT. CB$_1$ and CB$_2$ cannabinoid receptors are implicated in inflammatory pain. *Pain.* 2002;96:253-260.
151. Valenzano KJ, Tafesse L, Lee G, et al. Pharmacological and pharmacokinetic characterization of the cannabinoid receptor 2 agonist, GW405833, utilizing rodent models of acute and chronic pain, anxiety, ataxia and catalepsy. *Neuropharmacology.* 2005;48:658-672.
152. Malan TP, Ibrahim MM, Deng H, et al. CB$_2$ cannabinoid receptor-mediated peripheral antinociception. *Pain.* 2001;93:239-245.
153. Nackley AG, Makriyannis A, Hohmann AG. Selective activation of cannabinoid CB$_2$ receptors suppresses spinal Fos protein expression and pain behavior in a rat model of inflammation. *Neuroscience.* 2003;119:747-757.
154. Quartilho A, Mata HP, Ibrahim MM, et al. Inhibition of inflammatory hyperalgesia by activation of peripheral CB$_2$ cannabinoid receptors. *Anesthesiology.* 2003;99:955-960.
155. Hohmann AG, Farthing JN, Zvonok AM, Makriyannis A. Selective activation of cannabinoid CB$_2$ receptors suppresses hyperalgesia evoked by intradermal capsaicin. *J Pharmacol Exp Ther.* 2004;308:446-453.
156. Ibrahim MM, Porreca F, Lai J, et al. CB$_2$ cannabinoid receptor activation produces antinociception by stimulating peripheral release of endogenous opioids. *Proc Natl Acad Sci USA.* 2005;102:3093-3098.
157. Ross RA, Coutts AA, McFarlane SM, et al. Actions of cannabinoid receptor ligands on rat cultured sensory neurones: implications for antinociception. *Neuropharmacology.* 2001;40:221-232.
158. Holt S, Comelli F, Costa B, Fowler CJ. Inhibitors of fatty acid amide hydrolase reduce carrageenan induced hind paw inflammation in pentobarbital-treated mice: comparison with indomethacin and possible involvement of cannabinoid receptors. *Br J Pharmacol.* 2005;146:467-476.
159. Calignano A, La Rana G, Giuffrida A, Piomelli D. Control of pain initiation by endogenous cannabinoids. *Nature.* 1998;394:277-281.
160. Beaulieu P, Bisogno T, Punwar S, et al. Role of the endogenous cannabinoid system in the formalin test of persistent pain in the rat. *Eur J Pharmacol.* 2000;396:85-92.
161. Notcutt W, Price M, Miller R, et al. Initial experiences with medicinal extracts of cannabis for chronic pain: results from 34 'N of 1' studies. *Anaesthesia.* 2004;59:440-452.
162. Noyes R, Brunk SF, Baram DA, Canter A. Analgesic effect of delta-9-tetrahydrocannabinol. *J Clin Pharmacol.* 1975;15:139-143.

163. Noyes R, Brunk SF, Avery DH, Canter A. Analgesic properties of delta-9-tetrahydrocannabinol and codeine. *Clin Pharmacol Ther*. 1975;18:84-89.
164. Pertwee RG. Cannabinoids and multiple sclerosis. *Pharmacol Ther*. 2002;95:165-174.
165. Wade DT, Robson P, House H, Makela P, Aram J. A preliminary controlled study to determine whether whole-plant cannabis extracts can improve intractable neurogenic symptoms. *Clin Rehabil*. 2003;17:21-29.
166. Zajicek J, Fox P, Sanders H, et al. Cannabinoids for treatment of spasticity and other symptoms related to multiple sclerosis (CAMS study): multicentre randomised placebo-controlled trial. *Lancet*. 2003;362:1517-1526.
167. Gauter B, Rukwied R, Konrad C. Cannabinoid agonists in the treatment of blepharospasm - a case report study. *Neuroendocrinol Lett*. 2004;25:45-48.
168. Brady CM, DasGupta R, Dalton C, Wiseman OJ, Berkley KJ, Fowler CJ. An open-label pilot study of cannabis-based extracts for bladder dysfunction in advanced multiple sclerosis. *Mult Scler*. 2004;10:425-433.
169. Svendsen KB, Jensen TS, Bach FW. Does the cannabinoid dronabinol reduce central pain in multiple sclerosis? Randomized double blind placebo controlled crossover trial. *BMJ*. 2004;329:253-257.
170. Iwamura H, Suzuki H, Ueda Y, Kaya T, Inaba T. In vitro and in vivo pharmacological characterization of JTE-907, a novel selective ligand for cannabinoid CB_2 receptor. *J Pharmacol Exp Ther*. 2001;296:420-425.
171. Lavey BJ, Kozlowski JA, Hipkin RW, et al. Triaryl bis-sulfones as a new class of cannabinoid CB_2 receptor inhibitors: identification of a lead and initial SAR studies. *Bioorg Med Chem Lett*. 2005;15:783-786.
172. Lunn CA. Immune modulation by cannabinoids: targetting the cannabinoid CB_2 receptor. Symposium on cannabinoid receptors: pharmacological opportunities for obesity and inflammation: New York Academy of Sciences, 2004; Available at: http://www.nyas.org/ebriefreps/main.asp?intSubsectionID=1406.
173. Costa B, Colleoni M, Trovato AE, Comelli F, Franke C, Giognoni G. Anandamide transport and hydrolysis as targets for the treatment of neuropathic pain: Effects of AM404 and URB597 in rats with chronic constriction injury of the sciatic nerve. 2005 Symposium on the Cannabinoids; June 24-27; Clearwater Beach, FL. Burlington, VT: International Cannabinoid Research Society.; 2005:33.
174. Mestre L, Correa F, Arévalo-Martin A, et al. Pharmacological modulation of the endocannabinoid system in a viral model of multiple sclerosis. *J Neurochem*. 2005;92:1327-1339.
175. Pryce G, Ahmed Z, Hankey DJR, et al. Cannabinoids inhibit neurodegeneration in models of multiple sclerosis. *Brain*. 2003;126:2191-2202.
176. Baker D, Pryce G, Croxford JL, et al. Cannabinoids control spasticity and tremor in a multiple sclerosis model. *Nature*. 2000;404:84-87.
177. Brooks JW, Pryce G, Bisogno T, et al. Arvanil-induced inhibition of spasticity and persistent pain: evidence for therapeutic sites of action different from the vanilloid VR1 receptor and cannabinoid CB_1/CB_2 receptors. *Eur J Pharmacol*. 2002;439:83-92.
178. Wilkinson JD, Whalley BJ, Baker D, et al. Medicinal cannabis: is Δ^9-tetrahydrocannabinol necessary for all its effects? *J Pharm Pharmacol*. 2003;55:1687-1694.
179. Lyman WD, Sonett JR, Brosnan CF, Elkin R, Bornstein MB. Δ^9-tetrahydrocannabinol: a novel treatment for experimental autoimmune encephalomyelitis. *J Neuroimmunol*. 1989;23:73-81.
180. Wirguin I, Mechoulam R, Breuer A, Schezen E, Weidenfeld J, Brenner T. Suppression of experimental autoimmune encephalomyelitis by cannabinoids. *Immunopharmacology*. 1994;28:209-214.
181. Croxford JL, Miller SD. Immunoregulation of a viral model of multiple sclerosis using the synthetic cannabinoid $R(+)$WIN55,212. *J Clin Invest*. 2003;111:1231-1240.
182. Arévalo-Martin N, Vela JM, Molina-Holgado E, Borrell J, Guaza C. Therapeutic action of cannabinoids in a murine model of multiple sclerosis. *J Neurosci*. 2003;23:2511-2516.

183. Vaney C, Heinzel-Gutenbrunner M, Jobin P, et al. Efficacy, safety and tolerability of an orally administered cannabis extract in the treatment of spasticity in patients with multiple sclerosis: a randomized, double-blind, placebo-controlled, crossover study. *Mult Scler.* 2004;10:417-424.

184. Wade DT, Makela P, Robson P, House H, Bateman C. Do cannabis-based medicinal extracts have general or specific effects on symptoms in multiple sclerosis? A double-blind, randomized, placebo-controlled study on 160 patients. *Mult Scler.* 2004;10:434-441.

185. Killestein J, Hoogervorst ELJ, Reif M, et al. Safety, tolerability, and efficacy of orally administered cannabinoids in MS. *Neurology.* 2002;58:1404-1407.

186. Bifulco M, Laezza C, Valenti M, Ligresti A, Portella G, Di Marzo V. A new strategy to block tumor growth by inhibiting endocannabinoid inactivation. *FASEB J.* 2004;18: U320-U33.

187. Bifulco M, Laezza C, Portella G, et al. Control by the endogenous cannabinoid system of *ras* oncogene-dependent tumor growth. *FASEB J.* 2001;15:U100-U16.

188. Bifulco M, Di Marzo V. Targeting the endocannabinoid system in cancer therapy: a call for further research. *Nat Med.* 2002;8:547-550.

189. Portella G, Laezza C, Laccetti P, De Petrocellis L, Di Marzo V, Bifulco M. Inhibitory effects of cannabinoid CB_1 receptor stimulation on tumor growth and metastatic spreading: actions on signals involved in angiogenesis and metastasis. *FASEB J.* 2003;17:U458-U74.

190. Guzmán M. Cannabinoids: potential anticancer agents. *Nat Rev Cancer.* 2003;3:745-755.

191. Guzmán M. Effects on cell viability In: Pertwee RG, ed. *Cannabinoids, Handbook of Experimental Pharmacolology.* Heidelberg, Germany: Springer-Verlag; 2005;168:627-642.

192. Izzo AA, Coutts AA. Cannabinoids and the digestive tract. In: Pertwee RG, ed. *Cannabinoids, Handbook of Experimental Pharmacolology.* Heidelberg, Germany: Springer-Verlag; 2005;168:573-598.

193. Panikashvili D, Mechoulam R, Beni SM, Alexandrovich A, Shohami E. CB_1 cannabinoid receptors are involved in neuroprotection via NF-κB inhibition. *J Cereb Blood Flow Metab.* 2005;25:477-484.

194. El Banoua F, Caraballo I, Flores JA, Galan-Rodriguez B, Fernandez-Espejo E. Effects on turning of microinjections into basal ganglia of D_1 and D_2 dopamine receptors agonists and the cannabinoid CB_1 antagonist SR141716A in a rat Parkinson's model. *Neurobiol Dis.* 2004;16:377-385.

195. Fernandez-Espejo E, Caraballo I, Rodriguez de Fonseca F, et al. Cannabinoid CB_1 antagonists possess antiparkinsonian efficacy only in rats with very severe nigral lesion in experimental parkinsonism. *Neurobiol Dis.* 2005;18:591-601.

196. Meschler JP, Howlett AC, Madras BK. Cannabinoid receptor agonist and antagonist effects on motor function in normal and 1-methyl-4-phenyl-1,2,5,6- tetrahydropyridine (MPTP)-treated non-human primates. *Psychopharmacology (Berl).* 2001;156:79-85.

197. Wagner JA, Varga K, Ellis EF, Rzigalinski BA, Martin BR, Kunos G. Activation of peripheral CB_1 cannabinoid receptors in haemorrhagic shock. *Nature.* 1997;390:518-521.

198. Kadoi Y, Hinohara H, Kunimoto F, Kuwano H, Saito S, Goto F. Effects of AM281, a cannabinoid antagonist, on systemic haemodynamics, internal carotid artery blood flow and mortality in septic shock in rats. *Br J Anaesth.* 2005;94:563-568.

199. Robson PJ. Human studies of cannabinoids and medicinal cannabis. In: Pertwee RG, ed. *Cannabinoids, Handbook Exp Pharmacol.* Heidelberg, Germany: Springer-Verlag; 2005: 719-756.

200. Robson PJ, Guy GW. Clinical studies of cannabis-based medicines. In: Guy GW, Whittle BA, Robson PJ, eds. *The Medicinal Uses of Cannabis and Cannabinoids.* London, UK: Pharmaceutical Press; 2005:229-269.

201. Consroe P, Musty R, Rein J, Tillery W, Pertwee R. The perceived effects of smoked cannabis on patients with multiple sclerosis. *Eur Neurol.* 1997;38:44-48.

202. Ware MA, Adams H, Guy GW. The medicinal use of cannabis in the UK: results of a nationwide survey. *Int J Clin Pract.* 2005;59:291-295.

203. De Vry J, Denzer D, Reissmueller E, et al. 3-[2-cyano-3-(trifluoromethyl)phenoxy]phenyl-4,4,4-trifluoro-1-butanesulfonate (BAY 59-3074): a novel cannabinoid CB_1 /CB_2 receptor partial agonist with antihyperalgesic and antiallodynic effects. *J Pharmacol Exp Ther.* 2004;310:620-632.
204. Rukwied R, Watkinson A, McGlone F, Dvorak M. Cannabinoid agonists attenuate capsaicin-induced responses in human skin. *Pain.* 2003;102:283-288.
205. Dvorak M, Watkinson A, McGlone F, Rukwied R. Histamine-induced responses are attenuated by a cannabinoid receptor agonist in human skin. *Inflamm Res.* 2003;52:238-245.
206. Cichewicz DL. Synergistic interactions between cannabinoid and opioid analgesics. *Life Sci.* 2004;74:1317-1324.
207. Holdcroft A, Smith M, Jacklin A, et al. Pain relief with oral cannabinoids in familial Mediterranean fever. *Anaesthesia.* 1997;52:483-488.
208. Pertwee RG. The pharmacology and therapeutic potential of cannabidiol. In: Di Marzo V, ed. *Cannabinoids.* New York, NY: Kluwer Academic/Plenum Publishers; 2004:32-83.
209. Mendelson WB, Basile AS. The hypnotic actions of the fatty acid amide, oleamide. *Neuropsychopharmacology.* 2001;25:S36-S39.
210. Pertwee RG, Ross RA. Cannabinoid receptors and their ligands. *Prostaglandins Leukot Essent Fatty Acids.* 2002;66:101-121.
211. Sim-Selley LJ. Regulation of cannabinoid CB_1 receptors in the central nervous system by chronic cannabinoids. *Crit Rev Neurobiol.* 2003;15:91-119.
212. Lichtman AH, Martin BR. Cannabinoid tolerance and dependence. In: Pertwee RG, ed. *Cannabinoids, Handbook of Experimental Pharmacolology.* Heidelberg, Germany: Springer-Verlag; 2005;168:691-717.
213. De Vry J, Jentzsch KR, Kuhl E, Eckel G. Behavioral effects of cannabinoids show differential sensitivity to cannabinoid receptor blockade and tolerance development. *Behav Pharmacol.* 2004;15:1-12.
214. Paria BC, Dey SK. Ligand-receptor signaling with endocannabinoids in preimplantation embryo development and implantation. *Chem Phys Lipids.* 2000;108:211-220.
215. Van Gaal LF, Rissanen AM, Scheen AJ, Ziegler O, Rossner S. Effects of the cannabinoid-1 receptor blocker rimonabant on weight reduction and cardiovascular risk factors in overweight patients: 1-year experience from the RIO-Europe study. *Lancet.* 2005;365:1389-1397.
216. Idris AI. van't Hof RJ, Greig IR, Ridge SA, Baker D, Ross RA, Ralston SH. Regulation of bone mass, bone loss and osteoclast activity by cannabinoid receptors. *Nat Med.* 2005;11:774-779.
217. Brown AJ, Ueno S, Suen K, Dowell SJ, Wise A. Molecular identification of GPR55 as a third G protein-coupled receptor responsive to cannabinoid ligands. Symposium on the Cannabinoids; June 24-27; Clearwater Beach, FL. Burlington, VT: International Cannabinoid Research Society; 2005:16.
218. Sjögren S, Ryberg E, Lindblom A, et al. A new receptor for cannabinoid ligands Symposium on the Cannabinoids; June 24-27; Clearwater Beach, FL. Burlington, VT: International Cannabinoid Research Society; 2005:106.
219. Hohmann AG, Suplita RL, Bolton NM, et al. An endocannabinoid mechanism for stress-induced analgesia. *Nature.* 2005;435:1108-1112.

Chapter 39
Further Advances in the Synthesis of Endocannabinoid-Related Ligands

Anu Mahadevan[1] and Raj K. Razdan[1]

Abstract Recent advances in the synthesis of endocannabinoid-related ligands for the period 2001–2004 are covered in this review. During this period the first solid phase synthesis of anandamide (AEA) analogs was developed, which allows modification at both the head group and the end pentyl chain. Synthesis of water-soluble prodrugs of noladin ether was reported, which are chemically stable, rapidly release noladin ether under enzymatic conditions and are shown to reduce intraocular pressure. The structure-activity relationships (SAR) of alkylcarbamic acid aryl esters and the discovery of potent archidonylsulfonyl derivatives as fatty acid amide hydrolase (FAAH) inhibitors are summarized. Recent synthetic developments in the controversial area of anandamide membrane transporter (AMT) inhibitors are also discussed.

Keywords endocannabinoids, synthesis, structure-activity relationship.

Introduction

The past decade has seen a sudden spurt of interest in the cannabinoid field.[1-5] Two types of cannabinoid receptors have been discovered: the CB1 receptor located both inside and outside the central nervous system (CNS), and the CB2 receptor located mainly in the periphery.[6,7] The CB1 receptor has been established to be a G-protein-coupled receptor. The first potent CB1 receptor antagonist SR141716A was reported by Rinaldi-Carmona et al,[8] who also reported the CB2 selective receptor antagonist SR144522.[8,9] Anandamide (AEA) was identified as the endogenous ligand for the CB1 receptor. Another important endogenous ligand is 2-arachidonyl-glycerol (2-Ara-Gl), which activates both CB1 and CB2 receptors. Both AEA and

---

[1] Organix, Inc, Woburn, MA 01801

Corresponding Author: Anu Mahadevan, Organix, Inc, 240 Salem Street, Woburn, MA 01801. Tel: (781) 932-4142; Fax: (781) 933-6695; E-mail: mahadevan@organixinc.com

2-Ara-Gl are found together with a family of related fatty acid glycerol esters and fatty acyl ethanolamides. It was found that the potency of 2-Ara-Gl was enhanced in the presence of the related 2-acyl-glycerols. This effect has been termed the "entourage effect," which probably represents the pathway for molecular regulation of endogenous cannabinoid activity.[10] Hanus et al[11] isolated yet another endogenous ligand "noladin ether" (2-arachidonylglyceryl ether) from porcine brain.[11] It binds to CB1 receptors and very weakly to CB2 receptors. During this review period 2 other endocannabinoids, virodhamine and N-arachidonyl dopamine, were discovered.[12,13] Virodhamine was found to be a CB1 receptor antagonist and partial agonist of CB2 receptor and N-arachidonyl dopamine was CB1 selective and also active at vanilloid VR1 receptors. The pharmacological activities of Δ^9-tetrahydrocannabinol (Δ^9-THC) and the endogenous ligand AEA are alike, however the onset of action of AEA is much faster and the duration of action is much shorter compared with Δ^9-THC. This has been attributed to the enzymatic hydrolysis of the amide bond in AEA; the enzyme involved in the metabolic degradation of AEA has been characterized as "fatty acid amide hydrolase" (FAAH). Several metabolically stable analogs of AEA have been synthesized that have greater binding affinities than AEA.[14,15] Makriyannis and coworkers[15] have improved the metabolic stability of the AEA part by incorporation of the methanandamide head group; our group has enhanced the metabolic stability by introduction of substituents on the carbon in the 2-position of the arachidonic acid part of AEA. AEA is produced from phospholipid precursors and it has been proposed that for its termination AEA is carried into the neurons by the anandamide membrane transporter (AMT) and then undergoes enzymatic hydrolysis into AEA and ethanolamine. The synthetic approaches to ligands that are associated with the endocannabinoid system, eg, AEA, 2-Ara-Gl, noladin ether, FAAH and AMT, have been discussed in detail in our previous review.[16] In this article we will be covering the chemistry and SAR, which have been developed subsequently in the above-mentioned areas.

AEA and 2-Ara-Gl Analogs

The structures of AEA and 2-Ara-Gl are shown in Fig. 39.1. The ethanol amine group is described as the head group moiety **a**; the arachidonyl backbone is moiety **b**; and the end pentyl chain is moiety **c**. During this period, no new chemistry was

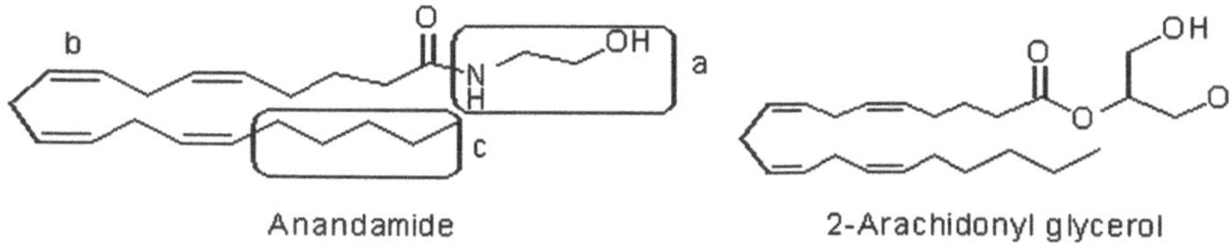

Anandamide   2-Arachidonyl glycerol

Fig. 39.1 Structures of AEA and 2-Ara-Gl.

described related to either the head group (moiety **a**) or the arachidonyl backbone (moiety **b**). Only a new route was described for the introduction of different substituents in moiety **c**.

Altundas et al[17] described a flexible route to the synthesis of AEA analogs with modifications in the end pentyl chain, which is moiety **c**. The key step in the strategy involves copper-catalyzed coupling of the bromo intermediate **1** (Fig. 39.2) with the appropriate acetylenic derivatives. The target amides in the AEA series were synthesized by hydrolysis of the esters **2a-d** (Fig. 39.2) to the acids using LiOH, followed by their conversion to the corresponding acid chloride and coupling with (R)-2-aminopropanol. Alternatively, the target amides in this series were also synthesized by the mixed anhydride procedure. The SAR studies of these compounds have not yet been published.

An important development is the report by Qi et al[18] on the first solid phase synthesis of AEA analogs. The synthetic route (Fig. 39.3) is very versatile and it involves attachment of 5-hexynoic acid to Wang resin via an ester linkage followed by repetitive copper-catalyzed coupling with propargylic alcohols to provide the tetrayne skeleton. Cleavage of the tetrayne was accomplished by treatment with TFA or AlMe$_3$/amine to furnish the corresponding acids and amides, respectively, which was then reduced with P-2 Ni as the catalyst to furnish the desired products. Advantages of this procedure are that it allows modifications at both the head group moiety **a** and the end pentyl chain moiety **c** and thus allows for the effective synthesis and SAR of several modified AEA analogs.

To examine the SAR in the arachidonyl alcohol series, Parkkari et al[19] synthesized several ester, carbonate, and carbamate derivatives of arachidonyl alcohol. The major hurdle that they encountered in the synthesis of archidonyl alcohol esters was its self-degradation and polymerization. In general, the synthesis of these

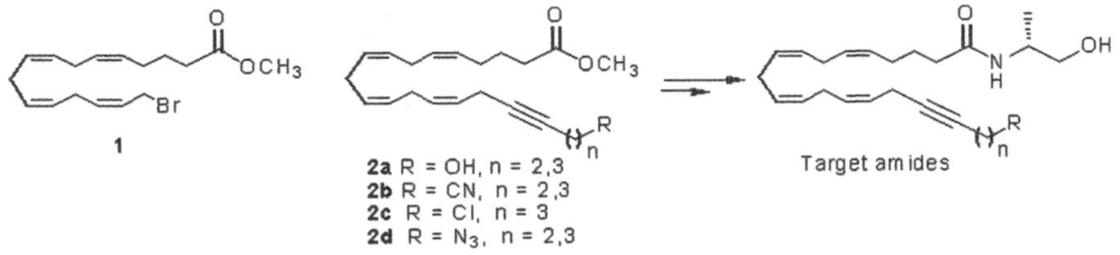

2a R = OH, n = 2,3
2b R = CN, n = 2,3
2c R = Cl, n = 3
2d R = N$_3$, n = 2,3

Target amides

Fig. 39.2 AEA analogs with modifications in the end pentyl chain.

R = alkyl, hydroxy alkyl
X = OH, NHR, N RR'

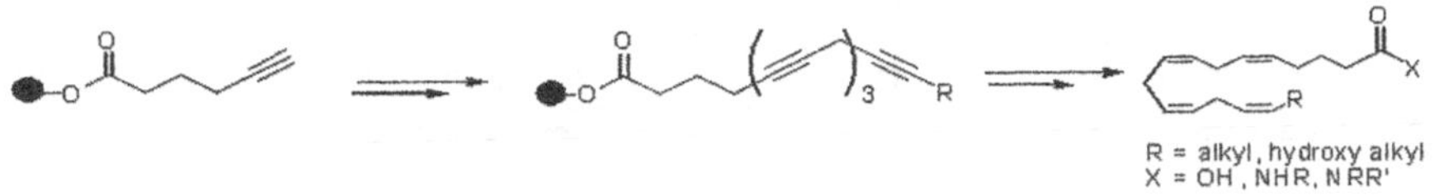

Fig. 39.3 Solid phase synthesis of AEA analogs.

analogs was accomplished by dicyclohexylcarbodiimide (DCC) coupling of the appropriate acid partners with arachidonyl alcohol. The silyl protecting groups, which were used to protect the alcohols, were deprotected using tetrabutyl ammonium fluoride (TBAF) in tetrahydrofuran (THF). The carbonates and the carbamates were synthesized via p-nitro-phenylchloroformate-activated intermediates as shown in Fig. 39.4. The results obtained from their SAR study indicate that among the different analogs that were tested only the ester analogs **3a** and **3b** (Fig. 39.4) showed some activity at the CB1 receptor, however even these compounds were found to be less potent and efficacious when compared with AEA.

Fangour et al[20] synthesized analogs based on 2-Ara-Gl and AEA template (Fig. 39.5) where one hydroxymethylene group of the glycerol moiety was replaced

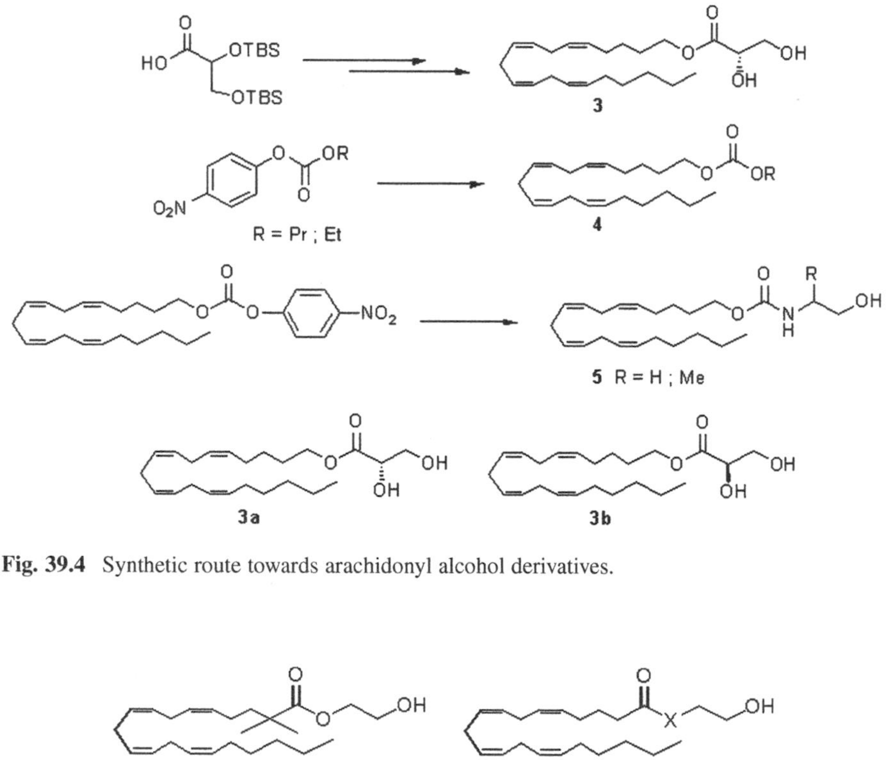

Fig. 39.4 Synthetic route towards arachidonyl alcohol derivatives.

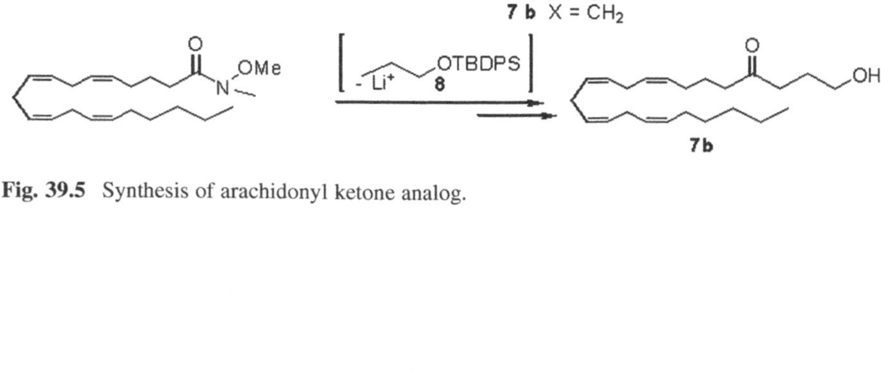

Fig. 39.5 Synthesis of arachidonyl ketone analog.

with hydrogen to give compound **7a**. The stability of the ester analog was improved by introduction of substituents on the carbon in the 2-position of the arachidonic acid part to give compound **6**. They also prepared the methylene-linked analog of AEA compound **7b** where the amide bond of AEA was replaced by a ketone functionality. The synthesis of the ketone analog **7b** was accomplished by treatment of Weinreb amide of arachidonic acid with the lithiated anion **8** to give the compound in an overall 27% yield. The analogs **6** and **7a** were prepared by standard procedures.[14] The affinity of these compounds for the CB1 receptor was investigated and it was found that the ketone analog **7b** showed moderate binding affinity (binding affinity [K_i] = 360 nM) to CB1 receptor, while the other two compounds **6** and **7a** were found to be inactive.

Noladin Ether

To increase the metabolic stability of 2-Ara-Gl, Mechoulam's group[14] synthesized noladin ether and it was later isolated from porcine brain as an endogenous cannabinoid ligand. To improve the aqueous solubility properties of these lipophilic compounds, Juntunen et al[21] synthesized water-soluble prodrugs of noladin ether. Monophosphate and diphosphate esters of noladin ether **9** and **10** (Fig. 39.6) were synthesized by treatment of noladin ether with dimethylchloro phosphate in the presence of pyridine as base. Juntunen et al found that both compounds **9** and **10** showed good chemical stability in buffer solutions at pH 7.4 and were also more soluble in aqueous solutions (>40 000-fold) when compared with noladin ether. These compounds rapidly converted into noladin ether under enzymatic hydrolysis conditions and the monophosphate ester **9** was able to reduce intraocular pressure in normotensive rabbits.

FAAH Inhibitors

A detailed discussion of the synthetic approaches and SAR of various classes of FAAH inhibitors can be found in our previous review.[16] Since then, the synthesis and SAR of alkylcarbamic acid aryl esters as FAAH inhibitors has been reported

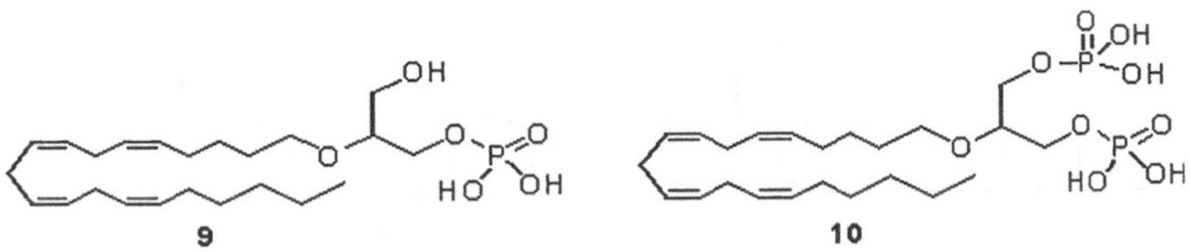

Fig. 39.6 Phosphate esters of noladin ether.

by Tarzia et al[22] and Mor et al.[23] One of the potent analogs, URB524, displayed profound anxiolytic-like properties in rats. The design of the alkylcarbamic acid aryl esters were based on the structural modifications of the known inhibitor of serine hydrolase acetylcholine esterase compound **11** (Fig. 39.7). In general these compounds were synthesized by addition of the appropriate alcohols or amines to isocyanatocyclohexane in the presence of triethyl amine as base. A brief summary of the SAR of this class of inhibitors is given below.

1. Replacement of the methyl group in **12** with the cyclohexyl group gave compound **13**, which showed a 60-fold improvement in inhibitor potency.
2. Modification of the carbamate function was found to be detrimental to its FAAH inhibitory activity. Ester and urea analogs were found to be inactive and replacement of the oxygen with sulfur to give the thiocarbamic acid derivatives was also found to be inactive.
3. Based on conformational analysis, Tarzia et al hypothesized that the shape of the aromatic substituent on the oxygen atom might be critical. Hence, they synthesized a series of analogs with different aromatic substituents in which they tried to mimic the "U-shaped" conformation of the fatty acid chain of AEA. The best inhibitor in this series was found to be URB524 (Inhibitor Potencies [IC_{50}] = 63 nM).
4. Modifications in which the aromatic substituents were replaced by alkyl chains were also found to be detrimental to the activity. Reversing the groups on the N- and O-substituents of URB524 gave compound **14,** which was found to be an inactive compound.
5. SAR was then conducted based on the structural template of URB524. The most potent compound in the series was URB597 (IC_{50} = 4.6 nM), which has a

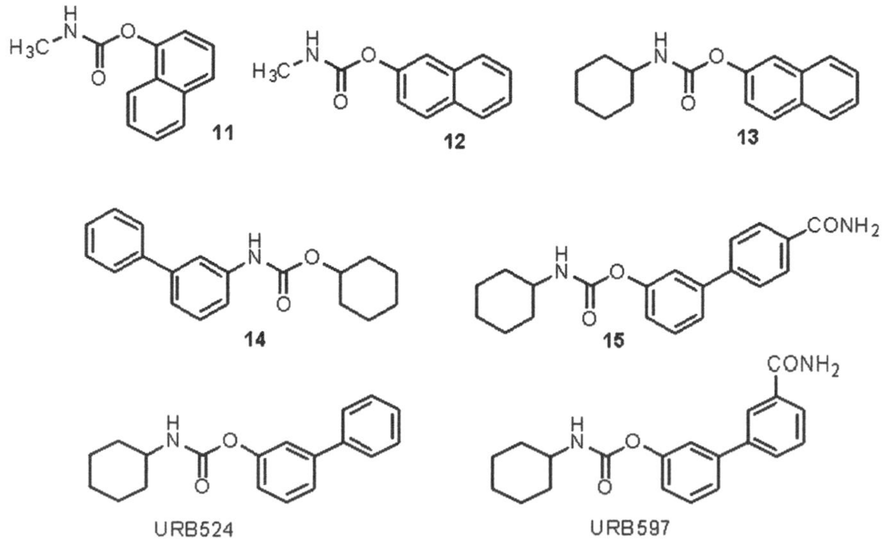

Fig. 39.7 Structures of Alkylcarbamic acid aryl esters.

substituent in the meta position of the distal phenyl ring. The meta-substituted compounds were in general found to be more active than the corresponding para isomers, for example compound **15** has an $IC_{50} = 5909\,nM$.

Arachidonylsulfonyl derivatives **16** and **17** (Fig. 39.8) were reported by Segall et al[24] as novel inhibitors of FAAH with the potency of **16** being similar to methyl arachidonyl-fluorophosphonate. The synthesis involves conversion of arachidonyl bromide into arachidonylsulfonyl chloride via Grignard reaction. Subsequent treatment of arachidonylsulfonyl chloride with tetrabutylammonium fluoride and ethanolamine provided compounds **16** and **17** respectively.

AMT Transporter Inhibitors

A comprehensive review of AMT inhibitors and their potential as drugs for CNS-related disorders was recently reported by Lopez-Rodriguez and Ortega-Gutierrez.[25] However, the AMT protein has not been isolated or cloned and the whole issue of AMT has since become controversial. Nevertheless, Di Marzo et al[26] synthesized a series of AMT transporter inhibitors based on arachidonyl **18b** and oleoyl templates **18a** (Fig. 39.9) where the head group moiety **a** contains different aromatic moieties.

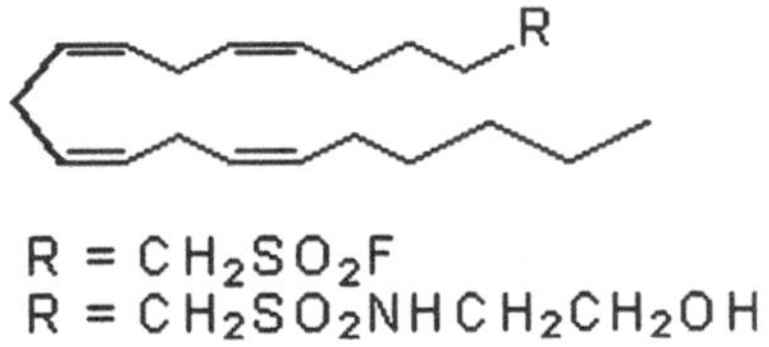
R
16 R = CH2SO2F
17 R = CH2SO2NHCH2CH2OH

Fig. 39.8 Structures of Arachidonylsulfonyl derivatives.

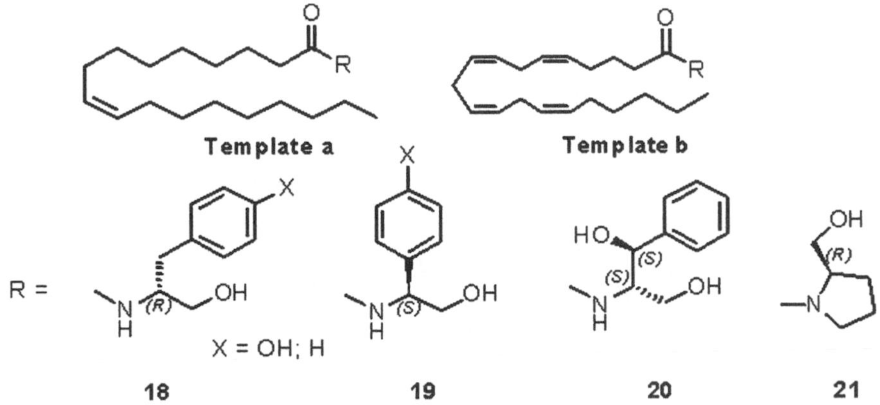
Template a
Template b
R =
X = OH; H
18
19
20
21

Fig. 39.9 AMT transporter inhibitors.

Their design is based on the observation that AMT transporter inhibitors, which have been designed to date, all contain aromatic moieties in the polar head group region. In general, the synthesis of these compounds has been accomplished by N-ethyl-N'-(3-dimethylamino propyl) carbodiimide (EDCI) coupling of the appropriate acids and amines to yield the desired products in good yields. The results obtained from their SAR study are summarized below.

1. Comparison of the arachidonyl template **b** and oleoyl template **a** show that the most potent and selective inhibitors in this series (**19a**, X=H K_i = 12.9 μM; **20a** K_i = 6.4 μM) have the oleoyl template.
2. Deletion of the phenolic hydroxyl from compounds **18a** and **18b** (for **18a** X = OH, K_i = 3.0 μM vs X = H, K_i = 11.1 μM) results in a decrease in the affinity for AMT. An opposite effect is seen in the compounds with general structure **19**. In the series of compounds with general structure **20** the (S,S)-diasteromer of oleic acid series shows an appreciable increase in activity with introduction of the hydroxyl group, however the trend is reversed in the arachidonic acid series where the (R,R)-diastereomer shows increase in activity.
3. Next, the restriction of the hydroxyalkyl group was investigated and it was observed that the conformationally restricted analogs **21** (both R and S) were found to be completely inactive.

Lopez-Rodriguez et al[27] synthesized a series of esters and amides with the general structural template **22** (Fig. 39.10) and explored the structure-affinity relationship between **22** and AMT. The compounds were synthesized from arachidonic acid by conversion to the acid chloride and coupling with the appropriate amine or alcohol or by direct DCC coupling of arachidonic acid with the appropriate amine or

X = CO, CH₂; Y = NH, NR, O, S; Z = N-CH₃, O, S; R₁ = H, CH₃; n = 0, 1.

23
AMT   inactive
FAAH IC_{50} = 12 μM

24
AMT IC_{50} = 0.8 μM
FAAH IC_{50} = 30 μM

25
AMT IC_{50} = 5 μM
FAAH IC_{50} = 34 μM

26
AMT IC_{50} = 21 μM
FAAH IC_{50} = 36 μM

27
AMT IC_{50} = 26 μM
FAAH IC_{50} = 28 μM

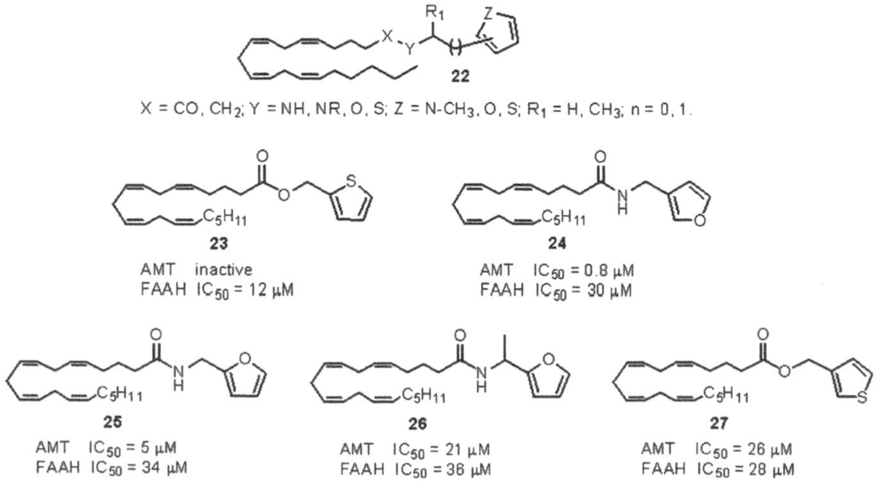

Fig. 39.10 Further examples of AMT inhibitors.

alcohol. From the results obtained, they concluded that there is no correlation between the effects on FAAH and on AMT. Compound **23** is a more potent FAAH inhibitor than compound **24**, however it is found to be inactive as an AMT inhibitor. Compounds **24 to 27** display similar FAAH inhibitory potencies, but differ in their ability to inhibit anandamide uptake (IC_{50} range from 0.8 to 26 µM). The most potent AMT inhibitor in this series is compound **24,** which is selective (CB1 K_i = 4700 nM; CB2 K_i = 67 nM; VR1 K_i > 5000 nM) except for moderate binding affinity to the CB2 receptor.

Conclusions

Since the discovery of the first endocannabinoids, anandamide and 2-arachidonyl glycerol, other endocannabinoids have been discovered, the pathway to their biosynthesis and degradation has been elucidated, and, as a result, the role of endocannabinoids in the brain has been firmly established. Progress is being made in understanding the full implications of their presence in the brain and the periphery, which may lead to the development of novel therapies in medicine.

References

1. Di Marzo V. *Cannabinoids*. New York: Plenum Publishers; 2004.
2. Di Marzo V, Bisogno T, De Petrocellis L, Melck D, Martin BR. Cannabimimetic fatty acid derivatives: the anandamide family and other "endocannabinoids." *Curr Med Chem.* 1999;6:721-744.
3. Pertwee RG, ed. *Cannabinoid Receptors*. London, UK: Academic Press Ltd; 1995.
4. Pertwee RG. Pharmacology of cannabinoid CB_1 and CB_2 receptors. *Pharmacol Ther.* 1997;74:129-180.
5. Pertwee RG. Pharmacology of cannabinoid receptor ligands. *Curr Med Chem.* 1999;6:635-664.
6. Devane WA, III, Dysarz FA, III, Johnson MR, Melvin LS, Howlett AC. Determination and characterization of a cannabinoid receptor in rat brain. *Mol Pharmacol.* 1988;34:605-613.
7. Munro S, Thomas KL, Abu-Shaar M. Molecular characterization of a peripheral receptor for cannabinoids. *Nature.* 1993;365:61-65.
8. Rinaldi-Carmona M, Barth F, Heaulme M, et al. SR141716A, a potent and selective antagonist of the brain cannabinoid receptor. *FEBS Lett.* 1994;350:240-244.
9. Rinaldi-Carmona M, Barth F, Millan J, et al. SR 144528, the first potent and selective antagonist of the CB2 cannabinoid receptor. *J Pharmacol Exp Ther.* 1998;284:644-650.
10. Martin BR, Mechoulam R, Razdan RK. Discovery and characterization of endogenous cannabinoids. *Life Sci.* 1999;65:573-595.
11. Hanus L, Abu-Lafi S, Fride E, et al. 2-Arachidonylglyceryl ether, an endogenous agonist of the cannabinoid CB1 receptor. *Proc Natl Acad Sci USA.* 2001;98:3662-3665.
12. Porter AC, Sauer JM, Knierman MD, et al. Characterization of a novel endocannabinoid, virodhamine, with antagonist activity at the CB1 receptor. *J Pharmacol Exp Ther.* 2002;301:1020-1024.

13. Huang SM, Bisogno T, Trevisani M. An endogenous capsaicin-like substance with high potency at recombinant and native vanilloid VR1 receptors. *Proc Natl Acad Sci USA.* 2002;99:8400-8405.
14. Sheskin T, Hanus L, Slager J, Vogel Z, Mechoulam R. Structural requirements for binding of anandamide type compounds to the brain cannabinoid receptor. *J Med Chem.* 1997;40:659-667.
15. Khanolkar AD, Makriyannis A. Structure-activity relationships of anandamide, an endogenous cannabinoid ligand. *Life Sci.* 1999;65:607-616.
16. Razdan RK, Mahadevan A. Recent advances in the synthesis of endocannabinoid related ligands. *Chem Phys Lipids.* 2002;121:21-33.
17. Altundas R, Mahadevan A, Razdan RK. A synthetic route to anandamide analogues carrying a substituent at the terminal carbon and an acetylene group in the end pentyl chain. *Tetrahedron Lett.* 2004;45:5449-5451.
18. Qi L, Meijler MM, Lee S-H, Sun C, Janda KD. Solid-phase synthesis of anandamide analogues. *Org Lett.* 2004;6:1673-1675.
19. Parkkari T, Savinainen JR, Rauhala AL, et al. Synthesis and CB1 receptor activities of novel arachidonyl alcohol derivatives. *Bioorg Med Chem Lett.* 2004;14:3231-3234.
20. Fangour SE, Balas L, Rossi J-C, et al. Hemisynthesis and preliminary evaluation of novel endocannabinoid analogues. *Bioorg Med Chem Lett.* 2003;13:1977-1980.
21. Juntunen J, Vepsalainen J, Niemi R, Laine K, Jarvinen T. Synthesis, in vitro evaluation, and intraocular pressure effects of water-soluble prodrugs of endocannabinoid noladin ether. *J Med Chem.* 2003;46:5083-5086.
22. Tarzia G, Duranti A, Tontini A, et al. Design, synthesis, and structure-activity relationships of alkylcarbamic acid aryl esters, a new class of fatty acid amide hydrolase inhibitors. *J Med Chem.* 2003;46:2352-2360.
23. Mor M, Rivara S, Lodola A, et al. Cyclohexylcarbamic acid 3'- or 4'-substituted biphenyl-3-yl esters as fatty acid amide hydrolase inhibitors: synthesis, quantitative structure-activity relationships, and molecular modeling studies. *J Med Chem.* 2004;47:4998-5008.
24. Segall Y, Quistad GB, Nomura DK, Casida JE. Arachidonylsulfonyl derivatives as cannabinoid CB1 receptor and fatty acid amide hydrolase inhibitors. *Bioorg Med Chem Lett.* 2003;13:3301-3303.
25. Lopez-Rodriguez ML, Ortega-Gutierrez S. The anandamide degradation system as potential targets for the treatment of central nervous system related disorders. *Curr Med Chem Cent Nerv Syst Agents.* 2004;4:155-160.
26. Di Marzo V, Ligresti A, Morera E, Nalli M, Ortar G. The anandamide membrane transporter. Structure-activity relationships of anadamide and oleoylethanolamine analogs with phenyl rings in the polar head group region. *Bioorg Med Chem.* 2004;12:5161-5169.
27. Lopez-Rodriguez ML, Viso A, Ortega-Gutierrez S, et al. Design, synthesis, and biological evaluation of new inhibitors of the endocannabinoid uptake: comparison with effects on fatty acid amidohydrolase. *J Med Chem.* 2003;46:1512-1522.

Chapter 40
Ajulemic Acid (IP-751): Synthesis, Proof of Principle, Toxicity Studies, and Clinical Trials

Sumner Burstein[1]

Abstract Ajulemic acid (CT-3, IP-751, 1',1'-dimethylheptyl-Δ^8-tetrahydrocannabinol-11-oic acid) (AJA) has a cannabinoid-derived structure; however, there is no evidence that it produces psychotropic actions when given at therapeutic doses. In a variety of animal assays, AJA shows efficacy in models for pain and inflammation. Furthermore, in the rat adjuvant arthritis model, it displayed a remarkable action in preventing the destruction of inflamed joints. A phase-2 human trial with chronic, neuropathic pain patients suggested that AJA could become a useful drug for treating this condition. Its low toxicity, particularly its lack of ulcerogenicity, further suggests that it will have a highly favorable therapeutic index and may replace some of the current anti-inflammatory/analgesic medications. Studies to date indicate a unique mechanism of action for AJA that may explain its lack of adverse side effects.

Keywords ajulemic acid, analgesia, anti-inflammatory, cannabinoid, IP-751

Background

A long-standing goal both in university and industrial laboratories has been to design a cannabinoid-derived drug that would show analgesic efficacy and have a low potential for abuse. The efforts were rationalized in large measure by the long history of the use of *Cannabis* preparations for the treatment of pain, inflammation, and a host of other medical needs. Literally hundreds of compounds have been synthesized and tested; however, few have reached the stage of human testing, and only one, nabilone, is currently used albeit in limited applications. Tetrahydrocannabinol (THC), the principal psychoactive component of *Cannabis*, is available as an oral

[1] Department of Biochemistry and Molecular Pharmacology, University of Massachusetts Medical School, 364 Plantation Street, Worcester, MA 01605

Corresponding Author: Sumner Burstein, Department of Biochemistry and Molecular Pharmacology, University of Massachusetts Medical School, 364 Plantation Street, Worcester, MA 01605. Tel: (508) 856-2850; Fax: (508) 856-2003; E-mail: sumner.burstein@umassmed.edu

R.S. Rapaka and W. Sadée (eds.), *Drug Addiction.*
© American Association of Pharmaceutical Scientists 2008

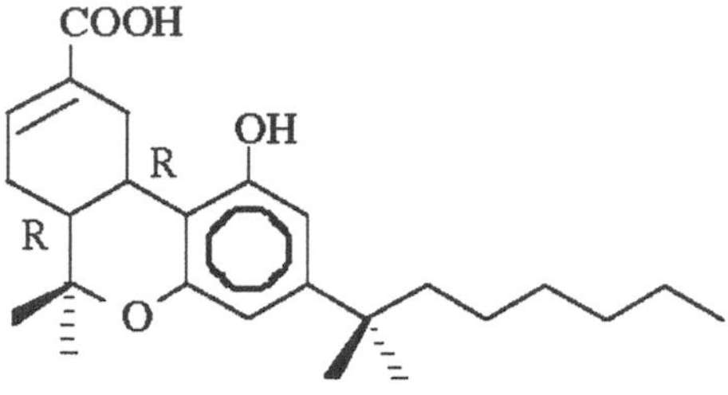

Fig. 40.1 Structure and physical properties. Ajulemic acid, $C_{25}H_{36}O_4$, is a white crystalline solid (molecular weight 400.55, melting point 96°C to 99°C) that is soluble in most organic solvents except hexane and is soluble in aqueous buffers above pH 8. It is also known as IP-751, CT-3, and 1', 1'-dimethylheptyl-Δ^8-tetrahydrocannabinol-11-oic acid.

medication (Marinol) for use as an anti-emetic and as an appetite stimulant for AIDS patients. However, its potential for abuse has discouraged its acceptance and use by physicians for a wider range of therapeutic applications. GW Pharmaceuticals has announced that mixtures of THC and cannabidiol (CBD) are currently awaiting approval in the United Kingdom and Canada for use in relieving pain and spasticity in patients with multiple sclerosis.

Ajulemic acid (AJA), which has a cannabinoid-derived structure (Fig. 40.1), is being developed to achieve the goal of providing a synthetic *Cannabis*-derived drug that will have a low potential for abuse.[1-4] The rationale used in designing the structure of AJA was based on several reports in the scientific literature relating to the metabolic transformations of THC.[5-9] As early as 1972, it was reported that a major route of metabolism for THC involves its stepwise oxidation to a series of carboxylic acid derivatives.[7] Unlike THC, the acids showed little activity in several studies of psychotropic responses in both animal models and in humans.[10] Thus, it was concluded that the acid metabolites are "inactive," and further studies of their potential pharmacological properties were not initiated.

This perception has changed following a series of reports showing that the acids do possess biological actions and that these could be exploited for therapeutic applications.[5,11-14] An advantage of cannabinoids as a class of drugs is their relative safety, especially when compared with analgesics such as the opiates and other narcotics. A downside of the acid metabolites is their low potency in the animal models; however, this deficiency has been successfully resolved with the discovery of AJA.[15] The recent completion of 2 studies in humans confirmed AJA's low abuse potential over the expected range of therapeutic doses.[16]

Manufacturing

Stereospecific syntheses of THC and its analogs follow a general scheme, and this has been applied to the production of AJA (Scheme 40.1). In this procedure an alkylated resorcinol is condensed with an appropriate, chirally pure, terpene such

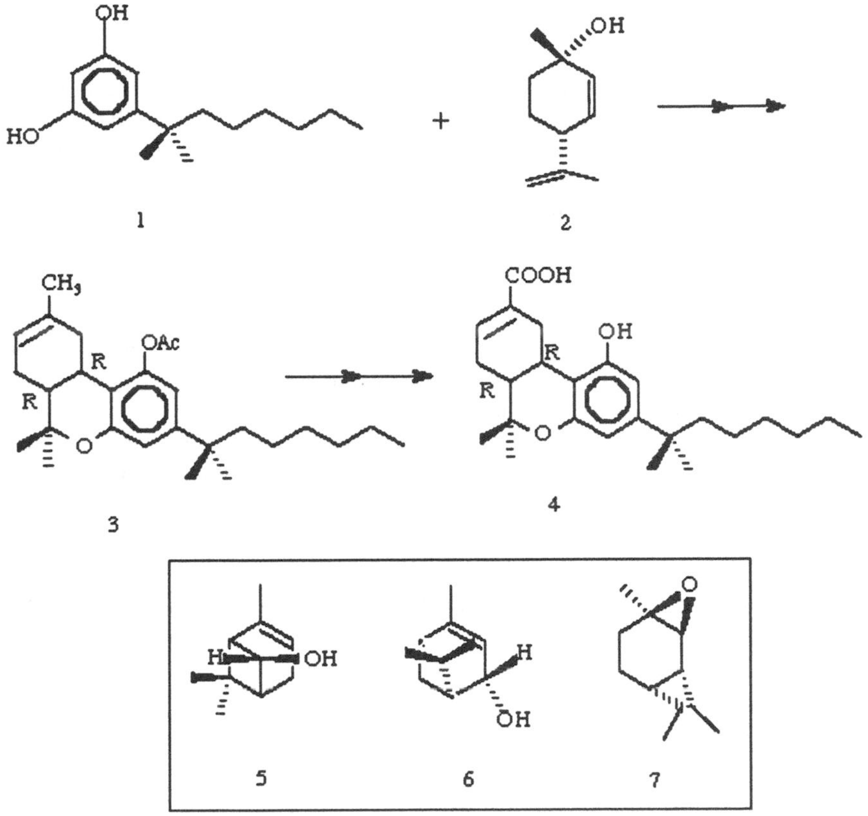

Scheme 40.1

as (+)-p-mentha-2,8-diene-1-ol (2), cis-chrysanthenol (5), cis-verbinol (6), or (+)-trans-2-carene oxide (7). The substituted resorcinol portion of the molecule is made by the reaction of 1,6-dimethoxyphenol with 1,1-dimethylheptanol in the presence of methane sulfonic acid. The product is then esterified with diethyl phosphite and triethylamine with cooling to yield the diethyl phosphate derivative. Reduction with lithium in liquid ammonia produces 1-(1',1'-dimethylheptyl) 3,5-dimethoxybenzene (1) that is used in the next step. This involves a condensation of the p-mentha-2,8-diene-1-ol (2) shown in Scheme 40.1 with dimethylheptyl resorcinol (1) catalyzed by p-toluenesulfonic acid to give the dimethylheptyl analog of Δ^8 — THC. Following conversion of the cannabinoid to the acetate (3), the allylic methyl group is oxidized to an aldehyde using selenium dioxide. Further oxidation to a carboxylic acid is accomplished by the use of sodium chlorite. Finally, free AJA (4) is obtained by saponification of the acetyl group with sodium carbonate in aqueous methanol.

Preclinical Studies

Significant progress in defining a mechanism of action for AJA has been made. On the one hand, modest binding to the known cannabinoid receptors, CB1 and CB2 has been reported,[17,18] and effects by receptor specific antagonists as well as stereo-specificity has been observed[15,19] suggesting a possible role for these receptors in the actions of AJA. On the other hand, the fact that AJA does not produce psycho-activity,[16] a process that is believed to require the activation of CB1, appears to be a contradiction. A possible explanation is that AJA, in addition to activating the receptor, selectively antagonizes a downstream event that is required for psycho-tropic activity but is not needed for anti-inflammatory actions. In general, the lack of data on the molecular events leading to cannabinoid-induced psychoactivity makes questionable any speculations on this subject.

Data have been obtained on several biochemical effects of AJA that may have relevance for its anti-inflammatory actions. Cannabinoid receptor binding in intact cell models causes the release of free arachidonic acid suggesting the activation of one or more phospholipases.[20] Recent findings show that AJA can likewise stimulate the release of arachidonic acid in human fibroblast-like synovial (FLS) cells.[21] The available data suggest complex effects by AJA on COX-2 activity,[22] and the expression levels of COX-2 mRNA.[21] All of these effects seem to depend very much on the model studied and the conditions of the experiment. AJA also inhibits 5-lipoxygenase (D. Morgan, unpublished data, February 22, 1993) but not COX-1[22] in agreement with its lack of ulcerogenicity[23] and its inability to prevent platelet aggregation.[24] Effects on specific cytokine levels and on the activation of nuclear factor-κB (NF-κB) have also been observed,[25] and it was reported that AJA binds directly and specifically to peroxisome proliferator-activated receptor-γ (PPAR-γ),[26] a pharmacologically important member of the nuclear receptor super family. Functional assays indicated that AJA initiates the transcriptional activity of both human and mouse PPAR-γ at pharmacological concentrations. Activation of PPAR-γ by AJA requires the AF-2 helix of the receptor, suggesting that AJA activates PPAR-γ through its ligand-dependent AF-2 region. Consistent with this, AJA binding enables PPAR-γ to recruit nuclear receptor coactivators. It was also found that AJA inhibits interleukin-8 promoter activity in a PPAR-γ-dependent manner, suggesting a link between the anti-inflammatory action of AJA and the activation of PPAR-γ. Finally, it was found that AJA treatment induces differentiation of 3T3 L1 fibroblasts into adipocytes, a process that is known to be mediated by PPAR-γ. Together, these data indicate that PPAR-γ is a molecular target for AJA under certain conditions, thus providing a possible mechanism for the anti-inflammatory activity of AJA, and perhaps other cannabinoid acids as well. These studies also suggest several possible additional therapeutic actions for AJA through the activation of PPAR-γ in multiple signaling pathways (eg, lipid metabolism, glucose homeostasis, cell differentiation).

AJA has been studied in a variety of preclinical in vivo models for anti-inflammatory activity, where it shows higher potencies than other cannabinoids.[13,19] As an example, orally administered AJA reduced the induction of paw edema in mice injected with arachidonic acid with an ED-50 of 0.02 mg/kg. A similar effect was seen when edema was induced by orally administered platelet-activating factor, where an ED-50 of 0.05 mg/kg was found.[13] A somewhat lower potency was seen with carrageenan-induced edema, where AJA inhibited the response at a higher dose showing an ED-50 of 2.2 mg/kg IV (Roche Center for Biological Research, Palo Alto, CA, unpublished data, June 16, 1997). In a different model, the migration of leukocytes into a subcutaneous air pouch following injection of tumor necrosis factor-α(TNFα) and interleukin-1β(IL1β) was markedly reduced at doses of 0.1 and 0.2 mg/kg.[22] AJA, at a dose of 0.2 mg/kg administered orally, reduced the effects of inflammation in an adjuvant-induced arthritis model in rats.[22] A dramatic effect was seen when histological examination of randomly selected specimens from this study was done, revealing a remarkable joint sparing effect in the AJA-treated animals when compared with vehicle/adjuvant treated controls (20% vs 80% ankylosis) (Fig. 40.2).

IL1β and TNFα are mediators of inflammation and joint tissue injury in patients with rheumatoid arthritis (RA). This prompted Zurier et al[27] to study human monocyte IL1β and TNFα responses after the addition of AJA to cells in vitro. Peripheral blood monocytes (PBM) and synovial fluid monocytes (SFM) were isolated from healthy subjects and patients with inflammatory arthritis, respectively, treated with AJA (0–30 μM) in vitro, and then stimulated with lipopolysaccharide. Cells were harvested for mRNA, and supernatants were collected for cytokine assay. Addition of AJA to PBM and SFM in vitro reduced both steady-state levels of IL1β mRNA and secretion of IL1β in a concentration-dependent manner. AJA did not influence TNFα gene expression in or secretion from PBM. Reduction of IL1β by AJA would contribute to the explanation of the joint sparing effects of AJA in the animal model of arthritis.[22]

Activation of T cells in the synovium can result in joint tissue injury in patients with RA. Bidinger et al[25] investigated the possibility that AJA would suppress human T-cell growth in vitro. T cells were isolated from peripheral blood of healthy volunteers and stimulated to proliferate with monoclonal antibodies to CD3 and CD4. They observed that T-cell proliferation was suppressed by AJA in a dose-dependent manner. Decreases in cell numbers also occurred following the addition of AJA to unstimulated cells. The involvement of apoptosis was detected by DNA fragmentation, caspase-3 activity, and microscopy, and AJA induced apoptosis of T cells in a dose- and time-dependent manner.[25] Apoptosis preceded loss of cell viability as measured by trypan blue dye exclusion, confirming that cell loss was due to programmed cell death rather than necrosis. T cells in the synovium of RA patients are resistant to apoptosis, further suggesting that a drug such as AJA may be a useful therapeutic agent for patients with RA.

The analgesic properties of AJA have been reported in a variety of animal models by several laboratories. Burstein et al[15,24] observed an antinociceptive action for AJA in the mouse hot plate assay at 55°C. Dajani et al[23] confirmed this finding and, under their conditions, reported an ED-50 of 6.7 mg/kg intragastrically that was equipotent to that observed with morphine. They also found a somewhat longer duration of activity for AJA when compared with morphine. In addition, they reported data using the tail clip assay in which an ED-50 of 4.4 mg/kg was determined.

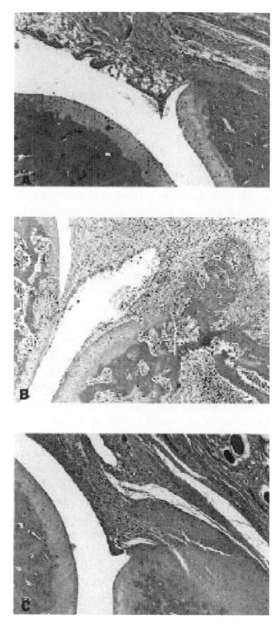

Fig. 40.2 AJA prevents bone damage in the rat adjuvant arthritis model. Histopathalogic findings: hind paw tibiotarsal joints at site of attachment to the anterior aspect of the tibia (hematoxylin and eosin stained, original magnification × 40); (A) Normal rat joint (no Freund's complete adjuvant [FCA]); (B) Joint from vehicle/FCA-treated rat on day 35. Synovitis with pannus formation is seen—exostosis seen at joint margin; (C) Joint from AJA/FCA-treated rat on day 35. Neither active pannus nor cartilage or bone damage is seen; Rx: AJA in safflower oil (0.1 mg/kg/day) given by mouth 3 times weekly. Adapted from Stebulis et al.[21]

Using the paraphenylquinone (PPQ) writhing assay, Burstein et al[24] found activity for AJA with an ED-50 of 1.24 mg/kg. They also reported inhibition in both the first and second phases of the mouse formalin test, indicating both centrally and peripherally mediated analgesia for AJA.

Walker et al[28] reported that allodynia induced by paw injection of platelet activating factor (PAF) in rats was completely reversed following the administration of 5 mg/kg of AJA. Higher doses resulted in analgesia as measured by increased tolerance to mechanical pressure. No effect on motor function (rotarod assay) was seen under the conditions of the assay. Analgesia was observed in a similar model following paw injection of either carrageenan or complete Freund's adjuvant (Atlantic Pharmaceuticals, New York, NY, unpublished data, July 15, 1998).

In a seemingly different model, Recht et al[19] demonstrated that AJA is highly effective in inhibiting the proliferation of several types of cancer cells. The effect on normal cells was lower and, in all cases, cell growth resumed upon withdrawal of the AJA. The involvement PPAR-γ was suggested by changes in lipid metabolism and prostaglandin synthesis that occurred concurrently; however, there is no direct evidence for this mechanism. In the same study, a modest but significant in vivo antitumor effect was seen in a subcutaneous mouse model at a dose of 0.2 mg/kg administered orally 3 times weekly. Cancer and inflammation are sometimes considered to be analogous processes, suggesting that AJA may act by similar mechanisms in reducing the course of these 2 conditions.

Side Effects

The use of many of the traditional anti-inflammatory agents such as aspirin and ibuprofen is limited by the formation of gastrointestinal ulcers attributed to their inhibition of COX-1 activity, which is required for gastric mucosal protection. For this reason, AJA was carefully examined[23] to detect any possible occurrence of ulcerogenicity. When given acutely to rats in doses up to 1000 mg/kg, no evidence for ulcer formation was seen. Chronic ig administration of up to 30 mg/kg likewise resulted in no ulcer formation, whereas the indomethacin control rats showed extensive formation of ulcers. This finding may be due to AJA's lack of inhibition of COX-1 as evidenced by its weak effect on human platelet aggregation.[24]

AJA's relationship to THC and its potent analgesic properties prompted a study for possible induction of opiate-like physical dependence in a 14-day rat study. None of the typical opiate withdrawal effects such as writhing, diarrhea, and wet dog shakes were observed (Atlantic, unpublished data, July 15, 1998), indicating that AJA has a low dependence liability. There were no effects on renal, cardiovascular, or gastrointestinal function and no signs of respiratory depression. Lethal doses were estimated following single doses in mice (600 mg/kg) and in rats (400 mg/kg). AJA was well tolerated in a 14-day study at doses up to 50 mg/kg. Three different standard tests for mutagenic potential gave negative findings, indicating a lack of carcinogenicity.

Clinical Trials

A phase 1, single-center, double-blind, randomized, placebo-controlled study of AJA was completed five years ago (Atlantic, unpublished data, May 8, 2000). The purpose of the study was to determine the safety, tolerability, and pharmacokinetics of a single oral dose of AJA in healthy adult male volunteers. A total of 32 subjects were given doses ranging from 0 to 10 mg and monitored for 24 hours following treatment. Pharmacokinetic measurements using mass spectrometry revealed that AJA is rapidly absorbed following oral administration and is eliminated with a terminal half-life of approximately 3 hours. The area under the curve (AUC) and C_{max} values showed a linear relationship when compared over the dose range of 1 to 10 mg/subject. Data from clinical laboratory tests, cardiovascular measurements, and tests for psychoactivity were also obtained. The latter consisted of a 12-item, yes/no questionnaire developed by the Addition Research Center at the National Institute on Drug Abuse, which is commonly referred to as the Addiction Research Center Inventory-Marijuana (ARCI-M) scale. It is designed to detect the full range of subjective responses experienced by marijuana users and has been validated by subjects following marijuana smoking. The subjects in the AJA study were told that they would receive a synthetic derivative of THC.

The data from all dose levels showed that AJA is safe and well tolerated. The scores obtained with ARCI-M scale showed no significant differences between placebo and AJA-treated volunteers. This finding is in agreement with the reported preclinical studies in rodents[5,15] and supports the conclusion that AJA does not produce a marijuana-like "high" at doses within the expected therapeutic range. This conclusion has recently been contested;[29] however, the basis for the assertion resides in one single-dose experiment in the mouse done at a level many-fold higher than the therapeutic dose. Burstein and Zurier have published a detailed reply to this claim pointing out the weaknesses of the arguments.[30]

The findings from a phase-2 trial to determine the efficacy of AJA for the treatment of chronic, intractable, neuropathic pain have been reported by Karst et al.[16] In a randomized, placebo-controlled, double-blind crossover trial, 21 patients (8 women and 13 men) with a mean age of 51 years who had a clinical presentation and examination consistent with chronic neuropathic pain with hyperalgesia (n = 21) and allodynia (n = 7) were recruited. The subjects were randomized into 2 7-day treatment groups in a crossover design. Two daily doses of AJA (4 10-mg capsules per day) or identical placebo capsules were given during the first 4 days, and 8 capsules per day were given in 2 daily doses in the following 3 days. After a washout and baseline period of 1 week each, patients crossed over to the second 7-day treatment period. The visual analog scale (VAS) and verbal rating scale scores for pain were used to determine the effect of AJA. The Trail-Making Test and the ARCI-M scale were used to detect possible cannabimimetic activity. The mean differences over time for the verbal analogic score (VAS) values in the AJA-placebo sequence measured 3 hours after intake of AJA differed significantly in favor of analgesia from those in the placebo-AJA sequence. Eight hours after intake of the drug, the pain scale differences between groups were less marked. There were no significant differences with respect to vital signs, blood tests, electrocardiogram, Trail-Making Test, and ARCI-M scale. In this preliminary study, AJA was effective in reducing chronic neuropathic pain compared with placebo, and no major adverse effects were observed.

In summary, the studies done with AJA demonstrate that naturally occurring cannabinoids can provide useful template molecules for the synthesis of analogs with potential anti-inflammatory activity. These could be expected to show a high therapeutic index since cannabinoids generally have minimal toxicity. It is also tempting to speculate that stable analogs of the endogenous cannabinoids such as anandamide may be discovered and will also exhibit high therapeutic indices.

Acknowledgments This publication was made possible by grants DA12178 and DA13691 from National Institute on Drug Abuse, National Institutes of Health, Bethesda, MD. Its contents are solely the responsibility of the author and do not necessarily represent the official views of the National Institute on Drug Abuse.

References

1. Burstein S. Therapeutic Potential of Ajulemic Acid (CT-3). In: Grontenhermen F, Russo E, eds. *Cannabis and Cannabinoids*. Binghamton, NY: Haworth Press Inc; 2002;381-388.
2. Burstein SH. Ajulemic acid (CT3): a potent analog of the acid metabolites of THC. *Curr Pharm Des*. 2000;6:1339-1345.
3. Burstein SH. The cannabinoid acids: nonpsychoactive derivatives with therapeutic potential. *Pharmacol Ther*. 1999;82:87-96.
4. Burstein SH, Karst M, Schneider U, Zurier RB. Ajulemic acid: a novel cannabinoid produces analgesia without a "high." *Life Sci*. 2004;75:1513-1522.
5. Burstein S, Hunter SA, Latham V, Renzulli L. A major metabolite of delta 1-tetrahydrocannabinol reduces its cataleptic effect in mice. *Experientia*. 1987;43:402-403.
6. Burstein S, Shoupe TS. Metabolic pathways for the transformation of delta 1-tetrahydrocannabinol in mouse hepatic microsomes. *Drug Metab Dispos*. 1981;9:94-96.
7. Burstein S, Rosenfeld J, Wittstruck T. Isolation and characterization of two major urinary metabolites of 1-tetrahydrocannabinol. *Science*. 1972;176:422-423.
8. Burstein SH, Kupfer D. Hydroxylation of trans-1-tetrahydro-cannabinol by a hepatic microsomal monooxygenase. *Chem Biol Interact*. 1971;3:316.
9. Burstein SH, Menezes F, Williamson E, Mechoulam R. Metabolism of delta 1(6)-tetrahydrocannabinol, an active marihuana constituent. *Nature*. 1970;225:87-88.
10. Perez-Reyes M. Pharmacodynamics of certain drugs of abuse. In: Barnett G, Chang CN, eds. *Pharmacokinetics and Pharmacodynamics of Psychoactive Drugs*. Foster City, CA: Biomedical Publishers; 1985:287-310.
11. Burstein S, Hunter SA, Latham V, Renzulli L. Prostaglandins and cannabis-XVI. Antagonism of delta 1-tetrahydrocannabinol action by its metabolites. *Biochem Pharmacol*. 1986;35:2553-2558.
12. Burstein SH, Hull K, Hunter SA, Latham V. Cannabinoids and pain responses: a possible role for prostaglandins. *FASEB J*. 1988;2:3022-3026.
13. Burstein SH, Audette CA, Doyle SA, Hull K, Hunter SA, Latham V. Antagonism to the actions of platelet activating factor by a non-psychoactive cannabinoid. *J Pharmacol Exp Ther*. 1989;251:531-535.

14. Doyle SA, Burstein SH, Dewey WL, Welch SP. Further studies on the antinociceptive effects of delta 6-THC-7-oic acid. *Agents Actions.* 1990;31:157-163.
15. Burstein SH, Audette CA, Breuer A, et al. Synthetic nonpsychotropic cannabinoids with potent antiinflammatory, analgesic, and leukocyte antiadhesion activities. *J Med Chem.* 1992;35:3135-3141.
16. Karst M, Salim K, Burstein S, Conrad I, Hoy L, Schneider U. Analgesic effect of the synthetic cannabinoid CT-3 on chronic neuropathic pain: a randomized controlled trial. *JAMA.* 2003;290:1757-1762.
17. Rhee MH, Vogel Z, Barg J, et al. Cannabinol derivatives: binding to cannabinoid receptors and inhibition of adenylylcyclase. *J Med Chem.* 1997;40:3228-3233.
18. Compton DR, Rice KC, De Costa BR, et al. Cannabinoid structure-activity relationships: correlation of receptor binding and in vivo activities. *J Pharmacol Exp Ther.* 1993;265:218-226.
19. Recht LD, Salmonsen R, Rosetti R, et al. Antitumor effects of ajulemic acid (CT3), a synthetic non-psychoactive cannabinoid. *Biochem Pharmacol.* 2001;62:755-763.
20. Hunter SA, Burstein SH. Receptor mediation in cannabinoid stimulated arachidonic acid mobilization and anandamide synthesis. *Life Sci.* 1997;60:1563-1573.
21. Stebulis JA, Burstein SH, Torres R, et al. Ajulemic Acid, an antiinflammatory nonpsychoactive cannabinoid acid, modulates activation of human synovial cells. Paper presented at: 2004 Symposium on the Cannabinoids. June 20, 2004; Paestum, Italy.
22. Zurier RB, Rossetti RG, Lane JH, Goldberg JM, Hunter SA, Burstein SH. Dimethylheptyl-THC-11-oic acid: a nonpsychoactive antiinflammatory agent with a cannabinoid template structure. *Arthritis Rheum.* 1998;41:163-170.
23. Dajani EZ, Larsen KR, Taylor J, et al. 1′,1′-Dimethylheptyl-delta-8-tetrahydrocannabinol-11-oic acid: a novel, orally effective cannabinoid with analgesic and anti-inflammatory properties. *J Pharmacol Exp Ther.* 1999;291:31-38.
24. Burstein SH, Friderichs E, Kogel B, Schneider J, Selve N. Analgesic effects of 1,1 dimethyl-heptyl-delta8-THC-11-oic acid (CT3) in mice. *Life Sci.* 1998;63:161-168.
25. Bidinger B, Torres R, Rossetti RG, et al. Ajulemic acid, a nonpsychoactive cannabinoid acid, induces apoptosis in human T lymphocytes. *Clin Immunol.* 2003;108:95-102.
26. Liú J, Li H, Burstein SH, Zurier RB, Chen JD. Activation and binding of peroxisome proliferator-activated receptor gamma by synthetic cannabinoid ajulemic acid. *Mol Pharmacol.* 2003;63:983-992.
27. Zurier RB, Rossetti RG, Burstein SH, Bidinger B. Suppression of human monocyte interleukin-1beta production by ajulemic acid, a nonpsychoactive cannabinoid. *Biochem Pharmacol.* 2003;65:649-655.
28. Walker JM, Owen K, Petros P, Huang SM. Antiallodynic and analgesic actions of ajulemic acid reversed by a cannabinoid antagonist. Paper presented at: Society of Neuroscientists; November 9, 2000; New Orleans, LA.
29. Sumariwalla PF, Gallily R, Tchilibon S, Fride E, Mechoulam R, Feldmann M. A novel synthetic, nonpsychoactive cannabinoid acid (HU-320) with antiinflammatory properties in murine collagen-induced arthritis. *Arthritis Rheum.* 2004;50:985-998.
30. Burstein SH, Zurier RB. Pain reduction and lack of psychotropic effects with ajulemic acid: comment on the article by Sumariwalla. *Arthritis Rheum.* 2004;50:4078-4080.

Chapter 41
Conformational Characteristics of the Interaction of SR141716A with the CB1 Cannabinoid Receptor as Determined Through the Use of Conformationally Constrained Analogs

Brian F. Thomas,[1] Yanan Zhang,[1] Marcus Brackeen,[1] Kevin M. Page,[1] S. Wayne Mascarella,[1] and Herbert H. Seltzman[1]

Abstract Interest in cannabinoid pharmacology increased dramatically upon the identification of the first cannabinoid receptor (CB1) in 1998 and continues to expand as additional endocannabinoids and cannabinoid receptors are discovered. Using CB1 receptor (CB1R) systems, medicinal chemistry programs began screening libraries searching for cannabinoid ligands, ultimately leading to the discovery of the first potent cannabinoid receptor antagonist, SR141716A (Rimonabant). Its demonstrated efficacy in treating obesity and facilitating smoking cessation, among other impressive pharmacological activities, has furthered the interest in cannabinoid receptor antagonists as therapeutics, such that the number of patents and publications covering this class of compounds continues to grow at an impressive rate. At this time, medicinal chemistry approaches including combinatorial chemistry, conformational constraint, and scaffold hopping are continuing to generate a large number of cannabinoid antagonists. These molecules provide an opportunity to gain insight into the 3-dimensional structure-activity relationships that appear crucial for CB1R-ligand interaction. In particular, studies in which conformational constraints have been imposed on the various pyrazole ring substituents of SR141716A provide a direct opportunity to characterize changes in conformation/conformational freedom within a single class of compounds. While relatively few conformationally constrained molecules have been synthesized to date, the structure-activity information is often more readily interpreted than in studies where entire substituents are replaced. Thus, it is the focus of this mini-review to examine the structural properties of SR141716A, and to use conformationally constrained molecules to illustrate the importance of conformation and conformational freedom to CB1R affinity, selectivity, and efficacy.

Keywords cannabinoid receptor, CB1, antagonists, SR141716A, structure-activity relationships, conformational analysis, molecular modeling

[1] Research Triangle Institute, Research Triangle Park, NC 27709-2194

Corresponding Author: Brian F. Thomas, Research Triangle Institute, PO Box 12194, 3040 Cornwallis Road, Research Triangle Park, NC 27709-2194. Tel: (919) 541-6552; Fax: (919) 541-6499; E-mail: bft@rti.org

R.S. Rapaka and W. Sadée (eds.), *Drug Addiction.*
© American Association of Pharmaceutical Scientists 2008

Introduction

With the discovery of the diarylpyrazole CB1 receptor (CB1R) antagonist/inverse agonist SR141716A (Rimonabant or Accomplia), researchers obtained a long-awaited and highly desirable molecular tool with which to further explore cannabinoid receptor function and signal transduction mechanisms. The remarkable phase 3 studies with SR141716A, demonstrating efficacy in both smoking cessation and obesity trials in humans, has continued to heighten interest in this class of compounds.[1] Several hundred analogs of SR141716A have since been designed, synthesized, and tested in a plethora of pharmacological assays, and compounds are continuing to be described with improved affinities, varying efficacies, differing receptor selectivities or unique pharmacological properties and clinical applications (see recent reviews by Muccioli and Lambert,[2] Padgett,[3] and Lange and Kruse[4]). These studies have helped characterize the conformational properties of SR141716A and the structure-activity relationships of cannabinoid antagonists and inverse agonists. Of particular relevance to the determination of the conformational requirements for receptor binding, receptor selectivity, and efficacy are studies where conformational constraints have been imposed on the various pyrazole ring substituents of SR141716A. Such studies can often define key conformational properties and relate changes in conformation/conformational freedom to ligand-receptor binding and G-protein coupling.

There are 4 torsion angles of rotation in SR141716A that can represent most of its key conformational characteristics (Fig. 41.1). Using quenched molecular dynamics simulations, it was possible to discern and compare the variety of conformational energies allowed by the structure of the molecule. For example, Fig. 41.2 shows that for the torsion τ_1, the molecule is confined energetically to

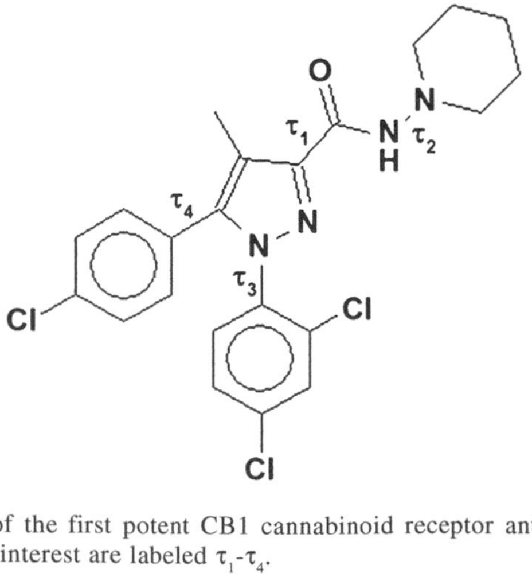

Fig. 41.1 Structure of the first potent CB1 cannabinoid receptor antagonist, SR141716A. The torsion angles of interest are labeled τ_1-τ_4.

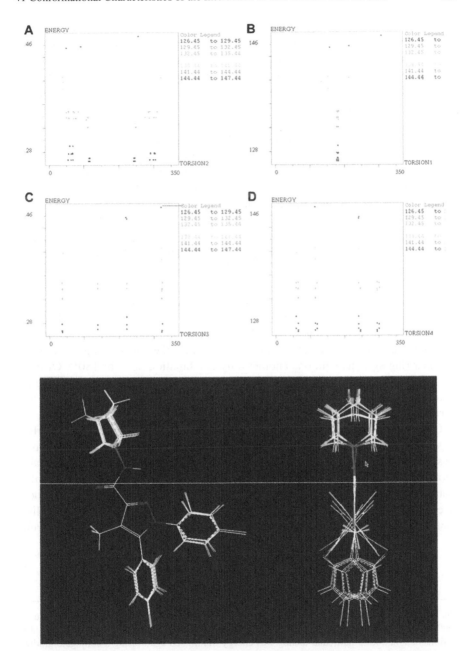

Fig. 41.2 (Top) Results of quenched molecular dynamics analysis of SR141716A plotted as graphs of conformational energy and torsion angle (τ_1, (B); τ_2, (A); τ_3, (C); and τ_4, (D)). (Bottom) Molecular dynamics were run up to 2000°K and snapshot conformations quenched using the MMFF94 force field within SYBYL (Tripos, St Louis, MO). This approach involves molecular dynamics simulations on each energy-minimized analog at 2000°K. During the molecular dynamics simulation, the molecule was heated from 0°K to 2000°K at 100°K steps lasting 10 picoseconds each, with snapshot conformations taken at 10-ps intervals.

an s-trans configuration of the carboxamide oxygen group as it connects to the pyrazole. While other conformational minima are possible, they are of considerably higher energy [~40 kJ/mol]. Torsion τ_2 describes the orientation of the amino-piperidine ring and reveals that 4 energetically preferred geometries exist, with torsion values of ~60°, 120°, 240°, and 300°. With these conformations, the energy differences are such that all 4 conformations are equally likely, but the symmetry of the piperidine ring makes the 60° and 240°, and the 120° and 300° conformations, identical. Despite this symmetry, this torsion angle, combined with the flexibility of the piperidine ring substituent, represents one of the areas of greatest conformational freedom for this molecule. The other 2 ring substituents are rigid aromatic ring systems, with each aryl substituent having 4 low energy conformations: torsion τ_3's energy minima are at ~40°, 140°, 220°, and 320°; τ_4's energy minima are at ~60°, 120°, 240°, and 300°. Because of the symmetry of the p-chloro ring system, the τ_4 torsion angle at 60° is equivalent to 240°, and 120° is the equivalent of 300°. These 2 torsion angles, τ_3 and τ_4, are "cogged," such that if τ_4 is at 60°/240°, τ_3 falls into energy minima at 40° or 220°, but if τ_4 is at 120°/300°, τ_3 has its energy minima at 140° and 320°. These interdependent conformational characteristics are quite apparent from the molecular dynamics simulations, and the energy plot obtained through a grid search of these 2 torsion angles (Fig. 41.3). In the 3-dimensional plot, the 2 torsions have energetically unfavorable interactions when the torsion angles result in coplanar ring systems with one another (any combination of 0° or 180°). Of interest, τ_4 appears to be the most energetically constrained system, despite its lacking the larger chlorine substituent in the ortho position as in the τ_3 system, pointing to a steric effect of the lone methyl group substituent on the pyrazole ring.

Using x-ray crystallography, s-trans geometry of τ_1 was observed in SR141716A crystals (telephone conversation from Clifford George, June, 2004),[5] as it was in crystals of an aryl ring constrained analog of SR141716A synthesized in our laboratory.[6] The importance of the carboxyhydrazine heteroatoms and the trans configuration of τ_1 in SR141716A for recognition and inverse agonist activity has been investigated by Reggio and colleagues through the use of molecular modeling, conformationally restricted analogs, and site-directed mutagenesis.[5] Molecular

---

Fig. 41.2 (continued) Upon reaching 2000°K, the molecule was held at this temperature for 1000 ps, while additional snapshots were acquired at 10-ps intervals. Each of the snapshot conformations obtained for a particular analog was energy minimized again using a conjugate gradient of 0.01 kcal/mol or a maximum of 100 000 iterations as termination criteria, yielding a group of 139 energy-minimized conformers per compound. After these simulations had been performed, all conformations from each of the analogues were overlaid using a single template molecule. Because the pyrazole ring system of SR141716 had a reasonably close corresponding central ring system in most of the analogues, the pyrazole ring atoms were used for atom-by-atom root mean square distance minimization. This alignment positioned all of the molecules in the same 3-dimensional space and superposed the central ring systems to as great an extent as possible.

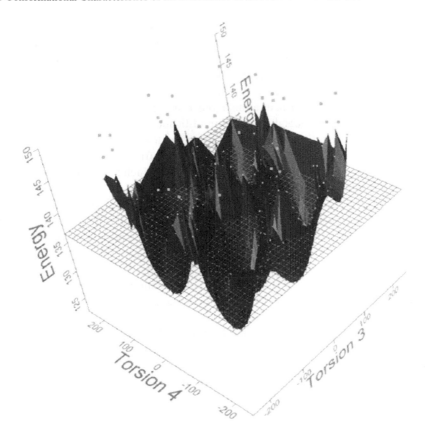

Fig. 41.3 Conformational energy profile for rotations about τ_3 and τ_4 of SR141716A. Energy minimization of the various permutations of $10°$ increments of τ_3 and τ_4 performed in SPARTAN using the MMFF94 force field (Wave Function).

modeling and receptor docking studies suggested a critical interaction with lysine K3.28(192) and this substituent. Based on this hypothesis, synthesis of a vinyl-cyclohexyl analog and 4 additional compounds differing in the presence, the orientation, or both of potential hydrogen-bond forming heteroatoms was performed. In studies using wild-type receptors, the binding affinity of the vinyl-cyclohexyl SR141716 analog (VCHSR) was reduced as compared with SR141716A. A similar decrease in binding affinity was observed with SR141716A when the lysine K3.28 was mutated to a nonhydrogen bonding residue (K3.28A) in the CB1R. However, an additive effect (or greater) was not observed when the VCHSR analog was tested in the K.328A mutation, consistent with a single (H-bonding) interaction between the carboxyhydrazine and the K3.28(192) residue. Although their modeling results suggest that it is the carboxamide oxygen of SR141716A that interacts with K3.28(192), the mutant cycle calculations could not identify the specific K3.28(192) hydrogen bonding site within the C3 substituent of SR141716A. It does seem apparent that the piperidine nitrogen is not necessary for high affinity binding, because the cyclohexyl analog has been shown to possess affinity similar to SR141716A. The authors further hypothesized that hydrogen bonding of the SR141716A C3 substituent with K3.28 is responsible for its higher affinity for the inactive receptor state, leading to its inverse agonism. Consistent with this hypothesis, VCHSR acted as a neutral antagonist at the wild-type CB1R. Additional conformational constraint and structural modifications of this region were recently reported.[7] Of interest, these molecules constrained the carboxyamide oxygen atom in the s-cis position and still retained reasonable affinities. The most analogous molecule to SR141716A, compound 2b (Fig. 41.4), which has only hydrogen bond accepting capability, exhibited surprisingly high affinities despite the poor overlap of the piperidinyl groups in the low-energy conformer of SR141716. These results suggest that this analog may bind differently than SR141716 in hCB1-R, with the piperidinyl group in 2b occupying a separate hydrophobic pocket, distinct from that for the 1-piperidinyl group in SR141716, and the hydrogen bond accepting groups forming different networks of hydrogen bond interactions. Alternatively, the conformationally constrained molecules may induce conformational changes in the receptor to accommodate the piperidinyl rings in the same hydrophobic pocket as well as allow alternative hydrogen bond formation.

Ring constraint of torsion τ_2 has not been fully characterized. Instead, investigators have often elected to replace the piperidinyl ring system entirely. Even though the plane of symmetry in the piperidine ring simplifies the system, it is relatively flexible and can occupy an extended area of space through several conformational minima. Thus, it remains to be determined if there is a benefit to be gained by reducing the conformational mobility of this particular substituent, an approach that might be considered promising, because modification of this system has been

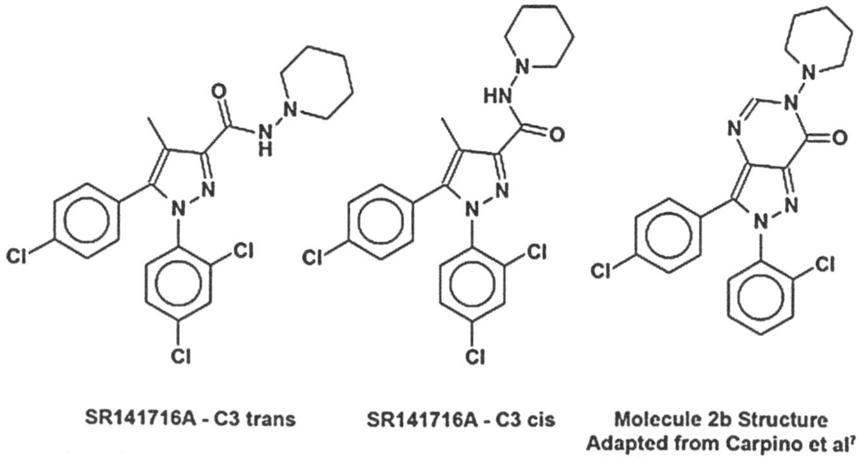

SR141716A - C3 trans   SR141716A - C3 cis   Molecule 2b Structure
                                                           Adapted from Carpino et al[7]

Fig. 41.4 S-trans (left) and s-cis (center) conformations of SR141716A and molecule 2b structure adapted from Carpino et al[7] (right).

shown to produce large changes in affinity as well alter receptor selectivity between CB1 and CB2.[6,8-11]

While τ_3 has 4 low energy torsion angles, and τ_4 has only 2 due to symmetry, these ring systems show coordinated movement such that modifications of the conformational freedom of one system typically have some implicit or quantifiable effect on the other. In addition, because of the symmetry of the molecule, several low energy nonsuperimposable mirror image conformations are possible, and these are not necessarily equivalent with regard to biological activity. It is possible that the chiral environment of the receptor binding site may preferentially permit high affinity interactions with only one of the mirror image conformations. Thus, constraint of these 2 aryl ring systems would be expected to provide additional information as to the nature of the interaction of these rings with the CB1R. Coplanarity of the diaryl ring systems can be forced via the structure shown in Fig. 41.5. This molecule was synthesized in our laboratory via a photocyclization reaction.[6] Its reduced affinity suggests that coplanarity is not an optimal configuration of the systems for interaction with CB1R, and/or that the o-chlorine contributes to the high affinity of SR141716A. An alternative approach to constrain τ_4 involved fusing the central pyrazole group of SR141716A with its 5-(4-chlorophenyl) to form a central indazole ring (Fig. 41.6).[12] However, this molecule does not constrain the overall geometry or conformation of the monochloro ring to a position that closely approximates that occupied by the same ring in SR141716A; thus its relatively low affinity (~500 nM) cannot be solely attributed to constraining the ring in the plane of the pyrazole. It would be interesting to examine additional analogs, such as the one proposed in Fig. 41.6, to better approximate the structure of

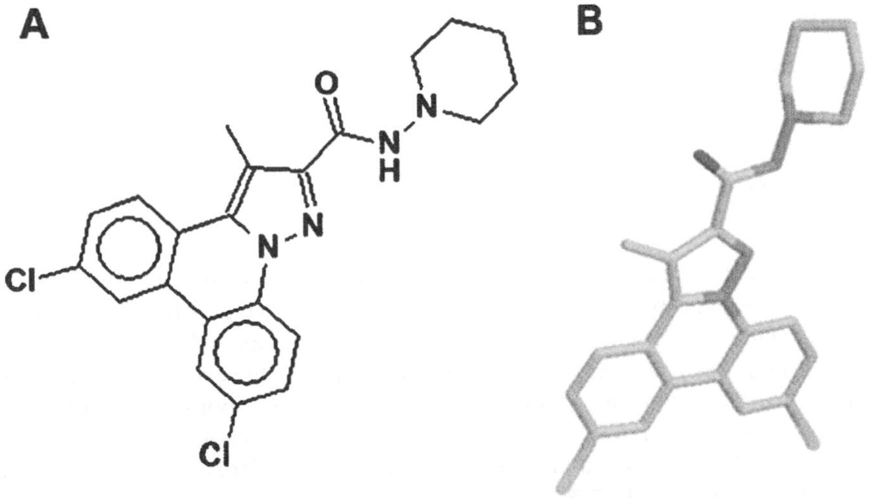

Fig. 41.5 Structure (A) and x-ray crystal structure (B) of pyrazole [1,5 f] phenanthridine analog adapted from Francisco et al.[6] Note the x-ray shows the transconfiguration of τ_1.

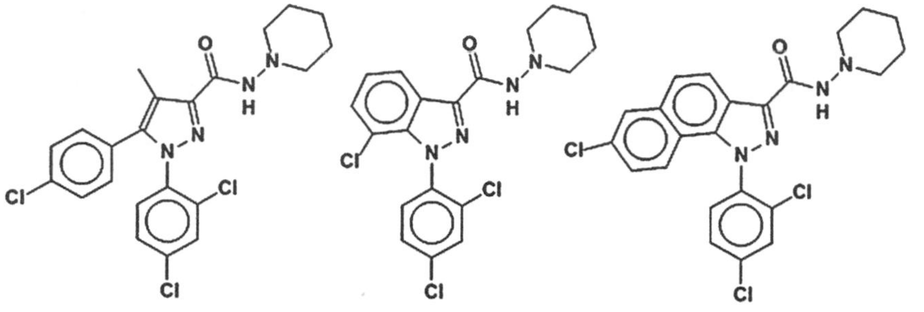

SR141716A | O-1248 Structure Adapted From Bass et al[12] | Hypothetical Ring-constrained Analog

Fig. 41.6 Structure of SR141716A (left), O-1248 structure adapted from Bass et al.[12] (center), and a hypothetical ring-constrained molecule (right).

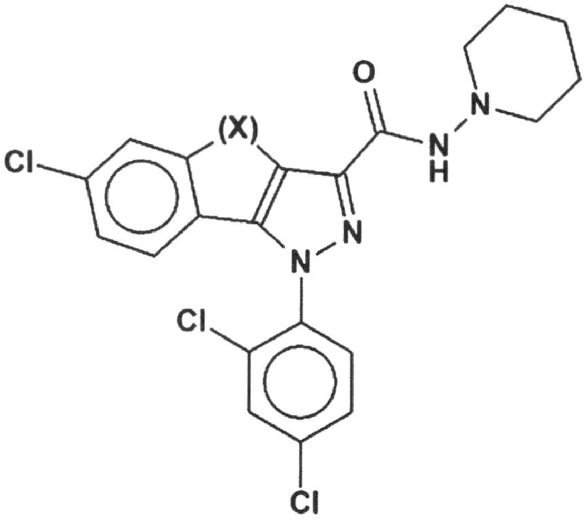

Fig. 41.7 Tricyclic pyrazole analogs.

SR141716A. The Stoit,[13] Mussinu,[11] and Murineddu[14,15] research groups used carbon bridges to reduce the conformational mobility of τ_4 (Fig. 41.7, Table 41.1). Initially, Stoit et al[13] reported the 3 carbon-bridged compound and found that it had lower affinity for the CB1R than SR141716A. However, Pinna and colleagues[11,13,14] varied the bridge length from 1 carbon to 3 carbons and reported that the 3 carbon bridged compound, NESS-0327, had fentomolar (fM) affinity as compared with the nanomolar (nM) affinity of SR141716A. Despite the large discrepancy between affinities, each group ascribed the changes in affinity to the conformational differences of the molecules as compared with those of SR141716A. Thus, in this particular instance, any interpretation must be tempered by the need

Table 41.1 Affinities of tricyclic pyrazole analogs for CB1 and CB2 receptors

X	K_i (CB1)	K_i (CB2)	Reference
1	2050 ± 90 nM	0.34 ± 0.06 nM	14
2	14.8 ± 0.43 nM	227 ± 5 nM	14
3	0.00035 ± 0.000005 nM	21 ± 0.5 nM	14
3	126 nM		13

*K_i indicates the concentration of the competing ligand that binds to half the binding sites at equilibrium.

to establish a more robust, reproducible estimation of the affinity and activity of these compounds, particularly the 3 carbon-bridged molecule. It is interesting to note that the research reported by Stoit et al[13] included in vivo administration of the 3 carbon-bridged compound by intraperitoneal (ip) and oral (po) routes, and the authors reported that no activity was detected, which would be more consistent with a compound that had decreased affinity as compared with SR141716A. However, it is not clear in their report what measures of pharmacological activity were measured, and as the authors pointed out, the bioavailability of the compounds could be quite different. Regardless of these difficulties, the conformational considerations of these bridged compounds are quite interesting.

As shown in Fig. 41.8, with 1 carbon atom as the bridge, the τ_4 torsion angle is drastically reduced in its range of motion, remaining almost coplanar with the pyrazole ring system. There is little range for torsional changes of τ_4, and the energy minima on each side are equivalent. Of interest, the one carbon-bridged molecule appears to pull the *p*-chloro-substituted aryl ring away from the dichloro aryl ring system, allowing free rotation across the entire 360 range of τ_3. The energy manifold shows a small energy barrier resulting from proton-proton steric interactions, and a somewhat larger energy barrier resulting from proton-chlorine interactions; however, these energy barriers are below 40 kJ/mol. Increasing the bridging carbon atoms to 2 appears to push the aryl ring systems closer together, making it energetically more difficult for τ_3 to rotate through its entire range. While it is clear that the energy barrier increases from the 1 to the 2 carbon-bridged compounds, particularly as the *o*-chlorine tries to pass by the *p*-chloro-substituted ring system, there is still a clear path for this transition that is below 40 kJ/mol. Finally, the barrier grows even further when the 3 carbon bridge is in place. Even here, however, there appears to be a path for transition (saddle point) at ~40 kJ/mol, so that τ_3 is in equilibrium across the full range of rotation at room temperature.

The effects on affinity and potency observed with these bridged compounds deserve further mention. First, the 1 carbon-bridged compound has significantly lower affinity (equilibrium dissociation constant (K_i) of ~2000 nM) than SR141716A (K_i of ~1 nM), or when the aryl rings are fused as in the pyrazole [1,5 f] phenanthridine analog (K_i ~50 nM).[6] Thus, constraining the rotation of τ_4 with the 1 carbon bridge, so that the ring is in the plane of the pyrazole ring system, is detrimental to binding affinity. However, if the constraint of τ_4 is done by forming the pyrazole [1,5 f] phenanthridine analog, the additional constraint of τ_3 appears to attenuate the

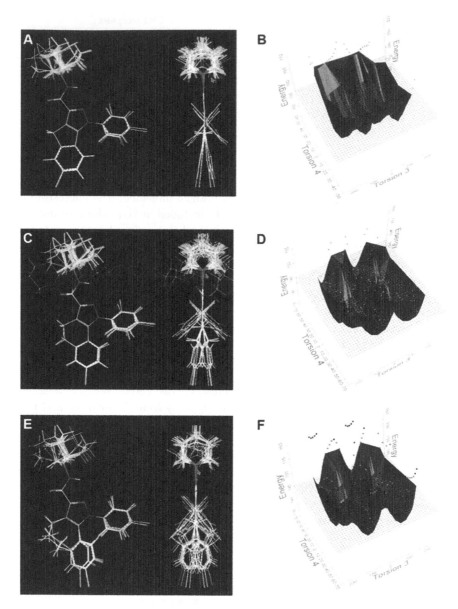

Fig. 41.8 Orthographic views of the minimum energy conformations (A,C,E) and energy surface for the rotation of τ_3 and τ_4 (B,D,F) for 1 (A,B), 2 (C,D), and 3 (E,F) carbon-bridged analogs reported by Stoit et al[13] and Murineddu et al.[14]

decrease in affinity seen with the 1 carbon-bridged molecule. Second, in the 2 carbon-bridged compound, τ_4 has somewhat greater flexibility and deviates from coplanarity with the pyrazole ring, and τ_3 can still freely rotate at room temperature; the affinity of this compound is intermediate (~14 nM). Finally, in the 3 carbon-bridged molecule, τ_3 can obtain positions similar to those available for SR141716A, and τ_4 can access all of the energy minima at torsions also in close proximity to the minimum energy torsion angles for SR141716A. Thus, based on similarity of conformational shape to SR141716A, it might be expected that the 3 carbon-bridged analog would have similar affinity to SR141716A. However, if the conformational constraint restrains the ring system to a bioactive conformation around τ_4, a more potent compound would be anticipated. Alternatively, a less potent compound would be anticipated if τ_4 and τ_3 were being constrained to angles outside of the bioactive conformation, which would still be quite energetically accessible with SR141716A's free rotation of τ_4. Because the barrier for free rotation does not exceed 40 kJ/mol, a compound of roughly the same affinity might be expected. However, the fact that 2 laboratories have reported such divergent values for the affinity of the 3 carbon-bridged molecules complicates our ability to make firm conclusions on what is the bioactive conformation of SR141716A.

Conclusion

The conformational properties of SR141716A are readily modeled and have been further characterized by the use of conformational constraint. However, the degree of conformational constraint that has been described to date has not been extensive. Some studies have indicated that the s-trans configuration of the amino-piperidine ring substituent is important in hydrogen bonding with the cannabinoid receptor, while others have illustrated the importance of the orientation of the aryl ring systems. Still, while some systematic changes in the conformation of the monochloro ring system have been imposed and tested, very little is known regarding the conformational considerations involved in the interaction of the dichloro ring system within the cannabinoid receptor binding site(s). It remains to be determined if molecules can continue to be synthesized that impose unique conformational constraints, that when tested, can further define the conformational requirements for optimal interaction with the cannabinoid receptor.

Acknowledgments Research funding for this study was provided by a grant from the National Institute on Drug Abuse, National Institutes of Health, Bethesda, MD (grant No. DA019217).

References

1. Cleland JG, Ghosh J, Freemantle N, et al. Clinical trials update and cumulative meta-analyses from the American College of Cardiology: WATCH, SCD-HeFT, DINAMIT, CASINO, INSPIRE, STRATUS-US, RIO-Lipids and cardiac resynchronisation therapy in heart failure. *Eur J Heart Fail.* 2004;6:501-508.
2. Muccioli GG, Lambert DM. Current knowledge on the antagonists and inverse agonists of cannabinoid receptors. *Curr Med Chem.* 2005;12:1361-1394.
3. Padgett LW. Recent developments in cannabinoid ligands. *Life Sci.* 2005;77:1767-1798.
4. Lange JH, Kruse CG. Keynote review: medicinal chemistry strategies to CB1 cannabinoid receptor antagonists. *Drug Discov Today.* 2005;10:693-702.

5. Hurst DP, Lynch DL, Barnett-Norris J, et al. N-(piperidin-1-yl)-5-(4-chlorophenyl)-1-(2,4-dichlorophenyl)-4-methyl-1H-pyrazole-3-carboxamide (SR141716A) interaction with LYS 3.28(192) is crucial for its inverse agonism at the cannabinoid CB1 receptor. *Mol Pharmacol.* 2002;62:1274-1287.

6. Francisco ME, Seltzman HH, Gilliam AF, et al. Synthesis and structure-activity relationships of amide and hydrazide analogues of the cannabinoid CB(1) receptor antagonist N-(piperidinyl)-5-(4-chlorophenyl)-1-(2,4-dichlorophenyl)-4-methyl-1H-pyrazole-3-carboxamide (SR141716). *J Med Chem.* 2002;45:2708-2719.

7. Carpino PA, Griffith DA, Sakya S, et al. New bicyclic cannabinoid receptor-1 (CB(1)-R) antagonists. *Bioorg Med Chem Lett.* 2006;16:731-736.

8. Rinaldi-Carmona M, Barth F, Millan J, et al. SR 144528, the first potent and selective antagonist of the CB2 cannabinoid receptor. *J Pharmacol Exp Ther.* 1998;284:644-650.

9. Wiley JL, Jefferson RG, Grier MC, Mahadevan A, Razdan RK, Martin BR. Novel pyrazole cannabinoids: insights into CB(1) receptor recognition and activation. *J Pharmacol Exp Ther.* 2001;296:1013-1022.

10. Thomas BF, Francisco ME, Seltzman HH, et al. Synthesis of long-chain amide analogs of the cannabinoid CB1 receptor antagonist N-(piperidinyl)-5-(4-chlorophenyl)-1-(2,4-dichlorophenyl)-4-methyl-1H-pyra zole-3-carboxamide (SR141716) with unique binding selectivities and pharmacological activities. *Bioorg Med Chem.* 2005;13:5463-5474.

11. Mussinu JM, Ruiu S, Mule AC, et al. Tricyclic pyrazoles. 1. Synthesis and biological evaluation of novel 1,4-dihydroindeno[1,2-c]pyrazol-based ligands for CB1 and CB2 cannabinoid receptors. *Bioorg Med Chem.* 2003;11:251-263.

12. Bass CE, Griffin G, Grier M, Mahadevan A, Razdan RK, Martin BR. SR-141716A-induced stimulation of locomotor activity: a structure-activity relationship study. *Pharmacol Biochem Behav.* 2002;74:31-40.

13. Stoit AR, Lange JH, Hartog AP, et al. Design, synthesis and biological activity of rigid cannabinoid CB1 receptor antagonists. *Chem Pharm Bull (Tokyo).* 2002;50:1109-1113.

14. Murineddu G, Ruiu S, Loriga G, et al. Tricyclic pyrazoles. 3. Synthesis, biological evaluation, and molecular modeling of analogues of the cannabinoid antagonist 8-chloro-1-(2′,4′-dichlorophenyl)-N-piperidin-1-yl-1,4,5,6-tetrahydrobenzo[6,7]cyclohepta[1,2-c]pyrazole-3-carboxamide. *J Med Chem.* 2005;48:7351-7362.

15. Murineddu G, Ruiu S, Mussinu JM, et al. Tricyclic pyrazoles. 2. Synthesis and biological evaluation of novel 4,5-dihydro-1H-benzo[g]indazole-based ligands for cannabinoid receptors. *Bioorg Med Chem.* 2005;13:3309-3320.

Chapter 42
Activation of G-Proteins in Brain by Endogenous and Exogenous Cannabinoids

Steven R. Childers[1]

Abstract The biological response to cannabinoid agonist begins when the agonist-bound receptor activates G-protein G_α subunits, thus initiating a cascade of signal transduction pathways. For this reason, information about cannabinoid receptors/G-protein coupling is critical to understand both the acute and chronic actions of cannabinoids. This review focuses on these mechanisms, predominantly examining the ability of cannabinoid agonists to activate G-proteins in brain with agonist-stimulated [^{35}S]guanylyl-5′-O-(γ-thio)-triphosphate ([^{35}S]GTPγS) binding. Acute efficacies of cannabinoid agonists at the level of G-protein activation depend not only on the ability of the agonist to induce a high affinity state in G_α for GTP, but also to induce a low affinity for GDP. When several agonists are compared, it is clear that cannabinoid agonists differ considerably in their efficacy. Both WIN 55212-2 and levonantradol are full agonists, while Δ^9-tetrahydrocannabinol is a weak partial agonist. Of interest, anandamide and its stable analog methanandamide are partial agonists. Chronic treatment in vivo with cannabinoids produces significant tolerance to the physiological and behavioral effects of these drugs, and several studies have shown that this is accompanied by a significant loss in the ability of cannabinoid receptors to couple to G-proteins in brain. These effects vary across different brain regions and are usually (but not always) accompanied by loss of cannabinoid receptor binding. Although the relationship between cannabinoid receptor desensitization and tolerance has not yet been established, these mechanisms may represent events that lead to a loss of cannabinoid agonist response and development of tolerance.

Keywords G-protein, Efficacy, Signal transduction, Anandamide, Delta-9-tetrahydrocannibinol, Levonantradol, Desensitization

[1] Department of Physiology and Pharmacology, Center for the Neurobiological Investigation of Drug Abuse, Wake Forest University School of Medicine, Winston-Salem, NC 27157

Corresponding Author: Steven R. Childers, Department of Physiology/Pharmacology, Wake Forest University School of Medicine, Medical Center Blvd, Winston-Salem, NC 27157. Tel: (336) 716-3791; Fax: (336) 716-0237; E-mail: childers@wfubmc.edu

R.S. Rapaka and W. Sadée (eds.), *Drug Addiction.*
© American Association of Pharmaceutical Scientists 2008

Introduction

When Howlett first reported the existence of specific cannabinoid receptors,[1] the crucial discovery depended on the fact that cannabinoid agonists inhibited adenylyl cyclase through a G-protein-coupled mechanism. Therefore, it was clear from the beginning that these receptors were members of the G-protein-coupled receptor superfamily. Subsequent studies demonstrated that cannabinoid receptors were indeed coupled to effectors that were modulated by the $G_{i/o}$ class of G-proteins.[2-4] This finding was followed by cannabinoid receptor radioligand binding,[5] receptor localization,[6] and cloning and sequencing of the brain cannabinoid receptor CB_1.[7] The cloning of a peripheral cannabinoid receptor, CB_2, from spleen cells[8] showed that there are at least 2 major types of cannabinoid receptors. Both receptor types are typical of the 7 transmembrane-domain superfamily of receptors, with 44% homology between CB_1 and CB_2 receptors. CB_1 is larger than CB_2, with an additional 72 amino acid residues in the N-terminal region, 15 additional residues in the third extracellular loop, and 13 additional residues in the C-terminal region. The highest degree of homology between CB_1 and CB_2 occurs in the transmembrane regions TM2, TM3, TM5, and TM6; of interest, the homology in other regions is not particularly striking.

From these findings, it is clear that cannabinoid receptors operate by many of the same principles that govern the other receptors in this family of proteins. But cannabinoid receptors also have several properties that make them unique among G-protein-coupled receptors, at least at this stage of our understanding. For example, CB_1 receptors exist in brain at levels higher than most other G-protein-coupled receptors,[5,6] approaching levels observed for amino acid receptors. This fact not only demonstrates the importance of CB_1 receptors in regulating brain activity in a variety of ways, but also has importance in regulating the efficacy of cannabinoid agonists.

Another unique aspect of cannabinoid receptors is the fact that their endogenous ligands represent a class of lipophilic compounds based on the general structure of modified arachidonic acid derivatives. The first of these compounds, arachidonyl ethanolamide or anandamide, was isolated in 1992,[9] followed later by other arachidonyl endogenous cannabinoids including arachidonyl glycerol.[10] Among endogenous agonists at G-protein-coupled receptors, anandamide is unique in that it is a partial agonist at CB_1 receptors, as will be discussed in detail later.

Acute Effects of Cannabinoids in Activating G-proteins

As observed above, cannabinoid receptors share many of the same properties of G-protein coupling and activation as other members of the GPCR superfamily. For example, guanine nucleotides inhibit cannabinoid agonist binding in a manner typical of G-protein-coupled receptors.[5] Moreover, cannabinoid binding sites can be solubilized from membranes together with G-proteins,[11] and recent evidence suggests that multiple cannabinoid ligands can activate different populations of

G-proteins.[12] Cannabinoid receptor activation of G-proteins in isolated membranes can be measured by agonist-stimulated [35S]guanylyl-5′-O-(γ-thio)-triphosphate ([35S]GTPγS) binding.[13] The technique was originally developed in purified systems,[14-16] and in membranes from heart,[17] brain,[18] and cultured cells[19] as a measure of specific receptor-stimulated G-protein activation. An important application for [35S]GTPγS binding is the quantitative estimate of agonist efficacy at the level of G-proteins, first studied with β-adrenergic receptors[20,21] and now applied to a large number of other G-protein-coupled receptors.

Agonist-induced stimulation of [35S]GTPγS binding to G_α is based upon the G-protein activation cycle. The critical step in the [35S]GTPγS assay is addition of excess GDP to shift the G-protein into the inactive state. This step is crucial because spontaneously active G-proteins will bind [35S]GTPγS, increasing the basal level of activity and making agonist-stimulated [35S]GTPγS binding undetectable. After the addition of GDP, [35S]GTPγS and agonist are added to activate those G-proteins coupled to the receptor of interest. Receptor activation decreases the affinity of G_α for GDP and increases its affinity for [35S]GTPγS. In cells, this increase in GTPγS affinity can be 100- to 300-fold.[22] In vivo, the α subunit GTPase hydrolyzes GTP to GDP; however, in vitro, [35S]GTPγS is useful because it is resistant to hydrolysis. Although first developed in isolated membranes, these same principles can be applied (with several technical changes) to brain sections to localize receptor activity in different brain regions. The development of [35S]GTPγS autoradiography represented the first in vitro method to provide a neuroanatomical localization of a receptor-coupled intracellular signal transduction system.[23]

The Scatchard plot in Fig. 42.1 shows the dramatic effect of WIN 55212-2 on activation of G-proteins as measured by [35S]GTPγS binding. This experiment

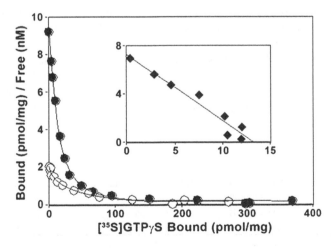

Fig. 42.1 Scatchard plot of cannabinoid activation of [35S]GTPγS binding in rat cerebellar membranes, showing basal (open symbols) and activated (closed symbols) [35S]GTPγS binding, as determined with 3μM WIN 55212-2. Inset shows net agonist-stimulated [35S]GTPγS binding, with a high affinity of 2.7nM compared with an affinity of 540nM in the basal state. Adapted from Sim et al.[24]

shows the affinities of G_α for [^{35}S]GTPγS in cerebellar membranes in the presence and absence of the agonist. Under basal conditions, in the absence of WIN 55212-2, most of G_α subunits in these membranes display low affinity for [^{35}S]GTPγS, with an equilibrium dissociation constant (K_D) of 540 nanomolar (nM). When WIN 55212-2 is added, there is an appearance of a substantial high affinity site for [^{35}S]GTPγS, with a K_D of 2.7 nM. Thus, WIN 55212-2 produces a 200-fold increase in the affinity of G_α for GTP.[24] The energy associated with this change in affinity is largely responsible for activation of receptor-mediated signal transduction.

In brain membranes, cannabinoid-stimulated [^{35}S]GTPγS binding is especially high because of the relatively large number of cannabinoid receptors in brain.[25] However, the number of receptors present does not always directly translate into a larger response because of the phenomenon of catalytic amplification between receptors and G-proteins. Several studies have shown that one receptor can couple to many different G-proteins to amplify agonist response. For example, in brain, cannabinoid receptor coupling to G-proteins is relatively inefficient[26,27]: in striatum, each cannabinoid receptor activates only 3 G-proteins compared with 20 G-proteins for each μ and δ opioid receptor (Table 42.1). It is possible that this relatively low amplification is related to the high number of CB_1 receptors; since these receptors exist in such high number in the brain, a high amplification between the receptor and transducer may not be necessary. A detailed brain regional analysis of cannabinoid amplification[27] showed that the amplification between CB_1 receptors and G-proteins varied widely between regions, with the smallest amplification factor of 2 in regions such as frontal cortex, cerebellum, and hippocampus, and the largest amplification factor of 7 in hypothalamus (Fig. 42.2). These results suggest that different behavioral effects of cannabinoids that are mediated in different brain regions may be less related to the number of receptors present, but rather to the level of coupling between receptors and signal-transduction systems.

Agonist-stimulated [^{35}S]GTPγS binding can also be used to determine differences in agonist efficacy at the level of G-protein activation.[26,28] Using this technique in brain membranes,[24,29,30] WIN 55212-2 and levonantradol are full agonists, while anandamide produces partial efficacy, and Δ^9-tetrahydrocannabinol (Δ^9-THC) is

Table 42.1 Catalytic Amplification Factors for Opioid- and Cannabinoid-Stimulated G-Protein Activation in Rat Striatal Membranes*

Receptor	Receptor B_{max} pmol/mg	G-Protein B_{max} pmol/mg	Amplification Factor
μ Opioid	0.30	5.15	17
δ Opioid	0.29	6.27	22
Cannabinoid	3.56	10.05	3

*Amplification factors were calculated as ratios of B_{max} values of receptor binding to agonist-stimulated [^{35}S]GTPγS binding assays in rat striatal membranes. Adapted from.[26]

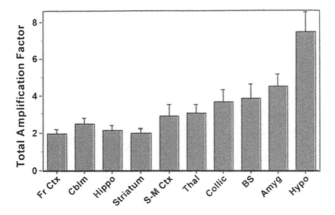

Fig. 42.2 Brain regional variation in catalytic amplification of cannabinoid-activated G-proteins in rat brain. Amplification factors were calculated by comparing the ratios between B_{max} values of [^{3}H]SR141716A binding and WIN 55212-2-stimulated [^{35}S]GTPγS binding in membranes from various rat brain regions. Fr Ctx indicates frontal cortex; Cblm, cerebellum; Hippo, hippocampus; S-M cortex, sensomotor cortex; Thal, thalamus; Collic, superior colliculus; BS, brainstem; Amyg, amygdala; and Hypo, hypothalalmus. Adapted from Breivogel et al.[27]

a weak partial agonist (Fig. 42.3). The discovery that anandamide is a partial agonist was surprising; traditionally, endogenous agonists in any neurotransmitter-receptor system are considered, by definition, full agonists. It is important to note that the lower efficacy of anandamide is not related to the metabolic instability of anandamide, since its metabolically stable analog methanandamide also produces the same partial efficacy as anandamide itself.

The efficacies of both exogenous and endogenous cannabinoids in activating G-proteins is related not only to the drugs ability to convert G_α into a high affinity state for GTP, but also to their ability to shift G_α into a low affinity state for GDP.[24] This principle is illustrated in Table 42.2, where the efficacies of several cannabinoids (E_{max}) are related to their ability to shift G_α into low affinity states for GDP in cerebellar membranes. In the basal state, [^{35}S]GTPγS binding sites have 2 affinity states for GDP, 33 nM and 1147 nM. Additions of agonists have no effect on the high affinity GDP binding, but the efficacies of various cannabinoid agonists are directly related to their ability to shift the GDP low affinity state into even lower affinity. For example, the full agonist WIN 55212-2 shifts the GDP affinity from 1147 nM to 8210 nM, a decrease in affinity of 7.1-fold. A low efficacy partial agonist such as Δ^9-THC produces very little effect on the GDP affinity, decreasing affinity from 1147 nM to 1330 nM (1.2-fold shift). As predicted from its moderate efficacy, methanandamide produces a moderate change in the affinity for GDP, decreasing affinity from 1147 nM to 6570 nM (5.7-fold shift). These results confirm that anandamide is simply unable to produce a maximal activation of G-proteins, either by shifting G_α into a high affinity state for GTP, or shifting G_α into a low

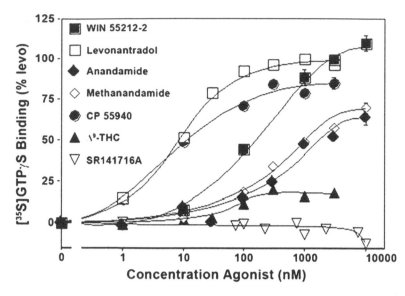

Fig. 42.3 Cannabinoid agonist efficacies in activating G-proteins, as measured by agonist concentration-effect curves in stimulating [^{35}S]GTPγS binding in rat cerebellar membranes. Data are expressed as percentage of stimulation by the full agonist levonantradol. Adapted from Sim et al.[24]

Table 42.2 Relationship Between Cannabinoid Efficacy in Stimulating [^{35}S]GTPγS Binding, and Decreasing Affinities of GDP*

Cannabinoid Agonist	E_{max} Values (% levo)	GDP K_i Values (nM)	
		High Affinity	Low Affinity
None (basal)	N/A	33 ± 5.1	1147 ± 141
Levonantradol	100 ± 5.9	34 ± 2.3	7730 ± 1030
WIN 55212-2	107 ± 2.3	39 ± 7.6	8210 ± 1190
CP 55940	81 ± 2.5	ND	ND
Anandamide	70 ± 5.8	ND	ND
Methanandamide	68 ± 2.1	33 ± 5.6	6570 ± 2540
Δ^9-THC	21 ± 0.7	20 ± 6.2	1330 ± 372

*Data compare the efficacies (E_{max} values) of various cannabinoid agonists determined from concentration-effect curves, with the affinity of GDP in displacing [^{35}S]GTPγS binding in the presence and absence of agonists. [^{35}S]GTPγS binding was performed in rat cerebellar membranes. Adapted from Sim et al.[24]

affinity state for GDP. This phenomenon is not just observed at the level of G-protein activation but also in the ability of anandamide to inhibit adenylyl cyclase[31] and affect ion channel function.[32,33] Why an endogenous ligand such as anandamide does not produce full efficacy at its receptor remains an unanswered question at this point. It is possible, however, that the relatively low efficacy of anandamide is counteracted by the large number of CB$_1$ receptors present in brain. Classical pharmacology predicts that partial agonists will exhibit full efficacy in the presence of a large receptor reserve, where less than full occupancy can produce a full agonist response.

There is a discrepancy in the actions of the CB_1 receptor antagonist SR141716A in [^{35}S]GTPγS experiments[24]; in rat cerebellar membranes, SR141716A is a neutral antagonist, with no effect on [^{35}S]GTPγS binding except at concentrations 10 000 times greater than its affinity at CB_1 receptors (Fig. 42. 3), while in CB_1 receptor-transfected cells, SR141716A is an inverse agonist, producing relatively potent inhibition of basal [^{35}S]GTPγS binding.[34] The signal of inverse agonists to reduce spontaneous activity of G-proteins is directly related to the number of receptors present, so that the detection of such activity is much more straightforward in transfected cells than in normal brain membranes. This fact demonstrates that findings of inhibition of basal [^{35}S]GTPγS binding in brain membranes by high concentrations of cannabinoid antagonists should be interpreted with caution.

Cannabinoid receptor activation of G-proteins influences multiple effector systems. Cannabinoid inhibition of adenylyl cyclase has been demonstrated in several cell types,[1,35,36] and in brain membranes.[31,37] In addition to inhibiting adenylyl cyclase, cannabinoids have been shown to stimulate cAMP accumulation.[38] As with other receptors coupled to $G_{i/o}$ proteins, activation of CB_1 receptors decreases Ca^{2+} conductance[32,39] and increases K^+ conductance.[40] Although beyond the scope of this review, retrograde signaling has been well documented as a mechanism of endogenous cannabinoid modulation of neuronal cell firing.[41]

Chronic Effects of Cannabinoids in Activating G-proteins

Chronic administration of cannabinoids to animals results in tolerance to many of the acute effects of Δ^9-THC, including memory disruption,[42] decreased locomotion,[43] and analgesia.[44] Several groups have attempted to correlate behavioral tolerance with biochemical alterations, and several studies have shown that brain cannabinoid receptor levels usually decrease after prolonged exposure to agonists,[45,46] although some studies have reported increases[47] or no changes[43] in receptor binding in brain. Appropriate controls have demonstrated that downregulation of cannabinoid receptors is homologous, and not simply due to neurotoxicity. Differences among studies may depend on the treatment agonist used, brain region examined, or treatment time. Despite these contradictory reports in vivo, there is general agreement that relatively short exposure of transfected cells in culture with cannabinoid agonists produces significant receptor internalization and trafficking.[48]

Another reason why reports of cannabinoid receptor downregulation have been contradictory is because receptor downregulation is only one consequence of receptor desensitization. For all G-protein-coupled receptors, the first step in desensitization is uncoupling of the receptor from G_α, thus reducing the agonist response. Therefore, the best place to look for chronic agonist-induced changes in receptor function is at the coupling between receptors and G-proteins. Chronic

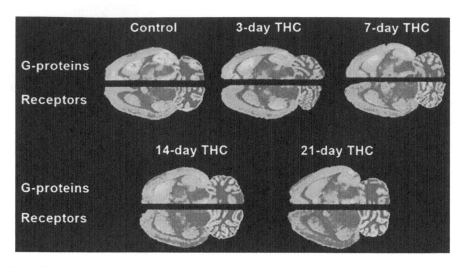

Fig. 42.4 Effect of chronic treatment of rats with Δ^9-THC on WIN 55212-2-stimulated [^{35}S]GTPγS binding (top) and [^{3}H]SR141716A binding, determined by autoradiography of brain sections. Rats were treated with 10 mg/kg Δ^9-THC for 3 to 21 days. Note the time-dependent reductions in [^{35}S]GTPγS binding in hippocampus, caudate, globus pallidus, and cerebellum. Adapted from Breivogel et al.[49]

Δ^9-THC treatment produces significant desensitization of cannabinoid-activated G-proteins in several rat brain regions, as determined by cannabinoid-stimulated [^{35}S]GTPγS autoradiography.[30] These studies showed significant reduction in cannabinoid-stimulated [^{35}S]GTPγS binding in virtually every brain region (Fig. 42.4), although the actual amount of desensitization varied across brain regions, with a maximum of 75% reduction in hippocampus. Moreover, the time course of the decrease in cannabinoid-stimulated [^{35}S]GTPγS binding varied across brain regions.[49] For example, the rate of desensitization was relatively fast in hippocampus, where significant reductions in cannabinoid-stimulated [^{35}S]GTPγS binding were observed after only 3 days of treatment with Δ^9-THC. A slower rate of desensitization was observed in cerebellum, where 7 days of treatment was required to see significant desensitization, while the slowest results were obtained in globus pallidus, where 14 days of chronic Δ^9-THC treatment were required for significant cannabinoid/G-protein desensitization. Such brain regional variation is consistent with the fact that tolerance to chronic drug exposure often develops at different rates for different behavioral effects. Other studies have confirmed the reduction in cannabinoid-activated G-proteins in brain following chronic treatment with several cannabinoid agonists, including Δ^9-THC,[50-52] WIN 5521-2,[51] and CP-55940.[53] Of interest, in a study comparing the chronic effects of Δ^9-THC and WIN 55212-2, both agonists produced significant reduction in cannabinoid-stimulated [^{35}S]GTPγS binding throughout brain, with chronic Δ^9-THC even producing somewhat more desensitization than chronic WIN 55212-2 in some brain regions,[51] despite the fact that WIN 55212-2 has more efficacy than Δ^9-THC in activating G-proteins.

The relationship between in vivo tolerance and the uncoupling of cannabinoid receptors to G-proteins observed after chronic administration of cannabinoid agonists is not yet clear.[54] The phenomenon of tolerance is complex and involves not only specific cannabinoid receptor mechanisms, but also interactions between cannabinoid systems and other neurotransmitters in brain circuitry. Nevertheless, the loss of receptor/G-protein coupling represents a fundamental alteration of cannabinoid-induced signal transduction and is consistent with the loss of agonist response that characterizes cannabinoid tolerance.

Acknowledgments Research cited from the author's laboratory was partially supported by Public Health Service (PHS) grant DA-06784 from the National Institute on Drug Abuse, National Institutes of Health, Bethesda, MD.

References

1. Howlett AC. Inhibition of neuroblastoma adenylyl cyclase by cannabinoid and nantradol compounds. *Life Sci.* 1984;35:1803-1810.
2. Howlett AC, Fleming RM. Cannabinoid inhibition of adenylate cyclase: pharmacology of the response in neuroblastoma cell membranes. *Mol Pharmacol.* 1984;26:532-538.
3. Howlett AC. Cannabinoid inhibition of adenylate cyclase: biochemistry of the response in neuroblastoma cell membranes. *Mol Pharmacol.* 1985;27:429-436.
4. Howlett AC, Qualy JM, Khachatrian LL. Involvement of G_i in the inhibition of adenylate cyclase by cannabimimetic drugs. *Mol Pharmacol.* 1986;29:307-313.
5. Devane WA, Dysarz FAI, Johnson MR, Melvin LS, Howlett AC. Determination and characterization of a cannabinoid receptor in rat brain. *Mol Pharmacol.* 1988;34:605-613.
6. Herkenham M, Lynn AB, Johnson MR, Melvin LS, de Costa BR, Rice KC. Characterization and localization of cannabinoid receptors in rat brain: a quantitative in vitro autoradiographic study. *J Neurosci.* 1991;11:563-583.
7. Matsuda LA, Lolait SJ, Brownstein MJ, Young AL, Bonner TI. Structure of a cannabinoid receptor and functional expression of the cloned cDNA. *Nature.* 1990;346:561-564.
8. Munro S, Thomas KL, Abu-Shaar M. Molecular characterization of a peripheral receptor for cannabinoids. *Nature.* 1993;365:61-65.
9. Devane WA, Hanus L, Breuer A, et al. Isolation and structure of a brain constituent that binds to the cannabinoid receptor. *Science.* 1992;258:1946-1949.
10. Mechoulam R, Ben-Shabat S, Hanus L, et al. Identification of an endogenous 2-monoglyceride, present in canine gut, that binds to cannabinoid receptors. *Biochem Pharmacol.* 1995;50:83-90.
11. Houston DB, Howlett AC. Solubilization of the cannabinoid receptor from rat brain and its functional interaction with guanine nucleotide-binding proteins. *Mol Pharmacol.* 1993;43:17-22.
12. Mukhopadhyay S, Howlett AC. Chemically distinct ligands promote differential CB_1 cannabinoid receptor-Gi protein interactions. *Mol Pharmacol.* 2005;67:2016-2024.
13. Selley DE, Stark S, Sim LJ, Childers SR. Cannabinoid receptor stimulation of guanosine-5'-O-(3-[^{35}S]thio)triphosphate binding in rat brain membranes. *Life Sci.* 1996;59:659-668.
14. Kurose H, Katada T, Haga T, Haga K, Ichiyama A, Ui M. Functional interaction of purified muscarinic receptors with purified inhibitory guanine nucleotide regulatory proteins reconstituted in phospholipid vesicles. *J Biol Chem.* 1986;261:6423-6428.

15. Florio VA, Sternweiss PC. Mechanisms of muscarinic receptor action on G_o in reconstituted phospholipid vesicles. *J Biol Chem*. 1989;264:3909-3915.
16. Asano T, Pedersen SE, Scott CW, Ross EM. Reconstitution of catecholamine-stimulated binding of guanosine 5'-O-(3-thiotriphosphate) to the stimulatory GTP-binding protein of adenylate cyclase. *Biochemistry*. 1984;23:5460-5467.
17. Hilf G, Gierschik P, Jakobs KH. Muscarinic acetylcholine receptor-stimulated binding of guanosine 5'-O-(3-thiotriphosphate) to guanine-nucleotide-binding proteins in cardiac membranes. *Eur J Biochem*. 1989;186:725-731.
18. Lorenzen A, Fuss M, Vogt H, Schwabe U. Measurement of guanine nucleotide-binding protein activation by A_1 adenosine receptor agonists in bovine brain membranes: stimulation of guanosine-5'-O-(3-[^{35}S]thio)triphosphate binding. *Mol Pharmacol*. 1993;44:115-123.
19. Lazareno S, Farries T, Birdsall NJM. Pharmacological characterization of guanine nucleotide exchange reactions in membranes from CHO cells stably transfected with human muscarinic receptors M1–M4. *Life Sci*. 1993;52:449-456.
20. Levy FO, Zhu X, Kaumann AJ, Birnbaumer L. Efficacy of β_1-adrenergic receptors is lower than that of β_2-adrenergic receptors. *Proc Natl Acad Sci USA*. 1993;90:10798-10802.
21. Birnbaumer L, Levy FO, Zhu X, Kaumann AJ. Studies on the intrinsic activity (efficacy) of human adrenergic receptors. *Tex Heart Inst J*. 1994;21:16-21.
22. Breivogel CS, Selley DE, Childers SR. Acute and chronic effects of opioids on delta and mu receptor activation of G-proteins in NG108-15 and SK-N-SH cell membranes. *J Neurochem*. 1997;68:1462-1472.
23. Sim LJ, Selley DE, Childers SR. In vitro autoradiography of receptor-activated G-proteins in rat brain by agonist-stimulated guanylyl 5'-[γ-[^{35}S]thio]-triphosphate binding. *Proc Natl Acad Sci USA*. 1995;92:7242-7246.
24. Breivogel CS, Selley DE, Childers SR. Cannabinoid receptor agonist efficacy for stimulating [^{35}S]GTPγS binding to rat cerebellar membranes correlates with agonist-induced decreases in GDP affinity. *J Biol Chem*. 1998;273:16865-16873.
25. Kuster J, Stevenson J, Ward S, D'Ambra T, Haycock D. Aminoalkylindole binding in rat cerebellum: selective displacement by natural and synthetic cannabinoids. *J Pharmacol Exp Ther*. 1993;264:1352-1363.
26. Sim LJ, Selley DE, Xiao R, Childers SR. Differences in G-protein activation by mu and delta opioid, and cannabinoid, receptors in rat striatum. *Eur J Pharmacol*. 1996;307:97-105.
27. Breivogel CS, Sim LJ, Childers SR. Regional differences in cannabinoid receptor/G-protein coupling in rat brain. *J Pharmacol Exp Ther*. 1997;282:1632-1642.
28. Selley DE, Sim LJ, Xiao R, Liu Q, Childers SR. Mu opioid receptor-stimulated [^{35}S]GTPγS binding in rat thalamus and cultured cell lines: signal transduction mechanisms underlying agonist efficacy. *Mol Pharmacol*. 1997;51:87-96.
29. Burkey TH, Quock RM, Consroe P, et al. Relative efficacies of cannabinoid CB_1 receptor agonists in the mouse brain. *Eur J Pharmacol*. 1997;336:295-298.
30. Sim LJ, Hampson RE, Deadwyler SA, Childers SR. Effects of chronic treatment with Δ^9-tetrahydrocannabinol on cannabinoid-stimulated [^{35}S]GTPγS autoradiography in rat brain. *J Neurosci*. 1996;16:8057-8066.
31. Childers SR, Sexton T, Roy MB. Effects of anandamide on cannabinoid receptors in rat brain membranes. *Biochem Pharmacol*. 1994;47:711-715.
32. Mackie K, Devane WA, Hille B. Anandamide, an endogenous cannabinoid, inhibits calcium currents as a partial agonist in N18 neuroblastoma cells. *Mol Pharmacol*. 1993;44:498-503.
33. Shen M, Piser TM, Seybold VS, Thayer SA. Cannabinoid receptor agonists inhibit glutamatergic synaptic transmission in rat hippocampal cultures. *J Neurosci*. 1996;16:4322-4334.
34. Landsman RS, Burkey TH, Consroe P, Roeske WR, Yamamura HI. SR141716A is an inverse agonist at the human cannabinoid CB_1 receptor. *Eur J Pharmacol*. 1997;334:R1-R2.
35. Felder CC, Joyce KE, Briley EM, et al. Comparison of the pharmacology and signal transduction of the human cannabinoid CB_1 and CB_2 receptors. *Mol Pharmacol*. 1995;48:443-450.
36. Pacheco M, Ward SJ, Childers SR. Identification of cannabinoid receptors in cultures of rat cerebellar granule cells. *Brain Res*. 1993;603:102-110.

37. Bidaut-Russell M, Devane WA, Howlett AC. Cannabinoid receptors and modulation of cyclic AMP accumulation in the rat brain. *J Neurochem*. 1990;55:21-26.

38. Glass M, Felder CC. Concurrent stimulation of cannabinoid CB1 and dopamine D2 receptors augments cAMP accumulation in striatal neurons: evidence for a G_s linkage to the CB1 receptor. *J Neurosci*. 1997;17:5327-5333.

39. Caulfield MP, Brown DA. Cannabinoid receptor agonists inhibit Ca currents in NG108-15 neuroblastoma cells via a pertussis toxin-sensitive mechanism. *Br J Pharmacol*. 1992;106:231-232.

40. Mackie K, Lai Y, Westenbroek R, Mitchell R. Cannabinoids activate an inwardly rectifying potassium conductance and inhibit Q-type calcium currents in AtT20 cells transfected with rat brain cannabinoid receptor. *J Neurosci*. 1995;15:6552-6561.

41. Diana MA, Levenes C, Mackie K, Marty A. Short-term retrograde inhibition of GABAergic synaptic currents in rat Purkinje cells is mediated by endogenous cannabinoids. *J Neurosci*. 2002;22:200-208.

42. Deadwyler SA, Heyser CJ, Hampson RE. Complete adaptation to the memory disruptive effects of delta-9-THC following 35 days of exposure. *Neurosci Res Commun*. 1995;17:9-18.

43. Abood ME, Sauss C, Fan F, Tilton CL, Martin BR. Development of behavioral tolerance to Δ^9-THC without alteration of cannabinoid receptor binding or mRNA levels in whole brain. *Pharmacol Biochem Behav*. 1993;46:575-579.

44. Adams IB, Martin BR. Cannabis: pharmacology and toxicology in animals and humans. *Addiction*. 1996;91:1585-1614.

45. Fan F, Tao Q, Abood ME, Martin BR. Cannabinoid receptor down-regulation without alteration of the inhibitory effect of CP 55,940 on adenylyl cyclase in the cerebellum of CP 55,940-tolerant mice. *Brain Res*. 1996;706:13-20.

46. Rodríguez de Fonseca F, Gorriti MA, Fernandez-Ruiz JJ, Palomo T, Ramos JA. Downregulation of rat brain cannabinoid binding sites after chronic Δ^9-tetrahydrocannabinol treatment. *Pharmacol Biochem Behav*. 1994;47:33-40.

47. Romero J, Garciá L, Fernández-Ruiz JJ, Cebeira M, Ramos JA. Changes in rat brain cannabinoid binding sites after acute or chronic exposure to their endogenous agonist, anandamide, or to Δ^9-tetrahydrocannabinol. *Pharmacol Biochem Behav*. 1995;51:731-737.

48. Coutts AA, Anavi-Goffer S, Ross RA, et al. Agonist-induced internalization and trafficking of cannabinoid CB1 receptors in hippocampal neurons. *J Neurosci*. 2001;21:2425-2433.

49. Breivogel CS, Childers SR, Deadwyler SA, Hampson RE, Vogt LJ, Sim-Selley LJ. Chronic Δ9-tetrahydrocannabinol produces a time-dependent loss of cannabinoid receptors and cannabinoid receptor-activated G-proteins in rat brain. *J Neurochem*. 1999;73:2447-2459.

50. Breivogel CS, Scates SM, Beletskaya IO, Lowery OB, Aceto MD, Martin BR. The effects of delta9-tetrahydrocannabinol physical dependence on brain cannabinoid receptors. *Eur J Pharmacol*. 2003;459:139-150.

51. Sim-Selley LJ, Martin BR. Effect of chronic administration of R-(+)-[2,3-Dihydro-5-methyl-3-[(morpholinyl)methyl]pyrrolo[1,2,3-de]-1,4-benzoxazinyl]-(1-naphthalenyl)methanone mesylate (WIN55,212-2) or delta(9)-tetrahydrocannabinol on cannabinoid receptor adaptation in mice. *J Pharmacol Exp Ther*. 2002;303:36-44.

52. Corchero J, Romero J, Berrendero F, et al. Time-dependent differences of repeated administration with Delta9-tetrahydrocannabinol in proenkephalin and cannabinoid receptor gene expression and G-protein activation by mu-opioid and CB1-cannabinoid receptors in the caudate-putamen. *Brain Res Mol Brain Res*. 1999;67:148-157.

53. Rubino T, Vigano D, Costa B, Colleoni M, Parolaro D. Loss of cannabinoid-stimulated guanosine 5'-O-(3-[(35)S]thiotriphosphate) binding without receptor down-regulation in brain regions of anandamide-tolerant rats. *J Neurochem*. 2000;75:2478-2484.

54. Sim-Selley LJ. Regulation of cannabinoid CB1 receptors in the central nervous system by chronic cannabinoids. *Crit Rev Neurobiol*. 2003;15:91-119.

Chapter 43
2-Arachidonoylglycerol (2-AG) Membrane Transport: History and Outlook

Anita Hermann,[1] Martin Kaczocha,[1] and Dale G. Deutsch[1]

Abstract Only a few studies have addressed the transport of 2-arachidonoylglycerol (2-AG), a naturally occurring agonist for cannabinoid receptors. Based upon saturation kinetics, these early reports have proposed that 2-AG enters the cell by a specific 2-AG transporter, via the putative anandamide transporter, or by simple diffusion. In this review, the uptake of 2-AG is discussed in light of the recent advances that have been made for anandamide transport, where the mechanism appears to be rate-limited diffusion through the membrane. Endocannabinoids may be a distinct class of agonists since they are hydrophobic and neutral, exhibiting similar biophysical properties to some anesthetics that freely diffuse through the membrane.

Keywords anandamide, 2-AG, 2-arachidonoylglycerol, cannabinoids, endocannabinoid, transport

Introduction

The discovery that 2-arachidonoylglycerol (2-AG) is an endogenous cannabinoid receptor ligand was described in 1995 by Sugiura et al[1] and Mechoulam et al.[2] In the central nervous system, the synthesis of 2-AG has been reported to occur in mature brains on postsynaptic membranes, while the main enzyme reported to degrade 2-AG is presynaptically localized in cytosol and in the intracellular membranes (for recent reviews see Piomelli,[3] Jonsson et al,[4] and Di Marzo[5]). There have been only a handful of studies addressing the mechanism by which 2-AG is transported into the cell (Fig. 43. 1), and these are reviewed here and compared with arachidonoylethanolamide (anandamide) (AEA) transport, which has been more extensively studied.

[1] Department of Biochemistry and Cell Biology, State University of New York at Stony Brook, Stony Brook, NY

Corresponding Author: Dale G. Deutsch, Department of Biochemistry and Cell Biology, State University of New York at Stony Brook, NY 11795-5215. Tel: (631) 632-8595; Fax: (631) 632-8575; E-mail: DDeutsch@notes.sunysb.edu

R.S. Rapaka and W. Sadée (eds.), *Drug Addiction*.
© American Association of Pharmaceutical Scientists 2008

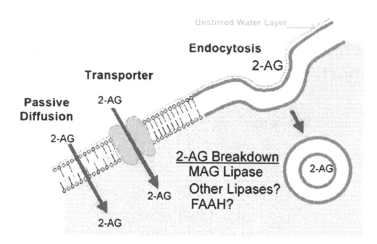

Fig. 43.1 Possible routes for 2-AG transport.

History of 2-AG Transport Studies

The cellular uptake of 2-AG in rat basophilic RBL-2H3 and mouse neuroblastoma N18TG2 cells was described in 1998 by Di Marzo et al[6] and Ben-Shabat et al.[7] Both groups independently observed accumulation of 2-AG in those cells with concurrent disappearance from the incubation media. Di Marzo et al[6] concluded that there was no evidence for a facilitated-diffusion process for the uptake of 2-AG. In addition, Ben-Shabat et al[7] studied 2-linoleoyl-glycerol and 2-palmitoyl-glycerol, 2 acyl-glycerols, which are present together with 2-AG in brain, gut, and spleen. These 2 compounds did not bind to CB1 or CB2 receptors, but they potentiated the binding of 2-AG to CB1 and CB2 receptors. Co-incubation of 2-AG with 2-linoleoyl-glycerol reduced 2-AG loss from the media, while 2-palmitoyl-glycerol was without effect.

In 1999, Piomelli et al.[8] showed evidence for a possible protein transporter for 2-AG. They observed saturable 2-AG uptake in human astrocytoma cells with a Michaelis-Menten constant (Km) of $0.7 \pm 0.1\,\mu mol/L$ and a Vmax of $28 \pm 6\,pmol/min/mg$ of protein, comparable to that shown for AEA transport. In these assays the clearance of radioactive material from the incubation medium was followed over a course of 20 minutes. The authors concluded that 2-AG may be internalized by the AEA transporter into these cells (Fig. 43.1).

These results were replicated in 2000 by Beltramo and Piomelli.[9] [³H]2-AG accumulation was inhibited by unlabeled 2-AG with a half-maximal inhibitory concentration (IC$_{50}$) of $5.5 \pm 1\,\mu mol/L$ and $100\,\mu mol/L$ 2-AG reduced [³H]2-AG accumulation to $24\% \pm 1\%$ of the control. AEA inhibited [³H]2-AG accumulation with an IC$_{50}$ of $4.2 \pm 0.3\,\mu mol/L$ and exhibited a maximal effect of 100%. AM404, a putative AEA transport inhibitor, also interfered with [³H]2-AG uptake (IC$_{50}$ of

1.8 ± 0.1 μmol/L). Several substrates and inhibitors of lipid transport systems had no effect on 2-AG uptake, but 100 μmol/L arachidonic acid significantly reduced 2-AG uptake in astrocytoma cells as did 10 μmol/L triascin C (an acyl-CoA synthetase inhibitor). BTNP ((E)-6-(bromomethylene) tetrahydro-3-1-naphthalenyl)-2H-pyran-2-one), a nonspecific fatty acid amide hydrolase (FAAH) inhibitor, had no effect on 2-AG uptake at 5 μmol/L. The authors concluded that a common carrier-mediated transport system is responsible for the internalization of 2-AG and AEA based on 4 key observations: (1) the similar kinetic properties of 2-AG and AEA uptake; (2) 2-AG and AEA competing with each other's uptake; (3) the blocking of [^{3}H]2-AG uptake by the putative AEA transport inhibitor AM404; and (4) the insensitivity of 2-AG and AEA transport to substrates and inhibitors of other known lipid transporters that are Na^+ and energy independent.

In 2001 Bisogno et al[10] studied the transport of AEA and 2-AG in rat C6 glioma cells at 37°C and 4°C at different time intervals and concentrations. Uptake was time- and temperature-dependent and saturable. The Km for 2-AG uptake was 15.3 ± 3.1 μmol/L and Bmax was 0.24 ± 0.04 nmol/min/mg protein. When 2-AG and AEA were co-incubated, only the uptake of 2-AG was significantly decreased. The authors suggested that if there is an AEA transporter, its efficacy with 2-AG is lower than with AEA, or that there are 2 different transporters involved. AM404 and linvanil (which is a capsaicin homolog[11]) inhibited the uptake of 2-AG with similar potency, K_i = 10.2 ± 1.7 and 6.4 ± 1.2 μmol/L, respectively. Bisogno et al[10] also found that nitric oxide donors increase the uptake of 2-AG as well as AEA. In conclusion, these authors provided evidence for a 2-AG/AEA transporter that may be identical or distinct from the putative AEA membrane transporter.

In 2004, Hajos et al.[12] also observed that 2-AG uptake in primary rat cortical neurons was temperature dependent and saturable. Uptake of [^{3}H]2-AG decreased with increasing concentrations of 2-AG and AEA and also with AM404. From these data the authors concluded that there is a common transporter for the 2 endocannabinoids.

Perspectives

The neuromodulatory functions of 2-AG require regulation of its synthesis, uptake/release, and inactivation. As a retrograde transmitter, 2-AG is believed to be synthesized postsynaptically[13] and translocated to the presynaptic cell by an unknown mechanism, where it signals via CB_1 and is then inactivated by being taken into the cell and metabolized mainly by monoacylglycerol lipase (MGL).[14,15] Owing to the structural and functional similarities between AEA and 2-AG, studies examining the mechanism of 2-AG transport pose similar challenges and limitations that have been observed for AEA uptake.

Because of the lipophilicity of 2-AG, future studies should address the degree of nonspecific interactions of this compound with plastic culture dishes and tips as has been performed for AEA.[16,17] In this regard, bovine serum albumin (BSA) should be included in incubation media to reduce nonspecific interactions and stabilize 2-AG in solution. The binding affinity of AEA to BSA is known,[18,19] and its uptake as a function of free/unbound AEA has been determined.[20] Owing to its structural similarity with AEA, 2-AG may bind BSA with similar affinity, reaching unbound concentrations in the nanomolar range. Determination of the dissociation constant (K_d) of 2-AG from BSA will enable calculation of free 2-AG that is available for uptake.

By plotting the uptake rate of unbound 2-AG with increasing 2-AG concentrations, it may be possible to elucidate the processes governing its accumulation. If 2-AG uptake exhibits linear kinetics, it would suggest simple diffusion across the plasma membrane. However, apparent saturable 2-AG uptake may be interpreted in 2 ways: (1) the saturation of an endocannabinoid transporter or (2) the resistance to uptake caused by the unstirred water layer surrounding the cells.[21]

Unlike most other neuromodulators, 2-AG and AEA are hydrophobic and uncharged. Uptake of 2-AG may show saturation owing to the unstirred water layer surrounding cells, and this may limit 2-AG permeation into the membrane in a manner similar to that found for AEA (Fig. 43.1).[20,21] Such apparent saturation of 2-AG uptake may preclude the use of transport kinetics as a criterion to define carrier-mediation because of the inability to distinguish between protein-mediated transport and rate-limited permeation of 2-AG through the unstirred water layer. Therefore, in all of the studies cited above that showed saturation of 2-AG uptake, the interpretation of the results may be confounded. Furthermore, in all experiments conducted to date, the free 2-AG concentrations are unknown because the solubility of 2-AG in aqueous buffers was not determined.

All of the 2-AG uptake studies have used incubation conditions longer than 1 minute. For AEA, it is known that such long incubation times are unable to distinguish uptake independent of downstream metabolism and sequestration.[20-24]

Since 2-AG accumulation has only been examined in the steady-state, it is not known whether the same kinetics will be observed when shorter incubation times are employed. As was found for AEA,[20,23,25,26] downstream metabolism of 2-AG by MGL may promote its accumulation in the steady-state. Consistent with this idea, competitive inhibitors of 2-AG inactivation have been found to reduce its cellular accumulation.[7] Selective inhibitors of MGL augment 2-AG levels in brain[27,28] and may likewise reduce 2-AG uptake in the steady-state in a manner similar to AEA. This action would delay the clearance of 2-AG from the plasma membrane and prolong CB_1 signaling to produce physiological effects.[27-29]

Conclusion

During the last decade there has been great emphasis on AEA uptake and its putative transporter. However, as discussed above, only a few studies investigated the cellular uptake of 2-AG. Conclusions from these studies are ambiguous. Although one report suggested simple diffusion, most have shown that transport occurs by facilitated diffusion. These reports indicated either a common transporter for 2-AG and AEA or individual carriers. It has also been suggested that there are 2 transporters, one of which is solely for AEA, while the other is a cotransporter for 2-AG and AEA. Most soluble neurotransmitters such as serotonin are hydrophilic and require a transporter to pass through the hydrophobic membrane. Similarly, some hydrophobic transmitters require a membrane transporter because of their charge. An example of the latter is the prostaglandins, whose transporter has been cloned, and whose uptake displays time and concentration dependence and is blocked by specific inhibitors.[30] AEA and 2-AG may be in a special class of agonists as they are lipophilic and in terms of transport may behave like some anesthetics that freely diffuse through the membrane. To date, the identification and cloning of an endocannabinoid transporter has yielded negative results. Of course, if one were discovered it would resolve some of the recent controversies surrounding the mechanisms of AEA and 2-AG transport. Efficient uptake of these lipids may involve different mechanisms, including rate-limited simple diffusion, uptake through a putative membrane transporter, or lipid raft-mediated endocytosis depending upon the cell type (see Fig. 43.1).[31,32]

Acknowledgments We thank the National Institute of Drug Abuse for support (NIDA grant numbers DA 9374 and DA 16419).

References

1. Sugiura T, Kondo S, Sukagawa A, et al. 2-Arachidonoylglycerol: a possible endogenous cannabinoid receptor ligand in brain. *Biochem Biophys Res Commun.* 1995;215:89-97.
2. Mechoulam R, Ben-Shabat S, Hanus L, et al. Identification of an endogenous 2-monoglyceride, present in canine gut, that binds to cannabinoid receptors. *Biochem Pharmacol.* 1995;50:83-90.
3. Piomelli D. The challenge of brain lipidomics. *Prostaglandins Other Lipid Mediat.* 2005;77:23-34.
4. Jonsson KO, Holt S, Fowler CJ. The endocannabinoid system: current pharmacological research and therapeutic possibilities. *Basic Clin Pharmacol Toxicol.* 2006;98:124-134.
5. Di Marzo V. A brief history of cannabinoid and endocannabinoid pharmacology as inspired by the work of British scientists. *Trends Pharmacol Sci.* 2006;27:134-140.
6. Di Marzo V, Bisogno T, Sugiura T, Melck D, De Petrocellis L. The novel endogenous cannabinoid 2-arachidonoylglycerol is inactivated by neuronal- and basophil-like cells: connections with anandamide. *Biochem J.* 1998;331:15-19.
7. Ben-Shabat S, Fride E, Sheskin T, et al. An entourage effect: inactive endogenous fatty acid glycerol esters enhance 2-arachidonoyl-glycerol cannabinoid activity. *Eur J Pharmacol.* 1998;353:23-31.
8. Piomelli D, Beltramo M, Glasnapp S, et al. Structural determinants for recognition and translocation by the anandamide transporter. *Proc Natl Acad Sci USA.* 1999;96:5802-5807.
9. Beltramo M, Piomelli D. Carrier-mediated transport and enzymatic hydrolysis of the endogenous cannabinoid 2-arachidonylglycerol. *Neuroreport.* 2000;11:1231-1235.
10. Bisogno T, Maccarrone M, De Petrocellis L, et al. The uptake by cells of 2-arachidonoylglycerol, an endogenous agonist of cannabinoid receptors. *Eur J Biochem.* 2001;268:1982-1989.
11. De Petrocellis L, Bisogno T, Davis JB, Pertwee RG, Di Marzo V. Overlap between the ligand recognition properties of the anandamide transporter and the VR1 vanilloid receptor: inhibitors of anandamide uptake with negligible capsaicin-like activity. *FEBS Lett.* 2000;483:52-56.

12. Hajos N, Kathuria S, Dinh T, Piomelli D, Freund TF. Endocannabinoid transport tightly controls 2-arachidonoyl glycerol actions in the hippocampus: effects of low temperature and the transport inhibitor AM404. *Eur J Neurosci*. 2004;19:2991-2996.
13. Bisogno T, Howell F, Williams G, et al. Cloning of the first sn1-DAG lipases points to the spatial and temporal regulation of endocannabinoid signaling in the brain. *J Cell Biol*. 2003;163:463-468.
14. Dinh TP, Kathuria S, Piomelli D. RNA interference suggests a primary role for monoacylglycerol lipase in the degradation of the endocannabinoid 2-arachidonoylglycerol. *Mol Pharmacol*. 2004;66:1260-1264.
15. Dinh TP, Carpenter D, Leslie FM, et al. Brain monoglyceride lipase participating in endocannabinoid inactivation. *Proc Natl Acad Sci USA*. 2002;99:10819-10824.
16. Fowler CJ, Tiger G, Ligresti A, Lopez-Rodriguez ML, Di Marzo V. Selective inhibition of anandamide cellular uptake versus enzymatic hydrolysis: a difficult issue to handle. *Eur J Pharmacol*. 2004;492:1-11.
17. Karlsson M, Pahlsson C, Fowler CJ. Reversible, temperature-dependent, and AM404-inhibitable adsorption of anandamide to cell culture wells as a confounding factor in release experiments. *Eur J Pharm Sci*. 2004;22:181-189.
18. Bojesen IN, Hansen HS. Binding of anandamide to bovine serum albumin. *J Lipid Res*. 2003;44:1790-1794.
19. Bojesen IN, Hansen HS. Membrane transport of anandamide through resealed human red blood cell membranes. *J Lipid Res*. 2005;46:1652-1659.
20. Kaczocha M, Hermann A, Glaser ST, Bojesen IN, Deutsch DG. Anandamide uptake is consistent with rate-limited diffusion and is regulated by the degree of its hydrolysis by FAAH. *J Biol Chem*. 2006;281:9066-9075.
21. Bojesen IN, Hansen HS. Effect of an unstirred layer on the membrane permeability of anandamide. *J Lipid Res*. 2006;47:561-570.
22. Glaser ST, Kaczocha M, Deutsch DG. Anandamide transport: a critical review. *Life Sci*. 2005;77:1584-1604.
23. Glaser ST, Abumrad NA, Fatade F, Kaczocha M, Studholme KM, Deutsch DG. Evidence against the presence of an anandamide transporter. *Proc Natl Acad Sci USA*. 2003;100:4269-4274.
24. Hillard CJ, Jarrahian A. Cellular accumulation of anandamide: consensus and controversy. *Br J Pharmacol*. 2003;140:802-808.
25. Deutsch DG, Glaser ST, Howell JM, et al. The cellular uptake of anandamide is coupled to its breakdown by fatty-acid amide hydrolase. *J Biol Chem*. 2001;276:6967-6973.
26. Day TA, Rakhshan F, Deutsch DG, Barker EL. Role of fatty acid amide hydrolase in the transport of the endogenous cannabinoid anandamide. *Mol Pharmacol*. 2001;59:1369-1375.
27. Hohmann AG, Suplita RL, Bolton NM, et al. An endocannabinoid mechanism for stress-induced analgesia. *Nature*. 2005;435:1108-1112.
28. Makara JK, Mor M, Fegley D, et al. Selective inhibition of 2-AG hydrolysis enhances endocannabinoid signaling in hippocampus. *Nat Neurosci*. 2005;8:1139-1141.
29. Quistad GB, Klintenberg R, Caboni P, Liang SN, Casida JE. Monoacylglycerol lipase inhibition by organophosphorus compounds leads to elevation of brain 2-arachidonoylglycerol and the associated hypomotility in mice. *Toxicol Appl Pharmacol*. 2006;211:78-83.
30. Chi Y, Khersonsky SM, Chang YT, Schuster VL. Identification of a new class of prostaglandin transporter inhibitors and characterization of their biological effects on prostaglandin e2 transport. *J Pharmacol Exp Ther*. 2006;316:1346-1350.
31. McFarland MJ, Porter AC, Rakhshan FR, Rawat DS, Gibbs RA, Barker EL. A role for caveolae/lipid rafts in the uptake and recycling of the endogenous cannabinoid anandamide. *J Biol Chem*. 2004;279:41991-41997.
32. Bari M, Battista N, Fezza F, Finazzi-Agro A, Maccarrone M. Lipid rafts control signaling of type-1 cannabinoid receptors in neuronal cells: implications for anandamide-induced apoptosis. *J Biol Chem*. 2005;280:12212-12220.

Chapter 44
Endocannabinoid Mechanisms of Pain Modulation

Andrea G. Hohmann[1] and Richard L. Suplita, II[1]

Abstract Cannabinoids are antinociceptive in animal models of acute, tissue injury–, and nerve injury–induced nociception. This review examines the biology of endogenous cannabinoids (endocannabinoids) and behavioral, neurophysiological, and neuroanatomical evidence supporting the notion that cannabinoids play a role in pain modulation. Behavioral pharmacological approaches, in conjunction with the identification and quantification of endocannabinoids through the use of liquid and gas chromatography mass spectrometry, have provided insight into the functional roles of endocannabinoids in pain modulation. Here we examine the distribution of cannabinoid receptors and endocannabinoid-hydrolyzing enzymes within pain modulatory circuits together with behavioral, neurochemical, and neurophysiological studies that suggest a role for endocannabinoid signaling in pain modulation. This review will provide a comprehensive evaluation of the roles of the endocannabinoids 2-arachidonoylglycerol and anandamide in stress-induced analgesia. These findings provide a functional framework with which to understand the roles of endocannabinoids in nociceptive processing at the supraspinal level.

Keywords 2-arachidonoylglycerol, anandamide, CB1, fatty acid amide hydrolase, monoacylglycerol lipase, periaqueductal gray, rostral ventromedial medulla

Introduction

The discovery, cloning, and characterization of cannabinoid receptors,[1-3] along with the isolation of endogenous ligands for these receptors, such as anandamide[4] and 2-arachidonoylglycerol (2-AG),[5,6] established the existence of an endocannabinoid

[1]Neuroscience and Behavior Program, Department of Psychology, University of Georgia, Athens, GA 30602-3013

Corresponding Author: Andrea G. Hohmann, Neuroscience and Behavior Program, Department of Psychology, University of Georgia, Athens, GA 30602. Tel: (706) 542-2252; Fax: (706) 542-3275; E-mail: ahohmann@uga.edu

R.S. Rapaka and W. Sadée (eds.), *Drug Addiction.*
© American Association of Pharmaceutical Scientists 2008

neuromodulatory system. Cannabinoid receptors occur in high densities in the rodent brain (>1 pmol/mg protein).[2] The heterogeneous distribution of cannabinoid receptors in the central nervous system[2,7] suggests a neuroanatomical basis for the profound behavioral effects induced by exogenous cannabinoids. The cannabinoid system is thus a major neurochemical system whose functional significance has only recently been explored. Cannabinoid receptors are localized in neuroanatomical regions subserving transmission and modulation of pain signals, such as the periaqueductal gray (PAG), the rostral ventromedial medulla (RVM),[2,7] and the dorsal horn of the spinal cord.[7] These findings suggest that endocannabinoids play a key role in central nervous system modulation of pain signaling. This review will focus on elucidating the pain modulatory functions of cannabinoids and endocannabinoids mediated primarily at the supraspinal level.

Cannabinoid Receptor Subtypes

Two subtypes of cannabinoid receptors—CB_1 and CB_2—have been identified. CB_1 is enriched in the brain.[3,8,9] By contrast, CB_2 is mainly expressed in immune tissues, including the spleen, tonsils, monocytes, and B and T cells[10-12] and is found only at low levels in neurons of the central nervous system.[8,9,11] In pathological pain states, CB_2 messenger RNA (mRNA) is also detected in the lumbar dorsal horn concurrently with the appearance of activated microglia.[13] CB_1 is negatively coupled to adenylate cyclase through Gi/o proteins.[14,15] Activation of these receptors inhibits N- and P/Q-type calcium channels[16,17] and activates inward rectifying potassium[18] and potassium A[19] channels. CB_2 is also negatively coupled to adenylate cyclase but is not coupled to calcium channels.[14] These signal transduction properties suggest that activation of CB_1 suppresses neuronal excitability and neurotransmitter release by modulating calcium and potassium conductances.

This review will examine evidence suggesting that endocannabinoids act at CB_1 receptors in the central nervous system to modulate pain processing. A more extensive review of the role of CB_1 receptor activation in modulating acute and sustained nociception at spinal and peripheral levels is available elsewhere.[20,21] A role for peripheral CB_1 and CB_2 receptors in modulating acute,[22] tissue injury–,[23-29] and nerve injury–induced[30] nociception has recently been demonstrated following systemic and local hind paw injections of CB_2-selective agonists. Interested readers are referred to recent reviews of peripheral cannabinoid antinociceptive mechanisms.[20,31-34]

Endocannabinoids

Several putative endocannabinoids have been isolated in the brain, including anandamide, 2-AG, noladin ether, virodhamine, and N-arachidonoyldopamine (NADA). Other endogenous cannabinergic compounds include the related fatty acid derivatives oleamide, palmitoylethanolamide, and a novel family of arachidonoyl amino acids. These substances lack affinity for cannabinoid receptors but appear to facilitate endocannabinoid function. The functional roles of these latter compounds remain poorly understood and are beyond the scope of this review. Because anandamide and 2-AG are the best characterized of the endocannabinoids isolated thus far, this review will focus on understanding the role of these endocannabinoids in pain modulation.

Anandamide[4] and 2-AG[5,6,35] are thought to be produced upon demand (ie, by activity-dependent or receptor-stimulated cleavage of membrane lipid precursors) and to be released from cells immediately after their production (for review, see Piomelli[36]). Anandamide is synthesized in vitro in a 2-step process (Fig. 44.1; for review, see Piomelli[36]). First, the phospholipid precursor N-arachidonoyl-phosphatidylethanolamine (NAPE) is formed from phosphatidylethanolamine through a mechanism that is both Ca^{2+} and cyclic AMP dependent, and catalyzed by the enzyme N-acyltransferase. Second, NAPE is believed to be hydrolyzed by a NAPE-specific phospholipase D—an enzyme that remains molecularly uncharacterized—to generate anandamide and the metabolic intermediate phosphatidic acid. Anandamide shows preferential affinity for CB_1 (K_i [CB_1 vs CB_2] = 89 vs 371 nM)

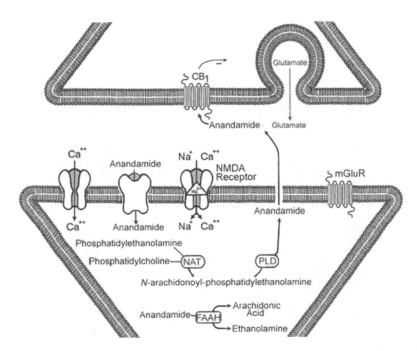

Fig. 44.1 Hypothetical model showing pathways of anandamide formation and deactivation. FAAH indicates fatty acid amide hydrolase; mGluR, metabotropic glutamate receptor; NAPE, N-arachidonoyl-phosphatidylethanolamine; NAT, N-acyltransferase; NMDA, N-methyl-D-aspartic acid; and PLD, phospholipase D.

in vitro and acts as a low-affinity agonist at vanilloid TRPV1 receptors.[37-39] Systemic administration of exogenous anandamide produces antinociception, suggesting that the endocannabinoid may also suppress pain under physiological conditions. This effect, however, is not reliably blocked by the selective CB$_1$ antagonist SR141716A (rimonabant),[40,41] likely owing to the fact that anandamide is readily metabolized in vivo by fatty acid amide hydrolase (FAAH) into ethanolamine and arachidonic acid.

In vitro experiments suggest that 2-AG formation (for review, see Piomelli[36]) occurs via successive activation of 2 enzymes (Fig. 44.2). First, the 2-AG precursor 1,2-diacylglycerol (DAG) is formed from phospholipase C–mediated hydrolysis of membrane phosphoinositides. Newly formed DAG may subsequently be hydrolyzed by DAG-lipase (DGL) to yield 2-AG. DAG can alternatively be phosphorylated by DAG kinase to yield phosphatidic acid. Therefore, DGL-mediated hydrolysis of DAG is likely the first committed step in 2-AG biosynthesis (for review, see Piomelli[36]). In brain slices and cultured cells, 2-AG formation may be stimulated by neural activity,[35] membrane depolarization,[42] or pharmacological activation of G protein-coupled receptors such as group I metabotropic glutamate receptors.[43] 2-AG is a naturally occurring 2-monoacylglycerol that activates both CB$_1$ and CB$_2$ receptors.[5,6] Although brain concentrations of 2-AG are 170-fold higher than those of anandamide,[35] the role of endogenous 2-AG in pain modulation is just beginning to be appreciated. 2-AG has been postulated to be the true natural ligand for cannabinoid receptors, with cannabinoid receptors serving primarily as

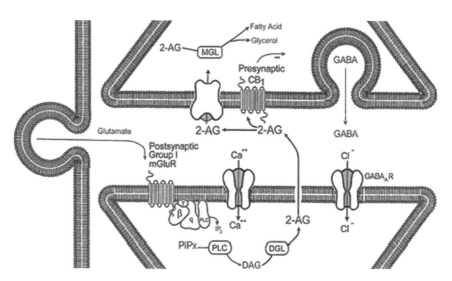

Fig. 44.2 Hypothetical model showing pathways of 2-AG formation and deactivation. 2-AG indicates 2-arachidonoylglycerol; DAG, diacylglycerol; DGL, diacylglycerol lipase; GABA, MGL, monoacylglycerol lipase; mGluR, metabotropic glutamate receptor; PLC, phospholipase C, and PIPx, phospholipid precursors.

2-AG receptors.[44,45] Exogenous 2-AG, administered systemically, suppresses noxious stimulus–induced responding in the tail-flick assay,[5] suggesting that endogenous 2-AG may suppress pain responding under physiological conditions. Behavioral responses to 2-AG are also enhanced by related, endogenous 2-acylglycerols, which fail to show significant activity in any of the tests employed when administered alone.[46] This "entourage effect" is likely to help regulate the activity of endocannabinoids in the nervous system[46]: competing for the same enzyme for hydrolysis may potentiate endocannabinoid actions.

Endocannabinoid Degrading Enzymes

Three of the 5 putative endocannabinoids—anandamide, 2-AG, and NADA—are susceptible to degradation by FAAH,[47-50] although a second enzyme, monoacylglycerol lipase (MGL),[51] catalyzes hydrolysis of 2-AG in vivo.[52] Immunocytochemical methods have been employed to map the distribution of FAAH in the brain.[53-55] The anatomical correspondence of FAAH and CB_1 mRNA also supports the hypothesis that endocannabinoids act as retrograde messengers.[54] Recent electrophysiological studies have provided confirmation of this hypothesis.[56,57] Significantly, immunocytochemical studies have demonstrated FAAH expression in the ventral posterior lateral nucleus of the thalamus,[53-55] which is the termination zone of the spinothalamic tract. This pathway is the major source of ascending nociceptive information to the brain. Furthermore, FAAH has been identified in Lissauer's tract and in neurons of the superficial spinal cord dorsal horn (ie, in close proximity to the termination zone of nociceptive primary afferents). These observations confirm that a mechanism for endocannabinoid deactivation is present in regions of the central nervous system implicated in nociceptive processing and further support the notion that endocannabinoids play a role in pain modulation.

Although FAAH reportedly metabolizes 2-AG in vitro,[58] MGL is likely to play the predominant role in 2-AG deactivation.[51] MGL is a serine hydrolase that converts monoglycerides to fatty acids and glycerol. Northern blot, immunocytochemical, and in situ hybridization studies reveal that MGL is heterogeneously distributed in the rat brain, with the highest levels observed in the cortex, the thalamus, the hippocampus, and the cerebellum.[51] Ultrastructural studies suggest that MGL is localized predominantly if not exclusively on axon terminals.[59] The recent development of pharmacological inhibitors of MGL such as URB602 has provided pharmacological tools for studying the functions of endogenous 2-AG in pain modulation, as described later in this review.[52] In vitro studies suggest that overexpression of MGL attenuates 2-AG accumulation in rat cortical neurons without altering anandamide accumulation.[51] Moreover, virally mediated RNA silencing of MGL is associated with marked enhancements of both basal and Ca^{2+}-stimulated 2-AG levels in HeLa cells.[60] Activation of mGlu5 receptors stimulates the formation of 2-AG (but not anandamide) in cultured cells derived from rat corticostriatal and hippocampal slices.[43] This formation of 2-AG is calcium-dependent and catalyzed by phospholipase C and 1,2-diacylglycerol lipase.[43] Also, the metabotropic glutamate 5 (mGlu5) receptor antagonist 2-methyl-6-(phenylethynyl)-pyridine (MPEP) prevents 2-AG formation induced by the group I mGlu receptor agonist 3,5-dihydroxyphenylglycine (DHPG).[43] More work, however, is necessary to determine whether the same processes control 2-AG formation in vivo.

The antinociceptive effects of exogenous 2-AG are preserved in FAAH(−/−) mice,[61] suggesting that FAAH does not catalyze 2-AG deactivation in vivo. Unlike anandamide and oleamide, monoacylglycerol lipids such as 2-AG exhibited equivalent hydrolytic activity in FAAH(+/+) and (−/−) mice.[61] These observations formed the basis for the conclusion that FAAH is an important regulator but not mediator of fatty acid amide activity in vivo.[61]

Transgenic approaches involving FAAH and CB_1 knockouts have recently been used in conjunction with pharmacological approaches to better evaluate the role of endocannabinoids in pain modulation. Mutant mice lacking the CB_1 gene fail to show typical antinociceptive responses to prototypical cannabinoid agonists.[9,62] It should be acknowledged, however, that high doses of Δ^9-tetrahydrocannabinol do exhibit a CB_1-independent antinociception,[9] although the receptor mechanism underlying this effect has not been evaluated. Cravatt et al developed mice lacking the FAAH gene and observed that these animals exhibited enhanced antinociceptive behavior following exogenous administration of anandamide.[63] Importantly, these enhancements of antinociception were blocked by the selective CB_1 antagonist rimonabant, providing compelling evidence that a CB_1-dependent process is responsible for FAAH-mediated anandamide hydrolysis. Furthermore, Cravatt et al[63] observed tonic centrally mediated CB_1-dependent analgesia in FAAH(−/−) mice, an effect likely due to the absence of this key enzyme, which catalyzes hydrolysis of fatty acid amides such as anandamide.[63,64] The behavioral phenotype was associated with a 15-fold increase in endogenous brain levels of anandamide in the FAAH(−/−) mice relative to FAAH(+/+) mice.[63] When mice lacking FAAH were treated with exogenous anandamide, they exhibited profound CB_1-dependent behavioral responses, including hypomotility, analgesia, catalepsy, and hypothermia. The generation of mutant mice that are incapable of synthesizing or inactivating 2-AG should further elucidate roles of this endocannabinoid in pain modulation.

Cannabinoid Receptor Pharmacology and Exogenous Cannabinoid Ligands

The development of competitive antagonists[65] and selective agonists for CB_1 has provided important pharmacological tools for investigating the biological functions of cannabinoids in the nervous system. SR141716A (rimonabant) shows high affinity for cannabinoid receptors in the brain ($K_d = 0.23$ nM)[65] but displays negligible affinity for CB_2 (K_i [CB_1 vs CB_2] = 5.6 nM vs >1 μM).[66] At high concentrations, rimonabant has been shown to inhibit vanilloid TRPV1 (formerly VR1) receptors. AM251 is a selective, competitive CB_1 antagonist (K_i [CB_1 vs CB_2] = 7.5 nM vs >2 μM)[67] devoid of vanilloid activity. Potent cannabinoid agonists CP55940 (K_i = 0.6 nM at CB_1 and CB_2), HU210 (K_i [CB_1 vs CB_2] = 0.73 vs 0.22 nM), and WIN55212-2 (K_i [CB_1 vs CB_2] = 1.9 vs 0.3 nM) show high affinity for CB_1 and CB_2 and show marked improvements in potency compared with Δ^9-tetrahydrocannabinol (Δ^9-THC), the prototypic classical cannabinoid. Selective competitive antagonists and high-affinity agonists have been used both to characterize the roles of cannabinoids in pain signaling and to map the sites of endocannabinoid action within the nervous system.

Studies relying upon the delivery of exogenous compounds that directly activate or block cannabinoid receptors have been indispensable for the initial assessment of the functional role of cannabinoid receptor activation in pain modulation. However, these studies do not provide direct evidence that endocannabinoids mediate these same functions under physiological conditions. More recently, the development of drugs that inhibit the enzymatic degradation of endocannabinoids (ie, through inhibition of FAAH or MGL) has facilitated research examining the functional consequences of activation of the body's endogenous system. URB597[68] is a well-characterized irreversible inhibitor of FAAH (IC_{50} = 4.6 nM) that lacks significant affinity for CB_1 and CB_2 receptors and does not affect MGL, acetyl-cholinesterase, butyryl-cholinesterase, or the anandamide membrane transporter at concentrations up to 300 μM. Arachidonoylserotonin[69] is a novel FAAH inhibitor that inhibits anandamide hydrolysis (IC_{50} = 5.6 μM), lacks affinity for CB_1, and does not significantly affect the cellular uptake of anandamide at 25 μM. MGL can be inhibited by a variety of nonselective serine hydrolase inhibitors (eg, methyl arachidonoyl fluorophosphonate). More recently, 2 selective inhibitors of MGL, URB602[52] and URB754,[70] have been described. URB602 inhibits rat brain MGL (IC_{50} = 28 ± 4 μM) through a noncompetitive mechanism, does not affect FAAH activity or anandamide levels, does not affect the activity of lipid-metabolizing enzymes such as diacylglycerol lipase[35] and cyclooxygenase-2,[71] and does not influence the binding of [^{3}H]-WIN55212-2 to CB_1 or CB_2 receptors (IC_{50} ≥ 5 μM) or [^{35}S]-GTP-γ-S to rat cerebellar membranes.[52] The effects of URB754 on pain modulation have not been examined.

Cellular uptake of anandamide reportedly involves facilitated diffusion,[72] although a specific transporter has yet to be cloned. Kinetics studies suggest the presence of an anandamide membrane transporter,[72] and pharmacological studies using inhibitors of anandamide transport[52,72] have supported the notion that anandamide transport inhibition has a role in modulating endocannabinoid tone. Among the most commonly employed drugs of this class are AM404, which also inhibits FAAH activity,[73] and VDM11. While AM404[74] activates TRPV1 receptors at low concentrations, VDM11[75] does not. VDM11 inhibits the cellular uptake of anandamide (IC_{50} = 1–11 μM), does not affect FAAH, and does not bind cannabinoid receptors at biologically relevant concentrations. Recently, a potent new competitive inhibitor of anandamide uptake, LY2318912,[72] was used to radiolabel the anandamide transporter binding site in rat cerebellum. Systemic administration of LY2318912 also induced a 5-fold elevation in brain anandamide levels. Moreover, LY2318912 diminished nociceptive behavior in the formalin test, with no concomitant expression of gross motor deficits typical of administration of direct cannabinoid agonists.[72]

Antinociceptive Effects of Exogenous Cannabinoids

Preclinical behavioral studies using different types of noxious stimulation (ie, thermal, mechanical, and chemical; for review, see Walker and Hohmann[21]) have demonstrated that cannabinoids effectively induce antinociception. In 1899, Dixon[76] demonstrated that delivery of cannabis smoke to dogs produced a failure to respond to pin pricks. Seminal studies on cannabinoid-induced antinociception by Bicher and Mechoulam[77] and Kosersky et al[78] provided a foundation for subsequent work that verified the ability of cannabinoids to profoundly suppress behavioral reactions to acute noxious stimuli and inflammatory and nerve injury–induced pain. The potency and efficacy of cannabinoids in producing antinociception is comparable to that of morphine.[79,80] However, cannabinoids induce profound motor deficits, including immobility and catalepsy,[81] which are a confound for behavioral studies that assess motor responses to noxious stimuli. Many recent studies of cannabinoid antinociception compensate for this limitation by additionally assessing behavioral measures of immobility and catalepsy to provide intrinsic controls for cannabinoid-induced changes in motor responding. Nonetheless, behavioral studies alone are not sufficient to demonstrate that cannabinoids suppress the processing of nociceptive information. An extensive literature now demonstrates that cannabinoids suppress nociceptive transmission, thus providing a compelling argument for the existence of endocannabinoid mechanisms of pain modulation.

Studies employing the systemic administration of cannabinoids have been useful in characterizing the antinociceptive effects of cannabinoids in animal models of acute and persistent nociception. The antinociceptive effects elicited by natural, synthetic, and exogenously administered endocannabinoids, along with the blockade of these effects by pharmacological and genetic disruptions of CB_1 activity, strongly suggest that cannabinoids have a specific physiological role in modulating pain sensitivity. Limitations of these approaches include the inability to localize the sites of action of cannabinoids and the failure to identify which endocannabinoids are involved in pain modulation. To address the first limitation, several important studies have used site-specific microinjections of cannabinoids into brain regions implicated in the processing and regulation of nociceptive signals. The second limitation has been addressed directly by identifying and quantifying endogenous mediators by microdialysis and liquid and/or gas chromatography mass spectrometry and indirectly by site-specific administration of pharmacological agents that regulate endocannabinoid uptake or degradation.

Cannabinoid-Induced Suppression of Nociceptive Transmission

Electrophysiological and neurochemical studies provide convincing evidence that cannabinoids suppress nociceptive transmission in vivo.[82-90] Walker's laboratory first demonstrated that cannabinoids suppress noxious stimulus–evoked neuronal activity in nociceptive neurons in the spinal cord and thalamus.[84,85,88,91,92] This suppression is observed in nociceptive neurons, generalizes to different modalities of noxious stimulation (mechanical, thermal, chemical), is mediated by cannabinoid receptors, and correlates with the antinociceptive effects of cannabinoids.[84-86,88,91] Cannabinoids also suppress C-fiber-evoked responses in spinal dorsal horn neurons recorded in normal, inflamed, and nerve-injured rats.[82,87,90,93] In addition, cannabinoids suppress spinal Fos protein expression, a neurochemical marker of sustained neuronal activation,[94] in a variety of animal models of persistent pain[28,91,92,95-98] through CB_1- and CB_2-selective mechanisms. Most electrophysiological studies have focused on wide-dynamic-range and nociceptive-specific cells recorded at the level of the spinal dorsal horn and have provided convincing evidence that cannabinoids suppress the transmission of nociceptive information. In vivo electrophysiological studies of brainstem neurons implicated in the descending control of pain have also provided insight into the role of cannabinoids in pain modulation and will be discussed below.[89,99]

Cannabinoid Antinociceptive Efficacy in Tissue Injury Models of Persistent Pain

Studies using systemic administration of cannabinoids have demonstrated antinociception in multiple models of inflammatory nociception. Kosersky et al.[78] showed that systemic Δ^9-THC increases the threshold for paw pressure–induced vocalization following the induction of inflammation in the hind paw. Tsou et al.[92] used the formalin test to show that systemic cannabinoids suppress noxious stimulus–evoked Fos protein expression and pain-related behaviors. The formalin test assesses supraspinally organized pain behavior. Our laboratory demonstrated that neurotoxic destruction of descending noradrenergic projections to the spinal cord reduces the suppression of formalin-evoked Fos protein expression induced by WIN55212-2.[100] The contribution of peripheral and spinal sites of action to cannabinoid antinociception in tissue and nerve injury models of persistent pain is now well documented (for review, see Hohmann[20]). By contrast, the contribution of supraspinal sites to cannabinoid analgesic action in models of persistent pain has received less attention.

Cannabinoid Antinociceptive Efficacy in Nerve Injury Models of Persistent Pain

Antihyperalgesic and antiallodynic efficacy of cannabinoids has been demonstrated in several rodent models of experimental neuropathy. Bennett's group demonstrated antihyperalgesic and antiallodynic efficacy of a cannabinoid following a chronic constriction injury of the sciatic nerve.[101] The changes were blocked by systemic administration of a CB_1 antagonist.[101] Hyperalgesia and allodynia induced by tight ligation of the L5 spinal nerve is also attenuated by systemic administration of WIN55212-2; these effects were reversed by a CB_1 but not by a CB_2 antagonist.[102] Cannabinoid-induced antinociception remains effective in nerve-injured rats following repeated administration, suggesting that cannabinoids are superior to opioids in alleviating neuropathic pain.[103] The existence of a substantial population of spinal cannabinoid receptors that remain intact following rhizotomy[86,104] may have clinical relevance, especially for deafferentation pain that is refractory to treatment with conventional narcotic analgesics.[105] The experimental studies thereby support the idea that the cannabinoids have a novel therapeutic target in treating neuropathic pain.

One possible mechanism for the antihyperalgesic actions of cannabinoids in neuropathic pain is suggested by cannabinoid-induced suppression of windup and noxious stimulus–induced central sensitization.[90,106] Support for the idea that there are both central and peripheral sites of cannabinoid antihyperalgesic efficacy has recently been demonstrated in a rat model of neuropathy using intrathecal and intraplantar administration of cannabinoid agonists and antagonists.[107] Electrophysiological studies also provide evidence for plasticity of the spinal cannabinoid system following tight ligation of the L5/L6 spinal nerve. Plasticity of cannabinoid systems may contribute to cannabinoid therapeutic efficacy in neuropathic pain states.[106] However, less is known about the possible contribution of supraspinal sites of cannabinoid analgesic action to the control of neuropathic pain.

The nucleus reticularis gigantocellularis pars alpha is implicated in cannabinoid modulation of neuropathic pain.[108] In rats subjected to partial sciatic nerve ligation (Seltzer model), unilateral hind paw injections of formalin contralateral to the site of nerve damage showed a reduced behavioral response to formalin compared with control conditions in the absence of nerve injury.[108] Administration of rimonabant to the nucleus reticularis gigantocellularis pars alpha of nerve-injured rats increased behavioral responses to formalin.[108] Although these data are consistent with the hypothesis that nerve injury activates CB_1-mediated endogenous antinociceptive mechanisms from the nucleus reticularis gigantocellularis pars alpha in the formalin test, inverse agonist effects[109] can complicate interpretation of studies employing rimonabant to evaluate endogenous cannabinoid tone.[90,110] Further work is necessary to determine whether endocannabinoids mediate the observed effects and to identify a physiological role for a specific endocannabinoid in this effect.

Supraspinal Sites Implicated in Cannabinoid Modulation of Pain

Direct support for the notion that there are supraspinal sites of cannabinoid antinociception was initially revealed in studies assessing acute withdrawal responses to thermal stimulation. The antinociceptive[111] effects of Δ^9-THC in the tail-flick test are attenuated following spinal transection, providing indirect evidence that supraspinal sites play an important role in cannabinoid antinociceptive action. Electrophysiological studies[86] similarly suggest that the suppressive effects of systemically administered cannabinoids on noxious stimulus–evoked responses in spinal nociceptive neurons are attenuated following spinal transection. Direct evidence for supraspinal sites of cannabinoid analgesic action was derived from the observation that intraventricular administration of cannabinoids WIN55212-2, CP55940, and Δ^9-THC induces antinociception.[112,113] Consistent with these behavioral studies, intraventricular administration of WIN55212-2 also suppresses noxious stimulus–evoked responding in wide-dynamic-range neurons recorded in the spinal dorsal horn.[86] Using autoradiographic methods, a study employing intraventricular administration of [^{3}H]WIN55212-2 confirmed that the radiolabeled drug was confined to periventricular sites throughout the brain. These studies underscore the importance of periventricular structures in contributing to cannabinoid-mediated pain modulation.

Site-specific injections of cannabinoid agonists to various brainstem regions have been used to identify supraspinal sites of cannabinoid antinociception. Using the tail-flick test, additional studies demonstrated that microinjection of cannabinoids into sites such as the dorsolateral PAG, dorsal raphe nucleus, RVM, amygdala, lateral posterior and submedius regions of the thalamus, superior colliculus, and noradrenergic A5 region produces antinociception.[114-116] Lichtman et al demonstrated that administration of CP55940 in the vicinity of the posterior ventrolateral PAG/dorsal raphe also produced antinociception, catalepsy, and hypothermia that was selective for the active stereoisomer.[113] By contrast, administration of CP55940 to the caudate putamen produced catalepsy but failed to induce antinociception or hypothermia. Microinjection of the cannabinoid HU210 into the dorsal PAG also produces a CB_1-mediated suppression of formalin-evoked nocifensive behavior and attenuates formalin-evoked Fos protein in the caudal lateral PAG.[98] The intra-PAG injection of the cannabinoid also attenuated aversive defense behavior (ie, locomotor activation) elicited by dorsal PAG injections of the excitatory amino acid D,L-homocysteic acid.[98] Exogenous cannabinoids also modulate ultrasound-induced aversive responses in rats through actions in the dorsal PAG, although these effects were insensitive to blockade by rimonabant.[117] These studies provide support for the hypothesis that endocannabinoids may modulate pain and defense behaviors through actions in the PAG.

While the studies described above identify sites where exogenously administered synthetic cannabinoids induce antinociception, they do not elucidate which endocannabinoids play a role in pain modulation. Investigators commonly hypothesize the role of a particular endocannabinoid from data showing that the compound induces antinociception. This method assumes that appropriate stimulation conditions result in the in vivo release of the endocannabinoid and that the compound's net effect is sufficient to suppress pain sensitivity. In other studies, investigators correlate endocannabinoid levels or release, and the observation of antinociception. This method is informative but incapable of establishing causation. With these limitations in mind, the following sections review what is known about the role of particular endocannabinoids in nociceptive responding.

PAG

The PAG is a common neural substrate underlying both analgesia and aversive responses. Electrical stimulation of the PAG produces analgesia and defensive behavior[118,119] that depends upon the activation of specific subdivisions of the nucleus. Electrical stimulation of the ventrolateral PAG produces analgesia that is blocked by opioid antagonists such as naltrexone,[118] suggesting that there is mediation by endogenous opioid peptides. By contrast, electrical stimulation of the dorsal and lateral PAG produces analgesia that is insensitive to blockade by opioid antagonists,[118] mediated by endocannabinoids, and blocked by cannabinoid antagonists.[120] Walker's group showed that electrical stimulation of the dorsal and lateral PAG resulted in cannabinoid receptor-mediated stimulation-produced analgesia concurrent with the mobilization of anandamide.[120] These actions were blocked by systemic or intra-PAG microinjection of rimonabant, consistent with mediation by CB_1. We recently demonstrated that 2-AG and anandamide are elevated in dorsal midbrain fragments containing the entire PAG concomitantly with the expression of nonopioid stress-induced analgesia (SIA). We showed that exposure to a 3-minute continuous foot shock induced a CB_1-mediated SIA independent of endogenous opioids.[52] Moreover, microinjection of FAAH inhibitors such as URB597[52] and arachidonoylserotonin[121] also enhanced SIA in a CB_1-dependent manner. Microinjection of the MGL inhibitor URB602 into the PAG also induced a CB_1-mediated enhancement of stress antinociception and selectively elevated levels of 2-AG (but not anandamide) in this region.[52] These data identify a physiological role for endogenous 2-AG in pain modulation at the level of the midbrain PAG.

Not all effects of endocannabinoids are mediated by CB_1 receptors, and therefore, it is important to demonstrate that endocannabinoid actions are blocked by selective cannabinoid antagonists. Microinjection of the FAAH inhibitor URB597 into the ventrolateral PAG has been reported to elevate endocannabinoids (both anandamide and 2-AG) and induce biphasic effects on thermal nociception via activation of CB_1 and TRPV1 receptor mechanisms.[99] In this study, the TRPV1-mediated antinociception and CB_1-mediated nociception caused by URB597 correlated with enhanced or reduced activity of RVM off-cells, suggesting that these effects occur via stimulation or inhibition of excitatory PAG output neurons, respectively.[99] At the highest dose tested, however, URB597 (4 nmol/rat) and WIN55212-2 (25–100 nmol) caused only CB_1-mediated analgesia, correlating with stimulation (possibly disinhibition) of RVM off-cells.[99] Thus, anandamide but not 2-AG may affect the descending pathways of pain control by acting at either CB_1 or TRPV1 receptors in select PAG subregions.[99]

In vitro electrophysiological studies indicate that cannabinoids inhibit both gamma-aminobutyric acid-ergic (GABAergic) and glutamatergic synaptic transmission presynaptically in rat PAG through a CB_1-specific mechanism.[122] The cellular actions of cannabinoids are distinct from those of mu opioids because cannabinoids lack direct postsynaptic action on PAG neurons. Exogenous cannabinoids are likely to reduce the probability of transmitter release from presynaptic terminals via a Ca^{2+}-independent mechanism,[122] suggesting that endocannabinoids behave similarly under physiological conditions.

Metabotropic glutamate and N-methyl-D-aspartic acid (NMDA) receptors are required for cannabinoid antinociception at the level of the PAG.[123] Infusion of WIN55212-2 into the PAG produced dose-dependent increases in paw withdrawal latencies in the plantar test.[123] This antinociceptive effect was blocked by pretreatment with rimonabant, which at high doses also produced modest hyperalgesia. Blockade of mGlu5 metabotropic glutamate receptors but not mGlu1 receptors completely blocked the effects of WIN55212-2. Both mGlu5 and mGlu1 receptors belong to the group I class of metabotropic glutamate receptors, which are G-protein-coupled and positively coupled to phospholipase C. Pretreatment with antagonists for group II (which includes mGlu2 and mGlu3) and group III (which includes mGlu4, mGlu6, mGlu7, and mGlu8) metabotropic glutamate receptors, which are negatively coupled to adenylate cyclase and preferentially localized to presynaptic active zones associated with autoreceptors, also suppressed WIN55212-2-induced antinociception. In addition to these metabotropic glutamate receptors, a selective antagonist for ionotropic glutamate (NMDA) receptors also blocked the antinociceptive effects of WIN55212-2. More work is necessary to elucidate the role of metabotropic glutamate receptors in endocannabinoid mechanisms of pain suppression.

RVM

Researchers have targeted synthetic cannabinoids at other brainstem nuclei such as the RVM[108,116,124] and the nucleus reticularis gigantocellularis[108] to better characterize sites of cannabinoid-mediated antinociception. Walker's group demonstrated that site-specific administration of cannabinoids (WIN55212-2 and HU210) in the RVM produced antinociception in the tail-flick test.[116] Mediation by CB_1 receptors was evident because the antinociceptive effects of HU210 were blocked by rimonabant and the receptor-inactive enantiomer WIN55212-3 failed to induce antinociception following microinjection to the same site.[116]

Electrophysiological studies have provided functional insight into the mechanism mediating these antinociceptive effects. In vivo recordings provide direct evidence that cannabinoids modulate on- and off-cells in the RVM,[89,125] thereby demonstrating the ability of these ligands to control descending pain modulatory signaling via a process similar to that of morphine. In lightly anesthetized rats, on-cells exhibit a burst of activity before the tail-flick nociceptive reflex, enhancing nociceptive transmission, whereas off-cells show a suppression of firing before the tail-flick reflex, inhibiting nociceptive transmission. Cannabinoids increased ongoing off-cell activity and reduced both the off-cell pause as well as the on-cell burst that occurs just prior to the tail-flick reflex. These actions were mediated by a CB_1 mechanism that is not dependent upon endogenous opioids.[89] Pharmacological inactivation of the RVM with site-specific administration of the $GABA_A$ receptor agonist muscimol also blocked the antinociceptive effects but not the motor deficits of systemically administered WIN55212-2.[89] This work identifies a GABAergic link in cannabinoid antinociceptive mechanisms. At the cellular level, cannabinoids exert their physiological effects in the RVM by presynaptic inhibition of GABAergic neurotransmission.[124] Collectively, these results suggest that nociceptive responsiveness is modulated in the RVM by endocannabinoids, although the specific endocannabinoids mediating these actions remain to be identified.

The nucleus reticularis gigantocellularis pars alpha within the RVM represents a major source of descending control induced by cannabinoids and is also directly activated by noxious stimulation. Microinjection of WIN55212-2 to the nucleus gigantocellularis pars alpha produced antinociception in the tail flick and formalin tests in otherwise untreated rats.[108] These effects were blocked by a CB_1 antagonist. Microdialysis studies coupled with high-performance liquid chromatography mass spectrometry, together with site-specific administration of inhibitors of endocannabinoid degradation and synthesis, would be particularly useful in identifying which endocannabinoids mediate these effects.

Role of the Amygdala

The amygdala consists of a nuclear complex located in the limbic forebrain and plays a key role in the coordination of fear and defensive reactions. The amygdala is optimally positioned anatomically to receive and integrate sensory information from multiple modalities and, in turn, to mediate emotional, autonomic, and somatic motor reactions to salient stimuli (especially threatening stimuli).[126] Within the amygdala, CB_1 immunoreactivity has been detected in a subset of GABAergic interneurons in the basolateral complex,[127] a site implicated in the formation and storage of aversive memories.[128] Anandamide and 2-AG are elevated in the basolateral amygdala in a conditioned fear aversion paradigm,[127] supporting the hypothesis that endocannabinoids serve naturally to inhibit extinction of aversive memories. Endocannabinoids and CB_1 receptors in the basolateral nucleus of the amygdala are implicated in the long-term depression of GABAergic inhibitory currents, suggesting that endocannabinoids regulate aversive memory extinction via selective inhibition of local inhibitory networks in the amygdala.[127]

The amygdala also plays a critical role in modulating antinociception. Microinjection of cannabinoids into the basolateral nucleus of the amygdala produces antinociception in the tail-flick test.[96] Microinjection of μ opioid agonists into the basolateral nucleus of the amygdala similarly results in marked antinociceptive responding in the radiant heat tail-flick[129,130] and formalin tests.[131] Moreover, bilateral lesions of the amygdala rendered nonhuman primates less sensitive to the antinociceptive effects of the potent synthetic cannabinoid WIN55212-2.[132] In rodents, microinjection of the $GABA_A$ agonist muscimol into the central nucleus of the amygdala, but not into the basolateral nucleus of the amygdala, reduced the antinociceptive effects of systemic WIN55212-2.[133] Moreover, FAAH and MGL are localized to postsynaptic and presynaptic sites, respectively, in the basolateral and lateral amygdala.[53,55,59] These data indicate that mechanisms exist for deactivation of anandamide and 2-AG in the basolateral amygdala. Both conditioned[134,135] and unconditioned[136] SIA depend on intact functioning of the amygdala. These observations, together with the demonstration of cannabinoid-mediated antinociceptive effects following site-specific administration to the basolateral nucleus of the amygdala,[114] suggest that endocannabinoids may serve naturally to suppress environmentally induced pain by actions in the amygdala. Below, we provide evidence that endocannabinoids may specifically mediate antinociceptive effects induced by exposure to environmental stressors, through actions in the PAG and to a lesser extent in the RVM and spinal cord.

Behavioral Evidence for a Role of Endocannabinoids in SIA

Stress activates neural systems that suppress pain sensation. This adaptive response is known as SIA and depends on the recruitment of brain pathways that project from the amygdala to the midbrain PAG and descend to the brainstem RVM and dorsal horn of the spinal cord (for review, see Walker and Hohmann[21]). For years, it has been recognized that endogenous opioid peptides participate in this process,[137,138] but the inability of opioid antagonists to block stress antinociception elicited by distinct stressor parameters made it clear that other unidentified mechanisms were also involved.

We hypothesized that endocannabinoids might mediate nonopioid SIA induced by brief, continuous foot shock.[52] First, agonists of CB_1 receptors—the predominant cannabinoid receptor subtype present in the brain[2,7]—exert profound antinociceptive effects[21] and suppress activity in nociceptive neurons.[84,86,88,89] Second, CB_1 antagonists increase the activity of nociceptive RVM neurons[89] and enhance sensitivity to noxious stimuli,[23] which suggests that an intrinsic endocannabinoid tone regulates descending antinociceptive pathways.[21]

We quantified the poststress sensitivity to pain in rats using the tail-flick test after exposure to a 3-minute foot shock stressor.[52] As demonstrated previously,[138,139] this stimulation protocol caused a profound antinociceptive effect that was not altered by systemic injection of the opiate antagonist naltrexone but was virtually eliminated by systemic administration of the competitive CB_1 receptor antagonists/inverse agonists rimonabant and AM251. Moreover, in rats rendered tolerant to the antinociceptive effects of cannabinoids (by daily treatment with WIN55212-2 for 14 days) a marked attenuation in stress antinociception was observed.[52] It was unlikely that this change was due to altered opioid tone, because cannabinoid-tolerant rats showed no changes in antinociceptive responsiveness to morphine and rats tolerant to morphine showed no attenuation of nonopioid stress antinociception.[52]

Pharmacological blockade of TRPV1 via systemic administration of capsazepine also failed to alter stress analgesia in our testing paradigm,[121] suggesting that endocannabinoid-mediated stress analgesia was not dependent on TRPV1. The same dose of capsazepine that failed to affect endocannabinoid-mediated stress antinociception, however, reliably reduced capsaicin-induced antinociception in the tail-flick test.[121]

We reasoned that if endocannabinoid activation of CB_1 receptors mediates nonopioid SIA, then inhibition of endocannabinoid deactivation should enhance stress antinociception. To test this hypothesis, we administered FAAH inhibitors (URB597, arachidonoyl serotonin, or palmitoyl trifluoromethyl ketone) to rats and examined the resultant stress-induced antinociception in the tail-flick assay.[52,121] Regardless of the pharmacological method used to inhibit FAAH, postshock SIA was enhanced in animals treated systemically with FAAH inhibitors. In all cases, these effects were blocked by rimonabant, consistent with a CB_1-dependent mechanism of action.[52,121] Systemic administration of rimonabant also attenuates fear-conditioned antinociceptive responses in the formalin test, together with freezing behavior and defecation, suggesting that CB_1 receptors and endocannabinoids may also contribute to fear-conditioned analgesia.[140]

Sites of Action of Endocannabinoid-Mediated SIA

To further investigate the sites of action of endocannabinoids in mediating stress antinociception, we microinjected rimonabant at multiple levels of the neuraxis and quantified poststress sensitivity to pain in rats using the tail-flick test. We targeted brain structures involved in pain and stress responsiveness that contain CB_1 receptors and are implicated in cannabinoid antinociception, including the dorsolateral PAG, ventral PAG, RVM, basolateral nucleus of the amygdala, central nucleus of the amygdala, and lumbar spinal cord.[52,121,141] Rimonabant microinjection into the dorsolateral PAG produced the greatest suppression of SIA relative to all other sites surveyed (Fig. 44.3 and data not shown). These findings are consistent with the presence of CB_1 receptors in the PAG and suggest that this structure plays a pivotal role in nonopioid SIA.

Stress Mobilizes Endocannabinoids to Suppress Pain

To determine whether endocannabinoid release is involved in SIA, we measured anandamide and 2-AG levels in dorsal midbrain fragments (containing the intact PAG) of rats killed without exposure to or at various times after foot shock.[52] Liquid chromatography/mass spectrometry (LC/MS) analyses revealed that midbrain 2-AG levels were markedly increased 2 minutes after shock and returned to baseline ≈15 minutes later. This response preceded a sustained increase in anandamide levels, which peaked 7 to 15 minutes following the shock. No such changes were observed in the occipital cortex, a brain region that contains CB_1 receptors but is not considered part of the SIA circuit. The rapid poststress accumulation of 2-AG in the PAG suggests that endocannabinoid release, rather than intrinsic CB_1 activity, is responsible for SIA.

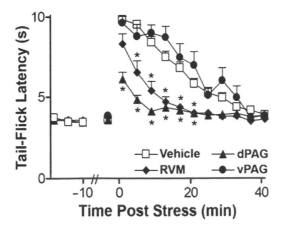

Fig. 44.3 The dPAG plays a pivotal role in nonopioid stress-induced analgesia. Rimonabant (2 nmol) microinjection into the dPAG induced a maximal suppression of stress antinociception ($F_{3,484} = 96.42$, $P < .0001$) relative to the vPAG, the RVM, or control conditions. SIA was assessed as the postshock (0.9 mA for 3 minutes) tail-flick latency by an investigator blinded to the experimental condition. Vehicle groups did not differ from each other and were pooled for all sites.[52,121] dPAG indicates dorsolateral PAG; RVM, rostral ventromedial medulla; SIA, stress-induced analgesia; and vPAG, ventrolateral PAG.

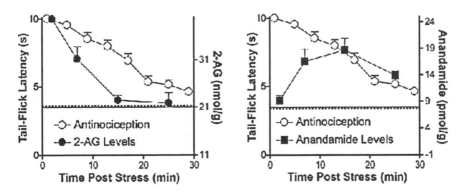

Fig. 44.4 Stress antinociception shows a temporal correspondence with 2-AG accumulation in midbrain periaqueductal gray. A significant correlation was observed between 2-AG ($r = 0.943$, $P < .03$) but not anandamide ($r = -0.479$, $P = .26$) accumulation and stress antinociception over the same time course. Stress antinociception was assessed as the postshock (0.9 mA for 3 minutes) tail-flick latency. (—) basal nociceptive threshold; (—) basal endocannabinoid level.[52] 2-AG indicates 2-arachidonoylglycerol.

We compared the time courses of endocannabinoid mobilization in the PAG with those of SIA. A strong temporal correspondence was found between these parameters ($r = 0.943$, $P < .03$), consistent with mediation by a common mechanism (Fig. 44.4). By contrast, anandamide was released with a strikingly dissimilar time course that does not closely correspond to that of 2-AG mobilization or SIA over the same interval (r = −0.479, P = .26). This temporal correlation points to 2-AG as a key mediator of nonopioid SIA.

Endogenous 2-AG Mediates SIA

If mobilization of 2-AG in the PAG mediates SIA, selective inhibitors of MGL should increase accumulation of 2-AG and enhance SIA.[52] Consistent with this prediction, microinjection of the novel MGL inhibitor URB602 into the dorsolateral PAG or ventrolateral PAG enhanced SIA.[52] Basal nociceptive thresholds in nonshocked rats were unaffected. The effect of URB602 was likely due to the accumulation of 2-AG in the PAG because the URB602-mediated enhancement of SIA was prevented by coadministration of rimonabant and accompanied by an elevation in midbrain 2-AG levels.[52] Microinjection of URB602 into the PAG increased accumulation of 2-AG in brains of rats exposed to the stressor relative to vehicle-treated controls without altering levels of anandamide. These findings indicate that the MGL inhibitor URB602 enhances both 2-AG accumulation and SIA. These studies suggest that endogenous 2-AG plays a physiological role in pain modulation.

Site-Specific Enhancement of Endocannabinoid Deactivation Enhances Stress Antinociception

Because the PAG serves key functions in both the descending control of pain[21,120] and the antinociceptive actions of cannabinoid agonists,[115] we examined the impact on stress antinociception of pharmacologically manipulating endocannabinoid deactivation using site-specific microinjections. Microinjection of either the FAAH inhibitor URB597[52] or arachidonoyl serotonin[121] to the dorsolateral PAG enhanced the magnitude and duration of endocannabinoid-mediated stress antinociception. These effects were blocked by coadministration of rimonabant, at a dose that was insufficient to reverse stress antinociception. It has recently been reported that site-specific microinjections of URB597 into the ventrolateral PAG enhance nociceptive behavior assessed in the plantar and tail-flick tests in otherwise naive rats,[99] despite producing enhanced anandamide and 2-AG levels. Consistent with our results, however, the highest dose of URB597 tested produced CB_1-mediated antinociception.

Cannabinoids microinjected into neural targets of the PAG in the RVM induce antinociception and suppress nociceptive processing.[98,116,125] Like opioids,[142] cannabinoids modulate on- and off-cells in the RVM,[89] demonstrating the ability of these ligands to control descending pain signaling. Based upon the anatomy of the midbrain-to-brainstem pain modulation circuit and upon the robust effects of blocking CB_1 receptors in the dorsolateral PAG or RVM in attenuating SIA,[52] we further reasoned that inhibition of endocannabinoid deactivation at the level of the RVM would enhance stress antinociception.[121] Pharmacological inhibition of

FAAH via site-specific microinjections of arachidonoyl serotonin into the RVM enhanced stress antinociception via a CB_1-specific mechanism.[121]

In rats, spinal transection reduces the antinociceptive[111] and electrophysiological[86] effects of cannabinoids. However, an enduring residual antinociception remains in spinally transected mice,[143] suggesting that endocannabinoids exert an analgesic effect at the spinal level as well as supraspinally. The localization of CB_1 receptors in the spinal dorsal horn[7,104] supports this view. Exogenously administered cannabinoids also produce antinociception when applied directly to the spinal cord[96,143-146] and suppress noxious stimulus–evoked neuronal activity in spinal nociceptive neurons,[82,85-87] suggesting that spinal cannabinoid receptors have a functional role in modulating nociceptive processing. Intrathecal administration of either rimonabant or CB_1 antisense oligonucleotides also elicits hyperalgesia,[147] suggesting that endocannabinoids may act tonically to suppress nociceptive responding.

To identify a physiological role for endocannabinoids at the spinal level, we bidirectionally manipulated endocannabinoid tone at CB_1 receptors in the lumbar spinal cord and assessed endocannabinoid mobilization in the lumbar spinal cord following exposure to a 3-minute continuous foot shock.[141] Stress antinociception was associated with the heightened release of endogenous 2-AG, whereas increases in anandamide mobilization were not detected,[141] perhaps because of greater variability and lower absolute levels of anandamide in these samples. Rimonabant failed to suppress endocannabinoid SIA when administered intrathecally to rats at a dose 10 times greater than that delivered to the PAG and RVM.[141] Nonetheless, pharmacological inhibitors of FAAH and MGL markedly enhanced the magnitude and duration of stress antinociception after intrathecal administration via a CB_1-specific mechanism.[141] Our results show that, at the level of the spinal cord, endocannabinoids regulate but do not mediate nonopioid SIA.

The activity of endocannabinoids in the descending neural pathway projecting from the PAG to the RVM to the spinal cord is implicated in the activation of endogenous pain suppression mechanisms in response to stress. We also examined neuroanatomically "upstream" centers responsible for activating this mechanism following exposure to a stressor. Situated in the limbic forebrain, the amygdala is implicated in both fear conditioning[148] and the affective[133,149] dimensions of pain. CB_1 immunoreactivity is dense in the basolateral nucleus of the amygdala (BLA)[2,150] but is reportedly absent in the central nucleus of the amygdala (CeA).[150] The anatomical localization of CB_1 in the BLA is consistent with electrophysiological data demonstrating that activation of these receptors presynaptically modulates GABAergic transmission.[150] The distribution of FAAH and MGL at this site also correlates well with the distribution of CB_1 receptors.[59] BLA efferents innervate the CeA, the main amygdaloid output nucleus, which sends projections to the PAG and other regions. Unilateral microinjection of cannabinoid agonists into the amygdala also induces antinociception in the tail-flick test,[114] supporting the notion that this structure plays a role in modulation of pain sensitivity.

Microinjections of rimonabant into the BLA, but not the CeA, suppressed nonopioid stress antinociception in our paradigm.[151] Our data are consistent with the observation that CB_1 agonists depress monosynaptic evoked inhibitory postsynaptic potentials in the BLA but not in the CeA.[150] Our results, therefore, suggest that CB_1 receptors in the BLA modulate local inhibitory networks in the BLA to ultimately regulate expression of SIA. Nonetheless, neither the FAAH inhibitor URB597 nor the MGL inhibitor URB602 enhanced SIA following microinjection into the BLA[151] at doses that markedly potentiated SIA following microinjection into the midbrain dorsolateral PAG.[52] These differences may reflect differential modulatory roles of distinct endocannabinoids in the ascending "affective" pain pathway compared with descending pain modulatory systems, or higher hydrolytic activity of endocannabinoid-degrading enzymes in the BLA relative to the PAG.

In sum, our results suggest that the coordinated release of 2-AG and anandamide in the PAG, RVM, and lumbar spinal cord mediates nonopioid SIA. The 2 endocannabinoids may act on local CB_1 receptors[2,7,122] to regulate glutamatergic and GABAergic transmission, ultimately disinhibiting descending pain control pathways. Three points are worthy of emphasis.[52] First, endocannabinoid-dependent stress antinociception is not affected by opioid antagonists or morphine tolerance, which implies that it may not require opioid activity. However, mutant CB_1 null mice also display reduced opioid-mediated responses to stress,[152] so opioid SIA need not be independent of endocannabinoids. Second, the residual antinociception observed in the presence of CB_1 antagonists leaves open the possibility that additional mediators of nonopioid SIA remain to be discovered. Third, stress mobilizes both 2-AG and anandamide in the dorsal midbrain, but these 2 endocannabinoids are released with distinctly dissimilar time courses. This observation underscores the existence of functional differences between these signaling molecules[36] that may be relevant to understanding endocannabinoid actions in other brain regions. The ability of both MGL and FAAH inhibitors to enhance endocannabinoid-dependent stress antinociception also highlights the significance of these enzymes as novel targets for the treatment of pain and stress- and anxiety-related disorders.[52,68]

Conclusions

Interest in the behavioral effects of cannabinoids has burgeoned since the cloning of cannabinoid CB_1 and CB_2 receptors and the isolation of endocannabinoids. The ability of cannabinoids to induce antinociception in virtually every animal model of acute or persistent pain evaluated has encouraged researchers to try to better understand this important nonopioid system of analgesia. Neuroanatomical studies have revealed that cannabinoid CB_1 receptors, endocannabinoids, and endocannabinoid-degrading enzymes are localized in central nervous system regions subserving the transmission and modulation of nociceptive signaling. Behavioral tests of acute nociception and tissue and nerve injury models of nociception have helped confirm the hypothesis that cannabinoids mediate antinociception via activation of CB_1 and CB_2 receptors. Recent studies have clarified the role of peripheral, spinal, and supraspinal sites in CB_1-dependent analgesia.

Cannabinergic agents may offer promise in clinical pain management both on their own and as adjuncts to conventional therapeutic agents. Cannabinoids may be particularly efficacious for pain syndromes that are intractable to conventional analgesics (eg, neuropathic pain)[153,154] and in patient populations where the emetic effects of opioids are poorly tolerated (eg, cancer patients, AIDS patients). Furthermore, inhibitors of endocannabinoid-degrading enzymes such as FAAH and MGL may function to selectively enhance CB_1-mediated neurotransmission only in nervous system areas where endocannabinoids are synthesized and released on demand, thereby precluding the induction of side effects associated with global CB_1 activation.[155] Moreover, synergism between cannabinoid and opioid analgesia has been demonstrated.[144,156] Collectively, these findings suggest that activation of cannabinoid receptors and inhibition of endocannabinoid deactivation may be promising targets for the clinical management of pain.

Acknowledgments A.G.H. was supported by DA14265 and DA14022. The authors are grateful to Nathan Bolton of the National Institute on Drug Abuse for his expert technical assistance with the figures.

References

1. Gerard CM, Mollereau C, Vassart G, Parmentier M. Molecular cloning of a human cannabinoid receptor which is also expressed in testis. *Biochem J*. 1991;279:129-134.
2. Herkenham M, Lynn AB, Johnson MR, Melvin LS, de Costa BR, Rice KC. Characterization and localization of cannabinoid receptors in rat brain: a quantitative in vitro autoradiographic study. *J Neurosci*. 1991;11:563-583.
3. Matsuda LA, Lolait SJ, Brownstein MJ, Young AC, Bonner TI. Structure of a cannabinoid receptor and functional expression of the cloned cDNA. *Nature*. 1990;346:561-564.
4. Devane WA, Hanus L, Breuer A, et al. Isolation and structure of a brain constituent that binds to the cannabinoid receptor. *Science*. 1992;258:1946-1949.
5. Mechoulam R, Ben-Shabat S, Hanus L, et al. Identification of an endogenous 2-monoglyceride, present in canine gut, that binds to cannabinoid receptors. *Biochem Pharmacol*. 1995;50:83-90.
6. Sugiura T, Kondo S, Sukagawa A, et al. 2-Arachidonoylglycerol: a possible endogenous cannabinoid receptor ligand in brain. *Biochem Biophys Res Commun*. 1995;215:89-97.
7. Tsou K, Brown S, Sanudo-Peña MC, Mackie K, Walker JM. Immunohistochemical distribution of cannabinoid CB1 receptors in the rat central nervous system. *Neuroscience*. 1997;83:393-411.
8. Buckley NE, McCoy KL, Mezey E, et al. Immunomodulation by cannabinoids is absent in mice deficient for the cannabinoid CB(2) receptor. *Eur J Pharmacol*. 2000;396:141-149.
9. Zimmer A, Zimmer AM, Hohmann AG, Herkenham M, Bonner TI. Increased mortality, hypoactivity, and hypoalgesia in cannabinoid CB1 receptor knockout mice. *Proc Natl Acad Sci USA*. 1999;96:5780-5785.
10. Galiegue S, Mary S, Marchand J, et al. Expression of central and peripheral cannabinoid receptors in human immune tissues and leukocyte subpopulations. *Eur J Biochem*. 1995;232:54-61.
11. Munro S, Thomas KL, Abu-Shaar M. Molecular characterization of a peripheral receptor for cannabinoids. *Nature*. 1993;365:61-65.
12. Schatz AR, Lee M, Condie RB, Pulaski JT, Kaminski NE. Cannabinoid receptors CB1 and CB2: a characterization of expression and adenylate cyclase modulation within the immune system. *Toxicol Appl Pharmacol*. 1997;142:278-287.

13. Zhang J, Hoffert C, Vu HK, Groblewski T, Ahmad S, O'Donnell D. Induction of CB2 receptor expression in the rat spinal cord of neuropathic but not inflammatory chronic pain models. *Eur J Neurosci.* 2003;17:2750-2754.

14. Felder CC, Joyce KE, Briley EM, et al. Comparison of the pharmacology and signal transduction of the human cannabinoid CB1 and CB2 receptors. *Mol Pharmacol.* 1995;48:443-450.

15. Howlett AC, Qualy JM, Khachatrian LL. Involvement of Gi in the inhibition of adenylate cyclase by cannabimimetic drugs. *Mol Pharmacol.* 1986;29:307-313.

16. Caulfield MP, Brown DA. Cannabinoid receptor agonists inhibit Ca current in NG108-15 neuroblastoma cells via a pertussis toxin-sensitive mechanism. *Br J Pharmacol.* 1992;106: 231-232.

17. Mackie K, Hille B. Cannabinoids inhibit N-type calcium channels in neuroblastoma-glioma cells. *Proc Natl Acad Sci USA.* 1992;89:3825-3829.

18. Mackie K, Lai Y, Westenbroek R, Mitchell R. Cannabinoids activate an inwardly rectifying potassium conductance and inhibit Q-type calcium currents in AtT20 cells transfected with rat brain cannabinoid receptor. *J Neurosci.* 1995;15:6552-6561.

19. Deadwyler SA, Hampson RE, Mu J, Whyte A, Childers S. Cannabinoids modulate voltage sensitive potassium A-current in hippocampal neurons via a cAMP-dependent process. *J Pharmacol Exp Ther.* 1995;273:734-743.

20. Hohmann AG. Spinal and peripheral mechanisms of cannabinoid antinociception: behavioral, neurophysiological and neuroanatomical perspectives. *Chem Phys Lipids.* 2002;121:173-190.

21. Walker JM, Hohmann AG. Cannabinoid mechanisms of pain suppression. In: Pertwee R, ed. *Cannabinoids—Handbook of Experimental Pharmacology.* Berlin, Germany: Springer; 2005:509-554.

22. Malan TP, Jr, Ibrahim MM, Deng H, et al. CB2 cannabinoid receptor-mediated peripheral antinociception. *Pain.* 2001;93:239-245.

23. Calignano A, La Rana G, Giuffrida A, Piomelli D. Control of pain initiation by endogenous cannabinoids. *Nature.* 1998;394:277-281.

24. Clayton N, Marshall FH, Bountra C, O'Shaughnessy CT. CB1 and CB2 cannabinoid receptors are implicated in inflammatory pain. *Pain.* 2002;96:253-260.

25. Hanus L, Breuer A, Tchilibon S, et al. HU-308: a specific agonist for CB(2), a peripheral cannabinoid receptor. *Proc Natl Acad Sci USA.* 1999;96:14228-14233.

26. Hohmann AG, Farthing JN, Zvonok AM, Makriyannis A. Selective activation of cannabinoid CB2 receptors suppresses hyperalgesia evoked by intradermal capsaicin. *J Pharmacol Exp Ther.* 2003;308:446-453.

27. Nackley AG, Makriyannis A, Hohmann AG. Selective activation of cannabinoid CB_2 receptors suppresses spinal fos protein expression and pain behavior in a rat model of inflammation. *Neuroscience.* 2003;119:747-757.

28. Nackley AG, 2nd, Suplita RL, 2nd, Hohmann AG. A peripheral cannabinoid mechanism suppresses spinal fos protein expression and pain behavior in a rat model of inflammation. *Neuroscience.* 2003;117:659-670.

29. Quartilho A, Mata HP, Ibrahim MM, et al. Inhibition of inflammatory hyperalgesia by activation of peripheral CB2 cannabinoid receptors. *Anesthesiology.* 2003;99:955-960.

30. Ibrahim MM, Deng H, Zvonok A, et al. Activation of CB2 cannabinoid receptors by AM1241 inhibits experimental neuropathic pain: pain inhibition by receptors not present in the CNS. *Proc Natl Acad Sci USA.* 2003;100:10529-10533.

31. Malan TP, Jr, Ibrahim MM, Vanderah TW, Makriyannis A, Porreca F. Inhibition of pain responses by activation of CB2 cannabinoid receptors. *Chem Phys Lipids.* 2002;121:191-200.

32. Rice AS, Farquhar-Smith WP, Nagy I. Endocannabinoids and pain: spinal and peripheral analgesia in inflammation and neuropathy. *Prostaglandins Leukot Essent Fatty Acids.* 2002;66:243-256.

33. Walker JM, Huang SM. Endocannabinoids in pain modulation. *Prostaglandins Leukot Essent Fatty Acids.* 2002;66:235-242.

34. Walker JM, Strangman NM, Huang SM. Cannabinoids and pain. *Pain Res Manag.* 2001;6:74-79.

35. Stella N, Schweitzer P, Piomelli D. A second endogenous cannabinoid that modulates long-term potentiation. *Nature.* 1997;388:773-778.
36. Piomelli D. The molecular logic of endocannabinoid signalling. *Nat Rev Neurosci.* 2003;4:873-884.
37. Gauldie SD, McQueen DS, Pertwee R, Chessell IP. Anandamide activates peripheral nociceptors in normal and arthritic rat knee joints. *Br J Pharmacol.* 2001;132:617-621.
38. Smart D, Gunthorpe MJ, Jerman JC, et al. The endogenous lipid anandamide is a full agonist at the human vanilloid receptor (hVR1). *Br J Pharmacol.* 2000;129:227-230.
39. Hogestatt ED, Zygmunt PM, Petersson J, et al. Vanilloid receptors on sensory nerves mediate the vasodilator action of anandamide. *Nature.* 1999;400:452-457.
40. Adams IB, Compton DR, Martin BR. Assessment of anandamide interaction with the cannabinoid brain receptor: SR 141716A antagonism studies in mice and autoradiographic analysis of receptor binding in rat brain. *J Pharmacol Exp Ther.* 1998;284:1209-1217.
41. Smith PB, Compton DR, Welch SP, Razdan RK, Mechoulam R, Martin BR. The pharmacological activity of anandamide, a putative endogenous cannabinoid, in mice. *J Pharmacol Exp Ther.* 1994;270:219-227.
42. Stella N, Piomelli D. Receptor-dependent formation of endogenous cannabinoids in cortical neurons. *Eur J Pharmacol.* 2001;425:189-196.
43. Jung K-M, Mangieri R, Stapleton C, et al. Stimulation of endocannabinoid formation in brain slice cultures through activation of group I metabotropic glutamate receptors. *Mol Pharmacol.* 2005;68:1196-1202.
44. Sugiura T. Evidence that the cannabinoid CB1 receptor is a 2-arachidonoylglycerol receptor. Structure-activity relationship of 2-arachidonoylglycerol, ether-linked analogues, and related compounds. *J Biol Chem.* 1999;274:2794-2801.
45. Sugiura T. Evidence that 2-arachidonoylglycerol but not N-palmitoylethanolamine or anandamide is the physiological ligand for the cannabinoid CB2 receptor. *J Biol Chem.* 2000;275:605-612.
46. Ben-Shabat S, Fride E, Sheskin T, et al. An entourage effect: inactive endogenous fatty acid glycerol esters enhance 2-arachidonoyl-glycerol cannabinoid activity. *Eur J Pharmacol.* 1998;353:23-31.
47. Cravatt BF, Giang DK, Mayfield SP, Boger DL, Lerner RA, Gilula NB. Molecular characterization of an enzyme that degrades neuromodulatory fatty-acid amides. *Nature.* 1996;384:83-87.
48. Deutsch DG, Chin SA. Enzymatic synthesis and degradation of anandamide, a cannabinoid receptor agonist. *Biochem Pharmacol.* 1993;46:791-796.
49. Di Marzo V, Bisogno T, Melck D, et al. Interactions between synthetic vanilloids and the endogenous cannabinoid system. *FEBS Lett.* 1998;436:449-454.
50. Huang SM, Bisogno T, Trevisani M, et al. An endogenous capsaicin-like substance with high potency at recombinant and native vanilloid VR1 receptors. *Proc Natl Acad Sci USA.* 2002;99:8400-8405.
51. Dinh TP, Carpenter D, Leslie FM, et al. Brain monoglyceride lipase participating in endocannabinoid inactivation. *Proc Natl Acad Sci USA.* 2002;99:10819-10824.
52. Hohmann AG, Suplita RL, Bolton NM, et al. An endocannabinoid mechanism for stress-induced analgesia. *Nature.* 2005;435:1108-1112.
53. Egertová M, Cravatt BF, Elphick MR. Comparative analysis of fatty acid amide hydrolase and cb(1) cannabinoid receptor expression in the mouse brain: evidence of a widespread role for fatty acid amide of endocannabinoid signaling. *Neuroscience.* 2003;119:481-496.
54. Egertov M, Giang DK, Cravatt BF, Elphick MR. A new perspective on cannabinoid signalling: complementary localization of fatty acid amide hydrolase and the CB1 receptor in rat brain. *Proc R Soc Lond B Biol Sci.* 1998;265:2081-2085.
55. Tsou K, Nogueron MI, Muthian S, et al. Fatty acid amide hydrolase is located preferentially in large neurons in the rat central nervous system as revealed by immunohistochemistry. *Neurosci Lett.* 1998;254:137-140.
56. Wilson RI, Nicoll RA. Endogenous cannabinoids mediate retrograde signalling at hippocampal synapses. *Nature.* 2001;410:588-592.

57. Wilson RI, Nicoll RA. Endocannabinoid signaling in the brain. *Science*. 2002;296:678-682.
58. Goparaju SK, Ueda N, Yamaguchi H, Yamamoto S. Anandamide amidohydrolase reacting with 2-arachidonoylglycerol, another cannabinoid receptor ligand. *FEBS Lett.* 1998;422:69-73.
59. Gulyas AI, Cravatt BF, Bracey MH, et al. Segregation of two endocannabinoid-hydrolyzing enzymes into pre- and postsynaptic compartments in the rat hippocampus, cerebellum and amygdala. *Eur J Neurosci*. 2004;20:441-458.
60. Dinh TP, Kathuria S, Piomelli D. RNA interference suggests a primary role for monoacylglycerol lipase in the degradation of the endocannabinoid 2-arachidonoylglycerol. *Mol Pharmacol*. 2004;66:1260-1264.
61. Lichtman AH, Hawkins EG, Griffin G, Cravatt BF. Pharmacological activity of fatty acid amides is regulated, but not mediated, by fatty acid amide hydrolase in vivo. *J Pharmacol Exp Ther*. 2002;302:73-79.
62. Ledent C, Valverde O, Cossu G, et al. Unresponsiveness to cannabinoids and reduced addictive effects of opiates in CB1 receptor knockout mice. *Science*. 1999;283:401-404.
63. Cravatt BF, Demarest K, Patricelli MP, et al. Supersensitivity to anandamide and enhanced endogenous cannabinoid signaling in mice lacking fatty acid amide hydrolase. *Proc Natl Acad Sci USA*. 2001;98:9371-9376.
64. Cravatt BF, Saghatelian A, Hawkins EG, Clement AB, Bracey MH, Lichtman AH. Functional disassociation of the central and peripheral fatty acid amide signaling systems. *Proc Natl Acad Sci USA*. 2004;101:10821-10826.
65. Rinaldi-Carmona M, Barth F, Heaulme M, et al. SR141716A, a potent and selective antagonist of the brain cannabinoid receptor. *FEBS Lett*. 1994;350:240-244.
66. Showalter VM, Compton DR, Martin BR, Abood ME. Evaluation of binding in a transfected cell line expressing a peripheral cannabinoid receptor (CB2): identification of cannabinoid receptor subtype selective ligands. *J Pharmacol Exp Ther*. 1996;278:989-999.
67. Palmer SL, Thakur GA, Makriyannis A. Cannabinergic ligands. *Chem Phys Lipids*. 2002;121:3-19.
68. Kathuria S, Gaetani S, Fegley D, et al. Modulation of anxiety through blockade of anandamide hydrolysis. *Nat Med*. 2003;9:76-81.
69. Bisogno T, Melck D, De Petrocellis L, et al. Arachidonoylserotonin and other novel inhibitors of fatty acid amide hydrolase. *Biochem Biophys Res Commun*. 1998;248:515-522.
70. Makara JK, Mor M, Fegley D, et al. Selective inhibition of 2-AG hydrolysis enhances endocannabinoid signaling in hippocampus. *Nat Neurosci*. 2005;8:1139-1141.
71. Kozak KR, Prusakiewicz JJ, Marnett LJ. Oxidative metabolism of endocannabinoids by COX-2. *Curr Pharm Des*. 2004;10:659-667.
72. Moore SA, Nomikos GG, Dickason-Chesterfield AK, et al. Identification of a high-affinity binding site involved in the transport of endocannabinoids. *Proc Natl Acad Sci USA*. 2005;102:17852-17857.
73. Jarrahian A, Manna S, Edgemond WS, Campbell WB, Hillard CJ. Structure-activity relationships among N-arachidonylethanolamine (Anandamide) head group analogues for the anandamide transporter. *J Neurochem*. 2000;74:2597-2606.
74. Beltramo M, Stella N, Calignano A, Lin SY, Makriyannis A, Piomelli D. Functional role of high-affinity anandamide transport, as revealed by selective inhibition. *Science*. 1997;277:1094-1097.
75. De Petrocellis L, Bisogno T, Davis JB, Pertwee RG, Di Marzo V. Overlap between the ligand recognition properties of the anandamide transporter and the VR1 vanilloid receptor: inhibitors of anandamide uptake with negligible capsaicin-like activity. *FEBS Lett*. 2000;483:52-56.
76. Dixon WE. The pharmacology of cannabis. *Indica Brit Med J*. 1899;2:1354-1357. PubMed
77. Bicher HI, Mechoulam R. Pharmacological effects of two active constituents of marihuana. *Arch Int Pharmacodyn Ther*. 1968;172:24-31.
78. Kosersky DS, Dewey WL, Harris LS. Antipyretic, analgesic and anti-inflammatory effects of delta 9-tetrahydrocannabinol in the rat. *Eur J Pharmacol*. 1973;24:1-7.

79. Bloom AS, Dewey WL, Harris LS, Brosius KK. 9-nor-9beta-hydroxyhexahydrocannabinol, a cannabinoid with potent antinociceptive activity: comparisons with morphine. *J Pharmacol Exp Ther*. 1977;200:263-270.

80. Buxbaum DM. Analgesic activity of 9-tetrahydrocannabinol in the rat and mouse. *Psychopharmacologia*. 1972;25:275-280.

81. Martin BR, Compton DR, Thomas BF, et al. Behavioral, biochemical, and molecular modeling evaluations of cannabinoid analogs. *Pharmacol Biochem Behav*. 1991;40:471-478.

82. Drew LJ, Harris J, Millns PJ, Kendall DA, Chapman V. Activation of spinal cannabinoid 1 receptors inhibits C-fibre driven hyperexcitable neuronal responses and increases [35S]GTPgammaS binding in the dorsal horn of the spinal cord of noninflamed and inflamed rats. *Eur J Neurosci*. 2000;12:2079-2086.

83. Harris J, Drew LJ, Chapman V. Spinal anandamide inhibits nociceptive transmission via cannabinoid receptor activation in vivo. *Neuroreport*. 2000;11:2817-2819.

84. Hohmann AG, Martin WJ, Tsou K, Walker JM. Inhibition of noxious stimulus-evoked activity of spinal cord dorsal horn neurons by the cannabinoid WIN 55,212-2. *Life Sci*. 1995;56:2111-2118.

85. Hohmann AG, Tsou K, Walker JM. Cannabinoid modulation of wide dynamic range neurons in the lumbar dorsal horn of the rat by spinally administered WIN55,212-2. *Neurosci Lett*. 1998;257:119-122.

86. Hohmann AG, Tsou K, Walker JM. Cannabinoid suppression of noxious heat-evoked activity in wide dynamic range neurons in the lumbar dorsal horn of the rat. *J Neurophysiol*. 1999;81:575-583.

87. Kelly S, Chapman V. Selective cannabinoid CB1 receptor activation inhibits spinal nociceptive transmission in vivo. *J Neurophysiol*. 2001;86:3061-3064.

88. Martin WJ, Hohmann AG, Walker JM. Suppression of noxious stimulus-evoked activity in the ventral posterolateral nucleus of the thalamus by a cannabinoid agonist: correlation between electrophysiological and antinociceptive effects. *J Neurosci*. 1996;16:6601-6611.

89. Meng ID, Manning BH, Martin WJ, Fields HL. An analgesia circuit activated by cannabinoids. *Nature*. 1998;395:381-384.

90. Strangman NM, Walker JM. Cannabinoid WIN 55,212-2 inhibits the activity-dependent facilitation of spinal nociceptive responses. *J Neurophysiol*. 1999;82:472-477.

91. Hohmann AG, Tsou K, Walker JM. Intrathecal cannabinoid administration suppresses noxious stimulus-evoked Fos protein-like immunoreactivity in rat spinal cord: comparison with morphine. *Acta Pharmacol Sin*. 1999;20:1132-1136.

92. Tsou K, Lowitz KA, Hohmann AG, et al. Suppression of noxious stimulus-evoked expression of FOS protein-like immunoreactivity in rat spinal cord by a selective cannabinoid agonist. *Neuroscience*. 1996;70:791-798.

93. Elmes SJ, Jhaveri MD, Smart D, Kendall DA, Chapman V. Cannabinoid CB2 receptor activation inhibits mechanically evoked responses of wide dynamic range dorsal horn neurons in naive rats and in rat models of inflammatory and neuropathic pain. *Eur J Neurosci*. 2004;20:2311-2320.

94. Hunt SP, Pini A, Evan G. Induction of c-fos-like protein in spinal cord neurons following sensory stimulation. *Nature*. 1987;328:632-634.

95. Farquhar-Smith WP, Jaggar SI, Rice AS. Attenuation of nerve growth factor-induced visceral hyperalgesia via cannabinoid CB(1) and CB(2)-like receptors. *Pain*. 2002;97:11-21.

96. Martin WJ, Loo CM, Basbaum AI. Spinal cannabinoids are anti-allodynic in rats with persistent inflammation. *Pain*. 1999;82:199-205.

97. Nackley AG, Makriyannis A, Hohmann AG. Selective activation of cannabinoid CB2 receptors suppresses spinal Fos protein expression and pain behavior in a rat model of inflammation. *Neuroscience*. 2003;119:747-757.

98. Finn DP, Jhaveri MD, Beckett SR, et al. Effects of direct periaqueductal grey administration of a cannabinoid receptor agonist on nociceptive and aversive responses in rats. *Neuropharmacology*. 2003;45:594-604.

99. Maione S, Bisogno T, de Novellis V, et al. Elevation of endocannabinoid levels in the vent-rolateral periaqueductal grey through inhibition of fatty acid amide hydrolase affects descending nociceptive pathways via both CB1 and TRPV1 receptors. *J Pharmacol Exp Ther*. 2005;316:969-982.

100. Gutierrez T, Nackley AG, Neely MH, Freeman KG, Edwards GL, Hohmann AG. Effects of neurotoxic destruction of descending noradrenergic pathways on cannabinoid antinociception in models of acute and tonic nociception. *Brain Res*. 2003;987:176-185.

101. Herzberg U, Eliav E, Dorsey JM, Gracely RH, Kopin IJ. NGF involvement in pain induced by chronic constriction injury of the rat sciatic nerve. *Neuroreport*. 1997;8:1613-1618.

102. Bridges D, Ahmad K, Rice AS. The synthetic cannabinoid WIN55,212-2 attenuates hyper-algesia and allodynia in a rat model of neuropathic pain. *Br J Pharmacol*. 2001;133:586-594.

103. Mao J, Price DD, Lu J, Keniston L, Mayer DJ. Two distinctive antinociceptive systems in rats with pathological pain. *Neurosci Lett*. 2000;280:13-16.

104. Farquhar-Smith WP, Egertova M, Bradbury EJ, McMahon SB, Rice AS, Elphick MR. Cannabinoid CB(1) receptor expression in rat spinal cord. *Mol Cell Neurosci*. 2000;15:510-521.

105. Arner S, Meyerson BA. Lack of analgesic effect of opioids on neuropathic and idiopathic forms of pain. *Pain*. 1988;33:11-23.

106. Chapman V. Functional changes in the inhibitory effect of spinal cannabinoid (CB) receptor activation in nerve injured rats. *Neuropharmacology*. 2001;41:870-877.

107. Fox A, Kesingland A, Gentry C, et al. The role of central and peripheral Cannabinoid1 receptors in the antihyperalgesic activity of cannabinoids in a model of neuropathic pain. *Pain*. 2001;92:91-100.

108. Monhemius R, Azami J, Green DL, Roberts MH. CB1 receptor mediated analgesia from the Nucleus Reticularis Gigantocellularis pars alpha is activated in an animal model of neuro-pathic pain. *Brain Res*. 2001;908:67-74.

109. Landsman RS, Burkey TH, Consroe P, Roeske WR, Yamamura HI. SR141716A is an inverse agonist at the human cannabinoid CB1 receptor. *Eur J Pharmacol*. 1997;334: R1-R2.

110. Rice AS, Beaulieu P, Bisogno T, et al. Role of the endogenous cannabinoid system in the formalin test of persistent pain in the rat. *Eur J Pharmacol*. 2000;396:85-92.

111. Lichtman AH, Martin BR. Spinal and supraspinal components of cannabinoid-induced anti-nociception. *J Pharmacol Exp Ther*. 1991;258:517-523.

112. Martin WJ, Lai NK, Patrick SL, Tsou K, Walker JM. Antinociceptive actions of cannabi-noids following intraventricular administration in rats. *Brain Res*. 1993;629:300-304.

113. Lichtman AH, Cook SA, Martin BR. Investigation of brain sites mediating cannabinoid-induced antinociception in rats: evidence supporting periaqueductal gray involvement. *J Pharmacol Exp Ther*. 1996;276:585-593.

114. Martin WJ, Coffin PO, Attias E, Balinsky M, Tsou K, Walker JM. Anatomical basis for cannabinoid-induced antinociception as revealed by intracerebral microinjections. *Brain Res*. 1999;822:237-242.

115. Martin WJ, Patrick SL, Coffin PO, Tsou K, Walker JM. An examination of the central sites of action of cannabinoid-induced antinociception in the rat. *Life Sci*. 1995;56:2103-2109.

116. Martin WJ, Tsou K, Walker JM. Cannabinoid receptor-mediated inhibition of the rat tail-flick reflex after microinjection into the rostral ventromedial medulla. *Neurosci Lett*. 1998;242:33-36.

117. Finn DP, Jhaveri MD, Beckett SR, Kendall DA, Marsden CA, Chapman V. Cannabinoids modulate ultrasound-induced aversive responses in rats. *Psychopharmacology (Berl)*. 2004;172:41-51.

118. Cannon JT, Prieto GJ, Lee A, Liebeskind JC. Evidence for opioid and non-opioid forms of stimulation-produced analgesia in the rat. *Brain Res*. 1982;243:315-321.

119. Reynolds DV. Surgery in the rat during electrical analgesia induced by focal brain stimula-tion. *Science*. 1969;164:444-445.

120. Walker JM, Huang SM, Strangman NM, Tsou K, Sanudo-Pena MC. Pain modulation by release of the endogenous cannabinoid anandamide. *Proc Natl Acad Sci USA.* 1999;96:12198-12203.

121. Suplita RL, II, Farthing JN, Gutierrez T, Hohmann AG. Inhibition of fatty-acid amide hydrolase enhances cannabinoid stress-induced analgesia: sites of action in the dorsolateral periaqueductal gray and rostral ventromedial medulla. *Neuropharmacology.* 2005;49:1201-1209.

122. Vaughan CW, Connor M, Bagley EE, Christie MJ. Actions of cannabinoids on membrane properties and synaptic transmission in rat periaqueductal gray neurons in vitro. *Mol Pharmacol.* 2000;57:288-295.

123. Palazzo E, Marabese I, de Novellis V, et al. Metabotropic and NMDA glutamate receptors participate in the cannabinoid-induced antinociception. *Neuropharmacology.* 2001;40:319-326.

124. Vaughan CW, McGregor IS, Christie MJ. Cannabinoid receptor activation inhibits GABAergic neurotransmission in rostral ventromedial medulla neurons in vitro. *Br J Pharmacol.* 1999;127:935-940.

125. Meng ID, Johansen JP. Antinociception and modulation of rostral ventromedial medulla neuronal activity by local microinfusion of a cannabinoid receptor agonist. *Neuroscience.* 2004;124:685-693.

126. Davis M, Whalen PJ. The amygdala: vigilance and emotion. *Mol Psychiatry.* 2001;6:13-34.

127. Marsicano G, Wotjak CT, Azad SC, et al. The endogenous cannabinoid system controls extinction of aversive memories. *Nature.* 2002;418:530-534.

128. Medina JF, Repa CJ, Mauk MD, LeDoux JE. Parallels between cerebellum- and amygdala-dependent conditioning. *Nat Rev Neurosci.* 2002;3:122-131.

129. Helmstetter FJ, Bellgowan PS, Poore LH. Microinfusion of mu, but not delta or kappa opioid agonists into the basolateral amygdala results in inhibition of the tail flick reflex in pentobarbital-anesthetized rats. *J Pharm Exp Ther.* 1995;275:381-388.

130. Helmstetter FJ, Bellgowan PS, Tershner SA. Modulation of spinal nociceptive reflexes by the microinjection of morphine into the amygdala. *Neuroreport.* 1993;4:471-474.

131. Manning BH, Mayer DJ. The central nucleus of the amygdala contributes to the production of morphine antinociception in the rat tail-flick test. *J Neurosci.* 1995;15:8199-8213.

132. Manning BH, Merin NM, Meng ID, Amaral DG. Reduction in opioid- and cannabinoid-induced antinociception in rhesus monkeys after bilateral lesions of the amygdaloid complex. *J Neurosci.* 2001;21:8238-8246.

133. Manning BH, Martin WJ, Meng ID. The rodent amygdala contributes to the production of cannabinoid-induced antinociception. *Neuroscience.* 2003;120:1157-1170.

134. Helmstetter FJ. The amygdala is essential for the expression of conditional hypoalgesia. *Behav Neurosci.* 1992;106:518-528.

135. Helmstetter FJ, Bellgowan PS. Lesions of the amygdala block conditional hypoalgesia on the tail flick test. *Brain Res.* 1993;612:253-257.

136. Bellgowan PS, Helmstetter FJ. Neural systems for the expression of hypoalgesia during nonassociative fear. *Behav Neurosci.* 1996;110:727-736.

137. Akil H, Young E, Walker JM, Watson SJ. The many possible roles of opioids and related peptides in stress-induced analgesia. *Ann N Y Acad Sci.* 1986;467:140-153.

138. Lewis JW, Cannon JT, Liebeskind JC. Opioid and nonopioid mechanisms of stress analgesia. *Science.* 1980;208:623-625.

139. Terman GW, Lewis JW, Liebeskind JC. Two opioid forms of stress analgesia: studies of tolerance and cross-tolerance. *Brain Res.* 1986;368:101-106.

140. Finn DP, Beckett SR, Richardson D, Kendall DA, Marsden CA, Chapman V. Evidence for differential modulation of conditioned aversion and fear-conditioned analgesia by CB1 receptors. *Eur J Neurosci.* 2004;20:848-852.

141. Suplita RL, II, Gutierrez T, Fegley D, Piomelli D, Hohmann AG. Endocannabinoids at the spinal level regulate, but do not mediate, nonopioid stress-induced analgesia. *Neuropharmacology.* 2005;262:25.

142. Heinricher MM, Morgan MM, Tortorici V, Fields HL. Disinhibition of off-cells and antinociception produced by an opioid action within the rostral ventromedial medulla. *Neuroscience.* 1994;63:279-288.

143. Smith PB, Martin BR. Spinal mechanisms of delta 9-tetrahydrocannabinol-induced analgesia. *Brain Res.* 1992;578:8-12.

144. Welch SP, Stevens DL. Antinociceptive activity of intrathecally administered cannabinoids alone, and in combination with morphine, in mice. *J Pharmacol Exp Ther.* 1992;262:10-18.

145. Welch SP, Thomas C, Patrick GS. Modulation of cannabinoid-induced antinociception after intracerebroventricular versus intrathecal administration to mice: possible mechanisms for interaction with morphine. *J Pharmacol Exp Ther.* 1995;272:310-321.

146. Yaksh TL. The antinociceptive effects of intrathecally administered levonantradol and desacetyllevonantradol in the rat. *J Clin Pharmacol.* 1981;21:334S-340S.

147. Richardson JD, Aanonsen L, Hargreaves KM. Antihyperalgesic effects of spinal cannabinoids. *Eur J Pharmacol.* 1998;345:145-153.

148. Cannich A, Wotjak CT, Kamprath K, Hermann H, Lutz B, Marsicano G. CB1 cannabinoid receptors modulate kinase and phosphatase activity during extinction of conditioned fear in mice. *Learn Mem.* 2004;11:625-632.

149. Bernard JF, Bester H, Besson JM. Involvement of the spino-parabrachio-amygdaloid and - hypothalamic pathways in the autonomic and affective emotional aspects of pain. *Prog Brain Res.* 1996;107:243-255.

150. Katona I, Rancz EA, Acsady L, et al. Distribution of CB1 cannabinoid receptors in the amygdala and their role in the control of GABAergic transmission. *J Neurosci.* 2001;21:9506-9518.

151. Connell K, Bolton N, Olsen D, Piomelli D, Hohmann AG. Role of the basolateral nucleus of the amygdala in endocannabinoid-mediated stress-induced analgesia. *Neurosci Lett.* 2005;12:22.

152. Valverde O, Ledent C, Beslot F, Parmentier M, Roques BP. Reduction of stress-induced analgesia but not of exogenous opioid effects in mice lacking CB1 receptors. *Eur J Neurosci.* 2000;12:533-539.

153. Atkinson JH, Slater MA, Wahlgren DR, et al. Effects of noradrenergic and serotonergic antidepressants on chronic low back pain intensity. *Pain.* 1999;83:137-145.

154. Portenoy RK, Foley KM. Chronic use of opioid analgesics in non-malignant pain: report of 38 cases. *Pain.* 1986;25:171-186.

155. Cravatt BF, Lichtman AH. Fatty acid amide hydrolase: an emerging therapeutic target in the endocannabinoid system. *Curr Opin Chem Biol.* 2003;7:469-475.

156. Yesilyurt O, Dogrul A, Gul H, et al. Topical cannabinoid enhances topical morphine antinociception. *Pain.* 2003;105:303-308.

Index

Color Plates

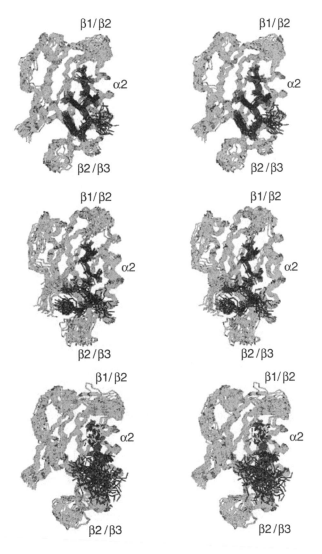

Fig. 9.2 Stereo views showing the NMR structures of the PDZ1 domain bound to Kv1.4 peptide (top), CRIPT (middle), and GluR6 (bottom). The conformers are superimposed for best fit of N, Cα, and carbonyl atoms. All the ligand's heavy atoms are shown for the fragment encompassing residues 0 and −5; carbons are depicted in dark green, oxygen in red, nitrogen in blue, sulfur in yellow. In the protein portion, only the superimposed atoms are shown as light green.

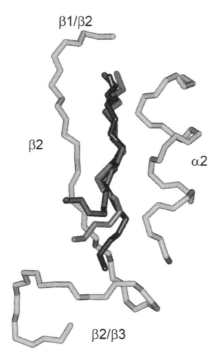

Fig. 9.3 Superposition of the last 6 C-terminal residues of Kv1.4 (dark green), CRIPT (blue), and GluR6 (magenta). The binding pocket of the PSD95/SAP90 PDZ1 domain is shown in light green.

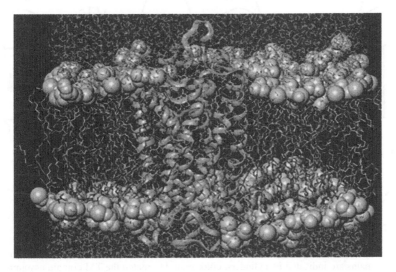

Fig. 17.3 Molecular model of the complete GPCR (rhodopsin) in an atomistic representation of its environment.

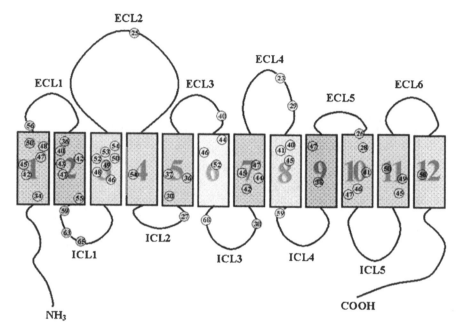

Fig. 18.1 Helical net topology scheme for discussed monoamine transporter mutations. The 12 TM domains are indicated by cylinders, color-coded to match the TM domain assignments of specific mutations listed in Table 18.1. Numbers inscribed in circles indicate specific positions of TM residues using the indexing system of Goldberg et al[17]; amino acid side chain assignments are listed in Table 18.1. Thus, the circled "34" in TM 1 refers to Position 1.34 in Table 18.1, in turn indicating that aspartic acid residues are found at this analogous position for the human DAT, NET, and SERT. Mutagenesis targets in the 6 extracellular loops (ECLs) and 5 intracellular loops (ICLs) are color-coded to indicate which of the flanking TM domains is used in the indexing system. Thus, the hDAT E218 residue in ECL 2 has been assigned Position 25 of TM 4 and is referred to as $E218_{4.25}$ in the text.

Table 18.1 Discussed Amino Acid Residue Mutagenesis Targets and Their Counterparts at Analogous Positions in the DAT, NET, and SERT.*

	1.34	1.42	1.45	1.47	1.48	1.50	1.56	2.36	2.40	2.42	2.43	2.47	2.55	2.59
DAT	D68 (h)	F76 (r)	D79 (r)	A81 (h)	N82 (h)	W84 (h)	C90 (h)	F98 (r)	Y102 (h)	L104 (m)	F105 (m)	A109 (m)	E117 (h)	G121 (h)
SERT	D87 (h)	Y95 (h)	D98 (h)	G100 (h)	N101 (h)	W103 (h)	C109 (h)	F117 (h)	Y121 (h)	I123 (h)	M124 (r)	G128 (h)	E136 (h)	G140 (h)
NET	D64 (h)	F72 (h)	D75 (h)	A77 (h)	N78 (h)	W80 (h)	C86 (h)	F94 (h)	Y98 (h)	L100 (h)	F101 (h)	A105 (h)	E113 (h)	G117 (h)

	2.63	2.65	3.46	3.48	3.49	3.50	3.52	3.53	3.54	4.25	4.54	5.27	5.30	5.36
DAT	R125 (h)	G127 (h)	V152 (h)	F154 (r)	F155 (h)	Y156 (h)	V158 (h)	I159 (h)	I160 (h)	E218 (h)	V247 (h)	K264 (h)	W267 (h)	P272 (r)
SERT	R144 (h)	G146 (h)	I172 (r)	S174 (h)	Y175 (h)	Y176 (r)	T178 (h)	I179 (h)	M180 (h)	R234 (h)	F263 (h)	K279 (h)	W282 (h)	P288 (h)
NET	R121 (h)	G123 (h)	V148 (h)	F150 (h)	Y151 (h)	Y152 (h)	V154 (h)	I155 (h)	I158 (h)	E215 (h)	V244 (h)	K261 (h)	W264 (h)	P270 (h)

	5.37	6.40	6.44	6.46	6.52	6.68	7.30	7.42	7.44	7.45	7.47	8.23	8.29	8.40
DAT	Y274 (h)	E307 (h)	W311 (h)	D313 (h)	C319 (h)	Y335 (h)	D345 (h)	S356 (r)	S359 (h)	S359 (r)	F361 (r)	D385 (h)	F390 (r)	P402 (h)
SERT	Y289 (h)	E322 (h)	W326 (h)	D328 (h)	F334 (h)	Y350 (h)	D360 (h)	S372 (r)	V374 (h)	S375 (r)	F377 (h)	A401 (h)	F407 (h)	P418 (h)
NET	Y271 (h)	E304 (h)	W308 (h)	D310 (h)	F316 (h)	Y332 (h)	D342 (h)	S354 (h)	V356 (h)	S357 (h)	F359 (h)	E382 (h)	F388 (h)	S399 (h)

	8.41	8.45	8.59	9.38	9.47	10.26	10.28	10.41	10.46	10.47	11.45	11.49	11.50	12.58
DAT	L403 (h)	W406 (r)	D421 (h)	T455 (r)	T464 (r)	D476 (h)	F478 (h)	E490 (r)	F513 (b)	W496 (r)	W523 (r)	S528 (h)	P529 (r)	M569 (h)
SERT	A419 (h)	F423 (h)	D437 (h)	C473 (h)	T482 (h)	E493 (h)	F495 (b)	E508 (h)	S513 (h)	W514 (h)	W541 (h)	S545 (r)	P548 (h)	F586 (h)
NET	G400 (h)	W404 (h)	D418 (h)	T453 (h)	T462 (h)	D473 (h)	F475 (h)	E488 (h)	S493 (h)	W494 (h)	W521 (h)	S525 (h)	P526 (h)	M566 (h)

* DAT indicates dopamine transporter; NET, norepinephrine transporter; and SERT, serotonin transporter. Residues are grouped by TM domain and color-coded to match the transmembrane (TM) domain in Figure 1. Individual residues are named by their one-letter amino acid code and position in the polypeptide chain of that transporter, parenthetically followed by the species employed in mutagenesis studies (eg, "D68 (h)" refers to the aspartic acid residue of the human DAT). Residues at the analogous position in the neurotransmitter:sodium symporter (NSS) family sequence alignment are collectively named using the indexing system described in the Introduction (from Goldberg et al[17]). Thus, hDAT D68, hSERT D87, and hNET D64 are found at Position 34 in TM 1. In many cases, only one monoamine transporter was mutated at the indicated position; the analogous residues in the other 2 transporters are shown as points of reference.

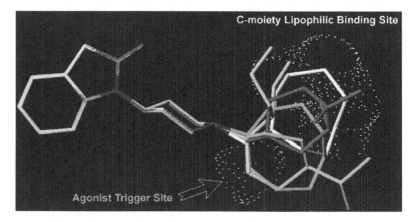

Fig. 24.4 Overlay of the dihydroindolinone-based agonists **20** (green), **23** (cyan), and **30** (yellow) with the antagonists **19** (white) and **26** (magenta). The lipophilic site that must be occupied by the C-moiety for good binding affinity is depicted by the white van der Waals surface. The green van der Waals surface represents the agonist trigger site, which when occupied by the agonists (eg **20**, **23**, **30**), triggers signal transduction leading to intrinsic activity. Antagonists **19** and **20** bind to the lipophilic site and have good affinity but do not interact with the agonist trigger site and therefore lack intrinsic activity.

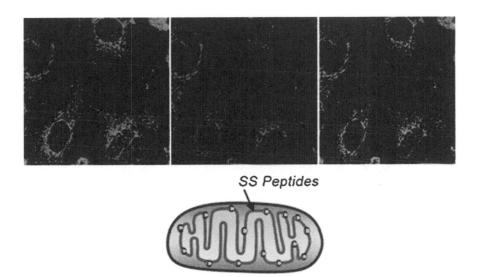

Fig. 31.5 Internalization and targeting of fluorescent SS peptide to mitochondria in living cells. Caco-2 cells were incubated with Dmt-D-Arg-Phe-atnDap-NH$_2$ (blue fluorescence) and TMRM (red fluorescence) at 37°C for 30 minutes and imaged by confocal laser scanning fluorescence microscopy.[16] Overlay of the 2 images shows colocalization of the fluorescent peptide and TMRM, suggesting mitochondrial targeting.

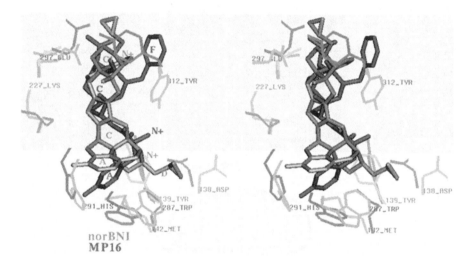

Fig. 33.5 Stereoview of the superposition of MP16 in the binding pocket of the agonist-bound conformation of KOR (red) and norBNI in the binding pocket of the antagonist-bound conformation of KOR (blue). Only ligands and several important residues from MOR: Asp138(3.32), Tyr139(3.33), Met142(3.35), Lys227(5.39), Trp287(6.48), His291(6.52), Glu297(6.58), and Tyr312(7.35) are shown. Pharmacophore elements are indicated by N+, A, C, C1, and F.

CPSIA information can be obtained at www.ICGtesting.com
Printed in the USA
LVOW05s1827071214

417657LV00004B/86/P

9 781441 926326